Neurology Board Review

An Illustrated Study Guide

Neurology Board Review

An Illustrated Study Guide

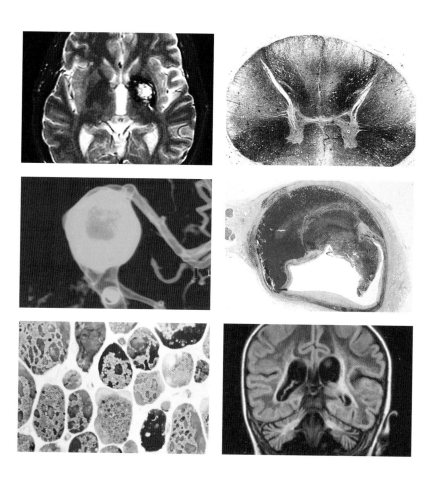

Editors

Nima Mowzoon, MD

Kelly D. Flemming, MD

MAYO CLINIC SCIENTIFIC PRESS

AND INFORMA HEALTHCARE USA, INC.

First published in 2007 by Informa Healthcare USA, Inc. This reissued edition published in 2011 by Informa Healthcare, London, UK.

Simultaneously published in the USA by Informa Healthcare, 52 Vanderbilt Avenue, 7th Floor, New York, NY 10017, USA.

Informa Healthcare is a trading division of Informa UK Ltd. Registered Office: 37–41 Mortimer Street, London W1T 3JH, UK. Registered in England and Wales number 1072954.

©2007 Mayo Foundation for Medical Education and Research. Reissued in 2011

No claim to original U.S. Government works

A CIP record for this book is available from the British Library.

Library of Congress Cataloging-in-Publication Data available on application

ISBN-13: 9780849337918

Orders may be sent to: Informa Healthcare, Sheepen Place, Colchester, Essex CO3 3LP, UK
Telephone: +44 (0)20 7017 5540
Email: CSDhealthcarebooks@informa.com
Website: http://informahealthcarebooks.com/

For corporate sales please contact: CorporateBooksIHC@informa.com
For foreign rights please contact: RightsIHC@informa.com
For reprint permissions please contact: PermissionsIHC@informa.com

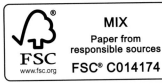

To my wife, Bita, whose everlasting love and support have made everything possible.
N. Mowzoon

To Michael and Julia.
K. Flemming

and
To the wonderful residents, fellows, and staff of Mayo Clinic Department of Neurology.

PREFACE

"To study the phenomenon of disease without books is to sail an uncharted sea, while to study books without patients is not to go to sea at all."

Sir William Osler

The elegance and complexity of the human nervous system continues to motivate many scholars and physicians in the fascinating field of neurology. The great many technological and research advances in this discipline have contributed to the ever-expanding volumes of textbooks often used as sources of reference by neurologists. Those studying for the American Board of Psychiatry and Neurology certification examination find it difficult to refer to many different sources for a complete review of the important topics and have been unable to be selective about the review material to be studied.

We now introduce *Neurology Board Review: An Illustrated Study Guide*. This book provides a comprehensive review of neurology and includes principles of basic neuroscience, neuroanatomy, neurophysiology, neuropathology, neuroradiology, molecular biology and genetics of the neurologic systems and syndromes, and a detailed and thorough review of different neurologic disorders in a succinct outline format. The purpose of this book is to provide a comprehensive review guide for those who wish to read a substantial amount of information in an efficient and timely manner. With more than 500 figures of pathology, neuroimaging, EEG tracings, EMG waveforms and nerve conductions, and illustrations of neuroanatomic pathways, this book is the first illustrated neurology board review book.

This review book is intended primarily for candidates seeking certification and recertification in neurology. Although it best serves the written portion of the neurology board examination and the Resident In-Service Training Examination of the American Academy of Neurology, the book can also be used as an easy reference and study guide throughout residency and fellowship.

Nima Mowzoon, M.D.

Kelly D. Flemming, M.D.

ACKNOWLEDGMENTS

The editors would like to thank the following individuals for their assistance and contributions to this project:

A. G. Engel, C. M. Harper, D. L. Renaud, G. A. Suarez, B. A. Crum, S. Kotagal, B. R. Younge, Y. E. Geda, K. A. Josephs, S. A. Cross, D. Selcen, C. J. Klein, W. N. Folger, S. Vernino, R. J. Spinner, P. J. Dyck, Jr., M. Tippmann-Peikert, O. H. Kantarci, G. R. Ghearing, M. L. Dodd, W. D. Freeman, M. L. Bell, J. A. Tracy, L. M. Lehwald, T. J. Young, D. H. Kilfoyle, L. K. Jones, S. C. Ahn, H. R.. Murali, G. A. Jicha, J. H. Uhm, and J. L. Corfits.

Special thanks to the Mayo Clinic Section of Scientific Publications, including Dr. O. Eugene Millhouse, editor, Roberta Schwartz, production editor, Virginia A. Dunt, editorial assistant, and Kenna L. Atherton, proofreader, to Media Support Services, including Karen E. Barrie, art director, James J. Tidwell, Paul W. Honermann, and Lynn Black, scientific illustrators, John V. Hagen and Carl G. Clingman, medical illustrators, JoLee J. Gruber, client service specialist, and James R. Hopfenspirger, medical photographer, and to Dr. Patrick H. Luetmer, Department of Radiology, and others who worked "behind the curtains," without whom this seemingly endless project would not have been possible.

CONTRIBUTORS

Sung C. Ahn, D.O.
Fellow in Neurology, Mayo School of Graduate Medical Education, Mayo Clinic College of Medicine, Rochester, Minnesota

Michael L. Bell, M.D.
Fellow in Neurology, Mayo School of Graduate Medical Education, Mayo Clinic College of Medicine, Rochester, Minnesota

Maryellen L. Dodd, M.D.
Senior Associate Consultant, Division of Inpatient Psychiatry and Psychology, Mayo Clinic, Rochester, Minnesota

Kelly D. Flemming, M.D.
Consultant, Department of Neurology, Mayo Clinic; Assistant Professor of Neurology, Mayo Clinic College of Medicine; Rochester, Minnesota

William D. Freeman, M.D.
Senior Associate Consultant, Department of Neurology, Mayo Clinic, Jacksonville, Florida

Yonas E. Geda, M.D.
Consultant, Department of Psychiatry and Psychology, Mayo Clinic; Assistant Professor of Psychiatry, Mayo Clinic College of Medicine; Rochester, Minnesota

Gena R. Ghearing, M.D.
Fellow in Neurology, Mayo School of Graduate Medical Education, Mayo Clinic College of Medicine, Rochester, Minnesota

Lyell K. Jones, M.D.
Fellow in Neurology, Mayo School of Graduate Medical Education, Mayo Clinic College of Medicine, Rochester, Minnesota

Orhun H. Kantarci, M.D.
Senior Associate Consultant, Department of Neurology, Mayo Clinic; Assistant Professor of Neurology, Mayo Clinic College of Medicine; Rochester, Minnesota

Dean H. Kilfoyle, M.B., Ch.B.
Fellow in Neurology, Mayo School of Graduate Medical Education, Mayo Clinic College of Medicine, Rochester, Minnesota

Lenora M. Lehwald, M.D.
Fellow in Neurology, Mayo School of Graduate Medical Education, Mayo Clinic College of Medicine, Rochester, Minnesota

Nima Mowzoon, M.D.
Former Fellow in Neurology, Mayo Clinic, Rochester, Minnesota; presently in Private Practice, Albany, New York

Hema R. Murali, M.B.B.S.
Fellow in Neurology, Mayo School of Graduate Medical Education, Mayo Clinic College of Medicine, Rochester, Minnesota

Deborah L. Renaud, M.D.
Consultant, Division of Child and Adolescent Neurology, Mayo Clinic; Assistant Professor of Neurology and of Pediatrics, Mayo Clinic College of Medicine; Rochester, Minnesota

Maja Tippmann-Peikert, M.D.
Senior Associate Consultant, Department of Neurology, Mayo Clinic; Instructor in Neurology, Mayo Clinic College of Medicine; Rochester, Minnesota

Jennifer A. Tracy, M.D.
Resident in Neurology, Mayo School of Graduate Medical Education, Mayo Clinic College of Medicine, Rochester, Minnesota

Steven Vernino, M.D., Ph.D.
Consultant, Department of Neurology, Mayo Clinic; Associate Professor of Neurology, Mayo Clinic College of Medicine; Rochester, Minnesota. Present address: Associate Professor of Neurology, University of Texas Southwestern Medical Center, Dallas, Texas

Timothy J. Young, M.D.
Fellow in Sleep Medicine, Mayo School of Graduate Medical Education, Mayo Clinic College of Medicine, Rochester, Minnesota

TABLE OF CONTENTS

How to Use This Book

This book is best suited for the written portion of the neurology board certification and recertification examinations administered by the American Board of Psychiatry and Neurology and the in-service examinations administered by the American Academy of Neurology. The long lists of topics covered in these examinations seem endless. Reading voluminous textbooks in an attempt to thoroughly review is often impossible, and many important topics are often missed by simply reviewing "high-yield" topics in undersized review texts. We now introduce a comprehensive source that provides detailed information in a succinct outline format. The guidelines sugggested below should be read before using the review text.

Before the Preparation: 8 to 12 Months Before the Examination

Our recommendation is to begin using this book as a reference guide at least 8 to 12 months in advance, making notes in the margins and referring to other sources. The text then becomes familiar and may be reviewed more easily in a short time before the examination. Tables, charts, anatomic drawings, index cards, and other such visual guides are often helpful in remembering complex topics. Candidates are encouraged to review these pictorial guides in the text and to prepare their own during the year before the examination. This text should not replace references to other standard textbooks and journals.

Initial Preparation: 4 Months Before the Examination

Formal preparation needs to be initiated at this time. Each day, 1 to 3 hours should be allocated to formal study. This can be modified depending on many factors, including how quickly a candidate can study, the candidate's schedule, the level of training and experience, and the examination itself. Part I of the neurology boards and the recertification examinations are designed for the general neurologist; however, there are often many questions on the written neurology board and in-service examinations that require detailed subspecialty knowledge. It is often the special attention to detail that separates those who excel in these examinations from those who simply "pass" the test. This text provides detailed information in each topic that can only be fully learned if the formal reviews are initiated several months in advance. Likewise, it is important for adult neurologists to allocate adequate time to cover pediatric neurology and psychiatry during this time because a thorough review of these topics is essential for part I of the neurology board examination. The topics important for pediatric neurology are found throughout the book, and psychiatry is discussed in a dedicated chapter.

Core Preparation: 1 to 8 Weeks Before the Examination

By this time, candidates should have studied most of the text and any other source that may be deemed useful. At this stage, candidates should review the chapters again, with emphasis on topics of weakness, answer questions at the end of each chapter, and refer to the text with each answer. In addition, question-and-answer books may be used, and reference should be made to the text. This facilitates "active learning," which is more effective than passively reading the text. Readers may also find the outline format more helpful for "active learning" than passively reading long paragraphs in most standard textbooks.

Last-Minute Reviews

Reviewing the "high-yield" boxes provided with each chapter, together with previously learned memory aids (tables, charts, index cards, etc.), will be helpful for "last-minute reviews." The candidates should emphasize the topics of relative weakness throughout the core preparation and review these again during the week before the examination. Finally, it is important to realize that one cannot (and is not expected to) know all of neurology.

N. Mowzoon

K. Flemming

Embryology and Developmental Disorders of the Nervous System

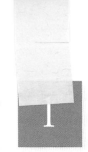

Nima Mowzoon, M.D.

I. Neurulation: Formation of the Neural Tube

A. Gastrulation

1. Primitive streak (Fig. 1-1)
   a. Formed from ectoderm
   b. Gives rise to the mesoderm, which is formed between the endoderm and ectoderm
   c. Hensen's node is at the end of the primitive streak
2. Notochord
   a. Mesodermal cells that induce the formation of the neural plate beginning at Hensen's node
   b. Gives rise to part of the vertebral column

B. Dorsal Induction

1. Transformation of neural ectoderm to neural tissue and formation of the neural plate and neural tube
2. Induction results from inactivation of bone morphogenetic proteins (BMPs), which normally act to change ectoderm to epidermis.
3. Hensen's node secretes factors, including chordin, noggin, and follisatin that inactivate BMPs and allow formation of the neural plate
4. Neural plate

Induction

Transformation of ectoderm into neural tissue

Formation of the neural plate

Results from the inactivation of bone morphogenetic proteins, which normally act to change ectoderm into epidermis

Results in formation of the neural tube

---

   a. First recognized in the middle of the third week after conception
   b. The first neural tissue formed from ectoderm under the influence of the underlying notochord
5. The ectoderm that transforms into the neural plate becomes columnar epithelium
6. The rest of the ectoderm becomes the skin and neural crest cells
7. Neural plate forms the neural tube (neurulation) (Fig. 1-1)
   a. Step 1: invagination along the midline axis
   b. Step 2: formation of the neural groove by the proliferation and migration of the surface ectodermal neural plate (cells at lateral edges proliferate more rapidly than those at the center)
   c. Step 3: formation and elevation of the neural folds, which approach each other and fuse
   d. This process is driven partly by proliferation of the underlying mesodermal tissue and the accumulation of contractile cytoskeletal filaments in the apical poles of the neural folds
   e. Step 4: neural folds fuse by day 24
      1) Fusion begins at the mid-cervical level and proceeds both caudally and cranially until the entire tube is closed
      2) The initially unfused areas are termed "neuropores"
      3) The anterior neuropore closes between days 24 and 26; the posterior neuropore between days 25 and 28
8. Folic acid is potentially important in neural tube closure
9. Primary neurulation: the formation of neural tube giving rise to brain and spinal cord through the future S2 level
10. Secondary neurulation: the formation of lower sacral and coccygeal segments, giving rise to the future conus medullaris and filum terminale
11. Closure of the neural tube occurs by end of the fourth week of gestation

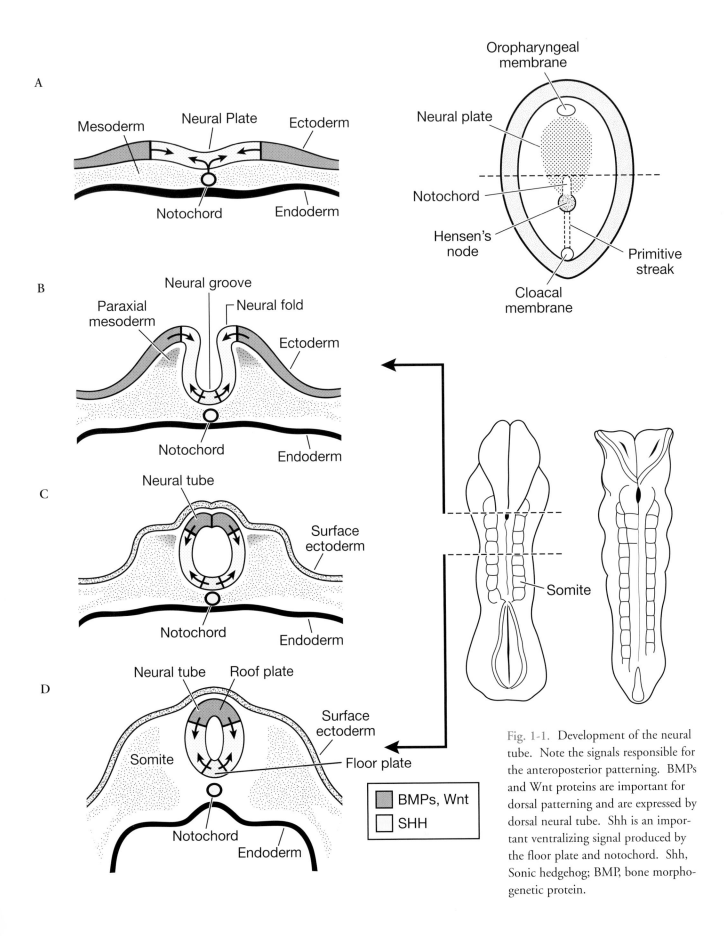

Fig. 1-1. Development of the neural tube. Note the signals responsible for the anteroposterior patterning. BMPs and Wnt proteins are important for dorsal patterning and are expressed by dorsal neural tube. Shh is an important ventralizing signal produced by the floor plate and notochord. Shh, Sonic hedgehog; BMP, bone morphogenetic protein.

C. Differentiation of the Neural Tube

1. Longitudinal differentiation: formation of forebrain, midbrain, and hindbrain and branchial arches and placodes (Fig. 1-2)

   a. With closure of neuropores, the neural tube is divided into three vesicles: forebrain (prosencephalon), midbrain (mesencephalon), and hindbrain (rhombencephalon) (Fig. 1-2)

   b. Prosencephalon forms telencephalon (cerebral hemispheres) and diencephalon

      1) Within the telencephalon, the dorsal zone gives rise to cerebral cortex and the ventral zone (ventral ganglionic eminence) produces basal ganglia

      2) The diencephalon becomes thalamus, hypothalamus, optic nerves, and pineal gland

   c. The mesencephalon forms the midbrain

   d. The rhombencephalon forms the metencephalon (pons and granule cells of cerebellum) and myelencephalon (medulla)

      1) Anteroposterior patterning of the hindbrain involves generation of segments of embryonic hindbrain called rhombomeres

      2) Homeobox (*Hox*) genes are responsible for anteroposterior patterning of hindbrain

      3) Arrangement of *Hox* gene on the chromosome correlates with and dictates the expression along the anteroposterior axis

      4) Activation of correct *Hox* gene and segmental expression require retinoic acid

2. Transverse differentiation of neural tube

   a. Proliferating neuroblasts accumulate in the lateral walls of neural tube, forming dorsolaterally situated alar plates and ventrolaterally situated basal plates, which are separated by sulcus limitans

   b. The middorsal and midventral portions of neural tube contain few proliferating neuroblasts and are termed roof plate and floor plate, respectively

      1) Alar plates give rise to afferent sensory structures in the brainstem and spinal cord, including dorsal horns

      2) Basal plates give rise to efferent motor structures in the brainstem and spinal cord, including anterior horns

   c. Signals involved in dorsoventral patterning

      1) Dorsal patterning

         a) Primary dorsalizing signals involved: BMP and Wnt

         b) Important for determination of alar plate and development of dorsal telencephalon and cerebellum, as well as dorsal brainstem and spinal cord

         c) Signals are derived from dorsal ectoderm, paraxial mesoderm, and roof plate

      2) Ventral patterning

         a) Primary ventralizing signal involved: Sonic hedgehog (Shh)

         b) Important for determination of basal plate and development of ventral telencephalon and diencephalon, as well as ventral brainstem and spinal cord

         c) Signals are derived from notochord and floor plate

D. Disorders of Neurulation (neural tube defects) and Related Conditions

1. Multifactorial disorders

2. Risk factors: family history, maternal risk factors (obesity, diabetes mellitus, hyperthermia, use of anticonvulsants, folate deficiency)

   a. Risk of spina bifida cystica in mothers taking valproate is 1% to 2 %

   b. Risk of spina bifida cystica in mothers taking carbamazepine is 0.5% to 1%

3. Detected by increased levels of α-fetoprotein (AFP) in maternal serum

4. If serum AFP is increased, ultrasonography is performed and amniotic fluid checked for AFP

5. Types of neural tube defects

   a. Craniorachischisis: congenital malformations of central nervous system due to defective neural tube closure

---

Segmentation and Patterning

Rostrocaudal: dependent on TGF-β family proteins
  Homeotic genes necessary for hindbrain patterning, depend on retinoic acid
Dorsoventral patterning
  Ventral patterning (secreted from floor plate and notochord): Sonic hedgehog protein
  Dorsal patterning (secreted from roof plate, dorsal ectoderm, and paraxial mesoderm): bone morphogenetic and Wnt proteins

---

Disorders of Neurulation

Detected by increased levels of α-fetoprotein in the maternal serum

Risk factors include family history and maternal risk factors, especially folate deficiency and use of anticonvulsants during pregnancy, particularly valproate and carbamazepine

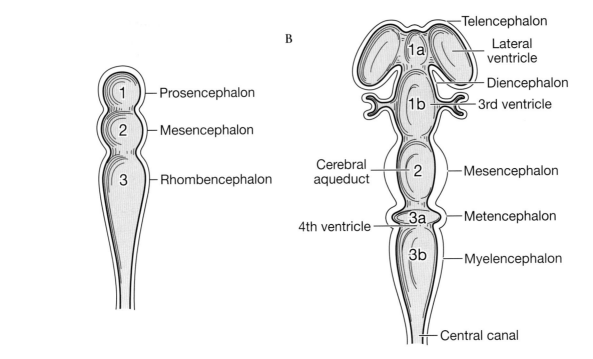

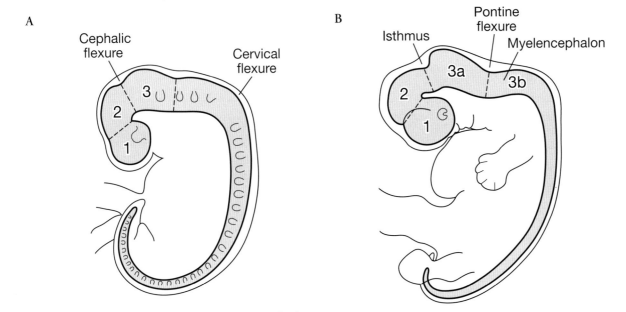

Fig. 1-2. Longitudinal differentiation of the neural tube.

during first trimester of pregnancy (usually between days 18 and 29 of gestation), producing contiguous exposure of brain and spinal column

b. Anencephaly (absence of a major portion of the brain, skull, and scalp)
   1) Due to failure of anterior neuropore closure
   2) Defective notochord induction of the neuroectoderm

3) More common in females
4) Occasionally familial; certain populations may be at higher risk (France, Wales, Ireland)
5) Replacement of most of the intracranial contents by area cerebrovasculosa (vascular mass of small blood vessels admixed with variable amounts of mature and immature neuronal and glial cells)

c. Meningomyelocele (spina bifida cystica)
   1) Herniation of spinal cord and meninges through a vertebral defect (Fig. 1-3 and 1-4)
   2) Is often seen in Chiari type II malformation and is associated with hydrocephalus
d. Spina bifida occulta
   1) A defect in one or more vertebral arches
   2) Spinal cord and meninges are normal
e. Cranium bifidum
   1) Defective fusion of cranial bones
   2) Most common in the occipital portion of the cranium
   3) Associated with herniated cerebral tissue and meninges (Fig. 1-5)
f. Encephalocele
   1) Extension of intracranial structures through the cranial vault from a defect in fusion of cranial bones
      a) Meningocele: herniated meninges through skull defect
      b) Meningoencephalocele: herniated brain tissue and meninges through skull defect
      c) Meningohydrocephalocele: herniated brain tissue, meninges, and ventricles through skull defect
   2) Most common in the occipital (less common in the parietal) area
      a) Herniated tissue is usually arranged haphazardly and hamartomatous
      b) Both intracranial and herniated contents may show signs of migration abnormalities such as heterotopias (see below)
      c) Occipital encephalocele often contains vascular structures and is associated with Meckel-Gruber syndrome (autosomal recessive condition associated with occipital encephalocele, polycystic kidneys, liver fibrosis, cleft palate, and polydactyly; is usually fatal)
6. Chiari malformations (cerebellar deformities)
   a. Chiari type I malformation (Fig. 1-6)
      1) Primary cerebellar ectopia: caudal displacement of cerebellar tonsils through the foramen magnum
      2) May be congenital or acquired condition caused by downward herniation of the brain in patients with low intracranial pressure
      3) Mean age at presentation: 41 years
      4) Upper limits of normal for the position of the cerebellar tonsils below the foramen magnum depends on age:
         a) 6 mm for first decade
         b) 5 mm for second and third decades
         c) 4 mm for fourth to eighth decades
         d) 3 mm for ninth decade
      5) Chiari type I malformation may be associated with
         a) Hydrocephalus
         b) Intermittent increase in intracranial pressure
         c) Syringomyelia, syringobulbia

Chiari Malformations

Chiari type I malformation: caudal displacement of cerebellar tonsils through the foramen magnum

Chiari type II malformation: caudal displacement of cerebellar tonsils, cervicomedullary junction, pons, fourth ventricle, medulla

Chairi type II malformation associated with
   Myelomeningocele
   Hydrocephalus
   Colpocephaly of the lateral ventricles
   Elongated fourth ventricle
   Interdigitating gyri (associated with hypoplastic falx cerebri)
   Skull abnormalities: lacunar skull, hypoplastic tentorium cerebelli, gaping foramen magnum

Chiari type III malformation: low occipital/high cervical encephalocele with herniation of the cerebellum, occipital lobes, pons, medulla

Chiari type IV malformation
   Likely a variant of Dandy-Walker malformation
   Hypoplastic brainstem and cerebellum

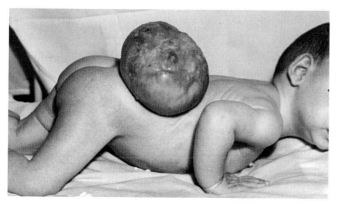

Fig. 1-3. Myelomeningocele (spina bifida cystica) is herniation of the spinal cord and meninges through a congenital defect in the vertebral arch. It is covered with skin.

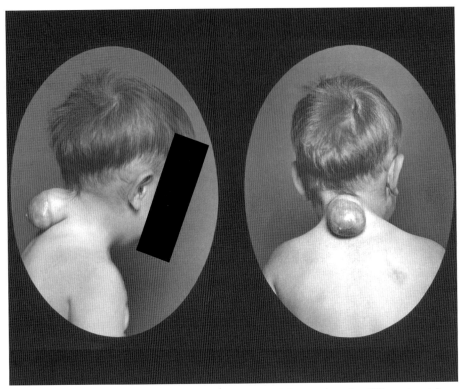

Fig. 1-4. Cervical spina bifida, associated with Chiari type I malformation. This needs to be differentiated from Chiari type III mal-formation, which is essentially herniated cerebellar and brainstem tissue.

   d) Klippel-Feil syndrome, basilar impression, and occipitalization of the atlas
   e) Compression of brainstem structures and some rostral extension of the medulla
  6) Presenting symptoms are due to any of the above asso-ciated abnormalities plus
   a) Headaches, especially brought on by neck exten-sion or the Valsalva maneuver (most common pre-senting symptom), sometimes associated with tinnitus, nausea, and vomiting
   b) Various cerebellar symptoms, lower cranial nerve dysfunction, diplopia and downbeat nystagmus, dissociated sensory loss (loss of pinprick and tem-perature sensation and relative preservation of large fiber modalities), and possibly pyramidal tract involvement
   c) May be asymptomatic
  7) Surgical treatment: early surgery for symptomatic patients and observation for asymptomatic ones
 b. Chiari type II malformation (Fig. 1-7 and 1-8)
  1) Caudal displacement of medulla, cervicomedullary junction, pons, fourth ventricle, and low cerebellar tonsils
  2) Usually associated with myelomeningocele and, rarely, spina bifida occulta

 3) Other major findings
  a) Medullary "spur" or "kink" as a result of caudally displaced, elongated medulla
  b) Extension of cerebellar tissue upward through the wide tentorium and anteriorly around the brain-stem, also posterior displacement of the tonsils
  c) Tectal "beaking" of the midbrain due to pressure from herniated cerebellum
  d) Elongated, tubular fourth ventricle
  e) Hydrocephalus in 90% of patients
  f) Colpocephaly of the lateral ventricles (enlargement of occipital horns)
  g) Enlarged massa intermedia (interthalamic adhe-sion) and absence of the septum pellucidum
  h) Interdigitating gyri (associated with hypoplastic falx cerebri)
 4) Skull and dural abnormalities
  a) Craniolacuna of the skull (lacunar skull, lücken-schädel), due to abnormal calvarial development
  b) Hypoplastic tentorium cerebelli with wide tentori-al incisura and concave petrous ridge
  c) Gaping foramen magnum
  d) Hypoplastic, fenestrated falx cerebri
 5) Associated with

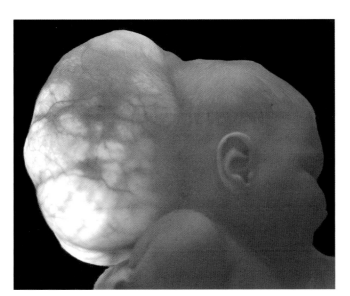

Fig. 1-5. Cranium bifidum. Defective fusion of the cranial bones, most commonly in the occipital part of the cranium. In this example, note herniation of the meninges with cerebrospinal fluid only (meningocele).

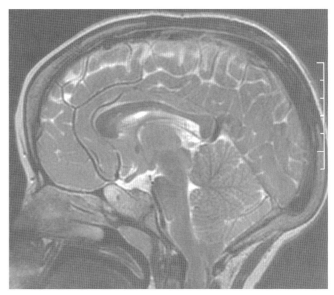

Fig. 1-6. Congenital Chiari type I malformation in a 35-year-old woman who presented with headaches. The primary manifestation is caudal displacement of the cerebellar tonsils below the foramen magnum.

     a) Dysgenesis or partial agenesis of the corpus callosum
     b) Microgyria
     c) Syringohydromyelia in up to 90% of patients
     d) Meningomyelocele in all cases
     e) Diastematomyelia
     f) Heterotopias
   6) Presentation
     a) Variable age at onset: usually neonatal to early childhood
     b) Neonatal presentation with rapid neurologic deterioration, including weak or absent cry, respiratory failure, stridor, apneic spells, swallowing difficulties from involvement of the medulla
     c) Hydrocephalus, weakness including facial weakness, lower cranial nerve abnormalities
   7) Treatment: surgical decompression and cerebrospinal fluid (CSF) shunt for hydrocephalus
 c. Chiari type III malformation
   1) Features of Chiari type II with herniation of the cerebellum, occipital lobes, and sometimes pons or medulla into a low occipital or high cervical encephalocele
   2) Most severe form, is usually incompatible with life
 d. Chiari type IV malformation
   1) Hypoplastic brainstem and cerebellum
   2) It is likely a variant of Dandy-Walker malformation

E. Disorders of Forebrain Induction and Midline Malformations
1. Midline malformations are due to either
 a. Deficient lateral growth of the cerebral hemispheres because of abnormal migration *or*
 b. Abnormal differentiation of the telencephalon from the lamina terminalis, which is formed by closure of the anterior neuropore
2. Holoprosencephaly (Fig. 1-9)
 a. Characterized by partial or complete failure of normal midline division of the two cerebral hemispheres, resulting in a single forebrain structure with one ventricle and continuity of gray matter across the midline
 b. Associated with many genetic mutations
   1) *SHH* gene on chromosome 7q36
   2) Patched (*PTC*) gene encoding for SHH receptor
   3) Gene coding for homeodomain-containing transcription factor Zic2 on chromosome 13q12
   4) Frequently associated with trisomy 13
 c. Associated with maternal diabetes mellitus
 d. Associated with midline defects and craniofacial anomalies
   1) Callosal agenesis
   2) Olfactory agenesis and arhinencephaly
   3) Craniofacial anomalies: cyclops, hypotelorism, and midline facial defects such as displaced nose
 e. Subtypes

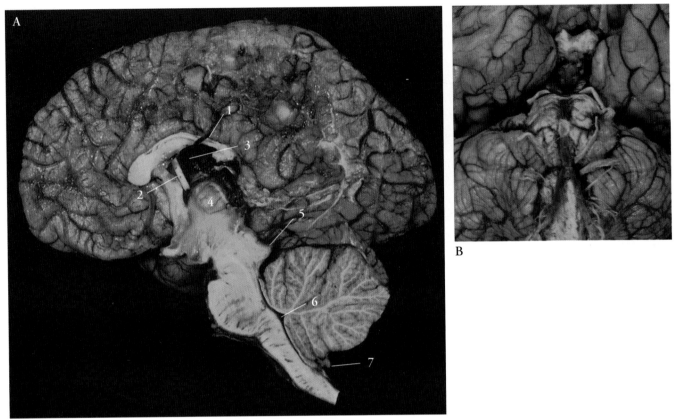

Fig. 1-7. *A*, Midsagittal and, *B*, ventral views of brain with Chiari type II malformation. This malformation results in caudal displacement of the medulla, cervicomedullary junction, pons, and fourth ventricle and low cerebellar tonsils (*7*). The cerebellar tonsils appear "kinked" because of being displaced through the foramen magnum. Note the cephalad displacement and anteromedial extension of the cerebellum around the brainstem (*B*). Associated findings (*A*) are beaking of the tectum (*5*), elongated tubular fourth ventricle (*6*), enlarged massa intermedia (*4*), absence of septum pellucidum (*3*), partial agenesis of corpus callosum (*1*), myelomeningocele, and hydrocephalus. (*2*), Cerebrospinal fluid shunt for treatment of hydrocephalus.

1) Alobar holoprosencephaly: single midline ventricle and continuity of cerebral cortex across the midline
2) Semilobar holoprosencephaly: incomplete interhemispheric fissure formed (more often, posteriorly with formed occipital lobes and occipital horns), partially separated thalami and basal ganglia, and partially formed falx cerebri
3) Lobar holoprosencephaly
   a) Less severe form
   b) Well-formed hemispheres and separated thalami and basal ganglia
   c) Interhemispheric fissure and ventricles are present, but septum pellucidum is absent
   d) Some fusion of the frontal cortices, including the cingulate gyri and indusium griseum
3. Septo-optic dysplasia
   a. Absence or dysgenesis of the septum pellucidum with hypoplasia of the optic nerve (sometimes involving the optic chiasm) and pituitary infundibulum
   b. May be associated with either
      1) Schizencephaly *or*
      2) Constellation of diffuse white matter hypoplasia, ventriculomegaly, and abnormal hypothalamic-pituitary function
4. Arhinencephaly: may present as isolated olfactory aplasia or in association with other developmental abnormalities such as holoprosencephaly or as part of Kallmann syndrome (X-linked or autosomal dominant anosmia, mental retardation, deficient gonadotropin hormones)
5. Colpocephaly (Fig. 1-10)
   a. Dilatation of the occipital horns out of proportion to the remaining ventricles due to
      1) Primary congenital anomaly
      2) Secondary congenital anomaly from agenesis of the

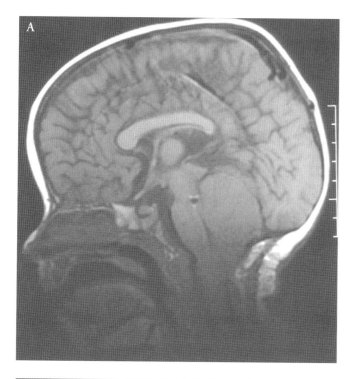

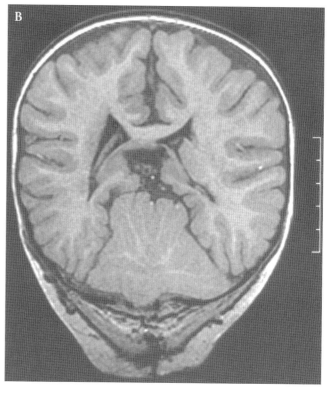

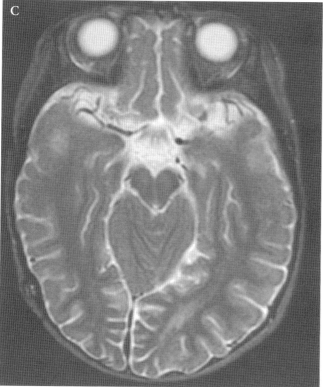

Fig. 1-8. *A*, Sagittal, *B*, coronal, and *C*, axial images of Chiari type II malformation in a 16-month-old infant after repair of a myelomeningocele. Note cephalad and caudal displacement of the cerebellum, tectal beaking, partial agenesis of the corpus callosum, enlarged massa intermedia, absence of septum pellucidum, and elongated tubular fourth ventricle. *A* and *B*, T1-weighted and, *C*, T2-weighted MRIs.

       splenium of the corpus callosum
       3) Acquired anomaly resulting from loss of periventricular white matter
    b. May also develop late in life from infarction and loss of deep, periventricular white matter posteriorly

II. NEUROGENESIS

A. Neural Determination

1. Both the neuronal and glial cell lineages originate from precursor cells (neural stem cells) through differentiation
2. This process is influenced by
    a. External signals in the microenvironment of the neural stem cells
    b. Intracellular signals and timed sequence of phenotypic expression determined genetically

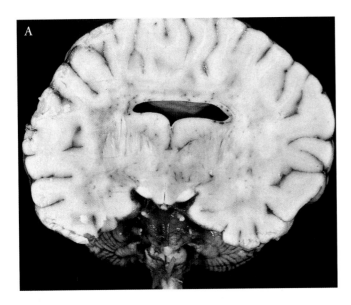
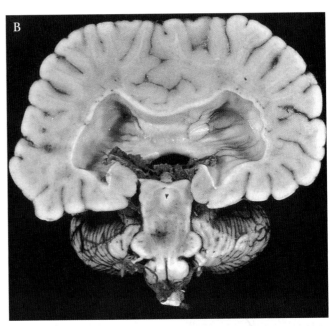

Fig. 1-9. *A* and *B*, Holoprosencephaly. It is characterized by, *A*, absence of the septum pellucidum and fused thalami and basal ganglia, and, *B*, well-formed occipital horns. Despite the appearance of gyral fusion on the surface (not shown), there is a well-formed inter-hemispheric fissure with a continuous band of cingulate gyrus crossing the midline and resting on the corpus callosum (*B*). (From Okazaki H, Scheithauer BW. Atlas of neuropathology. New York: Gower Medical Publishing; 1988. p. 288. By permission of Mayo Foundation.)

3. Differentiation starts in a cluster of precursor cells called the "proneural region"
   a. Intercellular interaction between the cells in this region is the inciting event for differentiation through the Notch signaling pathway (Fig. 1-11)
   b. Delta protein is necessary for differentiation into neurogenic lineage, and Notch protein for differentiation into both neurogenic and glial lineages
   c. Both Delta and Notch proteins are membrane-bound proteins
   d. Notch acts as a receptor for Delta protein
   e. The following is a hypothetical example of interaction of two neighboring cells (A and B) in the proneural region:
      1) Interaction of Delta protein of cell A with Notch receptor of cell B triggers intramembraneous proteolytic cleavage of Notch protein in cell B (carried out by presenillin-1, which is thought to be involved in a certain category of familial Alzheimer disease); the intracellular portion of Notch protein is transferred into the nucleus of cell B and binds to transcription factor CBF1 (C-promoter binding factor 1, homologue of the mammalian Suppressor-of-Hairless DNA-binding protein); CBF1 activates transcription of a repressor of proneural genes, *Hesl-5* in cell B, thus cell B will be of nonneuronal lineage (epidermal or glial cell)
      2) Notch signaling also acts to inhibit transcription of Delta protein in cell B, reducing production of peoneural factor Delta protein in cell B; this means reduced expression of the transmembrane Delta protein (which interacts with Notch protein in the neighboring cells); this reduces activation of the Notch receptor protein in cell A, making cell A a neuronal precursor (neuroblast), whereas cell B becomes a nonneuronal precursor
      3) Usually, a slight imbalance in the signaling between the neighboring cells triggers this cascade of differentiation
4. Differentiation of sympathetic neurons from neural crest cells depends on BMPs 2 and 4
5. Neural stem cells: earliest precursor cells, have excellent self-renewal capacity (as do neural crest cells), are multipotent, and responsible for multiple lineages
6. Neural stem cells give rise to progenitor cells that divide, proliferate, and produce specificity for different lineages under the influence of environmental factors

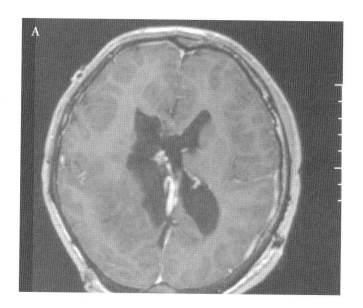

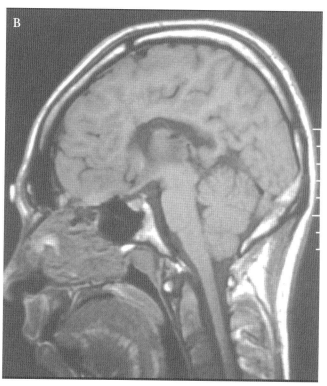

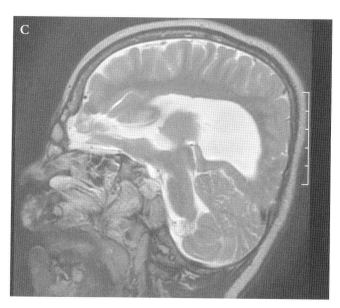

Fig. 1-10. *A* and *B*, MRI of a patient with developmental delay and intractable seizures. The T1-weighted, *A*, axial and, *B*, sagittal sequences show colpocephaly secondary to partial agenesis of corpus callosum (best seen in *B*). Also note periventricular aggregates of subcortical heterotopic gray matter. *C*, T2-weighted sagittal image showing colpocephaly in another patient.

III. NEOCORTICAL AND CEREBELLAR DEVELOPMENT (FIG. 1-12)

A. Ventricular Zone

1. Primary germinal zone of the neural tube
2. Responsible for initial proliferation of neuronal and glial cell precursors
3. Contains neuroepithelial cells with apical-basal (pial) polarity; the apical pole is at the ventricular surface
4. Neuroepithelial cells proliferate and differentiate into neuronal and glial cell lineages in the ventricular zone (greatest rate of mitosis: during first trimester)
5. Nuclei of neuroepithelial cells migrate throughout the cell cycle, but mitotic cells usually abut the ventricular surface
6. The orientation of the mitotic spindle determines the fate of daughter cells
   a. Vertical cleavage plane (perpendicular to the ventricular surface)

a. Neurogenins promote neuronal differentiation and inhibit differentiation of multipotent progenitor cells into glioblasts

b. Glial precursors destined for glial lineage differentiate into astrocytic precursor cells and O2A progenitor cells
   1) Platelet-derived growth factor promotes differentiation into O2A progenitor cells and ongoing proliferation
   2) With withdrawal of platelet-derived growth factor, O2A progenitor cells stop dividing and differentiate into astrocytes and oligodendrocytes

c. Ciliary neurotrophic factor promotes astrocytic differentiation

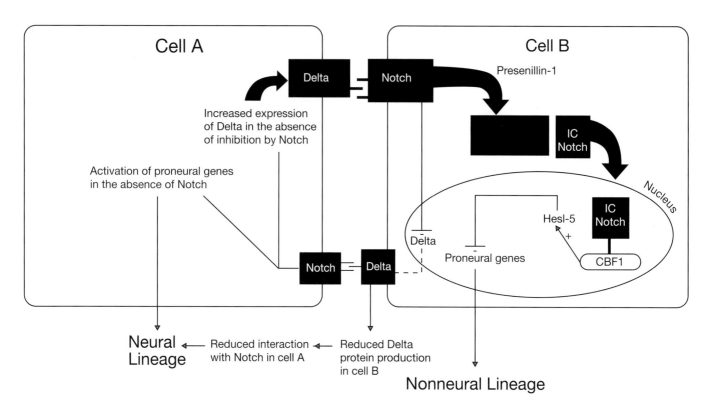

Fig. 1-11. Differentiation of neural and nonneural lineages. CBF1, C-promoter binding factor 1; IC, intracellular.

1) Symmetric division
2) The two daughter cells become neuroepithelial cells, maintain their apical connection, and reenter the cell cycle for further division
b. Horizontal cleavage plane (parallel to the ventricular surface)
1) Asymmetric division
2) The daughter cell closer to the ventricular surface (apical daughter cell) becomes another progenitor neuroepithelial cell and maintains its contact with the apical surface
3) The basal daughter cell loses its apical contact, migrates toward the cortical plate, and becomes a postmitotic neuroblast
c. The fate of the neuroepithelial cells is determined partly by the *numb* and *null* genes: with symmetric division, equal ratios of the products of both genes are passed on to the daughter cells; with asymmetric division, unequal ratios are passed on

B. **Preplate Zone**
1. Formed by postmitotic neuroblasts of ventricular zone around 4 weeks' gestation
2. Later separated from overlying marginal zone by developing cortical plate and forming subplate zone

C. **Subplate Zone**
1. Transient remnant of preplate zone, which appears at about 6 weeks' gestation as cortical plate develops
2. Important function in synaptogenesis and development of cortical and subcortical connections: migrating neuroblasts form connections with afferents from cortical and subcortical structures as they pass through the subplate zone

D. **Cortical Plate**
1. Formed by migrating neuroblasts (discussed below)
2. Migrating cells: younger neuroblasts migrate through the zones occupied by older neuroblasts and are eventually situated in the most superficial layer; as a result, youngest cells occupy the most superficial layers, and the oldest cells are in deepest layers (closer to ventricular surface)
3. Eventually forms neocortical layers II-VI

E. **Marginal Zone**
1. Eventually forms neocortical layer I

F. **External Granule Layer of the Cerebellum**
1. Secondary germinal zone

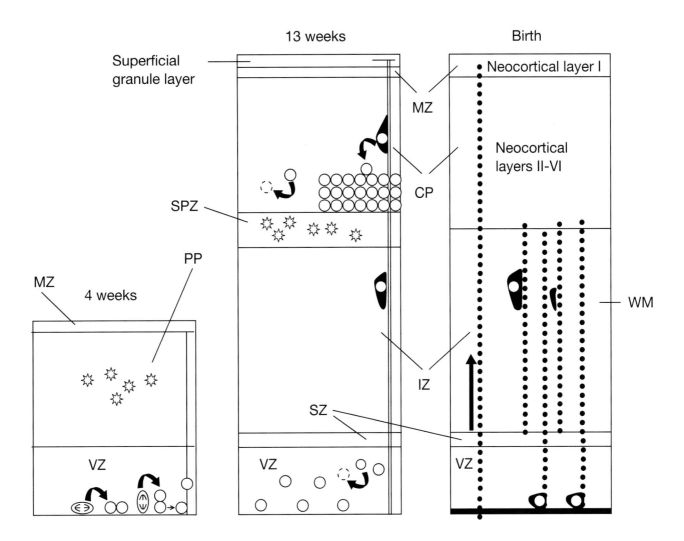

Fig. 1-12. Neocortical development: proliferation and migration. A cluster of progenitor neuroepithelial cells in the fetal ventricular zone (VZ) proliferate. Daughter cells with the mitotic axis parallel to the ventricular surface differentiate and migrate (via radial glia). Neuroepithelial cells migrate to the superficial layer of the cortical plate (CP); thus, younger cells are in the most superficial layer and older cells in deeper layers. Throughout this process, excess neuroepithelial cells degenerate via apoptosis. The preplate zone (PP) appears by 4 weeks of gestation and is eventually divided by the CP zone into a marginal zone (MZ) and a remnant of the PP zone, sometimes called the subplate zone (SPZ). This layer is transient; the MZ eventually becomes neocortical layer I. The cortical plate forms neocortical layers II through VI. By birth, the radial glia retract their processes, and the intermediate zone (IZ) becomes the white matter (WM). IZ acts primarily as a conduit for migrating cells and contains the radial glia. The subventricular zone (SZ) contains small interneurons and persists for several months postnatally.

2. Proliferative layer from which arise radial glial cells that migrate centripetally (continues throughout first year of life)
3. Granule neuroblasts are precursors of cerebellar granule cells, which form the external granule cell layer
4. After the initial proliferation of granule cells in the external granule cell layer at birth, the precursor cells migrate through the molecular and Purkinje cell layers

G. Migration of Progenitor Cells
1. Occurs soon after initial proliferation in the ventricular zone
2. Postmitotic cells migrate centrifugally from the ventricular zone to the cortical plate at the surface (except for centripetal migration of cells from the external granule cell layer of the cerebellum into the folia)
3. Migration usually occurs radially, but it can occur

Neocortical Development

Ventricular zone: the primary germinal zone of the neural tube

Neuroepithelial cells undergo mitosis and proliferate, some differentiate into neuronal and glial precursors and migrate centrifugally to the surface via radial glial cells (exception: granule neuroblasts in the cerebellum migrate centripetally throughout the first year after birth)

Differentiation of neuroepithelial cells depends on Notch and Delta proteins

Orientation of the mitotic spindles determines whether daughter cells again divide or migrate

tangentially (this can persist into adulthood, e.g., granule cells of the olfactory bulb)
4. Migration is responsible for the formation of gyri and sulci

H. Radial Glial Cells
1. Guide the migration of neuroblasts (centrifugally except for centripetal migration of cells from the external granule cell layer of the cerebellum)
2. Are produced in the ventricular zone in the early proliferative stage of gliogenesis
3. Are bipolar cells with cell bodies in the ventricular zone
4. Their processes extend from the ventricular surface to the pial surface and, thus, provide a scaffold for migrating cells
5. Neuroblasts migrate earlier than glioblasts, which can continue to migrate during the postnatal period
6. Initiation of migration depends on the cross-linking protein filamin-1 (encoded by the *FLN1* gene on chromosome Xq28), which binds actin
7. Microtubule-associated proteins doublecortin and LIS-1 are essential for migration: a mutation of the *LIS1* gene may be responsible for type 1 lissencephaly (Miller-Dieker syndrome)
8. Organization of laminae in the cerebral cortex depends on Reelin, which is secreted by the Cajal-Retzius cells
9. Contact between migratory cells and radial glial cells is established by factors such as astrotactin (encoded by gene on chromosome q25.2)
10. Migration of cells along the radial glia is facilitated by adhesion molecules

11. The initial wave of migration forms the cortical plate
12. Younger postmitotic cells migrate through the older cells already established in the cortical plate; thus, younger cells are located more superficially
13. After migration is completed, radial glial fibers retract and radial glia cells differentiate into astrocytes located in the white matter

I. Migration of Granule Neuroblasts in the Cerebellum
1. Granule cells arise from the neuroepithelium of the rhombic lip (rhombencephalon)
2. Purkinje cells arise from the ventricular neuroepithelium of the isthmus (junction between the mesencephalon and rhombic lip)
3. Migration of Purkinje cells
   a. Dependent on Reelin
   b. They migrate from the ventricular zone along radial glial fibers
4. Migration of granule neuroblasts
   a. A Reelin-independent process
   b. Occurs throughout first year after birth
   c. Occurs after rapid proliferation of the granule cells in the external granule cell layer at birth
   d. Granule neuroblasts migrate centripetally through the molecular and Purkinje cell layers to form the internal granule cell layer
   e. The superficial portion of the migrating cells remains in the external granule layer, forming the parallel fibers

J. Disorders of Migration
1. Lissencephaly (pachygyria-agyria) (Fig. 1-13)
   a. "Smooth brain": decreased or no formation of gyri and sulci, which normally occurs between 20 and 36 weeks (at midgestation, the brain of the normal fetus is smooth)
   b. Some authorities restrict the definition of "lissencephaly" to complete absence of gyral formation except for a short sylvian fissure (agyria), and reserve the term "pachygyria" for brains with relatively few gyri
   c. This condition may be acquired (intrauterine infection) or genetically determined
   d. Is associated with heterotopic gray matter and decreased amount of white matter
   e. *LIS1*–associated (see below): spares the cerebellum (four-layer cortex)
   f. Reelin-associated: lissencephaly with cerebellar hypoplasia (all cortical layers are present but in reverse order)
   g. Lissencephaly type 1
      1) Associated with deletion of chromosome 17p13.3

(*LIS1* gene); *LIS1* has also been associated with posterior-dominant subcortical band heterotopia
2) Histologically, the cortex has four layers:
   a) Layer one: molecular layer
   b) Layer two: corresponds to layers II to VI of normal neocortex
   c) Layer three: thin layer with sparse cellularity, persistent fetal subplate zone
   d) Layer four: deep, thick layer of cells that have not migrated completely and heterotopic nodules that sometimes form columns of cells in the persistent fetal intermediate zone
3) Neocortex and hippocampus are affected but cerebellum is relatively spared
4) Large deletions of *LIS1* gene result in Miller-Dieker syndrome
   a) Disorder of neuroblast migration causing agyria, mental retardation, intractable seizures, and spasticity
   b) Facial features: thin upper lip, high forehead, microcephaly, bitemporal hollowing, micrognathia, upturned nares, broad nasal bridge, and low-set ears
   c) Child usually dies before age 1 year
h. Lissencephaly type 2
   1) Poorly laminated, disorganized cortex with disoriented neurons
   2) Thickened cortex with an appearance resembling polymicrogyria ("cobblestone" appearance) and hypomyelination of the white matter
   3) Overmigration causing disrupted, discontinuous pia, and disoriented, disorganized neurons placed outside the pial surface, with no laminar organization
   4) Mental retardation, intractable seizures, hydrocephalus, death in infancy
   5) Associated with ocular anomalies such as retinal dysplasia
   6) Walker-Warburg syndrome
      a) Also called HARD ± E syndrome (**h**ydrocephalus, **a**gyria, **r**etinal **d**ysplasia, and, in some cases, **e**ncephalocele)
      b) Presentation is usually in neonatal period with marked hypotonia, later development of spastic quadriparesis

Disorders of Migration
Lissencephaly
   Type 1: disorder of *undermigration* associated with deletion of *LIS1* gene on chromosome 17p13.3, Miller-Dieker syndrome
   Type 2: disorder of *overmigration* causing poorly laminated, disorganized cortex, associated with Walker-Warburg syndrome, muscle-eye-brain disease, and Fukuyama muscular dystrophy
Polymicrogyria
   Usually occurs in context of intrauterine insult (usually ischemic)
   Also associated with intrauterine infections or in context of inherited metabolic disease

Heterotopia
   Isolated heterotopia
   Bilateral periventricular nodular heterotopia
   Subcortical band heterotopia

Schizencephaly
   Two types: closed lip and open lip
   Usually due to fetal ischemic insult

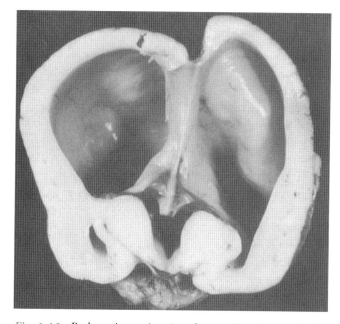

Fig. 1-13. Pachygyria, a migration abnormality characterized by little evidence of gyral development and secondarily enlarged ventricles. (From Okazaki H. Fundamentals of neuropathology: morphologic basis of neurologic disorders. 2nd ed. New York: Igaku-Shoin Medical Publishers; 1989. p. 288. By permission of Mayo Foundation.)

c) Seizures: may be neonatal presentation, or later development of infantile spasms, some with tonic seizures and development of Lennox-Gastaut syndrome

d) Electroencephalogram (EEG): fast alpha and beta activity with high-amplitude slow activity

e) Associated with agenesis of the corpus callosum, cerebellar dysplasia, Dandy-Walker malformation, polymicrogyria, hydrocephalus, posterior encephalocele

f) Associated with genital anomalies in males, cardiac anomalies, retinal dysplasia, and optic nerve hypoplasia

7) Muscle-eye-brain disease

a) Neonatal presentation with congenital myopathy; severe neonatal hypotonia with progression to spasticity; in addition to seizures, mental retardation, abnormal EEG with progression

b) Associated with retinal degeneration, optic atrophy, congenital glaucoma

8) Fukuyama muscular dystrophy: similar to Walker-Warburg syndrome and muscle-eye-brain disease, except with less prominent ocular involvement

2. Polymicrogyria (Fig. 1-14)
   a. Excessive, numerous small gyri
   b. May occur in combination with pachygyria
   c. Usually due to ischemic insult to the underlying parenchyma but can be due to defective migration
   d. Other acquired intrauterine insults include infections such as toxoplasmosis and cytomegalovirus (and others, including rubella and herpes simplex)
   e. Associated with X-linked dominant Aicardi's syndrome
   f. May occur in the context of specific inherited metabolic disorders, such as peroxisomal disorders (e.g., Zellweger's syndrome)
   g. Clinical presentation varies, depending on the associated condition
   h. If involvement is focal, patients may be asymptomatic or present with seizures

3. Heterotopia
   a. Isolated heterotopia (Fig. 1-10 A): group of cells that did not migrate because of damaged radial glial cells with retracted processes
   b. Bilateral periventricular nodular heterotopia (Fig. 1-15)
      1) X-linked, almost always occurs in females
      2) Nodules of periventricular heterotopic gray matter consisting of subependymal neuroepithelial cells that matured without having migrated
      3) Usually occurs bilaterally
      4) Nodules may appear to bulge into the lateral ventricles

5) Heterotopic cells usually vary in size and are haphazardly oriented, with no laminar organization

c. Subcortical band heterotopia ("double cortex") (Fig. 1-16)
   1) Associated with mutation of the *DCX* gene on chromosome X (encoding doublecortin, which is a microtubule-binding protein expressed in migrating neuroepithelial cells)
      a) Usually manifests in females and tends to be more severe in the anterior aspect of the brain (vs. the posterior-dominant subcortical band heterotopia seen with *LIS1* gene mutations)
      b) Hemizygous males with *DCX* mutation usually present with lissencephaly, although subcortical band heterotopia has been reported
      c) Variability of expression between the sexes may be due to random X inactivation and functional genetic mosaicism, producing two populations of neurons in the females (neurons with the abnormal chromosome manifest abnormal migration and form the subcortical band)
   2) Also associated with mutations in the *LIS1* gene on chromosome 17q13.3 (posterior-dominant subcortical band heterotopia)

4. Schizencephaly (Fig. 1-17)
   a. Not considered to be a primary migration disorder by some authorities
   b. May be genetic: associated with mutation of the *Emx2* gene
   c. May be sporadic: usually associated with fetal ischemic or vascular hypoxemic insult

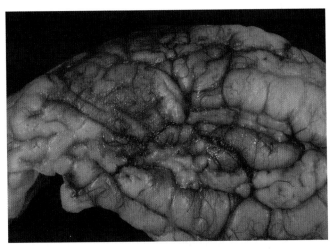

Fig. 1-14. Lateral view of cerebral hemisphere with polymicrogyri, a migration defect characterized by numerous, small gyri, usually a result of intrauterine ischemic or infectious insult.

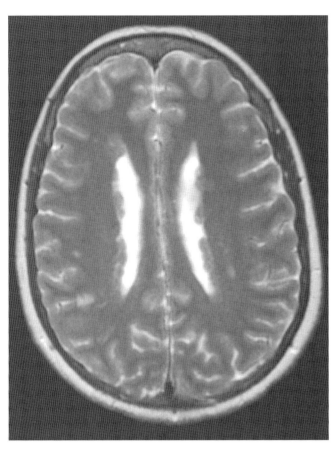

Fig. 1-15. Bilateral periventricular nodular heterotopia in an asymptomatic young female. The nodules are essentially heterotopic gray matter consisting of subependymal neuroepithelial cells that have matured but have not migrated. They are usually present bilaterally. (T2-weighted MRI.)

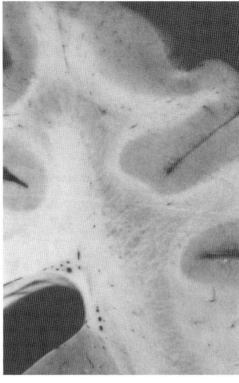

Fig. 1-16. Subcortical band heterotopia ("double cortex") likely due to a mutation of the *DCX* gene on the X chromosome encoding doublecortin. This occurs through abnormal migration of a group of neurons to form the subcortical band. (From Okazaki H. Fundamentals of neuropathology: morphologic basis of neurologic disorders. 2nd ed. New York: Igaku-Shoin Medical Publishers; 1989. p. 287. By permission of Mayo Foundation.)

d. Unilateral or bilateral cleft filled with CSF extends from the ependyma to pial surface
e. Typically, the walls of the cleft are lined with polymicrogyric cortex
f. Type I (closed lip): the "lips" of the cleft are in contact
g. Type II (open lip): the "lips" of the cleft are separated
h. A related anomaly with similar pathogenesis: porencephaly (smooth-walled cortical defect usually lined by gliotic white matter) (Fig. 1-18)
   1) Porencephaly is differentiated from schizencephaly by wall lining: gliotic white matter in porencephaly and heterotopic gray matter in schizencephaly
   2) Porencephaly is thought to occur from an insult to normally developed brain
i. Hypoxic or ischemic fetal insult may be related to an infection, maternal hypoxia, or poisoning, twinning, etc.

K. Other Disorders of Cortical Development
1. Megalencephaly
   a. Enlarged brain volume
   b. Increased volume of gray matter and white matter
   c. Broadening of gyri diffusely
   d. Primary causes
      1) Isolated familial megalencephaly (autosomal dominant or recessive)
      2) Isolated sporadic megalencephaly
      3) Associated with endocrine disorders, agenesis of corpus callosum, and achondroplasia
   e. Secondary causes
      1) Inborn errors of metabolism: GM_1 and GM_2 gangliosidoses, mucopolysaccharidoses, leukodystrophies such as Alexander disease and Canavan disease
      2) Neurocutaneous disorders such as neurofibro-

matosis 1, tuberous sclerosis, linear sebaceous nevus syndrome
2. Hemimegalencephaly
    a. Sometimes called "unilateral hemimegalencephaly"
    b. It is the unilateral enlargement of a portion or all of a cerebral hemisphere
    c. Pathologic features
        1) Defective migration: extensive heterotopia
        2) Defective differentiation: cortical dysplasia
        3) Ipsilateral ventriculomegaly
        4) Thickened cortical ribbon with poor differentiation of the gray-white matter junction and frequent heterotopic gray matter
    d. Presentation is variable: frequent associations are mental retardation, seizure disorder (infantile spasms, focal seizures), and hemihypertrophy
    e. Is associated with

1) Beckwith-Wiedemann syndrome
2) Linear sebaceous nevus syndrome
3) Wilms' tumor

L. Apoptosis
1. Process by which the excessive number of neuroblasts (normally produced during the proliferative stage) is decreased
2. Occurs prominently in the ventricular zone in early developmental stages
3. Cells that do not undergo synaptogenesis are vulnerable to apoptosis
4. Apoptosis depends on
    a. Deprivation of growth factors (e.g., nerve growth factor)
    b. Activation of caspases triggered by release of mitochondrial cytochrome c (relies on balance between antiapoptotic factor Bcl-2 and proapoptotic factor Bax protein)
    c. Activation of Fas receptor by Fas ligand
5. Agenesis of the corpus callosum: a disorder of apoptosis (Fig. 1-10 B)
    a. Caused by absence of the commissural plate (which normally acts to guide axons across the midline) or failure of degeneration of a portion of the commissural plate that normally allows the passage of axons
    b. The failure of apoptosis (cell death) of glial cells in the latter scenario acts as a barrier to the passage of axons
    c. Associated with bundle of Probst (large myelinated fiber bundle formed by aborted attempts of crossing axons)
    d. Associated with schizencephaly, holoprosencephaly, hydrocephalus, and migration defects

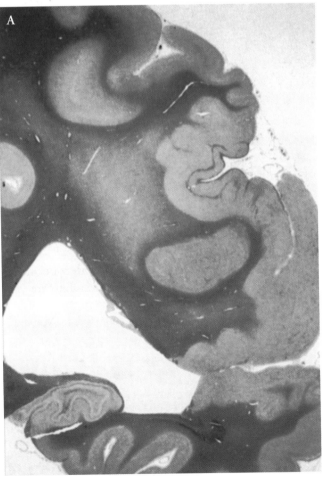

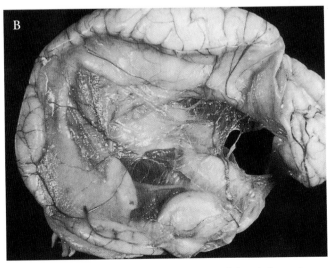

Fig. 1-17. Sporadic schizencephaly is usually associated with an in utero ischemic or hypoxic insult. The edges of the clefts are in contact in, *A*, type I ("closed lip") and, *B*, separated in type II ("open lip"). (From Okazaki H, Scheithauer BW. Atlas of neuropathology. New York: Gower Medical Publishing; 1988. p. 287. By permission of Mayo Foundation.)

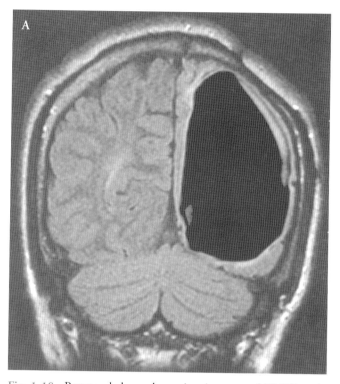

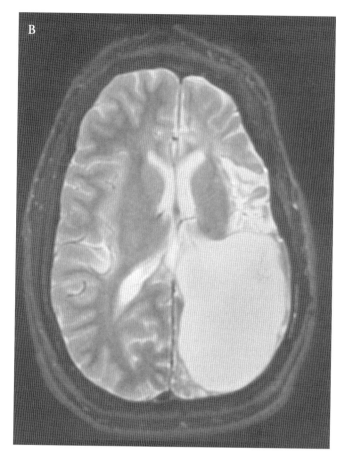

Fig. 1-18. Porencephaly, as shown in, *A*, a coronal FLAIR and, *B*, axial T2-weighted images. The lining of the cleft consists of gliotic white matter (as compared with the heterotopic gray matter lining the clefts of schizencephalic brains).

e. May be asymptomatic or present with mental retardation, learning disabilities, seizures arising from focal cortical dysplasias, hydrocephalus, microcephaly, or precocious puberty
f. Does not present with disconnection syndrome that often occurs with acquired lesions of the corpus callosum
g. Also associated with Aicardi's syndrome
  1) X-linked dominant inheritance, almost exclusively seen in girls (lethal in boys)
  2) Girls with infantile spasms
  3) Dorsal vertebral anomalies
  4) Chorioretinal lacunar defects
  5) Optic nerve colobomas
  6) Microphthalmos
  7) Associated with polymicrogyria
  8) Mental retardation
h. Associated with Andermann syndrome
  1) Autosomal recessive inheritance
  2) Mental retardation
  3) Agenesis of the corpus callosum
  4) Peripheral neuropathy

M. Axonal Growth and Dendritic Development
1. Axonal outgrowth is guided by a terminal structure, the growth cone
2. Growth cone: highly mobile structure that responds to environmental signals
3. Sheets of membrane at the edge of growth cones are called "lamellopodia" and fingerlike extensions are called "filopodia"
4. Dynamic changes of growing axons depend on changes in the internal structure and signals in the microenvironment of the growth cone
5. Signals in the microenvironment attract or repel the growth cone
6. The growth cone advances by ameboid motion over the surface
7. Growth cone movement depends on short- and long-range attractive and repulsive signals in the microenvironment
8. Axonal growth is guided by a concentration gradient of a chemotropic factor
   a. Microenvironmental cues may be diffusible (secreted

substances) or nondiffusable (adhesion molecules and components of the extracellular membrane)

  b. Short-range interactions are usually mediated by cell adhesion molecules such as laminin

    1) Short-range attractive signals: laminins (component of the basal membrane and potent attractant)

    2) Short-range repulsive signals: ephrins (expressed at the cell surface)

  c. Long-range attractive signals: netrins (important in development of spinal, hippocampal, and callosal commissural fibers, can also act as repellent of other axons such as the motor neurons of the trochlear nerve [CN IV])

  d. Long-range repulsive signals: semaphorins (secreted transmembrane proteins, also act as attractant for dendritic growth)

9. The motility of axons depends on actin polymerization at the leading edge of the growth cone and depolymerization with recycling of the actin monomer back to the leading edge (ready to be incorporated again into the actin polymer)

10. Simultaneously with actin polymerization at the growth cone, the cell membrane at the edge of the growth cone expands by ongoing exocytosis and fusion of vesicular membranes with the extracellular membranes

11. Intracellular signal for growth cone expansion is cytosolic calcium concentration: intracellular calcium levels above or below this optimal level impair motility

12. Axonal growth precedes dendritic development

13. In some cases of severe mental retardation without structural brain lesions, dendritic development and synaptic connections may be abnormal

N. Synaptogenesis

1. In neocortex: neocortical synaptogenesis occurs after migration of neuroblasts

2. In cerebellum: the superficial portion of the migrating granule cells remains in the external granule cell layer, becoming parallel fibers (parallel fibers form synapses with Purkinje cells before the granule cells migrate)

3. High degree of specificity of synapses

4. Depends on neurotransmitter receptor clustering in the postsynaptic membrane

  a. Likely influenced by the presynaptic nerve terminal

  b. The preference of the presynaptic nerve terminal for a specific portion of the target postsynaptic membrane indicates a high degree of synaptic selectivity

5. Plasticity: the process of modification or elimination of synaptic connections, sometimes involves neuronal apoptosis

O. Myelination of the Central Nervous System

1. Occurs in orderly spatial and temporal sequence: follows developmental milestones

2. Occurs as early as 14 weeks of gestation and continues to adulthood

3. Bulk of active myelination begins at third trimester and continues to about 2 years postnatally

4. Corticospinal tract myelinate throughout first 2 years of life: extensor plantar response is present at birth and disappears sometime during this development

5. Poor myelination of cortical pathways

  a. This is responsible for lack of cortical control over motor function at birth

  b. It is responsible for primitive reflexes present at birth, such as grasp reflex

6. Optic nerve myelinates postnally; most other cranial nerves myelinate prenatally

7. Certain subcortical association fibers (especially of frontal cortex) do not complete myelination until early adulthood

REFERENCES

Benarroch EE, Westmoreland BF, Daube JR, Reagan TJ, Sandok BA. Medical neurosciences: an approach to anatomy, pathology, and physiology by systems and levels. 4th ed. Philadelphia: Lippincott Williams & Wilkins; 1999.

Ellison D, Love S, Chimelli L, Roberts GW, Harding B, Vinters HV, et al. Neuropathology: a reference text of CNS pathology. London: Mosby International; 1998.

Hatten ME. Central nervous system neuronal migration. Annu Rev Neurosci. 1999;22:511-39.

Jessell TM, Sanes JR. Development: the decade of the developing brain. Curr Opin Neurobiol. 2000;10:599-611.

Kandel ER, Schwartz JH, Jessell TM, editors. Principles of neural science. 4th ed. New York: McGraw-Hill; 2000.

Northrup H, Volcik KA. Spina bifida and other neural tube defects. Curr Probl Pediatr. 2000;30:313-32.

Pilz DT. Subcortical band heterotopia: somatic mosaicism and phenotypic variability (commentary). Neurology. 2003;61:1027.

Ragsdale CW, Grove EA. Patterning the mammalian cerebral cortex. Curr Opin Neurobiol. 2001;11:50-8.

Sarnat HB, Flores L. Developmental disorders of the nervous system. In: Bradley WG, Daroff RB, Fenichel GM, Mardsen CD, editors. Neurology in clinical practice: the neurological disorders. Vol 2. 3rd ed. Boston: Butterworth-Heinemann; 2000. p. 1561-83.

Sicca F, Kelemen A, Genton P, Das S, Mei D, Moro F, et al. Mosaic mutations of the *LIS1* gene cause subcortical band heterotopia. Neurology. 2003;61:1042-6.

QUESTIONS

1. The developmental anomaly (Figure) is most likely a consequence of:
   a. Genetically determined factors associated with mutation of the *Emx2* gene
   b. Failure of normal apoptosis of glial cells
   c. Genetically determined disorder of migration and associated with mutation of the *LIS1* gene
   d. Intrauterine ischemic or vascular insult
   e. Abnormal synaptogenesis and dendritic development

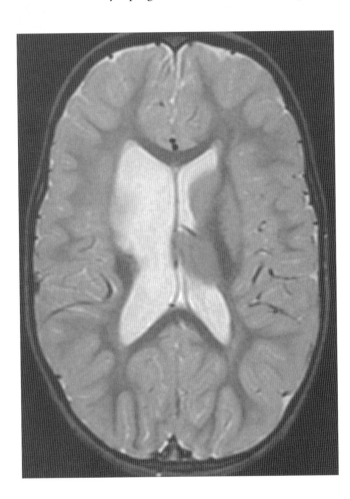

2. Which of the following is *not* true about the migration of neuroblasts?
   a. Migration of the granule and Purkinje cell neuroblasts of the cerebellum depends on Reelin and occurs centrifugally from the ventricular zone
   b. In neocortical development, when the mitotic spindle is perpendicular to the ventricular surface, both daughter cells become neuroepithelial cells and undergo further mitotic division
   c. The primary germinal zone of the neural tube is the ventricular zone
   d. Neuroblasts continue to migrate from the external granule cell layer of the cerebellum for 1 year after birth

3. Which of the following is true about schizencephaly?
   a. If genetically determined, it is usually associated with mutation of *LIS1*
   b. If genetically determined, it is usually associated with mutation of the *DCX* gene on the X chromosome
   c. If sporadic, it is usually associated with fetal ischemic or vascular insult
   d. May be associated with muscular dystrophy

4. Which of the following is/are true about Miller-Dieker syndrome?
   a. Disorder of neuronal migration associated with mental retardation, seizures, and facial anomalies
   b. Disorganized cerebral cortex with disoriented neurons, caused by "overmigration" of neuroblasts
   c. Associated with muscular dystrophy, optic nerve hypoplasia, and infantile spasms
   d. a and b are correct

5. Which of the following is *not* true about disorders of forebrain induction and midline malformations?
   a. May be due to abnormal migration
   b. May be associated with craniofacial anomalies such as hypertelorism or cyclops
   c. May manifest as a single midline ventricle, with continuity of cerebral cortex around the midline
   d. May be due to defective notochord induction of the neuroectoderm

ANSWERS

1. Answer: d.
In this T2-weighted MRI, the right caudate body is absent, the right thalamus is relatively small, and the internal capsule is indistinct. Note ex vacuo dilatation of the right lateral ventricle. These abnormalities are likely the result of an intrauterine vascular insult.

2. Answer: a.
Granule neuroblasts of the cerebellum migrate centripetally (neocortical neuroblasts and Purkinje cells migrate centrifugally); also, migration does not depend on Reelin and continues for the first year after birth.

3. Answer: c.
Sporadic schizencephaly is usually secondary to an intrauterine ischemic, hypoxic, or vascular insult.

4. Answer: a.
Miller-Dieker syndrome is lissencephaly type 1, associated with deletion of the *LIS1* gene. This is a primary disorder of "undermigration" in which the cortex usually consists of four layers, as compared with lissencephaly type 2, which is a primary disorder of "overmigration" in which the neurons are disoriented and neocortical lamination is poor.

5. Answer: d.
Anencephaly is the disorder of neurulation associated with failure of closure of the anterior neuropore and defective notochord induction of the neuroectoderm. Midline malformations are due to either abnormal lateral growth of the cerebral hemispheres because of abnormal migration or abnormal differentiation of the telencephalon from the lamina terminalis, which is formed by closure of the anterior neuropore.

Basic Principles of Neuroscience and Neurogenetics

2

Orhun H. Kantarci, M.D.

Gena R. Ghearing, M.D.

I. Molecular Neuroscience

A. Neuron Structure

1. Neurons have same components as other cells: endoplasmic reticulum, ribosomes, lysosomes, peroxisomes, mitochondria, nucleus, cell membrane
2. Characteristic features: axon and dendrites
3. Nucleus: large, spherical with a nucleolus
4. Cell membrane: a phospholipid bilayer
   a. Membrane proteins have hydrophobic regions usually made of alpha helices
   b. Spectrin-ankyrin network provides link between cytoskeleton and cell membrane
5. Integral proteins: span cell membrane (Fig. 2-1)
   a. Single transmembrane proteins
      1) Receptor tyrosine kinases
         a) Important in signal transduction
         b) Many are associated with receptors
      2) Cell adhesion molecules (CAMs)
         a) Important for direct interaction between cell membrane and intracellular and extracellular elements
         b) Critical for cell function, development, plasticity, myelination, response to injury
         c) Immunoglobulin (Ig) family: have extracellular Ig-like domains that may bind membranes to

---

surfaces or initiate signal transduction pathway
   i) May have one Ig-like domain, e.g., myelin protein P_O
   ii) Some have two Ig-like domains, e.g., Trk receptors that bind neurotrophic factors
   iii) This includes sialic-acid binding proteins such as myelin-associated glycoprotein (MAG) and Schwann cell myelin protein (SMP)
   iv) Responsible for calcium-independent cell adhesions: L1 and neural cell adhesion molecule (NCAM)
   d) Cadherins
      i) Transmembrane glycoproteins
      ii) Responsible for *calcium-dependent* adhesions (adherens junctions) of adjacent cells via homophilic interactions (dimerization) among cadherins of same kind
      iii) Important in cell-cell interactions and axonal growth
   e) Integrins: adhesions to extracellular matrix proteins (laminin, fibronectin, proteins of Ig family)
   f) Neuroligins
      i) Interact with β-neurexins of neuronal presynaptic membranes to form intercellular (interneuronal) junctions
      ii) Important for linking presynaptic and postsynaptic cells
   b. Multitransmembrane domain proteins: ion channels, pumps, transporters, connexins
      1) Ion channels: cysteine residue family, glutamate ionotropic family, G protein-coupled receptor family
6. Cytoskeletal proteins (Fig. 2-1)
   a. Microfilaments
      1) Polymers of actin: form double-stranded helix
      2) Found throughout cytoplasm: aggregate under cell membrane
      3) Found in growth cones, dendritic spines, axons: important in plasticity

---

Cell membrane: rich in phospholipids and gangliosides

Integral membrane proteins and connexins are involved in ion homeostasis, electrical activity, and signaling

Adhesion molecules are responsible for interactions of neurons with glial cells and extracellular matrix

Membrane proteins

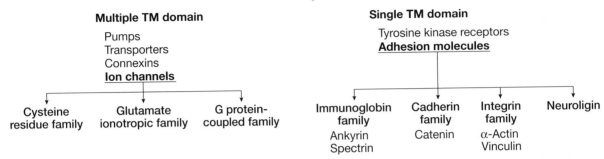

Multiple TM domain

Pumps
Transporters
Connexins
Ion channels

| Cysteine residue family | Glutamate ionotropic family | G protein-coupled family |

Single TM domain

Tyrosine kinase receptors
Adhesion molecules

Immunoglobin family	Cadherin family	Integrin family	Neuroligin
Ankyrin	Catenin	α-Actin	
Spectrin		Vinculin	

Cytoskeletal proteins

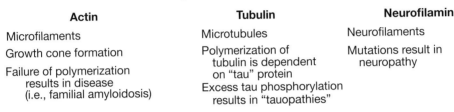

Actin

Microfilaments

Growth cone formation

Failure of polymerization results in disease (i.e., familial amyloidosis)

Tubulin

Microtubules

Polymerization of tubulin is dependent on "tau" protein

Excess tau phosphorylation results in "tauopathies"

Neurofilamin

Neurofilaments

Mutations result in neuropathy

Fig. 2-1. Structural proteins of neurons. TM, transmembrane.

4) Actin-binding proteins determine structural arrangement of actin microfilaments and cross-linking and interactions with cell membrane and extracellular matrix
   a) Spectrin: acts to cross-link actin oligomers and forms complex with ankyrin, actin, and other cytoskeletal proteins, forming stable submembranous cytoskeletal complex, stabilizing cell membranes
   b) Ankyrin
   c) Fibrin: may be important in formation of filopodia in growth cones
   d) Profilin: promotes actin polymerization
   e) Gelsolin: cytoplasmic, calcium-regulated, actin-modulating protein that binds to and severs existing actin filaments and can cap F-actin; mutations of gelsolin lead to familial amyloidosis type IV, Finnish type
b. Microtubules
   1) Polymers of α- and β-tubulin
   2) Action of guanosine triphosphatase (GTPase) is important for assembly and disassembly
   3) Critical role in intracellular transport: provide infrastructure for bidirectional axonal transport
   4) Microtubule-associated proteins
      a) Bind to microtubule polymers or monomers and facilitate polymerization and assembly
      b) Function: regulated by state of phosphorylation
      c) Kinesin and dynein: microtubule-associated proteins important for axonal transport (see below)
      d) Tau protein
         i) Six isoforms produced by alternative splicing of tau gene on chromosome 17
         ii) Three isoforms contain three microtubule-binding repeats: 3R (3-repeat) forms
         iii) Other three isoforms contain four microtubule-binding repeats: 4R (4-repeat) forms
         iv) Normal ratio of 3 tau:4 tau is 1:1
         v) Accumulation of a particular hyperphosphorylated tau isoform distorts the ratio and reduces microtubule binding, producing characteristic tau filamentous inclusions
         vi) Accumulation of hyperphosphorylated 4R tau yields paired helical filaments that form neurofibrillary tangles of Alzheimer's disease
         vii) Example of 3R tauopathy: Pick's disease
         viii) Examples of 4R tauopathies: corticobasal degeneration, progressive supranuclear palsy, argyrophilic grain disease
c. Neurofilament proteins
   1) Polymers of neurofilamin
   2) Neuron-specific intermediate filaments in axons

3) Determine axon caliber

4) Function depends on phosphorylation: undergo ongoing, extensive phosphorylation that slows their transport and obligates them to become an integral part of axonal cytoskeleton (important determinant of axonal caliber)

5) Important role in axonal growth (growth cones and collateral axonal sprouting) and axonal transport

6) Defects/mutations in neurofilament (*NEFL*) gene cause neuropathy (i.e., Charcot-Marie-Tooth [CMT] type 2e)

7. Perikaryon (soma, cell body): polymorphic; may be stellate, pyramidal, or globular

8. Dendrites: afferent component of neuron

a. Dendritic spines: critical sites of plasticity and depend on clustering of excitatory and inhibitory receptors (see below)

b. Growth cone dynamics depend on

1) Synaptic activity

2) Growth factors

a) Interact through receptor tyrosine kinase B (Trk B)

b) Include nerve growth factor (NGF), brain-derived neurotrophic factor (BDNF), neurotrophin 3 (NT3) and NT4/5

Microfilaments
    Subunit = actin
    Location = growth cone, dendritic spine, axons
    Associated proteins = spectrins, gelsolin, profilin, others
    Main function = interaction with membrane proteins
    Dynamic turnover
Microtubules
    Subunit = tubulin
    Location = soma, dendrites, axons
    Associated proteins = microtubule-associated proteins, tau
    Main function = axonal transport
    Dynamic turnover
Neurofilaments
    Subunit = Neurofilament proteins (NF)-L, NF-M, NF-H
    Location = axons
    Main function = maintenance of axon caliber
    No dynamic turnover

---

3) Ligands for Notch (cell membrane protein that promotes dendritic branching, but inhibits dendritic growth)

4) Rho GTPases: regulate actin cytoskeleton; control extension of growth cone (Rho GTPase–dependent transduction)

9. Axon

a. Functions

1) Conduction of action potentials

2) Synaptic transmission

3) Fast axonal transport: 200 to 400 mm/day

a) Anterograde: from cell body to axonal terminal

i) Transport of vesicles, organelles, receptors, and other proteins

ii) Involves motor protein kinesin

b) Retrograde: from terminal to soma

i) Important for membrane recycling and retrograde signaling

ii) Involves motor protein dynein

4) Slow axonal transport

a) Slow component A: 0.2 to 1 mm/day; transports microtubules and microfilaments

b) Slow component B: 2 to 8 mm/day; transports actin microfilaments and metabolic enzymes

5) Intermediate axonal transport: 50 to 100 mm/day

a) Bidirectional

b) Transports mitochondria

10. Myelin

a. Compacted myelin

1) Minor dense line or intraperiod line: formed by juxtaposed outer leaflets

2) Major dense line: composed of juxtaposed inner leaflets

3) Proteolipid protein (PLP) and myelin basic protein (MBP): myelin compaction in *central* nervous system (CNS)

4) Myelin protein zero (MPZ) and peripheral myelin protein (PMP)-22: myelin compaction in *peripheral* nervous system (PNS)

5) Defects or mutations in compact myelin proteins

Dendritic spines are dynamic structures that have a critical role in synaptic plasticity

Dendritic growth during development depends on synaptic activity, growth factors, ligands for Notch, and cytoskeletal changes triggered by Rho GTPase

lead to both CNS and PNS diseases
  a) PNS diseases: CMT1b (MPZ), CMT1a (PMP-22 duplication), hereditary neuropathy with liability to pressure palsies (PMP-22 deletion)
  b) CNS disease: Pelizaeus-Merzbacher disease (PLP, linked to chromosome Xq22)
b. Noncompacted myelin
  1) Lacks fusion of intracellular loops of myelin
  2) Present at paranodes and juxtaparanodes
  3) MAG mediates axon-glia adhesions important for myelination by Schwann cells (PNS) and oligodendrocytes (CNS); monoclonal anti-MAG antibodies occurs in neuropathies associated with paraproteinemias
  4) Connexin-32
    a) Gap junction protein at paranodal region (gene on chromosome X) that allows communication within periaxonal space and across myelin sheath
    b) Mutation of gene encoding connexin-32 protein is responsible for X-linked form of CMT (CMT-X)
c. Autoimmunity to myelin proteins and gangliosides cause PNS disease
  1) Demyelinating neuropathy: monoclonal anti-MAG antibodies
  2) Multifocal motor neuropathy: monoclonal anti-GM1 antibodies
  3) Acute motor axonal neuropathy: polyclonal anti-GM1 antibodies
  4) Miller Fisher variant of acute inflammatory demyelinating polyradiculopathy: polyclonal anti-GQ1B antibodies
11. Nodes of Ranvier

a. High concentration of voltage-gated sodium channels is important for saltatory conduction
b. Ankyrin G: linker protein that clusters voltage-gated sodium channels at these points
c. Also contain CAMs, Na^+/K^+ adenosine triphosphatases (ATPases), and GM1 gangliosides
12. Paranodal and juxtaparanodal region
a. Myelin loops are anchored to axon by contactin and contactin-associated protein (Caspr)/paranodin)
b. Express voltage-gated and inward rectifier potassium channels that have role in regulating axonal excitability
13. Internode
a. Length of internode varies proportionally with axon diameter
b. Covered by compacted myelin
14. Axonal growth or sprouting
a. Like dendritic growth cones, axons rely on synaptic activity, growth hormones, and Rho GTPases (Rho GTPase–dependent transduction)
b. Growth cone: finger-like extensions called filopodia, with lamellipodia in between these extensions
c. Growth cone guided by gradient of attracting agents (e.g., netrin, laminin), repelling agents (e.g., ephrin, semaphorin), or directing agents (e.g., Robo-Slit inhibits crossing midline)
d. MAG and proteins such as Nogo expressed by fully differentiated oligodendrocytes may inhibit regeneration of CNS axons

B.   Glial Cells
1. Astrocytes: large glial cells

Axonal transport
  Fast anterograde: transort of vesicular proteins (ion channels, neuropeptides) at 200-400 mm/day using kinesin

  Fast retrograde: transport of endocytic vesicles (nerve growth factor, toxin, virus) at 200-300 mm/day using dynein

  Slow: transport of microtubules, microtubule-associated proteins, neurofilaments, actin at 0.2-8 mm/day

  Intermediate: bidirectional transport of mitochondria at 50-100 mm/day

---

Myelin proteins
  Proteolipid protein (PLP) is involved in central myelin compaction; defect in this protein can lead to Pelizaeus-Merzbacher disease

  Defects of myelin protein zero (MPZ) and peripheral myelin protein (PMP)-22 in compacted peripheral myelin cause inherited neuropathies

  Noncompacted myelin proteins may be associated with inherited neuropathies (connexin-32 defect) or acquired neuropathies (anti-MAG-associated neuropathy)

  MAG, myelin-associated glycoprotein

a. Role in neuronal function
  1) Increase glycolysis and production of lactate (a fuel for neurons)
  2) Nitric oxide (NO)-mediated increased blood flow preferentially to active neuronal microenvironment
    a) NO: synthesized in neurons, glial cells, endothelial cells
    b) NO: rapidly diffusible and important in vasodilatation (e.g., penile erection), oxidative injury (acts as free radical), and neuronal plasticity
    c) NO: produced by NO synthetase (NOS)
    d) Arginine is substrate for NOS
    e) Astrocytes express arginine transporter and provide bulk of arginine supplies to neurons
    f) Influx of calcium into neuron through N-methyl-D-aspartate (NMDA) receptors (activated by glutamate) stimulates neuronal NOS to produce NO
    g) NO activates cytoplasmic guanylate cyclase, producing cyclic guanosine monophosphate (GMP)
b. Prevention of excitotoxicity (see below)
  1) Buffering extracellular potassium
  2) Uptake of excess glutamate and conversion to glutamine—neurons convert it back to glutamate
  3) Prevention of free radical-induced damage
    a) Glutathione source for mitochondrial antioxidation of H_2O_2
c. Role in neuronal networking
  1) Form neuronal migration paths away from ventricular layer during development (radial glial cells, Bergmann glia in cerebellum)
  2) Calcium wave propagation through interastrocytic gap junctions help networking between neurons supported by astrocytes
d. Formation of blood-brain barrier
e. Glial response to injury (gliosis)
2. Oligodendrocytes: myelin-forming cells in CNS
  a. Vimentin: marker of early oligodendrocyte development (oligodendrocyte progenitors and pre-oligodendrocytes)
  b. PLP and MBP: expressed only in mature oligodendrocytes
  c. May myelinate a segment of several axons
  d. Perineuronal oligodendrocytes are also in gray matter (function unclear)
3. Schwann cells: myelin-forming cells in PNS
  a. Nerve growth factor receptor (NGFRt): expressed in Schwann-cell precursors
  b. Myelinating Schwann cells express MBP, MPZ, PMP-22
  c. Unmyelinating Schwann cells express glial fibrillary acidic protein (GFAP) and NCAM
  d. One Schwann cell myelinates a segment of only one axon

e. Many small unmyelinated fibers may be invested by one Schwann cell
f. Peripheral nerve fibers have continuous basement membrane over Schwann cells
4. Ependymal cells
  a. Single layer of ciliated neuroepithelial cells lining the ventricles
  b. Connected by tight junctions to form selective barrier
5. Microglia
  a. Monocytic phagocytic cells
  b. Derived from mesoderm, not neuroepithelium
  c. Few in number, but proliferate rapidly after insult to nervous system (e.g., ischemia) and become macrophages, acting as scavenger cells to remove damaged tissue and debris
  d. No role in maintaining blood-brain barrier

C. Neuronal Microenvironment
1. Cerebral blood flow (CBF)
  a. About 750 mL/min
  b. Increased metabolic demand: proportionate increase in CBF of cortical gray matter
  c. Extrinsic regulators of CBF
    1) Dependent on cardiac output, systemic blood pressure, blood viscosity, and stimulation of baroreceptors in carotid sinus and aortic arch
    2) Sympathetic input from superior cervical ganglion causes vasoconstriction via norepinephrine, neuropeptide Y, and adenosine triphosphate (ATP)
    3) Parasympathetic input from sphenopalatine ganglion causes vasodilation via NO, acetylcholine (ACh), and vasoactive intestinal polypeptide (VIP)
    4) Sensory innervation arises from trigeminal ganglion

Glial cells

Astrocytes are important for potassium buffering, uptake of glutamate, and response to injury in central nervous system

Oligodendrocytes are myelin-forming cells in central nervous system

Schwann cells are myelin-forming cells in peripheral nervous system

Ependymal cells line the ventricles

Microglia are monocytic phagocytic cells

and releases substance P and calcitonin gene-related peptide (CGRP) to produce vasodilation

d. Intrinsic regulators of CBF

  1) Regional (local) metabolic regulation with vasodilator metabolites: cause vasodilatation and increased CBF (e.g., NO, amino acid metabolites, adenosine, potassium, oxygen free radicals)

  2) Regional (local) chemical regulation

    a) Cerebral blood vessels are very sensitive to any change in the local carbon dioxide tension ($PaCO_2$): increased $PaCO_2$ causes vasodilation, reduced $PaCO_2$ vasoconstriction (mediated primarily by change in extracellular pH)

    b) Change in local oxygen tension (PaO_2) causes opposite effect: increased PaO_2 produces vasoconstriction, reduced PaO_2 vasodilation (much less pronounced than $PaCO_2$ effect)

    c) Increased regional lactic acid levels in region of ischemia (low regional blood pH) induce regional vasodilation

    d) Hyperventilation may be used as temporary measure to reduce intracranial pressure by inducing a reduction in the $PaCO_2$ and causing vasoconstriction (this effect is short-lived and CBF usually returns to baseline and may overshoot)

  3) Autoregulation

    a) Ability to maintain stable CBF despite fluctuations in mean arterial blood pressure

    b) Occurs with fluctuations of systemic mean arterial blood pressures between 60 and 160 mm Hg, acting to preserve constant perfusion pressures to brain

    c) In patients with long-standing hypertension, both upper and lower limits of mean arterial pressure in which autoregulation occurs are raised

    d) Intraluminal pressure-responsive myogenic reflexive action of vascular wall: inducing vasoconstriction with increased intraluminal pressures and vasodilation with reduced intraluminal pressures

2. Blood-brain barrier

  a. Anatomy

    1) Endothelial cells: primary site of the barrier are relatively deficient in mechanisms for vesicular transport

    2) Tight junctions between endothelial cells (composed of occludin, claudins, cingulins, and zonula occludens proteins) make it necessary for substances to pass through the lipid bilayer membrane of endothelial cells (rather than in between endothelial cells)

    3) Layer of pericytes surrounds endothelial cells and is delineated by glial foot processes

  b. Blood-brain barrier absent in circumventricular organs (subfornicial organ, median eminence, neurohypophysis, vascular organ of lamina terminalis, pineal body, subfornical organ, area postrema)

  c. Passage through blood-brain barrier

    1) Highly lipid-soluble molecules (carbon dioxide, volatile anesthetics, circulating steroids, phenytoin, ethanol, nicotine) use simple diffusion through endothelial cell membranes

    2) Water-soluble compounds (glucose and amino acids) pass by carrier-mediated facilitated transport

    3) Glucose transporter isotype 1 (GLUT1)

      a) Responsible for transporting glucose down concentration gradient

      b) Driven by relatively higher plasma concentration of glucose

      c) Not energy-dependent

      d) GLUT1 deficiency: patients often normal at birth (may have microcephaly) and develop intractable seizures, developmental delay; treated with antiepileptic agents and ketogenic diet

    4) Large neutral amino acids use a sodium-independent, energy-independent transporter (transported down concentration gradient)

    5) Small nonessential amino acids use energy-dependent, sodium-dependent active transport

    6) Na^+/K^+ ATPase: energy-dependent ion channel located at endothelial cell membrane, responsible for energy-dependent exchange of extracellular potassium with intracellular sodium

    7) Proteins (insulin, transferrin, vasopressin) by transcytosis through saturable systems

    8) Vasogenic edema

      a) Accumulation of interstitial fluid that occurs with abnormal, leaky blood-brain barrier

      b) Malignant brain neoplasms: abnormal permeability of tumor endothelial cells

---

Neuronal Microenvironment Depends On
  Astrocytic network
    Buffers potassium
    Produces lactate and glutamine
  Cerebral blood flow
    Regulated by NO, amino acid metabolites, adenosine, and autonomic innervation
  Blood-brain barrier
    Formed by tight junctions

c) Meningitis: breakdown of blood-brain barrier from inflammatory response

d) Associated with early vacuolization and swelling of myelin sheaths

e) Often responsive to treatment with corticosteroids

f) In contrast, cytotoxic edema refers to primary neural or glial intracellular swelling, often not responsive to corticosteroids: movement of water molecules in extracellular space is limited and their diffusion is restricted, appearing as high signal in diffusion-weighted imaging

3. Cerebrospinal fluid (CSF)

a. Formed primarily by choroid plexus in lateral ventricles

b. Rate of production: 0.35 mL/min, about 500 mL/day

c. Estimated total CSF volume: 140 mL

d. Normal CSF pressure: between 80 and 180 mm H_2O

e. Course of flow: lateral ventricles through foramina of Monro into third ventricle and through cerebral aqueduct into fourth ventricle; exits fourth ventricle through single foramen of Magendie in midline and paired foramina of Luschka in lateral walls of fourth ventricle to enter subarachnoid space

f. CSF flows in thecal sac and around brain convexities and tracks along blood vessels into Virchow-Robin spaces

g. CSF is absorbed into superior sagittal sinus through arachnoid granulations (pacchionian granulations)

1) Clusters of villi are essentially protrusions of arachnoid membrane through dura mater into superior sagittal sinus

2) Functional one-way pressure valves: blood-brain interface with one-way flow of CSF and its contents into venous system, when CSF pressure is maintained above a certain threshold

h. Blood-CSF interface formed by cuboidal or columnar epithelial cells surrounding fenestrated capillaries

i. Apical surface of choroidal cells contains ATPase which acts to secrete sodium ions into ventricular CSF at the apical membrane in exchange for potassium

j. Carbonic anhydrase produces bicarbonate (from water and carbon dioxide), which is transported across apical membrane via bicarbonate-chloride exchange and acts to neutralize positive sodium charge

k. CSF production depends on active ion transport with secretion of sodium by Na^+/K^+ ATPase and chloride by the Cl^-/HCO_3 exchanger

l. Carbonic anhydrase inhibitors such as acetazolamide act to reduce CSF production

D. Trophic Factors and Neuronal Plasticity

1. Coincidence detection

a. Temporal coincidence (co-occurrence) of events strengthens synaptic connection: "neurons that fire together wire together," strengthening functionally relevant connections and eliminating exuberant connections

b. Sensory input can be critical during brief critical period

1) Harlow: demonstrated that isolated young monkeys could not form normal social interactions

2) Hubel and Wiesel: showed that monocular visual deprivation during a specific postnatal period decreased formation of axonal connections for deprived eye and prevented formation of normal eye dominance columns

c. Hebbian process

1) Repeated stimulation of specific receptors leads slowly to formation of "cell-assemblies" that can act as closed system after stimulation ends

2) High-frequency correlated activity produces long-term potentiation (LTP) (discussed below)

3) Low-frequency uncorrelated activity produces long-term depression (LTD) (discussed below)

4) Lack of long-term stimulation or use of network leads to loss of function and cell death: "use it or loose it"

2. Neurotrophism (Fig. 2-2)

a. Innervating neurons compete for limited supply of target-derived neurotrophic factors (e.g., NGF, BDNF, NT-3, cytokines)

b. Growth factor is released by the target and binds to receptors that transduce a signal, which is transmitted retrogradely to the cell body and is important for neuron's survival

c. Neurotrophic receptors

1) Receptor tyrosine kinases (Trk A, Trk B, Trk C) are

Occipital horn normally has a high degree of variability and asymmetry: most often rudimentary and not clinically significant

---

Innervating neurons compete for a restricted quantity of target-derived trophic factor

Neurotrophins control many critical decisions in development and death of neurons

Loss of neurotrophic support from a target of neural innervation may be responsible for many neurodegenerative diseases

low-affinity receptors when activated alone and relatively specific to individual growth factors

2) Common neurotrophin receptor (p75NTR) increases affinity of tyrosine kinases when activated together but is a nonspecific receptor

3) Specific cytokine receptors coupled with a receptor kinase

d. Neurotrophic pathways

1) Mitogen-activated protein kinase (MAPK)

a) Extracellular signal-regulated kinase (ERK 1/2): activated by growth factors

b) High osmolality glycerol-induced kinase (p38/HOG): activated by stress

c) C-jun N-terminal kinase/stress-activated protein kinase (JNK/SAPK): activated by stress

2) Phosphoinositide-3 kinase (PI_3K), phospholipase C (PLCγ), protein kinase C (PKC)

3) Janus kinase/signal transducer and activator of transcription (JAK/STAT)

3. Cell death (Fig. 2-2)

a. Necrosis

1) Often precipitated by energy failure

2) Cell swelling (cytotoxic edema) and membrane rupture

3) Likely to produce inflammatory response

b. Apoptosis

1) Normal developmental process of programmed cell death

2) Cellular and nuclear shrinkage (DNA fragmentation) but no membrane rupture

3) Does *not* produce inflammation

4) Involves activation of apoptotic receptors, activation of caspases, alteration of interaction and balance between proapoptotic and antiapoptotic factors, mitochondrial failure, and oxidative stress

5) Mitochondrial failure: increased intramitochondrial calcium, release of cytochrome *c* and other apoptotic factors into the cytosol

6) Cytochrome *c* activates Procaspase 9 via interaction with apoptosis activating factor-1 (Apaf-1)

7) Activation of caspase 9 is inhibited by inhibitor of apoptosis proteins (IAPs), which are in turn inhibited by mitochondrial-derived Smac (second mitochondrial activator of caspases)

8) Caspases eventually act to mediate DNA fragmentation and lipid peroxidation

c. Apoptotic receptors

1) Glutamatergic calcium channels: excitotoxicity

2) Death receptors (e.g., Fas, tumor necrosis factor receptor [TNFR], low-affinity nerve growth factor receptor [p75], TRAIL)

d. Apoptotic pathways

1) Calcium-induced excitotoxicity

a) DNA degradation via endonucleases

b) Phospholipase activation

c) Protein degradation via calpain

d) Lipid peroxidation via nitration (role of calcium/calmodulin and NOS) (see above)

i) NOS: activated by increased intracellular calcium (and calcium bound to calmodulin); calcium influx mediated by NMDA receptors

ii) NO reacts with superoxide (O_2^-), producing peroxynitrite ($ONOO^-$)

iii) Peroxynitrite acts as highly reactive radical

e) Mitochondrial energy failure via inhibition of Krebs cycle

2) Cellular effectors of apoptosis (caspase cascade)

a) Caspases (cysteine proteases)

i) Direct effector pathway for death receptors

ii) Caspases activate other caspases and cleave proteins leading to DNA destruction and lipid peroxidation

b) Bcl-2 family members

i) Proapoptotic members (Bad, Bax, Bid): form pores (MPT) in mitochondrial membrane; cytochrome *c* leaking out of mitochondria stimulates caspase cascade via Apaf 1

ii) Antiapoptotic members (Bcl-2, Bcl-X_L): inhibit cytochrome *c* leakage

3) Availability of glutathione via astrocytes stimulates conversion of H_2O_2 to H_2O and prevent respiratory chain failure–associated lipid peroxidation

a) Stimulation of poly (ADP-ribose) polymerase (PARP) induces NADP depletion and failure of conversion of H_2O_2 to H_2O, leading to lipid peroxidation

b) PARP also activates proapoptotic nuclear factor-kappa B and p53

4. Protein denaturation and folding (Fig. 2-3)

a. Heat shock proteins (HSPs)

1) Molecular chaperones responsible for preventing premature folding and destruction of native proteins

2) Usually expressed continually, but expression is induced at times of cellular stress (e.g., ischemia)

3) Transcription of *HSP* gene is mediated by binding of the heat shock factor to heat shock element (DNA sequence)

4) HSP-70 binds to misfolded or denatured proteins to prevent folding and destruction and induces ATP-dependent refolding of denatured proteins

b. Ubiquitin-proteasome system

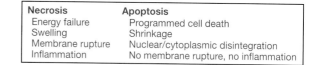

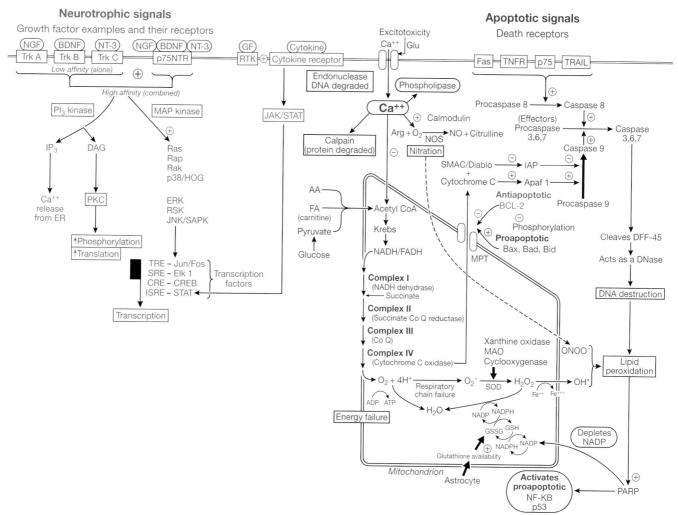

Fig. 2-2. Neurotrophism and cell death. Neurotrophic signaling pathways and apoptotic signaling pathways. The clustering of molecules does not necessarily represent the absolute sequence of involvement nor do molecules necessarily act in the same cell at the same time. AA, amino acid; ADP, adenosine diphosphate; Apaf 1, apoptotic protease-activating factor 1; ATP, adenosine triphosphate; Bad, bc12 antagonist of cell death; Bax, BCL2-associated x protein; BCL, B-cell lymphoma/leukemia protein; BDNF, brain-derived neurotrophic factor; Bid, bh3-interacting domain death agonist; CRE, cyclic AMP response element; CREB, cyclic AMP response element binding protein; DAG, dystrophin-associated glycoprotein; DEF45, DNA fragmentation factor 45; Diablo, direct IAP-binding protein with low pI; Elk 1, member of ETS oncogene family; ER, endoplasmic reticulum; ERK, extracellular signal-regulated kinase; FA, fatty acid; Fas, CD95; GF, growth factor; Glu, glutamate; GSH, reduced glutathione; GSSG, oxidized glutathione; IAP, inhibitor of apoptosis proteins; IP3, inositol triphosphate; ISRE, interferon-stimulated response element; JAK, Janus kinase; JNK/SAPK, c-Jun N-terminal kinases/stress-activated protein kinases; Jun/Fos family, avian sarcoma virus 17 oncogene homologue/fbj murine osteosarcoma viral oncogene homologue; MAO, monoamine oxidase; MAP kinase, mitogen-activated protein kinase; MPT, mitochondrial permeability transition; NADP, nicotinamide adenine dinucleotide phosphate; NADPH, reduced NADP; NAPH/FADH, reduced nicotinamide/flavin adenine dinucleotide; NF-KB, nuclear factor kappa B; NGF, nerve growth factor; NO, nitric oxide; NOS, nitric oxide synthase; NT-3, neurotrophin 3; p38, p38 MAP kinase; p53, transformation-related protein 53; p75 NTR, NGFR (nerve growth factor receptor); PI3 kinase, phosphatidylinositol 3-kinase; PKC, protein kinase C; RARP, poly(ADP-ribose) polymerases; RAS/RAB/RAK, Ras oncogene superfamily; RTK, receptor tyrosine kinase; SMAC, second mitochondria-derived activator of caspase; SOD, superoxide dismutase; SRE, sterol regulatory element; STAT, signal transducer and activator of transcription; TNFR, tumor necrosis factor receptor; TRAIL, tumor necrosis factor–related apoptosis-inducing ligand; TRE, 12-tetradecanoyl phorbol 13-acetate–responsive element; TRK, neurotrophic tyrosine kinase receptor.

1) Catalyzes degradation of damaged or misfolded proteins
2) Ubiquitination of proteins and ubiquitin-dependent degradation of cell proteins important for maintenance of cell cycle and apoptosis (ATP-dependent process)
3) Proteins are flagged for degradation by attachment of polyubiquinated chain
4) Three-enzyme system: protein undergoes activation (enzyme E_1), conjugation (enzyme E_2), ligation (enzyme E_3); mutation of the *PARK2* gene encoding parkin protein (an E_3 ubiquitin ligase) is responsible for an inherited parkinsonism with autosomal recessive inheritance
5) End result: polyubiquinated protein destined for 26 S proteasome, which in turn cleaves protein complex to ubiquitin and protein fragments
6) Protects against accumulation of denatured proteins and apoptosis

c. Abnormal inclusions in neurodegenerative disorders (Table 2-1)
   1) Aggregation of nascent proteins that have lost normal function and are resistant to degradation
   2) Abnormal ubiquitination and impaired ubiquitin-dependent degradation can cause aggregation of ubiquitin cellular inclusions characteristic of many neurodegenerative conditions (Alzheimer's disease and Parkinson's disease)

E. Synapses (Fig. 2-4)
1. Presynaptic component

a. Synaptic vesicles
   1) Small clear vesicles: γ-aminobutyric acid (GABA), glycine, glutamate, or ACh
   2) Intermediate-size vesicles: monoamines
   3) Large dense-core vesicles: neuropeptides
   4) Uptake of neurotransmitters in the nerve terminal is through vesicular protein ATPases specific to the neurotransmitter
b. Vesicle mobilization
   1) Synapsin binds vesicles to cytoskeleton at active zone
   2) Phosphorylation of synapsin allows mobilization of vesicles
   3) Rab 3 proteins are monomeric GTP-binding proteins implicated in control of regulated exocytosis
c. Docking, priming, fusion
   1) Depends on interaction between SNARE complex proteins
      a) Vesicular (V)-SNARE is synaptobrevin
      b) Transmembrane (T)-SNARE is syntaxin and SNAP-25
   2) Clostridial toxins hydrolyze SNARE proteins, preventing neurotransmitter release (Fig. 2-4): botulinum toxins (BTX) A and E cleave SNAP25; BTX C acts on syntaxin; BTX B and F cleave synaptobrevin
d. Exocytosis
   1) Depends on calcium influx through N and P/Q type calcium channels
   2) Synaptotagmin acts as calcium sensor for vesicle
e. Endocytosis and recycling
   1) Clathrin coats site of release, forming a pit
   2) Dynamin causes fission from cell membrane

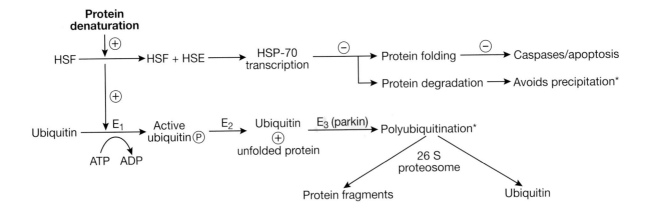

*Incomplete polyubiquitination → B pleated sheath formation

Fig. 2-3. Protein denaturation and folding. ADP, adenosine diphosphate; ATP, adenosine triphosphate; E_1, E_2, E_3, enzymes 1, 2, and 3 (e.g., parkin protein), respectively; HSE, heat shock element; HSF heat shock factor; HSP, heat shock protein.

Table 2-1. **Inclusion Bodies in Central Nervous System Neurodegenerative Disorders**

Inclusion (protein)	Cellular localization	Implicated disorder
Senile plaque (amyloid β protein)	Extracellular	Alzheimer's disease, aging
Neurofibrillary tangles (hyper-phosphorylated tau)	Neuronal soma	Alzheimer's disease
Hirano bodies (actin)	Neuronal soma	Alzheimer's disease
Globose tangles (tau)	Neuronal soma	Progressive super-nuclear palsy
Lewy body (α-synuclein)	Neuronal soma	Lewy body disease
Glial inclusions (α-synuclein)	Glial cytoplasm and nucleus	Multiple system atrophy
Spheroids (α-synuclein)	Neurons (axonal swellings)	NBID type I
Ballooned neurons (neurofilament proteins)	Neuronal soma	ALS, corticobasal degeneration
Bunina bodies (vimentin, HSP70)	Motor neurons	ALS
Rosenthal fibers (GFAP)	Astrocytes	Alexander's disease, pilocytic astro-cytoma
Prion plaque (prion protein)	Lysosomes	Prion disease (kuru, GSS)

ALS, amyotrophic lateral sclerosis; GFAP, glial fibrillary acidic protein; GSS, Gerstmann-Sträussler-Scheinker syndrome; NBID, neurodegeneration with brain iron depigmentation type I (formerly, Hallervorden-Spatz disease).

    a) This is regulated by endophilin, amphiphysin, and adaptins (clathrin adaptor proteins, which promote assembly of clathrin network)

    b) Synaptojanin and HSC-70 are involved in uncoating of vesicle to make it ready for neurotransmitter uptake

2. Postsynaptic component
    a. Anchoring of presynaptic and postsynaptic active zones: adhesion molecules anchor active zones together in junctional folds
    b. Nicotinic ACh receptors (nAChRs) in neuromuscular junction: clustered at postjunctional folds from multiple regulatory proteins
      1) Expression of nAChR: activated by neuroligins
      2) Clustering is triggered by agrin
      3) Laminin, MuSK (sarcoglycan in T-tubes), and rapsyn

Synaptic vesicles
    Small clear vesicles store and release γ-aminobutyric acid, glutamate, glycine, and acetylcholine

    Intermediate dense-core vesicles store and release monoamines

    Large dense-core vesicles store and release neuropeptides

Vesicle mobilization
    Storage of neurotransmitters depends on transporter-selective vesicular protein ATPases

    Synapsin phosphorylation facilitates vesicle mobilization

    Membrane docking, priming, and fusion depends on SNARE protein complex, which includes synaptobrevin, syntaxin, and SNAP-25

    Influx of calcium in depolarized axon terminal triggers exocytosis of vesicle through interaction with synaptotagmin

Vesicle endocytosis and recycling depends on
    Vesicle coating by clathrin

    Fission by dynamin

    Regulation by endophilin, amphiphysin, and synaptojanin

    (ankyrin in T-tube): also critical proteins for nAChR clustering
    4) Anti-MuSK antibodies have been associated with myasthenia gravis
    5) Different phenotypes of myopathies arise depending on type of regulatory protein deficiency or malfunction (Fig. 2-4)

F. **Ion Channels** (Fig. 2-5 *A*)
1. Basic electrophysiology
    a. The membrane potential (Vm)
      1) Vm: determined by the difference between intracellular and extracellular potentials

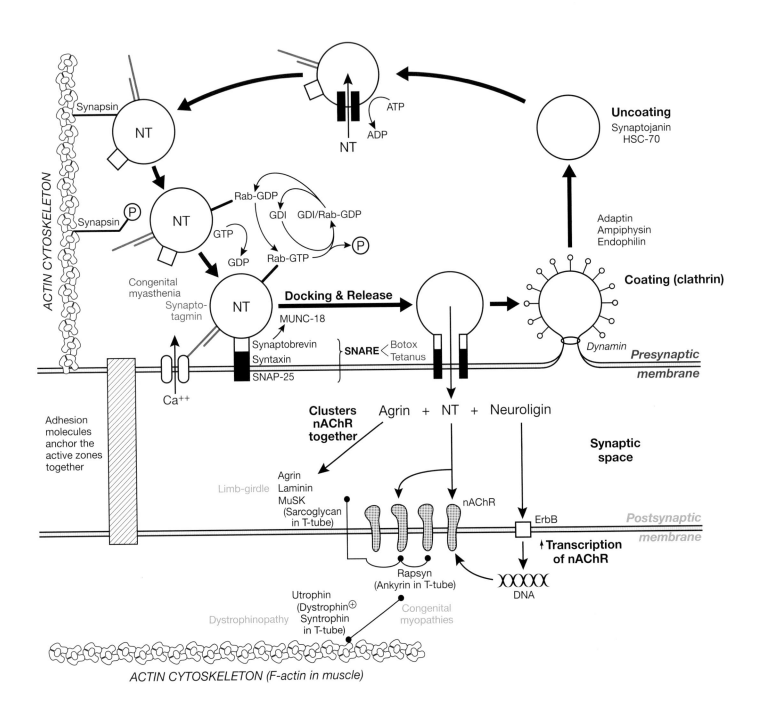

Fig. 2-4. Molecular events underlying vesicular recycling, neurotransmitter release, and presynatptic and postsynaptic membrane specialization. Different phenotypes of associated myopathies are indicated in green. ADP, adenosine diphosphate; ATP, adenosine triphosphate; GDI, guanosine nucleotide dissociation inhibitor; GDP, guanosine diphosphate; GTP, guanosine triphosphate; HSC-70, heat shock 70-Kd protein; MUNC-18, syntaxin binding protein; nAChR, nicotinic acetylcholine receptor; NT, neurotransmitter; Rab, Rab family of G proteins; SNAP-25, synaptosomal-associated protein 25; SNARE, SNARE complex.

2) Equilibrium potential of ion (E_{ion}): determined by ion's concentration gradient
   a) Sodium, calcium, and chloride: higher extracellular concentrations
   b) Potassium and other anions: higher intracellular concentrations
   c) Ionic gradient depends on ATP-driven ion pumps and regulation of neuronal microenvironment glial cells
   d) Nernst equation can be used to calculate E_{ion}:

$$E_{ion} = RT/zF \ln [ion]_o/[ion]_i = 58 \log [ion]_o/[ion]_i$$

   e) Vm can be determined by the Goldman equation:

$$Vm = \frac{RT}{F} \frac{\ln P_K[K^+]_o + P_{Na}[Na^+]_o + P_{Cl}[Cl^-]_i}{P_K[K^+]_i + P_{Na}[Na^+]_i + P_{Cl}[Cl^-]_o}$$

3) Resting membrane potential (RMP): Vm at steady state (no net flow of ions across the membrane)
   a) For neurons: between –60 and –80 mV
   b) For skeletal muscle: –85 to –95 mV
4) Opening an ion channel brings Vm closer to E_{ion} of that ion
   a) Opening a sodium channel with E_{Na} of +70 mV or a calcium channel with an E_{Ca} of +150 mV: depolarizes cell
   b) Opening a potassium channel with E_K of –100 mV: hyperpolarizes cell
   c) Opening a chloride channel with E_{Cl} of –75 mV: may hyperpolarize or depolarize cell
b. Action potential
   1) Once depolarization reaches the threshold for voltage-gated sodium channels, there is rapid depolarization (fast sodium spike)
   2) Any stimulus greater than threshold: produces action potential independent of its intensity; an all-or-none event
   3) Voltage-gated sodium channels rapidly inactivate
   4) Slow activation of potassium channels repolarizes membrane and produces transient hyperpolarization
   5) This transient hyperpolarization produces refractory period, preventing retrograde propagation of action potentials
   6) Propagation of the action potential depends on the resistance of the axoplasm and the outward leakage of current
   a) Length constant (λ): distance along dendrite where ΔVm has decayed to 37% of its value at the site of stimulation; usually between 0.1 and 1.0 mm

$$\lambda = \sqrt{r_m/r_a}$$

   b) Time constant (τ): amount of time for Vm to

Sodium channels
   Fast inactivating (tetrodotoxin sensitive) are responsible for spike of action potential

   Slow inactivating (tetrodotoxin resistant) are responsible for plateau or pacemaker potentials

Calcium channels
   L-type: slow depolarization and excitation-contraction coupling in skeletal muscle

   P/Q and N types: cause neurotransmitter release

   T type: produce low-threshold spike (oscillatory burst firing)

Potassium channels
   Delayed rectifying repolarization after action potential

   Type A (fast)

   2-Pore domain

   Slow calcium activated: sets excitability in response to neuron's energy state

   Inward rectifier: responsible for resting membrane potential

---

Ion channels are multimetric transmembrane proteins that form hydrophobic pores through which ions can passively flow

Activation of ligand-gated ion channels produces excitation or inhibition

---

move 63% of way to its final value
   c) Conduction velocity: higher in large diameter fibers because transverse membrane resistance is higher while longitudinal axoplasm resistance is lower
2. Voltage-gated channels (Fig. 2-5 *A*)
   a. Depolarization opens channel (sliding helix model)
   1) Four subunits: α subunit forms pore and determines ion selectivity and voltage sensitivity
   2) α unit of the voltage-gated sodium and voltage-gated calcium channels are made of four domains in tandem (TMI-IV), each composed of six transmembrane regions

A

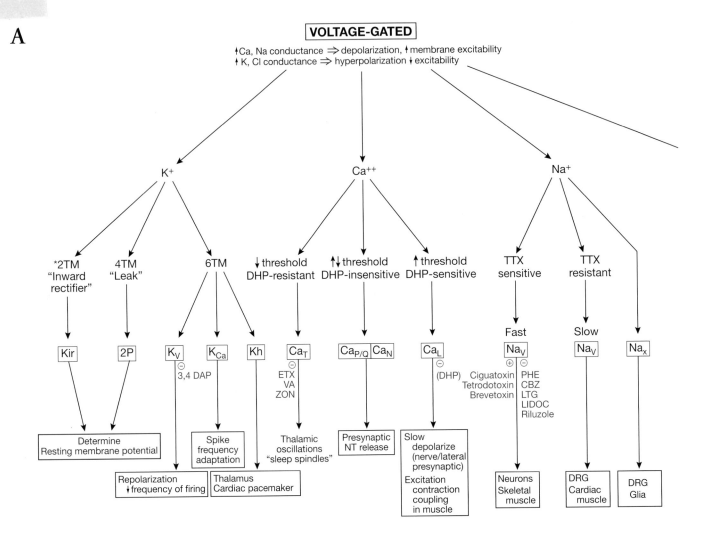

Channelopathies

Channel	Disorders
K⁺	Episodic ataxia type 1 (associated with myokymia)
	Isaac's syndrome (associated with neuromyotonia)
	Benign familial neonatal convulsions
	Increased QT syndrome
Ca⁺⁺	Lambert-Eaton myasthenic syndrome (associated with autoimmune antibodies to P/Q calsium channel subtype)
	Hypokalemic periodic paralysis type 1 (associated with mutation of *CACNL1AS* gene)
	Episodic ataxia type 2 (associated with mutation of *CACNA1A* gene)
	Familial hemiplegic migraine (associated with mutation of *CACNA1A* gene)
	SCA-6 (associated with mutation of *CACNA1A* gene)
Cl⁻	Myotonia congenita (associated with mutation of *CLCN1* gene)
Na⁺	Hyperkalemic periodic paralysis (associated with mutation of *SCN4A* gene)
	Paramyotonia (associated with mutation of *SCN4A* gene)
	Hypokalemic periodic paralysis type 2 (associated with mutation of *SCN4A* gene)
	Generalized epilepsy with febrile seizures

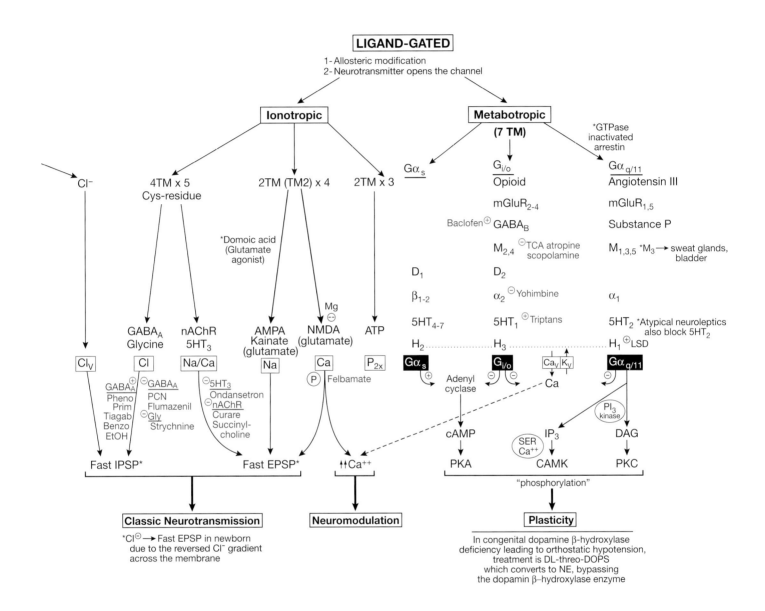

Disorders associated with ligand-gated channels

Channel	Disorders
Glycine	Familial hyperkplexia
nACHR	Autosomal dominant frontal lobe epilepsy
	Myasthenia gravis
	Botulism
	Congenital myasthenia
	Dysautonomia
	Tick paralysis
	Sea snake toxin

B

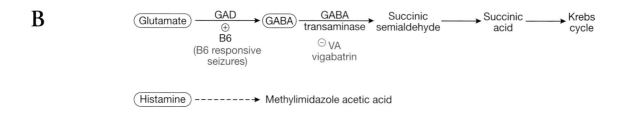

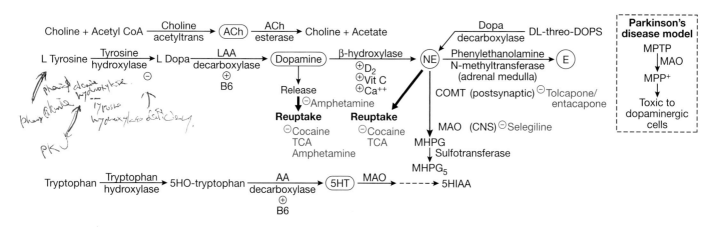

Fig. 2-5 *A,* Classification of ion channels and, *B,* neurotransmitter synthesis. AA, amino acid; AMPA, α-amino-3-hydroxy-5-methyl-4 isoxazolepropionate; ATP, adenosine triphosphate; Benzo, benzodiazepine; CACNA, voltage-dependent calcium channel subunit; CAMK, calcium/calmodulin-dependent protein kinase; cAMP, cyclic adenosine monophosphate; CBZ, carbamazepine; CLCN, chloride channel family; CNS, central nervous system; DAG, diacylglycerol; DAP, diaminopyridine; DHP, dihydropyridine; DRG, dorsal root ganglion; E, epinephrine; EPSP, excitatory postsynaptic potential; EtOH, ethanol; ETX, ethosuximide; GABA, γ-aminobutyric acid; GTP, guanosine triphosphate; H, histaminic; HIAA, hydroxyindoleacetic acid; 5HT, 5-hydroxytryptamine; IP$_3$, inositol 1,4,5-triphosphate; IPSP, inhibitory postsynaptic potential; LAA, L-amino acid; LIDOC, lidocaine; LSD, lysergic acid diethylamide; LTG, lamotrigine; M, muscarinic; MG, myasthenia gravis; mGluR, glutamate receptor; nAChR, nicotonic ACh receptor; NE, norepinephrine; NMDA, *N*-methyl-D-aspartate; PCN, penicillin; PHE, phenytoin; Pheno, phenobarbital; PI$_3$, proteinase inhibitor 3; PKA, protein kinase A; PKC, protein kinase C; Prim, primidone; SCA, spinocerebellar ataxia; SER, smooth endoplasmic reticulum; TCA, tricyclic antidepressant; Tiagab, tiagabine; TM, transmembrane; TOP, topiramate; TTX, tetrodotoxin; ZON, zonisamide; −, blocks receptor; +, activates receptor.

b. Potassium channels
  1) Responsible for hyperpolarization and reduction of neuronal excitability
  2) Categorized on basis of number of transmembrane domains
  3) Inward rectifier potassium channels (K$_{IR}$)
     a) Two transmembrane domains
     b) Responsible for maintaining resting membrane potential: when hyperpolarization of membrane potential "overshoots" below resting membrane,

Kir is activated and conducts K current into cell, bringing Vm toward E$_K$
     c) May be ATP-gated or G protein-coupled
  4) Two-pore (2P) domain potassium channels
     a) Four transmembrane domains
     b) Help to determine resting membrane, influences action potential duration, and important in modulation of neuronal excitability
     c) TASK channel currents: very sensitive to changes in extracellular pH

Vm is the elecrical potential inside the cell relative to the outside

Equilibrium potential is the voltage difference that offsets the tendency of an ion to move down its concentration gradient

Opening an ion channel brings the membrane potential toward the equilibrium potential of that ion (opening sodium and calcium channels causes depolarization; opening potassium channels causes hyperpolarization)

G protein-coupled receptors have neuromodulatory effects, which are determined by G protein molecular switch

G protein	Action	Receptors
$G\alpha_s$	cAMP production. Activation of PKA	β-adrenergic, D_1, 5-HT_{4-7}, H_2, VIP, CGRP
$G\alpha_{i/o}$	Opens potassium channels. Closes calcium channels	$GABA_B$, mGluR2-4, α_2-adrenergic, D_2, 5-HT_1, opioid, somatostatin; Y2, endocannabinoids
Gq/11	Activates PKC. Releases calcium from intracellular stores	mGluR1,5; M1; α_1-adrenergic; 5-HT_2; H_1; substance P; angiotensin II; bradykinin

CGRP, calcitonin gene-related protein; GABA, γ-aminobutyric acid; 5-HT, hydroxytryptamine; PKA, protein kinase A; PKC, protein kinase C; VIP, vasoactive intestinal polypeptide.

---

    d) TREK channel currents: cold-sensitive; may be important in neuroprotection against ischemia and seizures

    e) TRAAK channels: sensitive to change in cell volume, closed during extracellular hyperosmolarity

5) Type A potassium channels

    a) Contain six transmembrane domains

    b) Fast potassium channels: rapidly activated by depolarization and inactivated (produce a transient outward current, termed A-current)

    c) Located in paranodal regions of myelinated axons

    d) Responsible for prevention of repetitive firing of action potentials and prolong interspike interval (as with delayed-rectifier potassium channels discussed below)

    e) Examples: K_v 1.4 and K_v 1.7 (voltage-gated Shaker-related subfamily, encoded by *KCNA4* and *KCNA7*)

6) Delayed-rectifier potassium channels

    a) Contain six transmembrane domains

    b) Located primarily at nodes (and presynaptic), much less frequently at internodes

    c) Temporarily activated with depolarization

    d) Delayed activation, slow inactivation

    e) Act to prolong interspike interval, reduce frequency of action potentials, and prevent repetitive firing of action potentials: blocking or mutation of this channel can cause repetitive discharge of action potentials noted on needle electromyography (EMG) as myokymia or neuromyotonia

    f) Responsible for hyperpolarization afterpotential which activates Kir

    g) Predominantly voltage-gated Shaker-related subfamily (KCNA) members 1, 2, 3, and 6 (K_v 1.1, 1.2, 1.3, and 1.6, respectively): encoded by *KCNA*

1, 2, 3, and 6, respectively

    h) Mutations of K_v 1.1: responsible for episodic ataxia type 1 (EA 1), associated with myokymia (or neuromyotonia)

    i) Antibodies to K_v 1.6: associated with Isaacs' syndrome—hyperexcitability (often paraneoplastic) syndrome of excessive muscle twitching, fasciculations, cramps, stiffness, myokymia, and neuromyotonia

    j) Blocked by: 4-aminopyridine and phencyclidine

7) KCNQ family

    a) Responsible for M-current: low-threshold, non-inactivating, voltage-dependent K^+ current

    b) Slow delayed rectifier: activated in response to persistent depolarizing stimulus; limits repetitive firing

    c) Mutations of *KCNQ1* gene on chromosome 11p15.5: linked to long QT syndrome type 1

    d) Mutations of *KCNQ2* gene on chromosome 20q13.3 and *KCNQ3* gene on chromosme 8q24: linked to benign familial neonatal convulsions

8) Calcium-activated potassium channels (K_{Ca})

    a) Contain six transmembrane regions

b) Activated in response to depolarization-induced accumulation of intracellular calcium; and stay open for prolonged periods because of slow decay of intracellular calcium: responsible for slow afterhyperpolarization

c) May slow firing rate of action potentials in presence of continuous depolarizing stimulus

9) Hyperpolarization-gated potassium channels (K_H)

a) Contain six transmembrane domains

b) Hyperpolarization-gated, cyclic adenosine monophosphate (cAMP)-activated channels in thalamus and cardiac pacemaker cells

c. Voltage-gated calcium channels

1) L-type (long-lasting, large current) Ca channels (of Ca_v1 family)

a) High threshold of activation: activated with strong depolarization

b) Stay open for prolonged periods

c) Dihydropyridine (DHP) sensitive (e.g., nifedipine, nimodipine)

d) Responsible for slow depolarization in neurons and excitation-contraction coupling in myocytes

e) Mutation of *CACNL1AS* gene on chromosome 1q21-31, encoding α_1 subunit of muscle L-type calcium channel, is responsible for autosomal dominant familial hypokalemic periodic paralysis type 1

2) T-type (tiny or transient currents) calcium channels (of Ca_v3 family)

a) Low threshold of activation: activated with small depolarization (termed low-threshold spikes)

b) Voltage-dependent inactivation

c) Depolarization produced by activation of these channels, in turn, rapidly causes inactivation: produce oscillating pacemaker currents

d) Oscillatory pacemaker burst activity in thalamo-cortical relay neurons: responsible for spindles observed in electroencephalographic (EEG) recordings during non–rapid eye movement (NREM) sleep and 3-Hz spike-and-wave activity in EEG recordings of absence seizures

e) Blocked by zonisamide, ethosuximide, valproate

f) DHP-resistant

3) N-type calcium channels (of Ca_v2 family)

a) High threshold of activation: activated with strong depolarization

b) Slow inactivation

c) DHP-insensitive

d) Located in some presynaptic terminals; especially abundant in dorsal root ganglion neurons

e) Important in triggering neurotransmitter release

f) Blocked by ω-conotoxin GVIA

4) P/Q-type calcium channels (of Ca_v2 family)

a) Intermediate threshold of activation

b) Ubiquitous distribution, especially abundant in Purkinje cells

c) Occur in presynaptic terminals

d) Important in triggering neurotransmitter release (with N-channels)

e) Alternative splicing of *CACNA1A* gene on chromosome 19p13.1-2 encoding the α_1A subunits of channel gives rise to either P or Q channel

f) P channel: minimal rate of inactivation

g) Q channel: moderate rate of inactivation

h) Mutation of *CACNA1A* gene encoding α_1A subunits of channel: linked to episodic ataxia type 2 (EA-2), familial hemiplegic migraines (FHM), and spinocerebellar ataxia type 6 (SCA6) (the latter is due to increased CAG repeats in *CACNA1A*)

i) Lambert-Eaton myasthenic syndrome: due to action of autoantibodies against presynaptic P/Q- and N-types of calcium channels

d. Voltage-gated sodium channels (VGSCs)

1) Fast inactivating sodium channels (fast Na_v)

a) Most abundant VGSCs

b) Most sensitive to tetrodotoxin (TTX): exception is Na_v 1.4 in skeletal muscle (α subunit is encoded by *SCN4A* gene on chromosome 17q), which is not TTX-sensitive

c) Clustered at axon hillock and nodes of Ranvier by ankyrin B

d) Responsible for initiation of action potential in neurons and skeletal muscle

e) Blocked by local anesthetics, antiarrhythmics, and antiepileptics

f) Mutations of *SCN4A* gene is responsible for *hyper*kalemic periodic paralysis, *hypo*kalemic periodic paralysis type 2, paramyotonia congenita, myotonia fluctuans, myotonia permanens, and malignant hyperthermia: "gain of function" mutations, impaired inactivation of sodium channels causing membrane hyperexcitability

g) Sustained depolarization of muscle membrane and inactivation of normal sodium channels: possible mechanism for periodic paralysis in this setting

h) Mutation of *SCN1B* gene encoding the β_1-subunit of neuronal voltage-gated sodium channel: associated with generalized epilepsy with febrile convulsions plus (GEFS+)

2) Slow inactivating sodium channels (slow Na_v)

a) Resistant to TTX

b) Responsible for initiation of action potential in dorsal root ganglia and cardiac muscle

   3) Nax channels

     a) In dorsal root ganglia and glial cells

  e. Voltage-gated chloride channels (Cl$_v$, CLC channels)

   1) Together with ionotropic chloride channels (see below) are responsible for fast inhibitory postsynaptic potential (IPSP)

   2) CLCN1 proteins of skeletal muscle act as electrical buffer to maintain resting muscle membrane potential: any deviation from resting potential causes passive diffusion of negatively charged ions along electrochemical gradient, acting to return membrane potential to resting value

   3) Passive chloride current: limits duration of depolarization of T-tubular system

   4) Reduction in passive membrane chloride current: responsible for continous repetitive firing observed in needle EMG as myotonia

   5) Mutation of *CLCN1* gene on chromosome 7q: responsible for myotonia congenita

3. Ligand-gated ion channels (Fig. 2-5 *A*)

  a. Includes neurotransmitter-gated ion channels and sensory receptor channels

  b. Channels act as receptors for neurotransmitters; consist of several subunits arranged to form a central pore

  c. Binding of neurotransmitter to channel induces channel opening via allosteric modification and increases channel permeability to cations or anions conducted through the central pore, generating postsynaptic potentials (PSPs)

  d. Excitatory (depolarizing) postsynaptic potentials (EPSPs): produced by neurotransmitter-induced opening of cation channels

  e. IPSPs: produced by neurotransmitter-induced opening of anion channels

  f. Ionotropic channels

   1) Cysteine residue-containing family

     a) Pentamers of subunits (α, β, γ, δ, and ϵ) composed of four transmembrane domains

     b) Chloride channels

       i) GABA$_A$- and glycine-gated receptors

       ii) Responsible for fast IPSP: classic inhibitory neurotransmitters (discussed below)

       iii) In newborns: because of reversed chloride gradient, effect of these channels is one of fast excitation

     c) Cation channels

       i) nAChRs and 5-HT$_3$ serotonin receptors

       ii) Conduct sodium and calcium as well as potassium

       iii) Responsible for fast EPSP: classic excitatory neurotransmitters

   2) Ionotropic glutamate receptor family

     a) Tetramers of subunits with four transmembrane domains

     b) Sodium channels

       i) AMPA and kainate receptors

       ii) Conducts sodium more than calcium

       iii) AMPA receptors: four types of subunits GluR$_{1-4}$; low permeability to Ca^{2+} depends on presence of a GluR$_2$ subunit (coexpression of GLuR2 with GluR1 or GluR3 renders channels impermeable to calcium); synaptic current of rapid onset and decay

       iv) Antibodies to GluR3 have been associated with Rasmussen encephalitis, a progressive encephalopathy with seizures

       v) Kainate: five types of subunits GluR$_{5-7}$, and KA$_1$/KA$_2$ subunits

       vi) Responsible for fast EPSP: classic excitatory neurotransmitters

     c) Calcium channels

       i) NMDA receptors

       ii) Very permeable to calcium

       iii) Consists of NR1 and NR2 subunits

       iv) The ion channel is blocked by Mg^{2+} ions; removed by depolarization

       v) Requires binding of glycine and depolarization to remove magnesium blockade

       vi) Synaptic current of slow onset and even slower decay (likely due to high affinity of glutamate for receptor)

       vii) Responsible for fast EPSP and neuromodulation through controlling calcium pool within the neuron for LTP and LTD

       viii) Increased NMDA activation in patients with Parkinson's disease is likely explanation for levodopa-induced dyskinesias and motor fluctuations in the advanced disease; concomitant use of amantadine (NMDA-blocking agent) helps alleviate these symptoms

       ix) NMDA receptors and associated glutamate-triggered excitotoxicity have been targets of many pharmacologic agents; for example, memantine for Alzheimer's disease: memantine has low affinity for NMDA receptors, with rapid onset and offset of action, causing short-term activation thought to promote learning and memory (chronic low-grade NMDA activation promotes cell death)

3) P2X purinergic receptors: conduct ATP

g. Metabotropic G protein–coupled receptors (Fig. 2-5)

  1) Single polypeptide with seven transmembrane domains

  2) Common mechanism of action through three different types of G-protein coupling

    a) Receptors coupled to $G\alpha_s$-protein stimulate adenyl cyclase, cAMP production, and activation of protein kinase A: net effect is increased intracellular calcium and increased phosphorylation

    b) Receptors coupled to $G_{q/11}$ activate phospholipase C that activates phosphatidylinositol biphosphate (PIP_2), which activates diacylglycerol, thus activating proteinase C; PIP_2 also stimulates inositol triphosphate, which releases intracellular calcium and increases phosphorylation

    c) Receptors coupled to $G_{i/o}$ inhibits adenyl cyclase, opens potassium channels, closes calcium channels: net effect is decreased intracellular calcium and decreased phosphorylation

  3) Includes (Fig. 2-5)

    a) $GABA_B$ receptor

    b) Muscarinic cholinergic receptor

    c) Metabotropic glutamate receptor (mGluR)

    d) Most monoamine receptors

    e) Neuropeptide receptors

G. Neurotransmitters (Fig. 2-5 *B*)

1. Glutamate

  a. Major excitatory neurotransmitter in CNS

  b. Synthesis (two sources)

    1) Glutamine synthesized by astrocytes is converted to glutamate by glutaminase

    2) α-Ketoglutarate produced by Krebs cycle is converted to glutamate by glutamate dehydrogenase

  c. Vesicular storage

    1) In small, round clear vesicles

    2) Depends on vesicular glutamate transporter (GT-1)

    3) May be costored with zinc or *N*-acetylaspartylglutamate (NAAG), which modulates excitatory transmission

  d. Uptake

    1) Glutamate: rapidly cleared from synaptic cleft by high-affinity sodium- and potassium-coupled glutamate carriers, called excitatory amino acid transporters (EAATs)

    2) EAAT-1 and EAAT-2: occur in astrocytes; responsible for most of uptake

    3) EAAT-3: occurs in neurons (including all glutamatergic neurons) and some glia; responsible for smaller share of postsynaptic glutamate uptake

  e. Receptors

    1) Ionotropic glutamate receptors (AMPA, kainate, and NMDA, discussed above)

    2) Metabotropic glutamate receptors

      a) Group I

        i) mGluR1 and mGluR5

        ii) Coupled to $G_{q/11}$, generate inositol triphosphate and diacylglycerol

        iii) Increase glutamate release in presynaptic membrane

        iv) Potentiate NMDA responses in postsynaptic membrane

      b) Groups II and III

        i) Group II, mGluR2, mGluR3; group III, mGluR4 and mGluR6, 7, 8

        ii) Coupled to $G_{i/o}$; inhibit adenylyl cyclase, reduce calcium influx via L- and N-channels

        iii) Inhibit release of glutamate or GABA

  f. Role of glutamate in excitotoxicity

    1) With energy deprivation such as ischemia, function of Na^+/K^+ ATPase decreases as ATP stores are depleted

Neurotransmitter	Precursor	Synthesis enzyme	Transporter	Inactivation
Glutamate	α-KG glutamine	Glutamate dehydrogenase	VGAT	Reuptake (EAATs)
γ-Aminobutyric acid	Glutamate	Glutamic acid decarboxylase	VGAT	Reuptake
Acetylcholine	Choline	Choline acetyltransferase	VAChT	Acetylcholinesterase
Dopamine	Tyrosine	Tyrosine hydroxylase	VAMT-2	DAT/MAO_B > HVA
Norepineprhine	Dopamine	Dopamine-β-hydroxylase	VAMT-1	NET/MAO_A, COMT > MHPG
Serotonin	L-tryptophan	Tryptophan hydroxylase	VAMT-2	SERT/MAO_A > HIAA

2) Subsequently, increased concentration of sodium and calcium entering through AMPA and NMDA glutaminergic receptors

3) Increased intracellular calcium eventually leads to oxidative stress and cell death

4) Concurrently, with decreased Na^+/K^+ ATPase activity, extracellular potassium levels increase: causes depolarization that further activates voltage-dependent calcium channels, promoting further neurotransmitter release (especially glutamate)

5) Despite increased glutamate in synaptic cleft, glutamate reuptake mechanism is also damaged because it too is dependent on Na^+/K^+ ATPase

6) Result of this cascade: excessive glutamate release that acts further to upregulate excitatory AMPA, NMDA, and mGluRs

7) This upregulation further promotes increase in intracellular calcium levels, producing oxidative injury and disrupting plasma and mitochondrial membranes and cytoskeleton, eventually causing cell death

8) Increased glutamate levels also inhibit cystine-glutamate exchanger, which transports cystine into cell and exports equivalent level of glutamate from cell; inhibition of this transport mechanism leads to depletion of intracellular cystine stores, thus, oxidative stress

9) Other than ischemia, defective glutamate uptake and excitotoxicity are implicated in pathogenesis of degenerative diseases (amyotrophic lateral sclerosis, Huntington's disease)

10) Glutamate reuptake also impaired by increased ammonia levels in hepatic encephalopathy; this occurs through downregulation of EAAT-1 and EAAT-2 in astrocytes

g. NMDA receptor-dependent long-term depression (LTD) and long-term potentiation (LTP) in the hippocampus

1) LTP in hippocampus: caused by large, brief, high-frequency stimulus

a) High-frequency, large, and brief stimulation activates large number of AMPA receptors on CA1 cells, causing depolarization sufficient to activate NMDA receptors

b) Activation of NMDA receptors requires removal of the magnesium block and allosteric binding of two molecules of glycine

c) Early LTP: large, brief high-frequency stimulation of postsynaptic cells cause calcium-induced activation of the calcium-calmodulin–dependent protein kinase II (CaMKII) and protein kinase C

(PKC), which then phosphorylate GluR1 subunit of AMPA glutamate receptor

d) Activation of AMPA receptors promotes further expression of these receptors at the postsynaptic membrane, thus, increasing the postsynaptic currents responsible for LTP

e) Late LTP: involves protein synthesis and activation of protein kinases that phosphorylate (and activate) the respective transcription factors

2) LTD in hippocampus: caused by low-frequency, weak, and prolonged stimulus

a) Weak, prolonged presynaptic stimulation causes a small rise in intracellular calcium, activating calcineurin and subsequent dephosphorylation of GluR1 subunit of AMPA glutamate receptors in postsynaptic membrane, decreasing conductance of sodium current through these receptors

b) Inhibition of sodium current through AMPA receptors promotes endocytosis of AMPA receptors, further decreasing postsynaptic membrane depolarization

c) Reduction in depolarization of the postsynaptic membrane decreases the activation of the NMDA receptors, which is responsible for LTD

2. GABA

a. Main inhibitory neurotransmitter in brain

1) Present in inhibitory interneurons, cerebellar Purkinje cells, and basal ganglia output neurons

b. Synthesized from glutamate by glutamic acid decarboxylase (GAD)

c. Uptake by ATP-dependent GABA transporter (GAT) in GABAergic terminals and astrocytes; tiagabine inhibits this membrane transporter

d. Metabolized by GABA-transaminase (requires pyridoxal phosphate); vigabatrin inhibits this enzyme

e. Receptors

1) GABA$_A$

a) Ligand-gated chloride channels: activation causes rapid influx of chloride with lowering of membrane potential toward chloride ion equilibrium and net hyperpolarization

b) Result: fast IPSPs

c) Allosterically modulated by benzodiazepines, barbiturates, alcohol, and general anesthesia

i) These compounds (together with GABA) bind at different sites, but all act to enhance inhibitory synaptic transmission; each of these compounds potentiates action of GABA, and benzodiazepines bind better to a receptor bound to GABA

ii) Benzodiazepines bind to benzodiazepine-binding site and promote influx of chloride ions by increasing frequency of chloride channel opening; flumazenil is receptor antagonist

iii) Barbiturates bind to separate binding site on the channel and promote binding of GABA and GABA-induced chloride conductance

iv) Chronic alcohol use down-regulates GABA$_A$ receptors, which may be implicated in hyper-excitability and seizures associated with alcohol withdrawal

v) Endozepine stupor: recurrent coma or stupor with ictal EEG fast activity associated with increased levels of endogenous benzodiazepine, endozepine-4 (elevated serum and CSF levels); flumazenil reverses stupor or coma

vi) Abnormal activation of benzodiazepine GABA$_A$ receptor complex is implicated in hepatic encephalopathy; flumazenil may be used if withdrawal seizures not a concern

2) GABA$_B$
   a) Coupled to G$_{i/o}$
   b) Result: slow IPSPs via activation of inward rectifying potassium channels causing decreased excitability, and presynaptic inhibition of N- and P/Q channels causing decreased release of neurotransmitter
   c) Baclofen is agonist

3. Glycine
   a. Important inhibitory neurotransmitter in ventral horn and brainstem
   b. Minor excitatory role as coagonist for certain NMDA receptors lacking voltage-dependent magnesium block
   c. Glycine receptor (GlyR1): a ligand-gated chloride channel inhibited by strychnine
      1) Glycine receptor: activated by glycine and other amino acids
      2) Benzodiaepines and barbiturates do not allosterically modulate the receptor
      3) Missense mutation in α-subunit of glycine receptor causing reduced levels of inhibitory neurotransmitter in spinal cord has been implicated in pathogenesis of hyperekplexia, which is treated with benzodiazepines (e.g., clonazepam, which enhances GABAergic inhibition and compensates for deficient glycinergic inhibition)

4. Acetylcholine (Fig. 2-5 *B*)
   a. Synthesized from choline by choline acetyltransferase (ChAT): bioavailability of acetyl CoA is rate-limiting for ACh biosynthesis

b. Stored by vesicular ACh transporter (VAChT)
c. Vesicular secretion is calcium-dependent, 3,4-diaminopyridine prolongs depolarization (promoting calcium-dependent release) by blocking presynaptic potassium channels
d. Hydrolyzed by acetylcholinesterase (AChE)
   1) A sodium/ATP-dependent choline transporter is responsible for reuptake of free choline
   2) Cholinesterase inhibitors increase bioavailability of ACh, in synaptic cleft
      a) Physostigmine, neostigmine, and pyridostigmine bind AChE, rendering it incapable of hydrolyzing ACh
      b) Rivastigmine is noncompetitive inhibitor of enzyme
e. Receptors
   1) nAChRs
      a) Ligand-gated cation channel
      b) Mediate fast EPSPs and presynaptically increase neurotransmitter release
      c) Long-term exposure to ACh or nicotine leads to desensitization and upregulation of receptors
      d) Increased number of ACh receptors in brains of smokers: activation of nAChRs by nicotine enhances alertness, attention, memory, and learning, and improves cognitive performance in patients with Alzheimer's disease
      e) At neuromuscular junction: binding is blocked by depolarizing drugs such as succinylcholine (weak partial agonist acting to mildly activate nAChR and induce prolonged desensitization) and decamethonium; nondepolarizing competitive blockers such as d-tubocurarine, pancuronium, vecuronium, mivacurium, lophotoxin; δ-bungarotoxin
      f) Neuronal nicotinic receptors: diffusely in brain (especially thalamus and nucleus basalis of Meynert) and in sympathetic and parasympathetic ganglia; α7 homomeric receptors have high affinity for α-bungarotoxin and low affinity for nicotine; phencyclidine (PCP) and chlorpromazine are noncompetitive inhibitors; dimethylpiperazinium acts as agonist for this receptor
      g) Mutations involving neuronal nAChRs are responsible for autosomal dominant nocturnal frontal lobe epilepsy (ADNFLE): *CHRNA4* gene on chromosome 20q13.2 coding for α4 subunit of the nAChR, cluster of genes on chromosome 15q14 coding for α3, α5, and β4 subunits of nAChR, and *CHRNB2* gene on chromosome 1 coding for β2 subunit of nAChR

2) Muscarinic cholinergic receptors (mAChR)
 a) M1-type receptors
  i) Include M1, M3, and M5
  ii) Coupled to $G_{q/11}$ (second messenger system, IP_3/diacylglycerol [DAG])
  iii) Often located postsynaptically, may increase neuronal hyperexcitability and allow repetitive firing
  iv) In cerebral cortex, hippocampus, striatum, autonomic ganglia: postsynaptic mAChRs in CNS are usually M1
 b) M2-type receptors
  i) Include M2 and M4
  ii) Coupled to $G_{i/o}$
  iii) Inhibit neurotransmitter release presynaptically; produce prolonged hyperpolarization postsynaptically
 f. Cholinergic neurons (Fig. 2-6)
 1) Basal forebrain nuclei
  a) Major input: hypothalamus, prefrontal cortex

(attention); mesopontine tegmentum (arousal); neocortex, amygdala, nucleus accumbens (emotion)
 b) Major output: hippocampus, cingulate gyrus, cerebral cortex (learning–consolidation of memory and affect by potentiating excitatory effect of glutamate); limbic system (emotion)
 c) Medial component: arises from medial septum, diagonal band, and medial portion of nucleus basalis of Meynert; projects widely via fornix and cingulate bundle to cingulate gyrus
  i) Projections from medial septal nucleus to hippocampus: important in generation of memory
  ii) Cholinergic projections from nucleus basalis of Meynert to neocortex and amygdala: role in facilitation of attention and emotion via enhancement of sensory input and activation of prefrontal cortex
  iii) Input from amygdala to basal forebrain nuclei: provides information about affective aspects of stimuli

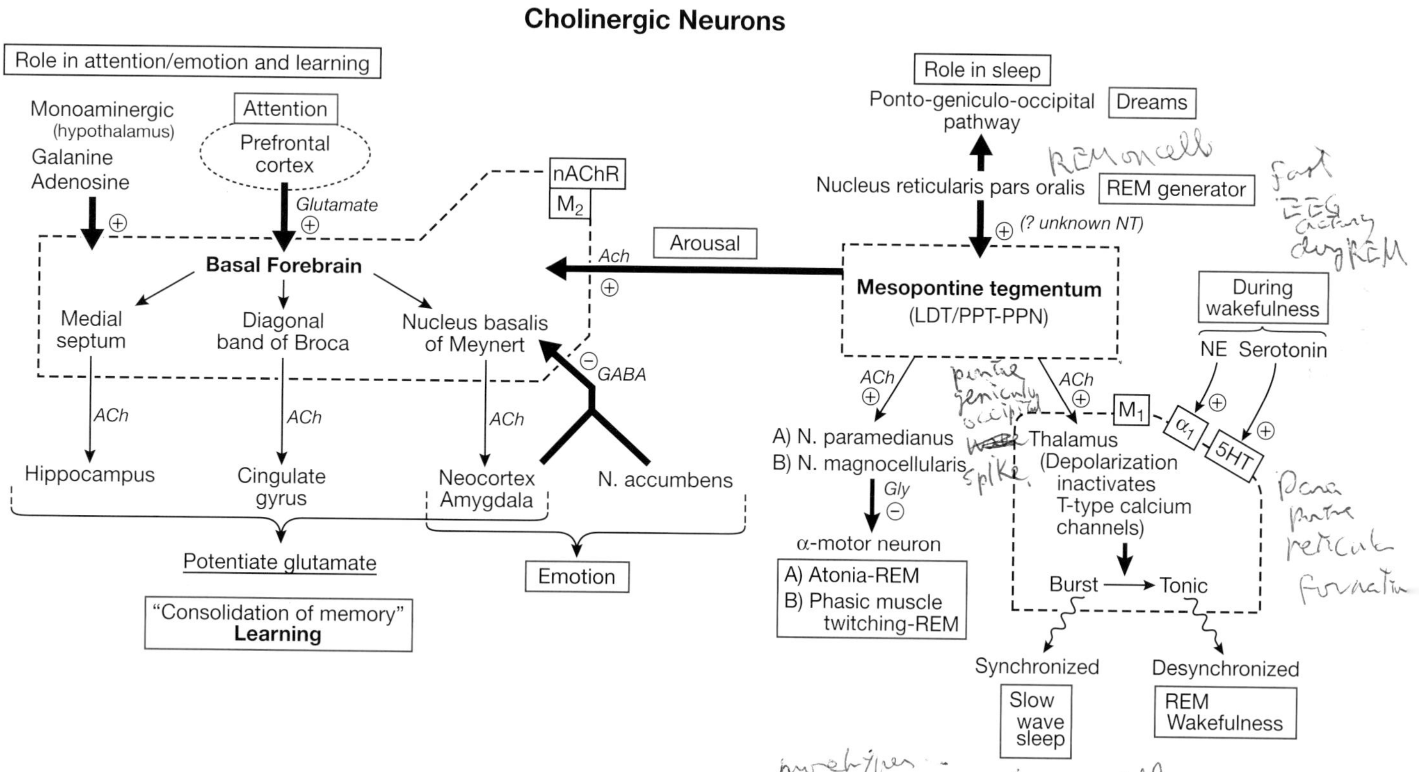

Cholinergic Neurons

Fig. 2-6. Cholinergic neurons (see text for the details). ACh, acetylcholine; GABA, γ-aminobutyric acid; Gly, glycine; 5HT, 5-hydroxytryptamine; LDT, laterodorsal tegmental nucleus; M1, M2, muscarinic receptors; nAChR, nicotinic ACh receptor, NE, norepinephrine; NT, neurotransmitter; PPT-PPN, pedunculopontine tegmental nucleus; REM, rapid eye movement.

   d) Lateral component: arises from lateral portion of nucleus basalis of Meynert and projects via external capsule to lateral cortex

   e) Cholinergic activation of thalamocortical projections occurs during wakefulness and REM sleep: responsible for low-amplitude high-frequency oscillations

   f) Loss of cholinergic neurons of nucleus basalis of Meynert in Alzheimer's disease

      i) Centrally acting anticholinesterase therapy (donezepil, rivastigmine, and galantamine): modest benefit

      ii) Donepezil: pure AChE inhibitor

      iii) Galantamine: allosteric presynaptic nicotinic receptor activator (promotes release of glutamate, GABA, ACh)

      iv) Rivastigmine: also inhibitor of butyrylcholinesterase

2) Mesopontine tegmentum

   a) Major input: nucleus reticularis pars oralis (REM sleep generator)

   b) Major output: basal forebrain (arousal); thalamus (sleep-wake cycle—activates thalamus and cortex during wakefulness and REM sleep); brainstem nuclei—nucleus paramedianus and nucleus magnocellularis (atonia and phasic muscle twitching during REM sleep)

   c) Contains caudal cholinergic neurons of laterodorsal tegmental nucleus and pedunculopontine tegmental nucleus

      i) Laterodorsal tegmental nucleus: projects to mediodorsal thalamic nucleus (has connections with prefrontal cortex) and anteroventral thalamic nucleus (has connections with hippocampus)

      ii) Pedunculopontine tegmental nucleus: projects to lateral thalamic nuclei (relay nuclei for sensory and cerebellar input to cerebral cortex)

      iii) Both nuclei project to reticular nucleus and intralaminar nuclei (most cholinergic innervation of reticular nucleus is from nucleus basalis of Meynert)

3) Brainstem-thalamocortical circuits in sleep (Fig. 2-6)

   a) Cholinergic input: primary modulator of thalamocortical projections

   b) Rhythmic burst activity during non-REM sleep

      i) Thalamocortical projections are hyperpolarized and "inactive"; this hyperpolarization removes inhibition of (and activates) T-type calcium channels and allows depolarization and rhythmic burst activity: this is manifested on EEG as sleep spindles, primarily in stage 2 non-REM sleep

      ii) Further hyperpolarization develops in deeper levels of non-REM sleep and sleep spindles disappear and give way to intrinsic cortical delta slowing

   c) Tonic activity during REM sleep and wakefulness

      i) Activation of thalamocortical projections by histaminergic input from hypothalamus

      ii) With depolarization of thalamocortical projections, T-current is inactivated and neurons fire in "tonic" mode, demonstrating high-frequency low-amplitude activity characteristic of wakefulness and REM sleep

      iii) Cholinergic neurons of laterodorsal tegmental and pedunculopontine tegmental nuclei implement events of REM sleep; nucleus reticularis pontis oralis contains cholinergic "REM-on" cells and their projections to intralaminar thalamic nuclei are responsible for fast EEG activity during REM sleep

      iv) Projections of pedunculopontine tegmental nucleus to parapontine reticular formation: implicated in stimulation of "burst cells" responsible for induction of quick saccades during REM sleep

      v) Projections of the pedunculopontine tegmental nucleus to thalamic lateral geniculate nucleus (which projects to occipital lobes): responsible for pontine-geniculate-occipital (PGO) spikes noted in EEG recordings

      vi) Cholinergic and glutaminergic projections of pedunculopontine tegmental nucleus to pontine and medullary reticular formation: responsible for inhibition of sensory input and motor output (atonia); resultant reticulospinal pathway activates glycinergic neurons in spinal cord, and glycinergic postsynaptic inhibition of motor neurons is ultimately responsible for atonia during REM sleep; inhibition of sensory input during REM sleep occurs through presynaptic GABAergic inhibition by reticular neurons

      vii) Degeneration of cholinergic and glutaminergic neurons in pedunculopontine tegmental nucleus and their projections to reticular formation: responsible for loss of atonia in REM sleep behavior disorder

      viii) Aminergic "REM-off" cells: primarily serotonergic and noradrenergic; are responsible for modulation of the thalamocortical neurons during wakefulness

4) Giant aspiny neurons of striatum: dopamine opposition during motor regulation

5) Loss of cholinergic input to cerebral cortex: a role in decreased plasticity, increased confusional state, dementia, and REM sleep behavior disorder

5. Dopamine (Fig. 2-5 B)

a. Synthesis

1) Produced from L-tyrosine, a dietary amino acid formed from phenylalanine (via enzyme phenylalanine hydroxylase) and actively transported across the blood-brain barrier

2) Classic phenylketonuria: deficiency of phenylalanine hydroxylase

3) Tyrosine hydroxylase catalyzes conversion to L-dopa, using tetrahydrobiopterin as cofactor

4) L-dopa is converted to dopamine by cytoplasmic pyridoxal phosphate-dependent enzyme L-amino acid decarboxylase

5) Carbidopa: peripheral inhibitor of this enzyme; this is clinically useful because peripheral conversion to dopamine is responsible for adverse effects such as nausea

6) Tyrosine hydroxylase deficiency

a) Autosomal recessive

b) Reduced levels of L-dopa and its metabolites

c) Parkinsonism and dystonia (presentation in infancy)

d) Improvement with oral L-dopa

b. Vesicular monoamine transporters: responsible for transport and packaging of catecholamines into vesicles; inhibited by reserpine and tetrabenazine

c. Uptake

1) Major method to stop synaptic effect

2) Depends on dopamine transporter, which depends on ATP and sodium gradient; dopamine transporter inhibited by cocaine

3) Amphetamines: inhibit dopamine uptake into vesicles and increase intracellular concentrations of dopamine

d. Metabolism

1) Intramitochondrial monoamine oxidase (MAO)-B (MAO_B) converts dopamine to dihydroxyphenylacetic acid; MAO_B produces hydrogen peroxidase and is inhibited by selegiline

2) MAO_A and MAO_B: equal efficacy for dopamine (but MAO_B preferentially acts on dopamine); MAO_A has stronger affinity for serotonin and norepinephrine and preferentially acts on these catecholamines

3) In Parkinson's disease model induced by MPTP, MAO converts MPTP to MPP, which is toxic to

dopaminergic cells

4) Catechol-O-methyltransferase (COMT) converts dihydroxyphenylacetic acid to homovanilic acid (HVA); COMT is inhibited by tolcapone and entacapone

e. Receptors

1) D_1 family (D_1 and D_5 receptors)

a) Coupled to G proteins (activate adenylyl cyclase to increase cAMP synthesis)

b) Modulate excitation

2) D_2 family (D_2, D_3, D_4 receptors)

a) Coupled to $G_{i/o}$ (inhibit adenylyl cyclase to reduce cAMP synthesis)

b) D_2 and D_3 receptors are located both presynaptically and postsynaptically, and all are found on postsynaptic membrane

c) Typical neuroleptics (phenothiazines and thioxanthenes) primarily block D_2 ($>D_1$) receptors and are associated with extrapyramidal adverse effects, including tardive dyskinesias

d) Atypical neuroleptics with less parkinsonian adverse effects primarily block D_3 and D_4 receptors; medicines of this class, including clozapine and olanzapine, are ideal treatments for tardive dyskinesias

e) Bromocriptine, pergolide, and pramipexole act as agonists on both D_2 and D_3 receptors with different affinities; bromocriptine is least potent dopaminergic agent

f) Bromocriptine and pergolide: ergot derivatives

3) Distribution of receptors

a) D_1 and D_2: greatest in caudate, putamen, nucleus accumbens, olfactory tubercle

b) D_3 and D_4: mostly in frontal cortex, amygdala, hippocampus

c) D_5: hippocampal formation, hypothalamus

f. Dopaminergic neurons and initiative and motor learning

1) Important roles in motor learning and control of agonist-antagonist muscle coordination during movement

a) All "cortical-based initiatives" of motor, limbic, and associative functions follow similar general loop starting from specific cerebral cortex → corpus striatum (caudate-putamen) → substantia nigra pars reticulata/internal segment of globus pallidus → specific thalamic nucleus → specific cerebral cortex (see Fig. 8-1 and Table 8-1)

b) Hyperdirect pathway of motor control

i) Bypasses striatum and substantia nigra and projects instead directly to subthalamic nucleus

ii) Subthalamic nucleus nonspecifically stimulates globus pallidus interna, which tonically inhibits VLo (ventral lateral, pars oralis) nucleus of thalamus, resulting in general background inhibition of all movements during motor activation

iii) Destruction of subthalamic nucleus: gross ballistic movements

c) Direct pathway of motor control (see Fig. 8-1): includes projections from motor cortex to putamen that specifically inhibit globus pallidus interna, thus releasing tonic inhibition it exerts on specific muscle group function coded in thalamus, allowing movement via projections back to motor cortex

d) Indirect pathway via putamen–globus pallidus externa–globus pallidus interna loop (see Fig. 8-1): possibly responsible for increased tonic inhibition of antagonist muscles during muscle activation

e) These direct and indirect pathways are targets of dopaminergic neurons (see below)

f) Role of dopaminergic neurons in motor learning and selective forgetting: increased firing of dopaminergic neurons in anticipation of reward and decreased firing after lack of reward (Schultz experiment) (see below)

2) Nigrostriatal system: projections of substantia nigra pars compacta to striatum

a) Act on medium spiny GABAergic striatal inhibitory output neurons with different effects depending on if neurons have "on" state (strong cortical activation of neuron) or "off" state (weak cortical activation of the neuron); this is important in organizing agonist-antagonist muscle coordination during movement

b) Implicated in parkinsonism and tardive dyskinesias (the pathophysiology of the latter is less clear)

3) Mesolimbic and mesocortical systems: dopaminergic projections from ventral tegmental area to limbic and cortical structures, respectively

a) Mesolimbic projections to the limbic structures (nucleus accumbens, septum, amygdala, hippocampus, and cingulate and entorhinal cortices): important for motivation, memory, reward, emotions; implicated in positive symptoms of schizophrenia (e.g., auditory hallucinations)

i) Nucleus accumbens: most important center to integrate and modulate input from the amygdala, hippocampus, entorhinal cortex, cingulate cortex; projects to ventral pallidum, hypothalamus, thalamus, brainstem tegmentum, and

anterior cingulate cortex

ii) Mesolimbic system: important in reward-dependent learning and arousal response associated with the anticipated reward and in mediating addiction to drugs of abuse

b) Stimulants (e.g., cocaine, nicotine, amphetamines)

i) Enhance dopaminergic levels in nucleus accumbens and other areas involved

ii) Cocaine and amphetamine inhibit reuptake of dopamine; nicotine acts on the presynaptic cholinergic receptors to increase dopaminergic release

iii) This enhancement of dopamine release causes euphoria, acting as positive reinforcement

iv) In addition to positive reinforcement, drug addiction involves tolerance and dependence: contingent on avoidance of withdrawal which is essentially a rebound decline in dopaminergic effects, among other mechanisms

c) Mesocortical projections to cortical areas (primarily prefrontal cortex): important for attention, working memory, executive functions, social behavior; are implicated in negative symptoms of schizophrenia

i) Normal prefrontal functioning relies on "balance" between the prefrontal "tonic" D_1 receptor activation (responsible for maintenance of information in working memory) and "phasic" D_2 receptor activation (responsible for updating this information)

ii) Excessive dopamine with chronic agonist use and chronic activation of tonic D_1 receptors causes maintenance of working memory and perseveration; reduced chronic dopamine levels with use of antagonists tips balance toward phasic updating, manifested as distractibility

iii) α_2-Adrenoreceptors in presynaptic dopaminergic terminals of prefrontal cortex (not striatum) are target of atypical neuroleptics (e.g., clozapine) that tend to spare nigrostriatal system

6. Norepinephrine and epinephrine (Fig. 2-5 *B*)

a. Synthesis

1) Dopamine β-hydroxylase in synaptic vesicles catalyzes conversion of dopamine to norepinephrine (with copper as cofactor)

2) Dopamine β-hydroxylase deficiency

a) Predominant presenting feature: orthostatic hypotension

b) Characterized by increased plasma levels of dopamine and undetectable plasma levels of

norepinephrine
  c) Treatment: DL-threo-3,4-dihydroxyphenylserine (DL-DOPS), which is converted directly to norepinephrine by dopa decarboxylase, bypassing dopamine β-hydroxylase
  3) L-threo-3,4-dihydroxyphenylserine (L-DOPS), a synthetic amino acid can also be converted to norepinephrine by L-amino acid decarboxylase (L-AADC); this may be used in patients with dopamine β-hydroxylase deficiency
  4) Adrenal medulla and few hindbrain neurons contain phenylethanolamine-*N*-methyltransferase which converts norepinephrine into epinephrine
b. Reuptake of released norepinephrine in synaptic cleft occurs by sodium-coupled norepinephrine transporter, which is inhibited by cocaine and tricyclic antidepressants
c. No reuptake mechanism for epinephrine
d. Norepinephrine transporter: not very specific for norepinephrine; also responsible for uptake of amphetamine and tyramine
  1) Amphetamine and tyramine can also replace stored norepinephrine, which is released into cytoplasm, most of which is released into synaptic cleft
  2) Amphetamine and tyramine enhance norepinephrine transmission
  3) Repetitive administration of amphetamines causes overall depletion of norepinephrine, and larger quantities of amphetamines will be needed to produce same affect—this may be physiologic basis for tolerance
e. As with other monoamines, vesicular monoamine transporters are responsible for packaging and storage into vesicles; reserpine, amphetamine, and tyramine inhibit vesicular monoamine transporters
f. Metabolism
  1) MAO$_A$ produces an aldehyde that is methylated by COMT to form main metabolite in CNS, 3-methoxy-4-hydroxyphenylglycol: this compound is excreted in urine and is a measure of norepinephrine metabolism in CNS
  2) In PNS, aldehyde dehydrogenase catalyzes oxidation of this aldehyde to form vanillylmandelic acid
g. Receptors
  1) α$_1$
    a) Coupled to G$_{q/11}$; linked to protein kinase C/PIP$_2$ pathway (diacylglycerol-activating protein kinase C) and inositol triphosphate, releasing calcium intracellularly (end result is increased intracellular calcium)

  b) Predominantly postsynaptic
  c) Found in postsynaptic nerve terminals throughout cerebral cortex and blood vessels
  d) Activated by phenylephrine, desglymidodrine, and phenylpropanolamine (agonists); inhibited by phenoxybenzamine, chloroethylclonidine, prazosin, or terazosin (antagonists)
  2) α$_2$
    a) Coupled to G$_{i/o}$, inhibition of adenylyl cyclase, decreased cAMP, opening of potassium channels, and closing of calcium channels
    b) Predominantly inhibitory presynaptic or somatodendritic receptors
    c) Autoreceptors and inhibitors of neurotransmitter release
    d) Found in presynaptic nerve terminals throughout brain
    e) Activated by clonidine and tizanidine and inhibited by yohimbine and mirtazapine
    f) α$_2$ Agonists may be effective in treating pain, spasticity, epilepsy, tics
  3) β
    a) All coupled to Gα$_s$ and stimulate production of cAMP (end result is increased cAMP)
    b) Abundant in cerebellum and cerebral cortex
    c) β$_2$ also important for relaxation of smooth muscles in blood vessels and bronchi
    d) Propranolol blocks both β$_1$ and β$_2$ receptors; atenolol and metoprolol block primarily β$_1$ receptors
    e) β$_1$ agonists (epinephrine = norepinephrine)
    f) β$_2$ agonists (epinephrine > norepinephrine)
    g) β$_1$ and β$_2$ both activated by isoproterenol; both inhibited by propranolol
    h) β$_2$ activated by terbutaline
    i) β$_1$ inhibited by metoprolol and atenolol
    j) β$_2$ inhibited by butoxamine
h. Adrenergic and noradrenergic neurons (Fig. 2-7 and Fig. 2-8)
  1) Locus ceruleus
    a) Most important source of norepinephrine
    b) Basal firing rate is low during sleep, elevated during wake state
    c) Upon presentation of stimulus (especially emotionally charged or nociceptive one), phasic activity of locus ceruleus increases, focusing attention on stimulus; high-frequency tonic activity of locus ceruleus causes inattention and distractibility
    d) Selective stimulus-induced phasic input of noradrenergic projections from locus ceruleus to

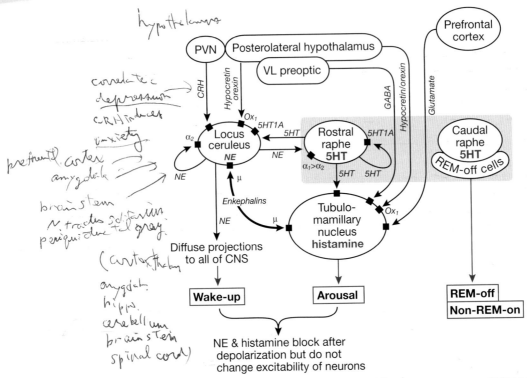

Fig. 2-7. Interaction of noreinephrine (NE), serotonin (5HT), and histamine in sleep regulation. CNS, central nervous system; CRH, corticotrophin-releasing hormone; GABA, γ-aminobutyric acid; Ox, orexin receptor; PVN, paraventricular nucleus; REM, rapid eye movement; VL, ventrolateral.

neocortex, cerebellum, hippocampus) inhibits baseline tonic activity, causing activation; this occurs by inhibiting afterhyperpolarization produced by calcium-dependent potassium channels
e) Provides noradrenergic input to spinal cord (together with pontine neuronal groups A5 and A7)
f) Primary regulatory input from medulla to nuclear portion of locus ceruleus: excitatory glutaminergic input from nucleus paragigantocellularis and inhibitory GABAergic input nucleus prepositus hypoglossi
g) Input to extranuclear portion of locus ceruleus: from hypothalamus (primarily preoptic, periventricular, lateral areas), brainstem (primarily nucleus tractus solitarius, periaqueductal gray), amygdala, neocortex (primarily prefrontal cortex); input mostly to extranuclear dendritic extensions of locus ceruleus neurons
h) Hypothalamic corticotrophin-releasing hormone (CRH) is excitatory to locus ceruleus: level of CRH correlates positively with depression, CRH induces anxiety in experimental animals

i) Widespread output: major ascending output to neocortex, thalamus, amygdala, hippocampus, cerebellum, and major descending output to brainstem and spinal cord
j) Postmortem examination of patients with Alzheimer's disease with depression: greater loss of locus ceruleus neurons than with normal aging
2) Brainstem projections
a) Ventral column (A1/C1): associated with nucleus ambiguus
   i) A1 neurons (noradrenergic) and C1 neurons (adrenergic) project to hypothalamus and amygdala
   ii) C1 neurons also project to spinal cord
b) Dorsal column (A2/C2): associated with nucleus solitarius and dorsal motor vagal nucleus; A2 neurons (noradrenergic) and C2 neurons (adrenergic) project to hypothalamus and amygdala
c) Pontine reticular formation (A5 and A7 groups): primarily provide descending projections and noradrenergic input to spinal cord
d) Ascending projections: dorsal and ventral bundles join medial forebrain bundle, which has ascending

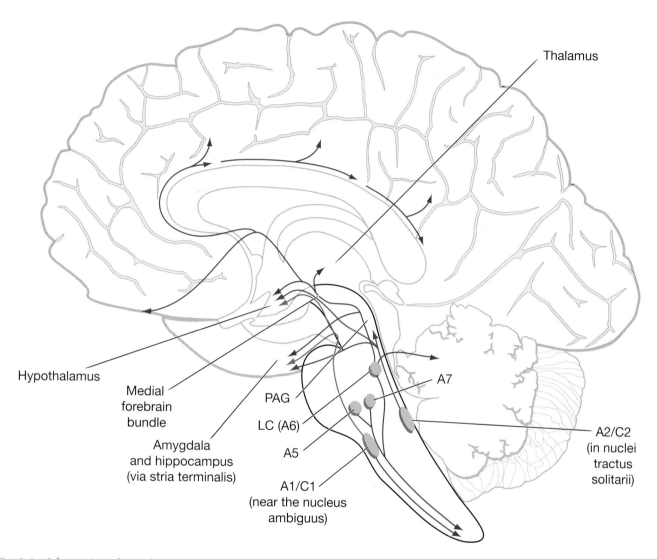

Fig. 2-8. Adrenergic and noradrenergic neurons. LC, locus ceruleus; PAG, periaqueductal gray matter.

connection with thalamus, cingulate cortex, neocortex, hippocampus (all primarily receiving input from locus ceruleus), amygdala (via stria terminalis), and hypothalamus

    e) Descending projections to spinal cord

      i) Noradrenergic (A5 and A7 groups, locus ceruleus)

      ii) Adrenergic (C1 group)

  3) Monoaminergic pathways important in maintaining arousal, wakefulness, vigilance (ascending arousal system) and response to novel stimuli; also regulation of cardiorespiratory reflexes via nucleus tractus solitarius, dorsal vagal motor nucleus, hypothalamus

7. Serotonin (Fig. 2-5 *B*)

  a. Synthesis

    1) Precursor is L-tryptophan, dietary amino acid; transported by energy-dependent active transport mechanism into brain; gabapentin also transported via this mechanism

    2) Tryptophan hydroxylase: rate-limiting step producing 5-hydroxytryptophan

    3) Tryptophan hydroxylase requires tetrahydrobiopterin and oxygen as cofactors

    4) Decarboxylation of 5-hydroxytryptophan is by L-amino acid decarboxylase, producing serotinin, called 5-hydroxytryptamine (5-HT)

  b. Stored by vesicular monoamine transporter

  c. Uptake by serotonin transporter: selective serotonin reuptake inhibitors inhibit serotinin transporter (e.g., fluoxetine)

1) Venlafaxine: inhibits both serotinin transporter and norepinephrine transporter
2) Vesicular transport inhibited by MDMA (3,4-methylene dioxymethamphetamine, "ecstacy")
d. Metabolism by MAO_A to 5-hydroxyindoleacetic acid (5-HIAA) (MAO_B is responsible for breakdown of other substrates such as dopamine)
e. Receptors
  1) $5\text{-}HT_1$
    a) Includes $5\text{-}HT_{1A}$, $5\text{-}HT_{1B}$, $5\text{-}HT_{1C}$, $5\text{-}HT_{1D}$
    b) Coupled to $G_{i/o}$ (second messenger cAMP, $5\text{-}HT_{1C}$ acts via IP_3/phospholipase C pathway)
    c) Autoreceptors and inhibitory presynaptic receptors
    d) Slow inhibitory response: activation of inward rectifying potassium channels by $5\text{-}HT_{1A}$ receptors in hippocampus and raphe nuclei and inhibition of calcium channels
    e) $5\text{-}HT_{1C}$ receptors in endothelial cells and choroidal plexus function in regulation of CSF production; those in limbic system regulate emotional behavior
    f) Agonists: buspirone (partial agonist at $5\text{-}HT_{1A}$), sumatriptan (agonist at $5\text{-}HT_{1B}$ and $5\text{-}HT_{1D}$ receptors)
    g) Inhibitors/antagonists: methysergide, cyproheptadine
  2) $5\text{-}HT_2$
    a) Includes $5\text{-}HT_{2A}$, $5\text{-}HT_{2B}$, $5\text{-}HT_{2C}$
    b) Coupled to $G_{q/11}$
    c) Occur throughout cerebral cortex, limbic system, basal ganglia; cortical receptors thought to be excitatory postsynaptic receptors
    d) Slow excitatory response via increasing intracellular calcium through IP_3/DAG second messenger system (also inhibition of potassium conductance)
    e) Agonist: lysergic acid diethylamide (LSD)
    f) Inhibitors/antagonists: trazodone, nefazodone, mirtazapine, risperidone, quetiapine, olanzapine, clozapine, methysergide, cyproheptadine
  3) $5\text{-}HT_3$
    a) Ligand-gated channel
    b) Fast excitatory response
    c) Expressed in area postrema (chemoreceptor trigger zone), stimulation of which causes projectile vomiting
    d) Serotonergic activation of $5\text{-}HT_3$ receptors in area postrema causes dopamine release: this effect may also be produced by dopamine agonists
    e) Antiemetic agents ondansetron and granisetron inhibit this receptor

4) $5\text{-}HT_{4\text{-}7}$ are coupled to Gs (second messenger system cAMP), associated with inhibition of potassium conductance
f. Serotonergic neurons
  1) Mostly in raphe nuclei
  2) Medullary serotonergic nuclei (groups B1-3, raphe magnus, raphe pallidus, raphe obscurus) project to lower brainstem and spinal cord
  3) Nucleus raphe magnus: in caudal pons; projects to dorsal horn (laminae I and II) and trigeminal nucleus to modulate pain perception
  4) Upper brainstem serotonergic nuclei (groups B4-9, pontine, dorsal, and median raphe nuclei) project to cerebral cortex, limbic system, cerebellum, basal ganglia, thalamus, hypothalamus
    a) Serotonergic projections from different raphe nuclei to telencephalic and diencephalic structures overlap
    b) Dorsal raphe nuclei have numerous, fine axons; axons arising from the median raphe nuclei are fewer in number and larger
8. Histamine
  a. Synthesized by histidine decarboxylase from precursor, L-histidine
  b. Metabolized by histamine-*N*-methyltransferase and monoamine oxidase to methylimidazoleacetic acid
  c. Histaminergic neurons are in lateral tuberomamillary nucleus (hypothalamus) and project diffusely to cerebral cortex, hypothalamus, limbic system, basal ganglia, brainstem, spinal cord
  d. Important role in arousal and wakefulness

II. LONGITUDINAL SYSTEMS

A. Sensory System
1. Sensory receptors
  a. Special cation channels (transduction receptors)
  b. Slowly adapting types discharge through stimulation period
  c. Rapidly adapting types discharge with any change in stimulus intensity
  d. Degenerin/epithelial sodium (DEG/ENA) channels: touch and proprioception (somatosensory) receptors, which contribute to 30% of large dorsal root ganglia neurons (DRGs) (see below); are also taste receptors
  e. TRP channels: pain, temperature, visceral (interoceptive) receptors, which contribute to 70% of DRG neurons (see below); also vestibular and hearing receptors
  f. CNG receptors: responsible for olfaction and

photoreception
2. Primary afferent neurons
   a. Primary afferent neuron: cell body in DRG, peripheral process, and central process
   b. Peripheral process: distal tip may be encapsulated, carrying information about proprioception and touch (somatosensory); may be a free nerve ending, carrying information about pain, temperature, visceral sensation (interoceptive)
   c. Type of receptor and size and conduction velocity of afferent fiber varies for different sensory modalities (Table 2-2)
   d. Fiber groups and names are based on these characteristics
3. Photoreception (Fig. 2-9)
   a. CNG receptors in retina
     1) Light travels through several layers before reaching photoreceptors (rods and cones)
     2) This distance likely serves as a tubular formation, limiting photoreceptor's field
   b. Cones
     1) Responsible for color vision under bright light (photopic or daylight)
     2) Located predominantly centrally (responsible for localization of more accurate color recognition in central retina)

     3) Different opsins determine color spectrum sensitivity
       a) S-cones: sensitive to blue spectrum (short wavelengths)
       b) M-cones: sensitive to green spectrum (medium wavelengths)
       c) L-cones: sensitive to red spectrum (long wavelengths)
   c. Rods
     1) More abundant than cones (24 rods for every cone)
     2) Responsible for dim light vision: convergence of signal from a group of rods onto a single bipolar cell ensures the response of the bipolar cell to the dim light signal, while compromising visual acuity of the periphery
     3) Produce black and white spectrum
     4) Predominant peripheral vision receptors
     5) Conduct slower than the cones
   d. Photoreception requires release of inhibition exerted by glutamate on "ON rod bipolar cells" stimulating "amacrine cells" stimulating "ON ganglion cells" and inhibiting "OFF ganglion cells" (dopaminergic): this is the only system where glutamate is inhibitory neurotransmitter
   e. Physiology of the rod photoreceptor "dark current"
     1) During darkness, there is an inward sodium and

Table 2-2. Sensory Receptors

Receptor type	Sensory detection	Fiber group	Fiber name	Conduction velocity, m/sec	Fiber size, μm
Mechanical nociceptor	Sharp, prickling pain (1st pain)	Aδ	III	25	1-6
Mechanical-thermal nociceptor	Burning pain	Aδ	III	4-36	1-6
Mechanical-thermal nociceptor	Freezing pain	C	IV	0.4-2.0	0.2-1.5
Polymodal nociceptor	Burning pain (2nd pain)	C	IV	0.4-2.0	0.2-1.5
Thermal receptor	Cool	Aδ	III	4-36	1-6
	Warm sensation	C	IV	0.4-2.0	
Meissner corpuscle	Touch	Aα, Aβ	Rapid adapting	72-120	12-20
Merkel disk	Pressure, texture	Aα, Aβ	Slow adapting	72-120	12-20
Pacinian corpuscle	Vibration	Aα, Aβ	Rapid adapting	72-120	12-20
Ruffini ending	Skin stretch	Aα, Aβ	Slow adapting	72-120	12-20
Golgi tendon organ	Muscle contraction	Aα	Ib	72-120	12-20
Muscle spindle receptor	Muscle length and speed	Aα	Ia	72-120	12-20
Joint capsule receptor	Joint angle	Aβ	II	36-72	6-12

Photoreception

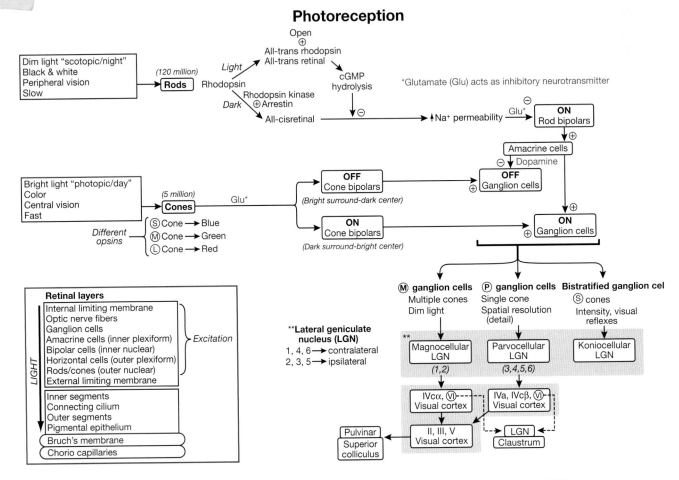

Fig. 2-9. Photoreception. See text. cGMP, cyclic guanosine monophosphate.

calcium current through the open cGMP-gated channels in the outer segment of rods, balanced by an outward calcium current via a Na$^+$-K$^+$-Ca^{2+} transporter in the outer segment and an outward sodium current by a Na$^+$-K$^+$ ATPase in the inner segment

2) Photoreceptor cells remain relatively depolarized in the baseline state while not exposed to light ("dark current")

3) Depolarized photoreceptor cell inhibits "ON rod bipolar cells" via glutamate

4) During darkness, the retinal portion of rhodopsin is present as 11-*cis*-isomer

f. Physiology of rod photoreceptor response to light

1) Retinal is transformed into an all-*trans* isomer with exposure to light

2) This conformational change in the rhodopsin molecule activates a phosphodiesterase, which catalyzes the conversion of cGMP to 5'-GMP

3) The latter reaction makes less cGMP available at the

photoreceptor, hence closing the cyclic nucleotide-gated cation channels and hyperpolarizing photoreceptor cells

4) Hyperpolarization of photoreceptor cells removes glutamate inhibition of the "ON rod bipolar cells"

g. Cones: contrast of center field compared with surrounding field determines transmission of information

1) Parallel information processing via on and off center cells helps cerebral cortex interpret contrast in a scene

2) "Dark surround-bright center" stimulus leads to hyperpolarization and release of inhibition on "cone bipolars," which in return stimulate "ON ganglion cells"

3) "Bright surround-dark center" stimulus leads to stimulation of "OFF ganglion cells"; this direct effect is in contrast to rods, which modify "cone ganglion cells" via intermediate "amacrine cells"

h. "M ganglion cells"

1) Receive input from multiple cones and rods, thus can

be activated in dimmer light) responses are rapid and transient (suitable for motion detection)

    2) Project to magnocellular portion of lateral geniculate nucleus of thalamus

  i. "P ganglion cells"

    1) Receive input from single cone

    2) Important in spatial resolution (detail); responses are sustained

    3) Project to parvocellular portion of lateral geniculate nucleus

  j. "Bistratified cells"

    1) Receive input from "S cones"

    2) Involved in intensity and visual reflexes

    3) Project to kineocellular portion of lateral geniculate nucleus

  k. Lateral geniculate nucleus: organized in layers

    1) Layers 1 and 2: magnocellular portion; project to visual cortex (M-channel)

    2) Layers 3-6: parvocellular portion; project independently to visual cortex (P-channel)

    3) Layers 1, 4, and 6 receive input from contralateral nasal retina; layers 2, 3, and 5 receive input from ipsilateral temporal retina

  l. Primary visual cortex or striate cortex (named after white matter stripe in layer IV)

    1) Transforms concentric center-surround information from ganglion cells into linear segments

    2) M-channel projects to layer IVc α, P-channel projects to layer IVc β; koniocellular layers project to cortical layers II and III

    3) Layer IV projects to layer VI, which projects to lateral geniculate nucleus and claustrum

    4) Layer IV also projects to layers II, III, V, which project to pulvinar and superior colliculus

  m. Information from primary visual cortex is processed in several steps through visual association cortices, which form dorsal visual stream ("where pathway") projecting to parietal and frontal lobes and ventral visual stream ("what pathway") projecting to temporal lobe (see Chapter 7, Part A)

4. Pain, temperature, and visceral sensation (Fig. 2-10 and Table 2-2)

  a. Mechanical nociceptor, bare nerve endings

    1) Activated by deep, noxious pressure applied to skin

    2) Results in sharp, prickling pain

    3) Felt immediately after stimulus: "first pain"

    4) Thinly myelinated Aδ-fiber type

    5) Conduction velocity: 5 to 30 m/s

    6) Neurotransmitter: L-glutamate

  b. Mechanical-thermal nociceptor

    1) Activated by extremes of temperature and mechanical stimuli

    2) Heat nociceptors (see below): activation results in burning pain, felt at extreme heat temperatures (>45°C); carried by Aδ fibers

    3) Cold nociceptors (see below): activation results in freezing pain, felt at temperatures lower than 5°C; carried by C fibers

  c. Polymodal nociceptor

    1) Activated by mechanical, thermal, chemical stimuli

    2) Results in slow, burning pain

    3) Felt sometime after stimulus and after the "first pain"; thus called "second pain"

    4) Unmyelinated axon, C fiber

    5) Conduction velocity: less than 2 m/s

    6) Neurotransmitters: substance P, calcitonin gene-related peptide

  d. Thermal receptor

    1) Tonic low rate of firing at rest and constant temperatures

    2) Changes in temperatures modulate firing of thermal receptors

    3) Cool receptors

      a) Aδ-fiber type: maintain low rate of tonic firing at resting constant termperatures of 5°C to 40°C, discharge maximally at skin temperatures of 25°C, do not respond to skin temperatures below 5°C

    4) Cold nociceptors—C-fiber type: respond to noxious cold (skin temperatures <5°C)

    5) Warm receptors—C-fiber type: maintain low rate of tonic firing at resting constant temperatures of 29°C to 45°C, discharge maximally at skin temperature of 45°C, do not respond to skin temperatures above 50°C

    6) Heat nociceptors—Aδ-fiber type: mechanical-thermal

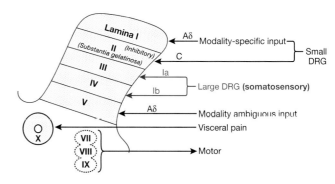

Fig. 2-10. Sensory input to Rexed's laminae. DRG, dorsal root ganglia neurons.

heat nociceptors, respond to noxious heat (skin temperatures >45°C)

   e. Visceral afferent

     1) Mechanical nociceptors activated by stretch within visceral organs: "silent nociceptors"

     2) Chemoreceptors also have role in visceral sensation

     3) Visceral afferents: travel in glossopharyngeal and vagus nerves to nucleus solitarius

5. Touch, vibration, and proprioception (Table 2-2)

   a. Touch and vibration

     1) Mechanoreceptors detect touch and vibration

       a) Superficial and deep receptors in skin

       b) Rapidly adapting receptors: detect motion of objects

       c) Slowly adapting receptors: detect shape and pressure of objects

     2) Superficial skin mechanoreceptors

       a) Meissner corpuscle

         i) Rapidly adapting

         ii) Activated by touch (burst of discharge at the beginning and end of touch)

         iii) Spatial and temporal discrimination: sensitive to change in the shape of objects (e.g., edges) and to moving objects

         iv) Fiber types: Aα, Aβ

       b) Merkel disk

         i) Slowly adapting

         ii) Important in contact recognition of objects

         iii) Activated by pressure, texture: increased discharge in response to convexities; no discharge in response to concavities; steady, low discharge in response to flat surfaces

         iv) Activated by raised letters

         v) Fiber types: Aα, Aβ

     3) Subcutaneous, deep skin mechanoreceptors

       a) Larger receptors and receptor fields (fewer in number) than superficial receptors

       b) Pacinian corpuscle

         i) Rapidly adapting

         ii) Lamellated capsule surrounding nerve ending

         iii) Detects vibration (rates >100 Hz), responds to rapid indentation of skin (not to constant pressure)

         iv) Fiber types: Aα, Aβ

       c) Ruffini ending

         i) Slowly adapting

         ii) Sense stretch of skin and bending of fingernails

         iii) Important in contact recognition of objects

         iv) Fiber types: Aα, Aβ

   b. Proprioception: limb position sense (stationary position)

and movement

     1) Golgi tendon organ

       a) Detects increased muscle contraction (proportional to force of muscle contraction)

       b) Tension feedback system important in preventing muscle stiffness: cause muscle relaxation by disynaptic inhibition of alpha motor neurons

       c) Aα fiber; Ib fiber type

     2) Muscle spindle receptors

       a) Detect muscle length and speed (stretch receptors on intrafusal fibers)

       b) Primary muscle spindle receptors: large diameter, fast-conducting type Ia afferent input from both nuclear bag and nuclear chain intrafusal fibers

       c) Secondary muscle spindle receptors (flower-spray endings): small diameter, slow-conducting type II afferent input from nuclear chain fibers only

       d) Responsible for stretch reflex

         i) Stimulation of Ia fibers by rapid lengthening of muscle spindle

         ii) Monosynaptic, direct activation of alpha motor neurons innervating the agonistic muscles (no interneurons)

         iii) Collateral inhibition of alpha motor neurons affecting the antagonistic muscles (via inhibitory interneurons)

         iv) Direct activation of the gamma motor neurons (concurrently with the alpha motor neurons) causes contraction of intrafusal fibers simultaneously with the extrafusal muscle, thus maintaining the proper length of the muscle

     3) Joint capsule mechanoreceptors

       a) Ruffini endings, Pacinian corpuscles, Golgi tendon organs

       b) Detect joint angle

     4) Cutaneous proprioception: Ruffini and Merkel cells

6. Spinal cord—dorsal horn

   a. Primary afferent fibers send central processes into spinal cord through dorsal root

   b. Dermatome: area of skin innervated by nerve fibers of a dorsal root

   c. Dorsal horn is divided into multiple laminae (Fig. 2-10)

   d. Dorsal horn neurons

     1) Nociceptive-specific neurons

       a) Superficial in dorsal horn

       b) Input: from only small myelinated and unmyelinated afferents

     2) Multiceptive neurons

       a) Deeper in dorsal horn

       b) Input: from all afferent fibers

c) Contribute majority of axons in spinothalamic projections; involved in producing referred visceral pain

7. Spinothalamic pathway (Fig. 2-11)
   a. Primary afferent fibers: responsible for pain and temperature sensation
      1) Enter dorsal horn and may ascend or descend 2 or 3 segments to form Lissauer's tract
      2) Terminate primarily in laminae I and V (but also II, IV, and VI) (Fig. 2-10)
         a) Lamina I: conveys primarily modality-specific information
         b) Lamina V: wide dynamic range neurons
         c) Laminae II (substantia gelatinosa) and III: role in segmental modulation of pain
      3) Cell bodies of primary afferents for face and head are in trigeminal ganglion; axons synapse in spinal trigeminal nucleus
   b. Spinothalamic tract
      1) Second-order neurons: axons across midline of spinal cord ventral to the central canal and ascend in contralateral anterolateral tract
      2) Second-order neurons: neurons in lamina I; project to ventral posterolateral nucleus of thalamus
      3) Dermatotopic representation of fibers: sacral segments are most lateral, with lumbar segments medial to sacral, then thoracic, and cervical segements most medial
      4) The second-order neurons carrying pain and temperature from ipsilateral face are in spinal trigeminal nucleus; their axons cross midline and ascend in trigeminothalamic tract (near the medial lemniscus)
      5) Indirect pathways
         a) Second-order neurons in laminae II and V involved in indirect paths
         b) Spinoreticular tract: axons from neurons in lamina V cross midline, join anterolateral tract, terminate in brainstem reticular formation
         c) From brainstem, fibers project to intralaminar and posterior thalamic nuclei
         d) Spinomesencephalic second-order neurons project to periaqueductal gray in midbrain
      6) Modulatory projections influencing nociceptive pathways
         a) Activation of interneurons of substantia gelatinosa (lamina II) inhibits nociceptive input (proposed mechanism for acupuncture)
         b) Enkephalin-containing neurons of midbrain periaqueductal gray project to and stimulate serotonergic raphe magnus nucleus and noradrenergic lateral tegmental nucleus, which directly inhibit dorsal horn cells responsible for nociception

   c) Posterior column axons send collaterals into substantia gelatinosa: activation of the posterior columns can facilitate inhibitory neurons (proposed mechanism for analgesia induced by dorsal column stimulation)
   c. Thalamus
      1) Spinothalamic tract ascends through lateral part of brainstem and synapses in ventral posterolateral nucleus of thalamus
      2) Trigeminothalamic tract, carrying information from the face, synapses in ventral posteromedial nucleus of thalamus
      3) Spinoreticular and spinomesencephalic pathways may synapse in intralaminar, medial dorsal, and posterior thalamic nuclear groups
   d. Cerebral cortex
      1) Third-order neurons in ventral posterolateral and posteromedial nuclei project to primary somatosensory cortex: this pathway predominantly carries information for localization of pain
      2) Medial dorsal nucleus of thalamus: projects to anterior cingulate gyrus and insula; important in emotional response to pain
      3) Intralaminar nuclei of thalamus: widespread projections to cerebral cortex for alerting related to painful stimuli
      4) Posterior nuclear group of the thalamus: projects to somatosensory association cortex

8. Dorsal column–medial lemniscus pathway (Fig. 2-12)
   a. Primary afferent fibers
      1) First-order neurons: cell bodies in dorsal root ganglia
      2) Central process enters dorsal funiculus and ascends ipsilaterally to medulla
      3) Dermatotopic organization of fibers for vibration and proprioception: fibers from T6 and below ascend in fasciculus gracilis, fibers above T6 ascend in fasciculus cuneatus
   b. Dorsal column–medial lemniscus
      1) Central processes in fasciculi cuneatus and gracilis synapse on second-order neurons in respective cuneate and gracile nuclei in caudal medulla
      2) Axons of second-order neurons sweep ventrally across midline as internal arcuate fibers and ascend as medial lemniscus
      3) Medial lemniscus projects to thalamus
   c. Thalamus
      1) Medial lemniscus synapses on third-order neurons in ventral posterolateral nucleus of thalamus
      2) Axons of these third-order neurons project to primary somatosensory cortex

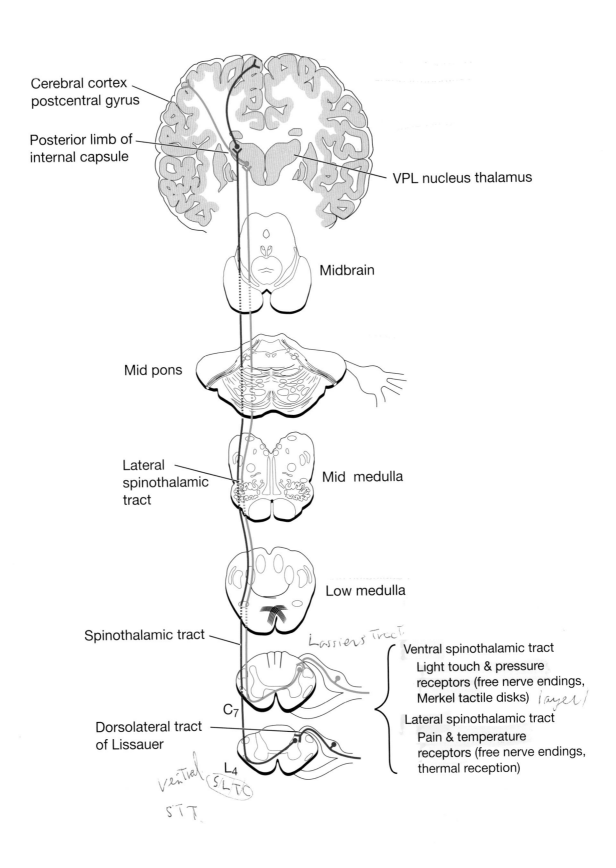

Cerebral cortex
postcentral gyrus

Posterior limb of
internal capsule

VPL nucleus thalamus

Midbrain

Mid pons

Lateral
spinothalamic
tract

Mid medulla

Low medulla

Spinothalamic tract

Lassiers Tract

Ventral spinothalamic tract
Light touch & pressure
receptors (free nerve endings,
Merkel tactile disks) layer l

Lateral spinothalamic tract
Pain & temperature
receptors (free nerve endings,
thermal reception)

Dorsolateral tract
of Lissauer

C₇

L₄

Ventral SLTC

STT

Fig. 2-11. The spinothalamic pathways. VPL, ventral posterolateral.

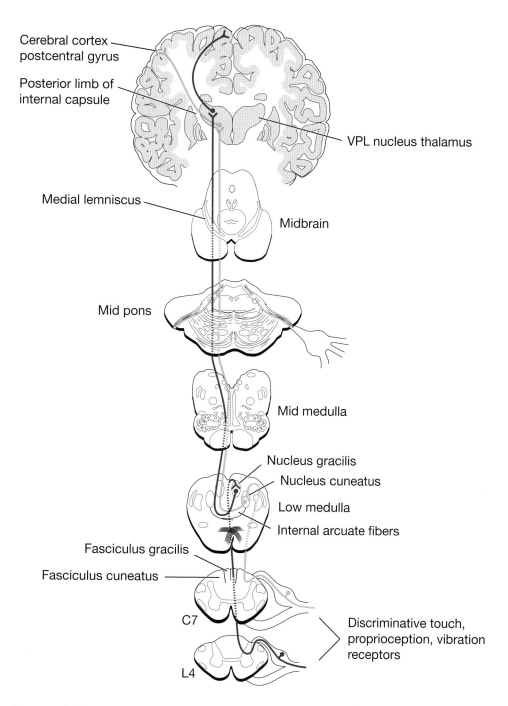

Fig. 2-12. The dorsal column–medial lemniscus pathway. VPL, ventral posterolateral.

d. Cerebral cortex
  1) Primary somatosensory cortex: postcentral gyrus, Brodmann areas 3, 1, and 2
  2) Each area of primary somatosensory cortex has a specific function, for example, proprioception from muscle spindle fibers is processed mainly in area 3a
9. Spinocerebellar pathways (Fig. 2-13) (discussed in

Chapter 9)
  a. Dorsal spinocerebellar tract (uncrossed tract)
    1) Responsible for unconscious proprioceptive information about muscle length and tension from *lower limbs* to the vermis and paravermis of cerebellum: receives input from muscle spindles, Golgi tendon organs, and pressure receptors

2) First-order neurons: large myelinated fibers (Ia and Ib) with cell bodies in dorsal root ganglia; synapse in ipsilateral thoracic nucleus of Clarke's column (segments T1-L3)

3) Second-order neurons: project from Clarke's column in ipsilateral lateral funiculus to inferior cerebellar peduncle, ending in cerebellar vermis and paravermis

b. Ventral spinocerebellar tract

1) Responsible for unconscious proprioceptive information about muscle length and tension from *lower limbs* to vermis and paravermis of cerebellum: receives input from muscle spindles, Golgi tendon organs, and pressure receptors

2) First-order neurons: large myelinated fibers (Ia and

Ib) with cell bodies in dorsal root ganglia; synapse on ipsilateral spinal border cells

3) Second-order neurons: axons decussate in the anterior white commissure to contralateral lateral funiculus; send mossy fiber projections to vermis and paravermis via superior cerebellar peduncle

c. Cuneocerebellar tract (uncrossed tract)

1) Responsible for unconscious proprioceptive information about muscle length and tension from *upper limbs* to vermis and paravermis of the cerebellum: receives input from muscle spindles, Golgi tendon organs, and pressure receptors

2) First-order neurons: large myelinated fibers (Ia and Ib) with cell bodies in dorsal root ganglia; axons

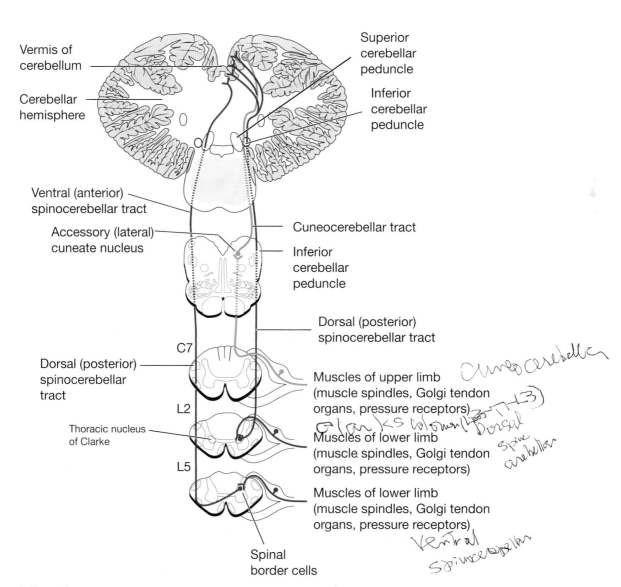

Fig. 2-13. The spinocerebellar pathways.

project directly via fasciculus cuneatus to accessory cuneate nucleus

   3) Second-order neurons: project to ipsilateral vermis and paravermis via inferior cerebellar peduncle

B. Motor System

1. Final common pathway: the motor unit
   a. Motor unit: an alpha motor neuron, its axon, and all the muscle fibers it innervates
   b. Neurotransmitter: ACh
   c. Alpha motor neurons: somatotopic organization in anterior horn or brainstem nuclei, with proximal muscles innervated by medial neurons, distal muscles by lateral neurons
2. Descending motor pathways—medial motor system (controls posture, muscle tone, and proximal muscles)
   a. Lateral vestibulospinal tract
      1) Origin: lateral and inferior vestibular nuclei
      2) Path: ipsilateral in ventral funiculus along entire length of spinal cord
      3) Functions: innervates antigravity extensor axial and proximal muscles and inhibits flexors; responsible for coordination of neck and eye movements
      4) Responsible for extensor (decerebrate) posturing in comatose patient: brainstem lesion caudal to red nucleus but rostral to the vestibular nuclei causes uninhibited hyperexcitability of extensor motor neurons by interrupting inhibitory descending input to vestibular nuclei
   b. Medial vestibulospinal tract
      1) Origin: medial vestibular nucleus
      2) Path: bilaterally, terminates in cervical cord
      3) Function: cervical posture
   c. Tectospinal tract
      1) Origin: superior colliculus
      2) Path: decussates in midbrain and ends in upper cervical cord
      3) Function: reflexive head turning to target visual stimuli
   d. Interstitiospinal tract
      1) Origin: interstitial nucleus of Cajal
      2) Path: descends in medial longitudinal fasciculus; synapses in cervical segments
      3) Function: cervical posture
   e. Reticulospinal tracts
      1) Pontine reticulospinal tract
         a) Origin: nucleus reticularis pontis caudalis, nucleus reticularis pontis oralis
         b) Path: descends in medial longitudinal fasciculus then ventral funiculus of spinal cord to terminate

in ventral horn; uncrossed pathway extending length of spinal cord
         c. Function: enhances extensor tone; head and body posture
      2) Medullary projections
         a) Origin: nucleus reticularis magnocellularis, nucleus reticularis gigantocellularis
         b) Path: descend bilaterally in ventral part of lateral funiculus and terminate in ventral horn of upper cervical cord
         c) Function: important for inhibition of postural reflexes that could interfere with voluntary movements; important for head posture
3. Descending motor systems—lateral motor system (control of contralateral limb movements)
   a. Corticospinal (pyramidal) tract (Fig. 2-14)
      1) Origin: cerebral cortex (2/3 from frontal lobe, 1/3 from parietal lobe)
         a) Primary motor cortex (Brodmann area 4)
            i) Somatotopic representation
            ii) Arm and face in middle cerebral artery territory; leg in anterior cerebral artery territory
         b) Premotor and supplementary cortex (Brodmann area 6)
         c) Postcentral gyrus (Brodmann areas 3, 1, 2)
         d) Superior parietal lobule (Brodmann areas 5, 7)
         e) Cingulate gyrus
      2) Course
         a) Axons from motor cortex (layer V Betz cells) and other cortical areas descend through corona radiata into posterior limb of internal capsule
         b) Fibers descend through midbrain (crus cerebri), pons (basis pontis), and medulla (medullary pyramids)
         c) At spinomedullary junction, 85% to 90% of corticospinal fibers cross midline: pyramidal decussation
         d) Fibers then descend in lateral funiculus, forming lateral corticospinal tract
         e) The 10% of fibers that do not cross continue ipsilateral in ventral funiculus of spinal cord
         f) Fibers terminate on anterior horn cells or interneurons at different levels of spinal cord
      3) Corticobulbar system
         a) Parallel to corticospinal tract
         b) Fibers originate in cerebral cortex but terminate in brainstem (bulb), synapsing in cranial nerve nuclei
         c) Origin: similar to that of corticospinal tract, but from lateral surace of cerebral hemisphere near face of homunculus

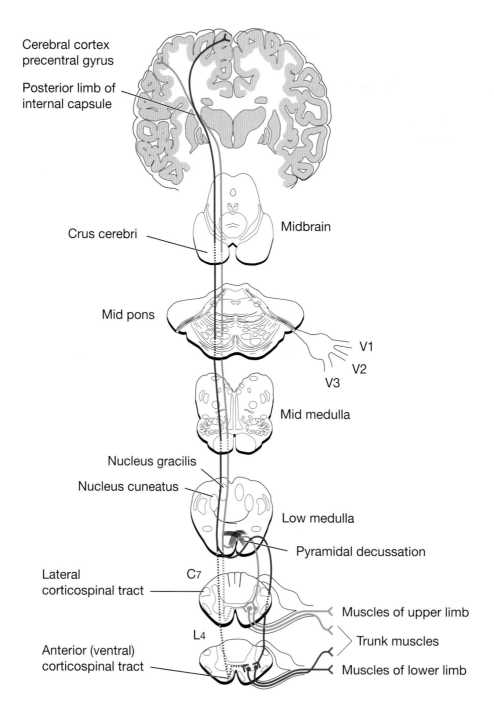

Cerebral cortex
precentral gyrus

Posterior limb of
internal capsule

Crus cerebri

Midbrain

Mid pons

V1
V2
V3

Mid medulla

Nucleus gracilis
Nucleus cuneatus

Low medulla

Pyramidal decussation

Lateral
corticospinal tract

C7

Muscles of upper limb

Trunk muscles

L4

Anterior (ventral)
corticospinal tract

Muscles of lower limb

Fig. 2-14. The corticospinal tracts. V1, V2, V3 are, respectively, the ophthalmic, maxillary, and mandibular divisions of the trigeminal nerve (cranial nerve V); VPL, ventral posterolateral.

d) Projections: motor nuclei of cranial nerves V, VII, IX, X (nucleus ambiguus), XI, XII
b. Rubrospinal tract
 1) Origin: red nucleus pars magnocellularis
 2) Path: decussates in midbrain; primarily ends at cervical level

3) Facilitates flexor movements of contralateral upper limb
4) Responsible for flexor (decorticate) posturing in comatose patient: lesion (upper brainstem or diffuse cortical localization) above the red nuclei cause uninhibited hyperexcitability of flexor alpha motor

neurons in upper limbs and flexor movements of arms (legs demonstrate extensor posturing because of weak rubrospinal influence in lower limbs and uninhibited hyperexcitability of vestibulospinal projections)

4. Cerebellum (see Chapter 9)
5. Basal ganglia (see Chapter 8)
6. Gaze control mechanisms and control of conjugate eye movements (see Chapter 3 and Fig. 2-15)

III. THALAMUS (FIG. 2-15, TABLE 2-3)

A. **Location:** thalamus extends from interventricular foramen anteriorly to posterior commissure (pineal body) posteriorly; medial to thalamus is third ventricle; lateral to thalamus is posterior limb of internal capsule

B. **Blood Supply:** via branches of posterior communicating and posterior cerebral arteries

C. **Function:** integrates and relays information for all sensory modalities (except olfaction), motor behavior, limbic system, and consciousness

D. **First-Order Relay Nuclei**
1. Each nucleus receives input from single modality or component of motor system and projects to a discrete area of cortex; usually, main input is from subcortical sensory or motor structure
2. Each nucleus has reciprocal connection with major projection site, allowing for regulation
3. Examples
   a. Motor relay nuclei: ventral anterior and ventral lateral (relay input from basal ganglia and cerebellum to motor cortices)

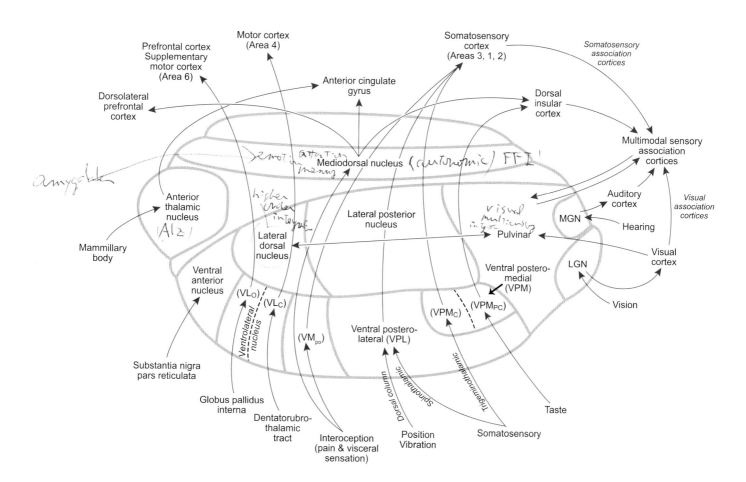

Fig. 2-15. Input and output of thalamic nuclei. LGN, lateral geniculate nucleus; MGN, medial geniculate nucleus; VL, ventral lateral nucleus (c, caudalis; o, oralis); VM_po, ventromedial posterior thalamic nucleus; VPM, ventral posteromedial (c, caudalis; pc, parvocellular).

Table 2-3. **Thalamic Nuclei**

Nucleus	Input	Output	Function
Anterior group			
Anterior	Mammillary bodies (via mamillothalamic tract) Medial temporal lobe (via fornix)	Posterior cingulate gyrus (via anterior limb internal capsule)	Limbic relay
Mediodorsal	Dorsal prefrontal cortex Substantia nigra Spinothalamic/trigemino-thalamic tracts	Dorsal prefrontal cortex Temporal lobe/amygdala (limbic) Anterior cingulate gyrus	Memory/executive function behavior Oculomotor behavioral basal ganglia circuits Emotional response to pain
Pulvinar and lateral posterior	Parietotemporal-occipital association areas Superior colliculus Retina	Visual association cortex Parietotemporal-occipital association areas	Role in integration of sensory information for visual attention; visual stimulus position
Ventral group			
Ventral posterolateral	Lemniscal/chief sensory of V	Primary somatosensory cortex	Sensory (touch/proprio-ception) relay
	Spinothalamic	Primary somatosensory cortex	Tactile pain sensory relay (body)
Ventral posteromedial (also called ventralis caudalis)	Nucleus solitarius Trigeminothalamic tracts	Insular cortex Primary sometosensory cortex	Gustatory sensory relay Tactile pain sensory relay (face)
Ventrolateral, oralis	Globus pallidus interna	Supplementary motor area Premotor cortex	Motor circuitry of basal ganglia
Ventrolateral, caudalis and ventrolateral, medialis (also called ventral intermedius)	Cerebellum (dentate nucleus)	Primary motor cortex	Cerebellar relay (coordi-nation of motor activity)
Ventral anterior (also called ventral rostralis)	Substantia nigra, pars reticularis	Frontal eye fields	Oculomotor basal ganglia circuitry
Posterior nuclear complex	Nociceptive input	Insular cortex	Pain relay
Metathalamus			
Lateral geniculate body	Retina	Primary visual cortex	Visual relay
Medial geniculate body	Auditory paths (especially inferior colliculus)	Primary auditory cortex	Auditory relay

b. Somatosensory relay nuclei: ventral posterolateral and ventral posteromedial (lesions of these nuclei are impli-cated in thalamic pain syndrome)

c. Auditory relay nucleus: medial geniculate

d. Visual relay nucleus: lateral geniculate

E. **Higher Order Relay** (association) **Nuclei**

1. Primary input and output: association cortices

2. Important for integration of sensory responses and emotional responses

3. Examples

a. Anterior nucleus

1) Important for memory

2) Component of posterior limbic circuit (input from mammillothalamic tract)

3) Involvement of anterior thalamic nucleus implicated in Korsakoff's amnesia

4) Thalamic amnesia is frequently anterograde and asso-ciated with confabulations

5) Development of amnesia usually requires bilateral lesions

b. Medial dorsal nucleus

1) Important in memory, attention, emotion

2) Component of anterior limbic circuit

3) Lesions may cause amnesia, apathy, inattention, behavioral dyscontrol and agitation, coma

c. Mediodorsal and ventral anterior thalamic nuclei are affected in fatal familial insomnia (see Chapter 7)

d. Lateral dorsal nucleus: may be involved in synthesis of higher order sensory function

e. Pulvinar nucleus: important for processing visual information and integration of multimodal sensory associations

F. **Nonspecific** (multimodal/diffuse projection) **Nuclei**

1. Project not only to cerebral cortex but to other thalamic nuclei

2. Likely important in arousal and consciousness

3. Examples include

   a. Midline and intralaminar nuclei: important for synchronization of thalamocortical signals; may contribute to sensorimotor control

   b. Centromedian/parafascicular complex: input from globus pallidus interna, output to caudate and putamen

G. **Reticular Nucleus of the Thalamus**

1. Thin layer of GABAergic neurons surrounding lateral thalamus proper

2. Corticothalamic projections and thalamocortical projections send collaterals to reticular nucleus

3. Projects to all other thalamic nuclei except nonspecific nuclei and anterior thalamus; projects to brainstem reticular formation

4. Involved in generation of sleep spindles

5. Function: modulate responses of thalamic neurons to cortical input

H. **Cortical Organization** (see Chapter 7)

I. **Limbic–Higher Cognitive–Memory System** (see Chapter 7, Part A)

1. Heteromodal sensory association cortices of temporo-parietal area, higher cognitive cortices, limbic system, and memory systems represent integrated circuitry

2. Primary motor and sensory areas (idiotypic cortices) have connections with unimodal association areas, which have projections with heteromodal association areas

3. Heteromodal association areas have connections with paralimbic regions (neocortex), which project to limbic regions (allocortex and corticoid)

4. Anterior limbic system: responsible for emotional responses

5. Posterior limbic system: responsible for declarative memory

6. Basic input to system is from somatosensory and interoceptive pathways through superior temporal gyrus, insula, multimodal association cortices, and pulvinar nucleus of thalamus

7. Within the system, similar organization to motor control is present, with integration through basal ganglia (Fig. 2-8)

8. Four functional loops make up the system

   a. Papez circuit: predominantly responsible for memory; center of this circuit is hippocampal formation

   b. Amygdaloid complex (amygdala, nucleus accumbens, ventral pallidum): core of limbic system; adds emotional content to memory; amygdala forms the center of this loop

   c. Disinhibition circuit: responsible for control of behavioral decisions; orbitofrontal cortex is the integrative center

   d. Cognitive-executive circuit: responsible for all initiative, executive, cognitive decisions made at highest level of the system; lateral (dorsolateral) prefrontal cortex is central cortical component of this system

9. Integration is through the following:

   a. Bidirectional interaction between hippocampal formation and amygdala

   b. Insular cortex and anterior cingulate gyrus input to amygdala

   c. Projections of amygdala to mediodorsal thalamus

   d. Cingulate fasciculus between anterior and posterior cingulate gyri

10. Output through fornix: to anterior cingulate gyrus, amygdaloid complex, and autonomic nervous system (via brainstem nuclei and hypothalamus)

IV. HYPOTHALAMUS AND CENTRAL INTEGRATION OF AUTONOMIC NERVOUS SYSTEM (FIG. 2-16 AND 2-17)

A. **Location**

1. Extends from optic chiasm and posteriorly to mammillary bodies

2. Hypothalamus is bordered medially by third ventricle and laterally by optic tracts

B. **Blood Supply**

1. Perforating arteries from A1 segment of anterior cerebral artery vascularize preoptic and supraoptic regions and lateral hypothalamus

2. Perforating arteries from P1 segment of posterior cerebral artery and posterior communicating artery vascularize mammillary body and tuberal regions

C. **General Functions of Hypothalamus:** integration of internal and external sensory inputs into appropriate

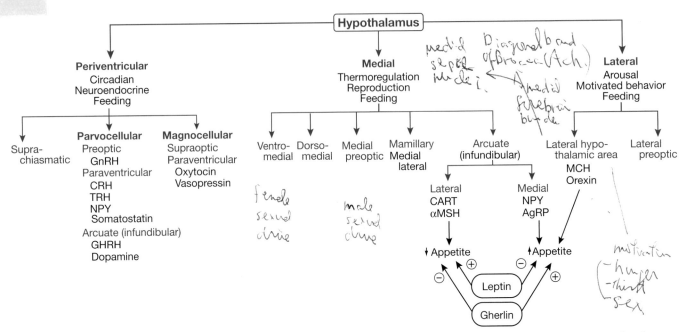

Fig. 2-16. Functional organization of hypothalamus. AgRP, agouti-related protein; CART, cocaine and amphetamine-regulated transcript; CRH, corticotrophin-releasing hormone; GHRH, growth hormone-releasing hormone; GnRH, gonadotropin-releasing hormone; MCH, melanin-concentrating hormone; MSH, melanocyte-stimulating hormone; NPY, neuropeptide Y; SS, somatostatin; TRH, thyrotropin-releasing hormone.

response (autonomic, endocrine, or behavioral)

1. Hormone release
2. Temperature regulation
3. Control of food and water intake
4. Sexual behavior and reproduction
5. Control of diurnal rhythms
6. Emotional response

D. **Hypothalamic Input**

1. Hippocampus (via fornix)
2. Amygdala (via stria terminalis)
3. Neurochemically specific cell groups (raphe nuclei, ventral tegmental area, locus ceruleus)
4. Humoral input (via circumventricular organs, e.g., lamina terminalis)

E. **Hypothalamic Output**

1. Medial forebrain bundle: sends information from lateral hypothalamus to septal region; serves as anatomic demarcation of medial and lateral hypothalamic zones
2. Releasing hormones released into hypophyseal portal system
3. Neurons directly release hormones in posterior pituitary gland
4. Mammillothalamic tract from mammillary bodies to

anterior nucleus of thalamus
5. Descending efferents to brainstem and spinal cord as part of autonomic nervous system

F. **Hypothalamic Nuclei**

1. Divisions: hypothalamic nuclei can be classified by rostrocaudal location or proximity to the third ventricle
   a. Proximity to third ventricle (Fig. 2-16)
      1) Periventricular
      2) Medial
      3) Lateral (divided from medial by fornix)
   b. Rostrocaudal
      1) Supraoptic (chiasmatic) (based on a coronal section through optic chiasm)
      2) Tuberal (based on coronal section through median eminence or tuber cinereum)
      3) Mammillary (based on coronal section through the mammillary bodies)
   c. Overview of nuclei (Table 2-4)
2. Endocrine function
   a. Hypothalamic influence on the posterior pituitary gland
      1) Hypothalamic nuclei: supraoptic and paraventricular (magnocellular) nuclei
      2) Axons from these nuclei extend to posterior pituitary and directly release hormones into blood vessels when

Table 2-4. Nuclei of the Hypothalamus

Nucleus	Function
Suprachiasmatic	Circadian rhythm
	Lesion: loss of diurnal rhythm
Supraoptic (magnocellular)	Secrete oxytocin and vasopressin (antidiuretic hormone)
Paraventricular (magnocellular)	Lesion: diabetes insipidus
Paraventricular (parvocellular)	Autonomic projections to brainstem and spinal cord
	Secretes corticotropin-releasing factor
	Involved in stress response
Medial preoptic nuclei	Secrete gonadotropin-releasing hormone (GnRH)
	Influence behavior related to sexual activity and feeding
	Thermoregulation
Lateral preoptic nuclei	Locomotion; arousal
Arcuate (infundibular)	Periventricular component: neuroendocrine
	Lateral component: satiety center
	Medial component: stimulates appetite
Ventromedial	Sexual behavior
	Cardiovascular function
	Previously thought to be satiety center, which is now thought to be related to arcuate nucleus
Dorsomedial	Emotion, stress response
	Stimulation: rage/aggression
Medial mammillary	Target of postcommissural fornix from hippocampus; start of mammillothalamic tract; memory/learning
	Lesion: Wernicke-Korsakoff syndrome; anterograde amnesia
Lateral mammillary	Merge with periaqueductal gray matter and midbrain reticular formation
	Emotion/pain
Lateral tuberal	Motivated motor activity
	Cortical arousal
Lateral hypothalamic	Feeding center; motivation
	Stimulation: stimulate feeding (via orexin and melanin-concentrating hormone)
	Lesion: anorexia

appropriately stimulated

3) Hormones: antidiuretic hormone (ADH) and oxytocin

4) ADH and oxytocin: synthesized in supraoptic and paraventricular nuclei, transported in axons of magnocellular neurosecretory neurons, are stored in secretory granules within axon terminals, released when stimulated

5) ADH increases reabsorption of water from renal tubules: destruction of supraoptic and paraventricular nuclei causes permanent diabetes insipidus

6) Oxytocin: involved in milk ejection of lactating females; uterine contraction; considered a "bonding" hormone in males and females

7) Supraoptic and paraventricular hypothalamic nuclei, supraopticohypophyseal tract, and posterior pituitary form a structural and functional unit

b. Hypothalamic influence on anterior pituitary gland

1) Hypothalamic nuclei: medial preoptic, paraventricular (parvocellular), and infundibular (arcuate)

2) Releasing hormones secreted from these hypothalamic nuclei into hypophyseal portal system: diffuse to anterior pituitary gland

3) Anterior pituitary gland, in turn, releases hormones affecting homeostasis

4) Hypophyseal portal system is supplied by inferior and superior hypophyseal arteries (branches of internal carotid artery)

5) Details of releasing hormones and anterior pituitary function are given in Table 2-5

3. Autonomic function

a. Hypothalamic nuclei: paraventricular nucleus, dorsomedial nucleus, lateral hypothalamic area

b. Output from these nuclei to regions involved with

Table 2-5. Hypothalamic Regulatory Hormones and Corresponding Anterior Pituitary Functions

Nucleus	Regulatory hormone	Effect on pituitary target cell	Function (effectors)
Medial preoptic	Gonadotropin-releasing hormone	Stimulate lutenizing hormone and follicle-stimulating hormone	Gonadal steroids
Paraventricular (parvocellular)	Corticotropin-releasing hormone	Stimulates corticotropin	Stress response
	Thyrotropin-releasing hormone	Stimulates thyroid-stimulating hormone	Thyroid hormones
	Neuropeptide Y	Stimulates prolactin	Prolactin release
	Somatostatin	Inhibits growth hormone	
Infundibular (arcuate)	Dopamine	Inhibits prolactin	
	Growth hormone-releasing hormone	Stimulates growth hormone	Bone growth, glucose, homeostasis

autonomic nervous system: ventrolateral medulla (sympathetic), dorsal vagal nucleus (parasympathetic), preganglionic sympathetic neurons
4. Behavioral function
  a. Lateral hypothalamic area: important in motivation and arousal, connections with limbic areas
  b. Functions: motivated behavior in response to thirst, hunger, reproduction
  c. Main output of lateral hypothalamus: via medial forebrain bundle to nuclei of diagonal band and the medial septal nuclei
  d. Ascending projections of reticular formation to cerebral cortex involve basal forebrain and medial forebrain bundle
5. Specific functions
  a. Thermoregulation: medial preoptic area
  b. Water metabolism
    1) Subfornical organ and organ vasculosum of lamina terminalis monitor plasma osmolality
    2) Angiotensin II, hypovolemia, osmolality: triggers for ADH release
    3) ADH increases water retention in kidneys
  c. Food intake
    1) Lesions of lateral hypothalamic area: decreased appetite
    2) Lesions of medial hypothalamic area: obesity
    3) Leptin
      a) Secreted by adipose tissue; acts on hypothalamus to stimulate satiety; reflection of degree of long-term fat storage
      b) Inhibits lateral hypothalamic area and medial arcuate (infundibular) nucleus
      c) Stimulates lateral arcuate (infundibular) nucleus
  d. Stress response: paraventricular nucleus is responsible for

integrated response to stress (main excitatory input to preganglionic sympathetic neurons)
  e. Reproductive function
    1) Hypothalamus responsible for reproductive hormone secretions, and sexual and parenting behaviors
    2) Regions of hypothalamus responsible for mediating sexual behavior: medial preoptic area in males and ventromedial nucleus in females (medial preoptic area contains twice as many neurons in men as in women)
    3) Medial preoptic area: responsible for parenting behavior in females
  f. Sleep-wake cycle
    1) Suprachiasmatic nuclei: role in diurnal variations and sleep-wake cycle
    2) Input: from retina via optic nerves
    3) Output: via sympathetic pathways eventually reaching pineal gland to activate melatonin synthesis

G. Components of Autonomic Nervous System (Fig. 2-17)
1. Insular cortex, anterior cingulate gyrus, central nucleus of amygdala, ventromedial prefrontal cortex: integrate interoceptive inputs with limbic-cognitive-memory circuits
2. Midline nuclei of thalamus: relay stations for input to the autonomic circuitry
3. Output of the system is through the paraventricular, dorsomedial, and lateral hypothalamic areas (Fig. 2-16)
4. Periaquaductal gray matter of the midbrain: coordinator of autonomic sensory and motor inputs
5. Parabrachial nucleus of the pons: relay station for converging somatosensory and interoceptive inputs to system
6. Nucleus tractus solitarius: relay for vagal visceral and taste afferents

7. Dorsal vagal nucleus and nucleus ambiguus: motor output of vagus for parasympathetic excitation
8. Ventrolateral medullary nuclei: responsible for sympathetic excitation
9. Descending sympathetic pathway descends through intermediolateral cell column
10. Most of the central integrative pathways of autonomic nervous system are reciprocal and glutamatergic

V.   NEUROGENETICS

A.   Nuclear DNA

1. 3×10^9 base pairs (nucleotides) on 22 pairs of autosomes and 1 pair of sex chromosomes form nuclear genome

2. Nucleotide bases in DNA are heterocyclic molecules derived from either pyrimidine or purine
   a. Purine bases: adenine (A) and guanine (G)
   b. Pyrimidine bases: thymine (T) and cytosine (C)
   c. Uracil (U) is present in RNA instead of T
   d. Three hydrogen bonds are formed between C and G; two are formed between A and T: results in complementary base pairs (G-C and A-T) through noncovalent bonds
3. Two antiparallel strands
   a. Nucleotide chain is formed by joining phosphate group at 5′ carbon to the hydroxyl group at 3′ carbon, producing a polar molecule
   b. Sequence of nucleotides on 5′ to 3′ strand of DNA is complementary to the other strand in the 3′ to 5′ direction

Components of the Autonomic Nervous System

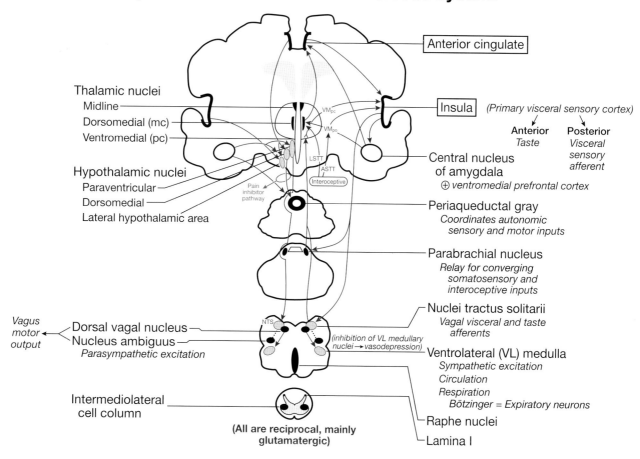

Fig. 2-17. Components of the autonomic nervous system. ASTT, anterior spinothalamic tract; LSTT, lateral spinothalamic tract; mc, magnocellular; NTS, nuclei tractus solitarii; pc, parvocellular; VM_pc, VM_po, ventromedial, pars caudalis and pars oralis. (Modified from Benarroch EE. Basic neurosciences with clinical applications. Philadelphia: Butterworth Heinemann/Elsevier. 2006. p. 726. By permission of Mayo Foundation.)

c. Sequence of nucleotides is written in the 5′ to 3′ direction by convention

B. Genes
1. Basic unit of heredity, or the original "factor" described by Mendel
2. Defined as contiguous region of DNA that contains protein-coding DNA (exons) and noncoding regions (introns)
3. Exons: 1% of DNA of eukaryotic cells; hybridizes with messenger RNA (mRNA)
4. Introns: 24% of DNA of eukaryotic cells that is transcribed initially, but then removed from the primary transcript
5. Intergenic sequence: 75% of eukaryotic DNA; composed mostly of repetitive sequences
   a. Tandem repeats are adjacent clusters of DNA sequences or "satellite" DNA
      1) Often located near centromere
      2) Considerable variability in length of tandem repeats among individuals; this has been used for identification purposes
      3) Minisatellites are small tandem repeats between 20 and 70 bp long
      4) Microsatellites are between 2 and 4 bp long
   b. Interspersed repeats are intergenic DNA clusters scattered throughout the genome
      1) Short interspersed nuclear elements include Alu repeats with no recognized function
      2) Long interspersed nuclear elements
      3) Includes mobile elements or transposons

C. Chromosomes
1. Consist of one double-stranded DNA molecule and proteins (histones and regulatory proteins)
2. Histones: five proteins; lysine and arginine rich; positively charged
3. Condensed chromatin is tightly folded
   a. Also called heterochromatin

b. Contains repetitive DNA sequences
c. Few or no active genes
4. Uncondensed chromatin or euchromatin contains active genes

D. Transcription: the synthesis of mRNA from information on the coding strand of DNA
1. The 3′ to 5′ strand: template for mRNA; it is the coding or antisense strand
2. The 5′ to 3′ strand: the noncoding or sense strand
3. mRNA: synthesized in the 5′ to 3′ direction, as below:
   5′-ATTGCCTTAAATT-3′: noncoding strand of DNA
   3′-TAACGGAATTTAA-5′: coding strand of DNA
   5′-AUUGCCUUAAAUU-3′: mRNA
4. DNA: organized in genes that begin at the transcription start site shortly beyond a TATA box
5. Formation of the initiation complex requires biding of RNA polymerase and other transcription factors
6. Methylation of DNA at cytosine residues is important in gene regulation
7. Primary mRNA transcript or pre-mRNA must undergo further processing
   a. Cap (7′ methyl guanosine)
   b. Polyadenylation at 3′ end
   c. Splicing allows multiple different transcripts per gene and is major source of gene diversity in humans, producing different isoforms
      1) Introns are spliced out and remaining sequences rejoined
      2) Splicing consensus sequences
         a) GT always starts intron (splice donor sites)
         b) AG always ends intron (splice acceptor sites)
      3) Complicated process that occurs at spliceosome made of small nuclear RNA molecules (snRNA)

E. Translation
1. Conversion of the nucleotides in mRNA to amino

Purine bases = adenine (A) and guanine (G)

Pyrimidine bases = thymine (T) and cytosine (C)

Uracil (U) is present instead of T in RNA

Complementary base pairs are formed between C and G and between A and T (G-C and A-T)

Exons	1% of DNA of eukaryotic cells
	Coding region of the genome
Introns	24% of DNA
	Noncoding regions that are removed from primary transcript
Intergenic sequences	75% of DNA Repetitive regions of DNA

acids; occurs in cytoplasm
2. Each codon of three nucleotides corresponds to an amino acid as well as the start and stop codons: this represents the genetic code
   a. Genetic code is universal and used by different organisms
   b. Genetic code is redundant, with different nucleotide codons coding for the same amino acid
3. Translation occurs in cytoplasm on ribosomes, with formation of an initiation complex made of mRNA, ribosome, and transcription RNA (tRNA)
   a. mRNA docks on ribosomal RNA (rRNA)
   b. Open reading frame on mRNA is recognized by tRNA, which carries a specific amino acid
   c. Bonds are formed between mRNA trinucleotide sequence (codon) and complementary tRNA nucleotide sequence (anticodon)
4. Three stages involved in polypeptide synthesis, as follows:
   a. Initiation: requires initiation factors and start codon (AUG) coding for methionine
   b. Elongation: requires codon recognition, peptide binding, and translocation to the next three nucleotides on mRNA
   c. Termination: when a stop codon (UAA, UGA, or UAG) is reached

F. Genetic Disorders
1. Chromosome disorders
   a. Often result in miscarriages
   b. Balanced chromosomal rearrangement (translocations) result in no chromosomal material being lost or added and usually do not result in disease
   c. Unbalanced rearrangements result in loss or gain of chromosomal material
      1) Numerical chromosomal abnormalities: individuals do not have the expected 46 chromosomes
         a) Aneuploidy: do not have a multiple of typical haploid set
            i) Turner syndrome (45, X): loss of paternal X chromosome
            ii) Trisomies increase with maternal age: trisomy 21 (Down syndrome), trisomy 18 (Edwards' syndrome), trisomy 13 (Patau's syndrome), trisomy 16 (most common autosomal trisomy in miscarriage)
         b) Polyploidy: abnormal number of chromosome sets instead of the expected two, for example, triploidy results in 69 chromosomes
      2) May also have genetic imbalance from chromosomal translocations, duplication, or deletion, while retaining 46 chromosomes
   d. Standard chromosomal analysis or karyotypes using G

banding detects large rearrangements (3-4 megabases)
   e. Smaller subtelomeric rearrangements are detected using molecular probes or fluorescence in situ hybridization (FISH)
2. Single-gene disorders
   a. Polymorphisms: variants in DNA sequences common in populations and represent different phenotypes (found >1% of a given population)
      1) Contribute to disease susceptibility; can influence drug responses
      2) Important for identifying alleles at a gene locus
   b. Mutation: alteration of DNA base sequence of one or both alleles of a gene that disrupt normal function of the gene's product
      1) Nonsense mutation: no functional gene product is encoded
      2) Missense mutation: codon is altered so a new amino acid is produced, but reading frame is unchanged; usually results in a milder phenotype
      3) Silent mutation: the sequence of amino acid produced is preserved
      4) Replicative errors
         a) DNA replication occurs by semiconservative method, with a new strand being synthesized by complementary base pairing
         b) Replicative errors occur at a rate of 1 in 10^5, but are reduced to a rate 1 in 10^7 or 10^9 by proofreading mechanisms
         c) Replication slippage: misalignment of DNA sequences during replication
         d) Predisposing factors are CAG repeats and secondary structure
         e) May be a forward slippage resulting in an insertion or backward slippage resulting in a deletion
         f) Deletion or insertion usually causes shift in reading frame or frameshift mutation; may result in a nonsense mutation
      5) Transposons: mobile regions of DNA
         a) Transposons are able to insert into new DNA location

---

Polymorphisms are common variants in the DNA sequence that may be related to disease susceptibility

Mutations are abnormalities in the DNA sequence that may be asymptomatic or produce disease

b) They may block transcription or cause altered transcripts

6) Point mutations: mutation types involving single nucleotides may result in substitutions or exchanges (transition vs. transversion)

   a) Transition: exchange of one purine for another purine or one pyrimidine for another pyrimidine

   b) Transversion: substitution of one purine for a pyrimidine or vice versa

c. Mendelian inheritance patterns

1) Autosomal dominant (AD): only one mutant copy of the gene on an autosomal (non-sex) chromosome will produce the disease

   a) Males and females are affected in 1:1 ratio

   b) Child of affected parent has a 50% chance of inheriting the disease

   c) May have variable expression between generations

   d) May occur sporadically or de novo

2) Autosomal recessive (AR): two mutant copies of the gene (one from each parent) are required to produce the disease

   a) Heterozygotes or carriers have one normal copy and one mutated copy of the gene; are usually asymptomatic

   b) Child of two carriers has 25% chance of being affected by the disease

3) X-linked recessive

   a) All males with X-linked mutation are likely to be affected clinically; these diseases are uncommon in females

   b) Affected father has a 100% chance of his daughters being carriers, but will not transmit it to his son

   c) Heterozygote female may be asymptomatic or have milder symptoms than affected male because of random inactivation of one of the X chromosomes (lyonization) in each cell

4) X-linked dominant

   a) Generally both male and female heterozygotes are affected, but lyonization may result in females being less affected

   b) An affected mother has a 50% chance of passing the mutation to her son or daughter

   c) An affected father has a 100% chance of transmitting the mutation to his daughter and a 0% chance of transmitting it to his son

d. Nonmendelian inheritance patterns

1) Mitochondrial DNA: some DNA resides in mitochondria in cytoplasm

   a) 2 to 10 copies of mitochondrial DNA are in each mitochondrion

   b) Mitochondrial DNA: derived from oocyte; is exclusively maternal

   c) 16.5 kb of circular DNA

   d) Overlapping genes

   e) No introns

   f) Codes for 2 rRNA, 22 tRNA, and 13 proteins involved in oxidative phosphorylation

   g) Mutation rate: 10× greater than that of nuclear DNA

   h) Mitochondrial proteins may be aggregates of nuclear and mitochondrial gene products

   i) Mitochondrial diseases can be caused by nuclear DNA defects (may involve substrate transport or utilization, Krebs cycle, oxidation-phosphorylation coupling, or respiratory chain)

     i) Autosomal recessive (e.g., pyruvate carboxylase deficiency, defects of Krebs cycle)

     ii) Autosomal dominant (e.g., myopathy with progressive ophthalmoplegia)

     iii) X-linked recessive (e.g., ornithine transcarbamylase deficiency)

   j) Mitochondrial disease can result from mitochondrial DNA defects

     i) Sporadic or transmitted large-scale mutations, point mutations, deletions

     ii) Transmitted only by the mother (maternal, nonmendelian inheritance)

     iii) More likely to affect single tissue than germline tissues (e.g., muscles)

     iv) Heteroplasmy: mutations accumulate in different mitochondria, cells contain differing proportions of affected mitochondria

     v) Examples of diseases caused by inherited mitochondrial DNA mutations or deletions: Kearns-Sayre syndrome (ophthalmoplegia,

---

Mitochondrial disease can occur from lesions
   Inherited in the nuclear DNA

   Inherited in mitochondrial DNA

   Acquired through aging or exposure to drugs

Mitochondrial DNA
   Is inherited from the mother

   Is circular

   Has no introns

conduction block); Leber's hereditary optic neuropathy; mitochondrial encephalomyopathy, lactic-acidosis with strokelike episodes (MELAS); myoclonic epilepsy and ragged red fibers (MERRF) syndrome; mitochondrial myopathy and cardiomyopathy; neurogenic muscle weakness with ataxia and retinitis pigmentosa; chronic external ophthalmoplegia; myoneurogastrointestinal (pseudo-obstruction) encephalopathy (MNGIE); and autosomal dominant mitochondrial myopathy with mitochondrial mutations in D-loop (type Zeviani)

   k) Mitochondrial disease can be acquired: Reye's syndrome, MPTP, zidovudine, aging

2) Trinucleotide repeats usually occur in groups of 5 to 35 repeats; may cause disease when a threshold is exceeded

   a) Type I trinucleotide diseases: expansion occurs in protein-coding region of gene producing a protein with neurotoxic properties

      i) Most are caused by expanded CAG repeats (polyglutamine tracts)

      ii) The repeat expansion tends to be shorter in length

      iii) Most of these are inherited in AD fashion

      iv) AD polyglutamine diseases: Huntington's disease; dentatorubral-pallidoluysian atrophy; spinocerebellar ataxia type 1 (SCA 1), SCA 2, SCA 3 (Machado-Joseph disease), SCA 6, SCA 7, SCA 17

      v) Spinobulbar muscular atrophy (Kennedy's disease): CAG repeat disease inherited in X-linked fashion

      vi) Oculopharyngeal muscular dystrophy: a type I triple repeat disease produced by expansion of GCG and may be AD or AR; results in expanded polyalanine

   vii) These are progressive neurodegenerative diseases with intraneuronal (often intranuclear) inclusions

   b) Type II diseases: characterized by expansions of CTG, GAA, GCC, CAG, or CGG within a noncoding region

      i) AD inheritance: CTG in myotonic dystrophy type 1, CTG in SCA 8, CAG in SCA 12

      ii) AR inheritance: GAA in Friedreich's ataxia

      iii) X-linked inheritance: GCC in fragile X syndrome type A (FRAXA), CGG in FRAXE, GCC in FRAXF

      iv) Expanded repeats may cause disease by different mechanisms in type II diseases: aberrant processing of RNA and silencing of neighbor genes may have role in myotonic dystrophy; hypermethylation may lead to the gene not being transcribed in FRAXA, FRAXE, and progressive myoclonic epilepsy type 1

      v) Jacobsen syndrome (FRA11B): caused by sporadic inheritance of CCG repeat

   c) Anticipation: expanded repeats often enlarge when passed to successive generations, producing more severe disease at earlier age of onset

      i) Anticipation: not seen in a few triple repeat diseases including oculopharyngeal muscular dystrophy, spinobulbar atrophy, SCA 6

      ii) Parent-of-origin effect: some diseases show preferential anticipation depending on which gender transmits the gene; most severe cases of congenital myotonic dystrophy are inherited from the mother; paternal inheritance is more likely to result in juvenile-onset Huntington's disease

   d) Other repeat expansion diseases have been found where the repeat unit is not a trinucleotide

      i) Tetranucleotide repeat disease: myotonic dystrophy type 2 is caused by repeat sequence CCTG inherited AD

Examples of diseases caused by mitochondrial DNA mutations include

Kearns-Sayre syndrome

Leber's hereditary optic neuropathy

Mitochondrial encephalomyopathy, lactic-acidosis with strokelike episodes (MELAS)

Myoclonic epilepsy and ragged red fibers (MERRF) syndrome

Expanded repeat diseases exhibit anticipation or a tendency to manifest at an earlier age and in a more severe form

Longer expanded repeats tend to produce more severe disease

Expanded repeats may occur in areas coding for proteins or in noncoding regions

    ii) Pentanucleotide repeat disease: SCA 10, expanded ATTCT inherited AD

    iii) Dodecanucleotide repeat disease: progressive myoclonic epilepsy type 1 produced by expansion of a 12-nucleotide repeat sequence inherited recessively

3) Imprinting diseases: result from deletions in certain chromosomal regions that only express maternal or paternal allele of a gene

    a) Prader-Willi syndrome: produced by deletion of chromosome 15 of paternal origin

    b) Angelman's syndrome: from deletion involving chromosome 15 of maternal origin

4) Multifactorial diseases or complex traits

    a) Do not follow mendelian inheritance and do not appear to be single-gene disease

    b) Gene-gene and gene-environmental interactions are likely important in the development of the disease

c) Multiple sclerosis: complex trait (as with many neurologic diseases)

    i) Increased risk to relatives: most are sporadic, but 1 in 7 patients has affected first-degree relative; child of affected individual has about 2% chance of inheriting the disease, and sibling of affected individual has about 3% chance; absolute risk is small, but relative risk is about 20× that of general population; monozygotic twin of someone with multiple sclerosis has about 30% chance of being affected, and dizygotic twin has about 5% chance

    ii) Presence of HLA DR2 (a polymorphism) increases susceptibility to multiple sclerosis, the effect is too small to be considered clinically useful (40% of multiple sclerosis patients will be negative and 15% of general population will be positive)

REFERENCES

Benarroch EE. Basic neuroscience with clinical applications. Philadelphia: Butterworth Heinemann/Elsevier; 2006.

Benarroch EE, Westmoreland BF, Daube JR, Reagan TJ, Sandok BA. Medical neurosciences: an approach to anatomy, pathology, and physiology by systems and levels. 4th ed. Philadelphia: Lippincott Williams & Wilkins; 1999.

Brazis PW, Masdeu JC, Biller J. Localization in clinical neurology. 3rd ed. Boston: Little, Brown; 1996.

Carpenter MB, Sutin J. Human neuroanatomy. 8th ed. Baltimore: Williams & Wilkins; 1983.

Chyung ASC, Ptacek LJ. Continuum: lifelong learning in neurology. Neurogenetics. April 2005;11:79-94.

Ensenauer RE, Reinke SS, Ackerman MJ, Tester DJ, Whiteman DA, Tefferi A. Primer on medical genomics. Part VIII. Essentials of medical genetics for the practicing physician. Mayo Clin Proc. 2003;78:846-57.

GeneTests [homepage on the Internet]. Seattle (WA): University of Washington; 2006. Available from: http://www.genetests.org.

Heurteaux C, Guy N, Laigle C, Blondeau N, Duprat F, Mazzuca M, et al. TREK-1, aK+ channel involved in neuroprotection and general anesthesia. EMBO J. 2004 Jul 7;23:2684-95. Epub 2004 Jun 3.

Kandel ER, Schwartz JH, Jessell TM, editors. Principles of neural science. 3rd ed. New York: Elsevier Science Publishing Company; 1991.

Noseworthy JH, Hartung H-P. Multiple sclerosis and related conditions. In: Noseworthy JH, editor. Neurological therapeutics: principles and practice. Vol 1. London: Martin Dunitz; 2003. p. 1107-8.

Passarge E. Color atlas of genetics. 2nd ed. New York: Georg Thieme Verlag; 2001.

Siegel GJ, Agranoff BW, Albers RW, Molinoff PB, editors. Basic neurochemistry. 6th ed. New York: Raven Press; 1996.

Tefferi A, Wieben ED, Dewald GW, Whiteman DA, Bernard ME, Spelsberg TC. Primer on medical genomics part II: background principles and methods in molecular genetics. Mayo Clin Proc. 2002;77:785-808.

QUESTIONS

1. The caliber of the axon is determined by:
   a. The state of phosphorylation of the neurofilaments
   b. The expression of myelin basic protein
   c. Rho-GTPase–triggered pathways
   d. Polymerization of tubulin

2. Clostridial toxins prevent vesicle fusion by:
   a. Blocking the presynaptic voltage-gated calcium channels
   b. Phosphorylating synapsin
   c. Hydrolyzing SNARE proteins
   d. Preventing the reuptake of acetylcholine

3. Hereditary neuropathy with liability to pressure palsies is caused by:
   a. Duplication of a noncompacted myelin protein gene
   b. Repetition of a noncompacted myelin protein gene
   c. Duplication of a compacted myelin protein gene
   d. Repetition of a compacted myelin protein gene

4. What would not be found at a node of Ranvier?
   a. Voltage-gated sodium channel
   b. Ankyrin G
   c. Dynein
   d. Na+/K+ ATPase
   e. GM1 gangliosides

5. The cysteine residue family of ligand-gated channels does *not* include:
   a. Nicotinic acetylcholine receptor
   b. 5-HT$_3$ receptor
   c. Glycine receptor
   d. P2X purinergic receptor
   e. GABA$_A$ receptor

6. Binding of acetylcholine to a presynaptic M2 receptor produces inhibition by:
   a. Activating adenylyl cyclase
   b. Initiating the phospholipase C cascade
   c. Opening potassium channels
   d. Generating acetylcholinesterase

7. Intranuclear inclusions in Parkinson's disease do not:
   a. Stain positive for ubiquitin
   b. Stain positive for synuclein
   c. Undergo degradation by the 26 S protease
   d. Include Lewy bodies

8. What would result from repetitive excitation of cell B by axon A if axon A followed Hebbian rules?
   a. Axon A would produce long-term depression of cell B
   b. Cell B would activate cysteine proteases
   c. Efficiency of axon A in exciting cell B would increase
   d. Only cell B would undergo growth or metabolic change

9. Hyperpolarization of a neuron's membrane would occur through:
   a. Outward flow of potassium ions
   b. Inward flow of potassium ions
   c. Closing of potassium channels
   d. Inward flow of sodium ions
   e. Opening of sodium channels

10. The number of myelin wrappings around a nerve fiber:
    a. Is proportional to membrane resistance
    b. Is inversely proportional to membrane capacitance
    c. Decreases the internode distance
    d. Is inversely proportional to the length constant

11. Glutamate is the neurotransmitter of all the neurons listed below *except*:
    a. Projection neurons of the cerebral cortex
    b. Input neurons of the cerebellum
    c. Output neurons of the striatum
    d. Sensory relay nuclei neurons

12. Activation of the NMDA receptor does *not* require:
    a. Binding of glutamate
    b. Binding of two molecules of glycine
    c. Hyperpolarization of membrane
    d. Removal of magnesium blockade

13. GABA$_B$ receptors are:
    a. Stimulated by baclofen
    b. Chloride channels
    c. Inhibited by bicuculline
    d. Modulated by benzodiazepines

14. Glycine receptors are:
    a. Located in the Purkinje cells of the cerebellum
    b. Inhibited by strychnine
    c. Anchored to the membrane by GRIP
    d. A tetrameric structure

15. Which of the following statements is false?
    a. The rate-limiting factor for the synthesis of acetylcholine is the action of choline acetyltransferase
    b. Chronic exposure to nicotine produces desensitization and upregulation of cholinergic receptors
    c. The basal forebrain cholinergic neurons project to the cerebral cortex
    d. The mesopontine cholinergic neurons project to the thalamus and brainstem

16. Which of the following statements is true?
    a. Mesolimbic dopaminergic neurons project to the subthalamic nucleus and globus pallidus
    b. D_2-like receptors activate adenylyl cyclase and decrease potassium conductance
    c. D_3 and D_4 receptors are concentrated in the striatum
    d. Midbrain dopaminergic neurons increase their firing rate in anticipation of an award

17. Serotonin and norepinephrine are both:
    a. Synthesized from L-tryptophan
    b. Restricted primarily to the locus ceruleus
    c. Implicated in mechanisms of depression and anxiety
    d. Taken up from the synaptic cleft by the same transporter

18. The primary method of synaptic inactivation does not depend on reuptake for which of the following neurotransmitters?
    a. Glutamate
    b. GABA
    c. Dopamine
    d. Norepinephrine
    e. Acetylcholine

19. Cerebral blood vessels are innervated by all the following *except*:
    a. Superior cervical ganglion
    b. Geniculate ganglion
    c. Sphenopalatine ganglion
    d. Trigeminal ganglion

20. Cerebrospinal fluid production
    a. Occurs at a rate of 90 mL/day
    b. Depends on the action of carbonic anhydrase

c. Requires the production of chloride
d. Occurs exclusively at the arachnoid granulations

21. A large dorsal root ganglion neuron:
    a. Has a C-type efferent fiber type
    b. Uses substance P as a neurotransmitter
    c. Depends on binding of GDNR to Ret+
    d. Depends on binding of NT-3 to Trk C

22. What is *not* true about vanilloid receptor 1?
    a. It is expressed in dorsal root ganglion neurons
    b. It has a binding site for endogenous cannabinoid
    c. It is activated by capsaicin
    d. It is inhibited by caspases

23. Thalamic neurons:
    a. That project from the relay nuclei are GABAergic
    b. Are typically in a tonic firing pattern during wake states
    c. Of the pulvinar nucleus are essential for sleep spindles
    d. In the suprachiasmatic nuclei control biologic rhythms

24. A 45-year-old man presents with progressive difficulty with memory and inability to function at work. On examination, he is noted to have small-amplitude choreiform movements and MRI shows generalized cerebral atrophy, with striking atrophy of the caudate nuclei. What genetic abnormality is most likely the cause of the patient's symptoms?
    a. Mitochondrial DNA point mutation
    b. Expanded CAG repeats on chromosome 4
    c. Duplication of *PMP22* gene
    d. Trisomy 16

25. The patient in question 24 has a genetic test for the suspected condition, and the result is positive; the family wants to have genetic testing for the patient's 8-year-old daughter, who is currently asymptomatic. What is the best way to proceed?
    a. Careful monitoring of the daughter and referral of family to a genetics specialist
    b. Reassure the family that the daughter cannot have inherited the mutation
    c. Proceed with genetic testing on the daughter
    d. Perform MRI of head to screen for caudate atrophy

ANSWERS

1. Answer: a.
Phosphorylation of the neurofilaments determines the caliber of the axon. Myelin basic protein is responsible for compaction of myelin at the major dense line. Rho-GTPase pathways regulate the actin cytoskeleton and are important in extension of the growth cone. Polymerization of tubulin is important in intracellular transport.

2. Answer: c.
Both botulism and tetanus toxins cleave synaptobrevins and other proteins important in vesicle fusion. Botulinum toxins prevent the release of acetylcholine, resulting in flaccid paralysis. Tetanospasmin blocks the release of inhibitory neurotransmitters, resulting in muscle spasms. Antibodies to presynaptic voltage-gated calcium channels are found in Lambert-Eaton myasthenic syndrome. Phosphorylation of synapsin is important for vesicle mobilization at the active zone.

3. Answer: d.
Charcot-Marie-Tooth disease type 1(CMT-1) and hereditary neuropathy with liability to pressure palsies (HNPP) are associated with different mutations in the same gene that encodes peripheral myelin protein 22 (PMP22). CMT-1 results from a duplication of this gene, and HNPP is seen with deletion of this gene. PMP22 is critical in compaction of peripheral myelin.

4. Answer: c.
The nodes of Ranvier are specialized for salutatory conduction and rely on the clustering of voltage-gated sodium channels by ankyrin. Gangliosides, sialic acid-containing glycosphingolipids, are enriched in neural tissue, and GM1 gangliosides are found at the nodes of Ranvier, where they may have a role in autoimmune peripheral nerve disorders. Patients with multifocal motor neuropathy (MMN) have high titers of monoclonal IgM anti-GM1 ganglioside antibodies. Polyclonal IgG anti-GM1 ganglioside antibodies are detected in acute motor axonal neuropathy. Dynein is a motor protein important for retrograde axonal transport.

5. Answer: d.
P2X purinergic receptors are ATP-binding receptors permeable to calcium. The other receptors listed belong to the ionotropic glutamate receptor family. These are pentamers of subunits containing four transmembrane regions.

6. Answer: c.
M2-type acetylcholine channels are coupled with $G_{i/o}$ proteins that inhibit adenyl cyclase, resulting in the opening of potassium channels and the closing of calcium channels.

7. Answer: c.
Lewy bodies stain positive for both ubiquitin and synuclein and are found in both idiopathic Parkinson's disease and Lewy body disease. These intranuclear inclusions are resistant to degradation by the ubiquitin-protease system.

8. Answer: c.
Under Hebbian rules, repetitive excitation of one neuron by another produces changes in both cells that lead to long-term potentiation.

9. Answer: a.
Opening potassium channels would result in the outward flow of potassium because concentration of potassium ions is higher intracellularly than extracellularly. This produces hyperpolarization because the membrane potential is brought closer to the equilibrium potential of potassium at −100 mV.

10. Answer: b.
Myelination decreases the capacitance of the axonal membrane and increases its resistance. This results in an increased conduction velocity and length constant. The resistance of the axon is determined by axonal diameter. Giant squid axons achieve higher conduction velocities through increased axonal diameter instead of myelination.

11. Answer: c.
Glutamate is the major excitatory neurotransmitter of the central nervous system and the neurotransmitter of the projection neurons of the cerebral cortex, thalamus, brainstem, and spinal cord. GABA is the neurotransmitter of inhibitory interneurons, cerebellar Purkinje cells, and output neurons of the basal ganglia.

12. Answer: c.
Opening of the NMDA channel depends on the binding of glutamate and glycine. At rest, there is a magnesium blockade that must be overcome by depolarization.

13. Answer: a.
Baclofen is an agonist of $GABA_B$ receptors. $GABA_A$ receptors are chloride channels activated by benzodiazepines and inhibited by bicuculline.

14. Answer: b.
Glycine receptors are expressed predominately in the spinal cord and are inhibited by strychnine. The glycine receptor is a pentameric chloride channel. AMPA glutamate receptors are anchored by GRIP, whereas inhibitory receptors such as

GABA$_A$ and glycine are anchored by gephyrin.

15. Answer: a.
The rate-limiting step in the synthesis of acetylcholine is the uptake of choline. Choline acetyltransferase synthesizes acetylcholine from choline. Prolonged exposure to acetylcholine or nicotine produces desensitization and upregulation of acetylcholine receptors.

16. Answer: d.
Mesolimbic dopaminergic neurons located in the ventral tegmental area of the midbrain are important in reward-mediated behavior and project to the amygdala, nucleus accumbens, and septal nuclei. Striatonigral dopaminergic neurons of the substantia nigra are important in the control of movement and project to the caudate and putamen. D$_2$-like receptors are coupled to Gi/o proteins that inhibit adenyl cyclase and open potassium channels. D$_1$ and D$_2$ receptors are concentrated in the striatum, whereas D$_3$ and D$_4$ receptors are located in the frontal cortex, amygdala, and hippocampus.

17. Answer: c.
Both serotonin and norepinephrine are implicated in mood and anxiety disorders, and many psychiatric medications affect these neurotransmitters. Tricyclic antidepressants, selective serotonin reuptake inhibitors, and newer antidepressants block the uptake of these two neurotransmitters and dopamine in varying amounts. Monoamine oxidase (MAO) is an intramitochondrial enzyme responsible for the breakdown of dopamine, norepinephrine, and serotonin; MAO inhibitors are another class of antidepressants.

18. Answer: e.
Acetylcholine is inactivated by acetylcholinesterase in the synaptic cleft. All the other neurotransmitters depend primarily on reuptake for inactivation.

19. Answer: b.
Geniculate ganglion neurons innervate taste buds on the tongue, the external auditory canal, a small patch of skin behind the ear, and the external tympanic membrane. Parasympathetic innervation from the sphenopalatine ganglion and sympathetic innervation from the superior cervical ganglion regulate cerebral blood flow. Cerebral blood vessels also receive innervation from the trigeminal ganglion.

20. Answer: b.
Cerebrospinal fluid is produced by the choroid plexus at a rate

of 500 mL/day. Production depends on the production of H$^+$ and HCO$_3^-$ by carbonic anhydrase.

21. Answer: d.
Axons of small neurons in the dorsal root ganglia are small myelinated A fibers and unmyelinated C fibers important for conduction of information about pain and temperature. Nonpeptidergic axons of the small dorsal root ganglion neurons depend on the production of GDNF. Large dorsal root ganglion neurons have large myelinated axons and depend on the production of NT-3.

22. Answer: d.
The vanilloid receptor is a calcium channel expressed in dorsal root ganglion neurons. It is activated by capsaicin and has a binding site for anandamide (an endogenous cannabinoid). Caspases are cysteine proteases important in apoptosis.

23. Answer: b.
The tonic firing of glutamatergic neurons in relay nuclei of the thalamus allows precise transmission of information to the cerebral cortex. Reticular neurons of the thalamic nucleus generate sleep spindles and may serve a gating function by producing rhythmic burst firing that prevents afferent information from reaching the cerebral cortex during sleep. The suprachiasmatic nucleus is located in the hypothalamus, not the thalamus.

24. Answer: b.
The triad of Huntington's disease includes chorea, cognitive decline, and various psychiatric symptoms. In 1983, a gene marker was localized near the tip of the short arm of chromosome 4, and it was cloned 10 years later. The gene located on chromosome 4p16.3 encodes a protein named "huntingtin." The mutation responsible for the disease consists of an unstable enlargement of the CAG (cytosine-adenine-guanine) repeat sequence in the gene. In unaffected persons, the number of repeats varies between 10 and 29 copies. In those with Huntington's disease, the gene contains 36 to 121 of these repeats. The intermediate-sized CAG repeats range from 30 to 35. Approximately 11% of patients with clinically suspected Huntington's disease have no family history of the disease; some of these patients may have de novo mutations.

25. Answer: a.
Huntington's disease is inherited in an autosomal dominant pattern. Thus, each offspring has a 50% chance of inheriting the gene. If no intervention is available to prevent the disease, then genetic testing is not appropriate for an asymptomatic minor.

Neuro-ophthalmology

3

William D. Freeman, M.D.

Nima Mowzoon, M.D.

I. VISUAL SYSTEM

A. Components

1. Retina, retinal nerve fiber layer, optic nerves, optic chiasm, optic tracts, lateral geniculate bodies, optic radiations, and visual cortices (Fig. 3-1)

B. Retina

1. Extends from ora serrata to optic nerve (Fig. 3-2)
2. Divided into four quadrants by the macula
   a. Vertical meridian: separates superior and inferior retina
   b. Horizontal meridian: separates nasal and temporal retina
3. Retina layers (Fig. 3-3)
   a. Retinal pigment epithelium
      1) Deepest layer of retina
      2) Forms outer blood-retinal barrier and supports photoreceptors physiologically
   b. Photoreceptor layer
      1) First neural elements in the retina to react to light
      2) Rod and cone cells contain light-sensitive pigment rhodopsin
      3) Photoreceptors hyperpolarize (membrane potential becomes more negative) in presence of light
      4) Rod cells are sensitive to low levels of light
         a) Minimal role in color vision (except blue spectrum)
         b) Rods are concentrated in peripheral retina
         c) No rods within the macula
      5) Cone cells respond to color
         a) Red, green, and blue
         b) Cones are densely concentrated in the macula
   c. Outer nuclear layer: contains cell bodies of photoreceptors
   d. Outer plexiform layer: contains synapses between photoreceptors and bipolar and horizontal cells
   e. Inner nuclear layer
      1) Amacrine cells are horizontally oriented, dopaminergic cells that modulate and convey photoreceptor information to ganglion cells

2) Bipolar cells convey photoreceptor information to ganglion cells
3) Horizontal cells provide antagonistic surround signals to bipolar cells
   f. Inner plexiform layer: contains synapses between bipolar and amacrine cells and ganglion cells
   g. Ganglion cell layer
      1) Most superficial retinal layer
      2) Ganglion cells divided into M and P cells
      3) M and P cell axons project to superior colliculus or lateral geniculate nucleus
      4) M cells lack color information, but have high contrast sensitivity, fast temporal resolution, low spatial resolution
      5) **M** cell axons project to **m**agnocellular neurons in layers 1 and 2 of lateral geniculate nucleus, and these neurons project to layer IVC alpha neurons in cortical area 17
      6) P cells have color opponency, low contrast sensitivity, and high spatial resolution
      7) **P** cell axons project to **p**arvocellular neurons in layers 3, 4, 5, and 6 of lateral geniculate nucleus, and these neurons project to layer IVC alpha neurons in cortical area 17
      8) Two types of signal processing
         a) ON center, OFF surround
            i) ON center: activated when light hits center of the receptive field
            ii) OFF surround: deactivated when light hits periphery of the receptive field
         b) OFF center, ON surround: center receptive field stimulation is OFF, and peripheral stimulation is ON
         c) ON-OFF signal processing helps establish sharp boundaries of objects in visual field
      9) Ganglion cell axons traveling to the optic nerve form the retinal nerve fiber layer

C. Retinal Nerve Fiber Layer

1. Papillomacular bundle: nerve fibers extending from

83

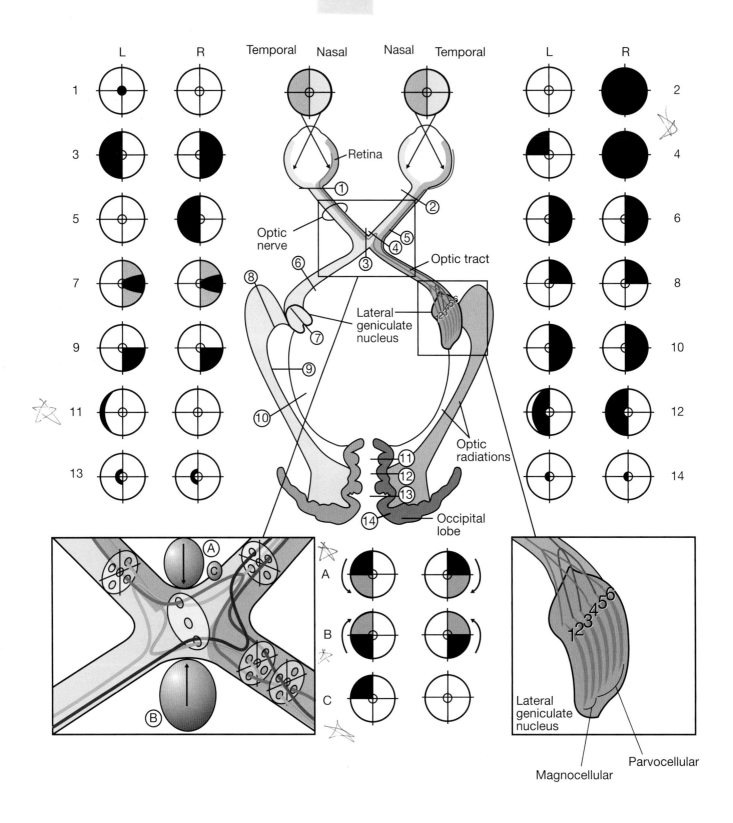

Fig. 3-1. Anatomy of the visual system and the associated visual field defects. *1*, Central scotoma from optic neuropathy. *2*, Unilateral blindness due to optic nerve transection. *3*, Bitemporal hemianopia from optic chiasmal lesion, may or may not be macular splitting (*left lower inset*): *A*, Lesion anterior to chiasm—more prominent defect in bitemporal upper quadrants early on and eventually evolving to full bitemporal field defect; *B*, lesion posterior to chiasm; more prominent defect in bitemporal lower quadrants early on and eventually evolving to full bitemporal field defect. *4*, Anterior chiasm or junctional syndrome: ipsilateral optic nerve defect and contralateral superior temporal field defect due to posterior optic nerve lesion involving the ipsilateral optic nerve and contralateral crossing fibers of Wilbrand's knee (contralateral lower nasal fibers representing upper temporal field) (also see Fig. 3-9); this is to be differentiated from junctional syndrome of Traquair, represented in lesion C. *5*, Unilateral nasal field defect due to ipsilateral lateral optic nerve lesion. *6*, Macular-splitting homonymous hemianopia from complete optic tract lesion. *7*, Complete (gray and black) homonymous hemianopia and incomplete (black only or gray only) field defects due to lateral geniculate body lesions (complete and incomplete lesions, respectively). Gray represents *quadruple sectoranopia* due to vascular lesions in the distribution of anterior choroidal artery; black represents *horizontal homonymous sector defect* due to vascular lesions in the distribution of posterior lateral choroidal artery. *8*, Right superior homonymous quadrantanopia ("pie in the sky") deficits from left temporal lesion affecting underlying optic radiations (lower bundle, called Meyer's loop as fibers pass lateral to temporal horn of lateral ventricle). *9*, Right inferior homonymous quadrantic ("pie on the floor") deficits from left parietal lesion affecting the underlying optic radiations (upper bundle). *10*, Macular-splitting homonymous hemianopia from lesion affecting both superior and inferior optic radiations (usually large hemispheric insults). *11*, Temporal crescent (half-moon) syndrome due to lesion at anterior tip of striate cortex. *12*, Macular-sparing homonymous hemianopia due to lesion involving entire medial occipital lobe, sparing the anterior tip (representing contralateral temporal crescent). *13*, Partial homonymous hemianopia (macular-sparing) affecting the most posterior portion of medial occipital lobe, sparing posterior poles (macular representation). *14*, Macular-splitting homonymous field defect limited to macular distribution and no involvement of peripheral visual fields (could be due to lesion of unilateral posterior occipital pole). Right lower inset: *1-6*, layers of lateral geniculate nucleus.

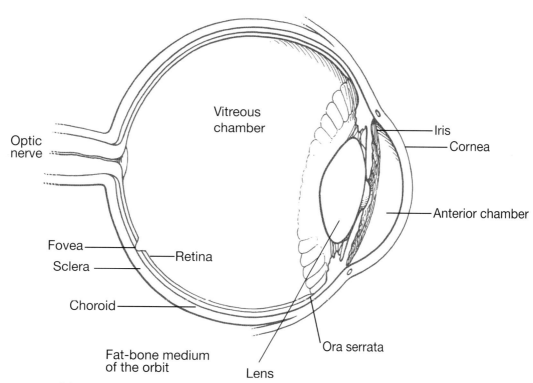

Fig. 3-2. Gross anatomy of the eye and retina.

macula to optic nerve
2. Temporal nerve fibers arch around papillomacular bundle to reach optic disc
3. Optic nerve creates a physiologic blind spot on visual field testing (temporal)
4. Scotomas ("blind spots"): areas of poor or absent vision within the visual field
5. Specific scotoma and visual field abnormalities may occur from optic nerve and retinal lesions based on arrangement of retinal nerve fiber layer
   a. Arcuate scotoma or defects: arch-shaped, characteristic of nerve fiber bundle defects (e.g., glaucoma) (Fig. 3-4)

b. Central scotoma (macular type of defect): a blind spot in the visual field represented by the macula (e.g., macular degeneration) (Fig. 3-5 *left*)
c. Centrocecal scotoma (optic nerve type of defect): affects the visual field in region of the macula and papillomacular bundle (Fig. 3-5 *right*)
d. Paracentral scotoma: affects retina and visual field just outside the macula (Fig. 3-6 *left*)
e. Ring scotoma: from combined superior and inferior retina and arcuate scotoma (Fig. 3-6 *right*)
f. Ring scotoma with a horizontal step: typically indicates retinal or nerve fiber layer lesion as opposed to ring

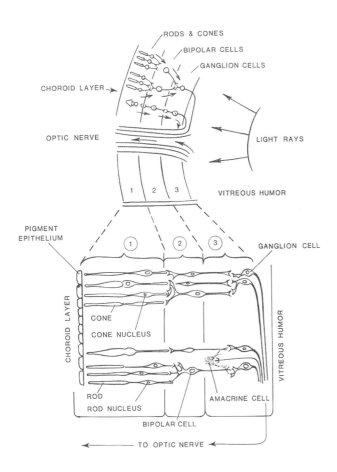

Fig. 3-3. The retina has three cell layers from outside to inside: rods and cones, the receptor cells *(1)*; the bipolar cells *(2)*; and the ganglion cells *(3)*. Note that the light rays have to pass through the inner layers to reach the receptor cells in the outer layer. (From Benarroch EE, Westmoreland BF, Daube JR, Reagan TJ, Sandok BA. Medical neurosciences: an approach to anatomy, pathology, and physiology by systems and levels. 4th ed. Philadelphia: Lippincott Williams & Wilkins; 1999. p. 583. By permission of Mayo Foundation.)

Monocular scotoma and noncongruous visual field abnormalities (especially monocular) occur from optic nerve and retinal lesions based on arrangement of retinal nerve fiber layer

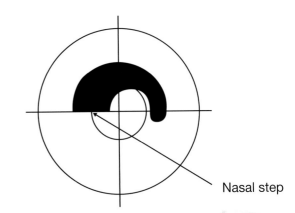

Fig. 3-4. Arcuate scotoma (Bjerrum's scotoma) in glaucoma.

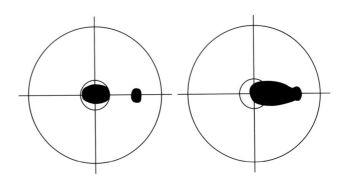

Fig. 3-5. Central scotoma (*left*) and centrocecal scotoma (*right*). The smaller circles represent the physiologic blind spot.

scotoma with a vertical step, which may indicate lesion in occipital lobe near calcarine fissure
  g. Enlargement of blind spot (e.g., optic disc swelling) (Fig. 3-7)
  h. Altitudinal defects: blind spots with a horizontal step; typically appear as an abrupt, monocular loss of superior or inferior visual field
  i. Sector scotoma or defects: typically caused by retinal lesion (e.g., retinal detachment) (Fig. 3-8)
  j. Noncongruous visual field defects: dissimilar monocular visual field patterns

D. Optic Nerve
1. Segments
  a. Intraocular segment (optic nerve head)
  b. Intraorbital segment
  c. Intracanalicular (optic canal) segment
  d. Intracranial segment

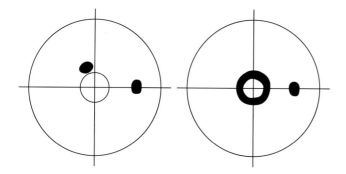

Fig. 3-6. Paracentral scotoma (*left*) and ring scotoma (*right*). The smaller circle on the right in each visual field represents physiologic blind spot.

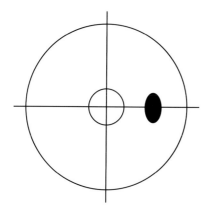

Fig. 3-7. Enlargement of blind spot (e.g., papilledema).

2. Topographic arrangement of nerve fiber layer within optic nerve
  a. Similar to topology of nerve fiber layer before entry into optic nerve
  b. Macular fibers (papillomacular bundle) are located peripherally (temporal aspect of the optic nerve) in the portion of optic nerve closest to the globe
  c. Macular fibers become more centrally located in more distal portion of optic nerve closest to the chiasm
  d. Peripheral retinal fibers travel peripherally
3. Monocular vision loss is usually due to disease of retina, optic disc, or optic nerve: anterior to optic chiasm
  a. Central field defects are caused by lesions that affect optic nerve, macula, or papillomacular bundle
    1) Unilateral central scotomas, for example, optic neuropathy, optic neuritis, or macular degeneration
    2) Bilateral central or centrocecal defects, for example, suggestive of bilateral optic neuropathies (hereditary, compressive, nutritional, inflammatory) or bilateral occipital lesions
  b. Unilateral temporal defects
    1) Lesion of nasal retina, optic nerve, or nasal optic nerve fibers at anterior optic chiasm (e.g., junctional scotoma of Traquair, see below)
    2) Monocular temporal crescent: retinal disease or lesion of anterior occipital lobe
  c. Altitudinal defects: characteristic of disease of the central retinal artery, with macular sparing (cilioretinal arteries) or posterior ciliary artery (anterior ischemic optic neuropathy)

E. Optic Chiasm
1. Nasal retinal nerve fibers: cross to contralateral optic tract at level of the optic chiasm (constitute about half of optic nerve fibers)

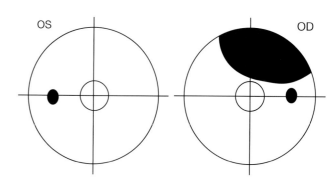

Fig. 3-8. Superior sector defect from inferior retinal detachment.

2. Inferior nasal fibers of one optic nerve cross ventrally into contralateral optic nerve proximally and are known as Wilbrand's knee (Fig. 3-1), (the existence of this anatomic entity has been questioned)
3. Temporal retinal nerve fibers remain ipsilateral in optic chiasm and optic tracts
4. Posterior to optic chiasm: pituitary stalk
5. Optic chiasm lesions: bitemporal field defects, almost never complete bitemporal field defects and exact field defect depends on localization of the compressive lesion
   a. Anterior chiasm (Fig 3-1)
      1) Compressive lesion anterior to optic chiasm generally causes bitemporal field defects involving the upper quadrants early on (may eventually evolve to more extensive bitemporal field defects)
      2) Junctional syndrome of Traquair
         a) Monocular superior temporal field defect in eye contralateral to the lesion
         b) Often due to early, anterior chiasmal compressive lesion limited to crossing fibers from inferonasal retina of contralateral eye (Wilbrand's knee), situated anterior to the ipsilateral inferonasal fibers (Fig. 3-1, *left lower inset, C*)
      3) Junctional syndrome
         a) Ipsilateral central scotoma with contralateral superior temporal defect
         b) Due to compression of Wilbrand's knee and ipsilateral optic nerve (Fig. 3-1, defect *4*, Fig. 3-9)

Nasal retinal fibers cross in the optic chiasm and temporal retinal fibers remain ipsilateral

Inferior nasal fibers of one optic nerve cross ventrally into the contralateral optic nerve proximally and are known as Wilbrand's knee

An isolated monocular temporal field defect affecting the contralateral optic nerve or Wilbrand's knee is called a junctional scotoma of Traquair

---

Junctional syndrome: an anterior chiasm lesion causes a central scotoma in one eye and a superior temporal visual field defect in the other eye (Fig. 3-9)

Bitemporal visual field defects are typical of a lesion affecting the body of the optic chiasm

---

      4) Bilateral superior temporal field defects due to early anterior compression of both inferonasal crossing fibers
   b. Body of the chiasm syndrome: typically bitemporal visual field defects (often incomplete, may be limited to central fields, peripheral fields, or both)
   c. Posterior chiasm syndrome
      1) Compressive lesion posterior to optic chiasm generally causes bitemporal field defects involving lower quadrants early on (may eventually evolve to more extensive bitemporal field defects)
      2) Bilateral temporal scotomas (involving central vision, peripheral fields spared)
      3) Bitemporal field defects primarily affecting inferior temporal fields due to early compressive lesions

F. **Optic Tracts**
1. Optic chiasmal fibers leading to lateral geniculate nucleus
2. Visual field defect related to lesion involving optic tract
   a. Complete (macular-splitting) homonymous hemianopia
   b. Wallerian degeneration and dying-back axonal loss causing ganglion cell fiber atrophy of contralateral nasal macula and nasal retina and ipsilateral temporal retina
   c. Contralateral relative afferent pupillary defect: optic tract lesion on one side may cause the contralateral eye to have a relative afferent pupillary defect (i.e., greater number of crossed vs. uncrossed fibers in chiasm, 53:47) and a temporal visual field defect
   d. This is the last post-chiasmal site for a relative afferent pupillary defect other than an asymmetric posterior midbrain lesion

G. **Lateral Geniculate Nucleus**
1. Has six layers (Fig. 3-1, *bottom right inset*)
2. Superior retinal fibers lie superomedial in the nucleus

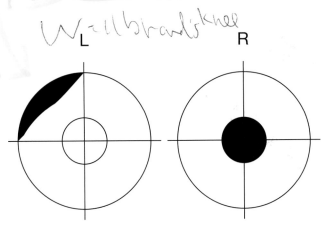

Fig. 3-9. Junctional syndrome.

3. Inferior retinal fibers lie lateral in the nucleus
4. Anterior choroidal artery occlusion causes a quadruple sectoranopia: homonymous defect affecting superior and inferior quadrants, with sparing of the horizontal sectors (Fig. 3-10 *A*)

5. Posterior lateral choroidal artery occlusion causes a horizontal homonymous sector defect: a homonymous defect of horizontal sectors (wedge- or triangle-shaped) (Fig. 3-10 *B*)

H. Optic Radiations

1. Optic radiations exit the lateral geniculate nucleus in three bundles, which course around the lateral ventricle through white matter to reach calcarine cortex (cortical area 17)
2. Three optic radiation bundles
   a. Upper bundle
      1) Originates from medial part of lateral geniculate nucleus
      2) Represents superior retina
      3) Passes deep in parietal white matter and ends in superior lip of the calcarine fissure
   b. Central bundle
      1) Originates from medial part of lateral geniculate nucleus
      2) Represents macular region
      3) Traverses posterior temporal and occipital white matter and ends on both lips of posterior part of the calcarine fissure
   c. Lower bundle
      1) Originates from lateral part of lateral geniculate nucleus
      2) Represents inferior retina
      3) Courses anteriorly from lateral geniculate nucleus and then turns around temporal horn of lateral ventricle (Meyer's loop) to end on inferior lip of the calcarine fissure
3. Superior homonymous quadrantic ("pie in the sky") defects may result from lesion of Meyer's loop (i.e., optic radiations that pass through temporal lobe to occipital lobe inferior to the calcarine fissure)
4. Inferior homonymous quadrantic ("pie on the floor") defects result from lesion of optic radiations that pass

A

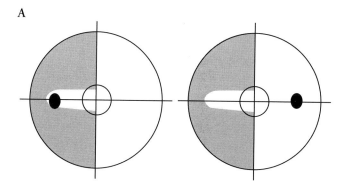

B

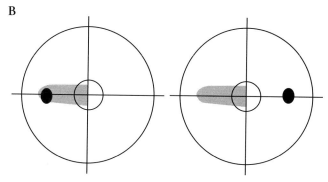

Fig. 3-10. *A*, Left quadruple sectoranopia from lateral geniculate body infarction caused by occlusion of right anterior choroidal artery. *B*, Horizontal homonymous sector defect from occlusion of right posterior lateral choroidal artery. The black dots represent the physiologic blind spots. The circles represent the fovea.

Superior retinal nerve fiber information travels in the superior optic radiations to the superior lip of the calcarine fissure

Inferior retinal nerve fiber information travels in the inferior optic radiations to the inferior lip of the calcarine fissure

---

Complete homonymous hemianopias indicate retrochiasmal disease (e.g., lateral geniculate nucleus, optic radiations, occipital cortex)

Visual field defects become more congruous (i.e., similar pattern in both eyes) from the lateral geniculate body toward the occipital lobe

A superior homonymous quadrantic ("pie in the sky") defect may result from a lesion of Meyer's loop in the temporal lobe or inferior occipital cortex

An inferior homonymous quadrantic ("pie on the floor") defect results from a lesion of the optic radiations traveling through the parietal lobe or superior occipital cortex

through parietal lobe to occipital lobe superior to the calcarine fissure

I. **Visual Cortex** (Fig. 3-11)

1. Striate cortex, or primary visual cortex, is Brodmann's area 17: located along superior and inferior banks of calcarine fissure
2. Central 10 to 15 degrees of vision represent a disproportionate amount of surface area (50%-60%) of occipital cortex
3. Homonymous quadrantic defects can occur from unilateral occipital lobe lesions; the visual field defects typically have a sharp horizontal edge
4. Medial occipital lesions cause congruous homonymous hemianopias, typically with macular sparing and are usually due to infarcts in territory of the posterior cerebral artery (absolute congruence in comparison with lesions of optic tracts or optic radiations, which are not as congruent)
5. Macular sparing is believed to be due to dual arterial supply (both posterior and middle cerebral arteries supplying the occipital pole responsible for macular vision) and also a larger cortical representation of the macular region
6. Striate cortex lesion localization
   a. Anterior lesion: causes a temporal crescent or half moon syndrome in contralateral eye (Fig. 3-1, defect *11*); the only retrochiasmal lesion that can cause a unilateral visual field defect
   b. Intermediate lesion: affects from 10 to 60 degrees in contralateral hemifield
   c. Posterior lesion: affects macular vision (central 10 degrees in contralateral visual field)
7. Cortical blindness: complete blindness or keyhole vision that may result from bilateral occipital lobe disease
8. Anton's syndrome: cortical blindness with denial of neurologic impairment

II. **OCULAR MOTOR SYSTEMS AND RELATED DISORDERS**

A. **Introduction**

1. Purpose of efferent visual system: direct and maintain the fovea toward target of interest
2. Efferent visual system has both slow and rapid visual tracking systems, with voluntary and reflex mechanisms
3. Efferent visual system: supranuclear, nuclear, infranuclear and internuclear neurons; neuromuscular junc-

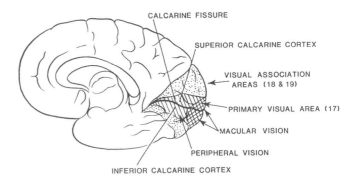

Fig. 3-11. Medial aspect of the occipital lobe showing primary visual cortex (area 17) and visual association areas (areas 18 and 19). The calcarine fissure separates the superior and inferior calcarine cortices. (From Benarroch EE, Westmoreland BF, Daube JR, Reagan TJ, Sandok BA. Medical neurosciences: an approach to anatomy, pathology, and physiology by systems and levels. 4th ed. Philadelphia: Lippincott Williams & Wilkins; 1999. p. 587. By permission of Mayo Foundation.)

> With lesions affecting the optic nerve or chiasm, patients may have decreased visual acuity, a relative afferent pupillary defect, and visual field defects—ophthalmoscopic findings are usually present
>
> With unilateral retrochiasmal lesions, patients typically have retained visual acuity, no relative afferent pupillary defect, a visual field defect, and usually normal ophthalmoscopic findings—an exception is an optic tract lesion

tion; ocular motor muscles

4. "Ocular motor" refers to cranial nerves (CNs) III, IV, and VI as a group
5. "Oculomotor" refers to CN III only

B. **Ocular Muscles** (Fig. 3-12 and Table 3-1): six muscles for each eye

1. Four rectus muscles (superior, inferior, medial and lateral)
2. Two oblique muscles (inferior and superior)

C. **Cranial Nerve III** (oculomotor nerve)

1. Neuroanatomy
   a. Oculomotor nuclear complex: located in midbrain at level of the superior colliculus; two unpaired and four paired columns of nuclei within the nuclear complex

A

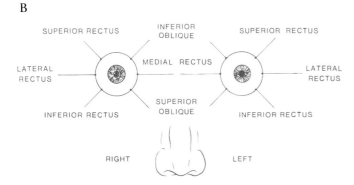

B

Fig. 3-12. *A*, Insertion of the ocular muscles on the globe. *B*, Movements of the globe produced by each ocular muscle. (From Benarroch EE, Westmoreland BF, Daube JR, Reagan TJ, Sandok BA. Medical neurosciences: an approach to anatomy, pathology, and physiology by systems and levels. 4th ed. Philadelphia: Lippincott Williams & Wilkins; 1999. p. 503. By permission of Mayo Foundation.)

Table 3-1. **Summary of the Extraocular Muscles, Innervation, and Action**

Muscle	Primary action	Secondary	Innervation (cranial nerve)
Superior rectus	Elevator	Intorsion*	Oculomotor (III)
Inferior rectus	Depressor	Extorsion†	Oculomotor (III)
Inferior oblique	Elevator	Extorsion†	Oculomotor (III)
Superior oblique	Depressor	Intorsion*	Trochlear (IV)
Lateral rectus	Abduction	...	Abducens (VI)
Medial rectus	Adduction	...	Oculomotor (III)

Intorsion of the right eye by the examiner's view appears as a clockwise rotation.
†*Extorsion of the right eye by the examiner's view appears as a counterclockwise rotation.*

Ocular muscle innervation mnemonic: "SO4 LR6"

SO = superior oblique innervated by cranial nerve IV

LR = lateral rectus, innervated by cranial nerve VI

Other ocular muscles are innervated by cranial nerve III

Superior muscles **in**tort or "SIN" mnemonic: the superior oblique (SO) and superior rectus (SR) muscles are **in**torters of the eye

---

1) Single caudal central nucleus (unpaired): innervates left and right levator palpebrae superioris muscles
2) Single visceral Edinger-Westphal nucleus (unpaired): most dorsal localization, provides parasympathic innervation of pupil (pupillary constrictors and ciliary muscle)
3) Medial nuclei (paired): each innervates superior rectus muscle ipsilaterally and sends decussating fibers (through contralateral medial nucleus) to contralateral superior rectus muscle (ablative lesion in one medial nucleus causes weakness in superior recti bilaterally); paired nuclei with decussating axons
4) Intermediate nuclei (paired): each innervates ipsilateral inferior oblique muscle
5) Dorsal nuclei (paired): each innervates ipsilateral inferior rectus muscle
6) Ventral nuclei (paired): each innervates ipsilateral medial rectus muscle

b. Fascicular arrangement is maintained similar to nuclear topology

c. Oculomotor fascicles travel ventrally, exit the interpeduncular fossa as the oculomotor nerve in the subarachnoid space

d. Subarachnoid space: oculomotor nerve passes between posterior cerebral and superior cerebellar arteries; near the uncus of temporal lobe (and in proximity to posterior communicating artery), it penetrates the dura mater into cavernous sinus (Fig. 3-13)

e. Cavernous sinus: oculomotor nerve is superior and lateral in cavernous sinus and exits the sinus to enter superior orbital fissure (Fig. 3-14)

f. Superior orbital fissure: after entering this fissure, oculomotor nerve divides into superior (innervates superior rectus and levator palpebrae superioris) and inferior (innervates medial and inferior recti and inferior oblique) divisions and provides parasympathetic input to ciliary ganglion

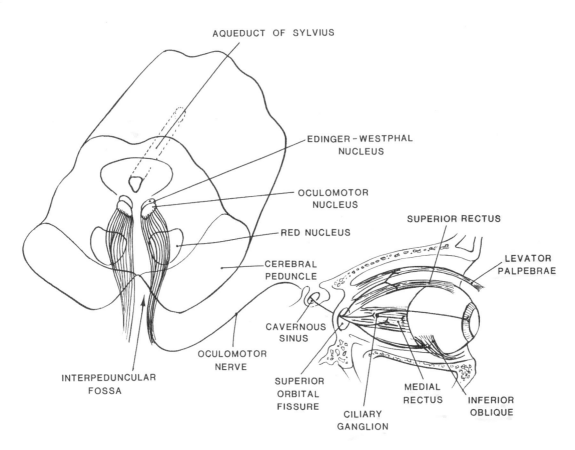

Fig. 3-13. Diagram of the oculomotor nerve and its course. (From Benarroch EE, Westmoreland BF, Daube JR, Reagan TJ, Sandok BA. Medical neurosciences: an approach to anatomy, pathology, and physiology by systems and levels. 4th ed. Philadelphia: Lippincott Williams & Wilkins; 1999. p. 495. By permission of Mayo Foundation.)

g. Orbit: oculomotor nerve divisions (superior and inferior)
2. Localization of third nerve palsy
    a. Nuclear lesions: ipsilateral complete pupil-involved third nerve palsy (including ptosis), contralateral eyelid ptosis, and superior rectus palsy
        1) Subnuclear lesions: rare, but can cause isolated muscle paresis (e.g, inferior oblique) or bilateral eyelid ptosis
        2) Nuclear lesions may spare Edinger-Westphal nucleus (pupil-sparing lesion)
        3) Differential diagnosis: focal hemorrhage, infarct, or mass (neoplastic, vascular malformation)
    b. Fascicular lesions
        1) Plus-minus syndrome (within midbrain): example of fascicular lesion causing ipsilateral ptosis and contralateral eyelid retraction (occurs with midbrain lesions involving fascicles supplying ipsilateral levator palpebrae and inhibitory projections to opposite subnucleus for contralateral levator palpebrae)

    2) Differential diagnosis: infarction, hemorrhage, mass, demyelination, infection
    3) Ipsilateral syndromes
        a) Weber's syndrome: ipsilateral third nerve palsy with contralateral hemiparesis due to involvement of CN III and cerebral peduncle
        b) Nothnagel's syndrome: ipsilateral third nerve palsy with ipsilateral ataxia (superior cerebellar lesion)
        c) Claude's syndrome: ipsilateral third nerve palsy and contralateral ataxia, due to involvement of the tegmentum, red nucleus, and CN III
        d) Benedikt's syndrome: clinical features of Claude's syndrome plus contralateral hemiparesis, latter due to involvement of cerebral peduncle
    c. Subarachnoid space lesions
        1) Posterior communicating artery aneurysm: usually involves pupils

        2) Uncal herniation
        3) Tumors and other mass lesions, arachnoid cysts
        4) Meningeal (inflammatory or infectious) disease (e.g.,

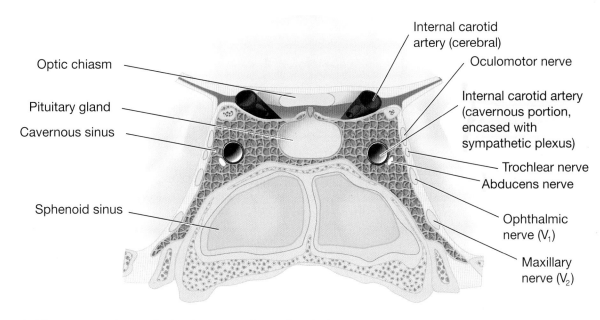

Fig. 3-14. The cavernous sinus and related structures (coronal section).

sarcoidosis, tuberculosis)

    5) Small-vessel ischemia in setting of diabetes mellitus (often pupil sparing, painful) or vasculitis

d. Cavernous sinus lesions (Fig. 3-14)

    1) Third nerve palsy with or without pain

    2) Third nerve palsy with some combination of other cavernous sinus constituents: CNs IV, VI, ophthalmic division of V (V_1) (and sometimes maxillary division of V [V_2] anatomy variable)

    3) Third nerve palsy and Horner's syndrome (sympathetic fibers along carotid artery)

    4) Masses of cavernous sinus may cause aberrant regeneration of CN III

    5) Differential diagnosis

        a) Compressive lesions: pituitary adenoma and other neoplastic compressive lesions, carotid-cavernous fistulas, pituitary apoplexy, aneurysm of intracavernous portion of internal carotid artery, cavernous sinus thrombosis

        b) Cavernous sinus infection with *Mucor* or *Aspergillus*, usually in setting of diabetes or immunosuppression

        c) Inflammatory (e.g., Tolosa-Hunt syndrome)

e. Superior orbital fissure lesions

    1) Third nerve palsy with possible palsies of CN IV, VI, V_1

    2) Differential diagnosis (similar to the cavernous sinus lesions): inflammatory (Tolosa-Hunt syndrome,

granulomatous disease often affecting superior orbital fissure), compressive lesions such as tumors (e.g., meningioma, metastatic tumor)

f. Orbital lesions

    1) Divisional third nerve palsy, optic neuropathy, proptosis, orbital injection, chemosis

    2) Differential diagnosis

        a) Compressive lesions (neoplastic, including meningioma and metastatic tumors, and vascular malformations)

        b) Trauma (orbital fractures)

        c) Inflammatory (idiopathic orbital pseudotumor)

g. Disorders of neuromuscular transmission

    1) Myasthenia gravis

    2) Lambert-Eaton myasthenic syndrome

h. Disorders of muscle

    1) Graves' ophthalmopathy (most often affecting inferior rectus muscle)

    2) Dystrophic myopathies (e.g., oculopharyngeal dystrophy)

    3) Ocular neuromyotonia: rare, episodic diplopia in setting of previous radiotherapy, usually in sellar or parasellar regions

i. Other nonlocalizing causes

    1) Miller Fisher variant of Guillain-Barré syndrome

    2) Ophthalmoplegic migraine: most frequently involving the oculomotor nerve and, commonly, the pupillary response and accommodation

3) Lyme disease with meningeal involvement
3. Pupillary involvement ("the rule of the pupil")
   a. Pupillomotor fibers are located superficially (peripherally) in CN III and tend to be spared by ischemic insults (which primarily affect deep fibers)
   b. Pupil-sparing third nerve palsy occurs with nerve infarction in setting of diabetes, giant cell arteritis, or systemic lupus erythematosus
   c. Compressive lesions generally tend to affect pupils (may be delayed)
   d. Exceptions to "the rule of the pupil": partial third nerve palsy or partial pupillary involvement
      1) Some ischemic lesions due to diabetes may produce minimal anisocoria
      2) Aneurysms presenting with partial oculomotor palsies may have minimal involvement of pupillomotor fibers (relative pupillary sparing)
      3) Certain cavernous sinus or subarachnoid partial compressive lesions involving only portions of CN III carrying no pupillary fibers
      4) The pupillary function is also spared by
         a) Some slow-growing tumors sparing pupillary fibers that tend to be more pressure-resistant than underlying oculomotor fibers
         b) Acute stage of a rapidly expanding mass (becomes more obvious later)

D. **Cranial Nerve IV** (trochlear nerve)
1. Neuroanatomy (Fig. 3-15)
   a. Nucleus: trochlear nucleus is at level of inferior colliculus
   b. Fascicles: travel posteriorly around cerebral aqueduct, decussate, and exit brainstem under the inferior colliculi
   c. Subarachnoid space
      1) CN IV: only cranial nerve to exit dorsally
      2) CN IV and CN III innervation of contralateral superior rectus muscle: only cranial nerves with axons that decussate
      3) CN IV travels through quadrageminal, ambient, crural, and pontomesencephalic cisterns
      4) CN IV travels in proximity to tentorium cerebellum: entrapment may occur at edge of the tentorium
   d. Cavernous sinus: CN IV enters cavernous sinus inferior to CN III, the lateral aspect of the clivus, and lies within lateral wall of cavernous sinus (Fig. 3-14)
   e. Superior orbital fissure: CN IV exits cavernous sinus and enters superior orbital fissure
   f. Orbit: within the orbit, CN IV innervates superior oblique muscle
2. Localization of fourth nerve palsy (differential diagnosis similar to third nerve palsy)
   a. Nuclear and fascicular lesions
      1) Contralateral fourth nerve palsy

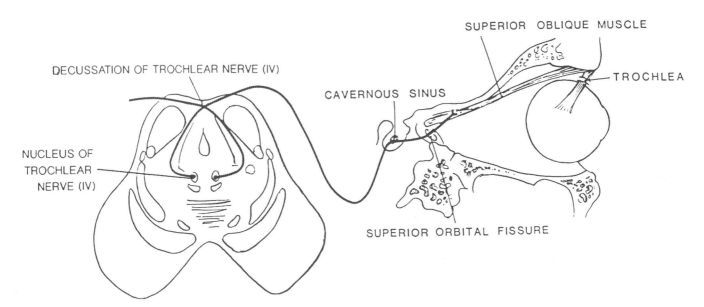

Fig. 3-15. Diagram of the trochlear nerve and its course. (From Benarroch EE, Westmoreland BF, Daube JR, Reagan TJ, Sandok BA. Medical neurosciences: an approach to anatomy, pathology, and physiology by systems and levels. 4th ed. Philadelphia: Lippincott Williams & Wilkins; 1999. p. 494. By permission of Mayo Foundation.)

2) Anterior medullary velum lesions: bilateral fourth nerve palsies (common cause in children is medulloblastoma)

b. Subarachnoid space (CN IV): ipsilateral fourth nerve palsy

c. Cavernous sinus: ipsilateral fourth nerve palsy with combination of deficits involving cavernous sinus constituents (CN III, VI, V_1, sympathetic innervation of orbit [Horner's syndrome])

d. Superior orbital fissure and orbit: ipsilateral fourth nerve palsy with possible combination of CN III, VI, or V_1

E. Cranial Nerve VI (abducens nerve)

1. Neuroanatomy (Fig. 3-16)

a. Nucleus: abducens nucleus is in pons and adjacent to floor of fourth ventricle

b. Fascicles: abducens fascicles travel ventrally through pons and emerge at pontomedullary junction

c. Subarachnoid space

1) Long intracranial upward course: CN VI travels through prepontine cistern subarachnoid space, enters Dorello's canal beneath petrosphenoidal ligament of Gruber to enter cavernous sinus

2) Lesion can cause "false localizing sign" (see below)

d. Cavernous sinus: CN VI lies inside cavernous sinus (Fig. 3-14)

e. Superior orbital fissure and orbit: CN VI exits cavernous sinus, passes through superior orbital fissure into orbit to innervate lateral rectus muscle

2. Localization of sixth nerve palsy (differential diagnosis similar to third nerve palsy)

a. Pons (nucleus and fascicles)

1) Ipsilateral sixth nerve palsy for discrete lesion

2) Foville's syndrome (see also Chapter 4)

a) Ipsilateral lower motor neuron facial paralysis

b) Ipsilateral gaze paralysis (abducens nucleus lesion)

c) Contralateral hemiparesis

3) Millard-Gubler syndrome (see also Chapter 4)

a) Ipsilateral lower motor neuron facial paralysis

b) Ipsilateral abducens paralysis

c) Contralateral hemiparesis

b. Subarachnoid space

1) Ipsilateral sixth nerve palsy

2) Gradenigo's syndrome (lesion of petrous apex or Dorello's canal)

a) Ipsilateral sixth nerve palsy: CN VI may be stretched over the petrous ridge

b) Ipsilateral facial pain

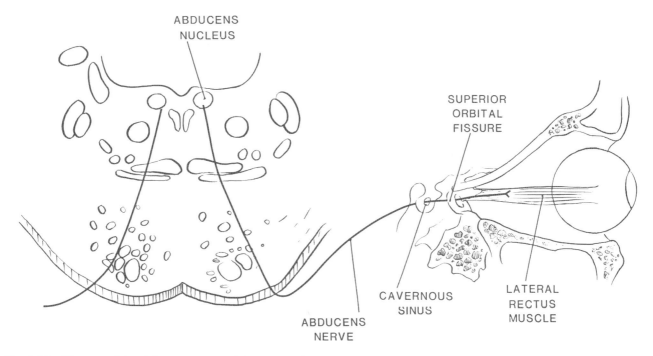

ABDUCENS NUCLEUS

SUPERIOR ORBITAL FISSURE

CAVERNOUS SINUS

LATERAL RECTUS MUSCLE

ABDUCENS NERVE

Fig. 3-16. Diagram of the abducens nerve and its course. (From Benarroch EE, Westmoreland BF, Daube JR, Reagan TJ, Sandok BA. Medical neurosciences: an approach to anatomy, pathology, and physiology by systems and levels. 4th ed. Philadelphia: Lippincott Williams & Wilkins; 1999. p. 488. By permission of Mayo Foundation.)

c) Ipsilateral deafnesss (CN VIII)

d) Due to compressive neoplastic or vascular malformation, inferior sinus thrombosis

3) False localizing sign in setting of increased intracranial pressure (e.g., hydrocephalus, pseudotumor cerebri)—CN VI has longest intracranial course of all cranial nerves and is more predisposed to stretch-induced injury, especially with shearing over the petrous ridge

c. Cavernous sinus: ipsilateral sixth nerve palsy for discrete lesion with possible involvement of CN III, IV, V$_1$ or Horner's syndrome

d. Superior orbital fissure and orbit: similar to cavernous sinus but may have orbital signs (e.g., proptosis, injection, chemosis)

F. **Smooth Pursuit** (Fig. 3-17)

1. Keeps an image on the fovea during slow movement of an object, such as a line moving slowly across an optokinetic drum

2. Cannot be created voluntarily

3. Must be slower than 5 degrees per second to maintain vision with high resolution and high visual acuity

4. Visual targets moving faster than 50 degrees per second induce voluntary fast saccades

5. Stimuli for smooth pursuits may be visual or nonvisual

a. Example of a nonvisual stimulus: proprioceptive input guiding the subject to make pursuit eye movements that follow movements of the limbs in the dark (or with eyes closed)

6. Temporary volitional anticipatory (predictive) pursuit movements also occur in response to predictable target motion, based on previously learned experience

a. Examples: predictive movements of the eyes in anticipation of onset of movement of the visual target (even in the absence of movement of the target) or predictive acceleration of the eye movements when the visual target actually moves

b. These depend on memory for previous tracking experiences

7. Afferent visual information is conveyed to striate cortex and then to occipitotemporal region called medial temporal (MT) and medial superior temporal (MST) areas

8. From MT/MST, information on speed and direction of moving target is conveyed ipsilaterally via arcuate fiber bundles to posterior parietal cortex and contralaterally through corpus callosum to contralateral MT/MST

9. Posterior parietal cortex: directs attention to moving visual stimuli

10. Frontal eye fields and supplementary eye fields

a. Have reciprocal connections with posterior parietal cortex and MT/MST

b. Both fields are responsible for predictive pursuit movements

11. Pursuit pathways: descend to dorsolateral and lateral pontine nuclei via internal capsule and cerebral peduncles

12. Nucleus of the optic tract

a. Pretectal localization in brachium of the superior colliculus

b. Receives retinal input from superior colliculus and cortical input from MT/MST and striate cortex

c. Projects to pontine nuclei and superior colliculus: important for initiating pursuit movements

13. Cerebellar flocculus and paraflocculus: important role in executing smooth pursuit eye movements and in gaze-holding

14. Impairment

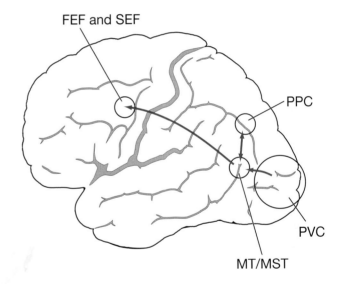

Fig. 3-17. Cortical pathways of the smooth pursuit system. FEF, frontal eye field; MT/MST, medial temporal (MT) and medial superior temporal (MST) areas; PPC, posterior parietal cortex; PVC, primary visual cortex.

Bilateral dysfunction of smooth pursuit system has many nonspecific causes (fatigue, medications, old age, dementia, bilateral smooth pursuit pathway lesions)

Smooth pursuit deficit toward one side usually indicates unilateral lesion(s)

a. With impairment of pursuit eye movements, compensatory catch-up saccades are produced, causing saccadic pursuit eye movements

b. Symmetric saccadic pursuit movements are nonspecific and may occur in several degenerative and toxic or metabolic conditions

c. Asymmetric or unilateral abnormalities of pursuit eye movements may indicate unilateral lesion somewhere in the pathway

d. Unilateral cerebral hemisphere lesions
1) May cause abnormal pursuit and/or impaired tracking of objects to the side of the lesion
2) Often may cause contralateral visual neglect after an acute lesion

G. Saccades

1. Fast (300-700 degrees per second) eye movements that bring visual images of interest onto the fovea

2. Types of saccades
a. Intentional saccades: bring an item quickly into vision
b. Antisaccades: intentional saccades made to look away from an object; requires suppression of saccade toward a novel stimulus and generation of a saccade away from the stimulus (frontal eye fields and prefrontal cortex are probably largely responsible)
c. Reflexive saccades: in response to sudden movement or sound
d. Spontaneous saccades: occur spontaneously at rest or with speech

3. Two mathematical elements of saccades
a. Pulse (velocity) command
b. Step (position) command

4. Pulse-slide-step: gradual transition from the end of the velocity command to a position command

5. Three cortical areas involved with creating saccades (Fig. 3-18)
a. Frontal eye field (Brodmann areas 4 and 6)
1) Intentional saccades help explore visual environment
2) Projects to superior colliculus: responsible for voluntary, intentional change in gaze in response to anticipated or learned experience
3) Lesion causes ipsilateral horizontal gaze deviation ("looks to the lesion"), whereas stimulation (e.g., focal seizure) causes eyes to deviate toward contralateral side
b. Parietal eye field
1) Visual attention and visually guided saccadic control
2) Projects to frontal eye field: contributing to initiation of saccades
3) Projects to superior colliculus: responsible for adjusting gaze and reflexive visual attention to a new visual

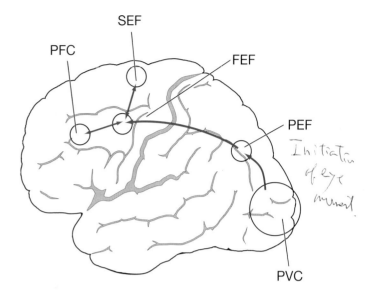

Fig. 3-18. Cortical pathways of the saccadic system. FEF, frontal eye field; PEF, parietal eye field; PFC, prefrontal cortex; PVC, primary visual cortex; SEF, supplementary eye field.

stimulus to explore the environment
c. Supplementary (frontal) eye fields
1) Located in posterior and medial aspect of superior frontal gyrus (supplementary motor cortex)
2) Responsible for motor programs (made of several saccades, complex saccades) as part of learned behavior

6. Other areas involved with saccades
a. Dorsolateral prefrontal cortex
1) Responsible for planning of saccades to target locations; controls inhibition of reflexive visually guided saccades
2) Degenerative disease of prefrontal lobe: patients have difficulty performing antisaccades or suppressing unwanted reflexive saccades (as may occur during visual field examination, "visual grasp reflex")
b. Posterior parietal cortex
1) Directing visual attention
2) Visual-spatial integration
3) Calculating saccadic amplitude
4) Projects predominantly to prefrontal cortex, only minor projections to frontal eye field
c. Medial temporal lobe: controls chronologic order of sequences of saccades
d. Pulvinar
1) Input from retina, superior colliculus, cortex
2) Projects to parietal cortex and guides shifting visual attention
3) Responds to movement of image on retina

4) Roles: maintains accuracy of saccades and directs visual attention to novel stimuli

e. Superior colliculus
   1) Responsible for reflexive visually guided saccades
   2) Receives input from parietal and frontal lobes
   3) Projects to burst cells in brainstem
   4) Frontal eye field and supplementary frontal eye field project directly to brainstem burst cells in parallel with superior colliculus projection

f. Basal ganglia: responsible for memory-guided and anticipatory saccades (relay for indirect projections of frontal eye field, supplementary eye field, and prefrontal cortex to superior colliculus)

g. Cerebellum
   1) Fastigial nucleus projects to brainstem (especially omnipause cells and burst cells) via uncinate fasciculus
   2) Destructive fastigial lesions: tend to be bilateral and produce severely hypermetric saccades in all directions
   3) Unilateral ablation of fastigial nucleus: hypermetria of ipsilateral saccades and hypometria of contralateral saccades
   4) Severe dysmetria (hypermetria) of saccades may give the appearance of macrosaccadic oscillations (may also be seen in patients with visual field defects who make excessive hypermetric saccades to explore defective visual field)
   5) Flocculus lesions: gaze-evoked nystagmus without saccadic pulse dysmetria (primary function affected is gaze holding)

7. Summary of anatomic projections responsible for saccades
   a. Parietal eye fields, prefrontal cortex, frontal eye field, supplementary eye field all project to superior colliculus
   b. Both supplementary eye field and frontal eye field project directly to superior colliculus and brainstem saccade centers
   c. Superior colliculus projects to brainstem saccade centers
   d. Frontal eye field and supplementary eye field also project indirectly to superior colliculus via basal ganglia

8. Brainstem regulation of saccades (Fig. 3-19)
   a. Excitatory burst neurons: responsible for the "pulse," the quick change in eye position
   b. Omnipause neurons
      1) Are located in midpons
      2) Send tonic inhibitory projections to burst cells
   c. Signals from frontal lobe and superior colliculus act to inhibit omnipause cells and initiate a saccade by allowing burst cells to fire
   d. Neural integrator

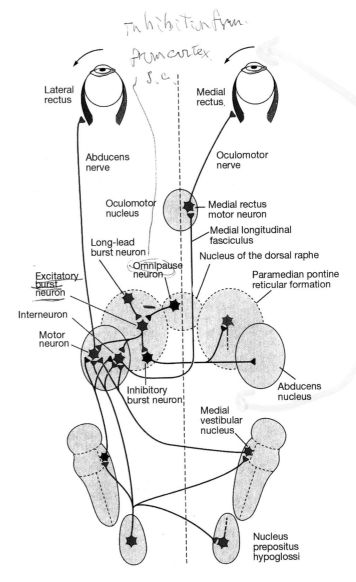

Fig. 3-19. Brainstem projections responsible for horizontal saccades. Signals from the frontal lobe and superior colliculus inhibit the omnipause cells and induce activation of the excitatory burst neurons in paramedian pontine reticular formation. The nucleus prepositus hypoglossi and medial vestibular nucleus are the horizontal gaze neural integrator responsible for gaze holding. Excitatory pathways are indicated with orange and inhibitory, gray. (From Goldberg ME. The control of gaze. In: Kandel ER, Schwartz JH, Jessell TM, editors. Principles of neural science. 4th ed. New York: McGraw-Hill; 2000. p. 783-800. Used with permission.)

1) Calculates eye velocity and stationary commands based on eye position and retinal information
2) Responsible for the "step" (i.e., the tonic discharge responsible for maintenance of eye position) after new position is obtained

e. Inhibitory burst neurons: inhibit saccades
9. Horizontal saccades
  a. Excitatory burst neurons
    1) Located in PPRF (Fig. 3-19)
    2) Project to ipsilateral abducens nucleus, which then projects to contralateral oculomotor nucleus via MLF
    3) Horizontal saccades are generated toward the side of the PPRF that initiates them
  b. Horizontal gaze neural integrators: nucleus prepositus hypoglossi and medial vestibular nucleus
  c. Inhibitory burst neurons for horizontal saccades
    1) Are caudal to abducens nucleus
    2) Inhibit contralateral abducens nucleus from initiating contralateral horizontal saccades
10. Horizontal conjugate gaze palsy
  a. Ablative lesions involving frontal eye field cause patient to "look at the lesion" in the acute phase
  b. Excitatory focus of frontal eye field causes patient to "look away from the lesion"
  c. Lesions involving the prefrontal cortex produce difficulty performing antisaccades or suppressing unwanted reflexive saccades
  d. Ablative pontine lesions involving excitatory burst neurons (PPRF) and horizontal gaze neural integrator causes patient to "look away from the lesion"
  e. Excitatory focus involving PPRF causes patient to "look toward the lesion"
11. Horizontal dysconjugate gaze palsy
  a. Internuclear ophthalmoplegia (INO) (Fig. 3-20)
    1) MLF lesion: weakness of ipsilateral medial rectus, especially evident when making horizontal saccades opposite the side of the paretic muscle
    2) This adductor paresis is often associated with jerk nystagmus in the abducting eye
    3) Slowing of the adducting saccade may be the only sign of partial INO
    4) Bilateral INOs (often asymmetric, partial) frequently seen with multiple sclerosis, but pontine infarct often causes unilateral complete INO
  b. One-and-a-half syndrome: combined unilateral conjugate gaze palsy and INO (Fig. 3-21)
    1) Horizontal gaze paresis in one direction plus medial rectus weakness, usually due to pontine lesions affecting abducens nucleus or PPRF *and* MLF ipsilateral to complete gaze paresis
    2) Often due to focal lesions of pons (e.g., multiple sclerosis, hemorrhage, infarct)
  c. Wall-eyed bilateral INO (WEBINO): marked bilateral exotropia caused by critical lesion of bilateral MLFs
12. Vertical saccades

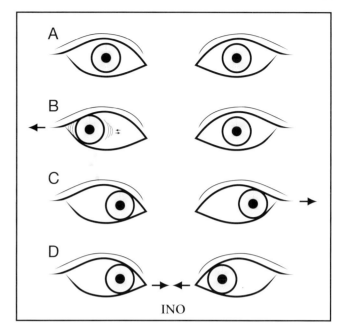

Fig. 3-20. Internuclear ophthalmoplegia (INO) of the left eye due to lesion of left medial longitudinal fasciculus. *A*, Normal primary gaze. *B*, When the patient is asked to look to the right, adduction of the left eye is paralyzed, associated with jerk nystagmus in the abducting eye. *C*, Normal gaze to the left. *D*, Normal convergence. *Arrows*, direction of gaze.

Vertical.

  a. Excitatory and inhibitory burst neurons for vertical and torsional saccades are in the midbrain in rostral interstitial nucleus of MLF
  b. Vertical neural integrator: interstitial nucleus of Cajal
  c. Axons from vestibular nuclei cross in MLF to contralateral interstitial nucleus of Cajal, rostral interstitial nucleus of MLF and trochlear and oculomotor nuclei to generate vertical gaze
  d. Interstitial nucleus of Cajal (vertical neural integrator) projects through posterior commissure to contralateral interstitial nucleus of Cajal and oculomotor and trochlear nuclei
13. Vertical conjugate gaze palsy
  a. Rostral brainstem lesions involving both interstitial nucleus of Cajal and rostral interstitial nucleus of MLF can produce vertical gaze palsies
    1) Thromboembolism at bifurcation of basilar artery can affect Percheron's artery (thalamic-subthalamic paramedian artery), with infarction involving medial thalami and rostral midbrain, including the rostral interstitial nucleus of MLF, bilaterally
    2) Bilateral thalamic involvement may cause coma

In. Top of basilar. pt. unable to look up

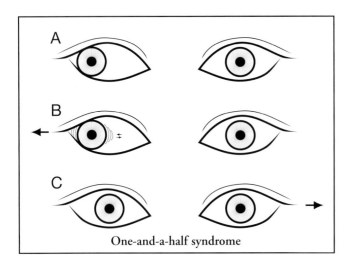

One-and-a-half syndrome

Fig. 3-21. Left one-and-a-half syndrome due to pontine tegmental lesion involving the left abducens nucleus (or left paramedian pontine reticular formation projecting to the abducens nucleus) and medial longitudinal fasciculus originating from the right abducens nucleus, sparing the latter. Because the left abducens nucleus gives rise to the left medial longitudinal fasciculus projecting contralaterally, the lesion essentially involves medial longitudinal fasciculus bilaterally and abducens nucleus ipsilaterally. *A,* Exotropia of the right eye at primary gaze. *B,* Apparent left internuclear ophthalmoplegia on rightward gaze. *C,* Complete saccadic palsy on attempted leftward gaze. *Arrows,* direction of gaze.

3) Bilateral rostral midbrain lesion may cause vertical gaze palsy (which may not be obvious in comatose patient)
b. Dorsal midbrain lesions affecting posterior commissure can cause vertical upward gaze palsy, often with downward ocular deviation
1) Vestibulocephalic vertical eye movements (doll's eyes) may be intact if other vertical gaze centers are intact
2) However, when lesions affect nuclear vertical gaze centers, vertical gaze paresis cannot be overcome by cold water caloric testing or doll's eyes maneuvers
3) Associated symptoms: light-near dissociation (poor-to-absent pupil reactivity to light with preservation of near reaction), absent or excessive convergence, convergence-retraction nystagmus, and Collier's sign (bilateral upper eyelid retraction)
4) This constellation of symptoms: dorsal midbrain syndrome (Parinaud's syndrome)
c. Right hemispheric strokes have been associated with bilateral ptosis (or apraxia of eyelid opening) and up-gaze palsies

d. Huntington's disease: increased saccadic latencies
e. Progressive supranuclear palsy
1) Vertical (especially downward) more than horizontal saccades affected earlier than pursuit movements
2) Slow and hypometric saccades: due to degenerative involvement of rostral interstitial nucleus of MLF (voluntary saccades to command often affected first and earlier than smooth pursuits)
3) Absence of Bell's phenomenon
4) Limitation of convergence and "wide-eyed stare" due to bilateral exophoria and bilateral lid retraction
5) Apraxia of eyelid movements (especially opening)
6) Saccadic intrusions on primary gaze and square wave jerks due to degenerative involvement of superior colliculus
7) Reduced vestibulo-ocular reflex (VOR) suppression
8) Reduced fast component of optokinetic nystagmus
9) Smooth pursuit movements may also be abnormal because of pontine involvement
10) Frontal lobe involvement may produce abnormal antisaccades
11) Eventually, complete bilateral ophthalmoplegia
f. Parkinson's disease: associated with abnormal smooth pursuit movements and hypometric saccades, especially late in disease course
g. Oculogyric crisis
1) Characterized by upward ocular deviation and mental status changes, sometimes accompanied by dystonic deviation of tongue and choreoathetosis
2) Most commonly due to medications such as neuroleptics
3) May also be seen (rarely) in Wilson's disease, acute bilateral thalamic lesions, paraneoplastic syndrome, rhombencephalitis, and several degenerative conditions
h. Setting sun sign: downward ocular deviation in preterm infants with intraventricular hemorrhage
i. Sustained upward ocular deviation in severe hypoxic encephalopathy
j. Paroxysmal upward ocular deviation may occur as epileptic phenomenon and also oculogyric crisis (discussed above)
14. Vertical dysconjugate gaze palsy
a. Skew deviation: vertical ocular misalignment due to supranuclear lesions, lesions involving projections from utricle to interstitial nucleus of Cajal, cerebellum, or different areas of brainstem
1) Ocular tilt reaction: skew deviation associated with conjugate ocular torsion or head tilt
a) Head tilt and ocular torsion are usually toward side

of hypotropic skewed eye

    b) This ipsiversive ocular tilt reaction results from lesion of ipsilateral otoliths, ipsilateral vestibular nerve, or ipsilateral vestibular nucleus disrupting otolithic input to interstitial nucleus of Cajal

    c) Lesions of interstitial nucleus of Cajal or rostral interstitial nucleus of MLF cause contraversive ocular tilt reaction

  2) Pretectal lesions may cause slowly alternating skew deviation, in which there is a cyclical swap of the ocular positions, such that the hypertropic eye falls as the hypotropic eye rises (may also occur with acute hydrocephalus, tentorial herniation, or Wernicke's encephalopathy)

  b. Vertical dysconjugate ocular misalignment: may be due to myasthenia gravis, Graves' thyrotoxicosis (most often affecting inferior rectus muscle), or isolated fourth nerve palsy or partial third nerve palsy

H. Vestibulo-ocular Reflex (VOR)

1. Moves eyes in direction opposite to rotation of the head (conjugate, equal eye movements) and acts to keep image stable on the retina
2. Three semicircular canals (on each side) send signals to vestibular nuclei
3. Bending of hair cells in vestibular labyrinth toward the kinocilium depolarizes axons in vestibular nerve
4. Turning head to the left causes endolymph to flow in opposite direction, activating hair cells in left horizontal canal (Fig. 3-22)
5. This activates ipsilateral lateral vestibular nucleus (which projects to ipsilateral oculomotor nucleus via ascending tract of Deiters) and medial vestibular nucleus (which projects to contralateral abducens nucleus, and this nucleus then projects to contralateral oculomotor nucleus, i.e., ipsilateral to the stimulated vestibular nuclei)
6. Result: excitation of ipsilateral CN III and contralateral CN VI and eye deviation to the right with left head turn
7. Downward head deviation activates left and right anterior semicircular canals and generates upward deviation of the eyes
8. Upward head deviation activates left and right posterior semicircular canals and generates downward deviation of the eyes when the gaze is fixed on an object
9. With pure vertical movements, torsional components are activated equally in opposite directions and block each other
10. Downward head deviation with torsional rotation activates ipsilateral anterior semicircular canal, ipsilateral superior rectus muscle, and contralateral inferior oblique muscle
11. Upward head deviation with torsional rotation activates ipsilateral posterior semicircular canal, ipsilateral superior oblique muscle, and contralateral inferior rectus muscle, producing depression and torsional movement of both eyes toward opposite side
12. VOR gain: ratio of eye velocity to head velocity (opposite directions); this ratio must equal 1 to keep vision stable
13. Ways to examine VOR gain
  a. Dynamic illegible E (or visual acuity) test (with rapid head shaking)
    1) Instruct patient to read a Snellen chart test while shaking the head at a steady rate between 2 and 3 Hz
    2) A decrease in visual acuity more than 2 lines indicates abnormal VOR gain (underactive or overactive)
  b. Ophthalmoscopic examination (with rapid head shaking): examiner concentrates on and follows the optic disc while shaking patient's head at 2 to 3 Hz

I. Convergence Spasm

1. Crossing eyes periodically with otherwise normal neuro-ophthalmologic examination (e.g., full ductions)
2. Characteristic finding: presence of miosis during the spasm
3. Most often occurs in the setting of psychogenic disease
4. The differential diagnosis: divergence weakness or esotropia/excess convergence due to posterior fossa lesions or acute thalamic hemorrhage

J. Other Causes of Ocular Motor Dysfunction

1. Botulism: extraocular muscle paresis like myasthenia gravis but also affects pupil reactivity and accommodation
2. Fisher syndrome (Miller Fisher syndrome)
  a. Rare variant of acute inflammatory demyelinating polyradiculopathy
  b. Clinical features: ataxia, ophthalmoplegia, and areflexia
3. Bell's phenomenon
  a. Physiologic upward (and oblique) rotation of globe with eye closure

> Lesions afffecting the pons generally cause horizontal gaze abnormalities
>
> Lesions affecting the midbrain generally cause vertical gaze abnormalities

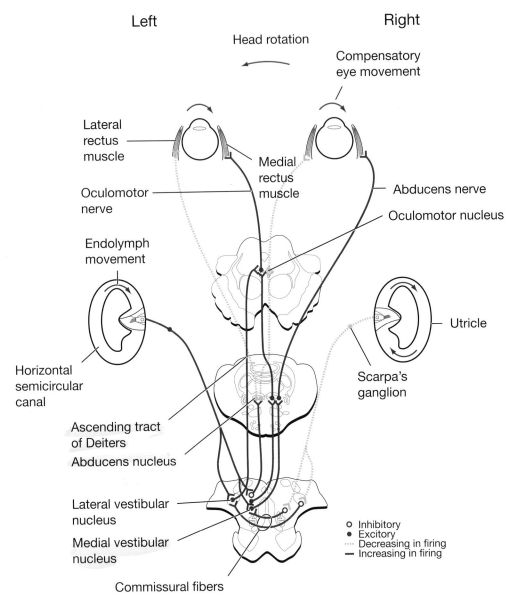

Left   **Right**

Head rotation

Compensatory
eye movement

Lateral
rectus
muscle

Medial
rectus
muscle

Oculomotor
nerve

Abducens nerve

Oculomotor nucleus

Endolymph
movement

Utricle

Horizontal
semicircular
canal

Scarpa's
ganglion

Ascending tract
of Deiters

Abducens nucleus

Lateral vestibular
nucleus

Medial vestibular
nucleus

○ Inhibitory
● Excitory
···· Decreasing in firing
— Increasing in firing

Commissural fibers

Fig. 3-22. Diagram of horizontal vestibulo-ocular reflex. Head rotation to the left excites left horizontal semicircular canal. This occurs because endolymph moves in the opposite direction (i.e., to the right), exciting hair cells in the vestibular labyrinth by deflecting stereocilia hair bundle toward the kinocilium. This depolarizes the hair cell and increases the firing of afferent fibers (i.e., vestibular nerve). The afferents project to the vestibular nuclei. The medial vestibular nucleus has excitatory projections to the contralateral abducens nucleus and inhibitory projections to the ipsilateral abducens nucleus. The medial longitudinal fasciculi project to the contralateral oculomotor nucleus. The net result of left head rotation is activation of the left medial rectus and right lateral rectus muscles, causing compensatory eye movements to the right.

b. Patients with psychogenic spells may have partial eye closure and opening showing the white of the eye as if rolling in the back of the head in the process of normal eye closure and may demonstrate Bell's phenomenon while forcefully attempting to close eyes against examiner's manual attempt to open eyelids

III. DISORDERS OF VISUAL PERCEPTION

A. Loss of Vision
1. History
   a. Loss of vision: monocular or binocular?
   b. Temporal profile of the loss of vision: transient or

persistent? progressive or nonprogressive? acute or gradual onset?

   c. Provoking events, positions, medications?

2. Transient monocular loss of vision

   a. Amaurosis fugax

      1) Most common cause of transient monocular loss of vision

      2) Results from transient ocular ischemia

      3) High-grade stenosis or complete occlusion of ipsilateral internal carotid artery can cause retinal or choroidal hypoperfusion

      4) More commonly, symptoms are due to thromboembolism to retinal circulation

      5) May be associated with Hollenhorst plaque (Fig. 3-23)

      6) Commonly a marker of systemic atherosclerosis and vascular disease

      7) Is a risk factor for cerebral infarction in distribution of ipsilateral internal carotid artery

   b. Occurrence on exposure to bright light suggests critical-grade carotid disease (photogenic claudication) or demyelinating disease (Uhthoff's phenomenon, often unilateral)

   c. Intrinsic ocular disease such as angle-closure glaucoma

   d. Transient visual obscurations associated with unilateral papilledema (subacute or chronic)

   e. Migraine (retinal migraine): possibly retinal artery vasospasm (debated) occurring with migraine headache (diagnosis of exclusion)

   f. Uhthoff's phenomenon: transient loss of vision often in demyelinating disease, due to increased body temperature (exercise, fever)

   g. Gaze-evoked amaurosis: loss of vision when looking in a certain direction or with reading; occurs with tumors near optic nerve or orbital disease, due to traction on nerve

   h. Duration of transient loss of vision may suggest cause

      1) Seconds: papilledema (transient obscurations and dimming of vision), optic disc anomaly, or Uhthoff's phenomenon in setting of an old optic neuritis

      2) Minutes: thromboembolic events, migraine, giant cell arteritis, carotid dissection, ocular ischemic syndrome, ocular or ophthalmologic disease

      3) Hours: carotid artery disease, migraine, thromboembolic disease

3. Acute onset and persistent monocular loss of vision

   a. Anterior ischemic optic neuropathy (arteritic and nonarteritic)

   b. Posterior ischemic optic neuropathy (much less common than anterior ischemic optic neuropathy): may occur with perioperative hypotension and shock

   c. Central retinal artery (or branch) occlusion

      1) Arteritic or nonarteritic

      2) Severe, permanent monocular loss of vision

      3) Ophthalmologic examination: pallor of inner retinal layers from ischemia, with relative preservation of fovea (supplied by choroidal artery), producing the appearance of cherry-red spot (Fig. 3-24)

   d. Central retinal vein occlusion: acute-onset monocular loss of vision and hemorrhagic retinopathy in setting of hypertension and diabetes mellitus

   e. Optic neuritis: usually idiopathic (almost always demyelinating); other causes include infectious (syphilis, Lyme disease, cat-scratch disease), inflammatory (e.g., sarcoidosis); less severe loss of vision than with anterior ischemic optic neuropathy

   f. Neuroretinitis

   g. Intrinsic ocular causes: retinal detachment, vitreous hemorrhage

   h. Traumatic: contusion of optic nerve or damage of nutrient arterial supply

   i. Leber's hereditary optic neuropathy: maternally inherited acute onset of severe optic neuropathy involving one or both eyes (often consecutively in the latter), linked to mitochondrial DNA

   j. Psychogenic

4. Transient simultaneous binocular loss of vision

   a. Most common cause: migraine-related phenomenon (aura) characterized by enlarging scotoma

   b. Transient basilar artery or bilateral posterior cerebral artery ischemia/hypoperfusion: thromboembolism (especially cardiogenic), systemic hypotension; hypercoagulability and hyperviscosity may contribute

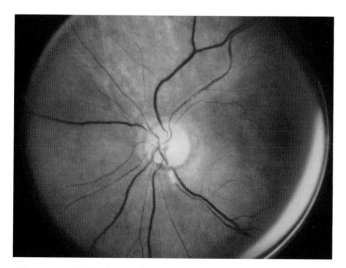

Fig. 3-23. Hollenhorst plaque.

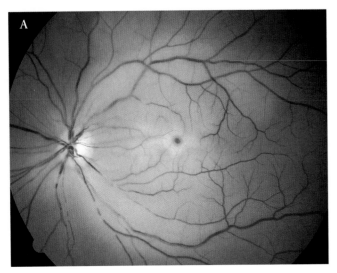
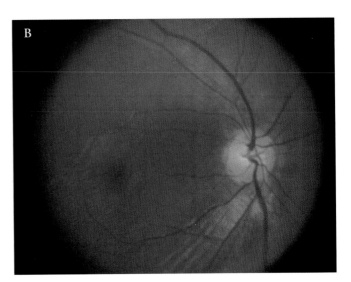

Fig. 3-24. *A,* Central retinal artery occlusion. Whitening of the retina and relative preservation of the fovea produces the appearance of a cherry-red spot. This is in contrast to the cherry-red spot in Tay-Sachs disease, in which there is no retinal whitening or pallor, *B.* (Courtesy of Brian R. Younge, MD.)

5. Acute-onset and persistent binocular loss of vision
   a. Bilateral occipital lobe infarcts: may present with Anton's syndrome (anosognosia for visual defects and confabulation, implicates right thalamic or parietal dysfunction; may also occur with ocular disease in dementia or altered mental status, to be differentiated from release phenomena or other visual hallucinations)
   b. Pituitary apoplexy
   c. Psychogenic: tested with observing normally evoked optokinetic nystagmus and normal eye movements looking at a moving mirror
6. Gradual onset and progressive loss of vision
   a. Compressive: neoplastic (e.g., optic nerve meningioma, sphenoid meningioma, intraorbital metastasis, craniopharyngioma), nonneoplastic (e.g., orbital pseudotumor, aneurysm, thyroid disease-related optic neuropathy)
   b. Infiltrative: neoplastic (e.g., lymphoma, optic nerve glioma, meningeal carcinomatosis), nonneoplastic inflammatory (e.g., sarcoidosis), paraneoplastic retinopathy
   c. Hereditary: autosomal dominant optic atrophy (Kjer's disease), Leber's hereditary optic neuropathy (the latter often presents acutely)
   d. Toxic/nutritional: alcohol-tobacco amblyopia, medications (ethambutol, isoniazid, chloramphenicol, vigabatrin, digitalis, chloroquine)
   e. Radiation-induced retinopathy

B. **Visual Acuity**
1. Retinal lesions do not affect visual acuity unless macula is affected

2. Optic nerve and optic chiasmal lesions impair visual acuity
3. Unilateral retrochiasmal lesions do not impair visual acuity

C. **Visual Field Defects** (permanent, nonprogressive, or progressive loss of vision)
1. Monocular loss of vision is usually due to disease of retina, optic disc, or optic nerve: anterior to optic chiasm
2. Binocular loss of vision may be due to bilateral optic neuropathies or chiasmal or retrochiasmal disease
3. Retrochiasmal homonymous visual field defects become more congruous the farther the lesion is from optic chiasm (i.e., the closer lesion is to occipital lobe)

D. **Disorders of Color Vision Perception**
1. Retinal lesions: affect blue more than red color perception
2. Optic nerve and optic chiasm lesions: impair red color perception
3. Retrochiasmal lesions: impair red color perception
4. Cerebral achromatopsia: lesion of nondominant occipitotemporal cortex affecting medial infracalcarine occipital gyri (fusiform and lingual gyri), often associated with superior quadrantanopia
5. Color agnosia
   a. Patient is not color blind and can read numbers from color plates
   b. Patient is unable to name colors or pick the correct color when prompted (intact general knowledge of colors on verbal cues, knows the color of the sky, etc.)

E.   **Disorders of Cortical Visual Function** (see Chapter 7)

F.   **Positive Visual Phenomena:** definitions
1. Irritative hallucinations may be epileptic, often due to underlying lesion
2. Release hallucinations often occur in association with impaired vision
3. Simple visual hallucinations
   a. Geometric shapes and simple patterns with seizures of occipital origin
   b. Migraine-associated aura (if no headache, called migraine equivalent)
      1) Photopsia (flashes of light)
      2) Fortification spectra, zig-zag lines
      3) Build up gradually over minutes and resolve slowly
      4) May be present for 5 to 30 minutes
      5) May move across visual field
4. Complex visual hallucinations: well-formed images of objects and people; may occur with epileptic foci in posterior temporal lobe
5. Visual hallucinations associated with medications (L-dopa, dopaminergic agonists, methysergide, lysergic acid diethylamide)
6. Visual hallucinations in acute confusional states, especially in the elderly: may be due to various toxic/metabolic abnormalities (e.g., delirium tremens with alcohol withdrawal)
7. Visual hallucinations in psychosis (aural hallucinations are more common in psychosis of primary psychiatric disease)
8. Visual hallucinations of brainstem origin
   a. Peduncular hallucinosis with acute insult to midbrain or thalamus
   b. Visual hallucinations associated with diffuse Lewy body disease (frequently visions of insects)
9. Hypnagogic or hypnopompic hallucinations
   a. Visual hallucinations occurring immediately before falling asleep (hypnagogic) or on awakening (hypnopompic)
   b. Occur in narcolepsy but also in normal subjects
10. Charles Bonnet hallucinations
   a. Well-formed release hallucinations thought to originate from occipitotemporal cortex as result of deprivation of visual sensory input
   b. Usually occur in the evening
   c. May be seen with central visual field defects or intrinsic ocular disease such as severe cataracts or glaucoma usually affecting both eyes
   d. Often consist of well-formed hallucinations of bright objects and people (sometimes animated)

   e. Patients often have reasonable insight and are usually aware that the visions are not real
11. Palinopsia: persistence of image after the stimulus has been removed from visual field; associated with occipitotemporal lesions (may be epileptic phenomenon)
12. Entoptic phenomena
   a. Simple visual experiences originating from peripheral ocular structures (e.g., floaters)
   b. May occur in normal subjects
   c. When excessive, may indicate pathologic state of ocular structures (e.g., retinal detachment)
13. Polyopia: persistance of an object in space, so that a single image may be seen multiple times (associated with migraine headaches)
14. Distortion of image in time and space (metamorphopsia, micropsia, macropsia), may be result of epileptic or migrainous phenomena

G.   **Other Associated Signs and Symptoms of Disorders of Visual Perception**
1. Relative afferent pupillary defect (RAPD)
   a. Retinal lesions do not cause RAPD unless macular involvement is severe
   b. Unilateral or bilateral asymmetric optic nerve disease causes RAPD (Marcus Gunn pupil) in affected optic nerve
   c. Optic tract disease may cause contralateral RAPD and macular splitting (complete) homonymous hemianopia
   d. Lateral optic chiasm lesions cause ipsilateral RAPD
   e. Retrochiasmal lesions do not cause RAPD
2. Optic disc edema (Fig. 3-25 and 3-26)
   a. Associated with loss of vision: papillitis, inflammation of optic disc
   b. Without loss of vision: papilledema (due to increased intracranial pressure)
   c. Unilateral: compressive (sphenoid or optic nerve sheath meningioma), optic neuritis (papillitis), ischemic optic neuropathy, infiltrative (lymphoma, leukemia, carcinomatosis, sarcoidosis); disc edema may not be present with acute optic neuropathy if primary involvement is retrobulbar
   d. Bilateral: papilledema often associated with increased intracranial pressure from hydrocephalus, intracranial lesions (e.g., tumor, infarct, hemorrhage), meningitis (infectious or inflammatory, carcinomatous), veno-occlusive disease with or without venous infarcts, idiopathic intracranial hypertension (pseudotumor cerebri), malignant hypertension, diabetic papillopathy
   e. Chronic papilledema: may lead eventually to atrophy and pallor of optic and nerve fiber layer (secondary optic atrophy) (Fig. 3-26)

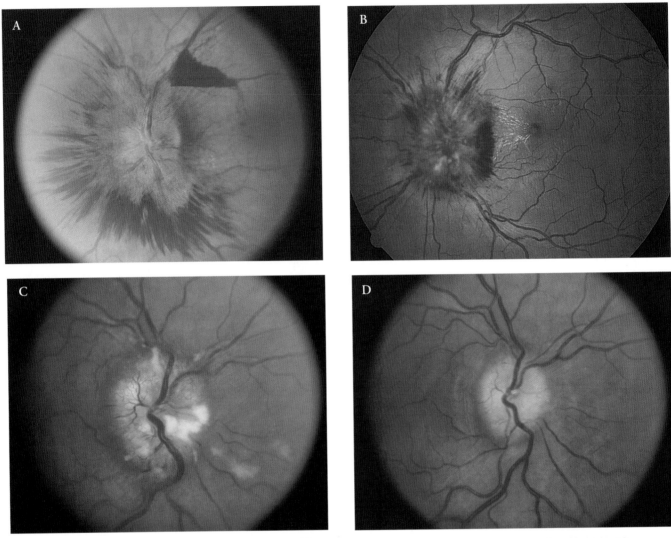

Fig. 3-25. *A,* Terson's syndrome: retinal subhyaloid and peripapillary hemorrhage in the hyperacute stage of presentation in a patient with increased intracranial presssure and subarachnoid hemorrhage. *B,* Severe acute (fully developed) papilledema emerges with progression: the disc appears hyperemic, with blurred margins, splinter hemorrhages, and engorged, dilated surrounding veins. There is early development of tiny hard exudates tracking along the maculopapular bundle. *C,* In the chronic stage, the disc has a pale appearance, and there is persistence of disc edema and cotton-wool spots and continued dilatation of the venous structures and capillaries. Note the appearance of neovascularization and disappearance of hemorrhages. *D,* Less severe papilledema in a patient with pseudotumor cerebri. (*A-D,* Courtesy of Brian R. Younge, MD.)

H. Specific Disorders of Visual Perception

1. Optic neuropathies: generalizations
   a. Optic neuropathy: impairment of optic nerve function
   b. Differential diagnosis: acquired (demyelinating, ischemic, toxic, traumatic, compressive, infiltrative) and hereditary
   c. Clinical features
      1) Unilateral: decrease in visual acuity, contrast sensitivity, and color perception; visual field defect; ipsilateral RAPD; optic disc edema or atrophy (unless acute retrobulbar cause)
      2) Bilateral: decrease in visual acuity, contrast sensitivity, and color perception; visual field defect; light-near dissociation in symmetric cases; optic disc edema or atrophy (unless acute retrobulbar etiology)
2. Optic neuritis
   a. Causes
      1) Demyelinating (most common)

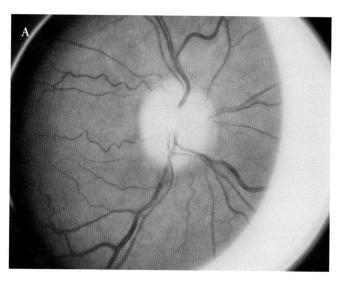 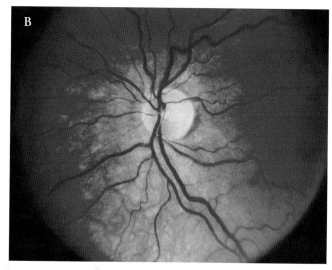

Fig. 3-26. End-stage papilledema is characterized by disc pallor due to optic atrophy and gliosis (atrophic papilledema); the disc margins remain indistinct (*A*). This is in contrast with the optic pallor seen chronically with traumatic transaction of the optic nerve (*B*) or chronic appearance of retrobulbar optic neuritis, in which the disc margins remain sharp and distinct. (Courtesy of Shelley A. Cross, MD.)

2) Other causes: inflammatory polyradiculopathies; infections such as cat-scratch disease, syphilis, Lyme disease, cytomegalovirus; systemic inflammatory disorders such as sarcoidosis, systemic lupus erythematosus; toxic causes such as bee stings, snake bites

b. Clinical features

1) Typically young (<40 years)

2) Acute, typically unilateral loss of vision with impaired visual acuity, contrast sensitivity, and visual field impairment

3) RAPD may be evident

4) Pain of the eye (90%); often worse with movement

5) Edema of optic nerve head (papillitis): one-third of cases

6) Normal optic nerve with retrobulbar involvement: two-thirds of cases

7) In most patients, visual recovery occurs in 2 to 4 weeks (may be delayed up to a year)

c. Treatment

1) Optic Neuritis Treatment Trial (ONTT)

a) Three arms: intravenous methylprednisolone 250 mg every 6 hours for 3 days, followed by oral prednisone (1 mg/kg daily for 11 days); oral prednisone (1 mg/kg daily for 14 days); oral placebo for 14 days

b) No long-term benefit after 1 year in the two treatment groups

c) Corticosteroids: hasten recovery in vision within first 2 weeks

> The diagnosis of optic neuropathy is clinical
>
> Clinical features of optic neuropathy include subjective findings of reduced visual acuity, color perception, and visual field deficit and objective findings such as a relative afferent pupillary defect and optic disc edema or pallor (except in retrobulbar cases)
>
> Bilateral symmetric optic neuropathies may have light-near dissociation

d) Despite low occurrence of immediate side effects in patients receiving oral prednisone, 30% in the prednisone group had recurrent attacks within the first 2 years (vs. 14% in methylprednisolone group), suggesting increased risk of recurrent attacks with oral corticosteroids

e) With 2-year follow-up, rate of development of multiple sclerosis was reduced with intravenous methylprednisolone, but this effect was not observed with 3-year follow-up

3. Ischemic optic neuropathy

a. Arteritic ischemic optic neuropathy

1) Cause: giant cell arteritis

2) Clinical features

a) Constitutional symptoms of polymyalgia rheumatica: malaise, shoulder and hip girdle aches, anorexia, weight loss
b) Headache: new onset, any type
c) Jaw claudication
d) Temporal artery abnormality (e.g, tenderness or beading)
e) May present with amaurosis fugax or transient diplopia
f) Acute, possibly severe monocular or binocular loss of vision
g) Age, older than 55 (mean age, 69); more than 90% of patients older than 60 years
h) Visual field defect: typically altitudinal
i) Optic disc edema: severe ("chalky white"), followed by optic pallor (in affected regions of optic nerve)
j) Concurrent retinal or choroidal ischemia or ischemic optic neuropathy occurring in both eyes simultaneously or consecutively: suggestive of giant cell arteritis (Fig. 3-27)
k) If untreated, 65% of patients have visual loss in other eye

3) Testing
a) Erythrocyte sedimentation rate (ESR) (>50 mm/1 hour) and C-reactive protein abnormal in 70% to 90% of patients
b) ESR may be normal in 10% to 30% of patients with giant cell arteritis
c) If ESR is normal but clinical suspicion remains high: perform temporal artery biopsy as soon as possible
d) Histopathologic confirmation of diagnosis: multinucleated giant cells and necrotizing arteritis seen in temporal artery biopsy specimen

4) Treatment
a) Corticosteroids: should be started the same day as onset of symptoms
b) Corticosteroid therapy should not be delayed for temporal artery biopsy
c) Intravenous corticosteroids considered for severe loss of vision or loss of vision in a monocular patient
d) Corticosteroid dose usually tapered over several months: ESR and clinical examination are used to monitor for recurrence of clinical symptoms

b. Nonarteritic ischemic optic neuropathy (usually anterior ischemic optic neuropathy)
1) Etiology
a) Small-vessel disease associated with vascular risk factors such as diabetes, hypertension, anemia
b) Postsurgical: posterior ciliary artery ischemia

2) Clinical features
a) Acute onset, persistent visual loss (may progress over hours to several days), typically painless (90%), typically in patients older than 50 years
b) Visual field defect: typically altitudinal
c) Optic disc edema with or without peripapillary hemorrhages, followed by optic pallor (regions of optic nerve affected)
d) Visual loss can affect other eye lifelong in 15% to 30% of patients, especially if other eye has small cup-to-disc ratio (0.2) (so-called disc at risk)
e) Visual loss may worsen over 1 to 2 weeks
f) Vision improves in slightly less than half of patients over months

3) Testing
a) ESR and C-reactive protein are normal (common presentation of giant cell arteritis that should always be considered in differential diagnosis)
b) If ESR and C-reactive protein are abnormal, consider giant cell arteritis or false-positive ESR (illness, infection, cancer, etc.)

4) Treatment
a) No known effective treatment to recover visual loss; prevention is key
b) Vasculopathic risk factor modification including blood pressure control, diabetes blood glucose stabilization, correction of lipid profile, and

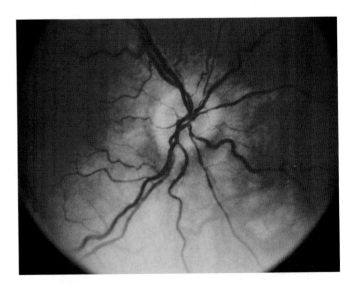

Fig. 3-27. Arteritic anterior ischemic optic neuropathy. Characteristic features are disc edema and associated retinal pallor. (Courtesy of Shelley A. Cross, MD.)

antiplatelet therapy with aspirin are recommended, assuming no contraindications

    c) Avoidance of nocturnal hypotension

4. Optic disc edema with macular star (ODEMS) and neuroretinitis (Fig. 3-28)

  a. Disorder characterized by optic disc edema, inflammatory peripapillary, macular hard exudates that appear in star pattern around macula ("macular star")

  b. Vitreous exudates usually present

  c. Etiology

    1) Idiopathic form: ODEMS

    2) Neuroretinitis refers to infectious or inflammatory causes such as cat-scratch disease or *Bartonella henselae* (most common), Lyme disease, syphilis, *Toxocara*, toxoplasmosis, tuberculosis; viral causes reported include hepatitis B, herpes zoster, Epstein-Barr virus; inflammatory causes include lupus erythematosus and sarcoidosis

  d. Clinical features

    1) Age: 6 to 50 years

    2) Males and females affected equally

    3) May have bilateral eye involvement

    4) Clinical manifestations of optic neuropathy (altered visual acuity, color vision, RAPD) in affected eye

    5) Optic disc edema may precede macular star formation by 1 to 2 weeks

    6) About 50% of patients have antecedent viral infection

    7) About 90% of patients have vitreous inflammatory cells

    8) Patients may have residual visual impairment after ODEMS or neuroretinitis

    9) ODEMS: not a risk factor for multiple sclerosis

  e. Testing

    1) *Bartonella henselae* serology

    2) Chest X-ray (tuberculosis, sarcoidosis, histoplasmosis)

    3) Histoplasmosis serology (especially in endemic areas or with exposure)

    4) Lyme serology

    5) Rheumatologic testing for sarcoidosis, lupus, autoimmune disease

    6) Syphilis testing with RPR or VDRL

    7) *Toxocara* and toxoplasmosis titers if clinical and funduscopic photos suspicious

    8) Tuberculosis testing (purified protein derivative [PPD])

  f. Treatment

    1) Treat any identified infection

    2) Corticosteroids have been used but benefit unknown

    3) In many cases, condition resolves even without treatment

5. Compressive optic neuropathy

  a. Etiology

    1) Brain or intraorbital tumor, either benign or malignant (e.g., meningiomas, gliomas, pituitary adenoma, metastases, lymphoma)

    2) Bone or meningeal disorders: extramedullary hematopoiesis, Paget's disease, idiopathic hypertrophic cranial pachymeningitis

    3) Vascular: arteriovenous malformation (AVM), carotid artery aneurysm, anterior communicating artery aneurysm, orbital hemorrhage

    4) Increased intracranial pressure: hydrocephalus, brain tumor

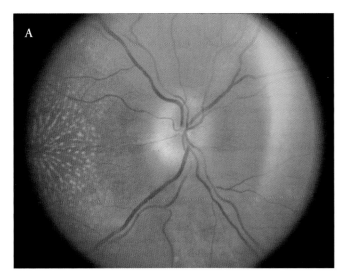 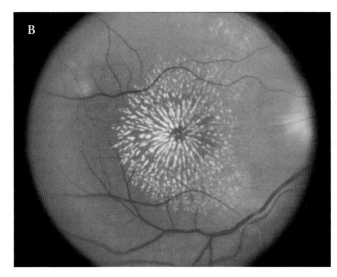

Fig. 3-28. Neuroretinitis with optic nerve edema (*A*) and macular star (*B*). (Courtesy of Brian R. Younge, MD.)

5) Orbital compression: thyroid ophthalmopathy, intra-orbital mass, vascular anomaly

b. Clinical features

1) Painless, progressive loss of vision characteristic of optic neuropathy (optic disc edema, followed by optic atrophy)

2) RAPD

3) Optociliary shunt vessels, indicative of collateral blood flow around chronic optic nerve compression

c. Testing

1) Magnetic resonance imaging (MRI) of brain and orbits with gadolinium and fat saturation sequence

2) Computed tomography (CT) of brain and orbits for acute hemorrhage or trauma, bone lesions, suspected thyroid ophthalmopathy

d. Treatment: directed at underlying cause

e. Foster Kennedy syndrome: papilledema of one optic nerve and optic atrophy of the other, associated with depression or loss of smell, usually due to a frontal lobe tumor or optic nerve meningioma

f. Pseudo-Foster Kennedy syndrome: papilledema of one optic nerve and optic atrophy of the other from ischemic, inflammatory, or infectious cause such as anterior ischemic optic neuropathy, optic neuritis, or syphilis

6. Hereditary optic neuropathies

a. May herald systemic or mitochondrial disorder that may or may not have other neurologic signs

b. Often confused for toxic or nutritional optic neuropathy but family history or genetic testing can help make diagnosis

c. Leber's hereditary optic neuropathy

1) Genetics

a) Mitochondrial DNA (mtDNA) mutations most commonly include 11778, 3460, 14484

b) Inheritance follows mitochondrial pattern: maternal carriers pass gene to all offspring but only up to 83% of men and 32% of women have loss of vision

2) Males affected, rarely females

3) Age at onset: generally 13 to 35 years, but varies (5 to 80 years)

4) Presentation: typically rapid, painless loss of vision progressing to blindness

5) Simultaneous bilateral or sequential loss of vision can occur

6) Spontaneous "remissions" in vision are reported for months to years

7) Signs and symptoms: those of subtle, progressive optic neuropathy (impaired visual acuity and color vision; visual field defects that are primarily central,

paracentral, or centrocecal; RAPD; optic atrophy); may also have telangiectatic microangiopathy and swelling of nerve fiber layer around the disc (pseudo-edema)

8) Dystonia may occur with 11778 and 3460 mtDNA mutations

9) Tremor occurs with all Leber's hereditary optic neuropathy mtDNA mutations

10) Cardiac conduction defects may be coexistent and require screening with electrocardiogram if signs or symptoms are present

d. Autosomal dominant Kjer's optic neuropathy

1) Onset in first decade of life

2) Signs and symptoms of optic neuropathy: impaired visual acuity and color vision; visual field defects that are primarily central or centrocecal; RAPD and optic atrophy

3) Slow progression of visual loss

e. Treatments

1) None proven to restore vision

2) Avoidance of factors that may worsen vision (toxic and nutritional factors)

7. Inflammatory and infiltrative optic neuropathies

a. Etiology: neoplastic (leukemia, lymphoma, carcinomatous meningitis, plasmacytoma); paraneoplastic retinopathy; infectious (human immunodeficiency virus, cryptococcal meningitis, *Aspergillus*, Lyme disease); inflammatory (sarcoidosis, Churg-Strauss angiitis, Wegener's granulomatosis)

b. Clinical features

1) Features of optic neuropathy

2) Inflammatory and neoplastic causes may appear (at least transiently) to be steroid-responsive

c. Testing

1) MRI of brain and orbit with gadolinium and fat suppression

2) Lumbar puncture with cytology, infectious cerebrospinal fluid (CSF) cultures, and serology

3) Complete blood count with differential, infectious serology screening based on history and physical examination

4) Autoimmune testing and chest X-ray may be considered

8. Toxic and nutritional optic neuropathies

a. Etiology

1) Mechanism is unclear

2) Possibly multifactorial such as ethanol and tobacco abuse

3) Questioned mechanisms: malnutrition (deficiencies in thiamine, vitamin B_{12}, folic acid, or a combination),

toxic effects (methanol, ethylene glycol, ethambutol, isoniazid, amiodarone, digitalis, chloramphenicol, metals, fumes, solvents) directly to optic nerve or accumulation of toxic agents causing vascular insult

b. Clinical features: vary with timing and pathophysiology of injury, but all result in optic nerve impairment or optic neuropathy (impaired visual acuity, impaired color vision, visual field defects, RAPD pupillary defect, optic disc edema or pallor)

c. Testing

  1) Serum vitamin B_{12} for pernicious anemia and red blood cell folate level, direct or indirect vitamin assays, serum protein concentrations, antioxidant levels; serologic testing for syphilis; heavy metals

  2) If clinically appropriate, MRI of optic nerves and chiasm with and without gadolinium may be helpful

d. Treatment

  1) Nutritional optic neuropathy

    a) Improved nutrition

    b) Well-balanced diet, supplemented with B vitamins (e.g., thiamine 100 mg orally twice daily, folate 1 mg orally, daily multivitamin), especially in patients abusing alcohol or tobacco

    c) For pernicious anemia, parenteral vitamin B_{12} supplementation may be necessary

  2) Tobacco-alcohol amblyopia

    a) Same as for nutritional optic neuropathy; vitamin B_{12} injections may help even when smoking continues

    b) Smoking or alcohol cessation with improved diet

    c) Elimination of causative agent (e.g., tobacco, alcohol)

  3) Toxic optic neuropathies

    a) Identify and remove offending agent

    b) Other than stopping offending agent, no specific treatment available for optic neuropathy caused by ethambutol

    c) Once this is accomplished, recovery may take weeks to months

    d) Rarely, vision may still decrease or fail to recover even when the drug is stopped

9. Traumatic optic neuropathies

  a. Etiology: damage to optic nerve(s) from head trauma or damage to orbit resulting in direct or indirect compression, optic nerve transection, or vascular insult to optic nerve

  b. Clinical features: vary with timing and pathophysiology of injury, but all result in optic nerve impairment or optic neuropathy (impaired visual acuity and impaired color vision, visual field defects, RAPD, pupillary defect, optic disc edema or pallor)

  c. Testing: CT is modality of choice for acute trauma, with emphasis on orbits and brain

  d. Treatment

    1) Corticosteroid therapy has been reported but efficacy uncertain

    2) Directed at discovering and remedying neuroanatomic lesion responsible for optic nerve impairment (e.g., decompressing optic nerve from compressed traumatic orbit)

IV. PUPILLARY DISORDERS AND HORNER'S SYNDROME

A. Neuroanatomy of Pupillary Light Reflex (Fig. 3-29)

1. Pupillary diameter: determined by opposing sympathetic (pupil dilating) and parasympathetic (pupil constricting) inputs

2. Parasympathetic component

  a. Afferent arm of reflex: via retina, optic nerve, optic chiasm to brachium of superior colliculus and dorsal midbrain—synapse in pretectal nuclei (Fig. 3-29 and 3-30)

  b. Interneuron: pretectal nucleus, which projects to ipsilaterally and contralaterally to Edinger-Westphal nucleus, the preganglionic parasympathetic neurons for miosis

  c. Efferent arm of reflex

    1) Preganglionic parasympathetic axons from Edinger-Westphal nucleus travel in oculomotor nerve to the orbit and synapse in ciliary ganglion

    2) Postganglionic parasympathetic axons from ciliary ganglion innervate iris sphincter and release acetylcholine, causing pupillary constriction

3. Sympathetic pupillary projections: three-neuron arc (Fig. 3-30)

  a. First-order (central): projections from posterior hypothalamus via dorsal longitudinal fasciculus (in brainstem reticular formation) to preganglionic sympathetic neurons

  b. Second-order: preganglionic sympathetic neurons in ciliospinal center of Budge (intermediolateral cell column at C8-T1)—axons travel via ventral root and paraspinal ganglionic chain traveling over lung apex and above subclavian artery, to synapse in superior cervical ganglion

  c. Third-order: postganglionic sympathetic neurons in superior cervical ganglion—axons travel along carotid artery intracranially as internal carotid plexus

  d. Postganglionic vasoconstrictor and sudomotor (sweat) fibers to face originate in superior cervical ganglion and travel via external carotid artery to the face (exception is

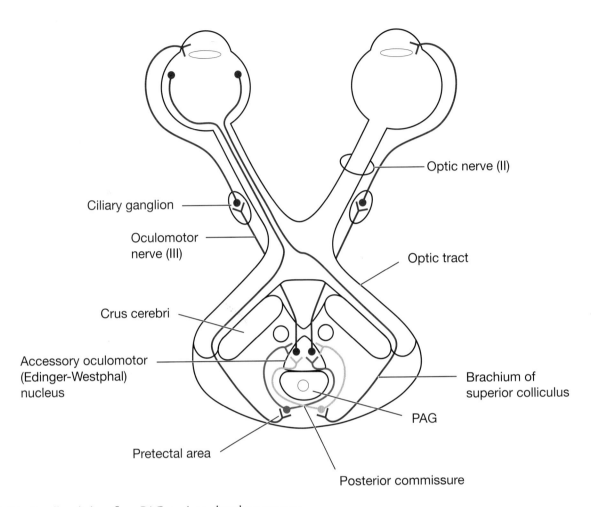

Fig. 3-29. Pupillary light reflex. PAG, periaqueductal gray matter.

forehead: sudomotor innervation of forehead is from terminal branches of internal carotid plexus)

e. Some sympathetic fibers of the carotid plexus also pass through the middle ear

f. Internal carotid plexus sends projections to ophthalmic division of CN V (V_1)

g. Long posterior ciliary nerve originates from the V_1 of the trigeminal nerve, and short ciliary nerves from the ciliary ganglion (without synapse): both supply innervation to the dilator of the pupil

h. Postganglionic sympathetic neurons release norepinephrine, which binds to α-adrenergic receptors on dilator of the pupil, causing pupillary dilatation

B. Horner's Syndrome

1. Causes: any lesion along the three-neuron arc
  a. First-order localization and causes
    1) Diencephalon and brainstem
    2) Occurs after brainstem infarction (e.g., lateral medullary syndrome of Wallenberg) and with brainstem hemorrhage, tumor or demyelination
    3) Lesions of cervical cord may interrupt descending (central) sympathetic projections (compressive lesions such as tumor or vascular malformations; syrinx; demyelination; trauma)
  b. Second-order localization and causes
    1) Root (radiculopathy, arteriovenous fistula, tumor)
    2) Chest (Pancoast's tumor or apical tumor, often lung cancer)
    3) Brachial plexus lesions (neoplasms, trauma)
    4) Cervical rib
    5) Anterior neck lesions (tumor, trauma, iatrogenic injury)
    6) Other head and neck compressive lesions spatially related to sympathetic pathways (e.g., mediastinal and hilar lymphadenopathy, thyroid adenoma, glomus tumors)
    7) Rowland Payne syndrome: preganglionic Horner's syndrome associated with vocal cord paralysis and phrenic nerve palsy

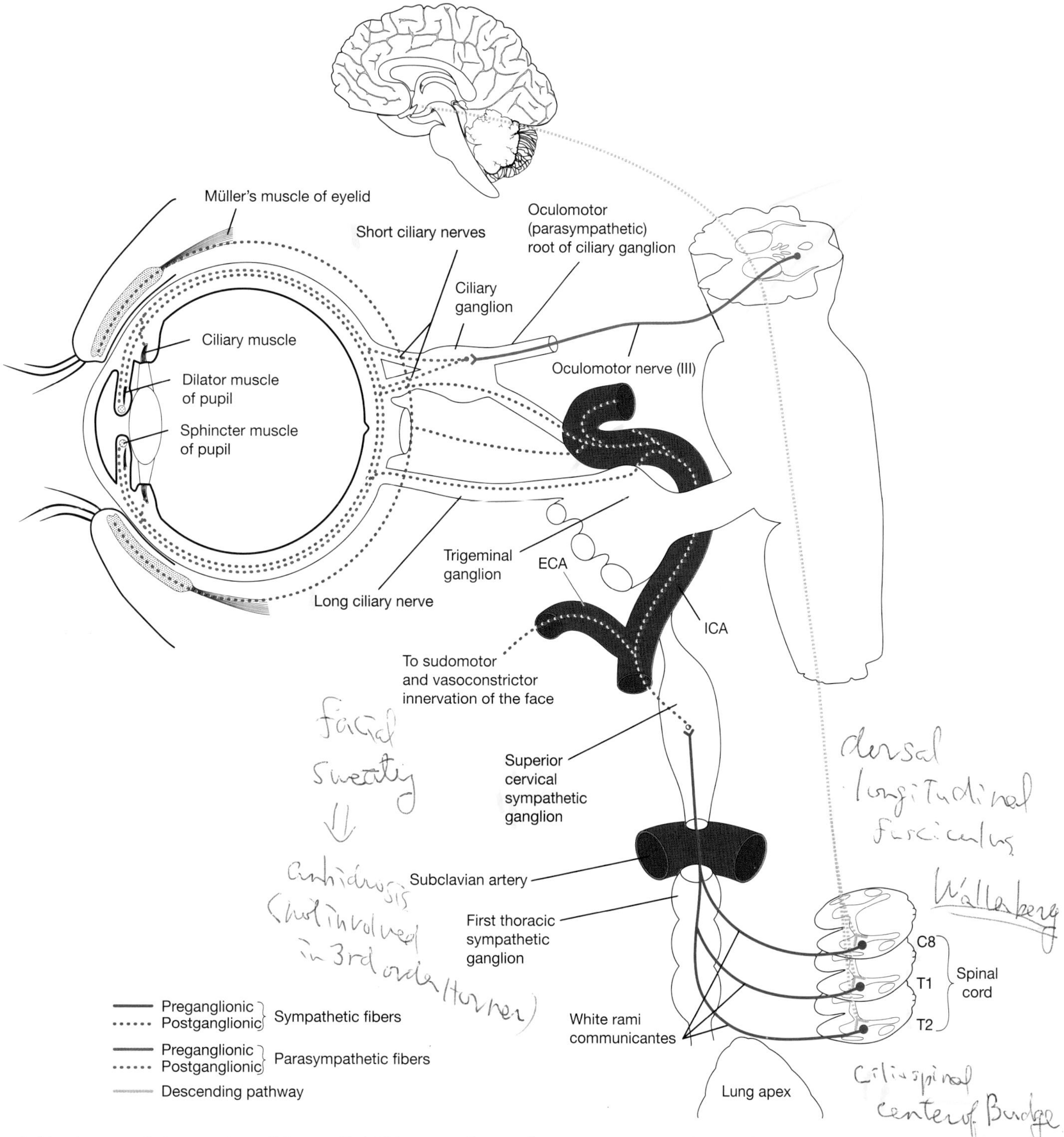

Müller's muscle of eyelid

Short ciliary nerves

Oculomotor
(parasympathetic)
root of ciliary ganglion

Ciliary
ganglion

Ciliary muscle

Dilator muscle
of pupil

Sphincter muscle
of pupil

Oculomotor nerve (III)

Trigeminal
ganglion

ECA

ICA

Long ciliary nerve

To sudomotor
and vasoconstrictor
innervation of the face

Superior
cervical
sympathetic
ganglion

Subclavian artery

First thoracic
sympathetic
ganglion

facial
sweating
↓↓
anhidrosis
(not involved
in 3rd order Horner)

dorsal
longitudinal
fasciculus

Wallenberg

C8

T1

T2

Spinal
cord

Ciliospinal
center of Budge

White rami
communicantes

Lung apex

———— Preganglionic ⎫ Sympathetic fibers
· · · · · Postganglionic ⎭

———— Preganglionic ⎫ Parasympathetic fibers
· · · · · Postganglionic ⎭

———— Descending pathway

Fig. 3-30. Autonomic innervation of the pupil. ECA, external carotid artery; ICA, internal carotid artery.

c. Third-order localization and causes
   1) Superior cervical ganglion (e.g., trauma)
   2) Internal carotid artery (e.g., dissection)
   3) Base of skull (e.g., nasopharyngeal carcinoma, tumor)

   4) Middle ear (tumor, trauma)
   5) Cavernous sinus (e.g., carotid-cavernous fistula,
      tumor such as pituitary adenoma, pituitary apoplexy,
      cavernous sinus thrombosis, intracavernous internal

carotid artery aneurysm, inflammation [Tolosa-Hunt syndrome])

6) Third-order Horner's syndrome does not involve anhidrosis of face (except for a small portion of forehead supplied by terminal branches of internal carotid plexus)

2. Clinical findings (ipsilateral)

   a. Ptosis: small (typically <2 mm), weakness of sympathetically innervated Müller's muscle (present in both upper and lower eyelids); affecting both upper and lower lids (latter deficit sometimes called upside-down ptosis)

   b. Miosis with dilation lag (pupil dilates slowly compared with normal eye, with greater anisocoria in 5 seconds than 15 seconds)

   c. Facial anhidrosis

3. Testing

   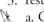 a. Cocaine test

      1) One drop of 10% cocaine solution in each eye, followed by the same after 1 minute

      2) In dark room 45 minutes after cocaine solution applied, examine pupils

         a) Normal pupil dilates, whereas sympathetically denervated (Horner's) pupil does not

         b) Warn patient that urine may test positive for cocaine for 48 to 72 hours

   b. Hydroxyamphetamine (paredrine) topical 1% test

      1) Performed at lest 48 hours after cocaine test

      2) Third-order Horner's pupil will not dilate

      3) First- and second (preganglionic)-order Horner's pupil will dilate

   c. No pharmacologic testing distinguishes between first- and second-order neuron Horner's pupil

C. Physiologic Anisocoria

1. Occurs in about 20% of normal population; pupil size may vary daily

2. Normal lids; pupil size difference is same in light and dark

3. Pupil size difference is typically less than 1 mm

D. Parasympathetic Dysfunction

1. Adie's (tonic) pupil

   a. Epidemiology

      1) Adie's pupil is common cause of anisocoria in women

      2) Female:male ratio is 3:1

      3) In women in third to fourth decade of life

      4) 80% of cases are unilateral

   b. Pathophysiology

      1) Tonic pupil occurs from damage to ciliary ganglion or short ciliary nerves (causing poor response to light),

followed by reinnervation and aberrant collateral sprouting

2) Initial stage (shortly after the primary injury): pupil becomes fixed and dilated, with loss of accommodation

3) Normal subjects: 30-fold higher postganglionic innervation of ciliary muscle than iris sphincter muscle

4) Reinnervation is haphazard and distributed more evenly between iris sphincter and ciliary muscle

5) This results in redirection (aberrant reinnervation) of some ciliary innervation to iris sphincter

6) Therefore, pupil remains large, poorly reactive to light, and irregular in shape, with vermiform (segmental constrictive) movements in response to light (because of haphazard reinnervation)

7) Chronic stage: accommodative response may recover and pupil become smaller

   c. Light reactivity of pupil is poor and segmental, and near response is tonic

   d. Anisocoria is greater in light

   e. One drop of 0.125% pilocarpine in both eyes causes Adie's tonic pupil to constrict, because of denervation and choline hypersensitivity, but normal pupil is not affected by this low concentration

   f. When associated with absent or diminished tendon reflexes, the condition is called Adie's syndrome or Holmes-Adie syndrome

   g. Treatment

      1) Adie's pupil is benign condition, with no treatment

      2) Patient reassurance is important

2. Ross syndrome: tonic pupils associated with hyporeflexia and segmental hypohidrosis

3. Association with third nerve palsy

4. Pharmacologic mydriasis: scopolamine, atropine, or phenylephrine usually causes a very large pupil, not segmentally affected (360-degree involved)

5. Argyll Robertson pupil

   a. Hallmark of neurosyphilis

   b. Both pupils are miotic, unreactive or poorly reactive to light, yet reaction may be asymmetric

   c. Light-near dissociation: no pupil constriction to bright light but brisk pupil constriction to near reaction

   d. Pupils are small, frequently irregular in shape, and have variable iris atrophy

   e. Pupils dilate poorly with pharmacologic mydriatic agents

   f. Vision in affected eye must be relatively normal

6. Causes of light-near dissociation

   a. Adie's pupil (discussed above)

   b. Argyll Robertson pupil of neurosyphilis (discussed above)

c. Dorsal midbrain syndrome

d. Wernicke's encephalopathy

e. Familial amyloidosis

f. Intraorbital lesion of ciliary ganglion or short ciliary nerves: trauma, tumors, iatrogenic (ocular surgery), viral ganglionitis

g. Related to peripheral neuropathy (inherited or acquired, the latter including neuropathies caused by long-standing diabetes, amyloidosis, alcohol and other toxins, vasculitis)

7. Preganglionic injury to oculoparasympathetic pathway (large, poorly reactive pupil)

a. Brainstem: ischemic or hemorrhagic lesion, mass lesion such as tumor or vascular malformation

b. Subarachnoid space: intraneuronal ischemia, aneurysm, basilar meningitis

c. Cavernous sinus: compressive lesion such as tumor (meningioma, pituitary adenoma), carotid-cavernous aneurysm and fistula, cavernous sinus thrombosis, inflammatory (Tolosa-Hunt syndrome)

V. NYSTAGMUS AND EYE OSCILLATIONS

A. Nystagmus

1. Definition: rhythmic, involuntary biphasic oscillation ("to and fro") of eyes that originates from and is perpetuated by pathologic slow eye movements

2. Description: trajectory, direction, frequency, amplitude, and latency

3. Trajectory: horizontal, vertical, rotatory (torsional), vertical, downbeat, upbeat

4. Direction: defined by the fast phase eye movement (e.g., slow rightward movement of the eyes with a fast eye movement to the left is a leftward horizontal nystagmus)

5. Conjugate nystagmus affects both eyes symmetrically

6. Disconjugate nystagmus may affect one (monocular) or both eyes (latter, asymmetrically)

7. Dissociated: refers to different nystagmus amplitudes in either eye

8. Pendular nystagmus: phases of equal velocity

9. Jerk nystagmus: phases of unequal velocity

10. Alexander's law: jerk nystagmus increases in amplitude with gaze toward direction of fast phase

B. Physiologic Nystagmus

1. End-position nystagmus—fatigue (prolonged deviation of eyes), nystagmus on extremes of gaze (right or left) that return to normal in primary gaze

2. Optokinetic nystagmus (OKN)

a. Combination of pursuit and saccadic eye movements to direct fovea on successive targets with the OKN stimulus

b. Abnormal when reduced: lesions of temporal and parietal lobes may cause impaired OKN toward side of lesion

c. To examine

1) OKN drum or tape with vertical lines that, when turned, creates line motion (often used)

2) The drum can be turned to create line motion, to the right, left, up, or down

d. OKN drum can be used to test for psychogenic blindness

e. May also bring out adduction lag in INO

3. Caloric nystagmus

a. Cold water injected into ear creates convection current within endolymph toward the ampulla, stimulating vestibular slow eye movement toward cold water and fast jerks away from cold water

b. Warm water creates the opposite slow and fast eye movements

c. COWS (**c**old **o**pposite, **w**arm **s**ame) indicates the side of the fast component

C. Specific Types of Nystagmus

1. Peripheral vestibular nystagmus

a. Unidirectional, uniplanar jerk nystagmus

b. Trajectory usually horizontal-torsional with complete labyrinthine destruction, or upbeat-torsional with selective involvement of a posterior semicircular canal (as with benign paroxysmal positional vertigo [BPPV])

c. Torsional component usually present

d. Fast component usually away from side of lesion: hypofunction of affected labyrinth in face of preserved contralateral labyrinthine function causes slow eye movements toward side of vestibulopathy and away from normal side, followed by a fast, corrective conjugate movement of the eyes away from side of lesion

e. Pure vertical or pure torsional trajectories often indicate a central origin

f. Nystagmus greatest toward direction of fast component (Alexander's law) or away from damaged vestibular organ

g. Nystagmus suppressed by visual fixation

h. Nystagmus exacerbated or induced by head movement (as with Dix-Hallpike maneuver, horizontal vigorous head shaking), hyperventilation, Valsalva maneuver, vibration of bony mastoid process, and, rarely, with loud auditory stimuli (latter three may occur in peripheral vestibulopathies related to perilymph fistula or superior canal dehiscence)

i. Nystagmus induced by Dix-Hallpike maneuver indicates BPPV: there is often a latency, and nystagmus tends to fatigue and fade during the same maneuver and with successive repetitive maneuvers

  j. Associated vestibulocochlear symptoms (tinnitus, hearing loss, vertigo) often present

2. Spasmus nutans

  a. Classic triad of pendular nystagmus, head nodding, and head turn (torticollis)

  b. Onset in first 18 months of life, resolves by 3 years

  c. Pendular, horizontal, or vertical low-amplitude high-frequency intermittent nystagmus, may be conjugate or disconjugate or monocular

  d. Unclear whether head nodding is a compensatory mechanism to reduce the nystagmus or a primary abnormality

  e. Diagnosis of exclusion; MRI is performed to exclude intracranial lesion

3. Bruns' nystagmus

  a. Heralds cerebellopontine angle mass compressing brainstem, with peripheral vestibular nerve involvement (e.g., acoustic neuroma, brainstem glioma, cerebellar tumor)

  b. Manifests as vestibular nystagmus and peripheral vestibular symptoms

  c. Two components

    1) Small-amplitude, rapid jerk gaze-evoked nystagmus when looking away from side of lesion (due to vestibular dysfunction)

    2) Slow, large-amplitude gaze-evoked nystagmus when looking toward side of lesion (due to abnormal gaze holding)

4. Congenital nystagmus

  a. Characteristic increasing velocity exponential slow phase on eye movement recordings

  b. Binocular and conjugate, with similar amplitude on both sides

  c. Uniplanar

    1) Plane or direction of nystagmus (usually horizontal): unchanged in all positions of gaze

    2) Seen in only three conditions: congenital nystagmus, peripheral vestibular nystagmus, periodic alternating nystagmus

  d. No oscillopsia (illusion of environmental movement) but may have head oscillation

  e. Dampened by convergence, increased by fixation effort

  f. Inversion of OKN (nystagmus is in opposite direction than expected)

5. Latent nystagmus

  a. Present since infancy

  b. Believed due to dysfunctional binocular vision early in life; associated with strabismus

  c. Arises (or enhanced) after one eye is covered

  d. Conjugate nystagmus with fast phase away from covered

eye, predominantly horizontal (with or without torsional and/or vertical components)

  e. Typically associated with esotropia

6. Dissociated nystagmus: example is abducting nystagmus in INO

7. See-saw and hemi-seesaw nystagmus

  a. Pendular (see-saw) nystagmus: cyclic eye movements, with elevation and intorsion of one eye and simultaneous depression and extortion of opposite eye, followed by complete reversal of the movement

  b. Jerk (hemi-seesaw) nystagmus: one-half of seesaw cycle

  c. Described in large parasellar tumors (most common) and brainstem lesions (including multiple sclerosis, syringobulbia, and Wallenberg's syndrome)

8. Convergence-retraction nystagmus (in Parinaud's syndrome)

  a. Eyes have asynchronous, adducting saccades

  b. Lid retraction (Collier's sign)

  c. Vertical gaze paresis

  d. Light-near dissociation

  e. Skew deviation

  f. Most likely cause in neonates: congenital aqueductal stenosis

9. Periodic alternating nystagmus

  a. Spontaneous horizontal nystagmus of the primary gaze

  b. Eyes display jerk nystagmus in primary position for 1 to 2 minutes, stop for a few seconds, nystagmus reverses direction in alternating fashion

  c. Poor suppression by visual fixation

  d. Etiology

    1) Congenital

    2) Posterior fossa anomalies (e.g., Arnold-Chiari malformation)

    3) Cerebellar degeneration, tumor, infection, demyelinating disease (multiple sclerosis)

    4) Brainstem encephalitis

    5) Ataxia-telangiectasia

    6) Anticonvulsant agents

10. Downbeat nystagmus

  a. Usually a central origin

  b. Present in primary gaze, central position

  c. Nystagmus usually worse on downward gaze

  d. Poor suppression by visual fixation

  e. May be exacerbated by changes in position of head or hyperventilation

  f. Etiology

    1) Craniocervical or posterior fossa anomalies (e.g., Chiari malformation)

    2) Cerebellar infarction, tumor, degeneration (e.g., spinocerebellar ataxia 6, multiple system atrophy)

3) Toxic (alcohol, thiamine deficiency, lithium, anticonvulsants, amiodarone, toluene)
4) Congenital
11. Upbeat nystagmus
   a. Most often, a central origin in its pure form
   b. Present on primary gaze, central position
   c. Nystagmus usually worse on upward gaze
   d. Poor suppression by visual fixation
   e. Etiology
      1) Cerebellar degeneration
      2) Arnold-Chiari malformation
      3) Brainstem infarction or hemorrhage
      4) Brainstem encephalitis
      5) Wernicke's encephalopathy
      6) Pelizaeus-Merzbacher disease
      7) Paraneoplastic syndrome
      8) Congenital cause

D. Gaze-Evoked Nystagmus

1. Does not occur in primary gaze and is nonspecific (multiple causes)
2. Etiology
   a. Posterior fossa disease
   b. Drugs (phenytoin, barbiturates)

E. Periodic Eye Deviations

1. Periodic alternating gaze deviation (see periodic alternating nystagmus above)
   a. Slow, conjugate eye deviation to one side for about 2 minutes then alternates to other side for the same time; this process cycles continuously
   b. Awake patients, generally with abnormalities of posterior fossa (usually involving cerebellum)
2. Ping-pong gaze (short-cycle periodic alternating gaze)
   a. Cyclic horizontal roving eyes similar to periodic alternating gaze deviation but a shorter cycle (2-8 seconds)
   b. Comatose patients, usually with bilateral cerebral dysfunction or damage
3. Ocular tilt reaction
   a. Rare, transient eye movement disorder
   b. Consists of head tilt, skew deviation (vertical eye misalignment), and conjugate eye torsion

F. Oculomasticatory Myorhythmia

1. Pathognomonic of Whipple's disease
2. Smooth rhythmic eye convergence, followed by return to primary position
3. Rhythmic elevation and depression of mandible

G. Monocular or Asymmetric Binocular Oscillations

1. Spasm nutans and mimickers
2. Monocular visual deprivation
3. Monocular downbeat or torsional nystagmus
4. Congenital nystagmus
5. Acquired monocular pendular nystagmus
6. Ictal monocular horizontal nystagmus
7. INO
8. Partial extraocular muscle paresis
9. Restrictive syndrome of extraocular muscles
10. Superior oblique myokymia

H. Saccadic Intrusions and Oscillations

1. Square wave jerks: small-amplitude left or right horizontal deviation, followed by return to primary gaze
2. Square wave oscillations: continuous square wave jerk activity
3. Macrosquare wave jerks: large-amplitude square wave jerks; may be seen in multiple sclerosis
4. Ocular flutter: biphasic oscillation, horizontal saccadic eye movement without intersaccadic interval
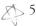
5. Opsoclonus
   a. Rapid, multivectorial, chaotic, fast eye movements
   b. Seen in neuroblastoma paraneoplastic effects in infants; in adults, result of encephalitis or paraneoplastic effect
6. Ocular dysmetria: ocular equivalent of limb dysmetria or past-pointing
7. Overshoot or hypermetric saccades are seen in cerebellar disease

I. Differential Diagnosis of Opsoclonus, Ocular Flutter

1. Encephalitis
2. Meningitis
3. Hydrocephalus
4. Kinsbourne's myoclonic encephalopathy, or dancing eyes and dancing feet
5. Neuroblastoma
6. Toxic: thallium, toluene, organophosphates, phenytoin, lithium, anticonvulsants
7. Paraneoplastic: small cell lung cancer, breast cancer
8. Congenital

J. Classification of Binocular Symmetric Eye Oscillations

1. Dysconjugate
   a. Vertical: seesaw nystagmus
   b. Horizontal
      1) Convergence retraction nystagmus
      2) Divergence nystagmus
      3) Oculomasticatory myorhythmia
      4) See-saw nystagmus

2. Conjugate nystagmus
   a. Two types: jerk and pendular nystagmus
      1) Jerk nystagmus
         a) Induced: optokinetic, rotational, caloric, positional, hyperventilation, and Valsalva maneuver
         b) Spontaneous: primary position
            i) Horizontal
            ii) Torsional
            iii) Vertical: upbeat and downbeat nystagmus
         c) Eccentric gaze (gaze-evoked)
      2) Pendular nystagmus
         a) Oculopalatal myoclonus
         b) Spasmus nutans
         c) Visual deprivation
         d) Pendular nystagmus
         e) Congenital nystagmus
3. Binocular symmetric jerk nystagmus: congenital nystagmus

VI. DISORDERS OF THE EYELIDS: PTOSIS, LID RETRACTION, AND LID LAG

A. Lid Anatomy and Physiology
1. Frontalis muscle: CN VII innervation
2. Orbicularis oculi muscle: CN VII innervation
3. Müller's muscle: sympathetic innervation
4. Levator palpebrae superioris: CN III innervation

B. Ptosis
1. Measured where eyelid imposes on iris or limbus, with normal position being 1.5 mm below the upper limbus
2. Ptosis is encroachment of eyelid from its normal position toward or on the pupil
3. Etiology
   a. Cortical or cerebral ptosis: typically lesion in right frontal lobe causing contralateral or bilateral ptosis
   b. CN III nucleus lesion may cause bilateral ptosis
   c. Third nerve palsy: ipsilateral moderate to severe ptosis
   d. Oculosympathetic dysfunction (Horner's syndrome): mild weakness of both upper and lower eyelids
   e. Myasthenia gravis
   f. Muscle and mechanical eyelid abnormalities

C. Lid Retraction and Lid Lag
1. Lid retraction may be present if upper eye sclera is observed between the lid margin in primary gaze
2. Lid lag may be present if similar findings are noted on down gaze
3. Etiology: thyroid eye disease is common cause of lid retraction; other causes, progressive supranuclear palsy, dorsal midbrain lesions, levator hyperactivity, proptosis, aberrant regeneration of CN III when adducting, myasthenia gravis, periodic paralysis

REFERENCES

Aragones JM, Bolibar I, Bonfill X, Bufill E, Mummany A, Alonso F, et al. Myasthenia gravis: a higher than expected incidence in the elderly. Neurology. 2003;60:1024-6.

Brazis PW, Lee AG. Part X. Neuro-ophthalmology. In: Evans RW, editor. Saunders manual of neurologic practice. Philadelphia: Saunders; 2003. p. 371-420.

Brazis PW, Masdeu JC, Biller J. Localization in clinical neurology. 4th ed. Philadelphia: Lippincott Williams & Wilkins; 2001.

Horton JC. Wilbrand's knee of the primate optic chiasm is an artefact of monocular enucleation. Trans Am Ophthalmol Soc. 1997;95:579-609.

Kline LB, Bajandas FK. Neuro-ophthalmology Review Manual. 4th ed. Thorofare, NJ: Slack, Inc; 1996.

Kolb H. How the retina works. Am Sci. 2003;91:28-35.

Krolak-Salmon P, Guenot M, Tiliket C, Isnard J, Sindou M, Mauguiere F, et al. Anatomy of optic nerve radiations as assessed by static perimetry and MRI after tailored temporal lobectomy. Br J Ophthalmol. 2000;84:884-9.

Kubis KC, Danesh-Meyer HV, Savino PJ, Sergott RC. The ice test versus the rest test in myasthenia gravis. Ophthalmology. 2000;107:1995-8.

Lee AG, Brazis PW. Clinical pathways in neuro-ophthalmology: an evidence-based approach. 2nd ed. New York: Thieme; 2003.

Lee AG, Hayman LA, Brazis PW. The evaluation of isolated third nerve alsy revisited: an update on the evolving role of magnetic resonance, computed tomography, and catheter angiography. Surv Ophthalmol. 2002;47:137-57.

Leigh RJ, Zee DS. The neurology of eye movements. 3rd ed. New York: Oxford University Press; 1999.

Miller NR, Newman NJ, editors. The essentials: Walsh & Hoyt's clinical neuro-ophthalmology. 5th ed. Baltimore: Williams & Wilkins; 1999. p. 85-100; 323-68.

The Optic Neuritis Study Group. Visual function 5 years after optic neuritis: experience of the Optic Neuritis Treatment Trial. Arch Ophthalmol. 1997;115:1545-52.

IMPORTANT WEB SITES

The William F. Hoyt Neuro-ophthalmology Collection. http://medstat.med.utah.edu/neuroophth/Hoyt/

Digre KB. Using the ophthalmoscope and viewing the optic disc. http://umed.med.utah.edu/neuronet/lectures/2002/Optic%20Disk.htm

North American Neuro-ophthalmology Society (NANOS) NOVEL updates. http://medstat.med.utah.edu/NOVEL/NOVEL_Updates/

North American Neuro-ophthalmology Society. Video clips. http://medstat.med.utah.edu/neuroophth/

Oculocephalic Reflex. http://medstat.med.uth.edu/kw/animations/hyperbrain/oculo_reflex/oculocephalic2.html

Online Vision Test (Visual Acuity. Color). http://www.richmondeye.com/visiontest.htm

Online Visual Field Test (Multifixation Campimeter). http://www.testvision.org/what_is.htm

Appendix. **Differential Diagnosis of Ocular Motor Nerve Palsies**

Nuclear lesions: focal hemorrhage, infarct, or mass (neoplastic, vascular malformation)

Fascicular lesions: infarction, hemorrhage, mass, demyelination, infectious and inflammatory (e.g., Bickerstaff encephalitis)

Subarachnoid space lesions: aneurysms (posterior communicating–internal carotid artery junction, posterior cerebral artery, superior cerebellar artery), uncal (temporal lobe) herniation and other compressive lesions such as tumors, hydrocephalus, meningeal disease (infectious, inflammatory, carcinomatous or lymphomatous meningitis), nerve infarction (in diabetes mellitus, giant cell arteritis, systemic lupus erythematosus), other inflammatory (e.g., Wegener's granulomatosis)

Cavernous sinus lesions: pituitary adenoma and other neoplastic compressive lesions, inflammatory (e.g., Tolosa-Hunt syndrome), carotid-cavernous fistulas, pituitary apoplexy, aneurysm of intracavernous portion of internal carotid artery, cavernous sinus thrombosis, cavernous sinus infection with *Mucor* or *Aspergillus* in diabetes mellitus or immunosuppression

Superior orbital fissure lesions: differential diagnosis similar to cavernous sinus lesions, i.e., inflammatory (Tolosa-Hunt syndrome), compressive lesions such as tumors (e.g., meningioma, metastatic tumor)

Orbital lesions: compressive lesions (neoplastic, including meningioma and metastatic tumors, vascular malformations), trauma (orbital fractures), inflammatory (idiopathic orbital pseudotumor)

Extraocular: myasthenia gravis, Graves' ophthalmopathy, myopathy (e.g., oculopharyngeal dystrophy, mitochondrial disease such as Kearns-Sayre syndrome), ocular neuromyotonia (rare, episodic diplopia in the setting of previous radiotherapy, usually in sellar or parasellar regions)

Questions

1. A 35-year-old woman has sudden painful loss of vision in her right eye. She comes to your office the next day, and a neuro-ophthalmologic examination documents 20/60 vision in the right eye, with a depressed monocular visual field. In the left eye, vision is 20/20 and the visual field is normal. Funduscopic examination shows optic disc swelling and an afferent pupillary defect of the right eye; the left eye is normal. Which of the following is the most likely diagnosis?
   a. Multiple sclerosis
   b. Optic neuritis
   c. Pseudotumor cerebri
   d. Anterior ischemic optic neuropathy
   e. Cat-scratch disease

2. A 35-year-old man presents with a 2-week history of loss of vision in his right eye. He drinks socially and smokes cigarettes. He reports that his brother went blind in middle age and is disabled and that no one could determine the cause of the brother's blindness. The neuro-ophthalmologic examination of the patient documents visual acuity 20/80 right eye, 20/20 left eye, a central visual defect of right eye visual field, and normal left eye visual field. Also, the right eye has a relative afferent pupillary defect, whereas the left eye is normal. The patient is able to read 7/10 HRR color plates on the right and 10/10 on the left. Optic nerve pallor of the right eye is evident with telangiectasias, and the left optic nerve appears normal. What is the most likely diagnosis?
   a. Nutritional optic neuropathy
   b. Optic neuritis
   c. Optic neuropathy, hereditary
   d. Compressive orbital tumor
   e. Ischemic optic neuropathy

3. A 69-year-old woman complains of new-onset headaches. She also describes pain in her jaw when chewing food. Three days before coming for medical help, she lost vision in her left eye. She comes for evaluation on a Friday afternoon. The neuro-ophthalmologic examination documents visual acuity of 20/30 in both eyes, with normal color vision and ocular motility in both eyes. Visual field testing shows an inferior altitudinal defect in the left eye. Funduscopic examination of the left eye discloses a pallid chalky-white optic disc on the superior margin of the optic nerve, and the optic nerve of the right eye appears normal, with a normal cup-to-disc ratio. The rest of the neuro-ophthalmologic examination is normal. Which of the following is the most appropriate management for this patient?
   a. Order an erythrocyte sedimentation rate, start 1 mg/kg oral prednisone, and order a temporal artery biopsy as soon as possible
   b. Order an erythrocyte sedimentation rate, start oral prednisone, and schedule a follow-up visit in 6 months
   c. Order an erythrocyte sedimentation rate for Monday, start oral corticosteroids, and schedule follow-up visit in 6 months
   d. First, perform a temporal artery biopsy, then start corticosteroid treatment
   e. Start corticosteroid treatment but request to have the temporal artery biopsy performed the same day so that the results are not altered by the treatment

4. A 75-year-old smoker with hypertension and hyperlipidemia complains of persistent visual impairment in his right eye for 2 weeks. Neuro-ophthalmologic examination shows a superior altitudinal visual field deficit in the right eye. Funduscopic examination shows a pale optic disc on the right and a small optic disc on the left (small cup-to-disc ratio). The erythrocyte sedimentation rate is 20 mm/h (normal). Which of the following is the most likely diagnosis?
   a. Giant cell arteritis with anterior ischemic optic neuropathy
   b. Branch retinal artery occlusion from a carotid embolus
   c. Nonarteritic anterior ischemic optic neuropathy
   d. Cerebral infarct in the occipital lobe
   e. Retinal detachment

5. An 18-year-old woman had a viral illness before vision was impaired in the left eye. One week after her vision was impaired, she is evaluated. Visual acuity is 20/40 in the left eye and 20/20 in the right eye. Funduscopic examination shows optic disc edema and peripapillary and macular hard exudates in the left eye. The right eye is normal. Which of the following is the most likely diagnosis?
   a. Optic neuritis
   b. Pseudotumor cerebri
   c. Papilledema
   d. Optic disc edema with macular star or neuroretinitis
   e. Pseudodisc edema (optic disc drusen)

6. A 29-year-old morbidly obese woman presents with severe pulsatile headaches. She also states that when she bends forward her vision goes out for a few seconds and then returns. The neurologic examination is normal except for 20/30 visual acuity in both eyes and bilateral papilledema. Visual field testing documents enlarged blind spots and mild dyschromatopsia on color testing. Results of magnetic resonance imaging and venography of the brain are normal. Opening pressure on lumbar puncture (left lateral decubitus position with legs extended) is 350 mm H_2O, with normal CSF constituents. Which is the most likely cause of this patient's symptoms?
   a. Migraine
   b. Pseudotumor cerebri
   c. Optic disc edema with macular star or neuroretinitis
   d. Hereditary optic neuropathy
   e. Optic neuritis with optic disc swelling

7. A 68-year-old man with a history of atrial fibrillation had a tooth extracted while off warfarin therapy. Two days after the tooth extraction, he found himself bumping into things on his left side. He was brought to the local emergency department for evaluation. His speech appears normal, and he has a left homonymous hemianopia with macular sparing on visual field testing. Where is the lesion localized?
   a. Left occipital lobe
   b. Right occipital lobe
   c. Right lateral geniculate body
   d. Left lateral geniculate body
   e. Right temporal optic radiations

8. A 40-year-old otherwise healthy woman describes sudden onset of double vision today and requests an urgent appointment. You examine her and find her neurologic examination is completely normal except for right horizontal gaze. The abnormality on right horizontal gaze indicates weakness of the left medial rectus muscle, and on testing saccadic eye movements on right gaze, a right abducting eye jerk nystagmus is noted. What disease most likely accounts for the patient's symptoms?
   a. Pontine infarct
   b. Congenital nystagmus with disconjugate nystagmus
   c. Midbrain infarct
   d. Multiple sclerosis causing an internuclear ophthalmoplegia
   e. Vestibular nystagmus

9. A 65-year-old man describes sudden left-sided neck pain that began 5 days ago. He is evaluated for neck pain. Neurologic examination shows anisocoria, with the left pupil being about 1 to 2 mm smaller than the right pupil. Pupil reactivity on the right is normal, but on the left, there is dilatory lag. Anisocoria is greater in darkness than in light. The patient has 1 to 2 mm of ptosis of the left eyelid greater than the right. No anhidrosis is evident. The rest of the neurologic examination is normal. Which of the following best explains the patient's symptoms?
   a. Sympathetic hyperactivity
   b. Brainstem infarction creating a left Horner's syndrome
   c. Horner's syndrome, possible carotid artery dissection
   d. Physiologic anisocoria
   e. Pupil-involved third nerve palsy

10. A 55-year-old man with history of diabetes mellitus describes an acute onset of diplopia associated with some mild pain around the right eye. He went to the local emergency department, where you are consulted to evaluate the patient for diplopia. The right eye has ptosis, and when you raise the eyelid, the eye is hypotropic and exodeviated ("down and out"). Ocular motility testing shows right adductor, elevator and depressor (in abducted eye) weakness, with left eye ductions appearing normal. Convergence is attempted and shows adduction weakness of the right eye. The right pupil is normal size and reacts normally, as does the left pupil. The rest of the neurologic examination is normal. Which of the following is the most likely diagnosis?
   a. Posterior communicating artery aneurysm compressing the right oculomotor nerve
   b. Diabetic (ischemic) right third nerve palsy
   c. Right-sided midbrain neoplasm
   d. Midbrain infarct
   e. Orbital tumor

11. A 25-year-old man was an unrestrained passenger in a motor vehicle collision. After being extracted from the car, he was taken to the emergency department. He has a broken clavicle, a broken fibula, and a scalp laceration on the vertex. Since the collision, he has noticed vertical diplopia. The emergency department physician orders computed tomography (noncontrast) of the head, which does not show any intracranial abnormality, hemorrhage, or stroke. You are consulted about the patient's diplopia. On examination, the

patient has a right hypertropia in primary gaze that is worse on left gaze and right head tilt. The rest of the neurologic examination is normal. What is the most likely diagnosis?

a. Right inferior rectus muscle weakness

b. Left superior rectus muscle weakness

c. Right inferior oblique muscle weakness

d. Skew deviation

e. Right fourth nerve palsy

12. A 17-month-old infant is brought to the pediatric neurology clinic because of jerking of the eyes. The infant has a small, rapid amplitude jerk nystagmus to the right in primary position. You use a toy to test for lateral gaze and find a slow left gaze-evoked nystagmus. The child has no head tilt or nodding. What is the cause of the nystagmus?

a. Spasmus nutans

b. Convergence-retraction nystagmus

c. Bruns' nystagmus

d. Congenital nystagmus

e. Opsoclonus

13. A 76-year-old man with a history of hypertension and hyperlipidemia comes to the emergency department because of an acute change in speech, binocular horizontal double vision, and left-sided extremity weakness. On examination, the patient has weakness of the right forehead, face, and mouth. He has a right abductor weakness on extraocular muscle testing. He has a left-sided hemiparesis, pronator drift, increased tendon reflexes, and Babinski sign. The rest of the neurologic examination is unremarkable. Which syndrome provides the most accurate localization?

a. Cavernous sinus syndrome

b. Foville's syndrome

c. Gradenigo's syndrome

d. Millard-Gubler syndrome

e. Pontomedullary lesion

14. A 75-year-old male smoker with hypertension is brought to the emergency department after experiencing a sudden severe headache. He noted double vision for several days before the severe headache. You are asked to see the patient emergently. In the emergency department, he is awake but complains of a severe headache. Neurologic examination shows ptosis of the left eye, and the eye is hypodeviated and exodeviated ("down and out"). On ocular motility testing, you note weakness of adduction and elevation of the left eye. The left pupil is large and unreactive to light compared with the right pupil. Funduscopic examination is shown in Figure 3-25 *A*. The patient becomes rapidly comatose. A noncontrast computed tomographic study of the brain shows, on multiple slices, blood in the subarachnoid space. Select the most likely diagnosis.

a. Pseudotumor cerebri with papilledema

b. Transtentorial herniation

c. Complete third nerve palsy, related to aneurysm

d. Bacterial meningitis

e. Nuclear third nerve palsy due to midbrain hemorrhage

15. A 70-year-old man describes intermittent double vision over the past 3 months. He first noticed double vision after long periods of reading, but it improved after he took a nap in his reading chair. Later, the double vision became worse and did not improve after he had a short nap but did improve after he slept through the night. He was concerned he had had a "ministroke" and comes for evaluation. On neurologic examination, the patient has a small right abductor weakness on rightward gaze. The rest of the neurologic examination is normal. What is the most likely diagnosis?

a. Right sixth nerve palsy

b. False localizing sixth nerve palsy

c. Breakdown of an existing phoria

d. Transient brainstem ischemia involving the abducens nucleus

e. Myasthenia gravis, ocular

ANSWERS

1. Answer: b.
The most likely diagnosis in this young woman is optic neuritis. Although optic neuritis may represent a forme fruste of multiple sclerosis and multiple sclerosis may develop in some patients after optic neuritis, the diagnosis of multiple sclerosis is premature until brain lesions are evident on magnetic resonance imaging. This patient does not have pseudotumor cerebri, which typically is associated with papilledema. Anterior ischemic optic neuropathy has two varieties: arteritic (giant cell arteritis) and nonarteritic. This patient does not have vascular risk factors for the nonarteritic variety nor should she have giant cell arteritis at her age. Cat-scratch disease can cause optic disc edema with macular star, producing optic neuritis-like features of sudden loss of vision and optic disc edema. This patient was not exposed to a cat, making the diagnosis less likely. Also, a macular star with neuroretinitis was not observed (although early), which is classic in *Bartonella* neuroretinitis.

2. Answer: c.
This patient's age and history of his brother's blindness suggest a hereditary disorder (Leber's hereditary optic neuropathy). The neuro-ophthalmologic examination findings are consistent with an optic neuropathy (impaired visual acuity, color vision, and visual fields and relative afferent pupillary defect). Nutritional optic neuropathy is often attributed to patients with a mitochondrial optic neuropathy such as Leber's hereditary optic neuropathy. Optic neuritis is a possibility, but the findings of optic disc telangiectasias support the diagnosis of Leber's optic neuropathy, not optic neuritis. A chronic compressive orbital tumor may cause optociliary shunt vessels, which provide collateral blood flow to the optic nerve, but these vessels are not seen in Leber's hereditary optic neuropathy. An ischemic optic neuropathy is unlikely because of the patient's age (too young for giant cell arteritis). The patient does smoke, which is a vasculopathic risk factor, but it would be unlikely to cause a nonarteritic anterior ischemic optic neuropathy at his age.

3. Answer: a.
The diagnosis is arteritic anterior ischemic optic neuropathy from giant cell arteritis. Ordering an erythrocyte sedimentation rate is standard practice, and the rate is elevated in more than 90% of cases of giant cell arteritis. Corticosteroids are the mainstay of therapy for giant cell arteritis. Some physicians prefer IV corticosteroids over oral corticosteroids once vision has been lost in giant cell arteritis. Corticosteroid treatment can be started about 3 to 5 days before temporal artery biopsy

is performed without interfering with the test results. Thus, choices d and e are incorrect. A temporal artery biopsy (not an erythrocyte sedimentation rate) is required to make the diagnosis of giant cell arteritis, thus making b and c incorrect. Also, follow-up at 6 months would be too long to monitor for symptoms of giant cell arteritis and the side effects of corticosteroids.

4. Answer: c.
This patient has vasculopathic risk factors and has an anterior ischemic optic neuropathy (AION). The question is whether the patient has arteritic (giant cell) or nonarteritic AION. On the basis of the vignette, this patient's vasculopathic risk factors and the normal erythrocyte sedimentation rate indicate the diagnosis of nonarteritic AION. Branch retinal artery occlusion can be seen on funduscopic examination and is not the diagnosis here. A cerebral infarct can cause visual deficit, but a monocular altitudinal visual field defect indicates a monocular cause (e.g., retinal, optic nerve). Retinal detachment can cause a sector defect in the visual field of one eye but there is no corroboratory history or funduscopic examination findings of retinal detachment.

5. Answer: d.
The prodromal viral illness and the classic findings on funduscopic examination indicate the diagnosis of optic disc edema with macular star, or neuroretinitis. The work-up for neuroretinitis includes serum laboratory testing for cat-scratch disease and other infectious causes. If the work-up is negative (idiopathic), then the term of optic disc edema with macular star is used. The patient did not have symptoms of increased intracranial pressure, which would make choices b and c incorrect. Optic disc drusen are buried material under the optic disc that can give the appearance of optic disc edema but do not represent true edema.

6. Answer: b.
Pseudotumor cerebri, or idiopathic intracranial hypertension, occurs in young (child-bearing years) obese women. The diagnosis was suspected in this patient because of the papilledema, signs and symptoms (transient obscurations of vision) of optic nerve-related visual loss, and headache. The diagnosis was confirmed by an opening pressure of more than 200 to 250 mm H_2O and cerebrospinal fluid analysis, magnetic resonance imaging, and magnetic resonance venography. The increased intracranial pressure signifies that the optic disc swelling is indeed papilledema (a term reserved for optic disc edema from increased intracranial pressure. Migraine causes headache but,

like hereditary optic neuropathy, does not cause papilledema. Optic disc edema with macular star or neuroretinitis may cause optic disc edema early before the appearance of a macular star but none of the patient's history is compatible with that disease (prodromal illness, history of cat scratch). Optic neuritis can cause swelling of the optic nerve and optic disc-related loss of vision or optic neuropathy, but the opening pressure would not be abnormal.

7. Answer: b.

Infarction of the right occipital lobe causes a left homonymous hemianopia, typically with macular sparing. (Infarction in the left occipital lobe causes a right homonymous hemianopia, typically with macular sparing.) Infarction of the lateral geniculate body occurs from either anterior choroidal artery or lateral choroidal artery ischemia or occlusion and results in a (homonymous) quadruple sectoranopia or horizontal homonymous sector defects, respectively. Neither visual field abnormality fits this patient's case. A lesion of the right temporal optic radiations would cause a left homonymous superior temporal ("pie in the sky") defect.

8. Answer: d.

This young woman has multiple sclerosis and a discrete lesion (demyelinating) affecting the left medial longitudinal fasciculus, which affects the left medial rectus. The abducting jerk nystagmus of the right eye on saccadic eye testing occurs from "overdrive" of the right lateral rectus muscle. The lack of any other brainstem (pons or midbrain) neurologic findings make brainstem infarction unlikely. Congenital nystagmus begins in children not adults, and vestibular nystagmus causes a jerk nystagmus but it is conjugate (both eyes), not disconjugate (one eye).

9. Answer: c.

Acute Horner's syndrome is carotid atery dissection until proven otherwise. Other causes of Horner's syndrome include brainstem infarction, spinal cord (around C8-T1) and brachial plexus lesions, and upper apex (Pancoast's) lung tumors. Anhidrosis may or may not be present and may suggest first- or second-order Horner's syndrome. The history and neurologic examination provided no findings to suggest brain, brainstem, or spinal cord disease. Physiologic anisocoria is approximately less than 1 mm and should not have any accompanying ptosis. There are no extraocular motor pareses suggestive of third nerve palsy. In pupil-involved third nerve palsy, the pupil is mydriatic because of parasympathetic denervation. In sympathetic hyperactivity, the pupil is larger, not smaller.

10. Answer: b.

Vasculopathic (ischemic) pupil-sparing third nerve palsy. A pupil-sparing third nerve palsy is the rule in diabetic (ischemic) third nerve palsy. Patients may be observed for 24 to 28 hours for pupil involvement, and if the pupil becomes involved, neuroimaging and angiography can be performed. Patients with pupil-involved third nerve palsy are considered to have an aneurysm until proven otherwise. Magnetic resonance imaging and magnetic resonance angiography (or computed tomographic angiography) should be considered in those cases. The patient has no neurologic findings of a midbrain neoplasm or infarct (Parinaud's syndrome, Weber's syndrome). An orbital tumor would not cause the presentation of acute pupil-sparing third nerve palsy.

11. Answer: e.

The fourth cranial nerve (CN IV) travels dorsally under the inferior colliculus around the brainstem under the tentorium cerebelli. During traumatic head injury, the free edge of the tentorium is thought to hit CN IV along its course from the brainstem. Isolated inferior rectus, superior rectus, or inferior oblique muscle weakness after trauma would be unusual unless it is part of an orbital fracture or blowout, causing ocular muscle entrapment. It also would be unusual to see a third nerve palsy with individual muscle weakness (inferior, superior recti, or inferior oblique muscle) unless orbit muscle entrapment is proven. The patient's physical examination and head computed tomogram did not suggest any major fractures around the orbit. Skew deviation is a vertical gaze misalignment due to a supranuclear cause.

12. Answer: c.

Bruns' nystagmus has two components: the first is a small-amplitude, rapid jerk nystagmus in primary position (fast phase is directed away from the side of the lesion) and the second component is a slow, gaze-evoked nystagmus directed toward the side of the lesion. This infant had both components of Bruns' nystagmus. The importance of Bruns' nystagmus is that it heralds a cerebellopontine angle mass. Therefore, patients with Bruns' nystagmus should have neuroimaging. Spasmus nutans, which may be confused with Bruns' nystagmus, begins within the first 18 months of life and resolves by 3 years. Spasmus nutans is characterized by the classic triad of pendular nystagmus, head nodding, and head turn (torticollis). Nystagmus in spasmus nutans is pendular, small amplitude, and high frequency and may be conjugate or disconjugate. Spasmus nutans is a diagnosis of exclusion, and magnetic resonance imaging is performed to exclude an intracranial lesion.

Congenital nystagmus is uniplanar (the plane or direction of nystagmus remains unchanged in all positions of gaze) and, thus, does not resemble Bruns' nystagmus. Opsoclonus is a chaotic, multivectorial, saccadic eye movement ("saccadomania") and can be due to paraneoplastic effects of neuroblastoma. In convergence-retraction nystagmus, the eyes have asynchronous, adducting saccades.

13. Answer: d.

Millard-Gubler syndrome is caused by a lesion in the anteroparamedial pons. This syndrome is manifested clinically as an ipsilateral sixth nerve palsy, seventh nerve palsy, and contralateral hemiparesis. A lesion in dorsolateral pons causes Foville's syndrome. Foville's syndrome consists of horizontal ipsilateral gaze paresis and facial weakness and contralateral hemiparesis and dysmetria. A lesion of the petrous apex or Dorello's canal causes Gradenigo's syndrome. Gradenigo's syndrome is characterized by an ipsilateral sixth nerve palsy, facial pain, and deafness (cranial nerve VIII). A cavernous sinus lesion could cause some combination of cranial neuropathies (cranial nerves III, IV, VI, V$_1$ and V$_2$) but would not cause a seventh nerve palsy. A pontomedullary lesion may cause a sixth nerve palsy but would have to extend far laterally to affect other cranial nerves such as CN VII.

14. Answer: c.

The patient most likely had an aneurysm of the posterior communicating artery on the left side that ruptured, causing a subarachnoid hemorrhage. The rupture or the aneurysm may be responsible for the third nerve palsy. The pupillomotor fibers are located in the periphery of the third nerve, and compression leads to a dilated pupil and weakness of the oculomotor muscles. Papilledema signifies increased intracranial pressure. Transtentorial herniation can cause third nerve palsy, but it was not seen on computed tomography. Pseudotumor cerebri may have papilledema, but it does not cause third nerve palsy. Bacterial meningitis can cause subarachnoid hemorrhage, increased intracranial pressure, and cranial nerve deficits. However, the patient did not present with signs or symptoms typical of bacterial meningitis (headache, neck stiffness, fever). A midbrain hemorrhage may cause a nuclear third nerve palsy and Parinaud's syndrome. A midbrain hemorrhage was not noted on computed tomography.

15. Answer: e.

Ocular myasthenis gravis is the most likely diagnosis because of the history of fluctuating diplopia and diurnal variation (better in morning) or improvement with rest. Myasthenia gravis can mimic any extraocular muscle weakness (third nerve, fourth nerve, and, in this case, sixth nerve innervated muscles). Myasthenia gravis does not affect the pupil musculature. False localizing sixth nerve palsy occurs with increased intracranial pressure. The patient had no symptoms of increased intracranial pressure (headache, nausea, vomiting, double vision). A breakdown (decompensation) of an existing phoria occurs when a latent strabismus (e.g., old sixth nerve palsy that improved) becomes manifest during illness or stress. There is no history of illness to report. None of the neurologic findings suggest pontine ischemia or stroke, making ischemia of the abducens nucleus unlikely.

DISORDERS OF THE CRANIAL NERVES

4

Kelly D. Flemming, M.D.

I. INTRODUCTION

A. General Remarks
1. Twelve pairs of cranial nerves (CNs): CN I–CN XII
2. This chapter reviews CNs I, V, VII, VIII, IX, X, XI, and XII; CNs II, III, IV, and VI are discussed in Chapter 3

B. Organization
1. Cranial nerves, like spinal nerves, contain sensory or motor fibers or a combination of sensory and motor fibers
2. The fibers are classified by their embryologic origin or common structural and functional characteristics
3. Motor fibers
   a. General somatic efferent (GSE) fibers: innervate muscles derived from somites (CNs III, IV, VI, and XII)
   b. Special visceral efferent (SVE) fibers: innervate muscles derived from branchial arches (CNs V, VII, IX, X, and XI)
   c. General visceral efferent (GVE) fibers: innervate structures derived from mesoderm or endoderm; parasympathetic (CNs III, XII, IX, and X)
4. Sensory fibers
   a. General somatic afferent (GSA) fibers: sensory information from body surface, joints, and mucosal membranes (CNs V, VII, IX, and X)
   b. General visceral afferent (GVA) fibers: sensory information from pharynx and endodermally derived structures such as viscera (CNs IX and X)
   c. Special visceral afferent (SVA) fibers: sensory information from taste and olfactory receptors (CNs I, VII, IX, and X)
   d. Special somatic afferent (SSA) fibers: sensory information from visual, auditory, and vestibular receptors (CNs II and VIII)
5. Cranial nerves and their components and functions are summarized in Tables 4-1 and 4-2
6. Cranial nerves and their attachments to the brain are shown in Figure 4-1
7. Cranial nerves and their brainstem nuclei are shown in Figure 4-2
8. Foramina of the skull through which cranial nerves pass are shown in Figure 4-3

II. CRANIAL NERVE I (OLFACTORY)

A. Olfactory Cranial Nerve
1. Type: SVA
2. Function: sense of smell
3. Receptor
   a. Chemoreceptor (olfactory receptor cell)
   b. A bipolar neuron unlike other sensory systems in which the receptor is distinct from the neuron
4. Pathway
   a. Cells of origin: bipolar neurons (olfactory receptor cells) within the nasal cavity; axons extend through the cribriform plate to the olfactory bulb
   b. Thalamic relay: none (unique feature)
   c. Course (Fig. 4-4)
      1) Olfactory receptor cell axons synapse with mitral cells or tufted cells in olfactory bulb
      2) Each mitral cell receives input from up to 1,000 olfactory nerve cells
      3) Mitral cell axons project to primary olfactory cortex (in piriform cortex—uncus and entorhinal cortex) and amygdala via olfactory tract and lateral olfactory stria
      4) Tufted and mitral cells may project to lateral, medial, and intermediate olfactory areas
      5) Medial olfactory stria passes to medial frontal lobe

---

Olfactory pathway is the only sensory pathway that does not synapse in the thalamus

---

Table 4-1.   **Summary of Cranial Nerve Components**

CN	GSE	SVE	GVE	GSA	SVA	SSA	GVA
I					Olfaction		
II						Vision	
III	Four extraocular m.		Pupil con-striction				
IV	Superior oblique m.						
V		Mastication		Facial sensation			
VI	Lateral rectus m.						
VII		Facial expression	Lacrimal gland Salivary glands	External ear sensation	Taste (ant 2/3 tongue)		
VIII						Equillibrium Hearing	
IX		Stylopharyn-geus m.	Parotid gland	External ear sensation	Taste (post 1/3 tongue)		Carotid body and sinus Pharynx
X		Palatal m. Laryngeal m.	Internal organs	External ear sensation	Taste (post pharynx)		Abdominal, thoracic viscera
XI		Sternocleid-omastoid, trapezius m.					
XII	Genioglossus m.						

ant, anterior; GSA, general sensory afferent; GSE, general somatic efferent; GVA, general visceral afferent; GVE, general visceral efferent; m., muscle(s); post, posterior; SSA, special somatic afferent; SVA, special visceral afferent; SVE, special visceral efferent.

and is thought to be involved with emotional response to odors

6) Some collaterals from mitral and tufted cells synapse in anterior olfactory nucleus near where olfactory bulb becomes olfactory tract

7) Axons from some neurons in anterior olfactory nucleus cross in anterior commissure to synapse in contra-lateral olfactory areas

8) Olfactory cortex interconnects with various autonomic and visceral centers (thalamus, hypothalamus, amygdala), perhaps explaining why odors can cause nausea, salivation, or increased gut motility

B. Differential Diagnosis of CN I Disorders

1. Terminology
   a. Anosmia/hyposmia: decreased or lack of smell/decreased sense of smell
   b. Dysosmia: smell perception is distorted; can occur with seizure disorders of temporal lobe
   c. Hyperosmia: increased sense of smell

d. Cacosmia: perception of a bad smell
e. Parosmia: sensation of smell in absence of appropriate stimulus

2. Disorders of CN I can occur anywhere along its pathway (Table 4-3)

III. CRANIAL NERVE V (TRIGEMINAL)

A. Overview

1. CN V has both sensory and motor components
2. Motor component: SVE, innervates muscles of mastication
3. Sensory components
   a. GSA: ipsilteral pain and temperature sensation of face and supratentorial dura mater
   b. GSA: vibration, proprioception, tactile sensation of ipsilateral face
   c. GSA: unconscious proprioception of jaw; reflexive chewing

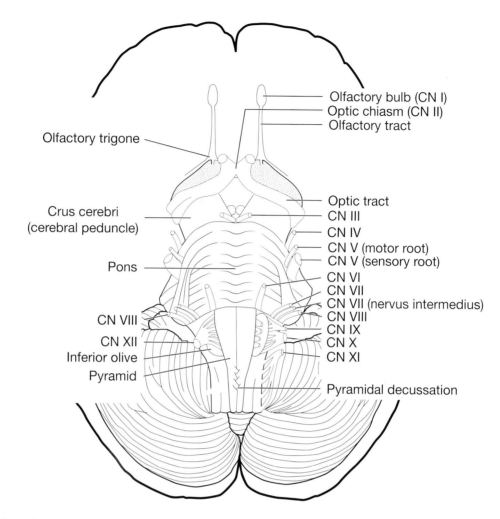

Fig. 4-1. Ventral surface of the brain showing the attachments of cranial nerve (*CN*) I to CN XII.

B. Motor Component of CN V

1. Type: SVE
2. Function
   a. Innervates muscles of mastication (temporalis, masseter, and medial and lateral pterygoid muscles); these muscles open (protract) the jaw, important in chewing
   b. Also innervates anterior belly of digastric, mylohyoid, and tensor tympani muscles
3. Nucleus: motor nucleus of V (midpons) (Fig. 4-2 *D*)
4. Course: axons exit brainstem laterally and travel with mandibular division (V$_3$) of CN V through foramen ovale to innervate skeletal muscle
5. Corticobulbar: bilateral corticobulbar input to motor nucleus of V
6. Dysfunction
   a. Upper motor neuron lesion: no pronounced weakness because of bilateral corticobulbar input

   b. Lower motor neuron lesion: jaw deviates to weak side

C. Sensory Components of CN V

1. General: sensory nuclei of V receive information from three separate divisions—ophthalmic (V$_1$), maxillary (V$_2$), and mandibular (V$_3$) (Fig. 4-5 and Table 4-4)
2. Cell bodies of V$_1$, V$_2$, and V$_3$ are in trigeminal ganglion (also called gasserian ganglion, semilunar ganglion) which lies in Meckel's cave in the middle cranial fossa
3. Spinal tract and nucleus of V (Fig. 4-6)
   a. Type: GSA
   b. Function: pain and temperature sensation of face, oral cavity, dorsum of head, including temporomandibular joint, supratentorial meninges, and teeth
   c. Receptors: cutaneous pain and temperature receptors (C fibers)
   d. Ganglion (first-order neuron): CN V (trigeminal

Table 4-2. **Summary of Cranial Nerves**

Cranial nerve	Type	Ganglion/nucleus	Function
I Olfactory	SVA	Olfactory receptor cells Olfactory bulb/tract	Sense of smell
II Optic	SSA	Retinal ganglion cells	Vision
III Oculomotor	GSE	Oculomotor nucleus	Innervates inferior, medial, and superior recti and inferior oblique muscles
	GVE	Edinger-Westphal nucleus Ciliary ganglion	Preganglionic parasympathetic to pupil and ciliary muscle
IV Trochlear	GSE	Trochlear nucleus	Innervates superior oblique muscle
V Trigeminal	SVE	Motor nucleus of V	Innervates muscles of mastication
	GSA	Trigeminal ganglion Spinal tract and nucleus of V	Ipsilateral pain and temperature sensation of face and supratentorial dura mater
	GSA	Trigeminal ganglion Principal sensory nucleus of V	Vibration, proprioception, tactile discrimination of ipsilateral face
	GSA	Mesencephalic nucleus of V	Unconscious proprioception of jaw, reflexive chewing
VI Abducens	GSE	Abducens nucleus	Innervates lateral rectus muscle
VII Facial	SVE	Facial nucleus (motor nucleus of VII)	Muscles of facial expression and stapedius muscle
	GVE	Superior salivatory nucleus Submandibular ganglion	Innervate submandibular and sublingual glands (salivation)
		Superior salivatory nucleus (lacrimal nucleus) Pterygopalatine ganglion	Lacrimation (tearing) and nasal mucosa
	SVA	Geniculate ganglion Nucleus solitarius (rostral)	Taste buds of anterior 2/3 of tongue
	GSA	Trigeminal ganglion Spinal nucleus of V	Somatic sensation of external ear
VIII Vestibulocochlear	SSA	Vestibular ganglion Vestibular nuclei	Control posture and movement of body and eyes relative to angular and linear acceleration
	SSA	Spiral ganglion	Hearing
IX Glossopharyngeal	SVE	Nucleus ambiguus	Innervates stylopharyngeus muscle
	GVE	Inferior salivatory nucleus Otic ganglion	Innervates parotid gland (salivation)
	GVA	Inferior ganglion Nucleus solitarius (caudal)	Input from carotid sinus baroreceptors and carotid body chemoreceptors Tactile input from posterior 1/3 of tongue, pharynx, middle ear, and auditory canal
	SVA	Inferior ganglion Nucleus solitarius (rostral)	Taste buds of posterior 1/3 of tongue
	GSA	Superior ganglion Spinal nucleus of V	Somatic sensation of external ear
X Vagus	SVE	Nucleus ambiguus	Innervates muscles of pharynx and larynx
	GVE	Dorsal motor nucleus of X	Preganglionic parasympathetic to viscera including heart, lungs, gastrointestinal tract

Table 4-2.   **(continued)**

Cranial nerve	Type	Ganglion/nucleus	Function
X Vagus (continued)			
	GVA	Inferior ganglion Nucleus solitarius (caudal)	Visceral sensation
	SVA	Inferior ganglion Nucleus solitarius (rostral)	Taste buds on epiglottis, pharyngeal wall
	GSA	Superior ganglion Spinal nucleus of V	Somatic sensation of external ear
XI Spinal accessory	SVE	Cranial: nucleus ambiguus Spinal: ventral horn cells (cervical)	Innervates muscles of larynx (with X) Innervates sternocleidomastoid and trapezius muscles
XII Hypoglossal	GSE	Hypoglossal nucleus	Tongue movement

GSA, general sensory afferent; GSE, general somatic efferent; GVA, general visceral afferent; GVE, general visceral efferent; SSA, special somatic afferent; SVA, special visceral afferent; SVE, special visceral efferent.

ganglion), CN VII (geniculate ganglion), CN IX (superior ganglion), and CN X (superior ganglion)
- e. Nucleus (second-order neuron): spinal nucleus of V (Fig. 4-2 *B*)
- f. Thalamic relay (third-order neuron): ventral postero-medial nucleus
- g. Course
    1) Sensory fibers enter the midpons and descend as spinal trigeminal tract in lateral brainstem
    2) Axons may terminate at low pons or medulla or descend as far as C2-3 (near zone of Lissauer) before synapsing
    3) Axons terminate in spinal trigeminal nucleus, which is medial to the tract
    4) Axons of second-order trigeminothalamic neurons decussate and form anterior trigeminothalamic tract
    5) This tract ascends through brainstem just posterior to medial lemniscus
    6) Tract synapses in ventral posteromedial thalamic nucleus (third-order neurons)
    7) Axons of third-order neurons terminate in ipsilteral primary somatosensory cortex (SI, Brodmann areas 3, 1, 2)
    8) Some collaterals of trigeminothalamic tract terminate in reticular formation and other thalamic nuclei; others are involved in local oral reflexes
- h. Dysfunction: ipsilateral loss of pain and temperature of the face
- i. Corneal reflex: bilateral blink in response to corneal stimulus
    1) Afferent arm: V_1

2) Interneuron: spinal nucleus of V
    3) Efferent arm: CN VII (Fig. 4-7)
4. Chief sensory nucleus of V (Fig. 4-6)
    - a. Type: GSA
    - b. Function: vibration, proprioception, and light touch/tactile discrimination sensation of face
    - c. Receptor: Pacinian corpuscle, Merkel cells, Meissner corpuscles
    - d. Ganglion (first-order neuron): trigeminal ganglion
    - e. Nucleus (second-order neuron): chief sensory nucleus (Fig. 4-2 *D*)
    - f. Thalamic relay nucleus (third-order neuron): ventral posteromedial nucleus
    - g. Course
        1) Axons from trigeminal ganglion enter midpons to synapse in chief sensory nucleus in pontine tegmentum
        2) Second-order axons cross midline and ascend in lateral brainstem to ventral posteromedial thalamic nucleus
        3) Axons from this nucleus terminate in ipsilteral primary somatosensory cortex
    - h. Dysfunction: ipsilateral loss of tactile discrmination
5. Mesencephalic nucleus of V
    - a. Type: GSA
    - b. Function
        1) Unconscous proprioception
        2) Muscle spindles in pterygoid, masseter, and temporalis muscles supply information about force of bite and/or stretch of muscle to mesencephalic nucleus of V, which forms a reflex circuit with motor nucleus of V to adjust and control force of bite

A

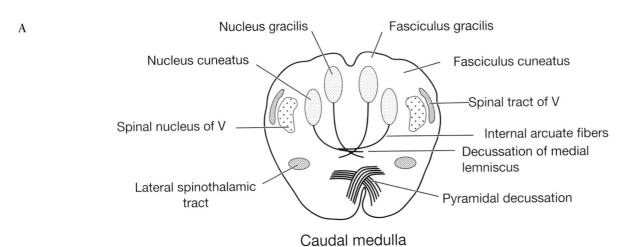

Caudal medulla

B

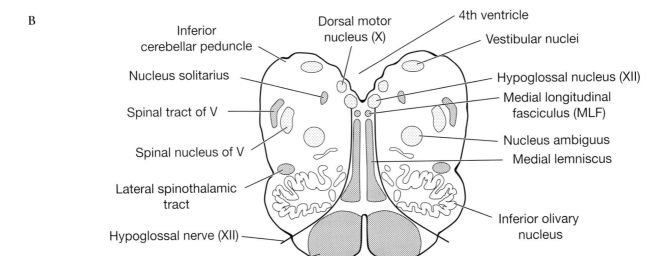

Upper medulla

C

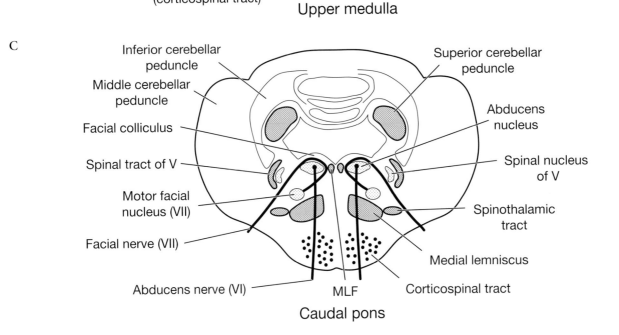

Caudal pons

D

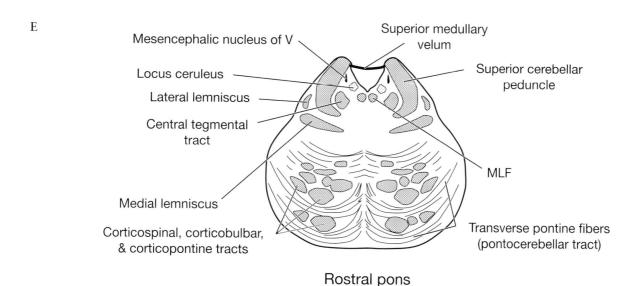

MLF

Middle cerebellar peduncle

Chief sensory nucleus of V

Trigeminal nerve (V)

Motor nucleus of V

Spinothalamic tract

Corticospinal, corticobulbar & corticopontine tracts

Medial lemniscus

Middle pons

E

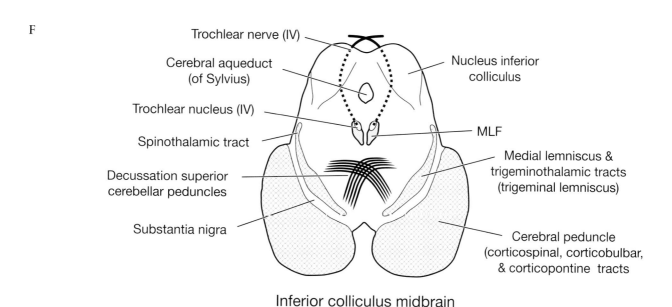

Mesencephalic nucleus of V

Superior medullary velum

Locus ceruleus

Superior cerebellar peduncle

Lateral lemniscus

Central tegmental tract

MLF

Medial lemniscus

Corticospinal, corticobulbar, & corticopontine tracts

Transverse pontine fibers (pontocerebellar tract)

Rostral pons

F

Trochlear nerve (IV)

Cerebral aqueduct (of Sylvius)

Nucleus inferior colliculus

Trochlear nucleus (IV)

Spinothalamic tract

MLF

Decussation superior cerebellar peduncles

Medial lemniscus & trigeminothalamic tracts (trigeminal lemniscus)

Substantia nigra

Cerebral peduncle (corticospinal, corticobulbar, & corticopontine tracts

Inferior colliculus midbrain

G

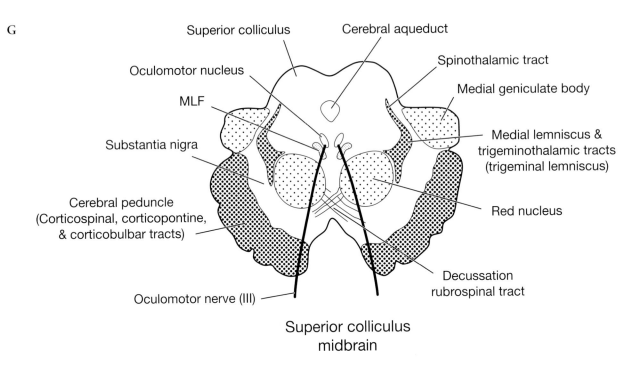

Fig. 4-2. Brainstem cross-sections. *A,* Caudal medulla; *B,* upper medulla; *C,* caudal pons; *D,* middle pons; *E,* rostral pons; *F,* caudal midbrain at the level of the inferior colliculus; *G,* rostral midbrain at the level of the superior colliculus. *MLF,* medial longitudinal fasciculus.

   c. Nucleus: mesencephalic nucleus of V—unique because it has no ganglion; unipolar neuron with cell body in midbrain

   d. Course

      1) Peripheral axon innervates muscle spindles

      2) Central axon terminates in the motor nucleus of V

   e. Jaw jerk

      1) Contraction of masseter and temporalis muscles when patient's lower jaw is tapped

      2) Afferent arm: peripheral axons of mesencephalic nucleus of V traveling with V3

      3) Efferent arm: central axons of mesencephalic nucleus of V synapse in motor nucleus of V and axons from this nucleus (traveling with V3) innervate muscles of mastication

      4) Lesions anywhere along this reflex arc cause depression of ipsilateral jaw reflex, and bilateral supranuclear lesions produce accentuated response

D. Differential Diagnosis of CN V Disorders
1. Disorders of CN V are listed in Table 4-5

E. Selected Disorders of CN V
1. Trigeminal neuralgia (see Chapter 18)

> The mesencephalic nucleus of V is unique. It is the only general somatic sensory pathway with a first-order neuron cell body in the central nervous system.

2. Idiopathic trigeminal sensory neuropathy

   a. Clinical findings

      1) Usually gradual onset

      2) Loss of sensation in a trigeminal distribution (generally V2 and V3, but can involve all three divisions)

      3) Pain is absent

   b. Pathology

      1) Thought to be inflammatory process primarily affecting trigeminal ganglion

      2) Pathology examination typically shows cell loss, lymphocyte infiltration, and fibrosis in trigeminal ganglion

   c. Diagnosis

      1) Rule out other causes of trigeminal nerve dysfunction (Table 4-5)

      2) Because trigeminal sensory neuropathy commonly associated with connective tissue disease, appropriate rheumatologic and serologic testing is important

      3) Nerve conduction studies may help establish involve-

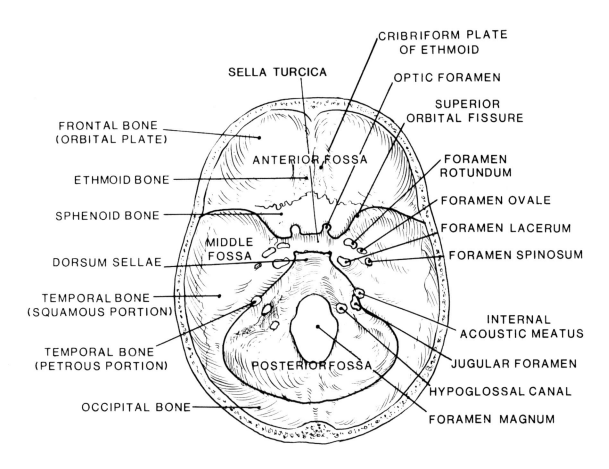

Fig. 4-3. Foramina of the skull. (From Benarroch EE, Westmoreland BF, Daube JR, Reagan TJ, Sandok BA. Medical neurosciences: an approach to anatomy, pathology, and physiology by systems and levels. 4th ed. Philadelphia: Lippincott Williams & Wilkins; 1999. p. 32. By permission of Mayo Foundation.)

ment of CN V
   d. Treatment
      1) No known specific treatment; corticosteroid therapy
        has been tried
      2) If V_1 distribution involved, protect cornea

IV. CRANIAL NERVE VII (FACIAL)

A. Overview
1. Organization and distribution of CN VII are shown in Figure 4-8
2. CN VII has both motor and sensory components: SVE, GVE, SVA, GSA
3. GVE, SVA, and GSA fibers form nervus intermedius

B. Motor Components of CN VII
1. Type: SVE

   a. Nucleus: facial (caudal pons) (Fig. 4-2 *C*)
   b. Function: innervates muscles of facial expression and stapedius muscle (functions to dampen sound)
   c. Course
      1) Axons go dorsally and sweep around the nucleus of CN VI, forming the facial colliculus, then exit the pons in the cerebellopontine angle
      2) Next, axons enter internal auditory meatus
      3) SVE fibers pass through facial canal of temporal bone, existing skull at stylomastoid foramen
      4) Before exiting at stylomastoid foramen, a small branch innervates stapedius muscle
   d. Corticobulbar input to facial nucleus
      1) Input to motor neurons controlling forehead muscles, including orbicularis oculi: bilateral
      2) Input to motor neurons controlling lower face muscles: unilateral (Fig. 4-9)
   e. Dysfunction

A
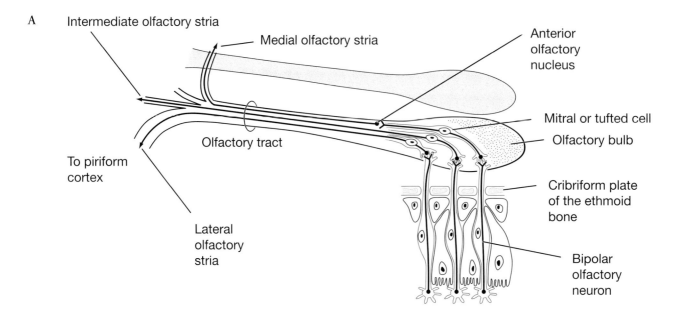

Intermediate olfactory stria
Medial olfactory stria
Anterior olfactory nucleus
Mitral or tufted cell
Olfactory bulb
Olfactory tract
To piriform cortex
Cribriform plate of the ethmoid bone
Lateral olfactory stria
Bipolar olfactory neuron

B
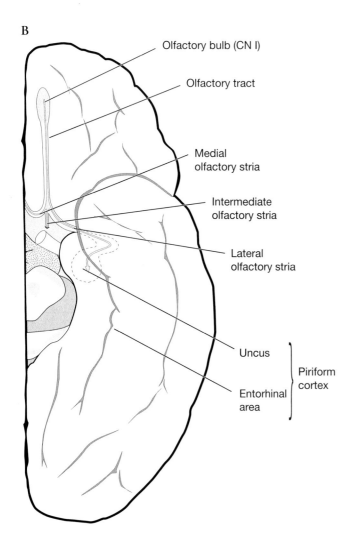

Olfactory bulb (CN I)
Olfactory tract
Medial olfactory stria
Intermediate olfactory stria
Lateral olfactory stria
Uncus
Entorhinal area
Piriform cortex

Fig. 4-4. Olfactory nerve (*CN I*). *A*, Olfactory neuron and olfactory bulb (see text). *B*, Olfactory cortex (see text). *CN*, cranial nerve.

1) Upper motor neuron: contralateral paralysis of lower face only
2) Lower motor neuron: paralysis of entire ipsilateral face
2. Type: GVE (parasympathetic motor component of CN VII)
   a. Preganglionic cells: superior salivatory nucleus
      1) Postganglionic cells: sphenopalatine (pterygopalatine) ganglion
      2) Function: innervation of lacrimal glands and nasal mucosa
      3) Course
         a) Parasympathetic motor fibers exit brainstem in nervus intermedius and enter internal acoustic canal
         b) Axons travel as greater petrosal nerve, exiting skull at greater petrosal foramen
         c) Axons then travel through pterygoid canal joining the deep petrosal nerve called nerve of the pterygoid canal
         d) Axons synapse in sphenopalatine (pterygopalatine) ganglion in the pterygopalatine fossa
         e) Postganglionic fibers innervate lacrimal gland and nasal mucosa
      4) Dysfunction: ipsilateral dry eye and dry nasal mucosa

Table 4-3.   **Causes of Anosmia and Hyposmia**

Location	Causes
First-order neuron	Nasal and paranasal sinus inflammatory disease
	Nasal neoplasms: esthesioneuroblastoma, melanoma, squamous cell carcinoma
	Head trauma
	Upper respiratory tract infection
	Drugs: cocaine
	Iatrogenic interventions (surgery, radiation)
Olfactory bulb	Intracranial neoplasms: olfactory groove or cribriform plate meningioma, frontal lobe glioma, other frontal or temporal lobe tumor—Foster Kennedy syndrome (ipsilateral reduction in smell, ipsilateral optic atrophy, and contralateral papilledema generally due to tumor affecting olfactory bulb and optic nerve)
	Developmental: Kallmann syndrome (hypogonadism, anosmia)
	Infectious: meningitides, syphilis
Other	Aging
	Degenerative disorders: Alzheimer's disease, Parkinson's disease, Huntington's disease
	Endocrine: diabetes mellitus, hypothyroidism, adrenal insufficiency, pseudohypoparathyroidism
	Metabolic: vitamin A, B_6, or B_{12} deficiency, zinc or copper deficiency, kidney and liver disease, malnutrition
	Toxins/drugs: cigarette smoking, benzene, carbon disulfide, chlorine, formaldehyde, solvents, sulfuric acid, lead, cadmium, nickel, silicon dioxide
	Medications (numerous): common offenders include chemotherapeutic agents, antipsychotics, certain antibiotics
	Irradiation of head and neck
	Epilepsy or migraine (olfactory aura)
	Psychiatric

Table 4-4.   **Sensory Divisions of the Trigeminal Nerve (Cranial Nerve V)**

Division	Innervation	Foramen
Ophthalmic (V_1)	Forehead, cornea, tip of nose	Superior orbital fissure
Maxillary (V_2)	Upper lip, cheek region	Foramen rotundum
Mandibular (V_3)	Lower lip, lower jaw region	Foramen ovale

b. Preganglionic cells: lacrimal nucleus (may be same nucleus as salivatory)

    1) Postganglionic cells: submandibular ganglia

    2) Function: salivation

    3) Course

        a) Preganglionic fibers exit brainstem in nervus intermedius

        b) Axons enter internal acoustic canal

        c) Axons continue as chorda tympani nerve, and join

        lingual branch of V_3

        d) Axons travel near inner surface of jaw and synapse in submandibular ganglion

        e) Postganglionic fibers innervate submandibular and sublingual glands

    4) Dysfunction: reduced salivation (dry mouth)

C. **Sensory Components of CN VII**

1. Type: SVA (taste sensation)

    a. Function: taste from anterior 2/3 of tongue

    b. Receptor: chemoreceptors (taste buds)

    c. Ganglion (first-order neuron): geniculate ganglion

    d. Nucleus (second-order neuron): rostral part of nucleus solitarius

    e. Thalamic relay (third-order neuron): ventral posteromedial thalamic nucleus

    f. Course

        1) Axons innervating taste buds on anterior 2/3 of tongue travel in ipsilateral chorda tympani nerve to petrous temporal bone, site of geniculate ganglion

        2) Axons enter brainstem and synapse in rostral part of nucleus solitarius

        3) Second-order neurons project to ipsilateral ventral posteromedial thalamic nucleus through central tegmental tract

        4) Ventral posteromedial nucleus projects to inferiormost part of primary sensory cortex near insula (Brodmann area 43)

    g. Dysfunction: decreased taste sensation from ipsilateral anterior 2/3 of tongue

2. Type: GSA (tactile sensation)

    a. Function: tactile sensation of skin of ear

    b. Ganglion (first-order neuron): geniculate ganglion

    c. Nucleus (second-order neuron): spinal nucleus of V

    d. Thalamic relay (third-order neuron): ventral posteromedial thalamic nucleus

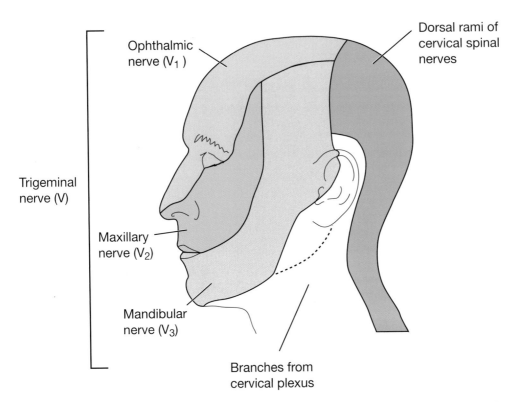

Fig. 4-5. Sensory innervation of the face and scalp. The three divisions of cranial nerve V are ophthalmic (V_1, yellow), maxillary (V_2, green), and mandibular (V_3, pink).

> Taste from anterior 2/3 of the tongue: CN VII
>
> General sensation from anterior 2/3 of the tongue: CN V

D. Differenial Diagnosis of Disorders of CN VII and Taste

1. Disorders of CN VII are listed in Table 4-6, and those of taste are listed in Table 4-7

E. Selected Disorders

1. Idiopathic Bell's palsy
   a. Epidemiology
      1) Incidence: 23/100,000 persons
      2) Equal occurrence in males and females
      3) Mean age at presentation: 40 years
   b. Clinical features
      1) Acute onset
      2) Unilateral (bilateral reported, but unusual) facial paralysis (lower motor neuron)
      3) May have abnormal ipsilateral tearing or taste
      4) May complain of ipsilateral ear pain or increase in sound

   c. Pathology
      1) Theory: latent herpes simplex virus reactivation may cause idiopathic Bell's palsy
      2) Lyme disease may also present with isolated facial paralysis
      3) Few pathology data available: in one autopsy case, inflammatory changes in geniculate ganglion extended from internal auditory canal to the stylomastoid process, with demyelinating changes in nerve
   d. Diagnosis
      1) Can be made on clinical basis
      2) Determine that paralysis is truly lower motor neuron
      3) Evaluate (history and examination) for involvement of any other cranial nerves
      4) Examine ear canal for any lesions suggestive of active herpes lesions, which may indicate diagnosis of Ramsay Hunt syndrome (see below)
      5) Evaluate (history and examination) patient for systemic symptoms suggesting more widespread disease (e.g., Lyme or neoplastic disease)
      6) Imaging recommended if other cranial nerves involved or symptoms progress or fail to improve; magnetic resonance imaging may show gadolinium enhancement of internal acoustic meatal segment of

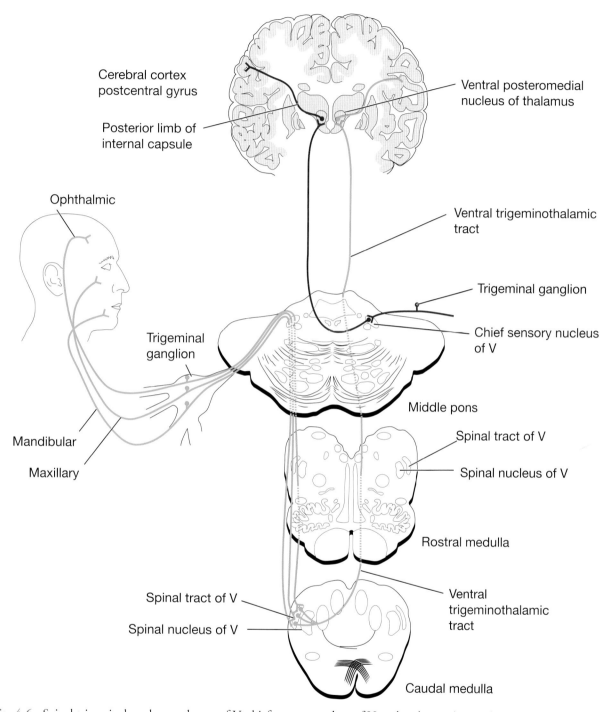

Fig. 4-6. Spinal trigeminal nucleus and tract of V, chief sensory nucleus of V, and pathways (see text).

CN VII on ipsilateral side
7) Nerve conduction studies and electromyography may be useful for prognostication
e. Treatment
1) Unclear because of lack of rigorous clinical trials
2) Corticosteroids (reduce nerve edema) and acyclovir (reduce viral replication) are generally considered for treatment and may increase number of patients with full recovery
a) Treat within 72 hours (up to 1 week)
b) Prednisolone 1 mg/kg daily for 1 week, then taper (maximum 80 mg/day) or 1 mg/kg prednisone (up to maximum of 70 mg/day) for 5 to 7 days, with subsequent taper

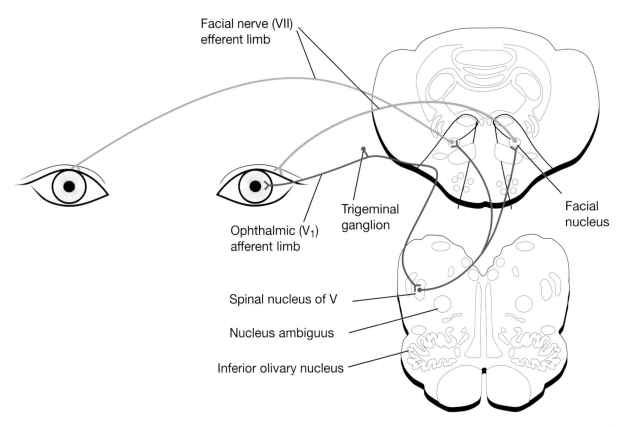

Facial nerve (VII) efferent limb

Ophthalmic (V₁) afferent limb

Trigeminal ganglion

Facial nucleus

Spinal nucleus of V

Nucleus ambiguus

Inferior olivary nucleus

Fig. 4-7. Corneal reflex. The afferent arm of the pathway is cranial nerve V (ophthalmic division), and the efferent arm is the facial nerve (VII).

    c) Acyclovir 1,000 to 2,400 mg/day in divided doses for 5 days (dose variable in studies)
   3) Controversial role for CN VII decompression
   4) There is a role for facial reconstruction and/or nerve graft operation if patient has complete paralysis after 1 year
  f. Prognosis
   1) Majority (70%) have complete recovery of facial paralysis within 3 to 6 months
   2) Some patients develop synkinesis, with facial muscle contracture or gustatory tearing as CN VII recovers
   3) Younger age, partial paralysis, and early recovery portend good prognosis
   4) Recurrence has been reported, but is unusual
2. Ramsay Hunt syndrome
  a. Characterized by herpes zoster oticus and ipsilateral facial nerve palsy
  b. Symptoms
   1) Rapid onset of facial palsy
   2) Ipsilateral ear pain, followed by development of herpetic vesicles in auditory canal
   3) Vestibulocochlear damage can occur, resulting in tin-

nitus, hearing loss, vertigo, and nystagmus
   4) Rarely, may involve other lower cranial nerves
  c. Pathophysiology
   1) Thought to be due to reactivation of varicella zoster within geniculate ganglion
   2) Viral inflammation leads to edema and nerve compression
  d. Treatment
   1) Acyclovir
   2) Prednisone
3. Möbius syndrome
  a. Congenital disorder
  b. Characterized by bilateral facial palsy that may occur in isolation but more commonly in association with other cranial nerve involvement, most frequently bilateral CN VI palsies (but can have CN IX, XII, and oculomotor involvement)
  c. Cranial nerve involvement due to nuclear hypoplasia
  d. Other congenital defects may include: limb malformations (syndactyly, polydactyly, brachydactyly), cranial malformations (bifid uvula, ear deformities, micrognathia), musculoskeletal system anomalies (Klippel-Feil

Table 4-5.   **Disorders of the Trigeminal Nerve (Cranial Nerve V)**

Location of lesion	Component affected	Cause
Upper motor neuron	SVE	No appreciable deficit because of bilateral corticobulbar input to motor nucleus of V
Nuclear or intramedullary	SVE	Lateral medullary or lower pontine stroke, demyelinating or mass lesion may cause dysfunction of spinal tract and nucleus of V
	GSA	Paramedian or lateral midpontine stroke, hemorrhage, demyelinating lesion, mass lesion (tumor, abscess), or syringobulbia may impair the chief sensory nucleus of V or motor nucleus of V
Trigeminothalamic tract	GSA	Mass lesion, stroke, hemorrhage, or demyelinating lesions may produce decreased sensation of contralateral face
Meningeal (nerve)	All	Vascular: dolichoectasia of vertebrobasilar system, aneurysm
		Inflammatory: sarcoidosis, Guillain-Barré syndrome; chronic inflammatory demyelinating polyradiculopathy, systemic lupus erythematosus, Sjögren's syndrome, mixed connective tissue disorder (trigeminal sensory neuropathy), Gradenigo's syndrome
		Infectious: basilar meningitides, herpes zoster, tuberculosis
		Neoplastic: schwannoma, meningioma, metastasis, lymphoma
		Toxic-metabolic: diabetes mellitus, vitamin B_{12} or B_6 deficiency, trichloroethylene
		Other: idiopathic trigeminal neuralgia, trigeminal autonomic cephalgias, cluster headache
Cavernous sinus	Sensory V_1, V_2	Vascular: carotid-cavernous fistula, cavernous sinus thrombosis, cavernous sinus aneurysm
		Mass lesion
		Tolosa-Hunt syndrome
		Trauma
Foramen ovale	Sensory V_3, motor V	Mass lesion can cause sensory loss in distribution of V_3 and ipsilateral jaw deviation
		Trauma
Foramen rotundum	Sensory V_2	Mass lesion can cause sensory loss in distribution of V_2
		Trauma
Superior orbital fissure	Sensory V_1	Mass lesions can cause sensory loss in distribution of V_1 and extraocular movement abnormalities
		Tolosa-Hunt syndrome
		Trauma
Extracranial distal nerve	V_1, V_2, or V_3	Jaw trauma
		Jaw surgery

GSA, general somatic afferent; SVE, special visceral efferent; V_1, ophthalmic division of cranial nerve V; V_2, maxillary division of cranial

anomaly, rib defects), cardiac anomalites, and, rarely, mental retardation

4. Melkersson-Rosenthal syndrome
   a. Thought to be either congenital or inherited
   b. Presents in childhood, usually second decade
   c. Characterized by recurrent facial palsy (alternating sides), ipsilateral facial edema, and tongue changes (lingua plicata)
   d. Some patients treated with corticosteroids and/or facial nerve decompression

V.   CRANIAL NERVE VIII (VESTIBULOCOCHLEAR)

A.   Anatomy of Vestibular Division

1. Type: SSA
2. Function
   a. Control of posture and movements of body and eyes relative to external environment
   b. Control of eye movements and posture to linear and angular acceleration through connections with ocular

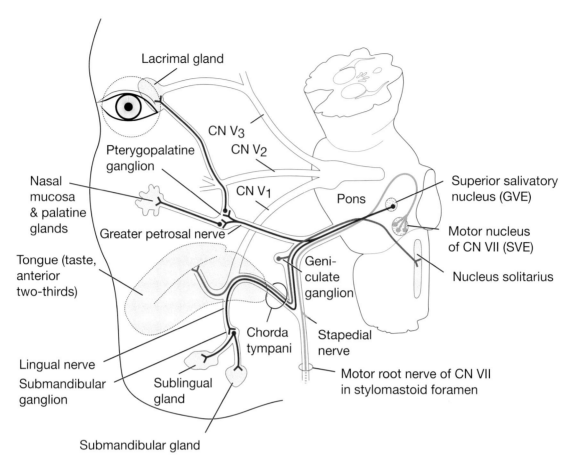

Fig. 4-8. Diagram of the facial nerve (*CN VII*). Parasympathetic motor (*GVE*) components (*red*) innervate the lacrimal gland (via pterygopalatine ganglia), submandibular, and sublingual glands (via submandibular ganglion). The motor (*SVE*) component of CN VII (*green*) innervates muscles of facial expression in addition to the stapedius muscle. Taste sensation (*SVA*) is transmitted from the anterior 2/3 of the tongue via the chorda tympani nerve to the rostral part of nucleus solitarius (*blue*). The somatic sensory component of CN VII is not shown. *CN*, cranial nerve; *GVE*, general visceral efferent; *SVA*, special visceral afferent; *SVE*, special visceral efferent; *V₁*, *V₂*, *V₃*, ophthalmic maxillary, and mandibular divisions, recpectively, of CN V.

motor system and vestibulospinal tracts
  c. Connections with thalamus and cortex (conscious awareness)
3. Receptors: hair cells in saccule and utricle (detect linear acceleration) and semicircular canals (detect angular acceleration)
4. Ganglion (first-order neuron): vestibular ganglion
5. Course
  a. Relation of vestibular system with extraocular eye movements is shown in Figure 4-10
  b. Vestibular system affects posture in relation to angular and linear acceleration via medial and lateral vestibulo-spinal tracts (Fig. 4-11)
  c. Information from vestibular nuclei also projects bilaterally to cerebral cortex (base of the central sulcus near the

motor cortex) via thalamus
6. Dysfunction
  a. Nystagmus
  b. Loss of postural tone
  c. Dysequillibrium, vertigo

B. Anatomy of Auditory Division
1. Type: SSA
2. Function: hearing
  a. Monaural (information about sounds at one ear): transmitted via contralateral pathways to inferior colliculus
  b. Binaural (information about differences between sounds at both ears): transmitted via superior olivary nuclear complex (information from both ears converge; important for sound localization)

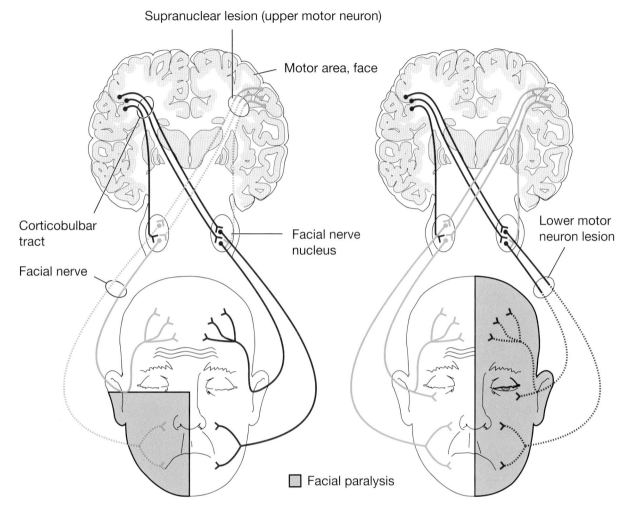

Fig. 4-9. Corticobulbar input to facial nerve (motor) nucleus and distribution of facial nerve to upper and lower muscles of facial expression. *Right*, A supranuclear (upper motor neuron) lesion produces paralysis of contralateral lower face. *Left*, A lower motor neuron lesion causes paralysis of ipsilateral upper and lower face.

3. Receptor: hair cells in organ of Corti
4. Ganglion (first-order neuron): spiral ganglion in cochlea
5. Nucleus (second-order neuron): cochlear nuclei (dorsal and ventral)
6. Thalamic relay: medial geniculate body
7. Course (Fig. 4-12)
   a. Cochlear nerve and nuclei
      1) Cochlear nerve (axons from spiral ganglion) synapse in ipsilateral dorsal and ventral cochlear nuclei
      2) Ventral and dorsal cochlear nuclei are at ponto-medullary junction
      3) Axons from ventral cochlear nucleus go ventral to inferior cerebellar peduncle to form trapezoid body
      4) Axons from dorsal cochlear nucleus travel dorsal to inferior cerebellar peduncle as the posterior acoustic stria and cross in pons to join lateral lemniscus
   b. Superior olivary nucleus and trapezoid body
      1) Crossing fibers from ventral cochlear nucleus travel through trapezoid body (myelinated fiber bundle) to terminate in contralateral superior olivary nuclear complex or ascend in contralateral lateral lemniscus
      2) Superior olivary nuclear complex
         a) Important sound localization and binaural sensation
         b) Contains two nuclei: lateral and medial superior olivary nuclei
         c) Projects via lateral lemniscus
   c. Lateral lemniscus
      1) Ascending fiber tract, but also contains two nuclei:

Table 4-6.   **Disorders of the Facial Nerve (Cranial Nerve VII)**

Location of lesion	Component affected	Cause
Upper motor neuron	SVE	Vascular: stroke Demyelinating disease Infection: abscess Neoplasm
Nuclear (facial nucleus)	SVE	Vascular Demyelinating disease Infection: abscess Neoplasm Syringobulbia Developmental: Möbius syndrome
Meningeal	All	Vascular: subrachnoid hemorrhage, dolichoectasia of vertebrobasilar system Infectious: basilar meningitides, Lyme disese, HIV Inflammatory: Guillain-Barré syndrome, sarcoidosis Neoplasms: schwannoma, meningioma Toxic-metabolic: diabetes mellitus, hypothyroidism, porphyria, arsenic Other: hemifacial spasm, amyloidosis
Internal acoustic meatus, ganglion	All	Inflammatory: Gradenigo's syndrome Idiopathic Bell's palsy
Stylomastoid foramen	SVE only	Mass lesion: squamous cell carcinoma, parotid neoplasm
Chorda tympani nerve	SVA; GVE	Mass lesion
Extracranial nerve	SVE	Facial trauma Parotid surgery Parotid neoplasm Botulinum toxin Melkersson-Rosenthal syndrome

GVE, general visceral efferent; HIV, human immunodeficiency virus; SVA, special visceral afferent; SVE, special visceral efferent.

anterior and posterior nuclei
2) Includes axons directly from cochlear nucleus, axons from superior olivary complex, and axons from nuclei of lateral lemniscus
3) Anterior nucleus: projects to inferior colliculus as part of monaural pathway
4) Posterior nucleus (input from superior olivary complex): conveys binaural information and axons terminate in inferior colliculus
5) Most ascending auditory pathways terminate in inferior colliculus
  d. Inferior collliculus
1) Lateral lemniscus projects to central nucleus of inferior colliculus
2) Central nucleus projects to medial geniculate body of thalamus
3) Paracentral nuclei of inferior colliculus: integrate attention, sensation, and auditory-motor reflexes through connections with superior colliculus, reticular formation, and precerebellar nuclei
  e. Medial geniculate body
1) Is medial to lateral geniculate body and lateral to pulvinar nucleus of thalamus
2) Anterior division: input from central nucleus of inferior colliculus; projects to primary auditory cortex (A1, Brodmann area 41)
3) Posterior division: input from paracentral nuclei of inferior colliculus; projects to auditory association areas of cerebral cortex
4) Medial division: projects to auditory association cortices, temporal and parietal association areas, and amygdala
  f. Auditory cortices
1) Primary auditory cortex: located in Heschl's gyrus;

Table 4-7.   **Disorders of Taste**

Infectious: oral infections

Inflammatory: Sjögren's syndrome, multiple sclerosis, Bell's palsy

Neoplastic: tumors of oral cavity or skull base along path of cranial nerve VII, IX, or X

Metabolic: vitamin B_{12} deficiency, zinc or copper deficiency, kidney or liver failure, adrenal insufficiency, diabetes mellitus, hypothyroidism, Cushing's syndrome

Toxins: solvents, benzene, chlorine, formaldehyde, sulfuric acid, chromium, lead, copper

Medications: numerous

Trauma

Irradiation

Oral appliances or procedures

Other: aging, migraine or seizure aura, psychiatric

tonotopic arrangement

   2) Secondary auditory cortex (A2, Brodmann area 42): located in second transverse temporal gyrus and planum temporale

   3) Left and right auditory cortices are connected reciprocally through corpus callosum

8. Dysfunction (Table 4-8)

   a. Lesion of CN VIII or cochlear nucleus: unilateral loss of hearing

   b. Unilateral lesion at mid pons or higher: no hearing loss

   c. Unilateral lesion at level of cerebral cortex: no hearing loss but sound localization may be impaired

D. Differential Diagnosis of Disorders of CN VIII

1. Disorders of CN VIII are listed in Table 4-9

E. Selected Disorder of CN VIII

1. Vestibular neuronitis

   a. Clinical features

      1) Rotary vertigo

      2) Nausea and/or vomiting

      3) Horizontal and rotatory nystagmus opposite to side of lesion

      4) Postural instability; patient leans toward side of lesion

   b. Pathogenesis

      1) Thought to represent either inflammation or infection of vestibular nerve

      2) Herpes simplex virus type 1 may be involved

   c. Treatment

      1) Recovery is spontaneous, wthin weeks to months

      2) Vestibular rehabilitation

VII. Cranial Nerve IX (Glossopharyngeal)

A. Overview

1. CN IX has motor and sensory components

2. Motor components

   a. SVE (innervates stylopharyngeus muscle)

   b. GVE (preganglionic parasympathetic neurons)

3. Sensory components

   a. GVA (carotid sinus baroreceptors; tactile sensation of pharynx)

   b. SVA (taste sensation from posterior 1/3 of tongue)

   c. GSA (tactile sensation from external ear)

B. Motor Components of CN IX

1. Type: SVE

   a. Function: innervates stylopharyngeus muscle of pharynx

   b. Nucleus: nucleus ambiguus

   c. Course

      1) Axons exit medulla dorsal to inferior olive (posterolateral sulcus of medulla)

      2) Axons join CN X and cranial portion of CN XI and exit through jugular foramen

   d. Corticobulbar input to nucleus ambiguus: bilateral

   e. Dysfunction: Stylopharyngeus muscles cannot be tested individually

2. Nucleus ambiguus (Fig. 4-2 *B*)

   a. Type: SVE (cell bodies for CN IX, X, and XI)

   b. Location: dorsal to inferior olivary nucleus

   c. Function: innervates striated muscles derived from branchial arches 3, 4, and 5

      1) CN IX: innervates stylopharyngeus muscle

      2) CN X: innervates palatal muscles (with contribution from CN V for tensor veli palatini), most pharyngeal muscles (with contribution from CN IX), laryngeal muscles, and striated muscles of esophagus

      3) CN XI: innervates laryngeal muscles (cranial portion)

   d. Corticobulbar input: bilateral

   e. Dysfunction

      1) Unilateral: nasal speech (palatine weakness), hoarse (laryngeal paralysis), uvula deviates to normal side

      2) Bilateral: dysphagia (difficulty swallowing), hoarseness, difficulty breathing (paralysis of laryngeal muscles)

3. Type: GVE (parasympathetic)

   a. Function: innervate parotid gland (salivation)

   b. Nucleus: inferior salivatory nucleus

   c. Postganglionic parasympathetic ganglion: otic ganglion

   d. Course

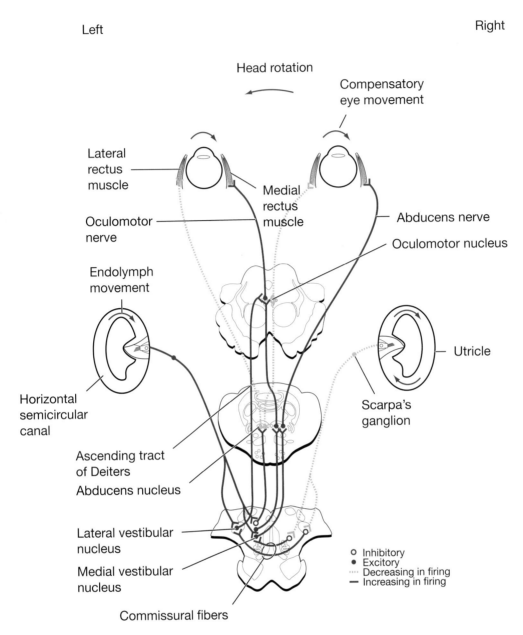

Fig. 4-10. Vestibulo-ocular connections. Each semicircular canal consists of a membranous labyrinth filled with endolymph and suspended within a bony labyrinth, filled with perilymph. One end of each semicircular canal is dilated, forming the ampulla. The ampulla contains a crista, a transversely oriented ridge of tissue. The cristae are composed of sensory hair cells (with cilia on the surface) embedded in a gelatinous material (the cupula). The group of cilia of each hair cell contains a single tall kinocilium on one end and an array of shorter cilia. Deflection of the cilia toward the kinocilium by movement of the endolymph excites the hair cell and deflection in the opposite direction decreases the response of the hair cell. The left and right sides are oppositely polarized. In this diagram, the head moves quickly to the left. The endolymph in the semicircular canal moves in the opposite direction and "lags behind" because of inertia. Thus, hair cells on the left side of the head are depolarized, and the signal is transmitted by cranial nerve VIII (vestibular nerve) to brainstem vestibular nuclei. The vestibular nucleus projects to the contralateral (*right*) abducens nucleus, which innervates the right lateral rectus muscle. Axons from the right abducens nucleus also project through the medial longitudinal fasciculus to the left oculomotor nucleus, which innervtes the left medial rectus muscle. Thus when the head is turned quickly to the left, the eyes conjugately turn to the right, maintaining fixation of a visual stimulus on the retina.

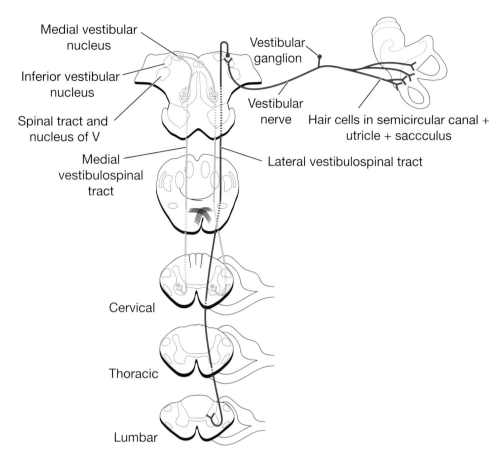

Fig. 4-11. Vestibulospinal tracts. The lateral vestibulospinal tract (*red*) originates in the lateral and inferior vestibular nuclei. It projects to the ipsilateral spinal cord in the anterior funiculus to terminate on the alpha and gamma motor neurons of the cervical and lumbar segments (termination in lumbar segment shown here). The medial vestibulospinal tract (*green*) originates in the medial vestibular nuclei and projects bilaterally to the cervical spinal cord alpha and gamma motor neurons that innervatre flexor and extensor muscles of the neck.

1) Axons exit dorsal to inferior olive (posteromedial sulcus)
2) Axons synapse in otic ganglion
3) Postganglionic axons innervate ipsilateral parotid gland
e. Dysfunction: decreased salivation

C. **Sensory Components of CN IX**
1. Type: GVA
   a. Function
      1) Input from carotid sinus baroreceptors and carotid body chemoreceptors
      2) Input from tactile receptors on posterior 1/3 of tongue, pharynx, middle ear, and auditory canal
   b. Ganglion (first-order neuron): inferior ganglion of CN IX
   c. Nucleus (second-order neuron): caudal part of nucleus solitarius
   d. Relay (third-order neuron): local reflex pathways, reticu-

lar formation, hypothalamus (indirect)
e. Dysfunction
   1) Carotid sinus reflex (Fig. 4-13)
      a) Increased blood pressure stimulates baroreceptors in wall of carotid sinus
      b) Afferent arms: CN IX (GVA fibers)
      c) Interneuron: caudal nucleus solitarius, which projects through reticular formation interneurons to dorsal motor nucleus of X
      d) Efferent arm: parasympathetic fibers in CN X project to heart
      e) Result: slowing of heart rate
      f) Inhibitory signals sent from nucleus solitarius to ventrolateral medulla (sympathetic region of medulla)
      g) Patients with hypersensitive carotid sinus reflex may present with recurrent syncope
   2) Glossopharyngeal neuralgia: irritation of CN IX may produce throat pain in addition to episodes of

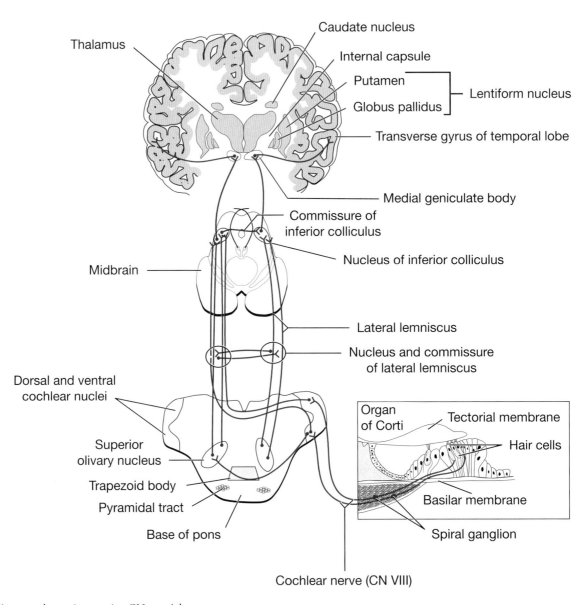

Fig. 4-12. Auditory pathway (see text). *CN*, cranial nerve.

syncope (carotid sinus reflex)
3) Gag reflex
   a) Touching posterior pharynx elicits gag response
   b) Afferent limb: CN IX (GVA fibers)
   c) Efferent limb: CN X (SVE from nucleus ambiguus)
2. Caudal part of nucleus solitarius
   a. Type : GVA
   b. Cranial nerves: CN IX (via inferior ganglion), CN X (via inferior ganglion)
   c. Function: mainly reflex responses to GVA input
3. Type: SVA (taste sensation)
   a. Function: taste sensation from posterior 1/3 of tongue

b. Receptor: chemoreceptors (taste buds)
c. Ganglion (first-order neuron): inferior ganglion of CN IX
d. Nucleus (second-order neuron): rostral part of nucleus solitarius
e. Thalamic relay (third-order neuron): ventral postero-medial thalamic nucleus
f. Sensory cortex: insular cortex (Brodmann area 43)
g. Dysfunction: decreased taste sensation in posterior 1/3 of ipsilateral tongue
4. Rostal part of nucleus solitarius
   a. Type: SVA
   b. Cranial nerves: CN VII (geniculate ganglion), CN IX (inferior ganglion), and CN X (inferior ganglion)

Table 4-8. **Auditory Pathway Lesions and Associated Clinical Syndromes**

Lesion	Clinical result
Cochlear nerve	Ipsilateral deafness (partial or complete), tinnitus
Unilateral brainstem	Because of binaural representation in ascending auditory paths above level of cochlear nuclei, unilateral brainstem lesions involving auditory paths do not impair audition
Bilateral brainstem	If severe bilateral brainstem lesions, bilateral hearing loss may occur
Unilateral auditory cortex	May have difficulty localizing sound
Unilateral dominant posterior temporal lesion or bilateral temporal lesion	Pure word deafness (auditory verbal agnosia): inability to understand spoken language despite normal auditory acuity and ability to read, write, and comprehend nonlanguage sounds
Bilateral auditory cortex	Range of disorders, including cortical deafness, auditory agnosia, pure word deafness, amusia

Table 4-9. **Disorders of the Vestibulocochlear Nerve (Cranial Nerve VIII)**

Location of lesion	Cause
Brainstem	Vascular: AICA stroke (cochlear), PICA stroke (vestibular)
	Mass: neoplasm, abscess
	Demyelinating disease
Cerebellopontine angle	Neoplastic: acoustic neuroma, meningioma, epidermoid, choroid plexus papilloma, lipoma, chordoma, craniopharyngioma, paraganglioma, metastasis
	Inflammatory: sarcoidosis
	Other: arachnoid cyst
Meninges, nerve	Vascular: dolichoectasia of vertebrobasilar artery, subarachnoid hemorrhage
	Infectious: meningitides, varicella-zoster, neuronitis, human immunodeficiency virus, cytomegalovirus, neurosyphilis, Lyme disease, herpes zoster oticus
	Inflammatory: Cogan's syndrome
	Neoplastic: carcinomatous meningitis
	Drugs: antibiotics, aspirin, quinine
	Toxic metabolic: kernicterus (hyperbilirubinemia), thiamine deficiency, organic mercury, uremia
	Genetic: otoferlin, Charcot-Marie-Tooth disease, cerebro-oculofacio-skeletal syndrome, Usher's syndrome
	Idiopathic
Vestibular organs	Benign positional vertigo
	Meniere's disease
	Vestibulitis

AICA, anterior inferior cerebellar artery; PICA, posterior inferior cerebellar artery.

c. Function: taste sensation from tongue, epiglottis, and pharynx (Fig. 4-14)
d. Course (Fig. 4-15): axons from CNs VII, IX, and X terminate
   1) In rostral part of nucleus solitarius
   2) This nucleus projects through solitariothalamic tract (uncrossed) in central tegmental tract

   3) Axons synapse in ventral posteromedial thalamic nucleus
   4) Axons project from thalamus to ipsilateral somatosensory cortex and anterior insular cortex
4. Type: GSA
   a. Function: tactile sensation of part of external ear
   b. Ganglion (first-order neurons): superior ganglion of CN IX

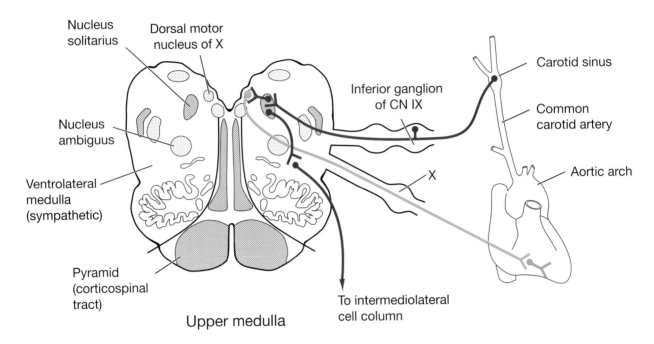

Fig. 4-13. Carotid sinus reflex (see text).

> Nucleus **am**biguus is a **m**otor nucleus.
>
> Nucleus **s**olitarius is a **s**ensory nucleus.

c. Nucleus (second-order neurons): spinal nucleus of V
d. Thalamic relay (third-order neurons): ventral posteromedial thalamic nucleus
e. Third-order axons synapse in ipsilateral somatosensory cortex

D. Differential Diagnosis of Disorders of CN IX
1. Disorders of CN IX are listetd in Table 4-10

E. Selected Disorders of CN IX
1. Glossopharyngeal neuralgia (see Chapter 18)
2. Carotid sinus hypersensitivity
   a. Recurrent syncope related to hypersensitive baroreceptor reflex
   b. Causes: tight clothing around neck, movement and/or stretching of neck, carotid body tumors, Takayasu's arteritis, certain medications, glossopharyngeal neuralgia
   c. Treatment
      1) Identify potential cause
      2) Consider muscarinic cholinergic blockage
      3) Some patients require placement of pacemaker

VIII. CRANIAL NERVE X (VAGUS)

A. Overview
1. CN X has motor and sensory components
2. Motor components
   a. SVE (innervates palatal and laryngeal muscles)
   b. GVE (preganglionic parasympathetic)
3. Sensory components
   a. GSA (tactile sensation from ear)
   b. GVA (viscerosensory)
   c. SVA (taste sensation from posterior pharynx)

B. Motor Components of CN X
1. Type: SVE
   a. Function: innervate muscles of pharynx and larynx
   b. Nucleus: nucleus ambiguus
   c. Course: medulla dorsal to inferior olive (posterolateral sulcus)
      1) Axons exit medulla dorsal to inferior olive (postero-lateral sulcus)
      2) Axons join CN X and cranial part of CN XI and exit through jugular foramen
   d. Corticobulbar input to nucleus ambiguus: bilateral
   e. Dysfunction (see section on nucleus ambiguus)
2. Type: GVE
   a. Function
      1) Parasympathetic innervation of visceral organs
      2) Vagal discharge may result in constriction of

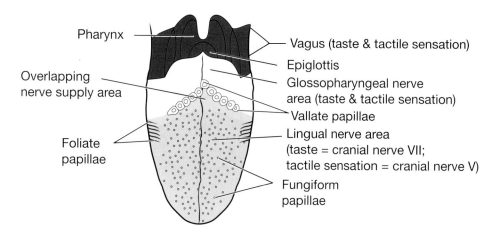

Fig. 4-14. Taste sensation from the anterior 2/3 of the tongue (*blue*) is carried by cranial nerve VII. Taste from the posterior 1/3 of the tongue (*yellow*) is carried by cranial nerve IX. Taste from the epiglottis (*red*) is carried by cranial nerve X.

bronchioles, decreased heart rate, increased blood flow, peristalsis, and increased secretions in gut
b. Nucleus: dorsal motor nucleus of X
c. Postganglionic parasympathetic ganglia: ganglia adjacent to or within walls of viscera (lungs, heart, digestive system, trachea)
d. Course
   1) CN X exits jugular foramen with CNs IX and XI
   2) Courses through neck in carotid sheath
   3) Enters thorax, passing anterior to subclavian artery on right and anterior to aortic arch on left
   4) Left and right CN X pass behind roots of lungs
   5) Left CN X continues on anterior side of right CN X on posterior side of esophagus to gastric plexus
   6) Fibers diverge from this plexus to duodenum, liver, biliary ducts, spleen, kidneys, and small and large intestine as far as splenic flexure

C. Sensory Components of CN X
1. Type: GVA
   a. Function: viscerosensory
   b. Receptors: visceral receptors, aortic baroreceptors, and chemoreceptors; tactile sensation from larynx, upper esophagus, pharynx
   c. Course
      1) Cell bodies in inferior ganglia of CN IX and CN X
      2) Central processes synapse in caudal portion of nucleus solitarius
      3) This nucleus projects to dorsal motor nucleus of X and other parts of brainstem and spinal cord involved in visceral reflexes
2. Type: SVA

a. Function: taste sensation from epiglottis and posterior pharynx
b. Receptor: chemoreceptors (taste buds)
c. Ganglion (first-order neuron): inferior ganglion of CN X
d. Nucleus (second-order neuron): rostral nucleus solitarius
e. Thalamic relay (third-order neuron): ventral postero-medial thalamic
f. Third-order neuron projects to insular cortex
g. Dysfunction: decreased taste sensation in epiglottis and posterior pharynx
3. Type: GSA
   a. Function: touch sensation on portion of external ear
   b. Ganglion (first-order neuron): superior ganglion of CN X
   c. Nucleus (second-order neuron): spinal nucleus of V
   d. Thalamic relay (third-order neuron): ventral postero-medial thalamic nucleus
   e. Third-order neuron projects to ipsilateral somatosensory cortex

D. Differential Diagnosis of Disorders of CN X
1. Disorders of CN X are listed in Table 4-11

IX. CRANIAL NERVE XI (SPINAL ACCESSORY)

A. Overview
1. CN XI has only a motor component (SVE)

B. Anatomy of CN XI
1. Type: SVE
2. Nucleus
   a. Cranial: nucleus ambiguus

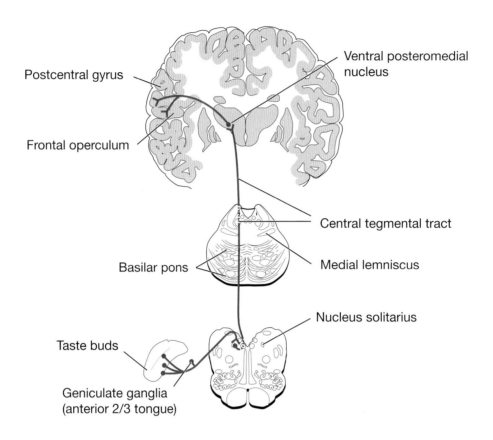

Postcentral gyrus

Ventral posteromedial nucleus

Frontal operculum

Central tegmental tract

Basilar pons

Medial lemniscus

Nucleus solitarius

Taste buds

Geniculate ganglia (anterior 2/3 tongue)

Fig. 4-15. Central taste pathways (see text).

b. Spinal: ventral horn cells (C1-6)
3. Function
  a. Cranial component: innervates muscles of larynx (with CN X)
  b. Spinal component: innervates ipsilteral sternocleidomastoid and trapezius muscles
4. Sternocleidomastoid muscle
  a. One head originates from medial third of clavicle and second head from sternum
  b. Muscle inserts on the mastoid bone
  c. Muscle contraction: turns chin to opposite side
  d. When both left and right muscles contract: draw the head forward
5. Trapezius
  a. Originates from external occipital protuberance, spinous processes C1 to T12
  b. Inserts on lateral clavicle, acromion, and superior spine of the scapula
  c. Muscle contraction: elevate shoulders and stabilize the scapula
6. Course

  a. Axons from cranial division exit medulla dorsal to inferior or olive and join CN X
  b. Axons from spinal division exit spinal cord, ascend through foramen magnum, and exit the skull through jugular foramen
7. Corticobulbar input
  a. Corticobulbar input to motor neurons innervating sternocleidomastoid muscle is ipsilateral
  b. Cortiobulabar input to motor neurons innervating trapezius muscle is contralateral
8. Dysfunction
  a. Upper motor neuron lesion: head may tilt ipsilateral (weak sternocleidomastoid) may be contralateral shoulder droop (weak trapezius)
  b. Lower motor neuron lesion: ipsilateral shoulder droop and head tilt on side opposite lesion (weak ipsilateral sternocleidomastoid muscle); fasciculations and atrophy may be seen
  c. Lower motor neuron (cranial portion): hoarseness

C. Differential Diagnosis of Disorders of CN XI
1. Disorders of CN XI are listed in Table 4-12

Table 4-10. Disorders of the Glossopharyngeal Nerve (Cranial Nerve IX)

Location of lesion	Cause
Medulla (nuclear)	Stroke Demyelinating disease Mass lesion: tumor, abscess Syringobulbia
Meninges	Infectious: meningitides, diphtheria, syphilis Inflammatory: Guillain-Barré syndrome Neoplastic: cerebellopontine angle tumors (see differential diagnosis for cranial nerve VIII) Metabolic: diabetes mellitus
Jugular foramen	Neoplasm: glomus jugulare (paraganglioma), schwannoma, metastases, chordoma Trauma Osteomyelitis
Retropharyngeal	Tumor Abscess Glossopharyngeal neuralgia

X. CRANIAL NERVE XII (HYPOGLOSSAL)

A. Overview
1. CN XII has only a motor component (GSE)

B. Anatomy of CN XII
1. Type: GSE
2. Nucleus: hypoglossal
3. Function
   a. Innervates intrinsic and extrinsic tongue muscles (except palatoglossus)
   b. Each genioglossus muscle pulls tongue anterior and medial
   c. When paired genioglossi work together, tongue protrudes
   d. If one side is weak, tongue deviates to that side
4. Course (Fig. 4-16)
   a. Axons exit ventral to inferior olive (anterolateral sulcus)
   b. Axons briefly travel through carotid sheath and exit skull via hypoglossal canal to innervate the genioglossus muscle
5. Corticobulbar input to hypoglossal nucleus: unilateral and crossed
6. Dysfunction
   a. Upper motor neuron: tongue deviates to side opposite the lesion
   b. Lower motor neuron: tongue deviates to side of lesion, with associated atrophy and fasciculations

C. Differential Diagnosis of Disorders of CN XII
1. Disorders of CN XII are listed in Table 4-13

XI. DISORDERS OF MULTIPLE CRANIAL NERVES

A. Anatomic Relations of Multiple Cranial Nerves
1. Contents of jugular foramen (Table 4-14)
2. Contents of carotid sheath (Table 4-15)
3. Contents of cavernous sinus
   a. CNs III, IV, VI, V_1, and V_2
   b. Cavernous portion of internal carotid artery
   c. Postganglionic traveling along the internal carotid artery

B. Clinical Brainstem Syndromes (Table 4-16)

C. Clinical Syndromes of Lower Cranial Nerves (Table 4-17)

D. Differential Diagnosis of Multiple Cranial Neuropathies (Table 4-18)
1. Selected disorders with multiple cranial nerve involvement
   a. Tolosa-Hunt syndrome
      1) Granulomatous inflammatory process involving cavernous sinus regions
      2) Clinical features
         a) Episodic attacks at recurrent intervals, with each attack lasting days to weeks
         b) Boring, steady retro-orbital pain, which may precede ophthalmoplegia
         c) Ophthalmoplegia usually involving CNs III, IV, and VI
         d) Trigeminal sensory (V_1) (reduced sensation) and

Table 4-11.   **Disorders of the Vagus Nerve (Cranial Nerve X)**

Location of lesion	Cause
Brainstem	Lateral medullary stroke (PICA)
	Demyelinating disease
	Mass lesions: tumor, abscess, syringobulbia
	Degenerative: multiple system atrophy, motor neuron disease
Meninges	Infectious: meningitides, sarcoidosis, Lyme disease, diphtheria
	Inflammatory: Guillain-Barré syndrome
	Neoplastic: schwannoma, carcinomatous meningitis
Jugular foramen	Neoplastic: glomus jugulare, schwannoma, metastases, chordoma
	Trauma
	Osteomyelitis
Retropharyngeal, vagus nerve	Vascular: carotid artery dissection
	Infectious: retropharyngeal abscess, diphtheria
	Neoplastic
	Toxic-metabolic: alcoholic neuropathy, vincristine neuropathy, neuritic beriberi
Recurrent laryngeal nerve	Neoplastic
	Intrathoracic lesion: mediastinal lymph node enlargement, carcinoma of bronchus or esophagus
	Neck lesion: head and neck cancers
	Surgery: carotid artery surgery, neck dissection, thyroid surgery
	Trauma: endotracheal tube placement
	Metabolic: diabetes mellitus
	Idiopathic

PICA, posterior inferior cerebellar artery.

Table 4-12.   **Disorders of the Spinal Accessory Nerve (Cranial Nerve XI)**

Location of lesion	Cause
Nuclear	Vascular
	Mass lesion: neoplasm, abscess
	Infectious/inflammatory: demyelinating disease, poliomyelitis
	Degenerative: motor neuron disease
	Syringobulbia
Jugular foramen	Neoplasm: glomus jugulare, schwannoma, metastases, skull base meningioma
	Trauma
	Osteomyelitis
Retropharyngeal, peripheral	Infection: abscess
	Head and neck tumors
	Neck irradiation
	Surgical procedure
	Trauma

sympathetics (Horner's syndrome) may be affected
- e) Optic nerve dysfunction less common but may indicate inflammatory process is also affecting orbital apex
- f) Secondary causes have been ruled out (aneurysms, trauma, neoplasm, and inflammatory and infectious processes)
- 3) Pathology: granulomatous inflammation reported by pathology studies
- 4) Differential diagnosis (Table 4-19 reviews other causes

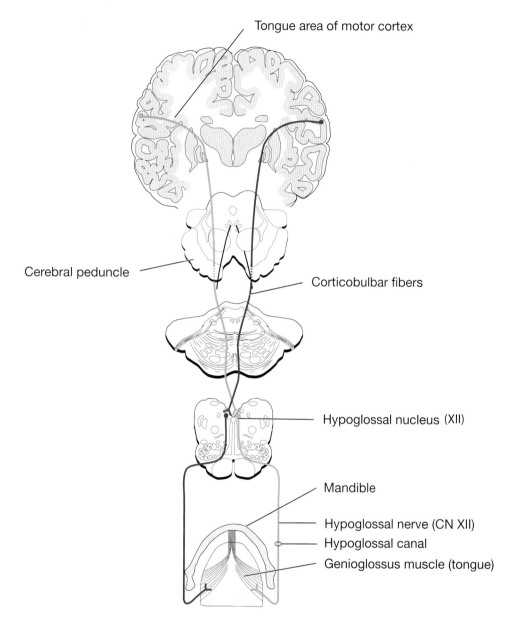

Fig. 4-16. The hypoglossal nerve innervates the ipsilateral genioglossus muscle of the tongue. The hypoglossal nucleus receives input from the contralateral cerebral hemisphere via the corticobulbar tract.

of painful ophthalmoplegia)

5) Diagnosis

   a) Rule out other cavernous sinus lesions with appropriate imaging

   b) Magnetic resonance imaging may demonstrate intermediate signal on T1-weighted image in area of cavernous sinus and enhancement with administration of gadolinium (this is nonspecif-

ic and could represent lymphoma or sarcoidosis)

   c) Cerebrospinal fluid studies to evaluate for chronic meningitides, sarcoidosis, lymphoma

   d) Serology studies to evaluate for vasculitides, sarcoidosis, and syphilis

   e) Biopsy may be necessary

6) Treatment

   a) Corticosteroids

Table 4-13. **Disorders of the Hypoglossal Nerve (Cranial Nerve XII)**

Location of lesion	Cause
Nuclear	Vascular: medial medullary ischemia, cavernous malformation
	Infectious/inflammatory: poliomyelitis, Guillain-Barré syndrome
	Mass lesion: tumor, abscess, syringobulbia
	Motor neuron disease
Meningeal	Vascular: vertebral artery aneurysm, vasculitis
	Infectious: chronic meningitides, mononucleosis
	Inflammatory: sarcoidosis
	Neoplastic: metastases, carcinomatous meningitis
	Metabolic: diabetes mellitus
	Developmental: Arnold-Chiari malformation
Hypoglossal canal	Neoplastic: glomus tumor, skull base meningioma, schwannoma, chordoma, cholesteatoma
	Infectious: osteitis
Carotid sheath, retropharyngeal region	Internal carotid artery dissection or internal carotid artery aneurysm
	Post-endarterectomy
	Retropharyngeal abscess
	Head and neck neoplasms
	Trauma
	Surgical procedures
Other	Idiopathic

Table 4-14. **Contents of the Jugular Foramen**

Cranial nerves IX, X, XI
Inferior petrosal sinus as it drains into jugular vein
Sigmoid sinus as it drains into jugular vein
Meningeal branch of ascending pharyngeal artery and
  meningeal branch of occipital artery

Table 4-15. **Contents of the Carotid Sheath**

Carotid artery
Jugular vein
Cranial nerves IX, X, XII
Note: the superior sympathetic ganglion is *outside* the
  carotid sheath

Table 4-16.   **Brainstem Clinical Syndromes**

Name	Picture	Localization	Vascular supply	Clinical symptoms (anatomy)
Midbrain syndromes				
Weber's syndrome		Medial midbrain	PCA perforators	Contralateral hemiparesis (cerebral peduncle) Ipsilateral CN III palsy (fascicles of CN III) Impaired ipsilateral pupillary reflex (CN III) and dilated pupil
Benedikt's syndrome		Midbrain tegmentum	PCA perforators	Ipsilateral CN III palsy usually with dilated pupil (CN III fascicles) Contralateral involuntary movements (red nucleus, subthalamic nucleus)
Claude's syndrome		Midbrain tegmentum (dorsal)	PCA perforators	Ipsilateral CN III palsy (CN III fascicles) Contralateral hemiataxia and dysmetria (dentatothalamic fibers within the superior cerebellar peduncle) Contralteral tremor (red nucleus)
Nothnagel's syndrome		Midbrain	PCA perforators	Ipsilateral CN III palsy (CN III fascicles) Contralateral hemiataxia (dentatothalamic fibers in superior cerebellar peduncle)
Pontine syndromes Millard-Gubler syndrome		Ventral pons	Basilar artery perforators, median and paramedian perforators	Ipsilateral lower motor neuron facial paralysis (CN VII) Ipsilateral abducens paralysis (CN VI fibers) Contralateral hemiparesis (corticospinal tract in basis pontis)
Foville syndrome		Dorsal pons tegmentum	Basilar artery perforators	Ipsilateral lower motor neuron facial paralysis (nucleus or fascicles of CN VII) Ipsilateral gaze paralysis (nucleus abducens palsy) Contralateral hemiparesis (corticospinal tract in basis pontis)

Table 4-16.   (continued)

Name	Picture	Localization	Vascular supply	Clinical symptoms (anatomy)
Ventral pontine syndrome		Ventral pons	Basilar artery: paramedian perforators	Ipsilateral CN VI palsy (CN VI fascicles) Contralateral hemiparesis (corticospinal tract in basis pontis)
Marie-Foix syndrome		Base of pons	Basilar artery perforators	Ipsilateral cerebellar ataxia (corticoponto-cerebellar fibers) Contralateral hemiparesis (corticospinal tract in basis pontis) Variable contralateral decrease in pain and temperature sensation (spinothalamic tract involvement)
Medullary syndromes Wallenberg syndrome		Lateral medulla	PICA	Ipsilateral hemiataxia (inferior cerebellar peduncle) Dysphagia, hoarseness, ipsilateral palatal weakness (nucleus ambiguus) Horner's syndrome (sympathetic) Ipsilateral face, contralateral body decrease in pain and temperature sensation (spinal tract and nucleus of V and lateral spino-thalamic tract)
Dejerine's syndrome (medial medullary syndrome)		Medial medulla	Vertebral artery perforators, anterior spinal artery	Contralateral hemiparesis (medullary pyramid) Contralateral decrease in vibration/proprio-ception sensation in limbs (medial lemniscus) Ipsilateral CN XII palsy

AICA, anterior inferior cerebellar artery; CN, cranial nerve; PCA, posterior cerebral artery; PICA, posterior inferior cerebellar artery.

Table 4-17. Clinical Syndromes of Lower Cranial Nerves

Syndrome name	Site of lesion	Cranial nerve IX	X	XI	XII	Sympathetics	Symptoms (cranial nerve)
Vernet's syndrome	Jugular foramen	■	■	■			Ipsilateral decrease in taste sensation of posterior 1/3 of tongue (IX) Ipsilateral soft palate weakness (X) Hoarseness (X) Ipsilateral SCM and trapezius muscle weakness (XI)
Collet-Sicard syndrome	Retropharyngeal space	■	■	■	■		Gag reflex decreased ipsilaterally (IX, X) Ipsilateral soft palate weakness (X) Hoarseness, dysphagia (X) Ipsilateral SCM and trapezius weakness (XI) Ipsilateral tongue weakness (XII)
Villaret's syndrome	Retropharyngeal space	■	■	■	■	■	All the above plus to ipsilateral Horner's syndrome

SCM, sternocleidomastoid.

Table 4-18. Differential Diagnosis of Multiple Cranial Neuropathies

Vascular	Vasculitis
Infectious	Viral: Epstein-Barr virus, cytomegalo-virus, varicella zoster virus, human immunodeficiency virus, hepatitis B Bacterial: Lyme disease, syphilis, diphtheria, *Listeria* Fungal meningitis Mycobacterium: tuberculosis
Inflammatory	Guillain-Barré syndrome and chronic inflammatory demyelinating polyradiculopathy Sarcoidosis Vasculitides: Wegener's granulomatosis, Sjögren's syndrome, systemic lupus erythematosus, Churg-Strauss syndrome Tolosa-Hunt syndrome
Neoplastic, paraneoplastic	Lymphoma Paraneoplastic Carcinomatous meningitis Paraproteinemias
Toxic-metabolic	Diabetes mellitus Porphyria Hypothyroid

Table 4-19. Differential Diagnosis of Painful Ophthalmoplegia

Localization	Cause
Cavernous sinus, parasellar region	Vascular: carotid cavernous fistula, carotid cavernous aneurysm, cavernous sinus thrombosis Infectious: bacterial sinusitis, periostitis, mucormycosis, syphilis, *Mycobacterium tuberculosis* Inflammatory: sarcoidosis, Wegener's granulomatosis, Tolosa-Hunt syndrome Neoplastic: pituitary adenoma, sarcoma, neurofibroma, epidermoid, craniopharyngioma, meningioma, chordoma, chondroma, giant cell tumor, metastases, lymphoma, carcinomatous meningitis
Orbital	Infectious: extension of sinusitis, mucormycosis Inflammatory: giant cell arteritis, idiopathic orbital inflammation (orbital pseudotumor) Neoplastic: metastases, lymphoma, leukemia Metabolic: multiple cranial neuropathies associated with diabetes mellitus
Other	Ophthalmoplegic migraine Trauma

REFERENCES

Benarroch EE, Westmoreland BF, Daube JR, Reagan TJ, Sandok BA. Medical neurosciences: an approach to anatomy, pathology, and physiology by systems and levels. 4th ed. Philadelphia: Lippincott Williams & Wilkins; 1999.

Dyck PJ, Thomas PK. Peripheral neuropathy. 4th ed. Philadelphia: Elsevier Saunders; 2005.

Gladstone JP, Dodick DW. Painful ophthalmoplegia: overview with a focus on Tolosa-Hunt syndrome. Curr Pain Headache Rep. 2004;8:321-9.

Grogan PM, Gronseth GS. Practice parameter: steroids, acyclovir, and surgery for Bell's palsy (an evidence-based review): report of the Quality Stanards Subcommittee of the American Academy of Neurology. Neurology. 2001;56:830-6.

Haines DE, editor. Fundamental neuroscience. 2nd ed. New York: Churchill Livingstone; 2002.

Kline LB, Hoyt WF. The Tolosa-Hunt Syndrome. J Neurol Neurosurg Psychiatry. 2001;71:577-82.

Moore JK. The human brainstem auditory system. In: Jackler RK, Brackmann DE, editors. Neurotology. 2nd ed. Philadelphia: Elsevier Mosby; 2005. p. 45-51.

Myssiorek D. Recurrent layngeal nerve paralysis: anatomy and etiology. Otolaryngol Clin North Am. 2004;37:25-44.

Piercy J. Bell's palsy. BMJ. 2005:330:1374.

Wrobel BB, Leopold DA. Clinical assessment of patients with smell and taste disorders. Otolaryngol Clin North Am. 2004;37:1127-42.

QUESTIONS

1. Which cranial nerves (CNs) are involved in gustatory sense (taste)?
   a. CNs III, VII, IX, X
   b. CNs V, VII
   c. CNs VII, IX, X
   d. CNs V, IX, X

2. A lesion of chorda tympani would result in deficits of which components of the facial nerve (CN VII)?
   a. SVA (taste) and GVE (parasympathetic output to submandibular and sublingual glands)
   b. SVE (motor of CN VII to ipsilateral face muscles)
   c. SVA (taste), GVE (parasympathetic output to submandibular and sublingual glands), and SVE (motor of CN VII to ipsilateral face muscles)
   d. GVE (parasympathetic output to lacrimal gland), GVE (parasympathetic output to submandibular and sublingual glands), SVA (taste)

3. A lesion at the foramen ovale would impair which divisions of CN V (trigeminal nerve)?
   a. Ophthalmic (V_1) and maxillary (V_2) sensory divisions
   b. Motor division of trigeminal nerve and V_2 sensory division
   c. Mandibular (V_3) sensory division
   d. Motor division of trigeminal nerve and V_3 sensory division
   e. All components (motor and sensory)

4. A patient presents with a 6-week history of gradual progressive hoarseness, dysphagia, weakness of the shoulder and dysarthria. Neurologic examination shows right-sided palatal weakness with reduced gag reflex and weakness and atrophy of the right sternocleidomastoid and trapezius muscles; when protruded, the tongue deviates to the right and is atrophic. This lesion localizes to:
   a. Cerebellopontine angle
   b. Carotid sheath
   c. Jugular foramen
   d. Retropharyngeal space

5. A patient presents with a 4-week history of left lower motor neuron facial weakness, bilateral sensorineural hearing loss, and lumbosacral radiculopathies. This lesion localizes to:
   a. Muscle
   b. Peripheral nerve
   c. Meningeal process
   d. Cerebellopontine angle

6. A patient presents with right tongue weakness and left arm and leg weakness in an upper motor neuron pattern. Where does the lesion localize?
   a. Right cerebral cortex
   b. Right medial medulla
   c. Meningeal process
   d. Hypoglossal canal
   e. Peripheral nerve

7. A patient presents with an ipsilateral decrease in smell, ipsilateral optic atrophy, and contralateral papilledema. The lesion producing this clinical syndrome is:
   a. Enesthesioblastoma
   b. Frontal lobe meningioma
   c. Acoustic neuroma
   d. Optic glioma

8. Cacosmia refers to:
   a. Increased sense of smell
   b. Perception of a bad smell
   c. Lack of sense of smell
   d. Perception of a pleasant smell

9. Tolosa-Hunt syndrome is characerized by:
   a. Petrous apex inflammatory syndrome resulting in dysfunction of CNs VII and VIII
   b. Ipsilateral anosmia and hypogonadism
   c. Congenital defect of CNs VI and VII bilaterally
   d. Painful ophthalmoplegia due to inflammation of cavernous sinus or parasellar region

10. A patient presents with ipsilateral hemiataxia, dysphagia, hoarseness, ipsilateral Horner's syndrome, and ipsilateral face but contralateral body decrease in pain and temperature sensation. The hoarseness and dysphagia are related to a lesion of what nucleus?
    a. Nucleus solitarius
    b. Dorsal motor nucleus of X
    c. Nucleus ambiguus
    d. Raphe nucleus

ANSWERS

1. Answer: c.
CNs VII (anterior 2/3 of tongue), IX (posterior 1/3 of tongue) and X (epiglottis). Information is relayed to rostral part of nucleus solitarius, which projects to ipsilateral ventral postero-medial thalamic nucleus.

2. Answer: a.
Taste from anterior 2/3 of tongue (SVA) and parasympathetic output to submandibular and sublingual glands (GVE).

3. Answer: d.
Motor division of trigeminal and V$_3$ sensory division.

4. Answer: d.
Retropharyngeal space (Collet-Sicard syndrome).

5. Answer: c.
Meningeal process (inflammatory, infectious, neoplastic). All cranial nerves and spinal nerves must exit the meninges before reaching the periphery. This would be the one location common to both.

6. Answer: a.
Medial medulla. If the tongue weakness were upper motor neuron, the tongue would deviate to the same side as the limb weakness. In this case, it deviates to opposite side. The lesion affects the exiting CN XII and nearby medullary pyramid.

7. Answer: b.
Foster Kennedy syndrome is typically due to a tumor affecting the olfactory bulb and optic nerve, with associated mass effect. This is seen most commonly with a frontal lobe meningioma.

8. Answer: b.
Perception of a bad smell.

9. Answer: d.

10. Answer: c.
Nucleus ambiguus. This case illustrates the clinical features of Wallenberg syndrome.

CLINICAL NEUROPHYSIOLOGY
PART A: ELECTROENCEPHALOGRAM (EEG)

Gena R. Ghearing, M.D.

I. INTRODUCTION

A. EEG

1. Physiologic measurement of brain electrical activity that aids in the diagnosis of spells and alterations of consciousness
2. EEG activity
   a. A recording of summated excitatory postsynaptic potentials (EPSPs) and inhibitory postsynaptic potentials (IPSPs) generated by synchronous activity at numerous synapses of cortical neurons
   b. Action potentials do not have an important role

B. Rhythmic EEG Activity: caused by oscillating EPSPs and IPSPs and is due to the following:

1. Intrinsic membrane properties of neurons
2. Synaptic connections of neurons
3. Thalamocortical inputs (sleep spindles are one of the best documented examples of rhythmic activity caused by projections of thalamic pacemaker cells in the nucleus reticularis)

II. BASIC EEG FREQUENCIES (FIG. 5-1)

A. Alpha Frequency (8-13 Hz)

1. Background activity of the wake state when eyes are closed
2. Present over posterior head region

Alpha activity is normal background wake activity

Beta activity is increased by benzodiazepines and barbiturates

Theta and delta slowing may indicate cerebral dysfunction

---

3. Attenuates with eye opening
4. May be blocked with sudden alerting or mental concentration
5. Maturation: 8 Hz reached by childhood, 9 to 12 Hz by adolescence
6. Absent in 11% of population: may be inherited, with autosomal dominant inheritance
7. Abnormality
   a. Asymmetry in amplitude between the cerebral hemispheres by more than 50% or more than 20 μV (higher amplitude of alpha activity over the right hemisphere is common)
   b. Failure of the rhythm to attenuate with eye opening (reactivity) unilaterally or bilaterally: may be due to structural lesions, e.g., occipital or pontine lesions in the absence of attenuation bilaterally (unilateral failure to attenuate usually indicates abnormality in ipsilateral occipital lobe or subcortical connections)
   c. Asymmetry in frequency: asymmetric slowing may occur with hypoperfusion
   d. Increases or decreases in frequency: may occur with metabolic conditions, drug use, or degenerative conditions
   e. Generalized alpha activity in context of coma or sedation: usually widespread with anterior predominance and not reactive
8. Variants
   a. Temporal alpha: independent rhythm over temporal regions as asynchronous bursts; normal in elderly
   b. Frontal alpha: predominant over anterior head regions; may be seen following arousal from sleep or toxic-metabolic insult
   c. Paradoxical alpha: alpha activity appearing with eye opening and mental alerting and disappearing with eye closure
      1) Occurs most commonly with sedation
      2) Occurs in context of awakening without immediate visual fixation

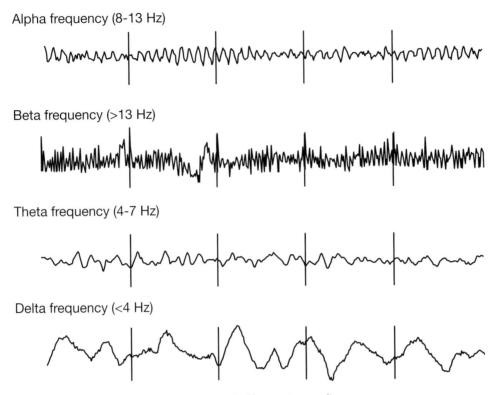

Fig. 5-1. Basic EEG frequencies (interval between two vertical bars = 1 second).

d. Slow variant: rhythm frequencies of 3.5 to 6.5 Hz which may be seen together with the normal alpha frequency, rare

e. Fast variant: rhythm frequencies of 14 to 16 Hz

B. Beta Frequency (>13 Hz)

1. Enhanced by drugs such as benzodiazepines and barbiturates
2. Low-voltage waves usually present over the frontal region
3. Beta rhythm often enhanced during drowsiness
4. Normal variants
   a. Frontal beta: predominantly over frontocentral head region; blocked by movement or intention to move
   b. Diffuse or generalized beta: present diffusely and not blocked by stimulus; induced by drugs
   c. Posterior beta: may be fast alpha variant and blocked by same maneuvers that block alpha rhythm

C. Theta Frequency (4-7 Hz)

1. Repetitive theta slowing
   a. May be sign of mild disturbance in cerebral function in awake adult
   b. Is normal in awake child or in states of drowsiness and sleep in adults
2. Young children (4 months-8 years): frontocentral predominance during drowsiness

3. Adolescents: anterior predominance during drowsiness
4. Adults: predominantly posterior head regions (and diffuse) during drowsiness

D. Delta Frequency (<4 Hz)

1. Normal in infants and during sleep
2. May represent moderate to severe disturbance of cerebral function

III. EEG RECORDING

A. **Recordings:** made from pairs of electrodes in different combinations over different areas of brain

B. **10-20 System of Electrode Placement:** most commonly used (Fig. 5-2)

1. Measurements made from the nasion to inion and between preauricular areas to determine position of electrodes
2. Electrodes are designated by an alphanumeric system
   a. F for frontal polar, P parietal or posterior temporal, T temporal, O occipital, C central, and Z midline areas
   b. Numbers increase with distance from anterior midline of the head

c. Odd numbers designate the left side, even numbers the right side
3. Standard recordings use 21 electrodes

C. Polarity Convention (Fig. 5-3)
1. If input to electrode 1 is negative in relation to electrode 2, pen moves upward
2. If input 1 is positive relative to input 2, pen moves downward

D. Bipolar Montage
1. Localizes focus of discharge by direction of pen deflection (phase reversal)
2. Uses three or more electrodes that may be linked in a transverse or longitudinal direction over the head
3. Best for viewing localized low to medium amplitude discharges

E. Referential Montage
1. Localizes focus of discharge by amplitude of deflection
2. Common electrode reference montage: the same electrode is used as input 2 of each amplifier; widespread high-amplitude activity is not filtered out, as it is in bipolar montage

a. Good for looking at asymmetry or electrode artifacts
b. Ear lobe reference: may be contralateral, ipsilateral, or combined
c. Vertex reference: helpful for temporal lobe abnormalities
3. Average reference montage: the reference is a sum of all electrodes in input 2 which is compared to each electrode in input 1
4. Weighted average reference montage
a. Gives a greater weight to electrodes closer to input 1 in the sum
b. Reduces the possibility of widespread activity tainting the reference of all channels

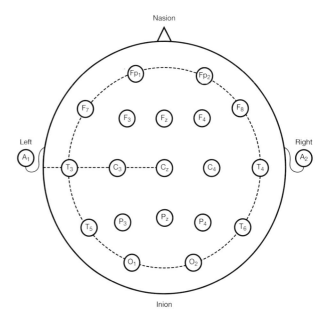

Fig. 5-2. 10-20 System of electrode placement.

Normal EEG		
Activity	Frequency	Area
Wake		
Beta	>13 Hz	Frontocentral
Alpha	8-13 Hz	Posterior
Theta	4-7 Hz	
Delta	<4 Hz	
Mu	7-12 Hz	Central
Lambda		Occipital
Sleep		
Spindles	10-14 Hz	Frontocentral, parietal
V waves		Vertex, frontocentral
K complex		Vertex, frontocentral
POSTS*		Occipital
Sawtooth waves		Central

*Positive occipital sharp transients of sleep

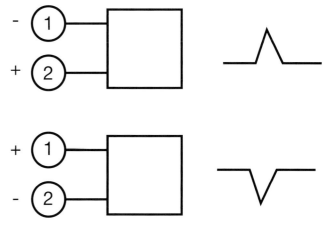

Fig. 5-3. Polarity convention.

5. Laplacian (source derivation) montage
   a. Used in digital recordings where one electrode is referenced to the sum of four surrounding electrodes C3- (T3+Cz+F3+P3)
   b. Good for detecting localized waveforms

F. Activation Procedures
1. Hyperventilation
   a. Normal responses include no change or generalized slowing
   b. Focal slowing can be seen in localized lesions
   c. Slowing that persists after the termination of hyperventilation may be seen in patients with syncopal attacks
   d. Buildup of slow waves minutes after end of hyperventilation may be seen in moyamoya disease
   e. May have prolonged slowing from hypoxia or hypoglycemia
   f. Activates epileptiform discharges in 30% to 50% of patients with absence seizures and 6% to 10% of patients with focal seizures
   g. Contraindications: heart and lung disease, sickle cell disease or trait, moyamoya disease, recent stroke, high-grade cerebral artery stenosis, intracranial hemorrhage, increased intracranial pressure
2. Photic stimulation
   a. Normally, occipital driving is at the same frequency as the stimulus
   b. Asymmetric responses suggest an occipital lesion (to less extent, posterior temporal)
   c. Occipital driving is similar morphologically to lambda waves
   d. No variability in the morphology (as compared with photomyogenic response, which shows variability in the morphology of the artifact's waveforms)
   e. Occipital driving is best elicited with the eyes closed or with stimulation using a red light
   f. Photomyogenic (photomyoclonic) response can be seen in drug withdrawal
   g. Photoparoxysmal (photoconvulsive) responses in 2% to 3% of patients, can be seen in renal disease
   h. Myoclonic seizures are the most common seizure type induced by photic stimulation
   i. Juvenile myoclonic epilepsy is the most common type of

> Hyperventilation activates epileptiform discharges in 30%-50% of patients with absence seizures
>
> A sleep recording increases the diagnostic yield in partial epilepsy

generalized epilepsy associated with photoparoxysmal (photoconvulsive) response
3. Sleep recording may identify abnormalities in 30% to 90% of patients who have normal wake recordings

G. Artifacts: noncerebral signals
1. Physiologic
   a. Patient movement
      1) Muscle artifact: high-frequency bursts
      2) Movement artifact: movement of head, or electrode wires (may be recognized in electrocardiographic [ECG] channel)
   b. Bioelectrical potential
      1) Eyes have a dipole, with the cornea relatively positive
         a) Upward eye movements produce downward deflection on a bipolar montage
         b) Are generally frontal and symmetric
      2) Tongue movements
         a) Produce a glossokinetic artifact that can be asymmetric
         b) Other oropharyngeal structures may have dipoles that create artifact
      3) Cardiac potential changes can be recorded
         a) Seen more commonly in obese patients
         b) Large artifacts may be seen in pacemakers
      4) Pulse wave artifact: precedes the heartbeat
   c. Skin resistance change: sweating, vasomotor activity
2. Nonphysiologic
   a. Electrode malfunction or other difficulties with the recording system (electrode popping is easily recognized example)
   b. External electrical interference

IV. NORMAL ADULT EEG

A. Wake
1. Lambda waves
   a. Occur with visual scanning (visual evoked potentials)
   b. Occipital positive sharp sawtooth transients that have amplitudes less than 50 μV
   c. Do persist in dark (may be related to eye movements)
2. Mu rhythm (Fig. 5-4)
   a. 7 to 11-Hz arch-shaped rhythm most obvious in centroparietal area
   b. Best observed in bipolar montage
   c. Attenuates with contralateral movement
   d. Enhanced by immobility and hyperventilation
   e. Seen in more than 10% of EEGs, predominately in young adults

f. Abnormalities include frequent trains of unilateral mu rhythm or marked asymmetry

3. Kappa rhythm
   a. Burst of low-amplitude alpha or theta activity
   b. May be associated with mental activity

B. Sleep

1. Stage 1: drowsiness (Fig. 5-5)
   a. About 5% of sleep time is spent in stage 1 sleep
   b. Slow eye movements (SEMs) which are less than 0.5 Hz
   c. Attenuation of background
   d. Dropout of alpha or replacement by theta activity
   e. Enhancement of beta activity

2. Stage 2: light sleep (Fig. 5-6)
   a. About 45% of time is spent in stage 2 sleep
   b. Characterized by sleep spindles and/or K complexes
   c. POSTS (positive occipital sharp transients of sleep)
      1) Triangular waves at irregular intervals (usually >1 second)
      2) Also called lamboid waves

Normal Adult Sleep EEG

Stage 1 sleep: attenuation of background and slow eye movements (SEMs)

Stage 2 sleep: spindles and V waves

Deep sleep (stages 3 and 4): delta activity

Rapid eye movement (REM) sleep: low-amplitude EEG, sawtooth waves, decreased muscle tone, increased heart rate

---

d. Vertex (V) waves
   1) Negative sharp transients at vertex with a frequency less than 2 Hz
   2) Occur rarely in wake persons who are startled
   3) May be more sharply contoured, appear in trains, or be located in midparietal region in children

e. Sleep spindles
   1) 11 to 15-Hz waveforms with more than 0.5 second duration
   2) Maximal centrally

f. K complexes
   1) Negative sharp waves similar to V waves
   2) Followed by slower positive component, more than 500 milliseconds

3. Stages 3 and 4: deep sleep
   a. 25% of time is spent in stages 3 and 4 sleep
   b. May still see POSTS, sleep spindles, K complexes
   c. Stage 3: less than 50% delta activity
   d. Stage 4: more than 50% delta

4. Rapid eye movement (REM) sleep (Fig. 5-7)
   a. 25% of time spent in REM sleep
   b. Low-amplitude EEG
   c. Sawtooth waves (medium amplitude, theta waves) over central region
   d. Decreased muscle activity
   e. Increased heart rate
   f. Epileptiform activity is most likely to be suppressed in REM sleep

C. Benign EEG Variants

1. Phantom spike-and-wave pattern (6-Hz spike-and-wave) (Fig. 5-8)
   a. 5 to 7-Hz spike-and-wave pattern in young adults
   b. Brief, bisynchronous bursts (lasting up to 2 seconds) of

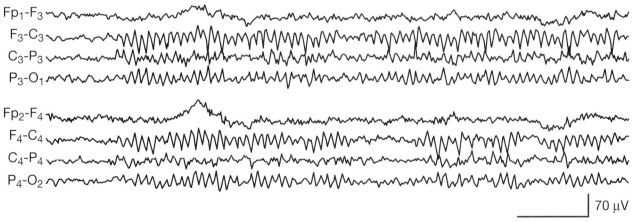

Fig. 5-4. Mu rhythm.

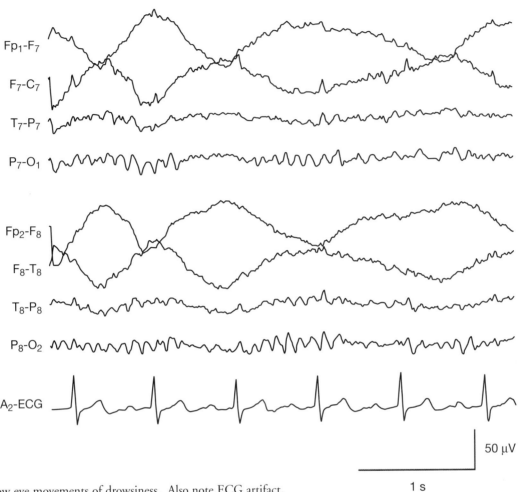

Fp$_1$-F$_7$

F$_7$-C$_7$

T$_7$-P$_7$

P$_7$-O$_1$

Fp$_2$-F$_8$

F$_8$-T$_8$

T$_8$-P$_8$

P$_8$-O$_2$

A$_2$-ECG

50 μV

1 s

Fig. 5-5. Slow eye movements of drowsiness. Also note ECG artifact.

Benign EEG Variants

Type	Age, y	Region
6-Hz spike-and-wave	10-20	Generalized
BSSS (benign sporadic sleep spikes)	>17	Temporal
14&6-Hz positive bursts	Young adults	Posterior
Wicket waves	Older adults	Temporal
RTTD (rhythmic temporal theta bursts of drowsiness)	Children & adults	Temporal
SREDA (subclinical rhythmic electrographic discharge of adults)	Adults	Diffuse

low-amplitude repeating spike and slow wave (the latter consisting of a higher amplitude and more widely distributed slow component than the small spike component, which may be buried in the slow wave)

   c. Higher incidence of epilepsy, especially in males with high-amplitude, anterior-predominant 6-Hz spike-and-wave waveforms occurring while awake (WHAM, see below)

   d. May be induced by the administration and withdrawal of sedatives and diphenhydramine

   e. Two variants: occipital form is usually benign, frontal form is commonly associated with epilepsy

      1) FOLD (female, occipital, low amplitude [<40 μV], drowsiness): benign, may be increased by diphenhydramine, prevalence of epilepsy about 30%

      2) WHAM (wake, high amplitude, anterior predominance, male): prevalence of epilepsy about 80%

2. Small sharp spikes (SSS), benign sporadic sleep spikes

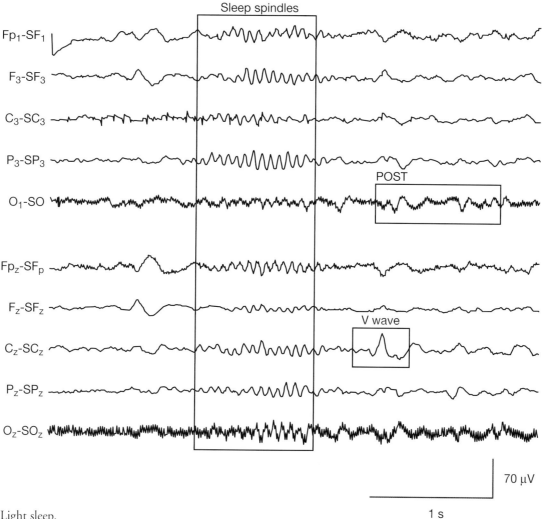

Fig. 5-6. Light sleep.

(BSSS), or benign epileptiform transients of sleep (BETS) (Fig. 5-9)
   a. Small amplitude, short duration (<65 milliseconds)
   b. Sharply contoured, one or two phases
   c. Unilateral or bilateral, noted predominantly in anterior and midtemporal regions
   d. Do not disturb background
   e. Disappear with deeper levels of sleep
3. 14&6 positive bursts (Fig. 5-10)
   a. Arch-shaped repetitive positive spikes at approximately 14 Hz or 6 Hz
   b. Most common in children and adolescents
   c. Amplitude less than 75 μV
   d. Maximal over posterior temporal area
   e. Occur with drowsiness and light sleep
   f. Nonspecific finding: observed in normal subjects or patients with anoxic or metabolic encephalopathy (including hepatic coma as in Reye's syndrome)

4. Wicket waves (Fig. 5-11)
   a. Single spike-like or 6 to 11-Hz mu-like waveforms
   b. Negative polarity, with an amplitude up to 200 μV
   c. Present over temporal regions
   d. Occur primarily in older adults during drowsiness and light sleep
5. Breach rhythm: enhancement of normal rhythms when recorded through a skull defect
6. Rhythmic temporal theta bursts of drowsiness (RTTD) (psychomotor-variant pattern)
   a. Flattopped or notched, monomorphic rhythmic waveforms of moderate amplitude, usually in theta frequency (4-7 Hz)
   b. Predominately over temporal regions, unilaterally or bilaterally
   c. Seen in relaxed wakefulness or drowsiness in adolescents and adults
7. Subclinical rhythmic electrographic discharge of adults (SREDA)

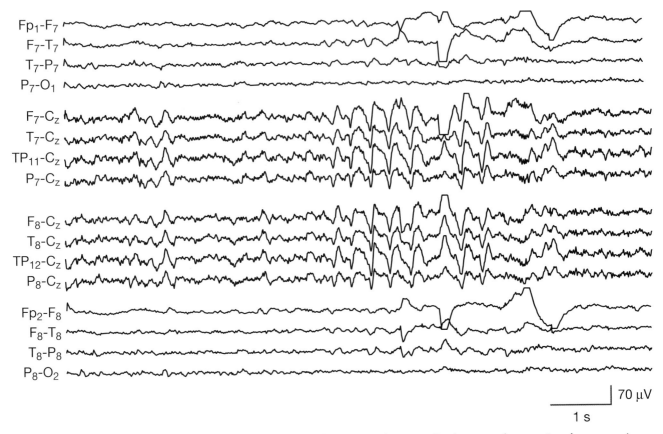

Fig. 5-7. Rapid eye movement (REM) sleep. Note the sawtooth waves, medium-amplitude sawtooth-appearing theta waves in frontal and central head regions and the REMs recorded in prefrontal electrodes, Fp1 and Fp2.

a. 5 to 7-Hz sinusoidal pattern lasting 40 to 80 seconds (sometimes a few minutes)

b. Occurs primarily in adults during wakefulness, hyperventilation, or sometimes sleep

c. Abrupt or stuttering onset

d. Occurs primarily in the elderly

e. May be distinguished from a seizure discharge by the following:

   1) May wax and wane
   2) Tendency to occur many times during the same recording and in subsequent recordings
   3) Maximum over parietal and posterior temporal regions
   4) Does not disturb background
   5) Not associated with a "postictal" EEG pattern
   6) Constant amplitude and rhythmic discharge that does not evolve into other frequencies

8. Photoparoxysmal response

   a. Generalized spike-and-wave discharges that may persist after the stimulus is turned off

b. May occur in patients without spontaneous seizures, but usually seen interictally in patients with generalized seizure disorder, especially juvenile myoclonic epilepsy

D. **Normal EEG Variants in Persons Older Than 60 Years**

1. Alpha rhythm

   a. Slows to an average of 9 Hz at 60 years, 8 to 9 Hz at 100 years
   b. This slowing may be demonstrated in serial EEGs of the same person
   c. Amplitude, persistence, and reactivity of the alpha rhythm may also decrease

2. Beta activity may be seen in half of those older than 60, more common in women

3. May see a slight increase in theta activity in persons older than 75 years

4. Temporal slowing of the elderly

   a. Bursts of theta or delta of medium to high amplitude
   b. Two-thirds have a left temporal onset

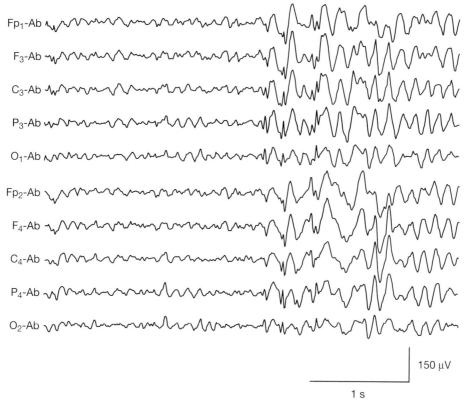

Fig. 5-8. Phantom spike-and-wave (6-Hz spike-and-wave) pattern (on the right side).

c. Delta slowing should be present in less than 1% of the recording

d. Theta slowing should be present in less than 10% of the recording

e. Increased prevalence in normal subjects during fifth and sixth decades

f. Facilitated by drowsiness

> **EEG of Premature Infants**
>
> Premature infants have active sleep and quiet sleep with a tracé alternant pattern
>
> May also see delta brushes, occipital slow waves, and frontal sharp transients in premature infants

V. NORMAL PEDIATRIC EEG

A. Neonatal EEG

1. Sleep activity
   a. Active sleep
      1) Bursts of REMs
      2) Body twitches and facial grimaces
      3) Diffuse, low-voltage EEG pattern
      4) Absence of chin myogram
      5) Irregular cardiorespiratory functions
   b. Quiet sleep
      1) No eye movements
      2) Reduced body movements
      3) Tonic activity of chin myogram
      4) Regular cardiorespiratory functions
      5) Slow-wave EEG and tracé alternant pattern

2. Premature infants less than 30 weeks of conceptual age
   a. Discontinuous tracing ("tracé discontinue")
      1) Bursts of medium- to high-amplitude, mixed frequency (mostly delta, may appear as occipital rhythmic delta activity) waves occurring in random, paroxysmal fashion, predominantly over posterior head regions
      2) These periods of EEG activity last less than 15 seconds and interrupt an almost flat background
   b. As brain matures, intervals between the bursts gradually

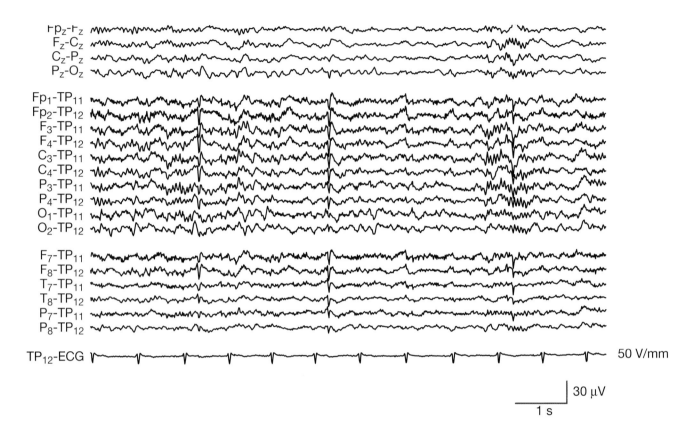

Fig. 5-9. Small sharp spikes, benign sporadic sleep spikes, or benign epileptiform transients of sleep.

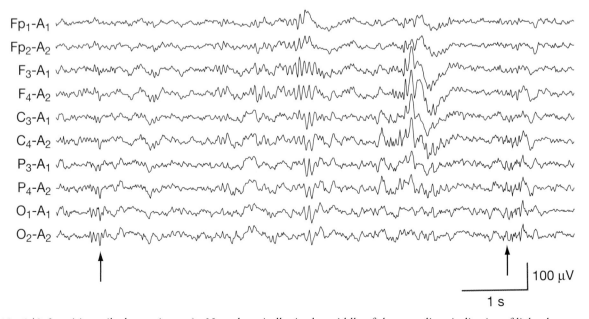

Fig. 5-10. 14&6 positive spike bursts (*arrows*). Note the spindles in the middle of the recording, indicative of light sleep.

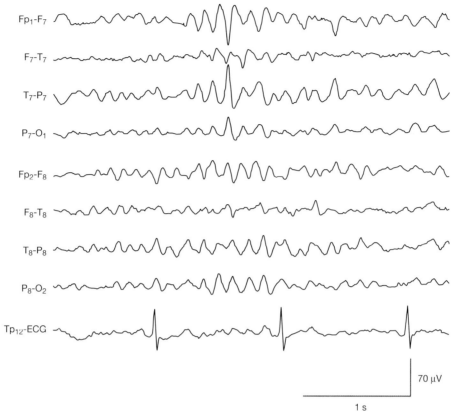

Fp₁-F₇

F₇-T₇

T₇-P₇

P₇-O₁

Fp₂-F₈

F₈-T₈

T₈-P₈

P₈-O₂

Tp₁₂-ECG

70 μV

1 s

Fig. 5-11. Wicket waves.

shorten, and the tracing changes into a less discontinuous pattern: the "tracé alternant" (periods between the bursts are shorter in duration)
1) As infant matures, the pattern becomes less prominent, but may be present until 1 month of age
2) This pattern usually occurs during quiet sleep
3) Generally regarded as abnormal if present after 1 month of age or during wakefulness
4) Waveforms appear more sharply contoured with longer interburst duration in more premature infants
c. Delta brushes (spindle delta bursts) over the occipital and central head regions appear by 26 weeks
1) Medium to high amplitude (25-200 μV) 0.3 to 1.5-Hz delta activity with superimposed 8 to 20-Hz fast activity, most prominently present during sleep
2) Delta brushes are maximally expressed at 35 to 36 weeks of conceptual age
3) May be present until 41 to 42 weeks, usually disappear in term infants
d. Paroxysmal temporal theta transients (theta activity over temporal head regions)
e. Little distinction between EEG patterns of wake and sleep

3. Premature infants of 31 to 32 weeks of conceptual age
a. Emergence of two different types of background activity
1) Discontinuous EEG activity with reduced body movements resembling *quiet sleep*
2) Continuous EEG activity with REM and increased body twitches resembling *active sleep*
b. Frequent delta brushes
c. Reduced paroxysmal temporal theta transients
d. Some degree of interhemispheric synchrony is present by this time: the waveforms (including bursts of tracé alternant) "time-locked" to less than 1.5-second difference
4. Premature infants of 33 to 36 weeks of conceptual age
a. Greater differentiation between active and quiet sleep
b. Active sleep (REM sleep): more continuous pattern
c. Quiet sleep: a discontinuous pattern, tracé alternant pattern
d. Tracé alternant pattern gradually replaces tracé discontinue pattern
e. Frequent delta brushes (spindle delta bursts)
f. Frontal sharp transients: biphasic sharply contoured frontal waveforms occurring most often during sleep
g. Multifocal sharp transients during sleep and wakefulness

h. Anterior rhythmic delta: short runs of bilateral rhythmic delta activity, often persisting into term
i. Occipital slow waves: moderate- to high-amplitude delta activity during sleep
j. More interhemispheric synchrony
k. Emergence of EEG reactivity: changes in EEG tracing induced by stimulation of infant

5. Premature infants of 37 to 38 weeks of conceptual age
   a. Wakefulness: characterized by a pattern of irregular low-amplitude theta and delta activity (activité moyenne)
   b. Quiet sleep: characterized by tracé alternant and delta slow waves
   c. Active sleep: characterized by continuous low-amplitude activity or mixed pattern of delta and theta activity
   d. Delta brushes continue
   e. Multifocal sharp transients are less abundant, but frontal sharp transients and anterior rhythmic delta continue, and interhemispheric synchrony is more prominent

6. Full-term infants of 39 to 42 weeks of conceptual age
   a. Interhemispheric synchrony continues such that by 40 weeks of conceptual age, almost all bursts of tracé alternant activity are synchronous
   b. Clearly defined wakefulness, active sleep, and quiet sleep
   c. Wake and active sleep
      1) Low-voltage, irregular pattern: characterized by continuous theta with intermittent superimposed low-amplitude delta-frequency activity
      2) This activity may be admixed with higher amplitude delta activity (termed mixed pattern), also occurring during active sleep and wakefulness.
   d. Quiet sleep: tracé alternant or high-voltage slow-wave pattern (characterized by continuous delta activity)
   e. Delta brushes continue, but infrequent (mainly during quiet sleep)
   f. Less frequent multifocal sharp transients and frontal sharp transients primarily during sleep

B. Pediatric EEG
1. First 3 months
   a. Tracé alternant disappears at about 46 weeks
   b. Wakefulness
      1) Characterized by delta and theta activity
      2) 5 to 6-Hz rhythmic central activity is present and represents a precursor of mu rhythm
      3) Also, a 3 to 4-Hz occipital rhythm, induced by passively closing the infant's eyes and blocked by eye opening, is present and represents a precursor of the alpha rhythm
   c. Majority of sleep starts in active sleep at term and quiet sleep by 46 weeks

d. Slow, high-amplitude sleep pattern
e. Rudimentary sleep spindles may be present at 40 weeks of conceptual age
   1) Are observed consistently by 8 to 12 weeks after birth and become more prominent by 3 months of age
   2) Can be asymmetric until 2 years
f. A photic driving response may be seen at lower flash frequencies (<3 Hz)

2. 4 to 6 months
   a. Better developed occipital and central rhythms
   b. Wake pattern reacts to stimulation
   c. Photic driving response present
   d. Rudimentary V waves and K complexes
      1) May be present at birth, become distinct by 3 to 5 months, appear well developed by age 2 to 3 years
      2) V waves often achieve high amplitudes and may be sharply contoured and occur in serial trains by age 3 to 5 years

3. 6 months to 2 years
   a. Central rhythms are often more prominent than occipital rhythms (of 6-8 Hz)
   b. Throughout childhood, the predominance of rhythmic background activity shifts from central to occipital head regions
   c. Drowsiness may be marked by hypnogogic hypersynchrony, paroxysmal drowsy bursts with spike-like morphology, seen in 8% of normal children from birth to 16 years
   d. Occipital diphasic slow-wave transients ("shut eye waves"): sharply contoured activity associated with eye blinks
   e. REM sleep (resembles low-amplitude activity of adult REM sleep)
      1) Replaces active sleep
      2) Presence of REM sleep (as a percentage of total sleep) changes from 50% to about 30% of sleep
   f. Non-REM sleep: characterized by generalized (posterior predominance) delta slow activity with intermittent large, monophasic or diphasic delta waveforms present over occipital regions (cone waves, "O" waves)

4. 2 to 5 years
   a. Central rhythm frequencies of 8 to 9 Hz and occipital alpha rhythm frequencies of 6 to 8 Hz by age 3 years
   b. Theta frequencies predominate
   c. 8-Hz alpha rhythm in most children by 3 years, less prominent than theta waves

5. 6 to 16 years
   a. Adult alpha frequency appears between ages 8 and 10 years, sinusoidal activity enhanced by eye closure develops from the background occipital rhythmic activity

b. Beta activity is rarely seen in normal children and adolescents; prominent over the occipital head region in children younger than 2 years and over anterior head regions in older children and adults

c. Rhythmic paroxysmal theta waves (during wakefulness)

   1) May be present over temporal and posterior head regions

   2) This activity may also appear over frontocentral head regions

d. Posterior slowing of youth (Fig. 5-12)

   1) Delta-like occipital slowing with superimposed alpha activity

   2) Posterior slowing attenuates with the alpha rhythm with eye opening or alerting and does not exceed alpha rhythm's amplitude by more than 1.5 times

e. Drowsiness in adolescence is marked by trains of monomorphic sinusoidal theta activity over frontal head regions

VI. ABNORMAL EEG PATTERNS

A. **Classified as Ictal or Interictal:** depends on whether the activity occurs during a seizure

B. **Slowing**

1. Theta slowing may reflect mild to moderate disturbance of cerebral function, may be focal or generalized

2. Polymorphic delta activity (PDA)

   a. Arrhythmic, irregular activity persisting throughout EEG recording

   b. Associated with white matter lesions

   c. May be generalized or focal

   d. Focal PDA usually signifies a focal lesion such as infarct, tumor, or abscess

   e. Focal PDAs are usually persistent through changes in physiologic states (nonreactive, present during sleep, and no attenuation with alerting), continuous (not intermittent), and with some variability in morphology of waveforms (appear irregular, not rhythmic)

   f. Focal slow waves usually appear maximally at onset of an acute insult and may either persist or become less prominent and disappear weeks to months after the insult

   g. Generalized PDA is usually seen in association with a diffuse encephalopathy or a degenerative cognitive disease

3. Intermittent rhythmic delta activity (IRDA)

   a. Medium to high amplitude, delta frequency bisynchronous slow waves

   b. Monomorphic, rhythmic, and intermittent (as compared with PDA, which is polymorphic, irregular, persistent)

   c. Enhances with drowsiness, attenuates with alerting, and disappears with sleep (whereas PDA usually persists through sleep and alerting)

   d. Distant rhythms originating from deep or midline structures projecting to the surface

   e. Lesions affecting these midline or deep structures (including subcortical gray matter, brainstem, diencephalon, mesial surfaces of frontal lobes, periventricular regions) by direct compression or distortion (e.g., herniation) may produce these bisynchronous slow waves

   f. May also been seen with increased *intraventricular* (not intracranial) pressure

   g. IRDA appearing maximal in the frontal areas is termed

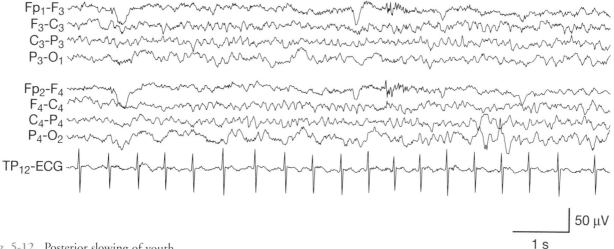

Fig. 5-12. Posterior slowing of youth.

"frontal intermittent rhythmic delta activity" (FIRDA) and may be seen in association with noncommunicating hydrocephalus, herniation syndromes causing pressure on deep midline structures, or diffuse cerebral processes affecting cortical or subcortical gray matter

h. IRDA appearing maximal in occipital areas is termed "occipital intermittent rhythmic delta activity" (OIRDA) and may be seen in association with lesions (e.g., medulloblastoma) involving posterior fossa structures

C. Asymmetry

1. Differences in amplitude between two homologous head regions
2. Amplitude may be decreased or, less often, increased on abnormal side
3. Persistent asymmetry of alpha activity by 50% or beta activity by 35% is considered abnormal
4. Usually caused by either unilateral lesions changing the underlying cortex producing the EEG activity or alteration in the media between cerebral cortex and recording surface
5. Examples of unilateral insults producing decreased amplitudes: cortical infarcts, tumors, trauma, transient ischemic attacks, migraine
6. Less commonly, cerebrovascular insults may paradoxically produce increased amplitudes (this may involve entire background activity or a specific background rhythm [e.g., alpha, beta, mu, or sleep activity])
7. Examples of asymmetry caused by alteration in the media between cerebral cortex and recording surface: skull defect produces increased amplitudes (termed "breach rhythm"), whereas local scalp edema, subdural hygroma, hematoma, or empyema may cause reduced amplitudes on ipsilateral side

D. Suppression

1. Loss of EEG activity, sustained cerebral activity less than 20 μV
2. May be focal or generalized

E. Epileptiform Discharges: definitions (Fig. 5-13)

1. Spike: duration less than 70 milliseconds, sharp ascending and descending limbs
2. Sharp wave: duration more than 70 milliseconds, potentials appear broader than spikes
3. Spike and wave: spike followed by slow wave
4. Paroxysmal fast activity: trains of spikes

F. Focal Epileptic Discharges

1. Interictal activity consisting of focal sharp waves or spikes

a. Usually asymmetric
b. Interrupt background activity
c. Usually have more than one phase
d. May be followed by a slow wave
e. May occur with focal cortical injury, diffuse insult, or no known lesion
f. Examples associated with specific conditions
   1) Occipital spikes in young children may correlate with visual difficulties and only 40% of patients have seizures, there is usually an underlying lesion in older patients
   2) Central-temporal (rolandic-sylvian) spikes (Fig. 5-14)
      a) Diphasic, high-amplitude, blunt spike followed by a wave
      b) Associated with benign seizures of childhood (4-12 years old)
      c) 60% to 70% have seizures
      d) Often start with facial twitching, followed by generalized seizure; occur at night
   3) Midline spikes may be associated with supplementary motor seizures
   4) Temporal spikes or slow waves: the most common interictal pattern in temporal lobe epilepsy

Spike

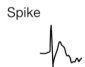

Slow wave

Spike and wave

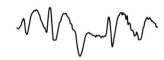

Multispike and wave

Fig. 5-13. Epileptiform discharges.

a) Most epileptogenic of focal waveforms (>95% have seizures)

b) Increased in sleep

2. Focal slowing

a. Temporal intermittent rhythmic delta activity (TIRDA)

1) Moderate-amplitude rhythmic delta activity in temporal area

2) Most prominent during drowsiness and non-REM sleep

3) Epileptogenic significance similar to temporal sharp waves

3. Focal seizures

a. Rhythmical activity with focal onset that evolves in shape, frequency, amplitude (Fig. 5-15)

b. May have secondary generalization (spread to involve all electrodes)

G. Generalized Epileptiform Patterns

1. Interictal patterns (last less than a few seconds)

a. Spikes or sharp waves may occur, but much less frequently than with focal disorders

b. Irregular, asymmetric theta and delta slowing may be seen in patients with tonic seizures

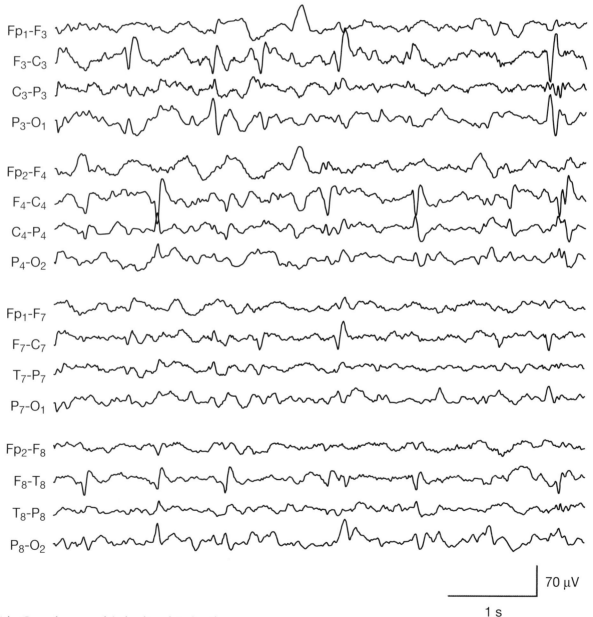

Fig. 5-14. Central-temporal (rolandic-sylvian) spikes.

c. 3-Hz spike-and-wave (typical spike-and-wave pattern) (Fig. 5-16)
1) High-amplitude spike or spikes, followed by high-amplitude wave
2) Stereotyped, symmetric spike-and-wave pattern
3) Variability in frequency: usually starts at fast frequency of 4 Hz and slows down to 2.5 Hz before ending
4) Maximal frontally
5) Readily enhanced by hyperventilation (and hypoglycemia): almost always detected (>98%) in a single recording with hyperventilation in patients not taking anticonvulsants

---

3-Hz spike-and-wave pattern is seen during absence seizures

Central-temporal spikes are seen in patients with rolandic epilepsy

Interictal temporal spikes or slow waves are commonly seen in temporal lobe epilepsy, especially during sleep

---

6) Also facilitated by alkalosis and drowsiness
7) Diminished during REM sleep
8) Usually associated with absence seizures in young children; often resolves after adolescence
9) May be associated with brief runs of 3-Hz slowing over occipital head regions
10) EEG pattern usually dramatically suppressed with use of anticonvulsants: interictal EEG can be used to determine the efficacy of treatment

d. Slow spike-and-wave
1) Similar to 3-Hz spike-and-wave pattern
2) Slow spike-and-wave discharges have the following characteristics (compared with 3-Hz spike-and-wave pattern):
   a) Frequency: 1 to 2.5 Hz, slower than typical 3-Hz spike-and-wave
   b) First component often resembles a sharp wave ("slow spike"), rather than the spike in the typical 3-Hz spike-and-wave pattern
   c) Distribution of activity may be asymmetric, focal, and may be shifting in emphasis or focal in one head region, persistently, whereas 3-Hz spike-and-wave pattern is usually symmetric, with only minor shifting asymmetries

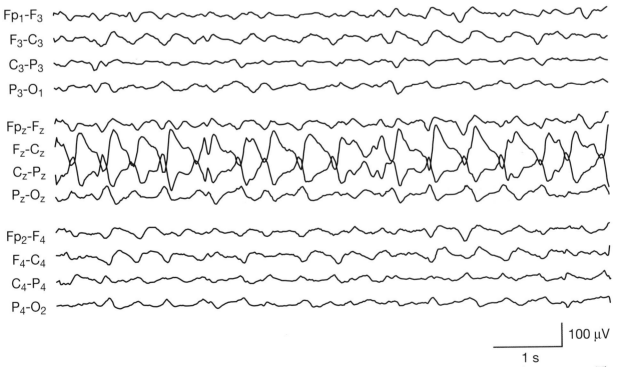

Fp_1-F_3
F_3-C_3
C_3-P_3
P_3-O_1

Fp_z-F_z
F_z-C_z
C_z-P_z
P_z-O_z

Fp_2-F_4
F_4-C_4
C_4-P_4
P_4-O_2

100 µV
1 s

Fig. 5-15. EEG recording from a 60-year-old man with multifocal seizures secondary to multiple embolic ischemic events. The tracing shows a seizure discharge in the midline leads (mainly C_z) associated with clonic movements of the feet. Note also generalized slowing of background activity in the delta range.

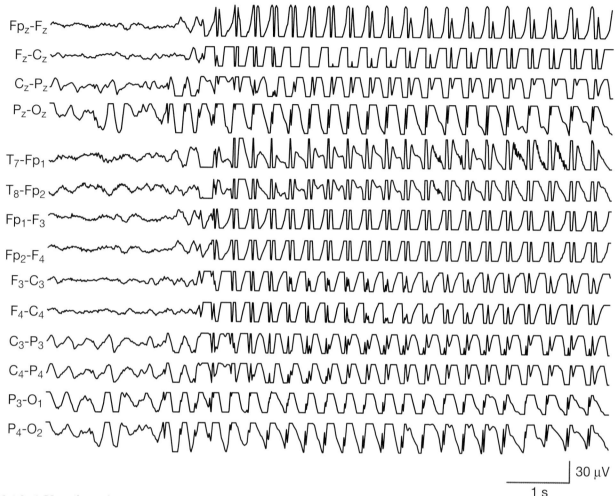

Fig. 5-16. 3-Hz spike-and-wave pattern (typical spike-and-wave pattern).

d) Associated with Lennox-Gastaut syndrome and several different seizures (tonic, tonic-clonic, atonic, myoclonic, atypical absence), but the 3-Hz spike-and-wave pattern is usually associated with childhood absence epilepsy

e) Usually not precipitated by hyperventilation or hypoglycemia (but may be activated with drowsiness), whereas typical 3-Hz spike-and-wave pattern is usually enhanced by hyperventilation and hypoglycemia

f) Neurologic examination: generally abnormal, often underlying cerebral lesion

3) Generalized discharges that are symmetric or asymmetric

4) Begins between 2 and 4 years of age, may persist into adolescence

5) Many patients have severe intractable seizure disorder (as mentioned above) and mental retardation

e. Atypical or irregular spike-and-wave
1) Occurs at varying frequencies between 4 and 6 Hz, may have multispike or polyspike components
2) Does not have rhythmic, stereotypic appearance of 3-Hz spike-and-wave pattern
3) May be asymmetric
4) Associated with different types of generalized seizures: tonic-clonic, myoclonic, atonic, and atypical absence seizures; associated with juvenile myoclonic epilepsy

f. Generalized paroxysmal fast activity
1) 2 to 4 seconds of sharp waves or spikes in the beta frequency (8-20 Hz)
2) Usually appears during sleep in patients with generalized epilepsy, may also be seen at onset of a generalized tonic-clonic seizure
3) Associated with tonic seizures
4) More common in patients with developmental delay

g. Hypsarrhythmia (Fig. 5-17)

1) High-amplitude activity that cannot be recorded at routine sensitivity settings, especially over posterior head regions
2) Irregular, multifocal, chaotic pattern of spikes, sharp waves, and slow waves
3) Usually appears between 6 months and 2 years (only rarely after 4 years of age), often a manifestation of severe cortical dysfunction
4) Sleep: intermittent hypsarrhythmia resembling a burst-suppression pattern, attenuation of pattern during REM sleep, and amplification of pattern during non-REM sleep
5) Classically associated with electrodecremental seizures
   a) Decrement of high-amplitude, chaotic pattern, which accompanies infantile spasms (discussed below)
   b) Patients also may have myoclonic jerks (shorter duration than infantile spasms) associated with generalized high-amplitude epileptiform activity (often spike or spike-and-wave discharges)
2. Ictal patterns
   a. Myoclonus
      1) Various forms of periodic complexes: sharp waves, spikes, or spike-and-wave discharges
      2) Spike-and-sharp-wave discharges coincide with myoclonic jerks
   b. 3-Hz spike-and-wave pattern
      1) Usually represents absence seizure

2) Morphology same as the interictal pattern
c. Electrodecremental pattern in setting of hypsarrhythmia
   1) Abrupt attenuation of background: usually preceded by generalized sharp and slow waves or high-amplitude slow waves most notable frontally
   2) Trains of fast activity may be observed during initial period of attenuation
   3) Associated with infantile spasms and West's syndrome, the clinical correlate to the electrodecremental pattern is usually infantile spasms (may occur in clusters)
d. Generalized tonic-clonic seizure
   1) Tonic phase
      a) Low-amplitude fast activity (>10 Hz), followed by higher amplitude and lower frequency rhythmic activity
      b) Lasts about 10 to 20 seconds
   2) Clonic phase
      a) High-amplitude spike or polyspike-and-wave complexes of 1 to 4 Hz
      b) Lasts about 30 seconds
      c) Postictal phase: low-amplitude, slow activity
e. Tonic seizure: may have trains of spikes, polyspikes, or rhythmic fast activity
f. Clonic seizures: usually associated with rhythmic spike-and-wave discharges, where spike correlates with clonic jerk

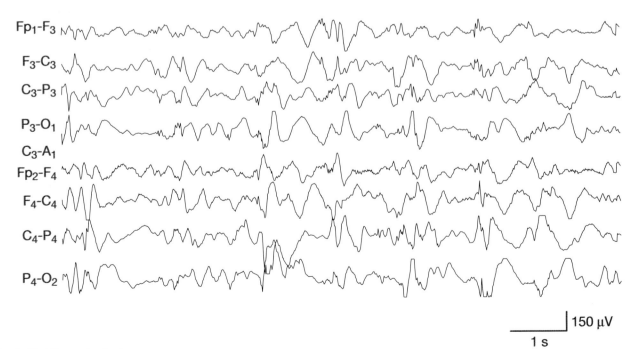

150 μV

1 s

Fig. 5-17. Hypsarrhythmia.

H. Status Epilepticus (see also Chapter 10)
1. EEG is important in making the diagnosis of status epilepticus
   a. Also aids in monitoring treatment
   b. Is critical in paralyzed patients
2. Nonconvulsive status epilepticus
   a. Clinical manifestation: alteration in consciousness or behavior with psychiatric symptoms
   b. Absence status epilepticus
      1) Less regular continuous 3-Hz spike-and-wave pattern than in typical absence seizures
      2) Common in elderly patients without previous history of absence seizures
      3) EEG and mental status rapidly improve with intravenous benzodiazepines
   c. Atypical absence status epilepticus
      1) Continuous or clusters of repetitive epileptiform generalized discharges, consisting of spike-and-wave (and polyspike-and-wave) and sharp-and-wave discharges, with no reactivity to stimuli
      2) Patient may be alert between clusters
   d. Simple partial status epilepticus
      1) May involve sensory or other regions of brain without causing motor activity
      2) Rhythmic focal activity, EEG may be normal
   e. Complex partial status epilepticus
      1) Intermittent alterations of consciousness, psychiatric manifestations, or automatisms
      2) Frontal and temporal rhythmic activity is most common
3. Generalized convulsive status epilepticus
   a. Consists of tonic-clonic, clonic, myoclonic, or tonic activity
   b. EEG shows continuous changes consistent with seizure type
4. Epilepsia partialis continua
   a. Continuous repetitive movement
   b. Rhythmic discharge over involved region, may be normal
5. Hemiconvulsive status epilepticus: often seen in young children as part of hemiconvulsion-hemiplegia-epilepsy

I. PLEDs (periodic lateralized epileptiform discharges) (Fig. 5-18)
1. Biphasic or multiphasic spikes, sharp waves, slow waves, or rhythmic fast activity
2. Occur in periodic or quasiperiodic fashion of 1 to 3 Hz
3. May evolve into seizure pattern
4. Usually resolve in 1 to 4 weeks
5. May occur in vascular insults, herpes simplex encephalitis, epilepsy, subdural hematoma, focal infection (abscess or cerebritis), and other disorders, including toxic-metabolic conditions such as hypoglycemia, uremia, alcohol withdrawal
6. PolyPLEDs: complex waveforms with polymorphic spikes and sharp waves or sharp-and-slow-wave complexes
7. BiPLEDs: independent PLEDs bilaterally over hemispheres, usually occur in diffuse or bilateral focal disease processes
8. Chronic PLEDs: rare and can occur with structural lesions, e.g., those associated with tuberous sclerosis

J. Encephalopathy
1. Generalized nonperiodic
   a. Slowing of alpha activity (nonspecific)
   b. Increase in theta activity (nonspecific)
   c. Polymorphic delta activity (nonspecific)
   d. Excess beta activity: medication effect
2. Generalized periodic activity
   a. Triphasic waves (Fig. 5-19)
      1) Not associated with seizures
      2) Large positive sharp wave with small negative wave before and after
      3) Frontal predominance (highest amplitude) with 1.5 to 2.5-Hz frequency, less commonly posterior predominance
      4) Sharply contoured, bilateral, and symmetric; often with an apparent anterior-posterior phase lag (time delay) of the second phase (less commonly posterior-anterior or side-to-side phase lag)
      5) Frequency of occurrence increases with aging
      6) Associated with hepatic coma (34%-50% of patients); other causes include renal failure, anoxia, electrolyte disturbances, encephalitis
      7) Lateralized triphasic waves (unilateral or asymmetric triphasic waves with asymmetry more than 50%) are more likely to represent epileptiform activity (than the symmetric bilateral triphasic waves), almost always associated with a structural abnormality rather than a metabolic-toxic disorder
      8) Impairment of reactivity and disruption of the background activity portend a worse prognosis
   b. Generalized periodic sharp waves (Fig. 5-20)
      1) Widespread, bisynchronous, sharp waves with one to three phases
      2) Duration: 0.25 to 0.5 second
      3) Occur at 0.5 to 1-second intervals
      4) Seen in Creutzfeldt-Jakob disease, metabolic encephalopathies (e.g., hypothyroidism), inflammatory

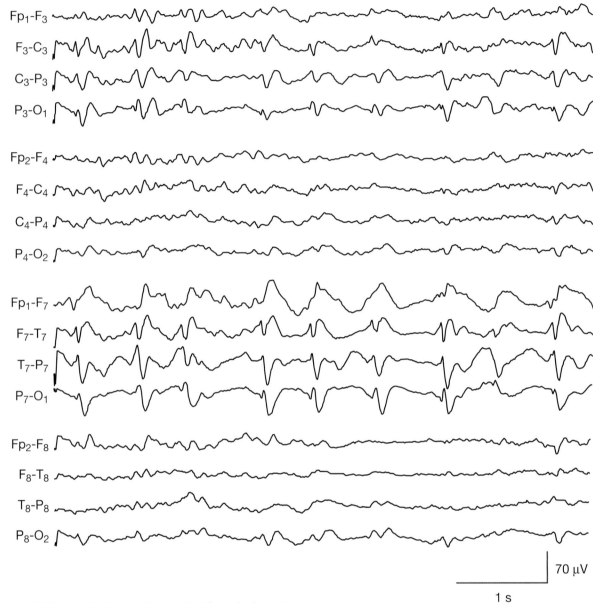

Fig. 5-18. PLEDs (periodic lateralized epileptiform discharges).

Triphasic waves are often associated with hepatic coma

Generalized periodic sharp waves are seen in Creutzfeldt-Jakob disease

---

disorders, hypoxia, and with use of baclofen, interferon, lithium, or ifosfamide

c. Generalized periodic epileptiform discharges
   1) May be seen in status epilepticus
   2) Also seen after cardiopulmonary arrest at a frequency of 1 to 2 Hz, often associated with myoclonus and a poor prognosis

d. Generalized periodic slow-wave complexes
   1) High-voltage slow-wave complexes lasting from 0.5 second to seconds and occurring every 4 to 15 seconds
   2) Seen in subacute sclerosing panencephalitis (SSPE)
   3) Occurrence of the complexes may be limited (and irregular initially), but eventually becomes generalized, symmetric, regular, and synchronous, although the firing frequency can vary during the course of the disease
   4) Morphology also changes with progression and is different between different patients

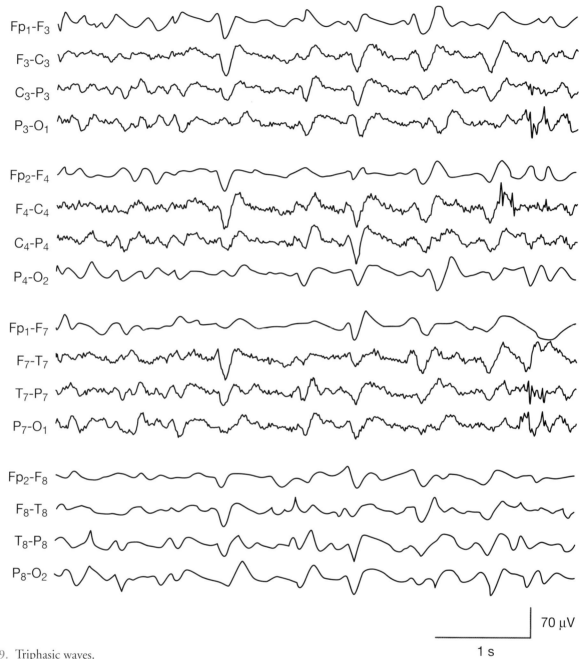

Fig. 5-19. Triphasic waves.

5) The complexes may be time-locked to myoclonic jerks
e. Burst-suppression pattern (Fig. 5-21)
   1) Burst of mixed frequency activity lasting 1 to 3 seconds, alternating with electrocerebral silence lasting longer than 1 second
   2) Most commonly occurs with cardiopulmonary arrest
     a) Portends a worse prognosis in this setting
     b) Has a mortality of 96% when seen after cardiopulmonary arrest

     c) The slower the frequency of the bursts, the worse the prognosis
   3) May also occur with deep anesthesia, drug overdose, or hypothermia—all of which are potentially reversible
   4) Often associated with myoclonus: neither the EEG nor myoclonus is significantly improved with antiepileptic treatment
   5) Poor prognostic indicators: absence of spontaneous

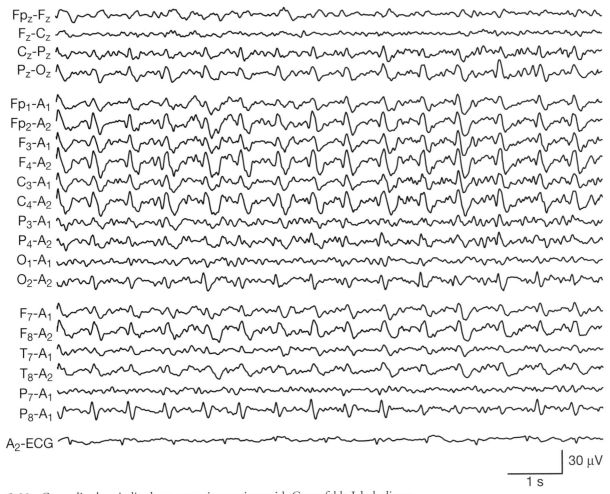

Fig. 5-20. Generalized periodic sharp waves in a patient with Creutzfeldt-Jakob disease.

variability, reactivity to external stimuli, progression to electrocerebral silence

3. Coma patterns
   a. Alpha coma
      1) Generalized, invariable alpha activity (unresponsive to external stimuli)
      2) Most often occurs 2 to 3 days after cardiopulmonary arrest, indicates a poor prognosis
      3) Can also be seen in brainstem strokes and drug overdose
      4) Posterior-dominant alpha coma pattern may be seen in setting of a brainstem lesion
      5) Anterior-dominant (or generalized) invariant alpha coma pattern may be seen in setting of a global insult such as cardiac arrest or bilateral thalamic infarcts
      6) Prognosis depends on etiology
   b. Beta coma
      1) Beta activity superimposed on delta
      2) Seen in drug overdose (often barbiturate or benzodiazepine intoxication)
   c. Spindle coma
      1) Resembles sleep EEG but little response to afferent stimuli
      2) Results from head trauma, brainstem lesions, drugs, hypoxia
      3) Associated with good prognosis (unlike most alpha coma patterns)
   d. Burst-suppression pattern (described above)

VII. BRAIN DEATH

A. No EEG Activity More Than 2 mV or Electrocerebral Silence Can Be Used to Help Confirm Brain Death

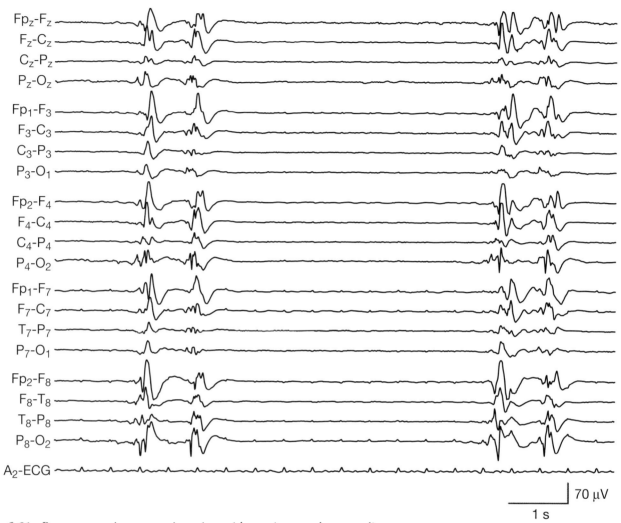

Fig. 5-21. Burst-suppression pattern in patient with anoxic coma due to cardiac arrest.

B. Criteria for Brain Death in Adults

1. Minimum of 8 scalp electrodes
2. Interelectrode impedances less than 10,000 Ω and more than 100 Ω
3. Sensitivity of a least 2 μV/mm for a least 30 minutes of recording
4. Test integrity of entire recording system by tapping on electrodes
5. Interelectrode distances of at least 10 cm
6. Appropriate filter settings
7. No EEG reactivity to external stimuli
8. Additional monitoring techniques (ECG, respirations) should be used when necessary
9. Performed by a qualified technologist
10. Exclusion of drug overdose, anesthetic agents, hypothermia

> Burst-suppression pattern or generalized periodic epileptiform discharges after cardiopulmonary arrest indicate a poor prognosis

QUESTIONS

1. Which of the following is true about alpha rhythm?
   a. It is predominant over the anterior region
   b. Asymmetry between the two sides of 20% is abnormal
   c. It is absent in 33% of the population
   d. Failure to attenuate with unilateral eye opening is abnormal

2. Which of the following does not enhance beta rhythm?
   a. Benzodiazepines
   b. Barbiturates
   c. Focal skull lesion
   d. Valproic acid
   e. Drowsiness

3. Which of the following is not a contraindication to hyperventilation?
   a. Chronic obstructive pulmonary disease
   b. Recent myocardial infarction
   c. Recent stroke
   d. Recent generalized seizure

4. EEG artifact from upward eye movements:
   a. Will produce an upward deflection on a bipolar montage
   b. Predominantly involves the occipital leads
   c. Is caused by the dipole of the eye, with the cornea relatively negative
   d. Occurs during blinking or closing the eyes

5. Lambda waves:
   a. Occur predominantly in the frontal head regions
   b. Are not present with darkness
   c. Occur with visual scanning
   d. Attenuate with contralateral movement

6. Non-REM sleep is associated with:
   a. Sawtooth waves
   b. Tonic muscle activity
   c. Low-amplitude EEG
   d. Increased heart rate

7. 6-Hz spike-and-wave pattern:
   a. Is usually seen in young adults
   b. Of the frontal form is not usually associated with seizures
   c. Does not disappear during deep levels of sleep
   d. Is usually unilateral

8. Which of the following is *not* true about SREDA?
   a. Occurs primarily in children
   b. May wax and wane
   c. Does not interrupt the background
   d. Monomorphic appearance of waveforms

9. Which EEG activity is not seen in neonates?
   a. Tracé alternant
   b. Delta brushes
   c. Anterior delta rhythm
   d. Posterior alpha rhythm

10. A developmentally normal 5-year-old has staring spells that last less than 20 seconds and can be induced by hyperventilation. The most likely EEG pattern is:
    a. 3-Hz spike-and-wave pattern
    b. Central-temporal spikes
    c. Periodic slow-wave complexes
    d. Slow spike-and-wave pattern

11. A 22-year-old man is febrile with new-onset seizures and an acute worsening encephalopathy. His pattern on the EEG would most likely be:
    a. RTTD
    b. PLEDs
    c. Periodic sharp waves
    d. Hypsarrhythmia

12. A comatose 72-year-old man develops myoclonus after a cardiac arrest. His EEG most likely reveals which pattern?
    a. Beta coma
    b. Alpha coma
    c. Triphasic waves
    d. Burst-suppression pattern

13. Criteria for EEG recordings of brain death include:
    a. EEG activity more than 2 μV
    b. Maximum of 3 scalp electrodes
    c. At least 15 minutes of recording
    d. Exclusion of hypothermia

ANSWERS

1. Answer: d.
Alpha rhythm predominates over the posterior head region, and failure to attenuate with unilateral or bilateral eye opening is worrisome for an underlying lesion. It may be absent in 11% of the population, and amplitude asymmetry more than 50% is abnormal.

2. Answer: d.
Valproic acid does not enhance beta activity.

3. Answer: d.
Hyperventilation is not contraindicated after a seizure but is contraindicated in the other conditions listed.

4. Answer: d.
During blinking, there is an upward movement of the eyes. The eyes have a dipole, with the corneas being relatively positive, and this upward movement produces a downward deflection on the EEG, which is usually in the frontal leads.

5. Answer: c.
Lambda waves are visual evoked potentials that generally occur in the posterior regions with visual scanning. They may occur in the dark.

6. Answer: b.
Non-REM sleep is associated with tonic muscle activity. Low-amplitude EEG activity, sawtooth waves, increased heart rate, and decreased muscle activity are associated with REM sleep.

7. Answer: a.
The 6-Hz spike-and-wave pattern is a bisynchronous pattern seen in adolescents and young adults. It usually disappears during deeper levels of sleep. The anterior high-amplitude variety is commonly associated with epileptic seizures.

8. Answer: a.
SREDA is a benign EEG pattern that occurs predominantly in elderly adults during wakefulness. It is a monomorphic pattern that does not interrupt the background and may wax and wane.

9. Answer: d.
A posterior alpha rhythm of about 6 Hz may be seen around 6 months, but an adult frequency is not fully developed until 8 to 10 years of age.

10. Answer: a.
The 3-Hz spike-and-wave pattern is associated with typical absence seizures.

11. Answer: b.
PLEDs, especially when seen first on one side and then on the other, are very suggestive of herpes simplex encephalitis. They may also be seen in other pathologic conditions such as stroke.

12. Answer: d.
Post-anoxic myoclonus is often associated with the burst-suppression EEG pattern.

13. Answer: d.
EEG activity more than 2 μV would be inconsistent with brain death. A minimum of eight scalp electrodes should be used to record for at least 30 minutes. Reversible causes such as drug overdose, the effects of anesthetic agents, and hypothermia must be excluded before a person meets criteria for brain death.

Nima Mowzoon, M.D.

I. NERVE CONDUCTION STUDIES

A. Introduction and Basic Instrumentation

1. Filter
   a. Limits and selects the desired signals from the amplifier
   b. Function
      1) To filter unwanted noise and help in resolving a waveform
      2) But filter may alter length and amplitude of waveforms (e.g., latency markings may change with different filter settings)
2. Differential amplifier removes noise by cancellation of activity common to both electrodes ("common mode rejection") (Fig. 5-22)
   a. For example, it produces upward deflection for a negative input on one lead and a downward deflection for same input on the second lead
   b. Summation of inputs, so that simultaneous inputs with opposite deflections cancel out
   c. Activity with wide field occurring simultaneously in both leads (noise) is removed
3. Amplifier impedance must be high to "amplify," by Ohm's law, low-voltage responses and allow recording of low-amplitude activity
4. Background electrical noise
   a. Larger in sensory potentials because of low amplitude of signal (low signal-to-noise ratio)
   b. Background noise from voluntary muscle activity needs to be minimized (high amplitude relative to signal)
5. Stimulus artifact is reduced by
   a. Proper skin preparation and electrode positioning
   b. Preventing electrode or sweat "bridging"
   c. Minimal duration and intensity of stimulus (just enough to obtain supramaximal response)
   d. Rotation of anode about the cathode
   e. Minimizing distance between stimulator and nerve to allow supramaximal depolarization with minimal possible current, reducing overstimulation and muscle artifact

6. Technique
   a. Cathode
      1) Negatively charged
      2) Depolarizes axons
      3) Action potential triggered if threshold is reached
   b. Anode
      1) Positively charged
      2) Hyperpolarizes axons
      3) Anodal block: action potential is blocked under anode
   c. Increased distance between cathode and anode causes deeper penetrance of underlying tissue by current
   d. Two types of stimulators used
      1) Constant current stimulators: the operator sets the current delivered by stimulator at a constant number and voltage is variable
      2) Constant voltage stimulators: the operator sets voltage at a constant number and current is variable
   e. Important factors
      1) Axon size: larger axons are stimulated more easily
      2) Myelin: myelinated axons are stimulated more easily than unmyelinated axons

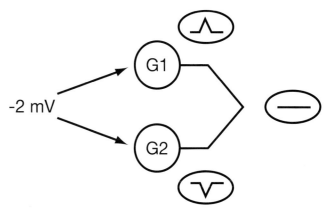

Fig. 5-22. Differential amplifier acts to remove noise by cancellation of simultaneous inputs with opposite deflections. G1 and G2, recording electrodes.

f. Submaximal stimulation: selectively activates larger myelinated fibers

g. Supramaximal stimulation: also activates smaller fibers

   1) As stimulus intensity is slowly increased from baseline of 0 mA, more axons are stimulated until all axons under the stimulus are depolarized, at which point the recorded response is maximized and a stronger stimulus does not produce further increase in the response (supramaximal response)

   2) Ensures that the potentials obtained are the summation of all axons at point of stimulation

   3) Ensures consistency for comparison with normal values (latency and amplitude of responses can vary depending on number and type of nerve fibers activated)

h. Segmental stimulation

   1) Stimulation of the nerve distal and proximal to lesion

   2) Important for identifying a focal lesion such as focal slowing or conduction block (e.g., focal demyelination or compression)

i. Sites of stimulation

   1) Sensory nerve action potential (SNAP) conduction is affected primarily by nerve conduction time; requires one site of stimulation

   2) Compound muscle action potential (CMAP) conduction affected by nerve conduction time, neuromuscular junction transmission, and the muscle

      a) More than one site of stimulation is required

      b) Nerve conduction velocity between the two sites is measured in the segment between the two sites of stimulation

j. Sliding

   1) After submaximal response is obtained, cathode and anode may be moved perpendicularly to course of the nerve for short distance to obtain larger responses

   2) Easier to obtain supramaximal response with minimal intensity

   3) Reduces stimulation artifact and spread of the stimulus to other nerves or a more distant site on same nerve

B. Sensory Nerve Conduction Studies

1. Technical considerations

   a. Strategies to isolate and study sensory nerve axons

      1) Stimulate and record a pure sensory nerve (e.g., sural nerve responses)

      2) Stimulate mixed motor and sensory nerve and record the action potential at the sensory branch of the nerve: antidromic technique

         a) Disadvantages of antidromic conduction study in hand: muscle artifact and volume conduction from lumbricals (with ring electrodes)

      3) Stimulate sensory portion of mixed motor and sensory nerve distal to branching point, and record proximally over mixed nerve: orthodromic technique

      4) Stimulate mixed motor and sensory nerve and record over the mixed nerve: palmar technique

   b. Only nerve axons are assessed (as compared with motor conduction studies, which measure conduction along motor nerve, neuromuscular junction, and muscle)

   c. Most sensory responses are very small: technical factors and electrical noise are important

   d. Technical factors that contribute to accuracy of the responses

      1) Anatomical variations (which obviate accurate localization of nerves)

      2) Background muscle activity (voluntary or involuntary)

      3) Skin temperature

      4) Age, height, sex, body mass

   e. Signal averaging

      1) Combines and averages different responses to eliminate background noise for small size potentials

      2) Improves signal-to-noise ratio

      3) Enhances, summates, enlarges activity that is time-locked to the stimulus, while eliminating or subtracting random noise

   f. Placement of electrodes and recording

      1) Two recording electrodes (G1 and G2) are placed over the nerve, 3.5 to 4 cm apart

      2) G1, the active recording electrode, is placed closer to stimulator

      3) Ground electrode: relatively large and placed between stimulating and recording electrodes

      4) Stimulator (two poles)

         a) Cathode

            i) Negatively charged

            ii) Depolarizes axon, generates action potential if

---

Segmental stimulation best used for identifying a focal lesion such as focal slowing or conduction block

---

Sensory nerve conduction studies assess sensory axons

Motor nerve conduction studies assess motor axons, neuromuscular junction, and muscle

depolarization is sufficient and axon reaches threshold
b) Anode
  i) Positively charged
  ii) Hyperpolarizes axon
5) Needle electrode: may need to be placed near nerve to provide adequate stimulation to deep nerves
  a) Advantages: more selective and less artifact
    i) Less shock artifact
    ii) Less spread along nerve
    iii) Less spread of stimulus to another nerve
  b) Disadvantages
    i) Discomfort
    ii) Potential for nerve damage
    iii) Exact site of stimulus may be uncertain
6) Sensory conduction studies require less current and have lower threshold than motor conduction studies
7) Current is increased slowly until sensory potential is maximized (SNAP)
2. SNAP characteristics (Fig. 5-23)
  a. Compound potential that is summation of individual nerve action potentials, may be biphasic or triphasic
  b. Usually more sensitive to both generalized and focal nerve disease than motor nerve conduction studies (e.g.,

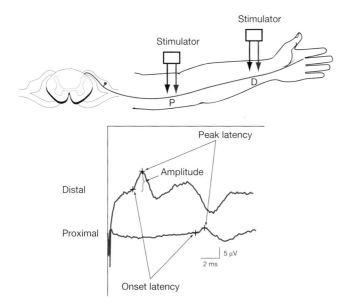

Fig. 5-23. Sensory nerve action potential (sensory antidromic technique). Conduction velocity is measured best with both proximal (P) and distal (D) stimulation as depicted. Note difference in waveform configurations because of dispersion and phase cancellation. Amplitude, in µV.

entrapment mononeuropathies such as carpal tunnel syndrome)
  c. SNAP abnormalities may be first abnormalities of a neuropathic process such as generalized sensorimotor neuropathy (earlier than motor studies) and may be selectively involved in sensory neuropathies
  d. Lack of collateral sprouting (limited reinnervation after axonal loss)
  e. Measurements
    1) Onset latency
      a) Time from stimulus to initial negative deflection for biphasic SNAPs or time to initial positive peak for triphasic SNAPs
      b) Onset latency at proximal site and onset latency at distal site are used to determine sensory conduction velocity
      c) Measures the fastest and largest conducting sensory fibers (cutaneous and sometimes Ia afferents from muscle spindles)
      d) Can be obscured by noise or stimulus artifact
      e) May be difficult to determine precise point of deflection from baseline
      f) May be mistaken for muscle artifact
    2) Peak latency
      a) Measured at midpoint of peak of first negative, or upward, deflection
      b) Nerve fibers studied by peak latency may be slower conducting fibers than those measured by onset latency
      c) Little variability among different electromyographers, more precise than onset latency measurements
      d) Used in distal latency determinations (normative data are available)
    3) Amplitude
      a) Measured from onset latency to peak latency
      b) Reflects the number of axons contributing to the potential
      c) Low SNAP amplitudes suggest a disorder of peripheral nerve (distal to or involving the dorsal root ganglion [DRG])
    4) Duration
      a) Measured from onset latency to first baseline crossing
      b) Usually shorter than CMAP duration, may be used to identify the potential as a nerve potential
    5) Conduction velocity
      a) Can be determined with one stimulation site (as compared with the motor conduction velocity that requires two stimulation sites)

b) May be measured by dividing distance traveled by onset latency: represents the speed of fastest, myelinated sensory fibers

c) Measurement of conduction velocity is most useful when proximal stimulation is used (Fig. 5-23)

d) Conduction velocity is calculated between proximal and distal sites:

$$\text{Conduction velocity} = \frac{\begin{array}{c}\text{Distance from distal to}\\\text{proximal stimulation}\\\text{sites in mm}\end{array}}{\begin{array}{c}\text{Proximal} - \text{distal (onset)}\\\text{latency in ms}\end{array}}$$

e) Represents speed of fastest conducting myelinated fibers if onset latency measurements are used to calculate conduction velocity (recommended by most authorities)

f) Represents speed of both large and medium-sized fibers if peak latency measurements are used to calculate conduction velocity

g) If distance is less than 10 cm, it is more appropriate to measure latency differences of the exact distances rather than divide the latency by a short distance

h) Proximal sensory studies result in smaller amplitude potentials and are difficult to perform

i) Greater proximally than distally

j) 3 to 6 m/s faster than motor conduction velocity

k) Nerve conduction velocities are approximately half the adult value in term infants, slower in premature infants, approximately adult values by age 2, but continue to increase slightly until age 5, and decrease after age 30

f. Special considerations

1) Antidromic technique (compared with orthodromic technique)

a) Stimulate nerve proximally and record distally (Fig. 5-23)

b) Amplitude of the responses is higher in antidromically conducted potentials because the recording electrodes (e.g., ring electrodes) are closer to underlying sensory nerves

c) Useful when recording small potentials in neuropathic conditions

d) Because a mixed motor-sensory nerve is stimulated, SNAP is usually followed by, and may be mistaken for, a volume-conducted motor response

2) Temporal dispersion and phase cancellation with proximal stimulation normally occur with SNAPs (Fig. 5-23)

a) Less prominent with distal stimulation and in motor responses

b) Affects duration, amplitude, and area of proximal potentials (not onset latency, which can be used to measure conduction velocity)

c) Temporal dispersion

i) Individual sensory fibers have different nerve action potential amplitudes and conduction velocities

ii) Lag time between faster and slower conducting fibers is exaggerated with proximal stimulation, leading to increased duration and decreased amplitude

d) Phase cancellation

i) Smaller potentials resulting from summation of different biphasic or triphasic single sensory fiber action potentials

ii) Occurs from overlap of negative phase of a single-fiber sensory action potential and positive phase of another sensory action potential

g. Clinical applications

1) May be normal in acute axonal injury, but amplitude of SNAP decreases in 4 to 6 days with axonal wallerian degeneration

2) Radiculopathy

a) Peripheral sensory nerve axons are from bipolar neurons with cell bodies in the DRG

b) With any lesion proximal to the DRG (such as spinal roots or in central nervous system) SNAPs are normal

c) Because the DRG of lower lumbar and upper sacral segments may be inside the spinal canal and axonal injury related to a compressive radiculopathy in these segments may be at or distal to the DRG, SNAPs potentially may be abnormal in lower lumbar or upper sacral radiculopathies

3) Axonal injury

a) Generally causes reduced amplitudes

Onset latency is not affected by temporal dispersion and phase cancellation and can be used to measure conduction velocity

---

With lesions proximal to dorsal root ganglion, SNAPs are normal

b) Relative preservation of conduction velocity and distal latency (unless severe enough to affect fastest and largest fibers)
c) Hyperacute axonal loss: normal sensory responses if assessed before wallerian degeneration
4) Focal demyelination
   a) Normal SNAPs distally
   b) Conduction block: reduced amplitudes across the site (proximal sensory responses may be absent)
   c) Focal slowing: slowed conduction velocity across the site and prolonged distal latency (if lesion is in distal segment)
   d) Focal slowing may not be appreciable with SNAPs (as seen in motor responses)
      i) Sensory amplitudes may decrease because of phase cancellation (motor amplitudes remain normal)
      ii) One exception is palmar orthodromic median sensory responses: phase cancellation is not important because of the short distance
5) Plexopathy
   a) Lateral antebrachial cutaneous sensory response useful for upper trunk or lateral cord distribution
   b) Superficial radial sensory response may be useful for middle trunk or posterior cord distribution
   c) Medial antebrachial cutaneous sensory response useful for lower trunk or medial cord distribution
6) Mononeuropathies
   a) Palmar orthodromic technique is more sensitive for determining focal slowing and prolongation of distal latency of median nerve across the carpal tunnel at the wrist because the distance is shorter and latency is compared with ulnar distal latency over the same distance
      i) Orthodromic technique: ideal for clinically mild median neuropathy at the wrist (greater sensitivity)
      ii) Antidromic technique: reasonable alternate for moderate to severe median neuropathy at the wrist (greater sensitivity is not needed)
   b) Ulnar sensory nerve is most commonly studied

> Conduction block causes normal sensory responses distally and absence of sensory responses proximally
>
> With antidromic studies, sensory amplitudes may decrease because of phase cancellation

with antidromic technique, with stimulation proximal to the wrist and above the elbow and recording at the fifth digit
   i) With pure conduction block of the ulnar nerve across the elbow, proximal sensory responses may be absent and distal sensory amplitudes and latencies may be normal

C. Motor Nerve Conduction Studies
1. CMAP: action potential recorded from a group of muscle fibers when motor axons are stimulated
2. CMAP: essentially an assessment of motor axons, neuromuscular junction, and muscle fibers
3. Motor nerve conduction studies may be used to assess motor neuron disease, but electrodiagnostic evaluation of central pathways requires evoked potential studies
4. CMAP may be normal in myopathy until disease is advanced and there is loss of muscle tissue
5. Technical considerations
   a. Motor responses are less affected by background noise and other technical factors than sensory responses (better signal-to-noise ratio)
   b. Gain is usually set at 2 to 5 mV per division
   c. Recording electrodes are placed over muscle of interest
   d. "Belly-tendon recording": active recording electrode (G1) is placed directly over the center of the muscle belly (over end-plate region) and reference electrode (G2) is placed distally over the muscle tendon
   e. G1 electrode directly over end-plate region records from origin of muscle action potential that spreads to rest of the muscle fiber
      1) Initial deflection from baseline is upward
      2) However, if initial deflection is downward, G1 is away from end-plate region or there is volume conduction from a distant muscle
   f. The stimulator is placed over the nerve, with the cathode closest to recording electrode
   g. Current is applied and slowly increased by 5 to 10 mA at a time to obtain supramaximal stimulation
6. CMAP characteristics (Fig. 5-24)
   a. Biphasic potential with initial negative, or upward, deflection from baseline
   b. Measurements
      1) Latency
         a) Time from stimulus to initial CMAP deflection from baseline
         b) Constituents
            i) Nerve conduction time: depends on distance, temperature, condition of nerve, patient characteristics (age, sex, height, body mass)

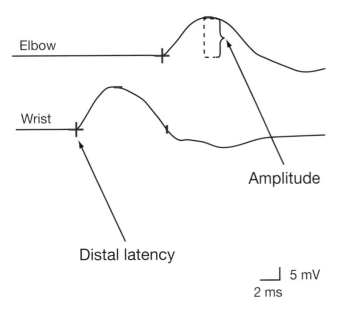

Elbow

Wrist

Amplitude

Distal latency

$\sqsupset$ 5 mV

2 ms

Fig. 5-24. Compound muscle action potential recorded from median nerve. Note the absence of dispersion and phase cancellation with the normal motor study, as compared with a sensory nerve action potential. Amplitude is expressed in mV (higher magnitude than sensory nerve action potential). Conduction velocity (47 m/s) is the conducted distance between the two stimulating sites (256 mm) divided by the conduction time, which is the difference between distal latencies (5.4 ms).

        ii) Neuromuscular transmission time (about 1 millisecond)
        iii) Muscle conduction time
  2) Amplitude
    a) Most commonly measured from baseline to negative peak
    b) Reflects summation of muscle fibers depolarized by the nerve
    c) May be reduced if denervation exceeds reinnervation, may be unaffected or less affected if reinnervation is adequate
    d) May be influenced by distance between recording electrode and underlying muscle, may be decreased with excess subcutaneous fat or edema
    e) Larger than SNAP amplitudes (expressed in mV, sensory responses are expressed in μV)
  3) Duration
    a) Is measured from initial deflection from baseline to first baseline crossing
    b) A measure of synchrony of activation of individual muscle fibers

    c) It increases in conditions that cause selective slowing of some motor nerve fibers but not others such as demyelinating conditions or decreased temperature
  4) Conduction velocity
    a) Determined by the fastest conducting motor axons
    b) Conduction velocity = $\dfrac{\text{Conducted distance in mm}}{\text{Conduction time in ms}}$
        i) Conduction time = proximal latency – distal latency
        ii) Conducted distance = distance between proximal cathode and distal cathode
    c) Latency is the only significant difference between normal CMAPs produced by proximal and distal stimulation
  5) Potential sources for error in measurements
    a) Incorrect distance measurements: distortion of skin, nonstandard positioning of body, simultaneous stimulation of adjacent nerves, incorrect placement and polarity of stimulating electrode
    b) Incorrect latency measurements: miscalculation of sweep speed, shock artifact that interferes with CMAP, incorrect electrode location, initial positive deflection from volume conduction
  6) If higher amplitude with proximal stimulation or initial positive deflection
    a) Technical errors: inadequate stimulus at distal site or excessive stimulus at proximal site (activating adjacent nerves)
    b) Physiologic: anomalous innervation
    c) Muscle atrophy
  7) If lower amplitude with proximal stimulation than distal
    a) Normal: 20% to 30% change observed in most nerves (40% in tibial)
    b) Conduction block (see below)
    c) Dispersion: compare amplitude/area, inspect waveform for increased duration, increased complexity, number of components
    d) Technical errors: understimulation at proximal site or overstimulation at distal site
 c. Clinical applications
  1) Conduction slowing
    a) Defined as prolonged distal latency, slowed conduction velocity, or prolonged F-wave latencies
    b) Segmental demyelination, axonal narrowing, and loss of large axons
  2) Conduction block (Fig. 5-25)
    a) Result of metabolic alteration in axonal membrane

or structural change in myelin, e.g., telescoping or segmental demyelination or dysfunction of axon at node of Ranvier

b) Implies intact axons are unable to conduct potentials

c) Larger diameter fibers are most sensitive to damage

d) May be total or partial (in which only some axons are able to conduct potentials)

e) Stimulation over short segments is more reliable for identifying conduction block because of temporal dispersion and phase cancellation that may occur with longer segments

f) Method of "inching": can better localize area of abnormality as indicated by greater decrease in amplitude between consecutive responses

g) Absent responses may also indicate hyperacute axonal damage that may mimic conduction block and become more obvious when there is wallerian

degeneration after approximately 4-6 days

h) Associated with clinical weakness and reduced recruitment on needle EMG

3) Temporal dispersion (Fig. 5-26) and phase cancellation

a) May be apparent with demyelinating lesions of motor fibers

b) More common in acquired demyelination with or without conduction block (less common in inherited demyelination)

D. Basic Patterns of Nerve Conduction Studies

1. Axonal loss (motor and sensory conduction studies)

a. Reduced amplitude at proximal and distal sites: but reduced amplitudes do not necessarily imply axonal loss

b. Conduction velocity and distal latency may be normal, assuming largest and fastest conducting axons are intact

c. Large reduction of amplitude and some slowing of

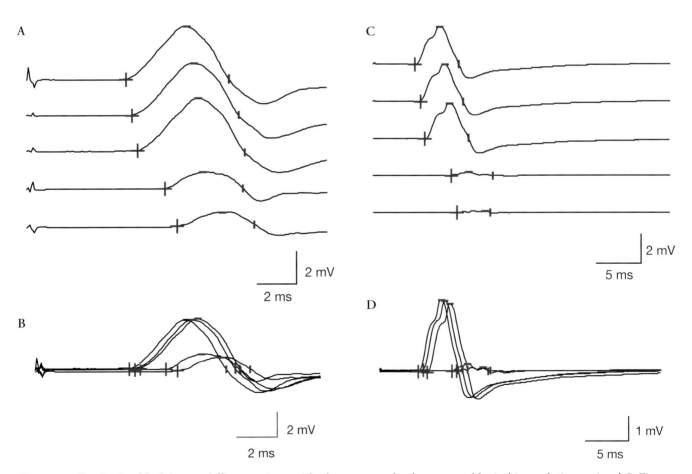

Fig. 5-25. Conduction block in two different patients with ulnar neuropathy demonstrated by inching technique. *A* and *B*, First patient has a partial conduction block, with an appreciable change in duration and area. *C* and *D*, Second patient has complete block and produces only trace response above the block. (Courtesy of W. Neath Folger, MD.)

conduction velocity or mild prolongation of distal latencies may indicate axonal loss, with relative loss of large fast-conducting fibers and relative preservation of slowly conducting fibers
  1) Conduction velocities may be decreased, but never less than 70% of lower limit of normal
  2) Distal latencies expected to be normal or slightly prolonged, but no more than 130% of upper limit of normal
  d. With hyperacute lesions, nerve conduction studies performed within first 4 to 6 days may be normal
  e. After 4 to 6 days, nerve segment distal to transection undergoes wallerian degeneration and distal and proximal amplitudes decrease
2. Demyelination (motor and sensory conduction studies)
  a. Slowing of conduction velocities: slower than 70% of lower limit of normal if amplitudes are preserved, 50% if amplitudes are decreased

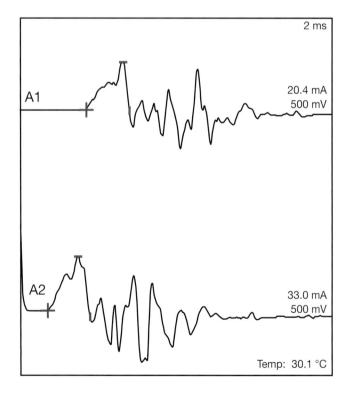

Fig. 5-26. Dispersion in a patient with demyelinating neuropathy. This response was recorded at the abductor hallucis muscle while stimulating the tibial nerve at the knee (A1) and ankle (A2). The conduction velocity was slowed, and there was an increase in the duration of the responses. Temp, temperature.

  b. Prolongation of distal latency
    1) Longer than 130% of upper limit of normal
    2) May result from focal slowing
  c. Any nerve conduction velocity slower than 35 m/s in the arms or 30 m/s in the legs (except regeneration of nerve fibers after axonal loss or injury)
  d. Focal slowing
    1) More than 10 m/s slowing over 10-cm segment
    2) More than 0.4-millisecond change in latency over 1-cm segment
  e. Motor conduction block and temporal dispersion
    1) Temporal dispersion and phase cancellation
      a) Increase in CMAP duration of more than 15% between proximal and distal sites
      b) May account for no more than a 50% change in amplitude between the two sites
    2) Complete block: loss of CMAP when stimulus is central to the lesion
    3) Partial block: definition is more controversial
      a) More than a 40% to 50% change in the area between proximal and distal sites of stimulation regardless of any change in duration or distance
      b) More than a 20% to 30% change in the area with a change in duration of less than 15% between proximal and distal sites regardless of distance
      c) More than a 10% change in the area if the distance between the two stimulation sites is less than 10 cm
  f. Inherited demyelinating polyneuropathies
    1) Usually all myelin is affected equally and demyelination is symmetric
    2) Slowing is uniform
    3) Dispersion and block are uncommon
  g. Acquired demyelinating polyneuropathies
    1) Patchy, multifocal, asymmetric demyelination with conduction block and temporal dispersion
    2) May show more dispersion with proximal stimulation than the hereditary causes

E. Normal Late Responses
1. Normal late responses (F waves and H waves) travel the entire length of peripheral nerve segment from muscle to spinal cord
2. F waves (Fig. 5-27)
  a. Definition
    1) Small muscle action potentials produced by antidromic stimulation of a small population of anterior horn cells
      a) Anterior horn cells backfire *and*
      b) Action potentials travel orthodromically to muscle

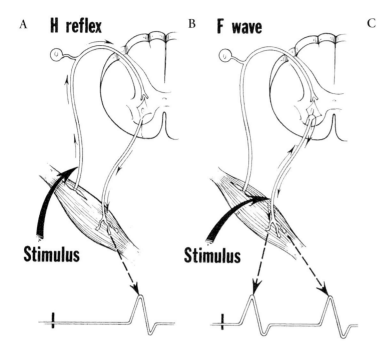

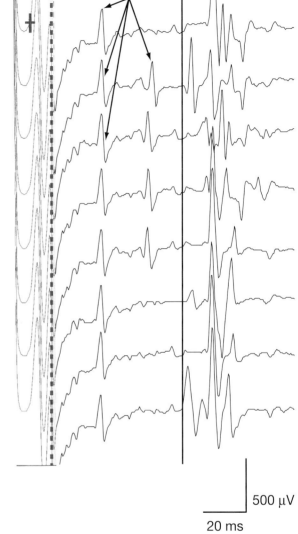

A waves

500 µV

20 ms

Fig. 5-27. Late responses. *A*, H reflex is a true monosynaptic reflex, with selective activation of Ia muscle spindle afferents (with low stimulus) and alpha motor neuron efferents supplying the gastrocnemius-soleus muscle group. *B*, In contrast, F wave is not a true monosynaptic reflex but represents antidromic stimulation of alpha motor neuron and a small population of anterior horn cells whose action potentials then travel ortho-dromically to the muscle. *C*, F response was obtained by stim-ulating tibial nerve. Responses on the left of solid line are A waves (axonal reflex). These responses are often repeated and almost identical in appearance. (*A* and *B* from Stolp-Smith KA. H reflexes. In: Daube JR, editor. Clinical neurophysiol-ogy. 2nd ed. New York: Oxford University Press; 2002. p. 375-81. By permission of Mayo Foundation.)

2) Named "F" because originally recorded from the foot
3) Both afferent and efferent arms are motor; no synapse involved
4) Not a true reflex
5) May be spared in conditions selectively involving sen-sory pathways or a relatively small number of motor axons
6) More commonly abnormal in demyelinating than axonal lesions
7) A different group of anterior horn cells may be stimu-lated with each response
   a) With advanced axonal loss and dropout of motor neurons, a smaller number of motor neurons is

left, thus higher chance for the same group of ante-rior horn cells to be stimulated
   b) Therefore, F waves may be repeated
8) Latency decreases with more proximal stimulation
9) Latency varies with limb distance
10) F-wave estimate
   a) Estimated F-wave latency if distal conduction velocity is applied to proximal nerve segment
   b) Calculated on basis of distal motor latency, con-duction velocity, and limb length
   c) Evoked F-wave latencies
      i) Should be within the normal range of F-wave estimates (within 3-5 milliseconds)

ii) If shorter than the estimated range of F-wave estimates: distal conduction is slower than proximal conduction (e.g., peripheral neuropathy)

iii) If longer than the estimated range of F-wave estimates: proximal conduction is slower than distal conduction (e.g., radiculopathy, polyradiculopathy)

b. Technique

1) Cathode is proximal to anode (rotate anode off the nerve at distal stimulation site)

2) Stimulus is supramaximal

3) Stimulation at distal site (wrist, ankle)

4) Recording electrodes are same as for routine motor conduction studies

5) Gain is increased to 100 to 500 μV

6) Measurements are made from the initial deflection from baseline

7) Muscle contraction and relaxation of other limbs may enhance F responses

8) Muscle noise from poor relaxation may obscure or be confused for F waves

c. Clinical applications

1) F waves span the entire length of nerve and are abnormal in disease states with abnormal distal motor latencies and conduction velocities

2) Useful in identifying demyelination that selectively affects proximal segments (e.g., inflammatory demyelinating polyradiculoneuropathy or inflammatory plexopathy)

3) Limited practical usefulness in processes predominantly involving axonal loss (e.g., motor neuron disease or radiculopathies)

3. H reflex (Fig. 5-27 *A*)

a. Obtained by stimulating tibial nerve in the popliteal fossa and recording the gastrocnemius-soleus muscle

b. Stimulus intensity is increased slowly from a low level in small increments

c. True monosynaptic reflex with Ia muscle spindle (sensory) afferents and alpha motor neuron efferents

d. May be abnormal with S1 radiculopathy or plexopathy

e. Long-duration, submaximal stimulus may selectively activate Ia afferents

f. Augmentation of stimulus intensity causes the following (Fig. 5-28):

1) Increase in amplitude and decrease in latency of H reflex

2) Further stimulation activates motor fibers and produces a motor (M) response

3) Further increase in stimulus activates more motor fibers and causes

a) Increased size of M response

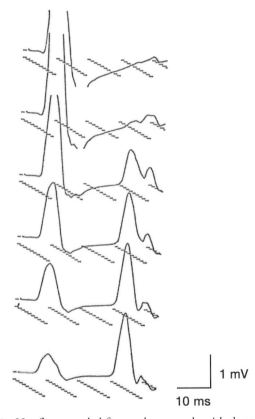

1 mV

10 ms

Fig. 5-28. H reflex recorded from soleus muscle with decreasing stimulus intensity. Maximal amplitude of the H reflex can be obtained with submaximal stimulation. (From Stolp-Smith KA. H reflexes. In: Daube JR, editor. Clinical neurophysiology. 2nd ed. New York: Oxford University Press; 2002. p. 375-81. By permission of Mayo Foundation.)

F-wave estimate = (2 × distance/conduction velocity) + distal latency

If measured F-wave latency longer than F-wave estimate: proximal slowing

Abnormal F waves but normal nerve conduction studies suggest proximal lesion

F-wave estimate is needed with abnormal nerve conduction studies

b) More antidromically conducted impulses in motor fibers to block orthodromic impulses of the H reflex and decrease in size of the H reflex

4) H reflex disappears with supramaximal stimulation

4. Blink reflexes (discussed below)

5. Jaw jerk (discussed below)

F. Abnormal Late Responses

1. Normal nerve conduction studies and abnormal late responses imply the lesion is proximal to the most proximal stimulation site used in the nerve conduction studies

2. Axonal reflex (Fig. 5-27 *C*)
   a. Not a true reflex
   b. Produced by impulse traveling antidromically (like F waves) to a branch point in the nerve and then ortho-dromically along the second branch (unlike F waves) toward the recording electrode to create an A-wave response
   c. May be seen in peripheral neuropathy, polyradiculopathy, or plexopathy
   d. Usually do not occur in normal subjects
   e. Initial antidromic impulse: latency *decreases* when stimulation site is moved proximally (as with F waves)

3. Satellite potentials
   a. Late components of a dispersed CMAP
   b. Constant location and configuration, in contrast to F waves
   c. Latency *increases* when stimulation site is moved proximally (in contrast to F waves)

G. Assessment of Neuromuscular Junction

1. Overview of neuromuscular junction physiology
   a. Collateral branches of the myelinated axons of the motor neurons end in the presynaptic nerve terminal which lies in a depression in the muscle membrane called the "synaptic cleft"
   b. The postsynaptic muscle membrane contains junctional folds containing acetylcholine receptors
   c. Synaptic vesicles are released into the synaptic cleft
   d. Each vesicle contains about 10,000 molecules of acetylcholine, a "quantum"
   e. Miniature end plate potential (MEPP): local, small depolarization of muscle membrane at the neuromuscular junction produced by a single quantum of acetylcholine
   f. Nerve action potential invades the terminal, releasing 60 to 100 quanta of acetylcholine
   g. These quanta generate an end plate potential (EPP) that triggers an action potential in the muscle fiber

h. Posttetanic potentiation or facilitation: potentiation or augmentation of the amount of acetylcholine released after brief repetitive exercise or rapid rate of stimulation (>10 Hz) (Fig. 5-29)
   1) Subsequent action potential occurring within 200 milliseconds after the preceding action potential causes more acetylcholine release
   2) Mechanism: increased calcium influx into nerve terminal through voltage-gated P/Q type calcium channels on presynaptic terminal
   3) In Lambert-Eaton myasthenic syndrome
      a) Antibodies to voltage-gated calcium channels reduce acetylcholine release
      b) Reduced acetylcholine release causes reduced postsynaptic EPP, often below threshold for neuromuscular junction transmission
      c) Result is low-amplitude CMAPs at rest and marked facilitation of amplitudes after brief exercise or rapid stimulation at 50 Hz (Fig. 5-30)
i. Decrement: reduction in amount of acetylcholine released with slow rates of repetitive stimulation (2-3 Hz), caused by depletion of acetylcholine stores in active zones of nerve terminal (Fig. 5-29)
   1) Normally, safety margin of neuromuscular transmission is large, and no decrement of CMAP occurs despite the decrease in EPP amplitude, which normally occurs with reduction of nerve terminal acetylcholine
   2) Myasthenia gravis
      a) Safety margin of EPP is reduced by acetylcholine receptor deficiency (Fig. 5-31)
      b) Repetitive stimulation at slow rates may cause lower subsequent EPPs that may not reach the threshold, causing transmission failure across neuromuscular junction and CMAP decrement
      c) CMAP decrement is greatest between first and second stimuli in a train of four stimuli
      d) Immediately after exercise, there is postactivation facilitation of CMAP amplitude and decrease in the decremental response
      e) There is a greater decremental response 4 minutes after exercise

2. Repetitive nerve stimulation technique
   a. Recording electrode: G1 over end plate and G2 over tendon
   b. The limb being studied should be immobilized
   c. Stimulus must be supramaximal to avoid any potential error caused by variation in the position of stimulating electrodes on nerve
   d. Trains of four stimuli separated by intervals of 500

milliseconds (2/second) may bring out any potential decrement due to neuromuscular junction disease

e. "Baseline" trains of repetitive stimuli are repeated at slow rates of stimulation (generally 2 Hz) to check for reproducibility of data

f. This is generally followed by brief (10 seconds) or more extended period (1 minute) of exercise—usually isometric contraction of hand muscles

g. If decrement is absent or questionable in "baseline" testing, patient should exercise for 1 minute

h. Brief period of exercise has same effect as rapid stimulation at 20 to 50 Hz, and is more tolerable

i. After brief exercise, four stimuli are given at 2 Hz immediately after exercise, and at 30, 60, 120, 180, and 240 seconds after exercise

j. Percentage decrement = $\dfrac{\text{(Amplitude of first response} - \text{Amplitude of fourth response)}}{\text{Amplitude of first response} \times 100}$

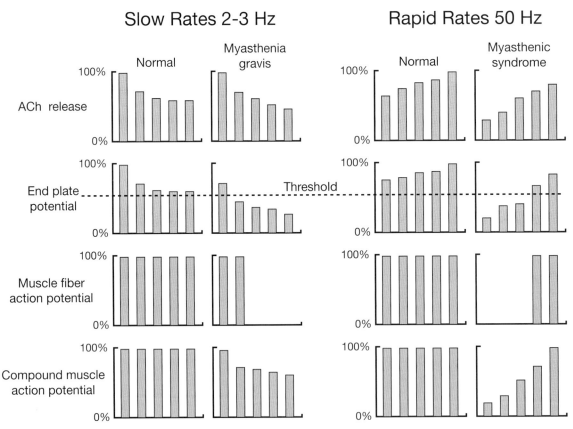

Fig. 5-29. Repetitive stimulation. On left, note decrement in compound muscle action potential (CMAP) amplitude with slow rates of repetitive stimulation (2-3 Hz) in myasthenia gravis. In normal subjects, a slow rate of stimulation reduces the release of acetylcholine (ACh), depletes ACh in nerve terminal, and induces a small decrease in amplitude of the end plate potential (EPP). In myasthenia gravis, safety margin for neuromuscular transmission is lower. In this situation, EPP is just above threshold for neuromuscular transmission, and a small decrease in EPP amplitude with repetitive stimulation (which normally occurs) results in low-amplitude EPPs below threshold that fail to produce a muscle fiber action potential, causing a decremental response in CMAP amplitude. In Lambert-Eaton myasthenic syndrome (on the right), defective presynaptic membrane causes reduced ACh release at rest, which is responsible for markedly low EPPs at rest that may not reach threshold for neuromuscular transmission, resulting in low-amplitude CMAPs. In this situation, posttetanic facilitation is observed with exercise or rapid rates of repetitive stimulation because increased ACh release causes higher amplitude EPPs that can reach threshold for neuromuscular transmission and produce higher amplitude CMAPs. (From Hermann RC Jr. Assessing the neuromuscular junction with repetitive stimulation studies. In: Daube JR, editor. Clinical neurophysiology. 2nd ed. New York: Oxford University Press; 2002. p. 268-81. By permission of Mayo Foundation.)

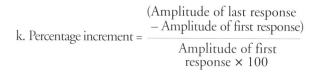

k. Percentage increment = $\dfrac{\text{(Amplitude of last response}}{\text{Amplitude of first}}$
$\dfrac{- \text{ Amplitude of first response)}}{\text{response} \times 100}$

l. Percentage facilitation = $\dfrac{\text{(Amplitude of last response)}}{\text{Amplitude of first}}$
$\dfrac{}{\text{response} \times 100}$

3. Interpretation of repetitive nerve stimulation studies and clinical correlation
   a. In normal subjects, no decrement should occur with 2-Hz stimulation
   b. Immediately after exercise, normal subjects may show small increments in responses caused by synchronized firing of motor units, usually with a decrease in duration and minimal net change in the area (termed "pseudofacilitation")

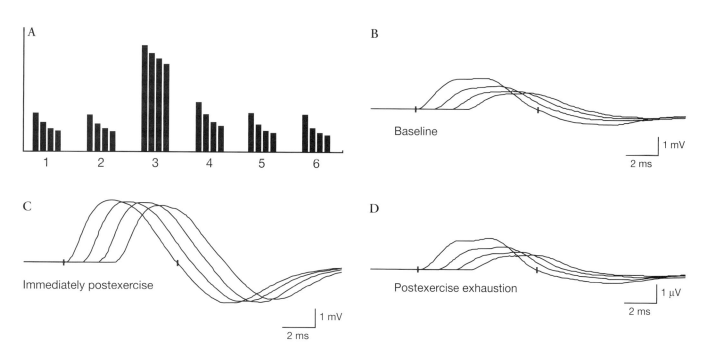

Fig. 5-30. Repetitive stimulation in Lambert-Eaton myasthenic syndrome. *A*, Histogram shows facilitation of amplitudes after brief exercise (bar graph 3). *B*, Baseline repetitive stimulation at 2 Hz demonstrates a decremental response, as in myasthenia gravis. *C*, Facilitation or increment of the amplitude of compound muscle action potential with brief exercise, as demonstrated in *A*, graph 3. *D*, This facilitation usually resolves by 60-120 seconds after exercise.

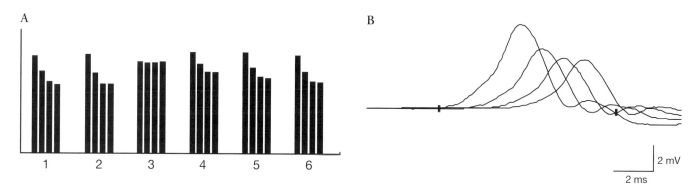

Fig. 5-31. Repetitive stimulation in myasthenia gravis. *A*, Histogram shows decremental response with 2-Hz repetitive stimulation with greatest decrement between first and second responses in the train of four responses (*B*). Postactivation facilitation of compound muscle action potential occurs with brief exercise (*A*, bar graph 3); decremental response is again observed some time after exercise.

c. Small decrements or poor sensitivity may result from technical problems
   1) Submaximal stimulation
   2) Poor relaxation with movement of stimulator away from nerve
   3) Voluntary contraction of target muscle during stimulation
d. How to identify technical problems
   1) Poor superimposition of baseline traces of four consecutive CMAPs
   2) Change in configuration of CMAP during train of stimuli
   3) Loss of smooth tapering pattern of decrement
e. Usually two or three baseline studies are performed to ensure reproducibility
f. Myasthenia gravis
   1) Normal resting CMAP (may be low in severe cases)
   2) Decrement with repetitive stimulation at 2 Hz
      a) Greatest relative change between the first and second response in the train of four stimuli
      b) Greatest absolute change between first and fourth
   3) Repair of decrement with or without postactivation facilitation with brief periods of exercise or rapid stimulation at 20 to 50 Hz
   4) Larger decrement noted 1 to 3 minutes after exercise
g. Lambert-Eaton myasthenic syndrome
   1) Low-amplitude resting CMAP
   2) Decrement with repetitive stimulation at 2 Hz, usually less prominent than in myasthenia gravis
   3) Marked increment (more than 100%) or facilitation (more than 200%) with rapid rates of stimulation or brief exercise
h. Botulism
   1) Low-amplitude resting CMAP
   2) Small decrement with slow rates of stimulation in some cases only
   3) Increment/facilitation with rapid rates of stimulation or brief exercise (less prominent but longer lasting than in Lambert-Eaton myasthenic syndrome)
i. Congenital myasthenic syndromes (see Chapter 23)
4. Single fiber electromyography (SFEMG)
   a. Selective technique of recording potentials from single muscle fibers within a motor unit
   b. Allows measurements of jitter and blocking, which reflect efficiency of neuromuscular transmission
   c. SFEMG electrode (recording surface diameter, 25 μm, approximates single muscle fiber diameter) with 500-Hz low-frequency filter: restricts recording field to 200 μm from recording surface
   d. Concentric electrode with 500-Hz low-frequency filter:

restricts recording field to 500 to 1,000 μm from recording surface
   e. Objective: to study simultaneously two single fiber potentials of same motor unit potential
   f. Nonspecific: may be abnormal with any lesion causing neuromuscular junction instability (e.g., denervation, myopathy, primary neuromuscular junction disorder)
   g. Highly sensitive: normal SFEMG finding in clinically weak muscle confirms stability of the neuromuscular junction and rules out a clinically important disorder of neuromuscular transmission (myasthenia gravis, Lambert-Eaton myasthenic syndrome, botulism, congenital myasthenic syndromes)
   h. Measurements specific to SFEMG
      1) Fiber density: represents number of muscle fibers within recording field
      2) Jitter (Fig. 5-32): interpotential variability
         a) Muscle fibers innervated by same motor neuron are activated almost simultaneously
         b) Disease of neuromuscular junction can cause variability in rise time of the EPP and, thus, time interval between two single fiber potentials in same motor unit
         c) Very sensitive measure of neuromuscular junction disease: findings are abnormal even in very mild disease
         d) Findings may be abnormal when repetitive stimulation studies are normal
      3) Blocking (Fig. 5-32)
         a) EPP may fail to reach threshold and may not cause an action potential, and the second single fiber potential in the "pair" fails to fire
         b) Occurs in more moderate to severe disorders of neuromuscular junction transmission
         c) Correlates with variable and unstable amplitude and configuration of motor unit potentials recorded with a concentric needle, and abnormal repetitive stimulation studies

II. NEEDLE ELECTROMYOGRAPHY

A. Basic Principles

1. All potentials are recorded from summated action potentials generated by individual muscle fibers
2. Motor unit potential (MUP): aggregate potential recorded from a group of muscle fibers innervated by a single lower motor neuron (anterior horn cell)
3. Innervation ratio: the number of muscle fibers innervated by one lower motor neuron (number of muscle fibers within a motor unit)

4. Cross-sectional diameter of the area containing muscle fibers of a single motor neuron is normally 5 to 10 mm
5. Type I motor neurons are activated easily with little effort (lower threshold), have a smaller MUP
6. Type II motor neurons are activated with greater effort (higher threshold), have a larger MUP

B. MUP Characteristics Recorded With Concentric Needle Electrodes (Fig. 5-33)
1. Duration
   a. Time between starting point (leaves baseline) and end point of MUP (returns to baseline)
   b. Influenced by number, size, spatial distribution of muscle fibers activated by the common motor neuron and by distance from recording electrode
   c. Determined primarily by the muscle fibers within 2.5 mm of recording surface
   d. Most accurate measure of disease
   e. Influenced by age of patient and temperature
   f. Normal values vary with individual muscles
   g. Increased with denervation and collateral reinnervation of muscle fibers

h. Decreased with loss of muscle fiber action potentials within motor unit
i. Short-duration MUPs may be seen in
   1) Myopathies: loss of muscle fibers or ability of muscle fibers to generate action potentials
   2) Disorders of nerve terminals: failure of neuromuscular transmission (e.g., myasthenia gravis) or neurogenic disease of terminal branches of axon
   3) Severe axonal loss with limited or very early reinnervation of target muscles
j. Long-duration MUPs: may be seen in conditions that increase spatial and temporal distribution of muscle fiber action potentials in a motor unit
   1) Axonal or motor neuron loss, with collateral or robust proximal-to-distal reinnervation of target muscles
   2) Chronic myopathies (e.g., inclusion body myositis)
2. Amplitude
   a. Measurement from positive peak to negative peak
   b. Heavily influenced by the muscle fibers closest to recording electrode (within 500 μm of recording surface), thus very sensitive to slight electrode movement
   c. Increased with collateral reinnervation, decreased

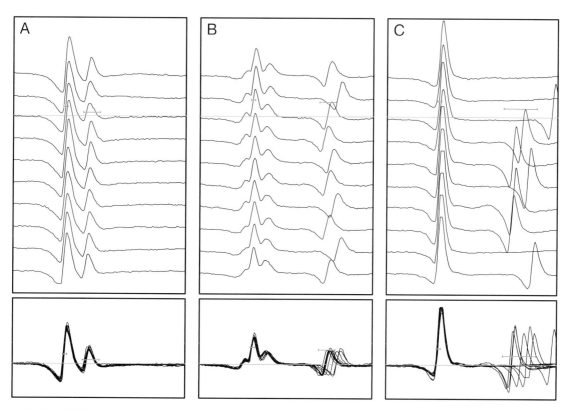

Fig. 5-32. Single fiber EMG recordings. *A*, Normal recording; *B*, increased jitter with no blocking; *C*, increased jitter with blocking. (Courtesy of W. Neath Folger, MD.)

temperature, and approximation of MUP to recording electrode

3. Area
   a. Measurement of surface area under the waveform (above and below baseline)
   b. Influenced by muscle fibers closest to recording electrode (within 1.5-2 mm of recording electrode)
   c. Difficult to measure accurately

4. Rise time
   a. The time between peak of the preceding positive deflection and peak of the largest negative deflection of the MUP
   b. Should be less than 0.5 millisecond to ensure comparison of MUP values with normal values
   c. Most accurate indication of the distance of muscle fibers from recording electrode

5. Phases
   a. Reflect the spatial and temporal distribution of recorded potentials within a MUP
   b. May be increased with loss of synchrony or change in fiber density in myopathic or neurogenic disease process
   c. Normal MUPs may have up to four phases and 15% polyphasic units
   d. Polyphasic MUPs
      1) May be seen with increased fiber density, fiber splitting, or fiber regeneration in a myopathic disease *or*
      2) May represent collateral or proximal-to-distal reinner-

vation in neurogenic disorders ("nascent potentials" appear as a result of early proximal-to-distal reinnervation after severe nerve injury and are often small and become highly polyphasic with reduced recruitment—see below)

6. Variation
   a. Refers to change in configuration and characteristics of MUPs during the same recording
   b. Reflection of instability of MUP amplitude, duration, and phase (i.e., dropout or addition of muscle fiber action potentials on consecutive discharges of MUP)
   c. Usually an indicator of abnormal neuromuscular junction which can occur in
      1) Primary disease of neuromuscular junction
      2) Immature and unstable neuromuscular junction due to early and ongoing reinnervation
   d. May also be seen in disorders of muscle fiber conduction (e.g., channelopathies such as periodic paralysis or myotonia congenita)

7. Recruitment
   a. Pattern of firing of MUPs with increasing voluntary activation secondary to anterior horn cell activation
   b. With increased voluntary contraction, MUPs fire at higher frequency and more MUPs are recruited
   c. Muscles with normal recruitment produce full interference pattern with maximal activity

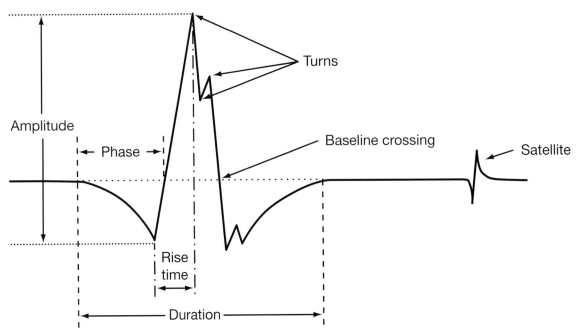

Fig. 5-33. Characteristics and measurements of a motor unit potential. (From Daube JR, editor. Clinical neurophysiology. 2nd ed. New York: Oxford University Press; 2002. p. 293-323. By permission of Mayo Foundation.)

d. Recruitment frequency: rate of firing of the first MUP at the time a second MUP begins to fire (normal, 9-11 Hz)

e. "Rule of Five": reduced recruitment if first MUP fires faster than 15 Hz before the second MUP appears or 20 Hz before third MUP appears

f. Reduced recruitment with loss of functioning MUPs
   1) Neurogenic disorders (e.g., axonal loss, conduction block)
   2) Very severe neuromuscular junction disease
   3) Some muscle disorders
      a) Severe destruction of muscle fibers (e.g., late in dystrophic myopathy)
      b) Severe loss of muscle electrical excitability (e.g., periodic paralysis during a spell)

g. Rapid recruitment: recruitment of many MUPs (near interference pattern, with minimal muscle contraction, always associated with reduction in size of MUPs)
   1) Usually seen in myopathies due to loss of individual muscle fiber action potentials within the MUP
   2) Also observed in disorders of nerve terminals (loss of conduction in terminal branches of axon or disorder of neuromuscular transmission with blocking of muscle fiber action potential)

h. Poor activation signifies poor voluntary effort or a central lesion

C. Analyzing MUPs

1. Isolation and measurement of at least 20 individual MUPs from each muscle group tested
2. Interference pattern analysis
3. Analysis by pattern recognition and semiquantitation

D. Insertional Activity

1. Increased insertional activity
   a. Normal variants: usually widespread distribution
      1) Brief trains of positive waves with regular firing pattern
      2) Brief bursts with irregular firing pattern
   b. Neuropathic conditions
   c. Myopathic conditions
2. Reduced insertional activity: seen in long-standing neuropathic or myopathic conditions in which muscle is replaced by connective tissue

E. Spontaneous Activity: during relaxation of the muscle

1. Assessment
   a. Morphology: often important in determining source of the potentials
   b. Stability of morphology: most potentials are stable in morphology
      1) Marked decrement of amplitude seen in neuromyotonia

      2) Waxing and waning of amplitude seen in myotonic discharges
   c. Firing rate and pattern (examples)
      1) Semirhythmic: normal MUPs (not spontaneous activity)
      2) Regular with steady change: fibrillation potentials, cramp discharges
      3) Regular with no change: complex repetitive discharges
      4) Regular with exponential waxing-and-waning amplitudes: myotonic discharges
      5) Irregular: end plate spike and fasciculation potentials
      6) Semiregular: myokymic discharge
   d. Firing rate
      1) Low (<20 Hz): fasciculation potentials
      2) Intermediate (>20 Hz and <100 Hz): myokymia, myotonia, end plate spikes, complex repetitive discharge
      3) High (>100 Hz): cramp discharge, neuromyotonia
2. End plate noise: normal
   a. Originates from neuromuscular junction
   b. Represents MEPPs produced by ongoing spontaneous quantal presynaptic release of acetylcholine, nonpropagating
   c. Small amplitude (10-50 µV), monophasic negative morphology, duration of 0.5 to 2 milliseconds
   d. Continuous firing ("hissing")
3. End plate spike: normal
   a. Muscle fiber action potentials triggered by mechanical stimulation of nerve terminal axons by the EMG needle
   b. Brief spike with biphasic morphology with initial negativity, amplitudes larger than MEPP (100-200 µV), duration of 3 to 4 milliseconds
   c. Rapid, irregular firing at frequency of 20 to 50 Hz ("fat in a frying pan")
4. Fibrillation potentials and positive waves (Fig. 5-34)
   a. Originate from single muscle fibers
   b. Produced by spontaneous depolarization of single muscle fibers due to separation or isolation of muscle fibers under study from their nerve supply
      1) Denervation and neurogenic injury: amyotrophic lateral sclerosis, radiculopathy, plexopathy
      2) Myopathic injury: muscle membrane irritability due to segmental necrosis, fiber splitting, vacuolar injury, or regenerating muscle fibers (e.g., myositis, muscular dystrophies, periodic paralysis, acid maltase deficiency)
      3) Severe neuromuscular junction disorders: due to complete blocking of neuromuscular junction, as in severe myasthenia gravis and botulism
   c. Regular firing rate (0.5-20.0 Hz), which may gradually slow down (rarely irregular)

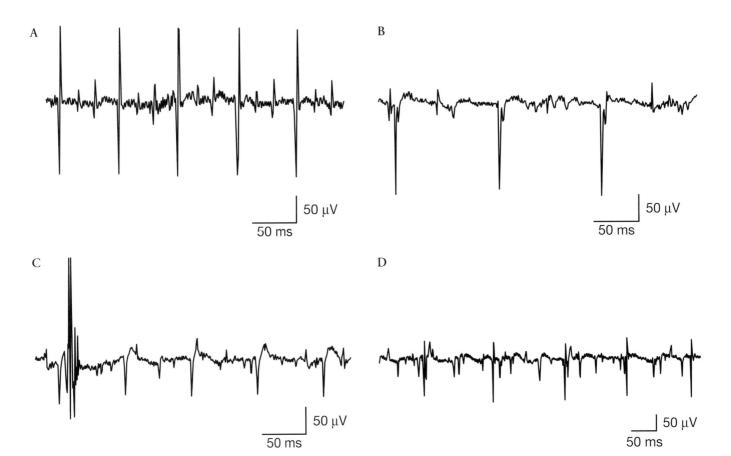

Fig. 5-34. *A-D*, Fibrillation potentials of different amplitudes and severity. Smaller amplitudes may occur with advanced muscle atrophy. Note regular firing of each waveform. Note also fasciculation potential at beginning of recording in *C*. This was recorded from anterior tibialis muscle in patient with amyotrophic lateral sclerosis.

d. May occur in two forms
   1) Brief biphasic or triphasic stable spikes: initial positivity and 20 to 200 μV in amplitude
   2) Positive waves: long duration and biphasic with brief initial positivity followed by long negativity (recorded at a distance or when electrode is next to a region of muscle membrane that is unable to conduct an action potential)
e. Amplitude decreases with muscle fiber atrophy
f. Brief, rapid (>50 Hz) train of positive waves may arise from an irritable single muscle fiber potential that does not propagate beyond the needle and is induced by needle movement—these rapid trains of positive waves may occur in absence of denervation (including normal muscle fibers)
g. Gradation
   1) 0: no fibrillation potential
   2) 1+: persistent single trains of potentials in two areas of muscle examined

   3) 2+: moderate number of different potentials in three or more areas
   4) 3+: many potentials in all areas of muscle tested
   5) 4+: completely fill baseline
5. Complex repetitive discharges (Fig. 5-35)
   a. Ephaptic transmission of action potentials to and between adjacent muscle fibers
   b. High frequency and regular firing rate (50-200 Hz) with abrupt onset and cessation
   c. Abrupt change in frequency and sound when adjacent ephaptic circuits become involved ("machinery sound")
   d. Nonspecific: may be seen in myopathic or neurogenic disorders or otherwise normal proximal muscles in elderly subjects
6. Fasciculation potentials (Fig. 5-34 *C*)
   a. Spontaneous involuntary discharge of a single MUP
   b. Originates from anterior horn cell, axon, or nerve terminal (usually)
   c. Single, random, irregular firing pattern, with variable rate

d. Morphology identical to a single MUP
e. May be seen in
1) Normal subject: benign fasciculations with cramps, fatigue, or overworked muscle
2) Metabolic disorders: thyrotoxicosis, tetany and hypocalcemia, anticholinesterase medications (e.g., pyridostigmine)
3) Neuropathic disorders: motor neuron disease, radiculopathy, plexopathy, peripheral neuropathy, disorders of peripheral nerve hyperexcitability (e.g., cramp-fasciculation syndrome, Isaacs' syndrome)

7. Doublets and multiplets
a. Spontaneous depolarization of two to five "time-locked" MUPs
b. Same clinical significance as fasciculation potential
c. May be seen in cramp-fasciculation syndrome, hyperventilation, tetany and hypocalcemia (as with carpopedal spasms), other metabolic conditions, and neuropathic conditions such as amyotrophic lateral sclerosis

8. Cramp potentials
a. Originate from a high-frequency discharge of axons, not the muscle
b. Associated with a rapid-onset, strong, painful, and involuntary muscle contraction
c. Firing rate rapidly accelerates from baseline to more than 100 Hz
d. Unique high-amplitude waveforms reproduced by stimulation of synchronized MUPs
e. Firing pattern may become irregular, especially at termination
f. May be a benign phenomenon or associated with same conditions associated with fasciculation potentials

9. Myokymic discharges (Fig. 5-36)
a. Spontaneous bursts ("marching soldiers") of 2 to 10 grouped potentials firing at 40 to 80 Hz in semiregular rhythm
b. Spontaneous discharges are essentially grouped depolarizations arising from same lower motor neuron or axon and sometimes from demyelinated segments of the nerve via ephaptic transmission
c. Essentially grouped fasciculations, but clinical significance different from fasciculation potentials
d. If recorded from facial muscles: multiple sclerosis, facial palsy due to brainstem neoplasm or idiopathic, or polyradiculopathy
e. If recorded from extremity muscles: radiation plexopathy, compression neuropathy (e.g., carpal tunnel syndrome), diffuse demyelinating disorders such as chronic inflammatory demyelinating polyradiculoneuropathy or disorder of peripheral nerve hyperexcitability (e.g., cramp-fasciculation syndrome, Isaacs' syndrome)

10. Myotonic discharges (Fig. 5-37)
a. Originate from the muscle fiber
b. Spontaneous, prolonged discharge of a group of muscle fibers induced by activation of sodium channels on muscle fiber membrane
c. Depending on underlying disorder, may be activated by various triggers: mechanical irritation of muscle fiber, changes in body temperature, voluntary activation, ischemia, changes in acid-base balance of microenvironment
d. Instability of diseased muscle membrane causes amplitude and frequency to wax and wane (due to alteration in one or more channels that affect membrane voltage [Na^+, Ca^{2+}, Cl^-])
e. Discharges have morphology of a positive wave when initiated by needle movement
f. May be seen in inherited channelopathies (myopathic

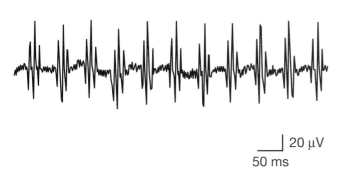

20 µV
50 ms

Fig. 5-35. Complex repetitive discharge recurring at 30-35 per second.

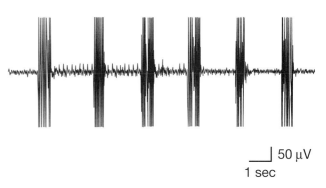

50 µV
1 sec

Fig. 5-36. Myokymic discharge recorded from patient with history of radiation-induced brachial plexopathy. (Courtesy of W. Neath Folger, MD.)

conditions associated with clinical myotonia, e.g., paramyotonia congenita or periodic paralysis), conditions with clinical myotonia (e.g., myotonic dystrophy), acquired disorders without clinical myotonia (e.g., inflammatory muscle disease or acid maltase deficiency)

11. Neuromyotonic discharges (Fig. 5-38)
    a. High-frequency (100-300 Hz) regular repetitive discharges of a single MUP characteristically wanes in amplitude and frequency
    b. Originates from terminal portion of motor axon
    c. Observed in disorders of peripheral nerve hyperexcitability, usually secondary to altered conductance of voltage-gated potassium channels (e.g., Isaacs' syndrome, cramp-fasciculation syndrome, some neuropathies)

III. BASIC PATTERNS

A. Axonal Loss or Injury

1. The following are general guidelines (see each disorder for discussion of specific conditions)
2. Hyperacute (<4-6 days old)
   a. Before wallerian degeneration occurs
   b. Stimulation distal to the lesion: normal conductions
   c. Stimulation proximal to the lesion: reduced or absent conductions (cannot differentiate between axonal loss and conduction block at this stage)
   d. Reduced recruitment (will persist)
   e. Normal MUP morphology and spontaneous activity
3. Acute (>4-6 days but <10 days)
   a. Nerve conduction studies: reduced amplitudes (proximal and distal to lesion) with relatively preserved conduction velocities and distal latencies

b. Reduced recruitment but no fibrillation potentials (inadequate time)
4. Early subacute (10-15 days)
   a. Increased spontaneous activity (increased insertional activity and possibly some fibrillation potentials)
   b. Reduced recruitment with normal MUP morphology
5. Late subacute (16-60 days)
   a. Development of fibrillation potentials (proportional to severity of axonal loss)
   b. Reduced MUP recruitment
   c. By 4 weeks, MUPs will likely have increased duration and be polyphasic
   d. Early denervation produces fibrillation potentials and may induce MUP variation due to instability of neuromuscular junction
   e. Reinnervation eventually produces long-duration, high-amplitude neurogenic potentials, which may become less polyphasic over time in absence of ongoing denervation
   f. By this stage, amplitudes of CMAPs (if preganglionic or postganglionic localization of lesion) and SNAPs (if postganglionic) may be reduced, with relative preservation of conduction velocities and distal latencies
6. Chronic axonal loss (after 180 days): in absence of ongoing denervation
   a. Nerve conduction studies are expected to be normal or show reduced amplitude, depending on severity of axonal injury and success of reinnervation (conduction velocities may be mildly reduced because reinnervated axons have smaller diameter and less myelin)
   b. "Nascent units" may be present with proximal-to-distal (not collateral) reinnervation (Fig. 5-39)
      1) This usually requires about 2 to 3 months and represents early reinnervation
      2) These potentials are often short duration, low ampli-

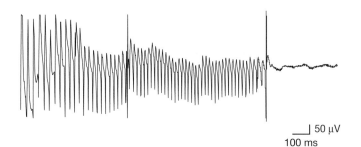

50 µV
100 ms

Fig. 5-37. Myotonic discharge recorded from patient with myotonic dystrophy. In addition, there were slow, tall fibrillation potentials (*arrows*) in the recording, two of which are shown here. The myotonic discharge ends with the second fibrillation potential represented in this segment.

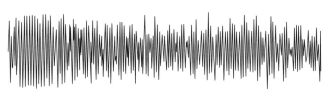

100 ms

Fig. 5-38. Neuromyotonic discharge firing at approximately 300 Hz.

tude, polyphasic, and varying (unstable) in morphology, with reduced recruitment
   3) The reduced recruitment differentiates these from myopathic units (which are expected to have early or rapid recruitment)
   4) Variability of the potentials is due to instability of neuromuscular junction
   5) Early on, the potentials have short duration, but with ongoing reinnervation, the duration increases (Fig. 5-39)
   c. Both collateral and proximal-to-distal reinnervation eventually result in long-duration, high-amplitude, stable MUPs with reduced recruitment, which may or may not be polyphasic (Fig. 5-40)
   d. Insertional activity is often normal, in absence of ongoing denervation
   e. Example: old poliomyelitis or old radiculopathy

B. Demyelination
1. The following are general guidelines (electrophysiologic properties of each condition are included with the discussion of that condition)
2. Focal proximal demyelination
   a. Normal distal sensory and motor conduction studies
   b. Stimulation across site of demyelination (if possible) demonstrates focal slowing or conduction block
   c. Abnormal late responses
   d. Normal MUP morphology (in pure demyelination)
   e. Reduced recruitment if conduction block; normal recruitment with focal proximal slowing
   f. If less than 4 days old, difficult to distinguish from hyperacute axonal loss

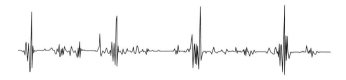

| 200 µV
50 ms

Fig. 5-39. "Nascent units." Early nascent units have short duration and low amplitude, but with ongoing reinnervation they become more polyphasic and duration increases, as seen here. Note the severely reduced recruitment that distinguishes these potentials from myopathic motor unit potentials. Also, there is variability of motor unit potentials due to neuromuscular junction instability.

3. Focal distal demyelination
   a. Distal nerve conduction studies may show conduction block or slowing, with less reduction of amplitude and abnormal late responses
   b. Reduced recruitment expected with conduction block
   c. MUP morphology otherwise normal in absence of secondary axonal injury
   d. This pattern may be seen in distal entrapment neuropathies

C. Polyneuropathy
1. The following are general guidelines (electrophysiologic properties of each condition are included with the discussion of that condition)
2. Common patterns
   a. Length-dependent: changes more severe distally
   b. Polyradiculoneuropathy: equal changes in proximal and distal regions of the body and segments of the nerve
   c. Mononeuritis multiplex
   d. Modality-specific: motor, sensory, autonomic
3. Axonal polyneuropathy
   a. Reduced CMAP and SNAP amplitudes, with relative preservation of distal latencies, conduction velocities, late responses
   b. Long-standing, slowly progressive polyneuropathies (as in the inherited conditions): minimal to no fibrillation (denervation) potentials
   c. Rapidly progressive polyneuropathies (mostly acquired): combination of denervation potentials and reinnervated neurogenic potentials
   d. Acute axonal polyneuropathies: may only see reduced recruitment in first 4 days (e.g., vasculitis or axonal polyradiculoneuropathy)
4. Demyelinating polyneuropathy
   a. Associated with prolonged distal latencies (>130% of upper limit of normal) and slowed conduction velocities (<70% of lower limit of normal)
   b. Inherited demyelinating polyneuropathies: usually symmetric and show uniform slowing of conduction velocities
   c. Acquired demyelinating polyneuropathies: may be symmetric or asymmetric because of multifocal demyelination; usually associated with conduction block, focal slowing, and temporal dispersion of motor responses

D. Neuropraxis
1. Transient loss of axonal conduction due to altered nodal function caused by
   a. Ischemia
   b. Metabolic dysfunction *or*
   c. Alteration of nodal architecture (demyelination,

mechanical distortion of node, alteration of axonal membrane in nodal region)
2. Conduction returns with repair of nodal function

E. Motor Neuron Disease
1. Nerve conduction studies
   a. May be normal or show abnormal motor responses with normal SNAPs
   b. Evidence of motor axonal loss
      1) Reduced CMAP amplitude with relative preservation of distal latency and conduction velocity
      2) Absence of conduction block
   c. Some slowing may be expected if larger, faster axons are affected
2. Needle examination
   a. Presence of large unstable MUPs with reduced recruitment (reinnervation) and poor activation if upper motor neuron involved
   b. Fibrillation potentials (ongoing or persistent denervation)
   c. Fasciculation potentials (irritability of motor axons)
   d. Diffuse distribution of abnormalities: cranial, cervical, thoracic, and lumbosacral segments (diagnostic criteria are discussed in corresponding section)

F. Radiculopathy
1. SNAPs are expected to be normal (except if DRG is inside spinal canal and axonal injury is distal to DRG, as at L5-S1 root level)
2. CMAP amplitudes are normal with mild axonal loss or in chronic cases with considerable collateral reinnervation
3. With severe axonal loss, CMAP amplitudes are reduced—if fastest axons are affected, conduction velocities may be slowed and distal latencies prolonged
4. H reflex may be absent with S1 radiculopathy (may also be absent in plexopathy or sciatic neuropathy)
5. The pattern of large MUPs with reduced recruitment on needle examination, including paraspinal muscles, localize the root in question

G. Brachial Plexopathy
1. SNAPs are abnormal in the distribution of involved segments (this includes asymmetric responses when compared with normal side)

A

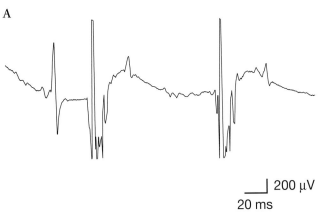

200 µV
20 ms

B

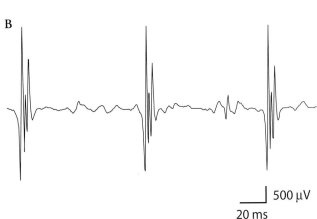

500 µV
20 ms

C

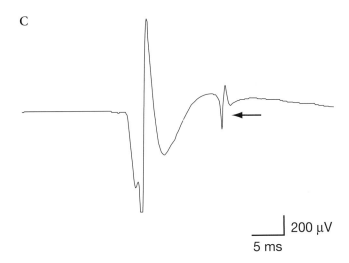

200 µV
5 ms

Fig. 5-40. Long-duration, high-amplitude motor unit potentials. *A,* A severely long-duration, high-amplitude complex motor unit potential with increased number of turns and severely reduced recruitment. *B,* Another example of long-duration, polyphasic, and stable motor unit potential with severely reduced recruitment. *C,* Motor unit potential also has long duration and is associated with a satellite potential (*arrows*), which is time-locked to the main component of the potential and is generated by a single muscle fiber in a distant end plate zone. (*C* courtesy of W. Neath Folger, MD.)

a. Upper trunk
1) Abnormal SNAPs: lateral antebrachial cutaneous (± median and radial sensory responses)
2) Neurogenic MUPs
    a) Supraspinatus and infraspinatus (direct branches of upper trunk)
    b) All (or some, with selective fascicular involvement) of the musculocutaneous-innervated muscles and C5, 6/axillary, radial, median-innervated muscles, including
        i) Deltoid muscle (axillary nerve, posterior cord, posterior division of upper trunk)
        ii) Biceps muscle (musculocutaneous nerve, lateral cord, anterior division of upper trunk)
        iii) Brachioradialis muscle (radial nerve, posterior cord, posterior division of upper trunk)
        iv) Pronator teres muscle (C6, 7) may be affected (median nerve, lateral cord, anterior division of upper trunk)
    c) Sparing of rhomboid muscles (C5 root/dorsal scapular nerve)
    d) Sparing of muscles innervated primarily by C7 root
b. Middle trunk
1) Abnormal SNAPs: median and radial nerves
2) Neurogenic MUPs: C7-innervated muscles (pronator teres, triceps brachii, etc.)
c. Lower trunk
1) Abnormal SNAPs: ulnar nerve
2) Neurogenic MUPs: all (or some, with selective fascicular involvement) of ulnar-innervated muscles, median- and radial-innervated muscles (C8/T1 distribution)
d. Lateral cord
1) Abnormal SNAPs: lateral antebrachial cutaneous and median nerves
2) Neurogenic MUPs: all (or some, with selective fascicular involvement) of musculocutaneous-innervated muscles (biceps) and C5-7/median-innervated muscles (if radial-innervated muscles affected, think upper trunk)
e. Posterior cord
1) Abnormal SNAPs: radial sensory, with normal median and ulnar SNAPs
2) Neurogenic MUPs: all (or some, with selective fascicular involvement) of the radial and axillary innervated muscles, as well as latissimus dorsi and teres major, directly innervated by the posterior cord
f. Medial cord
1) Abnormal SNAPs: ulnar and/or medial antebrachial cutaneous nerve (ulnar nerve may be spared)
2) Neurogenic MUPs: all (or some, with selective fascicular involvement) of ulnar-innervated muscles,

C8, T1, and median nerve-innervated muscles (if radial nerve-innervated muscles are also involved, localization to the lower trunk should be considered)
2. Median and ulnar CMAPs may show reduced amplitudes with axonal injury (most causes involve axonal injury rather than demyelination)
3. Sparing of paraspinal muscles (there may be root involvement with traumatic root avulsion, cancer, inflammatory plexopathies, etc.)
4. Lesions causing brachial plexopathy (e.g., Parsonage-Turner syndrome) may be multifocal (this may be reflected in patchy distribution of abnormality on the conduction studies and needle examination)

H. Mononeuropathy (for electrodiagnostic evaluation of mononeuropathies, including entrapment neuropathies, see Chapter 21)

I. Myopathy
1. Nerve conduction studies may be normal or CMAP amplitudes may be reduced when advanced
2. Normal or abnormal spontaneous activity
    a. Fibrillation potentials due to muscle fiber necrosis, splitting, or vacuolation, may also be positive sharp waves
    b. Complex repetitive discharges common with chronic myopathies, but nonspecific
    c. Myotonic discharges are more specific, may be seen in certain myopathies
3. Insertional activity: normal, increased, or decreased, depending on the myopathy, severity, and stage of progression
4. Rapid (early) recruitment: fewer muscle fibers per motor unit, thus activation of more motor units to generate the same force
5. Classic myopathic morphology
    a. Short-duration, low-amplitude (sometimes polyphasic) MUPs (Fig. 5-41)
    b. Chronic severe or end-stage myopathies may appear "neurogenic" (i.e., long duration, large amplitude, polyphasic), probably because of excessive motor unit remodeling that occurs with advanced disease of the muscle fibers

IV. EVOKED POTENTIALS

A. Brainstem Auditory Evoked Potentials (BAEPs)
1. Assessment of peripheral and central auditory pathways
2. May be performed in patients under general anesthesia or sedation

3. Useful as ancillary testing for multiple sclerosis or other neurologic disorders affecting central brainstem pathways (e.g., brainstem tumors)
4. Comparable in sensitivity to MRI as screening test for suspected acoustic neuroma (sensitivity is less for other cerebellopontine angle tumors)
5. Sensitivity for brainstem lesion is compromised if the lesion does not involve auditory pathways bilaterally
6. Absent in brain death
7. Technical considerations
    a. Monaural click stimulation used with contralateral masking noise to prevent stimulation of contralateral ear through bone conduction
    b. Stimulus needed for waveform detection: usually 60 to 70 dB above click hearing threshold
    c. Physiologic variables: age, sex, auditory acuity
    d. Greater stimulus intensity needed for patients with hearing loss
8. Waveform generators ("eight crows sing lullabies in my town") (Fig. 5-42)
    a. Wave I: eighth cranial nerve (CN VIII)
    b. Wave II: cochlear nuclei (and proximal CN VIII)
    c. Wave III: superior olivary nucleus
    d. Wave IV: lateral lemniscus
    e. Wave V: inferior colliculus
    f. Wave VI: medial geniculate body
    g. Wave VII: thalamocortical connections
9. Measurements (for normal values, see Appendix B)
    a. Normal absolute peak latencies: add 0.6 to 0.8 to the number of waveform (e.g., wave II has peak latency of 2.80)
    b. Interpeak latencies of waves I-III, I-V, and III-V (normal values in Appendix E)
        1) Prolongation of I-V interpeak latency is nonlocalizing

indicator of disease process affecting central auditory pathways
        2) I-III and III-V interpeak latencies useful in localizing a central lesion
    c. Amplitude ratio of wave V:wave I
10. Clinical correlations
    a. Both peripheral and central lesions may potentially cause absence of all waveforms
    b. Central auditory conduction abnormalities
        1) Prolonged I-V interpeak latency (most common)
        2) Reduced amplitude ratio of wave V:I
        3) Poorly formed waves II to V, with relative preservation of wave I
        4) All waveforms may be absent
        5) Brainstem tumors: often bilateral BAEP abnormalities, prolonged interpeak latencies of waves III to V and I to V (Fig. 5-42)

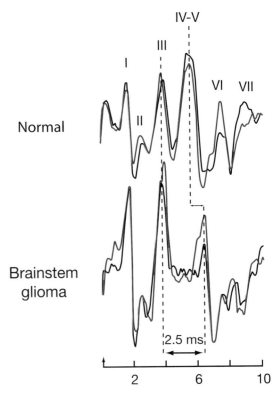

Fig. 5-42. Brainstem auditory evoked potentials from normal subject (*top*) and patient with brainstem glioma (*bottom*). In bottom tracing, note a prolonged III-V interpeak latency (dashed lines), indicative of abnormal central auditory pathways. (From Caviness JN. Brain stem auditory evoked potentials in central disorders. In: Daube JR, editor. Clinical neurophysiology. 2nd ed. New York: Oxford University Press; 2002. p. 204-13. By permission of Mayo Foundation.)

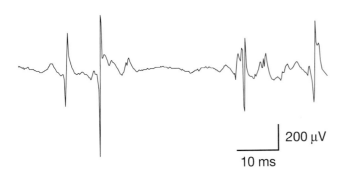

Fig. 5-41. Myopathic motor unit potentials.

6) Acoustic neuromas: prolonged ipsilateral waves I to V and I to III absolute interpeak latencies or poorly defined or absent waveforms (all)

7) Brain death
   a) Wave I should be present to ensure recording is technically adequate
   b) Waves II through V always absent

c. Peripheral auditory dysfunction (including laterally placed small acoustic neuromas)
   1) Prolongation of all absolute latencies with normal interpeak latencies (excluding processes affecting CN VIII peripherally)
   2) Wave I may be absent while other latencies are prolonged
   3) All waveforms may be absent

B. Visual Evoked Potentials (for normal values, see Appendix E)

1. Electrophysiologic assessment of central visual pathways
2. Monocular visual stimulation using a shifting checkerboard pattern (pattern reversal evoked potentials) projected on TV monitor
3. Pattern evoked stimulus: requires alert subject able to maintain fixation at center of TV monitor
4. Flash evoked stimulus
   a. May be used with young children, poorly cooperative or sedated adults, or patients under anesthesia
   b. Response obtained with this is less reliable than with pattern stimulus
5. Waveforms
   a. N1 (N75): initial negative deflection
   b. P1 (P100): positive deflection
   c. N2 (N145): second negative deflection
6. P100 peak latencies: most important measurement (Fig. 5-43)
   a. Generated in occipital lobe
   b. The size of the potential may be affected by size of checks in checkerboard pattern, pupil size, visual acuity, and age
   c. Latency is affected mainly by conduction in optic nerve and central visual pathways
   d. Use larger size checks for patients with poor visual acuity
7. Anterior visual pathway lesions (prechiasmal)
   a. High sensitivity for lesions of anterior pathway
   b. Unilateral P1 abnormalities
      1) Prolonged P1 latencies may indicate poor conduction such as demyelination (optic neuritis)
      2) Abnormal morphology or reduced amplitudes may indicate compressive lesion

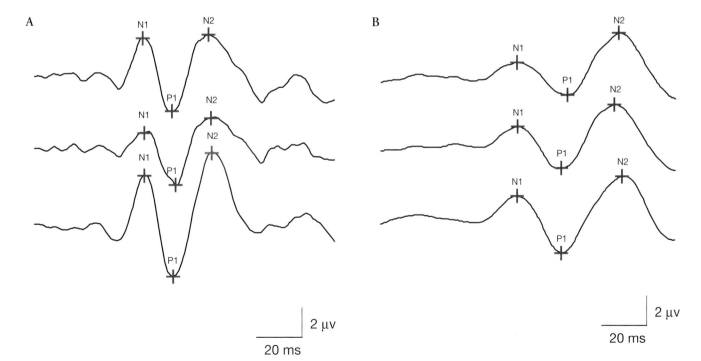

Fig. 5-43. Visual evoked potentials from patient with right optic neuritis due to multiple sclerosis. *A,* Recording from left eye is normal. *B,* Recording from right eye shows prolonged P1 latency.

c. Bilateral P1 abnormalities
  1) Nonlocalizing
  2) May be seen with chiasmal, postchiasmal, or bilateral prechiasmal lesions
8. Poor sensitivity for lesions of postchiasmal and cortical visual pathways
9. Patients with relatively focal cortical visual dysfunction usually have normal visual evoked potentials
10. Normal visual evoked potentials in a blind person can indicate cortical blindness or functional visual loss

C. Somatosensory Evoked Potentials (for normal values, see Appendix D)

1. Electrophysiologic assessment of large-fiber sensory pathways of peripheral nerves, spinal cord, and brain
2. Responses recorded with stimulation of upper extremity nerves (usually median or ulnar nerve at wrist)
   a. N9: Erb's point
   b. N13: cervical neck
   c. N20: scalp
3. Responses recorded with stimulation of lower extremity nerves (usually tibial or peroneal nerve)
   a. N22: lumbar cord
   b. N30: cervical neck
   c. N38: scalp
4. Generated mainly in sensory pathways of dorsal column and medial lemniscus and primary somatosensory cortex and, to lesser extent, in spinocerebellar pathways
5. Interpeak latencies primarily reflect conduction in proximal peripheral nerve segments and central nervous system
6. Clinical use
   a. Detect or confirm myelopathy in asymptomatic subjects or symptomatic subjects with negative or equivocal findings on neurologic examination or imaging
   b. Demyelinating or dysmyelinating diseases tend to affect interpeak latencies
   c. Compressive or axonal diseases tend to reduce amplitudes
   d. Often, considerable overlap and lesion may not always be predicted
   e. Cervical myelopathy: low-amplitude or absent N13 with prolonged N9-N20 interpeak latencies in upper limb somatosensory evoked potential and/or absent N30 with prolonged N22-N38 interpeak latencies in lower limb somatosensory evoked potential
   f. Brain death (scalp potentials may be lost): bilateral loss of N20 scalp response and preservation of N13 cervical neck response (Fig. 5-44) (may also be seen in drug intoxication and diffuse cerebral edema)
   g. Monitoring in spine surgery

D. Cranial Reflexes

1. Blink reflex
   a. Electrophysiologic assessment of trigeminal (CN V) and facial (CN VII) nerves and their central connections
   b. May be helpful in assessing cranial neuropathies, polyradiculoneuropathies, brainstem lesions
   c. Electrical stimulation of trigeminal nerve at supraorbital notch and recording motor responses at orbicularis oculi bilaterally
   d. Afferent limb: trigeminal nerve, ophthalmic division (V1)
   e. R1 response
     1) Afferent input synapses in principal sensory nucleus of CN V
     2) Interneuron connections and input to ipsilateral facial motor nucleus (oligosynaptic, i.e., only a few synapses)
   f. R2 response
     1) Afferent input to spinal nucleus of CN V
     2) Interneuron connections and input to facial motor nuclei bilaterally (longer course, polysynaptic, many synapses)

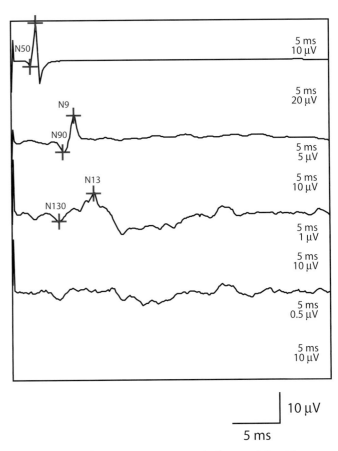

Fig. 5-44. Median somatosensory evoked potentials with absence of scalp recordings in patient with brain death due to severe anoxic injury.

g. Efferent limb: facial nerve branches supplying the orbicularis oculi
h. Clinical correlation
   1) Trigeminal neuropathies (Fig. 5-45)
      a) Stimulation of involved side: delayed or absent responses (ipsilateral R1 and R2 and contralateral R2)
      b) Stimulation of uninvolved side: normal responses
   2) Facial neuropathies (Fig. 5-46)
      a) Stimulation of involved side: delayed or absent ipsilateral R1 and R2 responses
      b) Stimulation of uninvolved side: delayed or absent contralateral R2 response
   3) Pontine lesion selectively involving principal sensory nucleus of CN V and interneurons
      a) Ipsilateral stimulation: delayed or absent R1 responses with preservation of remaining responses
      b) Contralateral stimulation: normal responses
   4) Medullary lesions
      a) R1 responses: normal
      b) R2 responses: vary depending on exact anatomy of lesion
   5) Synkinesis
      a) May be seen with hemifacial spasms or aberrant regeneration of facial nerve after facial nerve palsy
      b) Stimulation of supraorbital branch of trigeminal nerve may cause ipsilateral synkinetic response recorded at orbicularis oris
2. Masseter reflex (jaw jerk)
   a. Monosynaptic reflex arc
   b. Afferent limb of reflex arc: input from muscle spindles in masseter muscle (Ia proprioceptive fibers) traveling via the mandibular division of CN V to the mesencephalic nucleus (pseudounipolar neurons) to synapse in motor nucleus of CN V
   c. Efferent limb: from motor nucleus of CN V via mandibular motor division of CN V to masseter muscle
   d. Recording electrodes placed over masseter muscle, and patient's chin tapped with a reflex hammer containing a microswitch that triggers the response

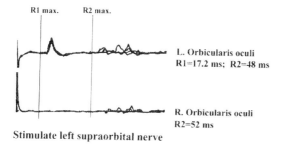

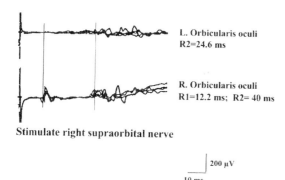

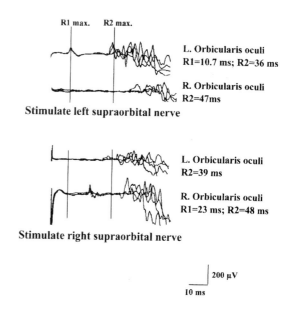

Fig. 5-45. Blink reflex studies in a patient with a lesion of left trigeminal nerve. Stimulation of the right side produces normal responses, whereas stimulation of the left side produces delayed responses. *R1 max* and *R2 max* are the upper limit of normal for the onset of the R1 and R2 responses, respectively. (From Auger RC, Stevens JC. Cranial reflexes. In: Daube JR, editor. Clinical neurophysiology. 2nd ed. New York: Oxford University Press; 2002. p. 382-93. By permission of Mayo Foundation.)

Fig. 5-46. Blink reflex studies in a patient with a lesion of the right facial nerve. Stimulation of the right side produces delayed ipsilateral R1 and R2 responses, while stimulation of the left side produces a delayed contralateral R2 response. *R1 max* and *R2 max* refer to the upper limit of normal for the onset of the R1 and R2 responses, respectively. (From Auger RC, Stevens JC. Cranial reflexes. In: Daube JR, editor. Clinical neurophysiology. 2nd ed. New York: Oxford University Press; 2002. p. 382-93. By permission of Mayo Foundation.)

e. Tends to be preserved in ganglionopathies because the cell body of afferent limb is in central nervous system (unlike the DRG for spinal reflexes)

f. May be useful in detecting central brainstem lesions or trigeminal neuropathy

g. Normal latencies: between 6 and 10 milliseconds (one usually looks for presence or absence of response)

3. Masseter inhibitory response

a. Proprioceptive inhibitory reflex arc with inhibitory function to control force of bite to avoid injury

b. Inhibitory response is recorded as silent period (SP) and is elicited by mechanical tap or electrical stimulation of chin (or any surface innervated by V2 or V3) during active muscle contraction (clenching teeth)

c. Recording electrodes over masseter muscle

d. Mechanical tap: one silent period recorded (SP1), usually 11 to 15 milliseconds after stimulus

e. Electrical stimulation: two silent periods recorded
   1) SP1 as above
   2) SP2 usually 30 to 60 milliseconds after stimulus

f. May be abnormal in trigeminal neuropathies, tetanus, some basal ganglia disorders

References

Aminoff MJ, editor. Electrodiagnosis in clinical neurology. 4th ed. New York: Churchill Livingstone; 1999.

Beaussart M. Benign epilepsy of children with Rolandic (centro-temporal) paroxysmal foci: a clinical entity: study of 221 cases. Epilepsia. 1972;13:795-811.

Blume WT, Kaibara M. Atlas of adult electroencephalography. New York: Raven Press; 1995.

Blume WT, Kaibara M. Atlas of pediatric electroencephalography. 2nd ed. Philadelphia: Lippincott-Raven; 1999.

Chatrian GE, Bergamasco B, Bricolo A, Frost JD Jr, Prior PF. IFCN recommended standards for electrophysiologic monitoring in comatose and other unresponsive states: report of an IFCN committee. Electroencephalogr Clin Neurophysiol. 1996;99:103-22.

Daly DD, Pedley TA, editors. Current practice of clinical electroencephalography. 2nd ed. New York: Raven Press; 1990.

Daube JR, editor. AAN Continuum Issue on Clinical Neurophysiology. Vol 4, No 5; 1998.

Daube JR, editor. Clinical neurophysiology. 2nd ed. New York: Oxford University Press; 2002.

Fisch BJ. Fisch and Spehlman's EEG primer: basic principles of digital and analog EEG. 3rd ed. Amsterdam: Elsevier; 1999.

Fisch BJ, Klass DW. The diagnostic specificity of triphasic wave patterns. Electroencephalogr Clin Neurophysiol. 1988;70:1-8.

Gibbs FA, Gibbs EL, editors. Atlas of electroencephalography. Vol 4. Cambridge (MA): Addison-Wesley Press; 1978.

Gibbs FA, Rich CL, Gibbs EL. Psychomotor variant type of seizure discharge. Neurology. 1963;13:991-8.

Hughes JR. Two forms of the 6-sec spike and wave complex. Electroencephalogr Clin Neurophysiol. 1980;48:535-50.

Klass DW, Westmoreland BF. Nonepileptogenic epileptiform electroencephalographic activity. Ann Neurol. 1985;18:627-35.

Lebel M, Reiher J, Klass D. Small sharp spikes (SSS): electroencephalographic characteristics and clinical significance [abstract]. Electroencephalogr Clin Neurophysiol. 1977;43:463.

Markand ON. Electroencephalography in diffuse encephalopathies. J Clin Neurophysiol. 1984;1:357-407.

Niedermeyer E, Lopes da Silva F, editors. Electroencephalography: basic principles, clinical applications, and related fields. 4th ed. Baltimore: Williams & Wilkins; 1999.

Noachtar S, Binnie C, Ebersole J, Mauguière F, Sakamoto A, Westmoreland B. A glossary of terms most commonly used by clinical electroencephalographers and proposal for the report form for the EEG findings. Electroencephalogr Clin Neurophysiol. 1999;52 Suppl:21-41.

Preston DC, Shapiro BE. Electromyography and neuromuscular disorders: clinical-electrophysiologic correlations. Boston: Butterworth-Heinemann; 1998.

Schaul N. The fundamental neural mechanisms of electroencephalography. Electroencephalogr Clin Neurophysiol. 1998;106:101-7.

Stockard-Pope JE, Werner SS, Bickford RG. Atlas of neonatal electroencephalography. 2nd ed. New York: Raven Press; 1992.

Synek VM. Prognostically important EEG coma patterns in diffuse anoxic and traumatic encephalopathies in adults. J Clin Neurophysiol. 1988;5:161-74.

Tan FC. EMG secrets. Philadelphia: Hanley & Belfus; 2004.

Westmoreland BF. Clinical EEG manual: Mayo Clinic clinical neurophysiology course; 2004.

Westmoreland BF. Clinical EEG Manual. Rochester (MN): Mayo Clinic; c2003 [updated 2003 Mar 31; cited 2005 Aug 31]. Available from: http://mayoweb.mayo.edu/man-neuroeeg/index.html.

Westmoreland BF, Klass DW, Sharbrough FW, Reagan TJ. Alpha-coma: electroencephalographic, clinical, pathologic, and etiologic correlations. Arch Neurol. 1975;32:713-8.

Wijdicks EF, Parisi JE, Sharbrough FW. Prognostic value of myoclonus status in comatose survivors of cardiac arrest. Ann Neurol. 1994;35:239-43.

Young GB. The EEG in coma. J Clin Neurophysiol. 2000;17:473-85.

Young GB, Kreeft JH, McLachlan RS, Demelo J. EEG and clinical associations with mortality in comatose patients in a general intensive care unit. J Clin Neurophysiol. 1999;16:354-60.

Appendix A. Normal Values for Motor Nerve Conduction Studies Used in Mayo EMG Laboratory

	Latency (side-side), ms	Amplitude (side-side), mV	Conduction velocity (side-side), m/s	Distal distance, cm
Median/APB	<4.5 (<1.0)	>4.0 (<10)	>48 (<5)	7
Median/lumb	<4.9 (<0.4)	>0.5 (>50%)	---	
Ulnar/ADM	<3.6	>6.0	>51 (<7)	6.5
Ulnar/FDI	<3.7	>7.0	>51	
Radial/EDC	<3.1	---	>67	
Musculo/biceps	<3.4	>4.0	>52	
Peron/EDB	<6.6	>2.0	>41	8.5
Peron/AT	<6.8	>5.1	>43	
Tibial/AH	<6.1	<4.0	>40	8
		AH ankle-to-knee amplitude difference <50%		
Tibial/ADMP	<7.4	>1.4	>40	
Facial/nasalis	<4.1 (<0.6)	>1.8		

ADM, abductor digiti minimi; ADMP, abductor digiti minimi pedis; APB, abductor pollicis brevis; AT, anterior tibialis; EDB, extensor digitorum brevis; EDC, extensor digitorum communis; FDI, first dorsal interosseous muscle.

Appendix B. Normal Values for Sensory Nerve Conduction Studies Used in Mayo EMG Laboratory

	Latency, ms	Amplitude, μV	Conduction velocity, m/s	Distal distance, cm
Median-II-anti	<3.6 (<0.5)	>15	>56	13
Median-uln-IV-anti	<0.4 diff		---	---
Med-rad-I-anti	<0.5 diff		---	---
Median palmar	<2.3 (<0.4 diff from uln)	>50	>56	8
Median ortho	<3.6	>10	>54	---
Ulnar-V-anti	<3.1	>10	>54	11
Ulnar-dorsal-anti	<2.6	>8	---	8
Ulnar palmar	<2.3	>15	>55	8
Ulnar ortho	<3.1	>0	---	---
Radial anti	<2.9	>20 (15 if age 60)	>49	10
Sural A	---	>15	---	7
Sural B	<4.5	>6 (if age <60)	>40	14
Sural C	---	>4.0	---	21
Superficial peroneal	<4.1	>0 (if age <55)	---	14
Medial plantar	<4.0	>7 (if age <55)	---	12
Lateral plantar	<4.6	>3 (if age <55)	---	12

anti, antidromic; ortho, orthodromic.

Appendix C. Normal Values for Blink Reflex Studies Used in Mayo EMG Laboratory

Sensory	Latency (side-side), ms	Amplitude (side-side), ms	Conduction velocity (side-side), ms
Blink reflex	R1 lat 8-13 (<1.5)	R2 lat ipsi 29-41 (<8)	R2 lat contra <44 (<8)

Appendix D. Normal Values for Somatosensory Evoked Potentials (SEPs) Used in Mayo EMG Laboratory

	Latency	Amplitude
Tibial SEP		
Lumbar N22	18-28	0-2.8
Cervical N30	24-37	0.4-1.5
Cortical P38	32-46	0.6-6.5
N22-N30	5.5-11.0	
N30-P38	5.0-12.0	
N22-P38	12.2-20.0	
Median SEP		
Clavicle N9	8.2-11.7	1.0-6.5
Cervical N13	11.3-15.5	0.9-3.0
Cortical N20	16.9-21.9	0.5-8.7
N9-N13	2.2-4.7	
N13-N20	4.7-6.6	
N9-N20	7.8-10.5	
Ulnar SEP		
Clavicle N9	9.2-12.8	0.6-3.1
Cervical N13	12.8-17	0.5-1.9
Cortical N20	18.1-22.7	0.8-5.8
N9-N13	3.3-4.5	
N13-N20	4.3-6.4	
N9-N20	8.2-10.6	

Appendix E. Normal Values for Brainstem Auditory Evoked Potentials (BAEPs) and Visual Evoked Potentials (VEPs) Used in Mayo EMG Laboratory

BAEP	Mean, ms	Range, ms	Interpeak latency, ms	Latency ULN, ms	VEP P100	Female	Male
Wave I	1.62	1.26-1.98	I-V <0.4 between sides	Female/ male (ms)	Age <60	<115	<120
Wave II	2.80	2.23-3.37	Age <60	<4.6/<4.65	Age >60	<120	<125
Wave III	3.75	3.25-4.26	Age >60	<4.7/<4.75		<10 ms side-side difference	
Wave IV	4.84	4.15-5.53	I-III	2.63			
Wave IV/V	5.27	4.61-5.93	I-IV/V	4.32			
Wave V	5.62	4.93-6.31	III-V	2.31			

ULN, upper limit of normal.

Appendix F. Normal Values for Parameters Defined by Needle Examination Used in Mayo EMG Laboratory

	0	±	+	++	+++	++++	Comments
Spontaneous activity							
Fibrilla-tion	None	Nonsustained or sustained in only 1 area	Sustained in ≥2 areas	Moderate numbers in all areas	Large numbers, close to filling baseline	Oblitera-tion of baseline	Positive waves & triphasic waves have same meaning
Fascicu-lation	None	Single, non-recurrent in 1 area	2 areas at freq of 2-10/min	10-50/min	50/100/min	>100/min	Grouped fascicu-lations may qualify as doublets or myo-kymic discharge
Voluntary activity							
MUP ampli-tude & dura-tion*	<3 SD of mean or <10% outside range	3-4 SD of mean or 10%-15% outside range	4-5 SD of mean or 15%-25% outside range	5-6 SD of mean or 25%-50% outside range	6-7 SD or 50%-90% outside range	7-8 SD or 90%-100% outside range	
Turns	1-2	3-4	5-6	7-8	8-10	>10	Phases—list as esti-mated % of poly-phasic on report
Reduced recruit-ment	If 1 MUP firing / If 2 MUPs firing / If 3 MUPs firing	Rate >10 Hz / Rate >15 Hz / Rate >18 Hz	Rate >15 Hz / Rate >18 Hz / Rate >20 Hz	Rate >20 Hz / Rate >25 Hz / Rate >30 Hz	Rate >25 Hz / Rate >30 Hz / Rate >40 Hz	Activation	Normal, MUP >20 Hz / Poor, no MUP >20 Hz / None, no MUP activity (may also say ++++ reduced recruitment)
Rapid recruit-ment	MUP with limb move-ment & no weakness	MUP with limb move-ment & weak-ness	MUP with joint move-ment & weakness	MUP with muscle but no joint movement	MUP with no visible muscle move-ment		

MUP, motor unit potential.

QUESTIONS

1-5. Match the description (questions 1-5) with the appropriate "late response" (choices a-d). Each choice may be used once, more than once, or not at all; each question may have more than one answer.

1. Response produced by antidromic stimulation of few alpha motor neurons which subsequently travels orthodromically to the muscle

2. A true monosynaptic reflex

3. Usually obtained with submaximal stimulus

4. Usually a late component of a dispersed compound muscle action potential

5. Latency decreases when the stimulus is moved proximally

a. H reflex

b. F waves

c. Satellite potentials

d. Axonal reflex

6. Increased jitter is expected in all the following *except*:
   a. Myasthenia gravis
   b. Steroid myopathy
   c. Amyotrophic lateral sclerosis (ALS)
   d. Rapidly progressive inflammatory myopathy
   e. All the above are usually associated with increased jitter

7. All the following originate from anterior horn cells, axons, or nerve terminals *except*:
   a. Fasciculation potentials
   b. Fibrillation potentials
   c. Myokymic discharges
   d. Neuromyotonic discharges
   e. All the above originate from anterior horn cells, axons, or nerve terminals

8. A lesion of the facial nerve causes:
   a. Delayed or absent R1 and ipsilateral R2 responses with stimulation of the involved side
   b. Delayed or absent R1 and ipsilateral and contralateral R2 responses with stimulation of the involved side
   c. Delayed or absent contralateral R2 responses with stimulation of the uninvolved side
   d. Delayed or absent ipsilateral and contralateral R2 responses only
   e. Both a and c

9. A 35-year-old woman with metastatic breast cancer presents with 4-day history of rapidly progressive asymmetric severe bilateral lower extremity weakness with absent reflexes and early urinary incontinence. The needle EMG of the affected muscle groups would be expected to show:
   a. Large polyphasic motor unit potentials and fibrillation potentials
   b. Reduced recruitment, unstable motor unit potentials, with dense fibrillation potentials in most muscles examined
   c. Rapidly recruited small motor unit potentials with no fibrillation potentials
   d. Reduced recruitment of motor unit potentials with normal morphology and relative absence of fibrillation potentials

10. Which of the following clinical diagnoses is likely in the patient in question 9?
    a. Cauda equina syndrome due to metastatic carcinoma
    b. Acute myopathy related to steroid use
    c. Bilateral lumbosacral plexopathies due to pelvic metastases

ANSWERS

1. Answer: b.

2. Answer: a.

3. Answer: a.

4. Answer: c.

5. Answer: b and d.

6. Answer: b.
Increased jitter is seen in the setting of disorder of neuromuscular transmission and may also be seen in active neurogenic or myopathic conditions associated with unstable motor unit potentials. Metabolic myopathies and steroid-induced myopathy often are not associated with increased jitter.

7. Answer: b.
Fibrillation potentials originate from muscle fibers. The rest of the responses originate from anterior horn cells, axons, or nerve terminals.

8. Answer: e.
Facial neuropathies will cause both delayed or absent R1 and ipsilateral R2 responses with stimulation of the involved side and delayed or absent contralateral R2 responses with stimulation of the uninvolved side.

9. Answer: d.
In the acute stage, there is often reduced recruitment of normal motor unit potentials. There has not been adequate time for development of fibrillation potentials, although there may be early fibrillation potentials in the most proximal muscle groups such as the paraspinal muscles.

10. Answer: a.
This patient likely has cauda equina syndrome. In this clinical setting, metastatic carcinomatous seeding of the cauda equina is likely.

BASIC PRINCIPLES OF PSYCHIATRY*

Maryellen L. Dodd, M.D.

Yonas E. Geda, M.D.

I. PSYCHOTIC DISORDERS

A. Schizophrenia

1. Introduction
   a. A prototype psychotic illness characterized by chronic course, deterioration in social and occupational functions, and positive (delusion, hallucination) and negative (flat affect, alogia, avolition) symptoms
   b. Probably the most devastating psychiatric disorder
   c. Affects 1% of the world population
   d. Contributes greatly to the world's economic burden
2. Overview of *Diagnostic and Statistical Manual of Mental Disorders, Fourth Edition, Text Revision* (DSM-IV-TR) diagnostic criteria
   a. The presence of at least two of five characteristic positive or negative symptoms for at least 1 month: delusions, hallucinations, disorganized speech, grossly disorganized or catatonic behavior, or negative symptoms—only need one of five if the delusions are bizarre or a voice or voices are keeping running commentary on the person's behavior or two or more voices are conversing
   b. Deterioration in social, occupational, and interpersonal relationships
   c. Continuous signs of the disturbance for at least 6 months (can include prodromal or residual symptoms like amotivation)
   d. Schizoaffective disorder and mood disorder with psychotic features have been ruled out
   e. Not due to effects of substances or general medical condition
3. Clinical findings and issues
   a. Psychotic symptoms: hallmarks of schizophrenia

(patients experience a confusion of boundaries between themselves and the world surrounding them, often called "a loss of ego boundaries")
   b. Positive symptoms (hallucinations and delusions)
      1) Hallucinations
         a) Perceptual experiences that have no external stimulus (e.g., hearing voices but no one is speaking)
         b) Auditory (e.g., voices commenting, arguing, repeating patient's thoughts), visual, tactile, gustatory, or olfactory—auditory hallucinations are the most common
      2) Delusions (Table 6-1)
         a) Disturbance of thought
         b) Firmly held false beliefs that can be bizarre or nonbizarre (beliefs unique to certain cultural or religious groups are not synonymous with delusions)
         c) Somatic, grandiose, paranoid, religious, nihilistic, sexual, persecutory, delusions of reference, delusions of thought (insertion, withdrawal, control, broadcasting)

Schizophrenia

Prototypical psychotic disorder

Affects 1%, M=F, M earlier onset than F

Hallmark:
   Positive symptoms: delusions, hallucinations, bizarre behavior

   Negative symptoms: blunting of affect, autism, ambivalence, social withdrawal, poverty of speech

Subtypes: Paranoid (best prognosis), disorganized, catatonic, undifferentiated, residual

At least 6 months of symptoms

---

*Portions of this chapter are from American Psychiatric Association. Diagnostic and statistical manual of mental disorders, fourth edition, text revision. Washington (DC): American Psychiatric Association; 2000. Used with permission.

Table 6-1. **Delusions**

Delusion	Definition
Erotomanic	de Clérambault's syndrome, theme that another person is in love with the individual
Grandiose	Conviction of having some great (but unrecognized) talent, insight, discovery, relationship, religious purpose
Jealous	Belief that one's spouse or lover is unfaithful
Persecutory	Person believes he or she is subject of conspiracy, is being spied upon, followed, poisoned, harrassed, etc.
Somatic	Involves bodily functions and sensations (e.g., emits foul odor, insects in skin, organs not functioning)
Capgras' syndrome	Belief that a person closely related to him or her has been replaced by a double
Fregoli syndrome	Identifies a familiar person in various other people he or she encounters; even if no physical resemblance, he or she maintains they are psychologically identical
Koro	Belief that penis is getting smaller and will disappear
van Gogh's syndrome	Self-mutilation driven by delusions
Thought insertion	Belief that thoughts can be implanted into brain
Thought withdrawal	Belief that thoughts can be withdrawn from brain
Thought control	Belief that someone can control one's thoughts
Thought broadcasting	Belief that one's thoughts can be heard by others

       d) Delusions with special reference (Capgras' syndrome, koro, prison psychosis, van Gogh's syndrome)

  c. Symptoms of disorganization

    1) Disorganized speech or thought

    2) Blocking of thought, clanging, distractibility, derailment, neologisms, poverty of speech and content of speech, preservation of thought, tangential speech

    3) Disorganized or bizarre behavior, catatonic supor or excitement, stereotypy (repeated purposeless movements), odd mannerisms, echopraxia

    4) Negativism, incongruous affect, inappropriate smiling

    5) Deterioration of social functioning, inappropriate social behaviors, unkempt in appearance, messy or has much clutter in surroundings

  d. Negative symptoms (3 per DMS-IV-TR)

    1) Alogia: speech that is empty or with decreased spontaneity

    2) Affective blunting: sparsity of emotional reactivity

    3) Avolition: unable to initiate or complete goals

    4) Other common negative symptoms: anhedonia (unable to experience pleasure), inability to concentrate or "attend," inappropriate affect, poor hygiene

  e. Other symptoms and associations

    1) Poor insight into illness

    2) Abnormalities of eye movements (increased frequency of blinking and abnormal saccades during test of smooth pursuits)

    3) Decreased stage IV sleep

    4) Loss of normal gracefulness of body movements

    5) Up to 25% may have shown schizoid traits before schizophrenia developed

    6) Tend to be less interested in sexual activity

    7) Up to 10% of schizophrenics commit suicide within first 10 years of their illness

    8) Up to 20% of schizophrenics drink excessive amounts of water, which may lead to chronic hyponatremia and possible water intoxication

    9) Alcohol and drug abuse is common, and schizophrenics smoke cigarettes three times more than the general population

 f. Subtypes of schizophrenia (paranoid, disorganized, catatonic, undifferentiated, residual)

    1) Paranoid (best outcome)

      a) Presence of delusions (often persecutory)

      b) Frequent auditory hallucinations

      c) Onset of illness (late 20s or 30s) later than for other subtypes

      d) More likely to marry and have children

    2) Disorganized (formally called hebephrenic)

      a) Display disorganized, nonproductive behaviors and demonstrate disorganized speech patterns

      b) Exhibit flat or inappropriate affect; grimacing is common

      c) Can act silly or childlike and burst out laughing for no reason

      d) Delusions and hallucinations are less organized and fragmentary

      e) Earlier onset

    3) Catatonic (less commonly seen now than in previous years)

      a) According to DSM-IV-TR, must have at least two of the following:

        i) Motoric immobility (catalepsy, stupor)

        ii) Excessive motor activity

iii) Extreme negativism

iv) Stereotypies, mannerisms, grimacing

v) Echolalia, echopraxia

4) Undifferentiated: these patients do not satisfy criteria for any other schizophrenia subtype

5) Residual: according to DSM-IV-TR, these patients no longer have any major psychotic symptoms but still exhibit evidence of the illness, with negative symptoms or at least 2 other odd or eccentric behaviors or perceptual experiences

6) Psychiatric terms and definitions are listed in Table 6-2

4. Course

a. Chronic, usually early onset, poor long-term outcome, devastating illness

1) Prodromal phase: often prolonged period of social withdrawal, delayed developmental milestones, awkward in motor skills, loss of interest in self-care

2) Active phase: psychotic symptoms appear, diagnosis is made more clear

3) Residual phase: similar to prodomal phase

b. Prognostic features and indicators

1) Good outcome

a) Acute onset, short duration, no previous psychiatric history, no family history of schizophrenia

b) Mood symptoms present, sensorium clouded

c) No obsessive-compulsive disorder, no assaultiveness

d) Premorbid functioning good, high socioeconomic class

e) Married, good psychosexual functioning

f) Normal findings on neuroimaging

2) Poor outcome

a) Insidious onset, chronic duration, psychiatric history present, positive family history of schizophrenia

b) Mood symptoms absent, sensorium clear

c) Obsessive-compulsive disorder is present, assaultiveness is present

d) Poor premorbid functioning, low socioeconomic class

Schizophrenia Prognostic Factors
Better prognosis: female, older onset, married, good premorbid functioning, acute onset, mood symptoms present, clouded sensorium, short duration

e) Never married, poor psychosexual functioning

f) Structural abnormalities present on neuroimaging

5. Epidemiology

a. Prevalence over lifetime is about 1.0% (no differences worldwide)

b. Average age at onset: men, 21 years (17-27 years); women, 27 years (17-37 years)

c. Male (M):Female (F) equal frequency

d. M>F in severity of illness, negative symptoms, suicide risk

e. F>M in mood comorbidity, better prognosis, better social functioning

f. Onset before age 10 and after age 45 are uncommon

6. Etiology

a. "Two-hit" or "multiple-hit" idea has strong support: the subject may have genetic predisposition to develop schizophrenia but does not manifest it unless other factors are encountered (e.g., environmental stressors)

b. Genetics

Table 6-2. **Psychiatric Terms and Definitions**

Circumstantiality	Cannot seem to get to the point because of excess of trivia or details
Clang	Thoughts proceed from one to another by sound of words, such as rhyming
Delusions	See Table 6-1
Echolalia	Repeating words just spoken
Flight of ideas	Thoughts seem to move quickly from idea to idea; often with pressured speech
Hallucinations	Perceptual abnormalities: auditory, tactile, gustatory, visual, olfactory, cenesthetic (visceral)
Ideas of reference	Belief that one is the topic or subject of media or other people's thoughts or conversations
Impaired abstraction	Concrete qualities to actions and/or objects
Loose associations	Rapid shift from one unrelated topic to another
Loss of ego boundaries	Cannot tell where one's mind/body end compared with another's mind/body
Neologisms	Use of "made-up" or new words
Perseveration	Thinking about something over and over
Tangentiality	Thoughts begin in logical fashions, then get further off track
Thought blocking	Train of thought stops, usually because of hallucinations
Word salad	Jumbled, unrelated words/phrases

> **Schizophrenia Genetics**
>
> Twin studies: nearly 50% monozygotic, 17% dizygotic
>
> Chromosomes implicated: 3p, 5q, 6p, 6q, 8p, 10p, 13q, 15q, 18p, 22q
>
> Trinucleotide repeat (CAG/CTG) on chromosomes 17 & 18

1) Siblings of schizophrenics: 10% develop schizophrenia
2) Children of parent with schizophrenia: 6% chance
3) Children of both parents with schizophrenia: 46% chance
4) Twins: nearly 50% chance for monozygotic and 17% chance for dizygotic twins
5) Multiple linkages (chromosomes 3p, 5q, 6p, 6q, 8p, 10p, 13q, 15q, 18p, 22q)
6) Large trinucleotide repeats: CAG/CTG on chromosomes 17 and 18

7. Neuroanatomical findings on imaging
    a. Most consistent finding is ventricular enlargement, especially third and lateral ventricles
    b. Selective reduction in size of frontal lobe, basal ganglia, thalamus, and limbic regions, including the hippocampus and medial temporal lobe
    c. Possible decrease in volume of neocortical and deep gray matter
    d. Sulcal widening, especially frontal and temporal areas
    e. Some studies indicate small but significant difference in brain and intracranial volume
    f. Increased incidence of
        1) Cavum septum pellucidum
        2) Partial callosal agenesis
8. Functional neuroimaging
    a. Hypofrontality (frontal and prefrontal cortex): negative symptoms and neurocognitive deficits
    b. Positron emission tomographic (PET) studies implicate frontal cortex (orbital, dorsolateral, medial), anterior cingulate gyrus, thalamus, several temporal lobe subregions, and cerebellum
    c. PET studies: anatomic substrate for visual hallucinations in schizophrenia
        1) Inferotemporal cortex is responsible for visual recognition of objects and faces
        2) Basal ganglia output (primarily substantia nigra pars reticulata) to inferotemporal cortex with relay in ventral anterior thalamic nucleus—influences visual processing and causes altered visual perception (hallucinations) as a result of increased dopaminergic activity in basal ganglia (may also be the mechanism of hallucinations in parkinsonian syndromes sensitive to dopaminergic agents [diffuse Lewy body disease more so than idiopathic Parkinson disease])
9. Neuropathology
    a. Decreased cell density in the dorsomedial nucleus of thalamus
    b. Displacement of interneurons in frontal lobe cortex
    c. Developmental issues
        1) History of injury at birth may contribute to development of schizophrenia
        2) Season of birth: more schizophrenics are born in early spring or winter
10. Neurochemical considerations
    a. Dopamine hypothesis: excess of dopamine linked to psychotic symptoms
        1) Dopamine-blocking drugs seemed to lessen psychotic symptoms (antipsychotics)
        2) Drugs stimulating dopamine release caused psychotic symptoms (amphetamine, cocaine)
        3) Five types of dopamine receptors: D_1, D_2, D_3, D_4, D_5
            a) D_1: located in cerebral cortex and basal ganglia
            b) D_2: located in striatum
            c) D_3 and D_4: high concentration in the limbic system
            d) D_5: located in thalamus, hippocampus, and hypothalamus
        4) Hyperactivity of dopamine system (especially D_2 receptor): thought important to positive symptoms of schizophrenia
    b. Postmortem findings in schizophrenics
        1) Increased dopamine or homovanillic acid in limbic areas and left amygdala (may be consequence of treatment with antipsychotics)
    c. PET used to measure receptor occupancy of antipsychotic medications
        1) Typicals: D_2 receptors (78% receptor occupancy), no obvious D_1 receptors
        2) Atypicals: D_2 receptors (48%), D_1 receptors (38%-52%), D_1 receptors are associated with fewer extrapyramidal symptoms
11. Clinical management (see PSYCHOPHARMACOLOGY AND OTHER TREATMENTS)
    a. Mainstay treatments: antipsychotics (D_2 receptor blockers [postsynaptic])
    b. Treatment
        1) First line, atypicals (may improve neurocognitive

impairment in schizophrenia): risperidone (Risperdal), olanzapine (Zyprexa), quetiapine (Seroquel), ziprasidone (Geodon), aripiprasole (Abilify)

    2) Second line: clozapine (Clozaril), is atypical, expensive, and needs monitoring because of the potential for severe agranulocytosis

    3) Typicals (may worsen neurocognitive functioning): chlorpromazine (Thorazine), thioridazine (Mellaril), perphenazine (Trilafron), loxapine (Loxitane), trifluoperazine (Stelazine), thiothixene (Navane), haloperidol (Haldol), fluphenazine (Prolixin)

  c. Maintenance therapy, for at least 1 to 2 years after the initial psychotic episode

  d. Alternative treatments

    1) Electroconvulsive therapy (ECT): schizophrenia does not typically respond to ECT, but it could be considered for catatonic schizophrenia

    2) Many benefit from benzodiazepines, mood stabilizers, antidepressants

12. Psychosocial intervention strategies

  a. Emphasis on outpatient treatment

  b. Partial hospitalization, day treatments, outpatient care

  c. Family therapy reduces relapse rate

  d. Self-help organizations

  e. Cognitive therapy techniques: the goal is to remediate the abnormal thought processes

  f. Social skills training: little effect on risk of relapse

  g. Psychosocial rehabilitation

    1) Restore the patient's ability to function in the community

  2) Appropriate/affordable housing, group homes

  3) Vocational training

  4) Assertive community treatment

B. Schizophreniform Disorder

1. Duration of clinical signs and symptoms is less than 6 months

2. Overview of DSM-IV-TR criteria

  a. At least two of the following: delusions, hallucinations, disorganized speech, disorganized behavior or catatonia, or negative symptoms

  b. Symptoms not caused by schizoaffective disorder, mood disorder with psychotic features, substance-induced disorders, or general medical condition

  c. Symptoms last at least 1 month, but less than 6 months

3. Clinical findings and issues

  a. Similar to schizophrenia except for duration

  b. 33% fully recover within 6 months

  c. 66% usually progress to schizophrenia or schizoaffective disorder

4. Course

  a. Good prognostic factors: onset of psychosis within 4 weeks after change of behavior/functioning, good premorbid functioning, positive symptoms, confusion and

---

Schizophrenia: Associated Neurologic Manifestations

Ventricular enlargement

Frontal lobe abnormality

Cerebellar vermis atrophy

Decreased volume: basal ganglia, limbic areas, hippocampus, thalamus, temporal regions, parahippocampal gyrus

Hypofrontalility: frontal lobe dysfunction

Increased D_2 receptor density in striatum & nucleus accumbens

Abnormal saccadic eye movements

Primitive reflexes

Schizophrenia: Neurotransmitters Implicated in Pathogenesis

Dopamine: excessive dopaminergic activity in mesolimbic areas

Serotonin: hyperactivity

Norepinephrine: hyperactivity

γ-Aminobutyric acid (GABA): loss of GABAergic neurons in hippocampus (decreased GABA, increased dopamine)

Schizophreniform Disorder

Like schizophrenia but duation <6 months

66% progress to schizophrenia/schizoaffective disorder

Prevalence: 0.2%

M=F

disorganization at peak of psychotic symptoms
   b. Depression is often comorbid: increases risk of suicide
5. Epidemiology: prevalence, 0.2%; M=F
6. Clinical management and psychosocial interventions: same as for schizophrenia

C. Schizoaffective Disorder

1. Prominent mood symptoms and at least 2 weeks of psychotic symptoms in the absence of mood symptoms
2. Overview of DSM-IV-TR criteria
   a. Uninterrupted period during which a mood disorder (major depression, mania, or mixed episode) coexists with symptoms of the active phase of schizophrenia.
   b. Must have delusions or hallucinations present for 2 weeks or more in absence of mood symptoms
   c. Meets criteria for a mood disorder for a substantial period of time during the illness (active and residual periods)
   d. Symptoms not due to substances, medications, or general medical condition
3. Course
   a. Prognosis: better than schizophrenia, but worse than major depression
   b. Suicide risk: 10%
4. Epidemiology: prevalence <1%
5. Clinical management: often symptom-based
   a. Antipsychotics: all are effective (clozapine is most effective but not without risk)
   b. Antidepressants: tricyclic antidepressants (TCAs) can worsen illness, selective serotonin reuptake inhibitors (SSRIs), and trazodone can be beneficial for mood component
   c. Others: benzodiazepines, lithium, anticonvulsants, ECT
   d. Psychotherapy (group, family, behavioral)

D. Delusional Disorder

1. Rare disorder

2. Characterized by nonbizarre delusions and does not affect other areas of a patient's life
3. Delusional disorder persecutory type is the relatively more common delusional disorder
4. Overview of DSM-IV-TR criteria
   a. Nonbizarre delusions for 1 or more months
   b. Active-phase symptoms of schizophrenia have not been met
   c. Functioning usually is not impaired, behavior is not odd
   d. If present, mood symptoms are brief in relation to period of illness
   e. Not caused by substances or general medical condition
5. Clinical findings and issues
   a. Delusions are persistent; there may also be tactile and olfactory hallucinations
      1) Delusions are frequently the only presenting symptom
      2) Types of delusions: persecutory (most common), erotomanic (more common in females), grandiose, jealous (more common in males), somatic
   b. Few cases are seen by psychiatry (strong denial of illness)
   c. Common defense mechanisms: denial, reaction formation, projection
6. Course
   a. Chronic, yet remission seen in 33% to 50% of patients
   b. Risk factors: increasing age, insidious onset, sensory deficits, F>M, neurologic injury, family history of psychotic disorders
7. Epidemiology: low prevalence, 0.03%; often starts in middle age (35-50 years), F>M
8. Etiology and pathophysiology
   a. Not related to schizophrenia or mood disorders
   b. Psychosocial stressors may be involved
   c. Genetic factors may be important
   d. Neurologic injury may precipitate or worsen the disorder
9. Clinical management (see PSYCHOPHARMACOLOGY AND OTHER TREATMENTS)

Schizoaffective Disorder

Prominent mood symptoms with psychosis

At least 2 weeks of psychosis without mood symptoms

Prognosis: better than schizophrenia, worse than mood disorder

Prevalence: <1%

Suicide risk: 10%

Delusional Disorder

Delusions are nonbizarrre, persistent

Difficult to treat: denial of illness, difficulty with trust

Prevalence: 0.03%, F>M, onset in middle age

Functioning usually not impaired

a. Patients typically do not seek help through mental health professionals

b. Patients often are noncompliant with treatment (denial of illness or fear of medications)

c. Hospitalization usually is not required

d. Collateral history is important

e. Complete medical work-up is essential

f. Psychologic testing can be helpful

g. Consider atypical antipsychotic agent or high-potency typical antipsychotic agent

   1) Usually helps with anxiety and intensity of delusion

   2) SSRIs can be helpful, even apart from depression

   3) Pimozide (Orap) is helpful for somatic delusional disorder

10. Psychosocial interventions

a. Psychotherapy: individual (supportive, cognitive, and behavioral); building trust, assurance of confidentiality, gentle/cautious questioning of validity of delusion are important considerations

b. Group therapy: often rejected (trust issues)

c. Family therapy: the family often has a difficult time dealing with the patient's delusions

E. Brief Psychotic Disorder

1. Shorter duration than other psychotic disorders, sudden onset and termination of symptoms

2. Is often precipitated by a stressor, may occur without an apparent antecedent

3. Overview of DSM-IV-TR criteria

a. At least one of the following symptoms for 1 or more days *but* less than 1 month: delusions, hallucinations, disorganized speech, grossly disorganized or catatonic behavior

b. Not a mood disorder with psychotic features, schizoaffective disorder, schizophrenia, substance-induced, or due to general medical condition

4. Clinical findings and issues

a. Most often, is precipitated by an acute identifiable event

---

Brief Psychotic Disorder

Psychotic symptoms last <1 month

Usually due to precipitating event

Brief, sudden onset of psychosis

Usually 20 to 30-year-old age group

---

b. Emotional turmoil and lability, overwhelming confusion

c. Rapid intervention is important

d. Occurs most often in the 20 to 30-year-old age group

e. More commonly seen in patients with personality (borderline or histrionic) and dissociative disorders

5. Course

a. Brief, sudden onset of psychosis, with full return to premorbid functioning within a month

b. Factors associated with good prognosis: sudden onset, short duration, severe stressor, prominent mood symptoms, maintenance of affective reactivity, prominent confusion at peak of psychosis

c. 50% to 80% completely recover, and in the other 20% to 50% schizophrenia or a mood disorder may be diagnosed

6. Epidemiology: 20 to 30-year-old age group (consider substance-induced in the differential diagnosis)

7. Clinical management (see: PSYCHOPHARMACOLOGY AND OTHER TREATMENTS)

a. Hospitalization is usually needed for safety, medical work-up

b. Antipsychotics and benzodiazepines for acute agitation

F. Substance-Induced Psychotic Disorder

1. Overview of DSM-IV-TR criteria

a. Presence of prominent hallucinations or delusions

b. Evidence points to substance or medication as a cause of symptoms

c. Not better accounted for by other psychotic disorder or as part of a delirium

2. Clinical findings and issues

a. Work-up for substance-induced psychosis

   1) Cocaine, amphetamines, ephedrine, other stimulants

   2) Alcohol, benzodiazepines, barbiturates

   3) Hallucinogens (lysergic acid diethylamide [LSD], phencyclidine [PCP], marijuana, mushrooms)

   4) Anticholinergic agents (jimson weed, trihexyphenidyl)

   5) Medications (glucocorticoids, belladonna alkaloids)

G. Psychotic Disorder Due to a General Medical Condition (e.g., delusions and hallucinations due to dementia)

1. Overview of DSM-IV-TR criteria

a. Presence of prominent hallucinations or delusions

b. Evidence points to consequence of medical illness causing symptoms

c. Not better accounted for by another mental disorder or as part of a delirium

2. Clinical management

a. Work-up for medical and neurologic causes, most commonly for the following:
   1) Temporal lobe epilepsy
   2) Structural brain changes (trauma, neoplasm, cerebrovascular accident, normal-pressure hydrocephalus)
   3) Thyroid disorders
   4) Multiple sclerosis
   5) Dementias
   6) Deficiencies (vitamin B_{12}, pellagra)
   7) Central nervous system (CNS) infections (human immunodeficiency virus [HIV], neurosyphilis, Creutzfeldt-Jakob disease, encephalitis)
   8) Parkinson's disease, Huntington's disease, Wilson's disease
   9) Systemic lupus erythematosus

H. Psychotic Disorder Not Otherwise Specified
1. Overview of DSM-IV-TR criteria
   a. Psychotic symptoms are present
   b. Not enough information to make a specific diagnosis
   c. May have contradictory information

II. MOOD DISORDERS

A. Introduction
1. Disorders include major depressive disorder, dysthymic disorder, bipolar I disorder, bipolar II disorder, cyclothymic disorder, substance-induced mood disorder, mood disorder due to general medical condition, mood disorder not otherwise specified
2. These disorders are common and costly to society
3. History
   a. Documented as far back as ancient Egypt and biblical times
   b. Hippocrates used terms "mania" and "melancholia" to describe moods
   c. Celsus described melancholia (melan = "black" and chole = "bile") as depression caused by black bile
   d. Kraepelin described manic-depression psychosis

B. Major Depressive Disorder
1. Characterized by severely depressed mood and/or anhedonia leading to deterioration and inability to function socially and occupationally
2. Overview of DSM-IV-TR criteria
   a. Must have at least five or more symptoms (one of which must be depressed mood or loss of interest/pleasure) from the following: depressed mood, loss of interest or pleasure, notable (5%) weight loss or gain, insomnia or hypersomnia, psychomotor agitation or retardation,

---

Depression
"**SIG E CAPS**" (useful mnemonic for depression)

S—**sleep** disturbance
I—loss of **interest**
G—**guilt**
E—loss of **energy**
C—loss of **concentration**
A—**appetite** change (gain/loss)
P—**psychomotor** agitation/retardation
S—**suicidal** ideations

Need five symptoms for 2 weeks, must also have depressed mood or anhedonia

---

fatigue or loss of energy, feelings of worthlessness or guilt, decreased concentration or inability to decide, recurrent thoughts of death or suicide
   b. Symptoms must be present for at least 2 weeks
   c. Symptoms do not meet criteria for a mixed episode
   d. Symptoms cause marked distress such as social or functional impairment
   e. Not due to general medical condition or bereavement
3. Clinical findings and issues
   a. Overview of DSM-IV-TR specifiers
      1) Single episode or recurrent episode
      2) Severity: mild, moderate, severe without psychotic features, severe with psychotic features, mood-congruent psychotic features, mood-incongruent psychotic features
      3) Chronic if full criteria are met for at least 2 years—clinically challenging!
      4) Partial remission or in full remission or unspecified
      5) Melancholic feature specifier
         a) Loss of pleasure in all or almost all activities or lack of reactivity to usually pleasurable stimuli *and*
         b) At least three of the following: distinct quality of depressed mood, mood worse in the morning, early morning awakening, marked psychomotor retardation or agitation, marked anorexia or weight loss, or excessive or inappropriate guilt
      6) Atypical feature specifier
         a) Mood reactivity: brightens in response to positive events *and*
         b) At least two of the following: considerable weight gain or increased appetite, hypersomnia, leaden paralysis, long-standing interpersonal rejection sensitivity

7) Catatonic feature specifier
   a) At least two of the following: motoric immobility, excessive motor activity, extreme negativism, peculiarities of voluntary movement, echolalia or echopraxia
8) Postpartum onset specifier
   a) Onset of episode within 4 weeks post partum
   b) Can be life-threatening to mother and child
   c) High rate of recurrence, 30% to 50%
   d) 1:500 to 1:1,000 births
9) Longitudinal course specifier
   a) With full interepisode recovery
   b) Without full interepisode recovery
10) Seasonal pattern specifier
   a) Temporal relation between onset of mood disorder and a particular time of year *and*
   b) Full remissions (or change from depression to mania or hypomania) also occur at a characteristic time of year
11) Rapid-cycling specifier
   a) At least four episodes of mood disturbance in 12 months
   b) Episodes have either remission or change to opposite polarity for at least 2 months between episodes

4. Course
   a. Most episodes clear spontaneously within 6 months
   b. Prognosis is usually quite good
   c. Some patients have recurrent episodes
   d. 20% of patients have chronic form of depression
   e. Risk factors: female, presence of dysthymic disorder, family history of mood disorder, stressors or losses, substance abuse, previous suicide attempt, medical issues, postpartum period, poor social support
   f. Suicide risk: the most serious complication
      1) 10% to 15% of patients commit suicide
      2) 50% to 87% of those who complete suicide have been depressed
      3) Females *attempt* suicide more frequently than males
      4) Males *complete* suicide more frequently than females
      5) The highest incidence of suicide is in May, then October
      6) Risk factors for suicide: advancing age, feeling hopeless, psychotic symptoms, severe agitation, substance abuse, chronic medical illness, living alone

5. Epidemiology
   a. Nearly 5% of the population has depression at any time
   b. Lifetime prevalence: 10% to 25% for females; 5% to 12% for males
   c. F>M 2:1
   d. Peak incidence is between ages 18 and 44 years

6. Pathophysiology

a. Neurotransmitters: biogenic amines—low levels of serotonin, norepinephrine (NE), or dopamine in the limbic region may result in depression
   1) Serotonin (5-hydroxytryptamine [5HT])
      a) Regulates mood, hunger, sleep, impulsivity, cognition, pain, sexual responsiveness

Major Depression: Epidemiology
Prognosis usually good

Suicide (10%-15%): completers (M>F), attempters (F>M)

Prevalence: 10%-25% for F, 5%-12% for M

Peak age: 18-44 years

Suicide Risk Factors

Decreased	Increased
No previous suicide attempts	Previous suicide attempt(s)
Younger	Older
Minimal substance use	Substance abuse
Not impulsive	History of rage, violence
Female	Male
African American	White
Married	Socially isolated
No family history of suicide	Family history of suicide
Catholic/Muslim	Jewish/Protestant
Relatively good health	Failing health or chronic illness

Major Depression
Neurotransmitters: low levels of serotonin, norepinephrine, dopamine in limbic areas

Genetics: 50% concordance rates in monozygotic twins, 10%-25% in dizygotic twins

Sleep: shortened latency of first rapid eye movement (REM) period, increased length of first REM period, increased REM density, increased REM sleep first part of night

b) 5HT metabolite levels in cerebrospinal fluid are usually low in suicidal patients

c) Those who complete suicide have fewer $5HT_2$ receptors

2) NE: maintains mood, energy, interest, motivation

    a) Nobel Prize winner, Julius Axelrod, proposed that NE deficit causes depression

3) Dopamine: important in motivation, drive, and pleasure and reward

4) Monoamine oxidase inhibitors (MAOIs): increase the levels of the above neurotransmitters

b. Genetics

    1) Family studies: first-degree relatives of patients with major depressive disorder are 2× to 3× more likely than controls to have major depressive disorder

    2) Adoption studies: biologic children of affected parents are at increased risk for the development of major depressive disorder

    3) Twin studies: 50% concordance rate in monozygotic and 10% to 25% rate in dizygotic twins

c. Psychosocial: stressors or losses often precede major depressive disorder (losing parent before age 11, loss of spouse, unemployment)

d. Sleep disturbances

    1) Sleep time is usually decreased in patients with major depressive disorder

    2) Patients have shortened latency of first rapid eye movement (REM) period

    3) Increased length of first REM period

    4) Increased REM sleep during first part of the night

    5) Increased REM density

e. Disorders associated with depression and mood disorders

    1) Cancer (especially pancreatic): 25% of cancer patients often develop depression

    2) Dementia: 11% of patients with Alzheimer's disease have depression

    3) Seizure disorders: up to 60% of patients with seizure disorders (especially temporal lobe epilepsy) develop depression

    4) Endocrine

        a) Thyroid dysfunction: 40% of hypothyroid patients have depression, hyperthyroidism can also lead to depression

        b) Corticosteroids

            i) Cushing's disease: up to 80% of patients have depression

            ii) Increasing levels of corticosteriods can induce mania or psychosis

            iii) Decreasing levels can result in depression

        c) Diabetes mellitus is often associated with depression

5) Collagen vascular disorders (systemic lupus erythematosus, rheumatoid arthritis) are associated with depression

6) Infections

    a) Depression reduces immune response, leading to increased susceptibility to infection

    b) Many infections can trigger depression (HIV/acquired immunodeficiency syndrome [AIDS], tuberculosis, neurosyphilis)

7) Nutritional factors associated with depression: deficiencies in vitamin B_{12}, folate, thiamine

8) Cardiac: depression is frequent after myocardial infarction

9) Cerebrovascular: depression often develops after stroke, especially left hemisphere brain injury or subcortical strokes and disorders

10) Movement disorders

    a) 50% of Parkinson's patients can have depression

    b) 40% incidence of depression among patients with Huntington's disease

    c) 20% incidence of depression among patients with Wilson's disease

11) Pain disorders

12) Hypercholesteremia

13) Substance abuse: alcohol, cocaine, opiates, marijuana, anabolic steroids

14) Medications: β-blockers, diuretics, corticosteroids, birth control pills with progesterone, cimetidine, disulfiram, sulfonamides, reserpine, methyldopa, glucocorticoids, benzodiazepines, barbiturates, digitalis, clonidine, phenytoin

7. Neuroanatomy and structural neuroimaging

a. PET and single photon emission computed tomography (SPECT) may show functional changes in brains of patients with major depressive disorder

    1) Limbic system: hypothalamus, amygdala, limbic striatum, cingulate cortex

        a) Possibly involved in development of depressive symptoms

        b) May be the site of action of antidepressants

    2) Hypothalamus: functioning is decreased in depression

        a) Changes in sleep, appetite, and libido

        b) Depression linked to hypothalamic-pituitary-adrenal axis and cortisol secretion abnormalities

        c) Depression linked to hypothalamic-pituitary-thyroid axis and thyroid hormone secretion abnormalities

    3) Basal ganglia: higher incidence of depression in patients with Parkinson's disease

4) Left frontal regions have less perfusion/metabolism in depressed patients

b. Computed tomography (CT)
1) Anterior left hemisphere strokes lead to dysphoria
2) Right hemisphere strokes lead to euphoria

c. MRI
1) Depressed patients may have increased number of focal signal hyperintensities in the white matter
2) Patients with major depressive disorder may have smaller caudate nuclei and frontal lobes

8. Clinical management (see PSYCHOPHARMACOLOGY AND OTHER TREATMENTS)
a. Antidepressants: SSRIs, TCAs, MAOIs, mixed-mechanism antidepressants
b. Mood stabilizers, antipsychotics, stimulants, ECT, exercise, sleep deprivation, alternative therapies, psychotherapies, repetitive transcranial magnetic stimulation, vagus nerve stimulation

C. Dysthymic Disorder

1. Features: less severe than major depressive disorder, insidious onset, chronic course, and no loss of social or occupational function

2. Overview of DSM-IV-TR criteria
a. Depressed mood more days than not during at least a 2-year period
b. At least two of the following: poor appetite or overeating, insomnia or hypersomnia, low energy or fatigue, low self-esteem, poor concentration, hopelessness
c. Useful mnemonic: ACHE2S—appetite, concentration,

Dysthymic Disorder

Depressed mood at least 2 years

"I've been depressed all my life"

Prevalence = 3%, F>M 2:1

"ACHE2S"

A—**appetite** (increased/decreased)
C—**concentration** down
H—**hopelessness**
E—**energy** down
E—**esteem** of self down
2—**2 years** (more days down than not)
S—**sleep** (increased/decreased)

Double depression = major depressive disorder + dysthymia

---

hopelessness, energy, esteem, sleep; "2" refers to 2 years and 2 symptoms beginning with "e"
d. Never without depressed mood for more than 2 months at a time
e. Not an episode of major depressive disorder, not a manic episode, does not occur with psychotic disorder
f. Not due to substances or general medical condition

3. Patients are often "depressed all my life," sarcastic, complaining, brooding, resistant to therapy—leads to negative countertransference by physician toward patient

4. "Double depression" = major depressive disorder + dysthymia

5. Comorbidities: major depressive disorder, anxiety, substance abuse, eating disorder, personality disorder, chronic pain

6. Epidemiology: lifetime prevalence is 3%, F>M 2:1

D. Bipolar I Disorder: bipolar I disorder, single manic episode; bipolar I disorder, most recent episode hypomanic; bipolar I disorder, most recent episode manic; bipolar I disorder, most recent episode mixed; bipolar I disorder, most recent episode depressed; and bipolar I disorder, most recent episode unspecified

1. Manic episode: overview of DSM-IV-TR criteria
a. At least 1 week of persistently elevated, expansive, or irritable mood (less duration if hospitalization is required)
b. At least three (four if mood is only irritable) of the following: grandiosity or inflated self-esteem, decreased need for sleep, pressured speech, flight of ideas or racing thoughts, distractibility, increased goal-directed activity, risky behaviors
c. Helpful mnemonic: DIG FAST, **d**istractibility, **i**nsomnia, **g**randiosity, **f**light of ideas, **a**ctivities increased, pressured **s**peech, **t**houghtlessness
d. Criteria not met for mixed episode, symptoms not due to substance use
e. Causes impairment in functioning, psychotic features exist, or hospitalization is required to ensure safety of the patient or others

2. Treatment of acute mania (see below, PSYCHOPHARMACOLOGY AND OTHER TREATMENTS): mood stabilizers, antipsychotics, ECT

3. Mixed episode: overview of DSM-IV-TR criteria
a. Criteria met for manic episode and major depressive episode except duration is at least 1 week
b. Causes impairment in functioning, psychotic features exist, or hospitalization is required to ensure safety of patient or others
c. Not due to substance use

Bipolar: Manic Episode
"DIG FAST"

   D—distractibility
   I—insomnia, decreased need for sleep
   G—grandiosity, inflated self-esteem
   F—flight of ideas
   A—activities or goals increased or displays
       psychomotor agitation
   S—pressured speech
   T—thoughtlessness, seeks pleasure without
       considering consequences

3 or more for at least 1 week

Treatments for acute mania

   FDA-approved: lithium, divalproex, chlorpromazine, haloperidol, aripiprazole, olanzapine,
   quetiapine, risperidone, ziprasidone, and ECT

   Others likely equally effective but not FDA-
   approved: carbamazepine, gabapentin, lamotrigine, oxcarbazepine

4. Hypomanic episode: overview of DSM-IV-TR criteria
   a. At least 4 days of persistently elevated, expansive, or irri-
      table mood
   b. At least three (four if mood is only irritable) of the fol-
      lowing: grandiosity or inflated self-esteem, decreased
      need for sleep, pressured speech, flight of ideas or racing
      thoughts, distractibility, increased goal-directed activity,
      risky behaviors
   c. Change in functioning uncharacteristic of person's usual
      behavior
   d. Changes are observable by others
   e. Not severe enough to cause impaired functioning, no
      psychotic features exist, and no hospitalization is
      required to ensure safety of the patient or others
   f. Not due to substance use
5. Bipolar I disorder, single manic episode: overview of
   DSM-IV-TR criteria
   a. Only one manic episode (see manic criteria above) and
      no past major depressive episode
   b. Not part of schizoaffective disorder, not superimposed
      on schizophrenia, schizophreniform disorder, delusional
      disorder, or psychotic disorder not otherwise specified
6. Bipolar I disorder, most recent episode hypomanic:
   overview of DSM-IV-TR criteria

   a. Patient is currently in a hypomanic episode (see hypo-
      manic criteria above)
   b. Past history of at least one manic episode or mixed
      episode
   c. Not better accounted for by one of the psychotic
      disorders
7. Bipolar I disorder, most recent episode manic:
   overview of DSM-IV-TR criteria
   a. Patient is currently or recently in a manic episode (see
      manic criteria above)
   b. Past history of at least one major depressive or mixed
      episode
   c. Not better accounted for by one of the psychotic
      disorders
8. Bipolar I disorder, most recent episode mixed:
   overview of DSM-IV-TR criteria
   a. Patient is currently or recently in a mixed episode (see
      mixed criteria above)
   b. Not better accounted for by one of the psychotic
      disorders
9. Bipolar I disorder, most recent episode depressed:
   overview of DSM-IV-TR criteria
   a. Patient is currently or recently in a major depressive
      episode
   b. Past history of at least one manic episode
   c. Not better accounted for by one of the psychotic disorders
10. Bipolar I disorder, most recent episode unspecified:
    overview of DSM-IV-TR criteria
    a. Criteria (except duration) met for manic, hypomanic,
       mixed, or major depressive episode
    b. Past history of a least one manic episode
    c. Causes marked impairment
    d. Not better accounted for by one of the psychotic
       disorders
    e. Not accounted for by substance abuse or general medical
       condition
11. Epidemiology
    a. Bipolar I disorder: lifetime prevalence is 1.0%, M=F
       1) Early onset is associated with more psychotic issues
       2) Peak manic episodes occur in summer
    b. Bipolar II disorder: lifetime prevalence is 0.5%
    c. Cyclothymic disorder: lifetime prevalence is 0.7%
12. Course and clinical findings
    a. Bipolar I disorder is episodic, noncurable, and has a vari-
       able course and outcome
    b. Risk factors leading to poorer prognosis: rapid cycling or
       mixed episodes, substance abuse, psychotic symptoms,
       male gender, poor socioeconomic/occupational status
    c. The patient is often quite creative during hypomanic
       periods

Bipolar Disorder

Prevalence: 1.0%, M=F

Early onset associated with increased psychotic issues

Episodic, noncurable, variable course and outcome

First episode between 20-25 years old

Highest rate of suicide completion is 15%-50%

Divorce rate 3 times higher

d. Mean age at first episode is between 20 and 25 years
e. Onset of manic episode is rapid
f. Untreated manic episode may last 3 to 4 months
g. Untreated depressive episode may last 6 to 9 months
h. Highest rate of suicide completion is 15% to 50%
i. Divorce rate is three times higher than for general population

E. Bipolar II Disorder (recurrent major depressive episode with hypomanic episodes)
1. Overview of DSM-IV-TR criteria
   a. History of at least one major depressive episode
   b. History of at least one hypomanic episode
   c. No history of manic episode or mixed episode
   d. Not better accounted for by one of the psychotic disorders
   e. Causes marked impairment

F. Cyclothymic Disorder
1. Overview of DSM-IV-TR criteria
   a. At least 2 years of periods of hypomania and periods of depressive symptoms that do not meet criteria for major depressive episode (1 year for children and adolescents)
   b. Never without symptoms for more than 2 months at a time
   c. No major depressive episode, manic episode, or mixed episode present during first 2 years of disturbance
   d. Not better accounted for by one of the psychotic disorders
   e. Not accounted for by substance abuse or general medical condition
   f. Causes marked impairment

G. Bipolar Disorder not Otherwise Specified
1. Disorders with bipolar features but not satisfying criteria completely

H. Mood Disorder due to General Medical Condition (specify condition)
1. Overview of DSM-IV-TR criteria
   a. Disturbance of mood predominating clinical picture (i.e., depressed, decreased interest, elevated, irritable moods)
   b. Evidence points to consequence of a general medical condition
   c. Not meeting criteria for adjustment disorder
   d. Not part of a delirium
   e. Causes marked impairment
2. Specifiers: with depressive features, with major depressive-like episode, with manic features, with mixed features

I. Substance-Induced Mood Disorder
1. Overview of DSM-IV-TR criteria
   a. Disturbance of mood predominates the clinical picture (i.e., depressed, decreased interest, elevated, irritable moods)
   b. Caused by substance intoxication or withdrawal
   c. Not better accounted for by other mood disorders
   d. Not part of a delirium
   e. Causes marked impairment

III. ANXIETY DISORDERS

A. Generalized Anxiety Disorder
1. Characterized by excessive worry
2. Overview of DSM-IV-TR criteria
   a. At least 6 months of excessive anxiety or worry about life circumstances
   b. Difficult for patient to control worry
   c. At least three of the following: restlessness, easily fatigued, poor concentration, irritability, muscle tension, sleep disturbance
   d. Anxiety that does not satisfy criteria for another Axis I disorder
   e. Causes marked impairment
   f. Not due to substance use or general medical condition
3. Clinical findings and issues
   a. Few seek treatment
   b. Comorbidities: 62% in major depressive disorder, 37% in alcohol dependence
   c. Increases suicide risk in patients with major depressive disorder
4. Course: chronic with fluctuating severity, 33% develop panic disorder
5. Epidemiology

> **Generalized Anxiety Disorder**
>
> Excessive worry of at least 6 months' duration
>
> Chronic, fluctuating course
>
> Prevalence: 4%-7%, F>M, onset in early 20s
>
> Norepinephrine ("fight or flight")
>
> Consider medical causes during work-up

    a. Lifetime prevalence is 4% to 7%
    b. F>M 3:2
    c. More frequent in African Americans and those younger than 30 years
    d. Onset is usually in early 20s
6. Etiology
    a. 25% of first-degree relatives of a patient with generalized anxiety disorder have the disorder
    b. Twin studies: genetic factors have a role, but nongenetic factors may be more important
    c. Neurotransmitters implicated: NE ("fight or flight"), γ-aminobutyric acid (GABA) (modulates anxiety reactions), 5HT (especially in frontal lobe, prefrontal cortex, amygdala, locus ceruleus, limbic system, hippocampus)
    d. Psychoanalytic theory of anxiety: unresolved unconscious conflicts or separation from important objects
    e. Psychosocial theory of anxiety: learned response from exposure to situations that induce anxiety
    f. Disorders related to anxiety
        1) Cardiovascular: congestive heart failure, myocardial infarction, angina, mitral valve prolapse, arrhythmias, labile hypertension
        2) Pulmonary: asthma, chronic obstructive pulmonary disease, pulmonary embolus, hyperventilation
        3) Endocrine: hyperthyroidism, carcinoid syndrome, pheochromocytoma, pituitary dysfunction, Cushing's disease
        4) Gastrointestinal: irritable bowel syndrome, porphyria
        5) Infectious diseases: pneumonia, hepatitis, encephalitis, influenza
        6) Neurologic: transient ischemic attack, cerebrovascular attack, tumor, traumatic brain injury, seizures, movement disorder, multiple sclerosis, migraines, subarachnoid hemorrhage
        7) Substance abuse and dependence: intoxication and withdrawal
        8) Medication induced: theophylline, caffeine, pseudoephedrine, thyroxine
        9) Inflammatory: lupus erythematosus, rheumatoid arthritis
      10) Systemic: hypoxia, anemia
      11) Psychiatric: depression, mania, psychotic disorders, other anxiety disorders
7. Clinical management (see PSYCHOPHARMACOLOGY AND OTHER TREATMENTS)
    a. Antidepressants: SSRIs, TCAs, mixed-mechanism antidepressants
    b. Benzodiazepines, buspirone, β-blockers
8. Psychosocial interventions: insight-oriented or supportive psychotherapy, interpersonal therapy, cognitive-behavioral therapy, group therapy, biofeedback, yoga, exercise

B. Panic Disorder With or Without Agoraphobia ("fear of the marketplace")
1. Panic attack: overview of DSM-IV-TR criteria
    a. Intense fear or discomfort
    b. At least four of the following: pounding heart, sweating, trembling, shortness of breath, feelings of choking, chest pain, nausea, dizziness, derealization, loss of control, fear of dying, paresthesias, chills or hot flashes
2. Agoraphobia: overview of DSM-IV-TR criteria
    a. Anxiety in settings in which escape may be difficult or help is not available
    b. Those settings/situations are avoided
3. Panic disorder: overview of DSM-IV-TR criteria
    a. Recurrent panic attacks
    b. At least 1 month of concern about having additional attacks, worry about implications of another attack, change in behavior related to attacks
    c. Absence of agoraphobia (panic disorder without agoraphobia) or presence of agoraphobia (panic disorder with agoraphobia)
    d. Not due to substance use or general medical condition
    e. Not better accounted for by another Axis I condition
4. Clinical findings
    a. Usually no precipitators
    b. Often prompts visit to emergency department and extensive, unnecessary work-up
    c. Usually, psychiatry is consulted after many other evaluations have been performed
    d. Panic: sudden onset, peaks in minutes, lasts 5 to 30 minutes, occurs several times per week
5. Course
    a. Usually considered chronic and lifelong, fluctuating in intensity
    b. 30% of patients recover fully
    c. 50% of patients have occasional symptoms but usually do well

Panic Disorder

"**PANIC**"

P—**palpitations**
A—**abdominal** distress, **anxiety**
N—**nausea**
I—**increased** perspiration, intense dread/doom
C—**chest** pain, **chills**, **choking**, lost **control**

Episodes: 5-30 minutes

Prompts frequent emergency department visits, unnecessary work-up

Prevalence: 2%-3% in F, 0.5%-1.5% in M

Onset in mid-20s, usually chronic or lifelong

30% recover fully

45% concordance monozygotic twins, 15% dizygotic twins

Increased catecholamine levels

Locus ceruleus likely affected

d. 20% of patients have marked dysfunction
e. Increases suicide risk when comorbid with major depressive disorder or substance abuse or dependence
6. Epidemiology
   a. 2% to 3% of women, 0.5% to 1.5% of men
   b. Females develop agoraphobia more often than males
   c. Onset is in mid-20s (onset after age 40 suggests underlying medical condition or major depressive disorder)
7. Etiology and pathophysiology
   a. Increased catecholamine levels
   b. Locus ceruleus possibly implicated in pathophysiology
   c. Carbon dioxide hypersensitivity: "false suffocation alarm"
   d. Family and twin studies strongly suggest genetic component: higher concordance rate among identical twins (45%) than among nonidentical twins (15%)

C. Specific Phobia

1. Stimulus or situation triggers panic or anxiety (Table 6-3)
2. Overview of DSM-IV-TR criteria
   a. Excessive, persistent, unreasonable fear in anticipation of object or situation
   b. Exposure to phobia leads to intense anxiety response

c. Patient recognizes the fear to be unreasonable or excessive
d. Situations or objects are avoided, causes marked impairment in function
e. At least 6 months in duration (if younger than 18 years)
f. Not better accounted for by another mental disorder
3. Clinical findings and issues
   a. Common specific phobias: blood, tunnels, bridges, heights, elevators, flying, enclosed places, injury, injections, animals, weather
4. Course
   a. Bimodal age of onset: childhood and early adulthood
   b. Tends to remit with age
   c. If phobia persists into adulthood, it is usually chronic but does not cause disability
5. Epidemiology
   a. Specific phobia is most common of the phobias
   b. Lifetime prevalence: 11% to 33%
   c. F>M
6. Etiology and pathophysiology
   a. Phobic disorders tend to "breed true"; those with specific phobias tend to have relatives with specific phobias and not socials and vice versa
   b. Twin studies are supportive of a heritable cause
7. Clinical management (see PSYCHOPHARMACOLOGY AND OTHER TREATMENTS)
   a. Benzodiazepines, propranolol
   b. Cognitive-behavioral therapy, biofeedback, exposure therapy

D. Social Phobia

1. Social anxiety disorder: exaggerated fear of social situations
2. Overview of DSM-IV-TR criteria
   a. Excessive, persistent, unreasonable fear in anticipation of performance or social situation, possible scrutiny by others, possible humiliation
   b. Exposure to social situation leads to intense anxiety response
   c. Patient recognizes the fear to be unreasonable or excessive
   d. Situations or objects are avoided
   e. Causes marked impairment in function
   f. At least 6 months in duration (if younger than 18 years)
   g. Not better accounted for by another mental disorder, substance use, or medical issue
3. Clinical findings and issues
   a. Patient avoids social interactions
   b. Patient is hypersensitive to criticism
   c. Patient has low self-esteem, poor social skills, poor eye contact
4. Course

Table 6-3. **Specific Phobias**

Phobia	Fear of
Animals	
Ailurophobia	Cats
Arachnophobia	Spiders
Cynophobia	Dogs
Entomophobia	Insects
Musophobia	Mice
Ophidiophobia	Snakes
Scoleciphobia	Worms
Selachophobia	Sharks
Natural environment	
Acrophobia	Heights
Keraunophobia	Thunder
Nyctophobia	Night
Phonophobia	Loud noises
Photophobia	Light
Pyrophobia	Fire
Blood, injection, injury	
Hemophobia	Blood
Odynophobia or algophobia	Pain
Poinephobia	Punishment
Situation	
Agoraphobia	Open market
Automysophobia	Being dirty
Claustrophobia	Closed spaces
Dentophobia	Going to dentist
Iatrophobia	Going to doctor
Taphephobia	Being buried alive
Thanatophobia	Death or dying
Tocophobia	Childbirth
Topophobia	Stage fright
Other	
Homophobia	Homosexuals
Theophobia	God

Modified from Andreason NC, Black DW. Introductory textbook of psychiatry. 3rd ed. Washington (DC): American Psychiatric Publishing, Inc.; 2001. p. 333. Used with permission.

Specific phobia
Most common of phobia disorders

Types: animal; blood, injection, injury; situational; natural environment; other

Prevalence: 11%-33%, F>M

Phobic disorders "breed true," have same phobia

---

    a. Develops slowly, is chronic, no precipitating stressor
    b. Waxes and wanes in intensity, complete remission is rare
5. Epidemiology
    a. High lifetime prevalence of 3% to 13%, yet often unrecognized
    b. Mean age at onset is 15 years, unlikely to start after age 30
    c. F≈M
6. Etiology and pathophysiology
    a. Phobic disorders tend to "breed true"; those with specific phobias tend to have relatives with specific phobias and not socials and vice versa
    b. Twin studies support heritable component
7. Clinical management (see PSYCHOPHARMA- COLOGY AND OTHER TREATMENTS)
    a. SSRIs: first line of treatment
    b. MAOIs, mixed-mechanism antidepressants, benzodiazepines
    c. Propranolol can help about 30 minutes before performance or test situation
    d. Most effective treatment: cognitive-behavioral therapy + medications

E. Obsessive-Compulsive Disorder
1. Characteristics: excessive, repetitive counting, checking, cleaning; behaviors are ego dystonic
2. Overview of DSM-IV-TR criteria
    a. Obsessions (thoughts)
       1) Recurrent or persistent thoughts, impulses, or images felt to be intrusive or inappropriate and that cause anxiety or distress
       2) Not simply excessive "real-life" worries
       3) Attempts are made to ignore and suppress or neutralize

---

Obsessive-Compulsive Disorder (OCD)
Counting, checking, cleaning: ego dystonic

Chronic, 85%; deteriorating, 10%

Prevalence: 2%-3%, F=M

Associated with Tourette's syndrome

35% OCD if relatives have OCD

May be observed in context of head trauma, epilepsy, Sydenham's chorea, Huntington's disease

Some patients have decreased caudate size

Hypermetabolism in frontal cortex

4) Patient recognizes these are products of his or her own mind
  b. Compulsions (behaviors)
    1) Repetitive behaviors: counting, checking, praying, repeating
    2) Behaviors aimed at preventing or reducing stress or preventing a perceived dreaded event from taking place
  c. Causes marked distress
  d. Not due to substance use or general medical condition
3. Clinical findings and issues
  a. Usually both obsessions and compulsions are present in 80% of patients
  b. Consumes a great deal of time
  c. Ego-dystonic
4. Course
  a. Chronic in 85% of patients, deteriorating in 10%
  b. Waxes and wanes in intensity
  c. Prognosis is better if obsessions only, a precipitating event is identified, episodic symptoms, and good overall social adjustment
  d. Prognosis is worse if yielding to compulsions, childhood onset, obsessions and compulsions are bizarre, hospitalization is required because of severity of symptoms
5. Differential diagnosis: schizophrenia, obsessive-compulsive personality disorder
6. Epidemiology
  a. Lifetime prevalence: 2% to 3%
  b. Typically starts in adolescence or early adulthood
  c. F≥M
  d. Males usually have earlier onset of illness than females
7. Etiology and pathophysiology
  a. Serotonergic dysregulation
  b. Genetics
    1) 20% to 35% of relatives of patients with obsessive-compulsive disorder have the disorder
    2) Tourette's syndrome and OCD have been linked in family studies
    3) Twin studies: higher concordance of OCD among identical twins
  c. Behavioral theory: obsessive-compulsive disorder is learned behavior (classical conditioning)
  d. Psychoanalytic theory: OCD is caused by unconscious conflicts (defensive, punitive) and show regression to anal phase of development; overactive superego leading to defense mechanisms such as "undoing," "reaction formation," and "displacement"
  e. Neurobiologic theory: occurs more often in patients with head trauma, epilepsy, Sydenham's chorea, Huntington's disease

8. Neuroanatomy and structural neuroimaging: OCD is associated with decreased size of caudate nuclei bilaterally
9. Functional circuitry and functional neuroimaging: OCD is associated with
  a. Increased blood flow to frontal lobes, basal ganglia, and cingulate cortex
  b. Hypermetabolism in frontal cortex
10. Clinical management (see PSYCHOPHARMACOLOGY AND OTHER TREATMENTS)
  a. SSRIs, TCAs (strongest serotonergic TCA is clomipramine)
  b. Behavioral therapy (flooding, implosion), supportive psychotherapy

F. Posttraumatic Stress Disorder

1. Key feature is catastrophic traumatic event leading to hyperarousal, withdrawal, flashbacks, survivor's guilt, numbing
2. Not all people who experience severe trauma develop posttraumatic stress disorder
3. Overview of DSM-IV-TR criteria
  a. Exposure to traumatic event—must have both of the following:
    1) Experienced or confronted with actual or threatened death or injury to self or others
    2) Response involved intense fear, helplessness, horror
  b. Traumatic event is reexperienced in at least one of the following:
    1) Recurrent and intrusive recollections of the event
    2) Recurrent and distressing dreams of the event
    3) Acting or feeling as if event were recurring
    4) Intense psychologic distress at exposure to triggers or cues related to the event

---

Posttraumatic Stress Disorder

Exposure to catastrophic or traumatic event

Symptoms: hyperarousal, withdrawal, reexperiencing event, flashbacks, avoidance/adaptation

May be chronic, intensity waxes & wanes

Prevalence: 8%, 30% Vietnam vets, 80% rape victims, F>M

Decreased rapid eye movement latency in stage IV sleep

Noradrenergic pathways implicated

5) Physiologic reactivity on exposure to triggers or cues symbolizing the event

c. Persistent avoidance and numbing as indicated by three of the following:
1) Efforts to avoid thoughts, feelings, or conversations associated with the traumatic event
2) Avoiding activities, places, or people that arouse memories of the traumatic event
3) Unable to recall important aspects of the trauma
4) Diminished interest or participation in important activities
5) Feelings of detachment from others
6) Restricted range of affect (i.e., unable to have loving feelings)
7) Feelings that one has a shortened future (i.e., not expecting to have a career, marriage, children, or normal life span)

d. Persistent symptoms of increased arousal
1) Problems falling asleep or staying asleep
2) Problems with irritability or anger outbursts
3) Problems concentrating
4) Hypervigilant
5) Exaggerated startle response

e. Duration of symptoms: longer than 1 month
f. Causes marked distress and decrease in functioning
g. Specifiers: acute (symptoms <3 months), chronic (symptoms >3 months), with delayed onset (onset of symptoms at least 6 months after stressor)

4. Clinical findings and issues
a. Common findings: "psychogenic amnesia," "psychic numbing," depressive symptoms, impulsivity, aggression, isolation, "survivor's guilt," marital strain, social and occupational difficulties
b. Often associated with wartime experiences: "shell shock" (from World War II), "combat fatigue," "combat neurosis," "post Vietnam syndrome," "post rape syndrome," "accident syndrome," "soldier's heart" (from U.S. Civil War)
c. Comorbidity with other psychiatric disorders is up to 80% for patients with posttraumatic stress disorder
d. High rates of somatization disorder in patients with posttraumatic stress disorder
e. Often, psychotic symptoms are associated with posttraumatic stress disorder

5. Course and prognosis
a. Symptom onset can be immediate or delayed
b. Intensity waxes and wanes (anniversaries of trauma may be worse)
c. Can be chronic, lasting 40+ years
d. Risk factors for developing posttraumatic stress disorder: person's age (very young and very old have difficulties),

past history of emotional disturbance, lack of social support, being female, genetic vulnerability to psychiatric illness, recent stressful life changes, recent excessive alcohol consumption, proximity to stressor (i.e., 80% of young children who suffered burn injury developed posttraumatic stress disorder 1 to 2 years after injury but only 30% of adults sustaining a similar injury develop posttraumatic stress disorder)

e. Better outcome for those with rapid onset of symptoms, short duration of symptoms, rapid intervention (Gulf War veterans received care more promptly than Vietnam veterans did), good premorbid level of functioning, good social support, no previous psychiatric or substance abuse history, high motivation for all treatment modalities, absence of other ongoing stressors)
f. If untreated, 30% recover

6. Epidemiology
a. Lifetime prevalence is 8% for the general population
b. 30% of Vietnam veterans
c. 80% of rape victims
d. F>M
e. Prevalence: 1.2% females, 0.5% males

7. Etiology and pathophysiology
a. Primary etiologic event is the stressor
b. Decreased REM latency in stage IV sleep found in persons with posttraumatic stress disorder
c. Biologic factors
1) Hypothalamic-pituitary-adrenal axis can be affected by high levels of arousal
2) NE pathways implicated (e.g., increased levels of epinephrine in veterans with posttraumatic stress disorder and in sexually abused girls)
3) Opioid system
4) 5HT pathways implicated: decrease in 5HT produces anxiety

8. Clinical management (see PSYCHOPHARMACOLOGY AND OTHER TREATMENTS)
a. Antidepressants: SSRIs (first line), TCAs, trazodone, MAOIs
b. Anxiolytics: benzodiazepines, buspirone
c. Mood stabilizers and antipsychotics
d. Psychotherapy: cognitive-behavioral therapy, insight-oriented, stress inoculation therapy, desensitization, group therapy, family therapy, marital therapy

G. Acute Stress Disorder
1. Symptoms: less than 4 weeks
2. Overview of DSM-IV-TR criteria
a. Exposure to traumatic event—must have both of the following:

1) Experienced or confronted with actual or threatened death or injury to self or others
2) Subject's response to include intense fear, helplessness, and horror

   b. During or after experiencing traumatic event, must have at least 3 of the following:

1) Feelings of numbing, detachment, absence of emotional response
2) Decreased awareness of surroundings
3) Derealization
4) Depersonalization
5) Dissociative amnesia (unable to recall important aspect of the trauma)

   c. Persistent reexperience of trauma by recurrent images, thoughts, dreams, illusions, flashbacks, reliving, distress when exposed to reminders of the trauma
   d. Avoidance of stimuli that may arouse recollections of the trauma
   e. Increased anxiety or arousal: difficulty sleeping, irritability, decreased concentration, hypervigilance, exaggerated startle response, restlessness
   f. Causes marked distress and functional impairment
   g. Duration: at least 2 days and less than 4 weeks
   h. Must occur within 4 weeks after the traumatic event
   i. Not associated with substance use or general medical condition

3. Epidemiology: 14% to 33% of those exposed to trauma
4. Clinical management (see management for posttraumatic stress disorder)

H. Anxiety Disorder Due to General Medical Condition (indicate condition)

1. Overview of DSM-IV-TR criteria
   a. Panic attacks, obsessions, or compulsions predominate clinical picture
   b. Evidence suggests the disturbance is due to general medical condition
   c. Not better accounted for by other mental disorder (e.g., adjustment disorder with anxiety) or delirium
   d. Causes notable distress or functional impairment
   e. Specifiers: with generalized anxiety, with panic attacks, with obsessive-compulsive symptoms
2. Epidemiology: very common
3. Clinical management (see PSYCHOPHARMACOLOGY AND OTHER TREATMENTS)

I. Substance-Induced Anxiety Disorder

1. Occurs in association with intoxication or withdrawal
2. Overview of DSM-IV-TR criteria

   a. Panic attacks, obsessions, or compulsions predominate clinical picture
   b. Evidence suggests the disturbance is due to at least one of the following:

1) Symptoms developed within 1 month after substance intoxication or withdrawal
2) Medication use etiologically related to the disturbance

   c. Not better accounted for by other anxiety disorder (e.g., adjustment disorder with anxiety) or delirium
   d. Causes marked distress or functional impairment
   e. Specifiers: with generalized anxiety, with panic attacks, with obsessive-compulsive symptoms, with phobic symptoms, onset during intoxication, onset during withdrawal

3. Epidemiology: very common
4. Clinical management (see PSYCHOPHARMACOLOGY AND OTHER TREATMENTS)

J. Anxiety Disorder not Otherwise Specified

1. Overview of DSM-IV-TR criteria
   a. Disorders with prominent anxiety or phobic avoidance not meeting criteria for a specific anxiety disorder, adjustment disorder with anxiety, or adjustment disorder with mixed anxiety and depressed mood
2. Clinical management (see PSYCHOPHARMACOLOGY AND OTHER TREATMENTS)

IV. Substance-Related Disorders (Table 6-4)

A. Overview of DSM-IV-TR Criteria for Substance Abuse

1. Maladaptive pattern of substance use
2. Leading to marked distress and impairment
3. At least one of the following during a 12-month period:
   a. Recurrent use leading to failure to fulfill obligations at home, work, school
   b. Recurrent use in hazardous situations (e.g., driving, operating machinery)
   c. Recurrent substance-related legal problems
   d. Continued use even when causing recurrent social or interpersonal problems
4. Symptoms have not met criteria for dependence

B. Overview of DSM-IV-TR Criteria for Substance Dependence

1. Maladaptive pattern of substance use
2. Leading to marked distress and impairment

Table 6-4. **Substance-Related Disorders**

| Substance | Epidemiology | Signs and symptoms | | Course | Emergency treatment |
		Intoxication	Withdrawal		
Alcohol	90%, have had drink Abuse: 5%-10% F 10%-20% M Dependence: 3%-5% F, 13% M	Cognitive deficit Ataxia Slurred speech Hypotension Decreased coordination Coma, death	Tremulousness Anxiety/agitation HTN, diaphoresis Hallucinations Delusions Delirium tremens Seizures	First intoxication: midteens Dependence: 20s-30s Rehab: 1-year abstinence rate of 45%-65%	Thiamine must be given before IV fluids with glucose! BZDs for withdrawal & delirium tremens
Amphetamine	Most common for ages 18-30 IV route common in lower SEC M>F 3-4:1 7% prevalence	Pupillary dilation Blood pressure changes Diaphoresis Nausea/vomiting Chest pain Arrhythmias Confusion Seizures Dyskinesias Coma Rapid "high"	Constricted pupils Fatigue Vivid dreams Sleep disturbance Increased appetite Agitation Retardation Intense "crash"	Dependence occurs rapidly Some chronic use Some episodic use	UDAS+ for 1-2 days BZDs for agitation Antipsychotics Supportive measures
Caffeine	M>F 80%-85% prevalence 85% use >200 mg/d	Restlessness Nervousness GI symptoms Muscle twitching Arrhythmia Agitation Diuresis Flushing	Headache Weight gain Lethargy Depression	Begins midteens Use increases in 20s-30s 40% of those who stop did so for treatment of side effects & health concerns	Analgesics for headaches Eliminate/taper from diet
Cannabis	Most commonly used illicit drug 32% have used M>F Most use during ages 18-30 Prevalence 5%	Conjunctival injection Increased appetite Dry mouth Tachycardia Decreased coordination Uncontrollable laughter Poor insight Poor judgment "Bad trips" Delusions Psychosis	None	Common among young people with conduct problems "Gateway" drug to other illicit drugs Use declines after age 35 Chronic use can cause a motivational syndrome	Sleep "Talk down" BZDs Antipsychotics UDAS+ for 7-10 days, 28 days in heavy users
Cocaine	Peaked in 1970s M>F 1.5-2.0:1 2% prevalence Highest use during ages	Pupillary dilation BP changes Diaphoresis Nausea/vomiting Chest pain	Constricted pupils Post-use "crash" Depression Malaise Fatigue	Episodic use Chronic use Rapid progression to abuse & dependence	UDAS+ for 1-3 days after single use, 7-12 days after repeated use BZDs

Table 6-4   (continued)

Substance	Epidemiology	Signs and symptoms		Course	Emergency treatment
		Intoxication	Withdrawal		
	18-25 years (5% cocaine, 1% crack)	Arrhythmias Confusion Seizures Dyskinesias Coma Euphoria then depression	Increased appetite Craving Vivid dreams Insomnia or hypersomnia Agitation or retardation		Antipsychotics Amantadine Bromocriptine Antidepressants Desipramine Behavioral therapy
Hallucinogens	First use in teens M>F 3:1 10% >12 years old have used 16% ages 18-25 have used Prevalence 0.6%	Illusions Hallucination Depersonalization Derealization Synesthesias Tachycardia Pupillary dilation Diaphoresis Palpitations Blurry vision Tremors Incoordination	None	Episodic vs. chronic use Tolerance possible Most stop as they age	UDAS+ for LSD
Inhalants	Begin ages 9-12 Peak in adolescence M>F Prevalence highest for ages 18-25, 11% 30% prison inmates	Dizziness Nystagmus Incoordination Slurred speech Ataxic gait Lethargy Depressed reflexes Tremor Weakness Blurry vision Coma/death Euphoria	None	Rapid onset Intoxication brief Younger children: several times/week Adults: several times/day Pattern may persist for years	Supportive care
Nicotine	Most common 55%-90% mental health patients smoke 25% are dependent 78% lifetime prevalence for those >35 years	None	Dysphoric mood Irritability Insomnia Agitation Anger Anxiety Poor concentration Restlessness Increased appetite Decreased heart rate	Use begins in teens 95% who smoke by age 20 become dependent 45% are eventually able to quit	Nonemergent treatment Hypnosis Aversive therapy Acupuncture Nicotine patches & sprays Clonidine Bupropion (Zyban)
Opioids	Analgesics: 9% for ages 18-25 Heroin 1% 0.7% opioid dependency M>F 3:1 for heroin F>M 1.5:1 for	Euphoria then apathy & dysphoria Pupillary constriction Drowsiness Coma	Dysphoric mood Nausea/vomiting Muscle aches Lacrimation Rhinorrhea Pupillary dilation Piloerection	Start in late teens/ 20s Dependence over period of many years Relapse common 2% mortality/y	Naloxone for overdose Support respiratory state with O_2, airway For gradual withdrawal: methadone UDAS+ 12-36 h

Table 6-4   **(continued)**

Substance	Epidemiology	Signs and symptoms		Course	Emergency treatment
		Intoxication	Withdrawal		
	nonheroin opioids 50% have anti-social personality disorder Common in health care workers/ physicians	Slurred speech Impaired attention Impaired memory	Diaphoresis Diarrhea Yawning Fever Insomnia	20%-30% achieve long-term abstinence	
Phencyclidine	Highest lifetime prevalence 4% for ages 26-34 3% of substance-related deaths due to phencyclidine M>F 2:1 Prevalence 2× higher in ethnic minorities	Nystagmus HTN Tachycardia Numbness Ataxia Dysarthria Muscle rigidity Seizures Coma Hyperacusis Euphoria Derealization Bizarre behaviors Paranoia Violent behavior Life-threatening organ break-down	None	Long-time users said to be "crystallized" (dulled thinking, decreased reflexes, memory loss, lethargy, depression) Average user is M mid-20s Usual pattern is 1/wk Some do "runs" of 2-3 days	UDAS+ >1 wk Acidification of urine Decrease stimulation BZDs Antipsychotics Recovery usually rapid Do not try to talk down!
Sedatives (BZDs & barbiturates)	F>M, increases with age Prevalence 6% for ages 26-34 90% of hospitalized patients have orders for these drugs	Respiratory depression Slurred speech Incoordination Unsteady gait Nystagmus Memory impairment Stupor Coma	Autonomic hyperactivity Tremor Insomnia Nausea/vomiting Hallucinations Agitation Anxiety Grand mal seizures May be life-threatening!	Teens, 20s Escalation of use as tolerance develops	UDAS+ 7 days Overdose: treat with emesis, gastric lavage, urine alkalization, hemodialysis, life support as needed Nonemergent treatment: taper using phenobarbital or BZD abused

BZD, benzodiazepine; GI, gastrointestinal; HTN, hypertension; IV, intravenous; LSD, lysergic acid diethylamide; SEC, Socioeconomic class; UDAS, urine drug abuse survey.

3. At least three of the following during a 12 month period:
   a. Tolerance
      1) Need for increased amounts to achieve intoxication or needed effects
      2) Diminished effect with same amount of substance
   b. Withdrawal
      1) Symptoms of withdrawal for that substance
      2) Need for same or similar substance to relieve symptoms of withdrawal
   c. Using more substance or over longer time than intended
   d. Unable to cut down or control substance use
   e. Lots of time spent getting the substances (e.g., multiple doctor visits, driving long distances)
   f. Social or recreational activities abandoned because of substance use

g. Continues to use substance despite knowing it is causing physical and psychologic problems

C. Overview of DSM-IV-TR Criteria for Substance Intoxication

1. Substance-specific reversible syndrome due to ingestion of substance
2. Maladaptive behavioral and psychologic changes due to effect of substance on the CNS (mood lability, belligerence, impaired judgment, cognition, functioning)
3. Symptoms not due to general medical condition or other mental disorder

D. Overview of DSM-IV-TR Criteria for Substance Withdrawal

1. Substance-specific syndrome due to cessation of (or reduction in amount of) substance after heavy, prolonged substance use
2. Causes marked distress and impaired functioning
3. Symptoms not due to general medical condition or other mental disorder

E. Alcohol (CAGE screening questions)

1. Introduction
   a. Alcohol causes a myriad of neuropsychiatric disorders: it is important to assess for alcohol use by all patients presenting with psychiatric symptoms
2. Definitions

Abuse vs. Dependence

Abuse: during 12 months, at least 1 of following:
   Failure at social obligations due to drug use
   Legal problems due to drug use
   Use even in hazardous situations
   Use despite having social problems

Dependence: during 12 months, at least 3 of following:
   Tolerance, increased amounts needed
   Withdrawal
   Need to use more
   Cannot cut down or control use
   Much time spent obtaining the drug
   Social activities relinquished as direct result of drug use
   Persistence of use despite being aware of harmful effects

---

a. "A drink" = 12 g pure alcohol = 1.5 oz 80-proof = 5 oz wine = 12 oz beer or wine cooler
b. "Moderate drinking" = 2 or less drinks/day for men younger than 65 ($\leq$1 drink/day for nonpregnant women and anyone >65 years)
c. "Dry drunk" = state of an alcoholic who is uncomfortable when not drinking (grandiose, impatience, overacting)
d. "Falling off the wagon" = resumption of drinking after a period of abstinence

3. Clinical findings and issues
   a. If you can smell alcohol on the person's breath, the likely level is greater than 0.125%
   b. Blood alcohol concentration and symptoms in nondependent persons
      1) 0.05%: "feeling good," sense of tranquility, a bit disinhibited, skin looks flushed
      2) 0.05% to 0.10%: problems thinking, more uncoordinated, considered mildly intoxicated
      3) 0.1% to 0.2%: noticeably intoxicated, having greater difficulty with cognition, exhibiting slurred speech and unsteadiness or ataxia
      4) 0.2% to 0.4%: often unconscious, with lowering of core body temperature; poor respiratory effort; hypotension; can progress to coma and death
      5) 0.4% to 0.5%: death rate as high as 50%; death is often secondary to respiratory failure or asphyxiation
   c. Tool for clinical testing: CAGE questions (CAGE questionnaire originally published in *American Journal of Psychiatry* in 1974 by the American Psychiatric Association)
      1) Two of four answered positively: 70%-80% indicative of alcohol dependence
      2) Four of four answered positively: 100% indicative of alcohol dependence
      3) C: "Have you ever tried to cut down your alcohol use?"

Drink Equivalents

12 g pure alcohol

1.5 oz 80-proof

5 oz wine

12 oz beer/wine cooler

"Moderate" drinking
   $\leq$2 drinks/d for men
   $\leq$1 drink/d for women and those >65 years

CAGE Questions for Alcohol Dependence
    C—tried to **cut** down?
    A—**annoyed** when others say cut back?
    G—feel **guilty** about your drinking?
    E—Need an **eye-opener**?

"Yes" for 2 of 4 = 70%-80% indicative of dependence

"Yes" for 4 of 4 = 100% indicative of dependence

  4) A: "Have you been annoyed by those asking you to cut back your alcohol use?"
  5) G: "Have you felt guilty for drinking?"
  6) E: "Do you ever require an eye-opener?"
d. Withdrawal symptoms
  1) Often starts with tremulousness
  2) Anxiety, agitation, aggressiveness
  3) Hallucination (most often visual), delusions
  4) Hypertension, respiratory depression, seizures, delirium tremens
  5) Death if symptoms are severe
  6) Symptoms can be reduced or cleared by alcohol or cross-tolerant agents (benzodiazepines, barbiturates) (see PSYCHOPHARMACOLOGY AND OTHER TREATMENTS and Table 6-4)
e. Possible positive effects of alcohol use (red wine thought to be best)
  1) One or two drinks per day: may lower risk of myocardial infarction or cerebrovascular accident (possibly by reducing platelet "stickiness") and can increase level of high-density lipoproteins ("good cholesterol")
f. Potential negative effects of alcohol use
  1) Increased morbidity and mortality
    a) Hypothermia: intoxicated person exposed to cold cannot constrict blood vessels adequately to conserve heat
    b) Alcohol intoxication: blood levels of 0.3 to 0.5% lead to respiratory depression, coma, death in nondependent persons
  2) Cardiovascular
    a) Initial decrease in blood pressure with increased heart rate
    b) Later, hypertension, tachycardia, risk of atrial fibrillation
    c) Increases risk for myocardial infarction
    d) Can lead to cardiomyopathy and congestive heart failure

  3) Central nervous system and neurologic complications (neurologic complications of alcohol abuse are discussed in Chapter 17)
    a) "Blackouts"; fragmented sleep, with deep sleep deficiency
    b) Wernicke's and Korsakoff's syndromes
    c) Dementing illness: Marchiafava-Bignami disease, alcohol-induced persisting dementia, pellagrous encephalopathy (pellagra = dementia, diarrhea, dermatitis)
    d) Cerebellar degeneration, peripheral neuropathy, decreased sensation of pain
  4) Dermatologic: rosacea, spider angiomas, telangiectases, palmar erythema, seborrheic dermatitis
  5) Endocrine
    a) Intoxication can lead to hypoglycemia
    b) Chronic alcohol use can lead to diabetes mellitus
    c) In males: testicular atrophy, gynecomastia (from increase in estrogen production), decreased erectile capability, increased or decreased sex drive
    d) In females: increased estrogen production, amenorrhea, decreased sex drive, infertility, spontaneous abortions, increase in male secondary sexual characteristics
  6) Gastrointestinal
    a) Esophagitis, varices, hemorrhages, Mallory-Weiss tears
    b) Gastritis, reflux disease, ulcers
    c) Hemorrhagic lesions of small bowel, diarrhea, increased intestinal motility with decreased absorption
    d) Acute and chronic pancreatitis, pancreatic pseudocyst, pancreatic cancer
  7) Hematologic
    a) Increase in mean corpuscular volume of erythrocytes, decreased erythrocyte production
    b) Leukopenia and thrombocytopenia
    c) Hyperplastic bone marrow, reticulocytopenia, sideroblastic changes
  8) Hepatic
    a) Increased gluconeogenesis, increased lactate acid production and accumulation
    b) Fats accumulate in liver cells, leading to "fatty liver"
    c) Alcohol-induced hepatitis
    d) Alcoholic cirrhosis (in up to 20% of alcohol-dependent persons): jaundice, ascites, potential for hepatic encephalopathy, asterixis, portal hypertension, possible coma and death
    e) Risk of hepatocellular carcinoma 10 times higher than for general public

f) Elevated serum transaminase levels, increased triglyccride levels

9) Malnutrition
   a) Poor absorption leading to multiple deficiencies: vitamins A, C, D, and E, also niacin, pyridoxine, riboflavin, and thiamine
      i) To prevent Wernicke's encephalopathy, must administer thiamine before any intravenous administration of glucose-containing fluids
   b) Hypomagnesemia and hypoalbuminemia common

10) Musculoskeletal
   a) "Alcoholic myopathy" (painful, swollen muscles with increased creatinine phosphokinase level, also muscle weakness is common
   b) Alterations of calcium metabolism can lead to increased risk of bone fractures, and especially osteonecrosis of femoral head

11) Oncologic: increased risk of cancers of head and neck (mouth, tongue, larynx), esophagus, stomach, liver, pancreas, breast

12) Oral: periodontal disease, parotid gland enlargement

13) Pulmonary
   a) Aspiration pneumonia is common
   b) Increased susceptibility to gram-negative infections and tuberculosis
   c) Recurrent bronchitis, asthma, chronic obstructive pulmonary disease

14) Renal
   a) Renal failure from hypertensive or diabetic effects on kidneys or from direct toxic effects of alcohol
   b) Decreased uric acid excretion, which can lead to gout

15) Splenic: alcohol use can lead to an enlarged spleen and sequestering of blood cells

16) Other
   a) Fetal alcohol syndrome: facial changes, small teeth, cardiac defects, microcephaly, mental retardation (10% of babies born to mothers who "drank excessively" during pregnancy)
   b) Increased risk of falls, fights, suicide
   c) Increased cortisol levels, abnormalities of vasopressin secretion based on either increasing or decreasing alcohol concentrations in blood

4. Course
   a. First episode of alcohol intoxication is likely to occur in midteens
   b. Age at onset of alcohol dependence: 20s to mid-30s
   c. Often, crisis prompts decision to stop, followed by short period of abstinence, then some controlled drinking, finally drinking escalates, again causing problems
   d. Most alcoholic patients have promising prognosis: after treatment, 45% to 65% of patients have 1 year of abstinence depending on their pretreatment level of functioning

5. Epidemiology
   a. 90% of U.S. population have had a drink, 60% to 70% are current drinker
   b. Lifetime prevalence of alcohol abuse: women, 5% to 10%; men, 10% to 20%
   c. Lifetime prevalence of alcohol dependence: women, 3% to 5%; men, 13%
   d. Up to 20% of primary care patients have their alcoholism go unnoticed
   e. Life expectancy can be decreased by up to 10 years from use of alcohol
   f. Alcohol is involved in more than 25% of those who die because of motor vehicle accidents (in some studies, up to 55%), drowning, suicide, homicide, or those who have suffered from abuse, assaults, or rape
   g. High rates of alcohol-use problems in whites more than in African Americans
   h. Higher prevalence in Native Americans
   i. Lesser prevalence in Asian Americans and Jews
   j. Age at onset of alcohol abuse in about 17 years and for dependence, about 22 years

6. Etiology
   a. Genetic
      1) Close relatives of alcohol-dependent persons have 3× to 4× higher risk of developing alcohol dependence
      2) Monozygotic twins have much greater risk of alcohol dependence than dizygotic twins
      3) Sons of severely alcoholic fathers have up to 90% chance of becoming alcohol-dependent in their lifetime
   b. Psychosocial and cultural
      1) Certain social settings and conditions reflect higher rates of alcohol-use disorders (college, military, the homeless, high school or college dropouts, the unemployed, those of low socioeconomic status)
      2) Certain cultural groups predispose to heavier drinking (adolescent Hispanics, Native Americans)
      3) Those with conservative religious beliefs have been found to have fewer alcohol-use disorders than those of other religious groups
      4) Some say they use alcohol to help with their anxiety, depressed mood, to tolerate psychotic symptoms, to "loosen up" and be "more social"
   c. Metabolism
      1) 90% of alcohol is metabolized by oxidation in the liver, 10% is excreted unchanged in the urine, sweat, air (thus the Breathalyzer test is useful)

2) Alcohol dehydrogenase breaks down alcohol to acetaldehyde, then aldehyde dehydrogenase breaks down acetaldehyde to acetic acid

3) Disulfiram (Antabuse) blocks aldehyde dehydrogenase, thus build up of toxic acetaldehyde

4) Because women have less aldehyde dehydrogenase in the gastric lining than men, they have a greater risk for intoxication with even small amounts of alcohol

5) Asians also have lower levels of alcohol dehydrogenase and aldehyde dehydrogenase, leading to greater potential for intoxication with small amounts of alcohol

7. Clinical management
   a. Management of withdrawal symptoms following intoxication
      1) Nutritional supplementation, food and hydration, monitoring
      2) Benzodiazepines, thiamine, folate, multivitamin, antipsychotics
   b. Rehabilitation, residential and outpatient treatment programs, Alcoholics Anonymous, individual and family therapy
   c. Disulfiram (Antabuse), naltrexone (ReVia, decreases craving for alcohol)

F. **Amphetamine** (speed, ice, meth, crank, crystal, go-fast, go, zip, Chris)
1. Definitions and criteria
   a. Amphetamine abuse (see criteria above for substance dependence)
   b. Amphetamine dependence (see criteria above for substance dependence)
   c. Amphetamine intoxication: overview of DSM-IV-TR criteria
      1) Recent use of amphetamine or related substance (e.g., methylphenidate)
      2) Maladaptive behavioral and psychologic changes surrounding use of amphetamine: euphoria, blunting, anxiety, tension, anger, impaired judgment and functioning
      3) At least two of the following: tachycardia or bradycardia, pupillary dilation, change in blood pressure, perspiration or chills, nausea or vomiting, weight loss, psychomotor agitation or retardation, weakness, respiratory depression, chest pain, arrhythmias, confusion, seizures, dyskinesias, dystonias, coma
      4) Symptoms not due to general medical condition or other mental disorder
   d. Amphetamine withdrawal: overview of DSM-IV-TR criteria

1) Discontinued use or reduction of amount of amphetamine after heavy and prolonged use

2) Dysphoric mood and at least two of the following occurring within hours or days after discontinued use or reduced amount of amphetamine after prolonged and heavy use:
   a) Fatigue
   b) Vivid, unpleasant dreams
   c) Insomnia or hypersomnia
   d) Increased appetite
   e) Psychomotor agitation or retardation

3) Symptoms cause marked distress or impairment of functioning

4) Symptoms not due to general medical condition or other mental disorder

2. Clinical findings and issues
   a. Amphetamine: route is oral, snorting, smoking, or intravenous injection
      1) Relatively cheap, longer lasting effects, can be made at home (*dangerous*)
      2) May cause life-threatening events: myocardial infarctions, cerebrovascular accidents, fatal arrhythmias
      3) Use can lead to loss of appetite and starvation for days and insomnia and may result in psychosis or manic-like presentation
      4) Common psychotic symptom is formication (sensation of crawling bugs, which may lead to excessive scratching until the skin is severely excoriated)
      5) Abuse of amphetamine-type medicines prescribed for treatment of obesity and sleep disorders led to regulation of distribution
   b. Methylphenidate: route is crushed, followed by snorting or intravenous injection
   c. Use of amphetamines can produce rapid onset of intense euphoria ("high" sensation)
   d. "Crash": marked withdrawal symptoms following a high-dose use ("speed-run"), including depression, suicidal thoughts, intense cravings, anxiety, irritability

3. Course (as described in DSM-IV-TR)
   a. Some start taking amphetamine-like substances for weight loss
   b. Dependence occurs rapidly
   c. Some use drug chronically (almost daily) and usually have gradual increase in dose over time
   d. Some use drug episodically (usually intensive high-dose use over weekend), separated by days of nonuse
   e. Tendency to decrease or stop use after 8 to 10 years (thought to be due to development of adverse mental or physical effects)

4. Epidemiology (as described in DSM-IV-TR)

a. Seen in all levels of society

b. Common among ages 18 to 30

c. Intravenous route is more common among lower socio-economic groups, M>F 3-4:1

5. Other neurologic complications

   a. Rhabdomyolysis and myoglobinuria: associated with seizures, fever, and altered mental status; rhabdomyolysis may also be seen in setting of serotonin syndrome, which has been associated with concomitant use of amphetamines with ecstasy

   b. Seizures with acute intoxication (mentioned above): usually generalized tonic-clonic seizures, less common than other psychostimulants such as cocaine

   c. Ischemic infarction and intracerebral hemorrhagic complications: may occur as a result of acute hypertension, vasoconstriction, and reversible vasospasm of the cerebral vasculature. Amphetamines may also cause a small vessel vasculitis, which may cause cerebral infarction, as well as intracerebral hemorrhage

   d. Movement disorders related to alteration of dopaminergic transmission: may yield (or exacerbate) akathisia, chorea, dystonia, tics, myoclonus. Repetitive chewing and tooth grinding were identified in the 1960s as characteristic observations in patients abusing amphetamines

G. Caffeine

1. Caffeine intoxication: overview of DSM-IV-TR criteria

   a. Recent use of caffeine, more than 250 mg

   b. At least five of the following: restlessness, nervousness, excitement, insomnia, flushed face, diuresis, gastrointestinal disturbance, muscle twitching, rambling thought and speech, tachycardia, arrhythmia, psychomotor agitation, periods of inexhaustibility

   c. Symptoms cause marked distress and impaired functioning

   d. Symptoms not due to general medical condition or other mental disorder

2. Course (as described in DSM-IV-TR)

   a. Usually begins in midteens, with increasing use in the 20s and 30s

   b. 40% of those who stopped using caffeine did so to alleviate side effects or because of health concerns

3. Epidemiology (as described in DSM-IV-TR)

   a. 80% to 85% of adults consume caffeine in a year

   b. 85% of caffeine users drink about 200 mg/day

   c. M>F

   d. Caffeine users in developing nations: average about 50 mg/day

   e. Caffeine users in Sweden, United Kingdom, Europe: average about 400 mg/day

H. Cannabis (pot, weed, reefer, herb, green, Mary Jane, MJ, joints, bong, toke)

1. History: hemp plant, use gained popularity in 1960s and 1970s

2. Cannabis intoxication: overview of DSM-IV-TR criteria

   a. Recent use of cannabis

   b. Maladaptive behavioral or psychologic changes surrounding use

   c. Within 2 hours after use, at least two of the following: conjunctival injection, increased appetite, dry mouth, tachycardia

   d. Symptoms not due to general medical condition or other mental disorder

3. Clinical findings and issues

   a. Route: usually smoked ("joint"), can be taken orally (made into tea, brownies)

   b. Intoxication is rapid, starts with a "high"

   c. Often accompanied by uncontrollable laughter, memory impairment (impairs transfer from immediate to long-term memory), decreased attention span, poor insight and judgment, distorted sensory perceptions, decreased coordination, depression, increased blood pressure and pulse rate, sedation, conjunctival injection, dry mouth, increased appetite and thirst, hypothermia, occasional "bad trips" (anxiety, panic attacks, paranoia, depersonalization, delusions, hallucinations)

   d. Suppression of REM sleep

   e. Prescription form of δ-9-tetrahydrocannabinol used for nausea control in cancer patients and for anorexia in AIDS patients

   f. Can be "spiked": phencyclidine or cocaine may be added by users to amplify the effect

   g. Does not produce physical dependence, thus no withdrawal syndrome

   h. Can be found in urine drug screen up to 30 days after chronic use

   i. There are scattered reports of both the anticonvulsant and proconvulsant properties of cannabis

4. Course (as described in DSM-IV-TR)

   a. Abuse and dependence develop over an extended time

   b. Progression to abuse and/or dependence is more rapid in young people with conduct problems

   c. Often considered a "gateway drug" to other substances

   d. Use usually declines after age 35

   e. Chronic use leads to "amotivational syndrome": apathy, inattentiveness, flat affect

5. Epidemiology (as described in DSM-IV-TR)

   a. World's most commonly used illicit substance; 32% of Americans have tried it

b. Used since ancient times as remedy for medical conditions and for psychoactive effects

c. Usual first drug of experimentation among teens

d. M>F

e. Most common for ages 18 to 30

f. Lifetime rate of abuse or dependence is 5%

6. Clinical management

a. Allow sleep, "talk down," benzodiazepines, neuroleptics (see PSYCHOPHARMACOLOGY AND OTHER TREATMENTS and Table 6-4)

I. Cocaine (coke, blow, crack, powder, sugar, nose candy, rock, base)

1. History: from leaves of coca plant from South and Central America

2. Definition and criteria

a. Cocaine intoxication: overview of DSM-IV-TR criteria

1) Recent use of cocaine

2) Maladaptive behavioral or psychologic changes surrounding use

3) At least two of the following: tachycardia or bradycardia, pupillary dilation, increased or decreased blood pressure, perspiration or chills, nausea or vomiting, weight loss, psychomotor agitation or retardation, muscle weakness, respiratory depression, chest pain, cardiac arrhythmia, confusion, seizures, dyskinesia, dystonia, coma (similar to amphetamines)

4) Symptoms not due to general medical condition or other mental disorder

b. Cocaine withdrawal: overview of DSM-IV-TR criteria

1) Discontinued use or reduction in amount of cocaine after heavy and prolonged use

2) Dysphoric mood

3) At least two of the following: fatigue, vivid dreams, insomnia or hypersomnia, increased appetite, psychomotor retardation or agitation

4) Symptoms not due to general medical condition or other mental disorder

3. Clinical findings and issues (as described in DSM-IV-TR)

a. Route: smoked ("crack cocaine"), intranasal ("snort"), or intravenous injection

b. "Speed balling": injecting combination of heroin and cocaine

c. Short-acting drug: rapid and powerful effects on CNS

1) Instant feelings of well-being, confidence, euphoria

2) Increased levels of dopamine and NE in brain

d. Persons often engage in criminal activity to get money for cocaine

e. Behavior can be aggressive, promiscuous, violent, extreme anger

f. Metabolite (benzoylecgonine) can be found in a urine drug screen 1 to 3 days after a single dose or 7 to 12 days after frequent use of high doses

g. Those who snort: sinusitis, perforated nasal septum, bleeding of nasal mucosa

h. Those who smoke: cough, bronchitis, pneumonitis, pneumothorax (from performing Valsalva-like maneuvers to better absorb inhaled cocaine)

i. Those who inject: "tracks" on forearms, high risk of HIV infection

j. Formication: feeling of bugs, "cocaine bugs"

4. Course (as described in DSM-IV-TR)

a. Various patterns from episodic to daily use

b. Episodic: use separated by 2 or more days, with "binges"

c. Chronic daily use: usually an increase in dose over time

d. Rapid progression to abuse and dependence: over weeks to months

5. Epidemiology (as described in DSM-IV-TR)

a. Affects all races, socioeconomic classes, ages, and both sexes

b. Started in more affluent populations in the 1970s and spread to all groups

c. M>F 1.5-2.0:1

d. Lifetime prevalence is 2%

e. Use peaked in the 1970s, then gradually declined until early 1990s

f. 10% of the population has used cocaine at some time

g. Highest rate was in 18 to 25-year-old group (5% for cocaine, 1% for crack)

6. Other neurologic complications (similar to amphetamines)

a. Ischemic or hemorrhagic stroke (as with amphetamines)

1) Cocaine is the most important cause of drug-related strokes

2) Mechanism is likely a combination of acute hypertension, vasospasm and vasoconstriction of cerebral vasculature (arterial occlusion), and platelet aggregation

3) Possible association with antiphospholipid antibodies

4) Cardiac complications of cocaine use such as cardiomyopathy, myocardial infarction, or cardiac arrhythmias may predispose to cardioembolic cause of strokes

5) Unlike amphetamines, this drug has not been established to cause CNS vasculitis

6) Asymptomatic subcortical white matter T2-hyperintense lesions are also more commonly observed in cocaine users

7) This may be due to cumulative hypertensive changes induced by the drug

b. Movement disorders related to alteration of dopaminergic transmission (as with amphetamines): may induce or exacerbate a movement disorder, including tics, myoclonus, dystonia, chorea, akathisias; known to exacerbate hallucinations in schizophrenics

    c. Acute seizures (as with amphetamines) usually observed within the first day after intoxication, and some may be due to cerebrovascular complications described above

7. Clinical management (see PSYCHOPHARMACOLO-GY AND OTHER TREATMENTS and Table 6-4)

    a. Benzodiazepines, antipsychotics (high potency), amantadine, bromocriptine, antidepressants, desipramine, behavioral therapy

J. Hallucinogens: LSD, mescaline (peyote cactus), methylenedioxymethamphetamine (MDMA) ("ecstasy," "XTC", "Adam," "wonder drug," "euphoria," "E"), methylenedioxyamphetamine (MDA) ("Eve"), psilocybin (mushrooms), dimethyltryptamine (DMT)

1. History

    a. Two naturally occurring plants (peyote and mescaline); most other forms are synthetic versions

    b. Became popular from 1960 to 1970s

    c. Thought by many to "expand their minds" or to "experience God"

    d. Often used in some religious practices (peyote used by Native Americans)

2. Definitions and criteria

    a. Hallucinogen intoxication: overview of DSM-IV-TR criteria

        1) Recent use of a hallucinogen

        2) Maladaptive behavioral or psychologic changes surrounding use

        3) Perceptual changes: illusions, hallucinations, depersonalization, derealization, synesthesias

        4) At least two of the following: tachycardia, pupillary dilation, sweating, palpitations, blurry vision, tremors, incoordination

        5) Symptoms not due to general medical condition or other mental disorder

    b. Hallucinogen persisting perception disorder: overview of DSM-IV-TR criteria

        1) Following cessation of hallucinogen, reexperiencing perceptual symptoms that were experienced during the intoxication with hallucinogens (flashbacks)

          a) Geometric hallucinations, flashes of color, intensified colors

          b) Halos around objects, macropsia, micropsia

        2) Symptoms cause marked distress or impaired functioning

        3) Symptoms not due to general medical condition or other mental disorder

    c. "Trip": first 4 hours after administration of the hallucinogen (as described in DSM-IV-TR)

        1) Physiologic changes: hypertension, tachycardia, pupillary dilation, sweating, tremors, blurry vision, incoordination

        2) Perceptual changes: heightened sensory experiences ("hearing" colors), hallucinations, illusions, delusions

        3) Psychologic changes: anxiety, depression, ideas of reference, derealization, depersonalization

        4) "Bad trip": intensely distressing or frightening experiences, perceptions, and sensations leading to panic, paranoia, and possibly suicide or homicide

3. Clinical findings and issues (as described in DSM-IV-TR)

    a. Often rapid alternation of moods, fearfulness, anxiety

    b. Dread of insanity or death

    c. Can result in injuries or death from motor vehicle accidents, fights, "attempting to fly" from high places

    d. Can cause increased levels of glucose, cortisol, ACTH, prolactin

    e. Can produce hallucinations in any of the five senses

    f. LSD is much more potent than other hallucinogens

    g. MDA and MDMA produce stimulant and hallucinogenic effects

4. Course (as described in DSM-IV-TR)

    a. May be brief and isolated event or may occur repeatedly

    b. Can develop tolerance

    c. Most stop using hallucinogens as they get older

5. Epidemiology (as described in DSM-IV-TR)

    a. First use is usually in adolescence

    b. M>F 3:1

    c. 10% of those age 12 and older have tried hallucinogens, 16% in ages 18 to 25

    d. Lifetime prevalence: 0.6%

6. Etiology and pathophysiology

    a. Hallucinogenic effect is likely produced by release of 5HT

7. Clinical management (see PSYCHOPHARMA-COLOGY AND OTHER TREATMENTS and Table 6-4)

    a. Haloperidol + lorazepam is effective

K. Inhalants (glue sniffing, sniffing, huffing)

1. Introduction

    a. Inhalants: aliphatic and aromatic hydrocarbons

        1) Gasoline, glue, paint thinners, spray paints, nail polish remover

        2) Cleaners, typewriter correction fluid, spray-can propellants

        3) Esters, ketones, glycols

    b. Active ingredients: toluene, benzene, acetone, tetrachloroethylene, methanol

2. Definitions and criteria
   a. Inhalant intoxication: overview of DSM-IV-TR criteria
      1) Recent use of an inhalant (intentional)
      2) Maladaptive behavioral or psychologic changes surrounding use
      3) At least two of the following: dizziness, nystagmus, incoordination, slurred speech, unsteady gait, lethargy, depressed reflexes, psychomotor retardation, tremor, generalized muscle weakness, blurry or double vision, coma, euphoria
      4) Symptoms not due to general medical condition or other mental disorder
3. Clinical findings and issues (as described in DSM-IV-TR)
   a. Methods: soaking rag and applying to mouth or nose ("huffing"), placing drug in bag and inhaling ("bagging"), spraying directly from can into mouth or nose
   b. Patients often present with auditory, visual, tactile hallucinations; perceptual disturbances; delusions; anxiety
   c. Often used by young in a group setting
   d. Physical signs might include "glue sniffers rash" around mouth or nose, conjunctival irritation, may see evidence of trauma or burns
   e. Pulmonary findings: airway irritation, increased airway resistance, pulmonary hypertension, acute respiratory distress, dyspnea, rales, cyanosis, pneumonitis
   f. CNS and peripheral nervous system findings (can be permanent): weakness, neuropathy, cerebral atrophy, cerebellar degeneration, white matter lesions (neurologic complications of inhalants are also described in Chapter 17)
   g. Hepatitis, chronic renal failure, bone marrow suppression
   h. "Sudden sniffing death": from acute arrhythmia, hypoxia, electrolyte disturbances
4. Course (as described in DSM-IV-TR)
   a. Rapid onset, peaks within minutes
   b. Intoxication is typically brief
   c. Younger children use several times per week
   d. Adults may use several times per day if severely dependent
   e. Pattern may persist for years, with recurrent need for treatment
   f. No specific withdrawal syndrome
5. Epidemiology (as described in DSM-IV-TR)
   a. 50% of Alaskan children have used solvents to get high
   b. Cheap and readily available: often the first drugs of experimentation
   c. Use may begin by ages 9 to 12, peak in adolescence, less common after age 35
   d. M>F, 70% to 80% of inhalant-related emergency department visits are by males
   e. 6% of Americans have tried inhalants

   f. Highest prevalence is in 18-to-25-year-old group, at 11%
   g. 30% of prison inmates have used inhalants
   h. High number of users among Latino and Native American populations, lower socioeconomic groups, children of alcoholic parents, and children from abusive or disruptive homes
6. Clinical management: supportive care

L. Nicotine
1. Definitions and criteria
   a. Nicotine dependence: overview of DSM-IV-TR criteria (see above summary of dependence)
   b. Nicotine withdrawal: overview of DSM-IV-TR criteria
      1) Several weeks of daily nicotine use
      2) Abruptly stops use or reduces use
      3) Within 24 hours after use of nicotine at least four of the following: dysphoric mood, insomnia, irritability, anger, anxiety, frustration, poor concentration, restlessness, decreased heart rate, increased appetite or weight gain
      4) Symptoms cause marked distress or functional impairment
      5) Symptoms not due to general medical condition or other mental disorder
2. Clinical findings and issues (as described in DSM-IV-TR)
   a. Craving: makes giving up nicotine so difficult
   b. Often, person craves sweets during withdrawal from nicotine
   c. Dependence develops quickly
   d. Smoking increases metabolism of many prescription medications; smoking cessation can lead to worrisome increases in blood levels of those medications
3. Course (as described in DSM-IV-TR)
   a. Nicotine use generally begins in the teens
   b. 95% of those who smoked by age 20 become regular, daily smokers
   c. 80% of smokers try to quit; less than 25% are successful on the first attempt to quit smoking
   d. 45% of smokers are eventually able to quit smoking
   e. Medical complications
      1) Implicated in lung, laryngeal, oral, esophageal, pancreatic, kidney, bladder, and cervical cancers
      2) Implicated in development of gastric and duodenal ulcers, respiratory diseases, cardiovascular diseases
      3) Oropharyngeal cancers: with snuff and chewing tobacco use
      4) Respiratory and cardiovascular disease: with second-hand smoke exposure
4. Epidemiology (as described in DSM-IV-TR)

a. Nicotine dependence is the most prevalent substance-related disorder

b. 55% to 90% of persons with mental disorders smoke (compared with 30% for the general population)

c. 25% of the general population may have nicotine dependence

d. Lifetime prevalence in the United States is highest among those older than 35 (78%)

e. Higher rates of nicotine dependence in schizophrenics and alcoholics

5. Etiology and pathophysiology (as described in DSM-IV-TR)

a. Smoking risk: 3× higher in first-degree biologic relatives of smokers

b. Twin and adoption studies: genetic factors contribute to age at onset and tendency to continue to smoke (similar to that seen in alcohol dependence)

6. Clinical management (see PSYCHOPHARMA-COLOGY AND OTHER TREATMENTS and Table 6-4)

a. Nicotine patches, sprays, inhalers

b. Clonidine

c. Bupropion (Zyban)

M. Opioids: morphine, heroin, hydromorphone (Dilaudid), meperidine (Demerol), methadone, propoxyphene (Darvon), codeine, levomethadyl (Orlaam)

1. History: commonly used for pain control (as described in DSM-IV-TR)

a. Naturally occurring: opium, morphine

b. Semisynthetic: heroin

c. Synthetic: methadone, codeine, hydromorphone, oxycodone, meperidine, fentanyl

d. Opioids: used as analgesics, anesthetics, antidiarrheal agents, cough suppressants

2. Definition and criteria

a. Opioid abuse: overview of DSM-IV-TR criteria (see above summary of abuse)

b. Opioid dependence: overview of DSM-IV-TR criteria (see above summary of dependence)

c. Opioid withdrawal: overview of DSM-IV-TR criteria (unlikely to be life-threatening)

1) Either

a) Cessation or reduction in use of opioid after heavy prolonged use *or*

b) Administration of opioid antagonist after period of opioid use

2) Within minutes to days after use, three or more of the following: dysphoric mood; nausea or vomiting; muscle aches; lacrimation or rhinorrhea; pupillary dilation, piloerection, or sweating; diarrhea; yawning; fever; insomnia

3) Symptoms cause marked distress or impaired functioning

4) Symptoms not due to general medical condition or other mental disorder

d. Opioid intoxication: overview of DSM-IV-TR criteria

1) Recent use of opioid

2) Maladaptive behavior or psychologic changes causing impaired judgment or functioning surrounding use of opioid (euphoria, then apathy, dysphoria)

3) Pupillary constriction (or dilation from anoxia from overdose) and one or more of the following: drowsiness or coma, slurred speech, impaired attention or memory

4) Symptoms not due to general medical condition or other mental disorder

3. Clinical findings and issues

a. Route: intravenous, intramuscular, subcutaneous, snorting, smoking, orally

b. Pharmacologic effects vary by receptor type bound by the opioid (mu, kappa, delta)

1) Analgesia: mu, kappa, delta receptors

2) Feelings of well-being or euphoria, decreased blood pressure, pulse, respiration, body temperature, decreased peristalsis (constipation), suppression of cough reflex, decreased pupil size (miosis), endocrine changes: mu, delta receptors

3) Release of histamine causing pruritus, vasodilation of skin vessels: mu, delta receptors

4) Dysphoria, endocrine changes: kappa receptors

5) Tolerance develops to some effects (euphoria, analgesia)

c. Opioid use causes release of dopamine (reward circuits): pleasurable effects

d. Heroin: illegal substance

1) Routes: intravenous ("mainlining"), intramuscular, subcutaneous, smoking ("chasing the dragon"), snorting, sniffing liquefied heroin ("shabanging"), oral administration, combined with cocaine ("speedballing" or "crisscrossing") or diazepam or alcohol

2) More toxic than morphine by sevenfold

3) Associated with HIV infection, hepatitis, endocarditis, septicemia, osteomyelitis

4. Course (as described in DSM-IV-TR)

a. Most commonly seen in late teens or early 20s

b. Dependence generally lasts over a period of many years

c. Relapse following abstinence is common

d. Up to 2% mortality rate annually

e. 20% to 30% may achieve long-term abstinence

5. Epidemiology (as described in DSM-IV-TR)
   a. Highest lifetime prevalence for inappropriate use of analgesics is in 18 to 25-year-old group (9%)
   b. Lifetime prevalence of heroin use is 1%
   c. 0.7% of adults had opioid dependence or abuse at sometime in their lives
   d. Increasing age is associated with decreasing prevalence
   e. M>F 1.5:1 for nonheroin opioids; M>F 3:1 for heroin
   f. Use is more common among physicians and health care professionals than among other occupations
   g. Up to 50% of opioid-dependent persons have antisocial personality disorder
6. Etiology and pathophysiology: family members of opioid-dependent persons often are more likely to have other psychopathology
7. Other neurologic complications
   a. Opioid-related movement disorders (uncommon, case reports)
      1) Dyskinesias (observed with fentanyl)
      2) Oculogyric crisis and generalized dystonia (intranasal heroin)
      3) Myoclonus (chronic use of meperidine)
      4) Tremor and chorea (methadone)
      5) Progressive spongiform leukoencephalopathy involving cerebral and cerebellar white matter and brainstem in chronic heroin abusers who inhale the vapor of heroin heated on metal
   b. Seizures: meperidine has been shown to lower seizure threshold
   c. No evidence of long-term cognitive impairment
8. Clinical management (see Table 6-4)

N. Phencyclidine (PCP, hog, tranq, angel dust, PeaCe pill, ketamine)
1. History
   a. Developed in 1950s as dissociative anesthetics generally used for animals
   b. Became a "street drug" in the 1960s
   c. Easy to manufacture, relatively cheap
   d. Often used to "lace" cigarettes or marijuana
2. Definition and criteria
   a. Phencyclidine dependence: overview of DSM-IV-TR criteria (see above summary of dependence)
   b. Phencyclidine abuse: overview of DSM-IV-TR criteria (see above summary of abuse)
   c. Phencyclidine intoxication: overview of DSM-IV-TR criteria
      1) Recent use of phencyclidine or related substance
      2) Maladaptive behavioral changes or impaired judgment or function shortly after use of phencyclidine

3) Within an hour after use, at least two of the following: vertical or horizontal nystagmus, hypertension or tachycardia, numbness or decreased pain sensation, ataxia, dysarthria, muscle rigidity, seizures or coma, hyperacusis
      4) Symptoms not due to general medical condition or other mental disorder
3. Clinical findings and issues (as described in DSM-IV-TR)
   a. Route: orally, intravenously, intranasally
   b. Rapid onset of action: 5 minutes, peaking in 30 minutes
   c. Euphoria, derealization, tingling, warmth
   d. Can see bizarre behaviors, myoclonic jerks, confusion, disorientation, coma, seizures
   e. Normal or smaller pupils are seen
   f. Can have long-term neuropsychologic damage
   g. Can lead to life-threatening organ system breakdown, hyperthermia, autonomic instability; use of physical restraints can lead to rhabdomyolysis
   h. Acidification of urine (ammonium chloride, vitamin C, cranberry juice) can help with urinary excretion of phencyclidine
4. Epidemiology (as described in DSM-IV-TR)
   a. Prevalence of phencyclidine dependence and abuse in general population is unknown
   b. Highest lifetime prevalence is found in 26 to 34-year-old age group (4%)
   c. Up to 3% of substance abuse–related deaths involve phencyclidine
   d. 3% of emergency department substance-related visits have phencyclidine as a problem
   e. M>F 2:1
   f. Prevalence is twice as high for ethnic minorities
5. Other neurologic complications
   a. Phencyclidine may have proconvulsant effects (primary or secondary to intracerebral hemorrhage or hypertensive encephalopathy secondary to hypertension)
   b. Hypertension (phencyclidine): may be seen in early or late stage of intoxication and may cause hypertensive encephalopathy, cerebral infarction, or hemorrhage
6. Clinical management (see PSYCHOPHARMACOLOGY AND OTHER TREATMENTS and Table 6-4)
   a. Benzodiazepines
   b. Antipsychotics

O. Sedatives, Hypnotics, Anxiolytics: benzodiazepines, barbiturates, ethchlorvynol, meprobamate, glutethimide, chloral hydrate
1. Introduction

a. All are cross-tolerant with one another and with alcohol
b. All are capable of physical and psychologic dependency and withdrawal
c. Two main categories of abusers (abuse potential is high)
   1) Teens to 20s: use drugs for recreational purposes, obtain them illegally
   2) Middle-aged women: prescribed by physicians for "nerves"
2. History
   a. 1903: barbital (first barbiturate) introduced
   b. 1960s: advent of benzodiazepines (safer, so they replaced barbiturates)
   c. 15% of the general population is prescribed benzodiazepines per year
3. Definitions and criteria
   a. Sedative, hypnotic, or anxiolytic dependence: overview of DSM-IV-TR criteria (see above summary of dependence)
   b. Sedative, hypnotic, or anxiolytic abuse: overview of DSM-IV-TR criteria (see above summary of abuse)
   c. Sedative, hypnotic, or anxiolytic intoxication: overview of DSM-IV-TR criteria
      1) Recent use of sedative, hypnotic, or anxiolytic
      2) Maladaptive behavioral or psychologic changes or impaired judgment or functioning surrounding use of sedative, hypnotic, or anxiolytic
      3) After sedative, hypnotic, or anxiolytic use at least one of the following: slurred speech, incoordination, unsteady gait, nystagmus, impaired memory or attention, stupor or coma
      4) Symptoms not due to general medical condition or other mental disorder
   d. Sedative, hypnotic, or anxiolytic withdrawal: overview of DSM-IV-TR criteria summarized
      1) Cessation of or reduction in use of sedative, hypnotic, or anxiolytic that has been prolonged and heavy
      2) Within several hours or days, at least two of the following: autonomic hyperactivity; increased hand tremor; insomnia; nausea or vomiting; transient visual, tactile, or auditory hallucinations or illusions; psychomotor agitation, anxiety, or grand mal seizure
      3) Symptoms cause marked distress or impaired functioning
      4) Symptoms not due to general medical condition or other mental disorder
4. Clinical findings and issues (as described in DSM-IV-TR)
   a. 20% to 30% of those with untreated withdrawal may develop grand mal seizures
   b. Intoxication can lead to accidental injury from falls and accidents
   c. In elderly, cognitive problems and falls

d. Some can become disinhibited and show aggressive behavior
e. Can be related to severe depression and suicide attempts or completions
f. Overdoses: deterioration in vital signs produce medical emergency
g. Classic test for degree of dependence: pentobarbital challenge test
   1) First, give 200 mg of pentobarbital by mouth
   2) In 1 hour, check for signs of intoxication (see above)
   3) If no signs of intoxication, give another 100 mg of pentobarbital and recheck in 1 hour; repeat until signs of intoxication or maximum of 500 mg
   4) When patient shows signs of mild intoxication, total amount given is the total daily dose
   5) Convert to phenobarbital by giving 30 mg phenobarbital for each 100 mg of pentobarbital given and divide that total into four daily doses for administration (similarly one may convert to a benzodiazepine such as diazepam using equivalence tables and proceed with a taper)
   6) Taper by about 10% per day which will complete detoxification in 10 to 14 days
5. Course (as described in DSM-IV-TR)
   a. Teens and 20s: escalation of occasional use until use meets criteria for dependence or abuse (intermittent party use leads to daily use at high levels or tolerance)
   b. When prescribed by physician for "nerves": tolerance develops, then gradual increase in dose and frequency
6. Epidemiology (as described in DSM-IV-TR)
   a. Women have higher risk of prescription drug abuse in this class of medications
   b. Up to 90% of hospitalized patients have orders for these types of medications
   c. Highest lifetime prevalence is in 26 to 34-year-old age group (6%)
   d. F>M, increases with age
7. Clinical management (see PSYCHOPHARMACOLOGY AND OTHER TREATMENTS and Table 6-4)
   a. Emergent: gastric lavage, emesis, urine alkalization, hemodialysis, life support
   b. Nonemergent: taper using phenobarbital or benzodiazepine of abuse

P. **Other Substances:** anabolic steroids, flunitrazepam (Rohypnol), γ-hydroxybutyrate (GHB), nitrate inhalants, nitrous oxide
1. Anabolic steroids ("roids")
   a. Abused by athletes, weight lifters
   b. Used to increase muscle mass and enhance athletic performance

c. Early: a sense of "well-being" is described

d. Later: decrease in energy, depressed mood, intense irritability (can lead to "roid rage")

e. Also possible: psychotic symptoms, liver injury, mania, grandiosity, hirsuitism, testicular atrophy

2. Flunitrazepam (Rohypnol): *illegal in the United States*

a. Has been used as a "date-rape drug" (intoxicate, rape)

b. A potent benzodiazepine; produces deep sedation that potentially can lead to respiratory depression and death

c. Associated with rapid tolerance and dependence

3. γ-Hydroxybutyrate ("liquid ecstasy"): *illegal in the United States*

a. Has been used as a "date-rape drug" (intoxicate, rape)

b. A potent CNS depressant: produces anterograde amnesia, respiratory depression, coma, death

c. Can cause hallucinations, euphoria

4. Nitrate inhalants ("poppers")

a. Intoxication: "fullness in head," euphoria, intensified sexual feelings, grandiosity, alteration of perception of time, visual distortions, aggression, violence

b. Often used by gay community

c. Can lead to impairment of immune system, headaches, vomiting, hypotension, irritation of respiratory system, slurred speech, ataxia, smooth muscle relaxation

5. Nitrous oxide ("laughing gas")

a. Intoxication: light-headedness, floating sensation, confusion, paranoia

V. PERSONALITY DISORDERS

A. Disorders Discussed

1. Cluster A "odd or eccentric" (paranoid, schizoid, schizotypal)

2. Cluster B "dramatic, emotional, erratic" (antisocial, borderline, histrionic, narcissistic)

3. Cluster C "fearful, anxious" (avoidant, dependent, obsessive-compulsive)

4. Physicians of all specialties are likely to encounter patients with personality disorder, particularly, patients with borderline personality disorder (BPD)

5. Patients with BPD are heavy users of the health care system

a. Examples: patient with BPD may present with recurrent self-mutilating behaviors such as cutting one's arm with razor blades on repeated occasions or may present to an emergency department after a near-lethal overdose on medications

b. Also, BPD makes up 30% to 60% of clinical samples of patients with personality disorders

B. General Diagnostic Criteria for Personality Disorder (DSM-IV-TR)

1. Enduring pattern of inner experience and behavior that deviates markedly from the expectations of the person's culture; this pattern is manifested in two (or more) of the following areas:

a. Cognition (i.e., ways of perceiving and interpreting self, other people, events)

b. Affectivity (i.e., range, intensity, lability, and appropriateness of emotional response)

c. Interpersonal functioning

d. Impulse control

2. The enduring pattern

a. Is inflexible and pervasive across a broad range of personal and social situations

b. Leads to clinically marked distress or impairment in social, occupational, or other important areas of functioning

c. Is stable and of long duration; its onset can be traced back at least to adolescence or early childhood

d. Is not better accounted for as a manifestation or consequence of another mental disorder

e. Is not due to direct physiologic effects of a substance (e.g., drug of abuse, medication) or general medical condition (e.g., head trauma)

C. Cluster A—paranoid personality disorder

1. Characterized by suspiciousness, distrust; interprets actions of others as threatening or "out to get them"

2. Overview of DSM-IV-TR criteria

a. Enduring, pervasive distrust and suspiciousness

b. Interprets intentions of others as harmful or exploitive

c. At least four of the following: suspects others are deceiving or exploiting, preoccupied with doubts regarding loyalty or trustworthiness of others, finds it difficult to confide in others, reads hidden meanings into words or situations, unforgiving and bears grudges, quickly reacts angrily if perceives character has been attacked, unjustified suspicions regarding fidelity of significant other

d. Not part of schizophrenia, psychotic mood disorder, or general medical condition

3. Epidemiology

a. Lifetime prevalence: 0.5% to 2.5% of general population

b. Males>females

4. Etiology: increased prevalence among those with relatives having chronic schizophrenia and delusional disorder, paranoid type

5. Hints for working with these patients

a. Few seek treatment; often they are forced into it by family or legal system

b. Challenge is building trust and a collaborative working

relationship
   c. Provider should be open, honest, and maintain strict boundaries
   d. Breaking or bending rules can lead these patients to litigation
   e. Maintain calm when met with anger or hostility
   f. Group therapy often should be avoided because the patients tend to misinterpret statements made by group members

D. Cluster A—schizoid personality disorder
1. Characterized by social detachment and limited emotional reactivity
2. Overview of DSM-IV-TR criteria
   a. Enduring, pervasive social detachment or isolation and limited emotional reactivity
   b. At least four of the following: no desire for close relationships, participates in solitary activities, minimal interest in sexual activity with others, very few activities bring pleasure, has very few close confidants, indifferent to opinions of others, limited emotional range
   c. Not a part of schizophrenia, psychotic mood disorder, or general medical condition
3. Epidemiology
   a. According to DSM-IV-TR, is uncommon in clinical settings
   b. Males>females
4. Etiology: increased prevalence among relatives of schizophrenics or those with schizotypal personality disorder
5. Hints for working with these patients
   a. Few seek treatment, often they are forced into it by family or legal system
   b. Challenge for providers is working with person with absence of response or emotional connection, which often leads to frustration
   c. Helpful to encourage social skills group participation only to level of engagement that they can endure, over time they often will build an attachment
   d. These patients generally lack the insight and motivation for individual psychotherapy

E. Cluster A—schizotypal personality disorder
1. Characterized by discomfort with close relationships, cognitive and/or perceptual distortions, and eccentric behaviors and beliefs
2. Overview of DSM-IV-TR criteria
   a. Enduring, pervasive pattern of deficits in social and interpersonal relationships, eccentric behavior, distortions of cognition and perception
   b. At least five of the following: ideas of reference; odd beliefs or magical thinking; unusual perceptual experiences; odd thinking and speech; suspiciousness or paranoia; affect is inappropriate; behavior or appearance is odd, peculiar, or eccentric; lacks close friends; social anxiety that contributes to negativity or paranoia
   c. Not a part of schizophrenia, psychotic mood disorder, or general medical condition
3. Epidemiology
   a. Prevalence: 3% in general population
   b. Often seen in females with fragile X syndrome
4. Etiology: increased prevalence in first-degree relatives with schizophrenia
5. Hints for working with these patients
   a. Few seek treatment, often they are forced into it by family or legal system
   b. Challenge for providers is to prevent pushing too hard, which can lead to increased anxiety or paranoia, and to build trust and minimize anxiety
   c. Providers often get frustrated, bored, overwhelmed with the odd, belabored discourses of schizotypal patients
   d. Try to get them into an environment structured to allow for achievement of greater success than they might have in the "outside world"
   e. Social skills training can be helpful, but group psychotherapies can be threatening to them

F. Cluster B—antisocial personality disorder
1. Characterized by pervasive disregard for and violation of the rights of others
2. Overview of DSM-IV-TR criteria
   a. Enduring and pervasive pattern of disregard for others, violation of the rights of others and occurring since age 15
   b. At least three of the following: unlawfulness, deceitfulness, impulsivity or failure to plan ahead, repeated physical assaults and irritability, reckless disregard for self or others, irresponsibility, indifferent to or rationalizes hurting others
   c. Must be at least 18 years old
   d. Previous history of conduct disorder before age 15
   e. Not part of schizophrenia or a manic episode
3. Epidemiology
   a. Prevalence: 3% of males and 1% of females in general population; higher prevalence rates associated with substance-abuse treatment settings
   b. Often associated with substance abuse, lower socioeconomic status, and urban locations
4. Etiology
   a. Increased prevalence in first-degree relatives with antisocial personality disorder
   b. Increased risk if previous diagnosis of conduct disorder

before age 10, together with attention-deficit/hyperactivity disorder
5. Hints for working with these patients
   a. Most often they are forced into treatment by legal system
   b. Provider will likely need to get collateral history for truth and accuracy
   c. These patients respect power and will not relate well to a "powerless" provider
   d. Provider will need to be uncompromisingly honest and make good on threats or promised consequences of inappropriate behavior
   e. One challenge is to help patient gain insight into his or her personal responsibility for problems encountered in life
   f. Cognitive-behavioral therapy has been used with some success; family and marriage counseling can be helpful

G. **Cluster B**—borderline personality disorder
1. Key feature is instability of mood, but these patients are also characterized by pervasive instability of affect, identity, marked impulsivity, chaotic interpersonal relationships, self-injurious behaviors, failed marriages, lost jobs, "black and white" thinking, "splitting" (one care provider valued and the other one is devalued, often causing strife among the providers)
2. Overview of DSM-IV-TR criteria
   a. Enduring and pervasive pattern of instability of interpersonal relationships, self-image, and affect as well as notable impulsivity
   b. At least five of the following: frantic efforts to avoid abandonment (real or imagined), unstable and intense relationships (alternating between idealization and devaluation), unstable self-image, impulsivity that is potentially self-damaging, recurrent suicidal gestures or self-injurious behaviors, intense and dramatic range of mood and affect, chronic feelings of emptiness, inappropriate anger, episodes of stress-related paranoia or dissociations
3. Epidemiology
   a. Prevalence: 2% of general population, 10% among persons seen in outpatient mental health clinics, about 20% among psychiatric inpatients, 30% to 60% of clinical populations with personality disorders
   b. Females>males, according to DSM-IV-TR, BPD is diagnosed predominantly (about 75%) in females, with female-to-male ratio of 4:1
4. Etiology
   a. Increased prevalence among those with early traumatic experiences (sexual abuse, neglect, hostility, parental loss)
   b. Five times more common in those with relatives having the disorder

5. Hints for working with these patients
   a. Often self-referred for treatment or referred by legal system
   b. These patients have knack for destructively disrupting entire systems
   c. They can be both treatment-demanding as well as treatment-resistant
   d. Challenge for providers is to consistently set limits, be involved, compassionate, and reliable and to examine countertransference feelings carefully because these patients provoke anger and feelings of helplessness in providers
   e. It is important to ensure that self-injurious behaviors exhibited by patients will not lead to secondary gain or gratification
   f. Dialectical behavioral therapy (DBT)
      1) An empirically validated therapy derived from cognitive behavioral therapy, the philosophy of dialectics, and the Buddhist concept of mindfulness
      2) Has become a standard treatment for BPD
      3) Is also widely used in management of recurrent suicidal and parasuicidal behaviors
      4) Results in reduction of self-harm behaviors and decreases hospitalization rates and anger dyscontrol

H. **Cluster B**—histrionic personality disorder
1. Characterized by excitable, emotional, colorful, flamboyant behavior and by inability to maintain long-lasting relationships
2. Overview of DSM-IV-TR criteria
   a. Enduring and pervasive pattern of emotionality and attention seeking
   b. At least five of the following: uncomfortable when not center of attention; often displays seductive, flirtatious, or provocative behavior; shallow expressions of emotion; draws attention by use of physical appearance; speech is excessively impressionistic; displays exaggerated expressions of emotion; easily influenced by others or situations; thinks relationships are more intimate than they really are
3. Epidemiology
   a. Prevalence: 2% to 3% of general population
   b. Females>males
4. Etiology: tends to run in families
5. Hints for working with these patients
   a. Often self-referred for treatment or referred by legal system
   b. Patients are inclined to seek approval by pleasing others, so initially may look like the "dream patient"
   c. Patients usually seek treatment during a life crisis, and once it is resolved, their motivation for change is greatly decreased
   d. Challenge for the provider is to maintain strict bound-

aries, to manage patient seductiveness and patient's tendency to avoid addressing relevant issues

    e. Provider should use clear treatment goals and strict limit-setting

    f. Traditionally, psychodynamic psychotherapy has been used, but others have found problem-based and cognitive-behavioral based therapies helpful, too

I. Cluster B—narcissistic personality disorder

1. Characterized by high sense of self-importance and uniqueness
2. Overview of DSM-IV-TR criteria
    a. Enduring and pervasive pattern of grandiosity, need for admiration, and lack of empathy
    b. At least five of the following: grandiose sense of self-importance; preoccupied with fantasies of success, power, brilliance, beauty, or love; believes self to be special or unique; needs excessive admiration; has high sense of entitlement; takes advantage of others; lacks empathy; envious of others; behaves arrogantly or haughtily
3. Epidemiology
    a. Prevalence: about 1% of general population
    b. Males>females
4. Etiology
    a. Higher risk for narcissistic personality disorder in offspring of narcissists
    b. Narcissists give their children an unrealistic sense of grandiosity
5. Hints for working with these patients
    a. Often self-referred for treatment or referred by legal system
    b. Patients are haughty, condescending to authority figures, have presumption of receiving "special treatment and special providers," display self-righteous indignation when questioned
    c. Patients have trouble seeking help because they view it as demeaning and unacceptable
    d. Challenge for the provider is to display genuine nondefensiveness and noncompetitiveness
    e. Provider will need to be firm and tactfully confront patient's grandiose sense of entitlement and arrogance while being sensitive to patient's potential for feeling tremendous shame if he or she perceives this as criticism directed toward them
    f. Several methods of therapy have been used with these patients with some success: psychodynamic, interpersonal, and cognitive-behavioral

J. Cluster C—avoidant personality disorder

1. Characterized by extreme sensitivity to rejection, shyness, need for uncritical acceptance

2. Overview of DSM-IV-TR criteria
    a. Enduring and pervasive pattern of feelings of inadequacy, sensitivity to negative evaluation, social inhibition
    b. At least four of the following: avoids situations and occupations that would involve a lot of interpersonal contact, only gets involved with someone if certain they will be liked, cautious regarding intimate relationships for fear of being shamed or ridiculed, preoccupied with criticism or rejection, feels inadequate, views self as inferior to others, reluctant to take personal risks in activities and relationships for fear of being embarrassed
3. Epidemiology
    a. Prevalence: 0.5% to 1% of general population
    b. Males=females
4. Etiology
    a. Infants with timid temperament may be prone to this disorder
    b. Disfigurement may predispose to this disorder
5. Hints for working with these patients
    a. Patients respond to kindness, any perceived irritability directed toward them can be intolerable
    b. Patients are generally motivated to change, but provider should be prepared for slow progress
    c. Patients rarely have social networks strong enough to help them during crises, so provider must guard against becoming overprotective or becoming a replacement for the patient's social relationships
    d. Challenge for provider is to develop trust and to display extreme patience, be nonthreatening and sympathetic, and take care about the patient's hypersensitivity so patient does not feel criticized or judged
    e. Helpful therapies: group therapy, assertiveness and social skills training, cognitive-behavioral therapy

K. Cluster C—dependent personality disorder

1. Characterized by excessive reliance on others for emotional support and decision-making
2. Overview of DSM-IV-TR criteria
    a. Enduring and pervasive pattern of excessive need to be taken care of, clinging behavior, fear of separation
    b. At least five of the following: needs excessive advice from others for decision-making, needs others to take responsibility for major things in his or her life, afraid to express disagreement, has difficulty initiating projects on his or her own because of lack of self-confidence, needs constant nurturance and support from others, has exaggerated fears of being unable to care for self, has a frantic need to establish another relationship when a close relationship comes to an end, preoccupied with fears of being left to care for self

3. Epidemiology
   a. Prevalence: 2% to 4% of general population; most frequent personality disorder
   b. Females>males; some say females=males
4. Etiology
   a. Predisposing factors may be chronic physical illness or separation anxiety disorder
5. Hints for working with these patients
   a. Patients are anxiously eager to please and often know they are dependent but do not view it as a problem
   b. Initially, patients seem easy to treat because they are attentive, cooperative, appreciative and usually compliant, but they tend to show their discomfort or disagreement by missing appointments or failing to complete treatment assignments
   c. Challenge for the provider is to prevent reestablishment of the dominant-dependent relationship that is seen in patient's other relationships
   d. Provider needs to adhere to clear professional limits and boundaries
   e. Cognitive-behavioral psychotherapy is helpful

L. Cluster C—obsessive-compulsive personality disorder
1. Characterized by preoccupation with orderliness, perfectionism, control to point of inflexibility
2. Overview of DSM-IV-TR criteria
   a. Enduring and pervasive pattern of preoccupation with orderliness, perfectionism, control
   b. At least four of the following: preoccupation with details, rules, and lists; inability to complete tasks because of focus on perfectionism; devoted to work at expense of leisure, friends, and family; inflexible when it comes to issues of morality, ethics, and values; unable to discard worthless or worn-out objects; has difficulty delegating tasks to others; hoards money; stubborn and rigid
3. Epidemiology
   a. Prevalence: 1% of general population
   b. Male-to-female ratio of 2:1
4. Etiology
   a. Predisposing factors may be linked to high central serotonergic function
   b. Some evidence to support that this can run in families
5. Hints for working with these patients
   a. Patients are careful to pay proper respect to authorities and are initially cooperative, polite, serious, and conscientious in treatment
   b. Over time patients can become consciously compliant but unconsciously oppositional
   c. Provider should exhibit ordinary kindness, patience, tolerance and be a good listener

d. Challenge for provider is to prevent going too quickly to emotional issues because patients are usually more business-like or problem-focused
e. Also, provider must guard against becoming bored and frustrated when listening to patients and then fail to recognize the emotional pain underlying the patient's strong defenses, such as isolation of affect, undoing, and regression
f. Recommended therapies: psychodynamic psychotherapy, cognitive-behavioral therapy

M. Clinical Management of Personality Disorder Symptoms (see PSYCHOPHARMACOLOGY AND OTHER TREATMENTS)
1. Aggression and impulsivity (see Antidepressants, Antipsychotics, Mood Stabilizers)
2. Mood dysregulation (see Antidepressants, Antipsychotics, Mood Stabilizers)
3. Anxiety (see Antidepressants, Antipsychotics, Benzodiazepines)
4. Psychotic symptoms (see Antipsychotics)
5. Psychosocial issues (see Psychotherapy and Psychosocial Treatments)

VI. PSYCHOPHARMACOLOGY AND OTHER TREATMENTS

A. Antidepressants: SSRIs, TCAs, MAOIs, mixed-mechanism antidepressants
1. Clinical uses: primary use is for depression, bipolar depression, panic disorder, agoraphobia, OCD, social phobia, generalized anxiety disorder, posttraumatic stress disorder, bulimia nervosa
2. SSRIs: citalopram (Celexa), escitalopram (Lexapro), fluoxetine (Prozac), fluvoxamine (Luvox), paroxetine (Paxil), sertraline (Zoloft)
   a. Most widely prescribed antidepressants since 1988, when fluoxetine (Prozac) was introduced
   b. Mechanism of action: SSRIs inhibit 5HT reuptake but do not act on NE or dopamine
   c. Fewer side effects, greater safety in medically ill and in overdose than TCAs and MAOIs
   d. Clinical uses: depression, dysthymia, seasonal affective disorder, bipolar depression, generalized anxiety disorder, panic disorder, OCD, posttraumatic stress disorder, eating disorder, personality disorder, paraphilia, chronic pain, premature ejaculation, neurotic excoriation, chronic fatigue syndrome
   e. Pregnancy: best studied is fluoxetine, thought to be safest SSRI in pregnancy, but potentially there may be

increased risk of perinatal complications (with use during third trimester)

f. Cytochrome P-450 drug interactions
  1) Fluoxetine and paroxetine, inhibitors of 2D6: potential for drug interactions with TCAs, haloperidol, antipsychotics, type 1C antiarrhythmics, trazodone
  2) Sertraline: inhibitor of 2D6—TCAs, haloperidol, antipsychotics, type 1C antiarrhythmics, trazodone; 2C—tolbutamide, diazepam; 3A4—carbamazepine
  3) Fluvoxamine: 1A2—theophylline, clozapine, haloperidol, amitriptyline, clomipramine, imipramine; 2C—diazepam; 3A4—carbamazepine, alprazolam, terfenadine, astemizol

g. Side effects
  1) Gastrointestinal: nausea, diarrhea or constipation, dry mouth, vomiting, weight gain
  2) CNS: increased migraine headaches, increased akathisias, anxiety, vivid dream, may produce hypomania and mania
  3) Endocrine: syndrome of inappropriate antidiuretic hormone, elevated prolactin and resultant galactorrhea, hyperglycemia
  4) Sexual function: reduced libido, delayed ejaculation, and anorgasmia (Table 6-5)

h. Discontinuation syndrome
  1) Transient dizziness and vertigo, lethargy, paresthesias (paroxetine), nausea, vivid dreams, irritability
  2) Treat by tapering dose

i. Apathy syndrome
  1) May sometimes occur months or years after successful treatment
  2) Reduced motivation, apathy, poor initiation; may be features of recurrent depression

j. Serotonin syndrome: dangerous, potentially life-threatening reaction to increased levels of 5HT in CNS, leading to altered mental status, agitation, tremor, hypotension, fever, ataxia, diarrhea, hyperreflexia, myoclonus (hypertoxicity, hyperthermia, rhabodomyolysis, renal failure may occur when severe)
  1) Concern with combining any agents that increase CNS 5HT levels (SSRIs, MAOIs, TCAs, mixed-mechanism antidepressants, psychostimulants, dopamine agonists, buspirone, sumatriptan, meperidine, dextromethorphan)
  2) MAOI + SSRI, L-tryptophan, dextromethorphan, meperidine, TCAs, trazodone, lithium, "ecstasy," or clonazepam
  3) SSRI + another SSRI, venlafaxine, dextromethorphan, buspirone, carbamazepine, lithium, mirtazapine, tramadol, nefazodone, sumatriptan, or "ecstasy"

Selective Serotonin Reuptake Inhibitors
Drugs
  Citalopram (Celexa): mild 2D6 inhibitor
  Escitalopram (Lexapro): mild 2D6 inhibitor
  Fluvoxamine (Luvox): potent 2C19 inhibitor
  Fluoxetine (Prozac): potent 2D6 inhibitor
  Paroxetine (Paxil): potent 2D6 inhibitor
  Sertraline (Zoloft): dose-dependent 2D6 inhibitor

Fewer side effects, safer in overdose

Indications:
  Major depressive disorder, dysthymia, seasonal affective disorder, bipolar affective disorder, generalized anxiety disorder, panic disorder, obsessive-compulsive disorder, posttraumatic stress disorder, eating disorder, personality disorder, chronic pain, premature ejaculation, neurotic excoriations, chronic fatigue syndrome

Serotonin syndrome—*life threatening*:
  Altered mental status, agitation, fever, hypotension, ataxia, hyperreflexia, myoclonus

High-yield facts
  Fluoxetine: longest half-life and active metabolite with longest half-life, side effects include reduced appetite
  Fluoxetine and fluvoxamine: best profile in regard to sexual side effects
  Sertraline: worst profile in regard to sexual side effects, most potent blocker of dopamine transporters, has active metabolite with short half-life
  Fluvoxamine and paroxetine: no active metabolites, more likely to cause discontinuation syndrome with abrupt withdrawal of drug
  Citalopram: most selective for 5HT
  Paroxetine: most potent SSRI, side effects include weight gain and somnolence

---

3. MAOIs: isocarboxazid (Marplan), phenelzine (Nardil), tranylcypromine (Parnate)
  a. Mechanism of action: irreversibly inhibit monoamine oxidase, blocking metabolism of monoamine neurotransmitters
  b. Clinical uses: atypical depression, panic disorder, social phobia, posttraumatic stress disorder, OCD, bulimia nervosa, pain management

c. Side effects: orthostatic hypotension, sedation or hyperstimulation, insomnia, dry mouth, weight gain, edema, sexual dysfunction (Table 6-5)

d. *Severe hypertension and complications of malignant hypertension* if taking MAOIs and tyramine-containing substance or food is ingested

e. Serotonin syndrome if MAOIs taken in combination with SSRIs or other antidepressants, over-the-counter medications, meperidine, stimulants, sympathomimetics

4. TCAs: amitriptyline (Elavil), clomipramine (Anafranil), desipramine (Norpramin), doxepin (Sinequan), imipramine (Tofranil), nortriptyline (Pamelor), protriptyline (Vivactil)

   a. Mechanism of action: block reuptake of NE and 5HT to varying degrees and all TCAs block muscarinic, histaminic, and α-adrenergic receptors

   b. Side effects: sedation, orthostatic hypotension, constipation, urinary hesitancy, dry mouth, visual blurring, weight gain, tremors, edema, myoclonus, restlessness, insomnia, nausea, vomiting, prolongation of cardiac conduction, withdrawal syndrome (Table 6-5)

   c. Clinical uses: better than SSRIs for melancholic depression, also used for insomnia, pain, obsessive-compulsive disorder, panic, anxiety

   d. Contraindications: recent myocardial infarction, bundle branch block, widened QRS, narrow-angle glaucoma, cardiac disease, prostatic hypertrophy, pregnancy/lactation

   e. Do not use with MAOIs (serotonin syndrome)

   f. Cytochrome P-450 2D6 interactions

      1) TCAs + alcohol, carbamazepine, phenytoin, cigarette smoking → increased metabolism of TCAs → subtherapeutic levels of TCAs

      2) TCA + neuroleptics, SSRIs (especially paroxetine and fluoxetine), cimetidine methylphenidate (Ritalin), quinidine, thyroid medications → decreased metabolism of TCAs → potentially toxic levels of TCAs

   g. Monitoring

      1) Some TCAs have established therapeutic levels that can be measured in blood (nortriptyline, imipramine, desipramine, amitriptyline)

         a) Nortriptyline: well-defined therapeutic window from 50 to 150 ng/mL and is found to be less effective at both very high and very low doses

         b) Imipramine: plasma imipramine + desmethylimipramine should exceed 200 ng/mL

         c) Desipramine: plasma levels should exceed 125 ng/mL

         d) Amitriptyline: therapeutic range is 75 to 175 ng/mL

            i) Clinicians must be aware of potential for toxicity

Table 6-5. Sexual Side Effects Associated With Antidepressant or Antipsychotic Medications*

Medication	Side effects
Antidepressants	
SSRIs: citalopram, escitalopram, fluvoxamine, fluoxetine paroxetine, sertraline	Nearly all can cause all listed sexual dysfunctions Paroxetine: most often implicated Sertraline: least often implicated Fluoxetine: priapism reported (rare)
Mixed-mechanism: bupropion, duloxetine, mirtazapine, nefazodone, trazodone, venlafaxine	Bupropion and nefazodone: least likely to cause any sexual dysfunction Duloxetine: some reports of sexual dysfunction (except for priapism) Mirtazapine: rare report of decreased libido Trazodone: decreased or increased libido, ejaculatory disturbances, priapism Venlafaxine: reports of the listed sexual dysfunctions, except for priapism
TCAs: amitriptyline, clomipramine, desipramine, doxepin, imipramine, nortriptyline protriptyline	Anticholinergic effects cause interference with erection and delayed ejaculation Some reports of painful ejaculations Desipramine: fewest effects reported Clomipramine: may increase libido
MAOIs: isocarboxazid, phenelzine, tranylcypromine	Phenelzine: rare reports of priapism, anorgasmia, erectile dysfunction, ejaculatory disturbances Tranylcypromine: rare reports of erectile dysfunction and ejaculatory disturbances
Antipsychotics	
Typicals: chlorpromazine, fluphenazine, haloperidol, loxapine, mesoridazine, molindone, thioridazine, thiothixene, trifluoperazine	Most all can cause decreased libido, anorgasmia, erectile and ejaculatory dysfunction Thioridazine, chlorpromazine, trifluoperazine, fluphenazine: retrograde ejaculation or ejaculatory dysfunction Chlorpromazine, mesoridazine, thiothixene, loxapine, haloperidol, fluphenazine: priapism
Atypicals: aripiprazole, clozapine, olanzapine, quetiapine, risperidone, ziprasidone	Most all can cause ejaculatory dysfunction Quetiapine, risperidone, ziprasidone: erectile dysfunction Clozapine, aripiprazole: rare priapism Risperidone, ziprasidone: anorgasmia

MAOI, monoamine oxidase inhibitor; SSRI, selective serotonin reuptake inhibitor; TCA, tricyclic antidepressant.
*Sexual dysfunctions include decreased libido, erectile dysfunction, ejaculatory disturbances, orgasmic disturbances.

at higher blood concentrations (can lead to delirium, seizures, cardiac arrhythmias) and be especially vigilant of possible cytochrome P-450 drug interactions that might affect blood concentrations of TCAs

5. Mixed-mechanism antidepressants: bupropion, duloxetine, mirtazapine, nefazodone, trazodone, venlafaxine
   a. Bupropion (Wellbrin)
      1) Dopamine-NE reuptake inhibitor: preferentially increases dopamine (weak inhibitor of dopamine reuptake)
      2) Clinical uses: FDA-approved for depression, smoking cessation; non-FDA–approved—attention deficit–hyperactivity disorder
      3) Side effects: headache, nausea, anxiety, tremors, insomnia, sweating, tinnitus, dizziness, visual hallucinations, nightmares, agitation, psychosis, mania, anorexia, and weight loss
      4) Can increase seizure risk at doses more than 450 mg/day
      5) Contraindications: patients with seizure disorders, eating disorders
   b. Duloxetine (Cymbalta)
      1) Clinical uses: FDA-approved for depression, diabetic peripheral neuropathic pain
   c. Mirtazapine (Remeron)
      1) Enhances release of NE and 5HT, inhibits $5HT_2$ and $5HT_3$ receptors, also potent histamine antagonist, moderate α_2-adrenergic antagonist
      2) Clinical uses: FDA-approved for depression; non-FDA–approved—improves appetite and sleep
      3) Side effects: early sedation, weight gain, possible agranulocytosis
      4) Mirtazapine is sedating even at lower doses
   d. Nefazodone (Serzone)
      1) Serotonin ($5HT_2$) receptor-antagonist, weak inhibitor of 5HT reuptake ($5HT_2$ antagonist/reuptake inhibitor)
      2) Clinical uses: depression
      3) Side effects: nausea, somnolence, dry mouth, glossitis, dizziness, constipation, asthenia, blurred vision, and watch out for *hepatotoxicity* (not seen with trazodone); hypoglycemia (not seen with trazodone); gait disturbance, nocturnal myoclonus, tremor, akathisia, paresthesias, tinnitus; agitation, confusion, disorientation, anxiety, panic, hypomania/mania, headaches and worsening of migraine headaches
      4) Cytochrome P-450 3A3/4 inhibitor, do not use with cisapride, MAOIs, pimozide, triazolam, terfenadine, astemizole; caution with alprazolam; many other interactions

---

Mixed-Mechanism Antidepressants

Bupropion (Wellbutrin): DA/NE reuptake inhibitor
  Indications: smoking cessation, MDD, adult attention deficit-hyperactivity disorder

Duloxetine (Cymbalta): 5HT/NE reuptake inhibitor
  Indications: MDD, diabetic peripheral neuropathic pain

Mirtazapine (Remeron): enhances NE and 5HT release via α_2-antagonism, potent histamine antagonist, antagonist of $5HT_2$, $5HT_3$ receptors
  Indications: MDD, improves sleep/appetite

Nefazodone: inhibitor of serotonin uptake and weakly of NE reuptake, antagonist of $5HT_{2A}$, may selectively activate $5HT_{1A}$
  Indications: MDD

Trazodone (Desyrel): blocks $5HT_2$ receptor, weak inhibitor of 5HT reuptake
  Indications: MDD, insomnia

Venlafaxine (Effexor): inhibits 5HT reuptake at low doses, NE/DA at higher doses
  Indications: MDD, GAD, social anxiety disorder

DA, dopamine; GAD, generalized anxiety disorder; 5HT, serotonin; MDD, major depressive disorder; NE, norepinephrine

---

   e. Trazodone (Desyrel)
      1) Serotonin ($5HT_2$) receptor-antagonist, weak inhibitor of 5HT reuptake ($5HT_2$ antagonist/reuptake inhibitor)
      2) Clinical uses: FDA-approved for depression; non-FDA–approved—insomnia
      3) Side effects: sedation; orthostatic hypotension; headache; nausea; dry mouth; in men, potential for priapism (can be irreversible, surgical emergency)
   f. Venlafaxine (Effexor)
      1) Inhibits 5HT reuptake at lower doses, inhibits NE reuptake at moderate doses, and dopamine reuptake at higher doses
      2) Clinical uses: FDA-approved for depression, generalized anxiety disorder
      3) Side effects: hyperstimulation, sexual dysfunction, transient withdrawal symptoms, hypertension, hypercholesterolemia, sedation, insomnia, anticholinergic side effects, and mania/hypomania (latter in 0.5%)

B. Antipsychotics: typicals and atypicals
1. History: chlorpromazine introduced in 1952 by Delay and Deniker
   a. Noted to have calming effects on agitated psychotic patients
   b. Next, found effective for schizophrenic patients, not curative but helpful
2. Typicals: chlorpromazine (Thorazine), mesoridazine (Serentil), thioridazine (Mellaril), fluphenazine (Prolixin), perphenazine (Trilafon), trifluoperazine (Stelazine), thiothixene (Navane), loxapine (Loxitane), haloperidol (Haldol), molindone (Moban)
   a. Haloperidol: high-potency agent
      1) Favorable side-effect profile (useful in emergency settings)
      2) Useful for positive symptoms but not negative symptoms of schizophrenia
      3) High potential for dose-dependent acute extrapyramidal side effects and sexual dysfunction
   b. Chlorpromazine and thioridazine: low-potency agents
      1) Low potential for acute extrapyramidal side effects because of anticholinergic properties
      2) Side effects: reduced seizure threshold, hypotension, anticholinergic side effects, weight gain, syndrome of inappropriate antidiuretic hormone, jaundice, cataracts, agranulocytosis, tardive dyskinesia, neuroleptic malignant syndrome, sudden death (Table 6-5)
      3) Thioridazine also has potential to cause retinitis pigmentosa, retrograde ejaculation, QTc prolongation
      4) Thioridazine is metabolized by cytochrome P-450 2D6, so check for drug interactions
   c. Thiothixene, perphenazine, trifluoperazine: medium potency agents
      1) Effective for positive symptoms, less effective for negative symptoms of schizophrenia
      2) Has a relatively favorable risk versus benefit ratio, so is widely used
3. Atypicals: clozapine, risperidone, olanzapine, quetiapine, aripiprazole, ziprasidone
   a. Clozapine (Clozaril): low-potency agent, for refractory schizophrenia
      1) Choice for patient with tardive dyskinesia or at high risk for tardive dyskinesia
      2) Effective for positive and negative symptoms of schizophrenia
      3) Should have had at least three failed trials of antipsychotics from different classes and at least one depot formulation trial
      4) Extrapyramidal side effects and tardive dyskinesia symptoms virtually absent

5) Side effects: sedation, weight gain, orthostatic hypotension, hypersalivation, eosinophilia, hypertriglyceridemia, hyperglycemia (Table 6-5)
      6) Serious side effects: agranulocytosis, seizures
   b. Risperidone (Risperdal): high-potency agent
      1) Effective for positive and negative symptoms of schizophrenia
      2) Reduced potential for acute or chronic extrapyramidal side effects
      3) Can significantly increase serum prolactin levels, more sexual dysfunction is possible (Table 6-5)
      4) May cause significant hypotension, agitation, anxiety, weight gain, increased appetite
   c. Olanzapine (Zyprexa): medium- to high-potency agent
      1) Is structurally similar to and acts like clozapine but with less risk for agranulocytosis and seizures
      2) Acute extrapyramidal side effects no more frequent than reported for placebo, low chance for chronic extrapyramidal side effects

---

Atypical Antipsychotics

Aripiprazole (Abilify): partial agonist D_2, $5HT_{1A}$ receptors and antagonist at $5HT_{2A}$ receptors

Clozapine (Clozaril): low potency, EPS/TD nearly absent, good with positive and negative symptoms
   Warning—agranulocytosis potential, seizures

Quetiapine (Seroquel): low potency, few EPS, less sexual dysfunction, no prolactin increase

Olanzapine (Zyprexa): medium/high potency, few EPS, high weight gain

Risperidone (Risperdal): high potency, few EPS, can increase prolactin, more sexual dysfunction

Ziprasidone (Geodon): good for positive and negative symptoms, improves cognition and depression, low EPS, not associated with weight gain
   Warning—can lead to QT prolongation

Indications:
   Psychotic disorders, schizophrenia, mood disorder with psychotic features, delirium, acute mania, aggressive behaviors, psychosis due to medical condition or substances

D, dopamine; EPS, extrapyramidal side effects; 5HT, serotonin; TD, tardive dyskinesia

3) Side effects: weight gain, hypertriglyceridemia, sedation, diabetes (?) , elevated liver function enzymes (Table 6-5)

4) Cigarette smoking reduces blood levels

d. Quetiapine (Seroquel): low-potency agent

1) Does not increase prolactin levels, less sexual dysfunction (Table 6-5)

2) Acute extrapyramidal side effects no more frequent than reported for placebo, low chance for chronic extrapyramidal side effects

e. Aripiprazole (Abilify): medium- to high-potency agent

1) Partial agonist at dopamine$_2$ (D$_2$) and 5HT$_{1A}$ receptors and antagonist at 5HT$_{2A}$ receptors

f. Ziprasidone (Geodon): adverse effects uncommon, no weight gain (Table 6-5)

1) Possible QT prolongation

2) It is a 5HT and NE reuptake inhibitor, so may have antidepressant effects

4. Clinical uses: psychotic disorders, schizophrenia, mood disorders with psychotic symptoms, psychotic disorders secondary to general medical condition, substance abuse, delirium, acute mania, for control of aggressive behaviors

5. Mechanism of action

a. Typicals bind to D$_2$ receptors, blocking dopamine at the site, more prone to extrapyramidal side effects

b. Atypicals are weaker D$_2$ receptor antagonists but are potent 5HT$_{2A}$ receptor antagonists and also have anticholinergic and antihistaminic activity

c. Central 5HT$_{2A}$ receptor antagonism: broadened therapeutic effects while reducing extrapyramidal side effects associated with D$_2$ antagonists (especially in nigrostriatal pathways)

6. Mesocortical and mesolimbic dopaminergic pathways are affected by antipsychotics

7. Haldol and clozapine blood levels can be monitored and be helpful

8. Adverse effects

a. Tardive dyskinesia: abnormal involuntary movements (usually mouth and/or tongue) after long-term use

1) Elderly, women, and those with mood disorders more susceptible to tardive dyskinesia

2) Can often help by switching to atypical antipsychotic

b. Parkinsonism (tremor, rigidity, hypokinesia): treat by lowering dose of antipsychotic or adding antiparkinsonian agent

c. Akathisia (subjective feelings of anxiety, tension, agitation): treat by lowering dose of antipsychotic, try β-blocker, clonidine, amantadine, or benzodiazepine

d. Acute dystonic reaction (sustained contraction of muscles of neck, mouth, tongue): treat with intravenous benztropine or diphenhydramine

e. Anticholinergic side effects (dry mouth, urinary retention, blurry vision, constipation, exacerbation of narrow-angle glaucoma): treat by reducing dose or change to more potent antipsychotic or to atypical antipsychotic

f. Agranulocytosis (associated with low-potency antipsychotics and especially clozapine; potentially fatal): requires weekly blood counts for first 6 months, then every 2 weeks thereafter

g. Neuroleptic malignant syndrome—*medical emergency*—(rigidity, high fever, delirium, autonomic instability, increased serum levels of creatine kinase and liver enzymes): treat by stopping offending drug, supportive care, try dantrolene or bromocriptine, ECT for severe cases

1) Other medications associated with neuroleptic malignant-like syndrome include metoclopramide, prochlorperazine, promethazine, droperidol, which all cause decreased dopamine receptor activation

2) Rapid removal of medications with dopaminergic properties such as those used to treat Parkinson's disease can also cause neuroleptic malignant-like syndrome

h. Other adverse effects: orthostatic hypotension, hyperprolactinemia, weight gain, retinitis pigmentosa, cholestatic jaundice, decreased libido

i. Antipsychotics are considered "safer" than benzodiazepines or mood stabilizers in pregnancy (haloperidol and trifluoperazine have lower incidence of teratogenic effects)

C. Anxiolytics, Sedative-Hypnotics: benzodiazepines, barbiturates, nonbarbiturate sedative-hypnotics, buspirone

1. Anxiolytics: most often prescribed psychotropic medications

2. Benzodiazepines and buspirone have best safety record

3. Benzodiazepines

a. Marketed in United States since 1964

b. Clinical uses: anxiety disorders (generalized anxiety, panic, social phobia, adjustment disorder with anxiety, depressive disorders with anxiety), sleep disorders, seizures, alcohol withdrawal, anesthesia induction

c. Mechanism of action

1) Bind to specific benzodiazepine receptors, which are linked to GABA receptors

2) Helps effects of GABA within limbic system to reduce anxiety symptoms

d. Long half-life: chlordiazepoxide (Librium), clonazepam (Klonopin), clorazepate (Tranxene), diazepam (Valium), flurazepam (Dalmane)

e. Medium half-life: estazolam (ProSom), lorazepam (Ativan), temazepam (Restoril)
f. Short half-life: alprazolam (Xanax), oxazepam (Serax), triazolam (Halcion)
g. Preferred benzodiazepines for the elderly: oxazepam, lorazepam, temazepam ("out the liver")
   1) Metabolized by glucuronide conjugation, have no active metabolites
   2) Relatively short acting (other benzodiazepines are metabolized chiefly by hepatic oxidation)
h. Adverse effects: CNS depression, drowsiness, somnolence, decreased coordination, memory impairment, potential for abuse and addiction, patients can have severe discontinuation symptoms
i. Safe for use in medically ill, elderly, pregnancy, but not for use during breast feeding or for those with sleep apnea
4. Other anxiolytics, sedative-hypnotics
   a. Buspirone (BuSpar)
      1) Used for generalized anxiety disorder: effects seen after 1 to 2 weeks
      2) Relatively nonsedating, no abuse potential
   b. Chloral hydrate (Somnote): sedative, hypnotic, for alcohol withdrawal
   c. Diphenhydramine (Benadryl): for insomnia, but watch for anticholinergic effects
   d. Zaleplon (Sonata): for insomnia, but watch for drug interactions with cimetidine, rifampin, phenytoin, carbamazepine, phenobarbital
   e. Zolpidem (Ambien): hypnotic, for insomnia

D. Electroconvulsive Therapy
1. Presented by Cerletti and Bini (Italy) in 1938
   a. Electric current applied across scalp electrodes, producing

Benzodiazepines
Potentiates actions of γ-aminobutyric acid → anxiolytic effect on limbic system

Benzodiazepines preferred for elderly or patients with liver failure: out the liver—oxazepam, temazepam, lorazepam

Indications: anxiety, generalized anxiety disorder, panic disorder, social phobia, seizure disorder, alcohol withdrawal, anesthesia induction, sleep problems, musculoskeletal disorders, other disorders with anxiety component

a grand mal seizure
b. Safe and effective treatment
c. Mechanism of action unknown: multiple effects on CNS and downregulation of β-receptors
d. Clinical use: treatment of depression, mood disorders, highly suicidal patients, mania, catatonia, neuroleptic malignant syndrome, acute forms of schizophrenia; psychotic/melancholic depression is *unresponsive to medications*
e. Clinical use in Parkinson's disease: ECT may improve both mood and motor symptoms of patients with advanced Parkinson's disease, but effects may be short-lived from days to weeks to 6 months, according to various studies
f. Clinical use in patients with cardiac conduction disturbances: ECT is considered to be safer than TCAs in these patients
g. Work-up: routine laboratory tests, complete blood count, electrolytes, urinalysis, electrocardiogram, physical examination
h. Possible contraindications: active pulmonary infection, recent myocardial infarction, unstable coronary artery disease, congestive heart failure, uncontrolled hypertension, space-occupying brain lesion, increased intracranial pressure, recent cerebrovascular accident, history of anesthesia complications, seizure disorder, reflux, aneurysms, venous thrombosis, recent bone fracture (especially cervical spine)
i. Procedure
   1) Patients must not have food or drink after midnight for treatment the next morning
   2) Patients are usually given their blood pressure, heart, and diabetic medications with a sip of water before treatment
   3) Patients are given short-acting anesthetic, oxygen, succinylcholine (muscle relaxant used to prevent full body convulsions during treatment), and atropine or glycopyrrolate (used to decrease secretions and prevent bradyarrhythmias)
   4) Electrodes are placed on the scalp: bitemporal, unilateral (thought to cause less cognitive impairment), or bifrontal
   5) Electrical stimulus is applied to cause a 30 to 60-second seizure
j. Adverse effects: brief episode of hypotension or hypertension, bradyarrhythmia or tachyarrhythmia, prolonged seizures, prolonged apnea (due to pseudocholinesterase deficiency), postictal confusion, headache, nausea, muscle pain, *memory impairment* (retrograde amnesia for short time surrounding hospitalization)
k. Response rate, 80%

Electroconvulsive Therapy
Safe & effective treatment

Indications: depression, mania, suicidal patients, neuroleptic malignant syndrome, acute schizophrenia, psychotic depression intractable to medical treatment (not chronic schizophrenia)

Absolute contraindications: unclear

Possible relative contraindications/concerns: recent myocardial infarction, unstable coronary disease, venous thrombosis, uncontrolled hypertension, space-occupying brain lesion, increased intracranial pressure, recent intracerebral hemorrhage

Mood Stabilizers

Lithium: inhibits inositol-1-phosphatase
  Indications: mania, augmentation of antidepressants, prophylaxis of mania/depression, schizoaffective disorder, aggression, impulsivity
  Concerns: thyroid/kidney, pregnancy (Ebstein's anomaly)

Valproate: enhances GABA
  Indications: mania, augmentation of antidepressants, alcohol withdrawal states, rapid cycling, mixed states
  Concerns: can increase liver function tests, agranulocytosis, life-threatening rashes, weight gain, alopecia, pregnancy (neural tube defects)

Carbamazepine: damping effect on kindling process
  Indications (non-FDA–approved): mania, rapid cycling, mixed states, schizoaffective, impulsivity, augmentation
  Concerns: agranulocytosis, life-threatening rashes, pregnancy (spina bifida, craniofacial defects)

Gabapentin: increases GABA, reduces glutamate

Lamotrigine: inhibits serotonin reuptake
  Indications: bipolar, rapid cycling, mania, depression
  Concerns: life-threatening rashes, toxic epidermal necrolysis, blurred vision, ataxia

Topiramate (non-FDA–approved): bipolar
  Concerns: hyponatremia, fatigue, headaches, blurred or double vision

GABA, γ-aminobutyric acid

E. Mood Stabilizers: lithium, valproate, carbamazepine, gabapentin, lamotrigine, oxcarbazepine, topiramate
1. Lithium: first-line treatment for bipolar disorder
   a. Lithium is a naturally occurring salt; first became available for clinical use in 1970
   b. In 1940s lithium was first noted to calm psychotic patients who were severely agitated
   c. Soon after, it was discovered to also relieve symptoms of mania
   d. Mechanism of action: inhibits inositol-1-phosphatase, thus decreasing cellular responses to neurotransmitters
   e. Onset of action is 5 to 7 days, effective plasma level is 0.9 to 1.4 mEq/L for mania, maintenance range is 0.4 to 0.6 mEq/L
   f. Clinical use: bipolar depression, augmentation of antidepressants for depressed patients, prophylaxis for manic and depressive episodes in bipolar patients, schizoaffective disorder, aggression (in mentally retarded, demented, impulsive personality disorders); concomitant use of benzodiazepines and/or antipsychotics is often required for treatment of acute manic episode, because it takes 10 days or longer for lithium to take effect
   g. Adverse effects: increased thirst, polyuria, tremor, diarrhea, weight gain, edema, hypothyroidism, can cause nephrogenic diabetes insipidus, tubulointerstitial nephropathy, nephrotic syndrome, worsening of acne and psoriasis, hair loss, sinoatrial node dysfunction, reversible leukocytosis, parkinsonian-like symptoms, distractibility, poor memory, confusion
   h. Contraindications: patients with renal disease, following myocardial infarction, myasthenia gravis (blocks release of acetylcholine), during pregnancy (can cause Ebstein's anomaly)
   i. Angiotensin-converting enzyme inhibitors, nonsteroidal anti-inflammatory drugs, and thiazide diuretics may increase lithium levels and potential for toxicity
2. Valproate (divalproex sodium [Depakote]): first-line treatment for bipolar disorder
   a. Common anticonvulsant
   b. Clinical use: manic phase of bipolar disorder (especially rapid cycling and mixed states), maintenance of bipolar disorder, augmentation of antidepressants in major depression, alcohol withdrawal states, now has replaced

lithium as first-line agent for patients with rapidly cycling bipolar disorder

c. Mechanism of action: increases GABA levels in CNS by increased synthesis and decreased degradation of GABA

d. Peak concentrations in 1 to 4 hours, 90% is protein-bound, effective plasma level is 50 to 125 μg/mL, onset of action is about 3 to 5 days

e. Adverse effects: nausea, poor appetite, vomiting, diarrhea, increased liver enzymes, weight gain, alopecia, tremors, sedation, rashes (Stevens-Johnson syndrome or erythema multiforme), agranulocytosis, polycystic ovaries, neural tube defects (during first trimester of pregnancy), coma, death from overdose, hematologic effects

f. Before treatment: complete blood count, liver enzymes (every 1-4 weeks for first 6 weeks, and every 6-24 months thereafter)

3. Carbamazepine (Tegretol)
   a. Common anticonvulsant
   b. Clinical use
      1) Even though non-FDA–approved for this, it is often used for bipolar mania, rapid cycling, and mixed episodes; also used as prophylaxis for bipolar disorder
      2) May be helpful in treatment of schizoaffective and impulse-control disorders
      3) May be used during alcohol withdrawal
      4) Often used to augment effects of neuroleptics, benzodiazepines, antidepressants
   c. Mechanism of action: affects CNS in several ways, but one theory proposes it slows or prevents the "kindling effect" (a process by which repeated exposure to stress can cause abnormal excitability of neurons in limbic system)
   d. Effective plasma level is 6 to 12 μg/mL, onset of action is about 5 to 7 days
   e. Adverse effects: sedation, confusion, dizziness, nausea, vomiting, diarrhea, ataxia, diplopia, rashes (dermatitis, Stevens-Johnson syndrome), hepatitis, agranulocytosis; has potential for teratogenic effects if used in first trimester of pregnancy (spina bifida, craniofacial defects, can lead to developmental delay)
   f. Before treatment: complete blood count (check every 2 weeks for first 2 months, then every 2-4 months), liver enzymes, renal function, pregnancy test, electrolytes, routine history and physical examination, electrocardiography
   g. Carbamazepine induces its own metabolism (gradually decreases level without dose change, therefore dose may need to be increased)

4. Gabapentin (Neurontin)
   a. Common anticonvulsant
   b. Clinical use: not FDA-approved for, but widely used for,

manic and depressive phases of bipolar disorder and for anxiety disorders, panic, and social phobia

c. Mechanism of action: resembles anxiolytics, increases synthesis of GABA, reduces levels of glutamate, it is an amino acid and is not metabolized and is not protein-bound

d. Does not require monitoring of plasma levels

e. Adverse effects: sedation, dizziness, weight gain, nystagmus, edema, it is safe in overdose

5. Lamotrigine (Lamictal)
   a. Common anticonvulsant
   b. Clinical use: bipolar disorder, especially rapid cycling, and manic and depressive phases of bipolar disorder
   c. Mechanism of action: inhibits 5HT reuptake
   d. Does not require monitoring of plasma levels
   e. Adverse effects: blurred vision, dizziness, ataxia, sedation, nausea, vomiting, rashes (including life-threatening dermatologic complications of Stevens-Johnson syndrome or toxic epidermal necrolysis)

6. Topiramate (Topamax)
   a. Common anticonvulsant
   b. Clinical use: not FDA-approved for, but widely used as an adjunct treatment for bipolar disorder
   c. Does not require monitoring of plasma levels
   d. Adverse effects: anorexia, weight loss, nephrolithiasis

F. Stimulants: amphetamine, dextroamphetamine, methylphenidate, modafinil

1. Amphetamine: introduced in 1930s, dextroamphetamine (Dexedrine), combination of amphetamine and dextroamphetamine (Adderall)
   a. Clinical use
      1) Narcolepsy and other sleep disorders, attention-deficit/hyperactivity disorder in children, obesity
      2) Has also been used for depression by augmenting antidepressant effects, neurasthenia, AIDS dementia, encephalopathy from brain injury
   b. Mechanism of action
      1) Causes direct release of dopamine and NE from neurons
      2) Blocks reuptake of catecholamines
      3) Peak plasma levels in 1 to 3 hours
   c. Effects: CNS stimulation, appetite suppression, vasoconstriction, hypothermia, tolerance can develop
   d. Adverse effects: stomach pain, anxiety, irritability, insomnia, tachycardia, arrhythmias, dysphoria, may worsen tics, psychosis, paranoia, delusions, delirium, seizures
   e. Monitor: blood pressure and pulse initially and after changes in dose, weight and height initially and several

times annually
2. Methylphenidate (Concerta, Ritalin): related to amphetamine, but milder stimulant (little or no abuse potential)
3. Modafinil (Provigil): novel stimulant for narcolepsy
4. Drug interactions
   a. Extreme caution if sympathomimetic used with MAOIs
   b. Sympathomimetic used with tricyclic or tetracyclic antidepressants, warfarin, primidone, phenobarbital, phenytoin, or phenylbutazone
      1) Decreased metabolism of these compounds produces increased plasma levels
   c. Sympathomimetics decrease efficacy of many antihypertensive agents, especially guanethidine (Ismelin) and guanethidine-hydrochlorothiazide (Esimil)

G. Psychotherapy and Psychosocial Treatments

1. Behavioral therapy: "change the behavior and feelings will follow"
   a. Goals: change the targeted behavior
   b. Patients: patients with alcohol and drug abuse, eating disorders, anxiety disorders, phobias, and obsessive-compulsive behavior
   c. Techniques: classic conditioning, operant conditioning, positive reinforcers, negative reinforcers, relaxation training, systematic desensitization, flooding, behavioral modification
2. Psychoanalysis
   a. Goals: personality reorganization, resolution of childhood conflicts
   b. Patients: psychoneuroses or mild to moderate personality disorders, high motivation, introspectiveness, able to tolerate frustration and therapeutic regression
   c. Techniques: four or five sessions/week, free association, use of couch, neutrality, analysis of defenses and transference, dream interpretation
   d. Length of treatment: 3 to 6 years or longer
3. Cognitive-behavioral therapy: has evidence-based support
   a. Developed by Albert Ellis and Aaron Beck
   b. Concept: a person's evaluation of a perceived adverse event largely determines the degree and type of emotional state experienced
   c. "Cognitive structures or schemas" shape the way people react and adapt to situations and encounters
   d. Goals: reduce symptomatic distress, enhance interpersonal skills, improve functioning at work and socially
   e. Patients: those with depression, anxiety, mood disorders, phobias, obsessive-compulsive disorder, generalized anxiety, panic disorder, eating disorders, substance abuse
   f. Techniques:

1) Identification of the emotion and how intense it has become (e.g., level of anxiety, depression, or hurt feelings)
2) Assessment of the event that activated these feelings (e.g., the boss embarrassed me in front of my coworkers)
3) Recognition of the patient's interpretation of the adverse event (e.g., "I'll get fired" vs. "it was embarrassing but I'll get through it")
4) Initiation of an intervention from a cognitive, behavioral, and emotional perspective
5) These steps described above use the "Socratic" questioning style
6) Patient must take an active role in the therapy
7) Goal is to restructure the "cognitive triad" (negative view of self, negative interpretation of the event, and negative view of the future)
8) Patient will eventually perceive reality in a less distorted way
   g. Length: one or two sessions/week, usually short-term and structured 3 to 6 months
4. Interpersonal therapy
   a. Harry Stack Sullivan proposed that mental illnesses may be the results of problems within relationships
   b. Goal: improve the patient's interpersonal relationships
   c. Patients: those with depression or personality disorders
   d. Techniques
      1) The "here and now" is emphasized
      2) Encourages patients to identify what problems are affecting their self-esteem and causing issues within their relationships
      3) Therapy lasts about 4 months
5. Supportive psychotherapy
   a. Goal: help patients get through difficult times
   b. Patients: appropriate for entire spectrum of psychiatric disorders
   c. Techniques: therapist functions as healthy, loving parent providing advise, direction, encouragement, praise associated with patient's current problem or situation
   d. Length: weekly sessions, may be brief or long-term
6. Group psychotherapy
   a. Goals: provide hope, help build social skills (often by modeling behavior and role playing), learning through receiving feedback from group members
   b. Patients: myriad of patient types and problems, can be very specific (e.g., Gulf War veterans)
   c. Techniques
      1) Usually led by physician, nurse, or social worker, but group member may be leader
      2) Share problems, give feedback, accountability, pre-

scribed exercises, establishing ground rules for group, resolve conflicts

    d. Length: variable, can be time-limited with specific goal

7. Marital therapy

    a. Goals: to improve the relationship between partners

    b. Patients: two people who are partners and willing to cooperate in the therapeutic process

    c. Techniques

        1) There must be a sense of fairness and impartiality throughout the process

        2) A specific problem is identified

        3) Changes are implemented over time

    d. Length: variable

8. Family therapy

    a. Goals: to improve the relationships within a family

    b. Patients: this often starts when a child with a particular problem is brought in by family members

    c. Techniques

        1) There must be a sense of fairness and impartiality

        2) There must still be respect for parental authority

        3) Parents are given suggestions to influence the child's behavior (such as positive reinforcement rather than criticism)

    d. Length: variable

REFERENCES

About, Inc. [home page on the Internet]. New York: New York Times Company; c2005 [cited 2005 Sept 29]. Psychology: phobias - abnormal fear. - Available from: http://psychology.about.com/library/bl/blphobia_a.htm.

American Psychiatric Association. Diagnostic and statistical manual of mental disorders, fourth edition, text revision. Washington (DC): American Psychiatric Association; 2000.

Andreasen NC, Black DW. Introductory textbook of psychiatry. 3rd ed. Washington (DC): American Psychiatric Publishing; 2001.

Brust JCM. Neurologic complications of substance abuse. Continuum: Lifelong Learning in Neurology. 2004 Oct;10:11-3.

Dewan MJ, Pies RW. The difficult-to-treat psychiatric patient. Washington (DC): American Psychiatric Publishing; 2001.

Dryden W, Mytton J. Four approaches to counselling and psychotherapy. New York: Routledge; 1999.

Ewing JA. Detecting alcoholism: the CAGE questionnaire. JAMA. 1984;252:1905-7.

Fadem B, Simring SS. High-yield psychiatry. 2nd ed. Philadelphia: Williams & Wilkins; 2003.

Ghaemi SN. Bipolar disorder and antidepressants: an ongoing controversy. Primary Psychiatry. 2001;8:28-34.

Hochman MS. Meperidine-associated myoclonus and seizures in long-term hemodialysis patients [letter]. Ann Neurol. 1983;14:593.

Kellner CH, Pritchett JT, Beale MD, Coffey CE. Handbook of ECT. Washington (DC): American Psychiatric Press; 1997.

Koenig HG, George LK, Meador KG, Blazer DG, Ford SM. Religious practices and alcoholism in a southern adult population. Hosp Community Psychiatry. 1992;45:225-31.

McCarron MM, Schulze BW, Thompson GA, Conder MC, Goetz WA. Acute phencyclidine intoxication: incidence of clinical findings in 1,000 cases. Ann Emerg Med. 1981;10:237-42.

Preskorn SH. Clinical pharmacology of SSRI's [monograph on the Internet]. Wichita (KS): Sheldon H. Preskorn, MD; 2005 [cited 2005 Sept 29]. Available from: http://www.preskorn.com/books/ssri_s1.html.

Sadock BJ, Sadock VA. Kaplan and Sadock's pocket handbook of clinical psychiatry. 3rd ed. Philadelphia: Lippincott Williams & Wilkins; 2001.

Sadock BJ, Sadock VA. Kaplan and Sadock's synopsis of psychiatry: behavioral sciences/clinical psychiatry. 9th ed. Philadelphia: Lippincott Williams & Wilkins; 2003.

Sadock BJ, Sadock VA, Jones RM, editors. Kaplan and Sadock's study guide and self-examination review in psychiatry. 7th ed. Philadelphia: Lippincott Williams & Wilkins; 2003.

Stern TA, Herman JB. Massachusetts General Hospital 1000 psychiatry questions and annotated answers. New York: McGraw-Hill; 2004.

Stern TA, Herman JB, editors. Massachusetts General Hospital psychiatry update and board preparation. 2nd ed. New York: McGraw-Hill; 2004.

Strahl NR. Clinical study guide for the oral boards in psychiatry. Washington (DC): American Psychiatric Publishing; 2001.

Tasman A, Kay J, Lieberman JA, editors. Psychiatry: therapeutics. 2nd ed. Chichester (England): John Wiley & Sons; 2003.

QUESTIONS

1. Good prognostic factors in schizophrenia include all the following *except*:
   a. Clouded sensorium
   b. Mood symptoms are absent
   c. Acute onset
   d. Married
   e. Short duration

2. Which of the following subtypes of schizophrenia has the best outcome and course?
   a. Paranoid
   b. Disorganized (hebephrenic)
   c. Catatonic
   d. Undifferentiated
   e. Residual

3. All the following statements are true about schizophrenia *except*:
   a. Lifetime prevalence is about 1%
   b. Males and females have equal frequency of developing schizophrenia
   c. Male age at onset of schizophrenia is generally younger than female age at onset
   d. Psychotic symptoms are thought to be caused by hyperactivity of the dopamine system
   e. Decreased size of the lateral and third ventricles in 10% to 50% of patients

4. Patients with schizoaffective disorder:
   a. Have a suicide rate that approaches 40%
   b. Have a prognosis that is worse than that for patients with schizophrenia
   c. Must have mood symptoms at the same time as psychotic symptoms for the duration of the illness
   d. Can have a good response to lithium
   e. Have a deteriorating course

5. All the following are true about delusional disorder *except*:
   a. Onset is generally in middle age (35-50)
   b. This disorder affects females more often than males
   c. Prevalence approaches 2% in the United States
   d. Jealous delusions are seen more often in men, whereas erotomanic delusions are seen more often in females
   e. These patients often are mistrusting of treatment and providers

6. What percentage of patients with major depression commit suicide?

   a. 5%
   b. 15%
   c. 25%
   d. 30%
   e. 40%

7. The most common mood disorder is:
   a. Bipolar I disorder
   b. Dysthymia
   c. Cyclothymia
   d. Major depressive disorder
   e. Bipolar II disorder

8. Features of generalized anxiety disorder include all the following *except*:
   a. Characteristic feature is "excessive worry"
   b. It has a chronic and fluctuating course
   c. Serotonin has been implicated in the "fight or flight" experience
   d. Major depression is comorbid in over 60% of patients with generalized anxiety disorder
   e. Females suffer from generalized anxiety disorder more often than males

9. In panic disorder, the panic attacks:
   a. Can be due to substances or general medical condition
   b. Can be precipitated only by exposure to a specific feared situation
   c. Usually last for several hours at a time
   d. Can be caused by carbon dioxide hypersensitivity
   e. Can happen only once or be recurrent

10. All the following are true about obsessive-compulsive disorder *except*:
    a. Obsessive-compulsive disorder and Tourette's syndrome have been linked in family studies
    b. Obsessive-compulsive disorder occurs more frequently in patients with head trauma or epilepsy
    c. Patients are ego-syntonic in regard to the illness
    d. Prevalence rate is 2% to 3%
    e. It has been noted that the caudate nuclei are decreased in size

11. In posttraumatic stress disorder, all the following are true *except*:
    a. Risks factors for developing posttraumatic stress disorder include age (very young and very old)

b. Previous psychiatric history does not increase the risk of developing posttraumatic stress disorder

c. Lifetime prevalence of posttraumatic stress disorder is 8%

d. The hypothalamic-pituitary-adrenal axis can be affected by high levels of arousal seen in posttraumatic stress disorder

e. Posttraumatic stress disorder is seen in 80% of rape victims

12. All the following statements are true about alcohol use *except*:

a. "One drink" is 8 oz of wine or 12 oz of beer

b. Women have less aldehyde dehydrogenase in their gastric stomach lining than men

c. Thiamine should be given before administering intravenous fluids with glucose when treating alcoholics

d. CAGE questions can help determine if a person is alcohol dependent

e. Complications of alcoholism include pancreatic cancer

13. A person can experience withdrawal from all the following substances *except*:

a. Alcohol

b. Nicotine

c. Opioids

d. Cannabis

e. Benzodiazepines

14. All the following are true *except*:

a. Duloxetine can be used for depression and diabetic peripheral neuropathic pain

b. Bupropion can be used for depression, smoking cessation, and eating disorders

c. Monoamine oxidase inhibitors and selective serotonin reuptake inhibitors should not be combined because it can lead to serotonin syndrome

d. Selective serotonin reuptake inhibitors are first-line antidepressants and can be used in obsessive-compulsive disorder, posttraumatic stress disorder, eating disorders, generalized anxiety disorders, and other disorders

e. Tricyclic antidepressants can be more effective than selective serotonin reuptake inhibitors for melancholic depression

15. First-line medication treatments for anxiety disorders might include each of the following *except*:

a. Paroxetine

b. Fluvoxamine

c. Venlafaxine

d. Lorazepam

e. Nefazodone

16. Which of the following has been found by most studies to be the most potent selective serotonin reuptake inhibitor (SSRI)?

a. Fluoxetine

b. Paroxetine

c. Citalopram

d. Sertraline

e. Fluvoxamine

17. A 35-year-old woman presented with a 3-year history of various gastrointestinal symptoms, chronic pelvic pain of unclear origin, chronic bilateral upper and lower extremity pain, complaints of diffuse paresthesias, and spells of dizziness. She was evaluated extensively. The examination findings and results of extensive testing were unrevealing. She most likely has:

a. Conversion disorder

b. Factitious disorder

c. Somatization disorder

d. Body dysmorphic disorder

e. Adjustment disorder

ANSWERS

1. Answer: b.
Mood symptoms are actually associated with better prognosis in schizophrenia. Good prognostic factors include acute onset, short duration, no previous psychiatric history, presence of mood symptoms, clouded sensorium, no symptoms of obsessive-compulsive disorder, no assaultiveness, good premorbid functioning, married, good psychosexual functioning, normal neurologic findings, no brain abnormalities, higher socioeconomic class, no family history of schizophrenia

2. Answer: a.
Paranoid schizophrenics most often have the best outcome and course compared with other subtypes. The patients are more likely to be older when affected, tend to marry and have children, and have better social support

3. Answer: e.
The lateral and third ventricles are enlarged in 10% to 50% of schizophrenic patients. Lifetime prevalence is 1%, and males = females in frequency. Onset in males is usually around age 21 and for females, about age 27. Excess dopamine has been thought to cause psychotic symptoms.

4. Answer: d.
Patients with schizoaffective disorder may be treated with antipsychotics, selective serotonin reuptake inhibitors, benzodiazepines, lithium, anticonvulsants, and electroconvulsive therapy with good benefit. These patients have a 10% suicide rate. Their prognosis is better than that for patients with schizophrenia but worse than that for those with major depression. They tend to have a nondeteriorating course.

5. Answer: c.
The prevalence of delusional disorder is only 0.03%. It is seen more often in females than males. Onset is usually in middle age (35-50), with a mean age of about 40. Jealous delusions are seen more frequently in men and erotomanic delusions, more frequently in females. The most common delusion for all is the persecutory type. Treatment is difficult because the patients strongly deny that anything is wrong and have difficulty trusting the treatment and providers.

6. Answer: b.
Suicide rate for depressed patients is 10% to 15%, and 50% to 87% of suicide completers had been depressed before committing suicide. Females attempt suicide more frequently, but males tend to complete suicide more often.

7. Answer: d.
Major depressive disorder has a lifetime prevalence of 10% to 20% for women and 5% to 12% for men. Bipolar I disorder has lifetime prevalence of 1.0%, dysthymia 3%, cyclothymia 0.4% to 1.0%, and bipolar II 0.5%.

8. Answer: c.
Norepinephrine is associated with "fight or flight" experience. Serotonin is also important in the pathophysiology of anxiety disorders. Generalized anxiety disorder has been thought of as having "excessive worry" as a key characteristic feature. The course is chronic and fluctuating in severity, and 33% of the patients eventually develop panic disorder. Females have generalized anxiety disorder more frequently than males, and the lifetime prevalence is 4% to 7%.

9. Answer: d.
Panic disorder DSM-IV-TR criteria specify that the person must have recurrent panic attacks, that the attacks are not caused by substance use or a general medical problem, and that there has been at least 1 month of concern or worry about having another attack. Panic attacks are thought to be related to increased catecholamine levels and abnormality of the locus ceruleus; they can be caused by carbon dioxide hypersensitivity, which can be thought of as triggering the "false suffocation alarm." The panic trigger does not have to be a specific feared situation, and in fact, there are usually no precipitators of the panic episode.

10. Answer: c.
There is thought to be a familial and perhaps genetic relationship between Tourette's syndrome and obsessive-compulsive disorder. Obsessive-compulsive disorder is noted to occur more frequently in patients who have suffered head trauma, have epilepsy, Sydenham's chorea, or Huntington's disease. Patients with obsessive-compulsive disorder are ego-dystonic, however, in regard to their illness. The prevalence rate is 2% to 3%, and the caudate nuclei have been noted to be decreased in size bilaterally in patients with obsessive-compulsive disorder.

11. Answer: b.
A previous psychiatric history does increase the risk for developing posttraumatic stress disorder. The very young and the very old often have difficulties with traumatic events and more often develop posttraumatic stress disorder than persons of other ages. The prevalence for posttraumatic stress disorder is 8%, but it is noted that 80% of rape victims and 30% of

Vietnam veterans experience(d) posttraumatic stress disorder. The hypothalamic-pituitary-adrenal axis is affected by the high levels of arousal, and increased levels of epinephrine are seen in veterans with posttraumatic stress disorder and in sexually abused girls. Noradrenergic and serotonergic pathways are implicated.

12. Answer: a.
One drink is considered to be 12 g of pure alcohol, 1.5 oz of 80-proof, 5 oz of wine, or 12 oz of beer or wine cooler. Women do have less aldehyde dehydrogenase in the stomach lining, so they are at greater risk for intoxication with even a small amount of alcohol. It is important to give thiamine before administering any intravenous fluids with glucose to alcoholics to prevent Wernicke's encephalopathy. The CAGE questions can detect alcohol dependence almost 100% if all four questions are answered positively. Complications of alcoholism include cirrhosis of the liver, throat cancer, liver cancer, pancreatic cancer, hypothermia, respiratory depression, coma, death, reflux, dementia, and many others.

13. Answer: d.
Withdrawal symptoms can be seen with the use of alcohol, amphetamine, cocaine, nicotine, opioids, sedatives. Withdrawal is not seen with use of cannabis, hallucinogens, inhalants, or phencyclidine.

14. Answer: b.
Bupropion is contraindicated for use in eating disorders because the risk for seizures increases. Duloxetine is a relatively new antidepressant, with indications for depression and diabetic peripheral neuropathic pain. Serotonin syndrome can be caused by the combination of any agents that increase serotonin levels in the central nervous system. Selective serotonin reuptake inhibitors are first-line antidepressants, with a myriad of indications. Tricyclic antidepressants can be more helpful than selective serotonin reuptake inhibitors for severe or melancholic depression and can also be used for insomnia, chronic pain, obsessive-compulsive disorder, panic, and anxiety.

15. Answer: d.
Antidepressants have become first-line treatments for anxiety disorders even though they take longer to work than benzodiazepines. They are much easy to taper and discontinue than benzodiazepines and have fewer adverse effects.

16. Answer: b.
Fluoxetine has been found to have the longest half-life of the SSRIs, making it less necessary to slowly taper this medication. Fluoxetine and fluvoxamine are considered to be the SSRIs with the least complaints of sexual side effects. Both fluvoxamine and paroxetine have no active metabolites and shorter half-lives, so are more likely to cause a discontinuation syndrome when treatment with them is stopped, so slow tapers are recommended. Citalopram has been found to be the most selective of the SSRIs, and paroxetine has been found to be most potent of the SSRIs.

17. Answer: c.
Conversion disorder is classically described as a sudden loss of function without clear medical explanation. Patients may be indifferent to the loss of function (*la belle indifférence*) and may have observed someone with real disease. Factitious disorder is defined as intentional feigning of physical or psychologic signs or symptoms, with motivation of assuming the sick role. Body dysmorphic disorder (although it sometimes may be considered a somatization disorder) is classically described as abnormal preoccupation with minimal (or absent) flaws in physical appearance, significantly impairing the individual's life. This is in contrast to the classic definition of somatization disorder, which is a chronic condition in which there are numerous physical complaints, often lasting for years and resulting in substantial impairment.

Nima Mowzoon, M.D.

I. ANATOMY OF CEREBRAL CORTEX (FIG. 7-1)

A. Anatomic Classification

1. Idiotypic primary cortex (sensory or motor, e.g., primary visual cortex)
   a. Initial cortical processing of afferent sensory input or source of primary motor efferents
   b. Modality-specific
   c. Directly connected with association cortices and subcortical modulating nuclei (e.g., basal ganglia, thalamus)
2. Homotypic unimodal association cortex
   a. Usually anatomically close to respective primary cortex; modulates the function of primary cortex
   b. Modality-specific
   c. Directly connected not only to respective primary cortex but also with heteromodal association cortex (convergence of pathways) and subcortical modulating nuclei (e.g., basal ganglia, thalamus)
3. Homotypic heteromodal (multimodal) association cortex
   a. Directly connected with each other and unimodal association cortices (including the limbic and paralimbic regions)
   b. Two major areas
      1) Anterior heteromodal association area (prefrontal cortex): concerned with planning of movements and executive functions
      2) Posterior heteromodal association area (parietotemporal

areas, junction between parietal, temporal, and occipital lobes): visuospatial perception and language
4. Limbic and paralimbic cortex
   a. Corticoid areas: basal forebrain (primitive organization without discernable lamination in some areas; least differentiated)
      1) Amygdala complex
      2) Septal nuclei
      3) Substantia innominata (basal nucleus of Meynert)
   b. Allocortex
      1) Hippocampal complex and piriform or primary olfactory cortex (paleocortex)
      2) One or two bands of neurons arranged in external and internal pyramidal layers
   c. Mesocortex (paralimbic structures)
      1) Parahippocampal region
      2) Orbitofrontal cortex
      3) Temporal pole
      4) Insula
      5) Cingulate cortex

B. Histology

1. Cell types
   a. Pyramidal cells
      1) Pyramidal-shaped cells with apical dendrites extending toward cortical surface
      2) "Projection neurons" involved in transmitting signals to other cortical, subcortical, or spinal areas
      3) Located mainly in layers III, V, and VI
      4) The neurotransmitter is glutamate (excitatory)
   b. Stellate cells
      1) Star-shaped neurons with dendritic extensions in all directions
      2) Found in all layers, but most common in layer IV
      3) Are local inhibitory interneurons; use γ-aminobutyric acid (GABA)
   c. Fusiform cells
      1) Found primarily in layer VI

Primary cortices do not communicate directly with each other

Heteromodal areas are responsible for integration of cortical processes and input from unimodal association areas, which in turn receive input from primary cortices

---

A

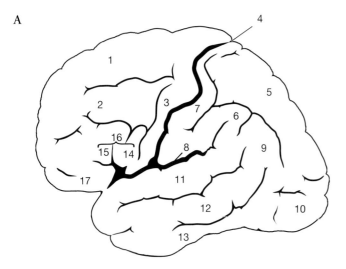

B

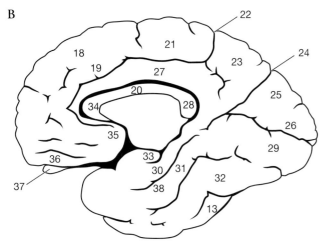

Fig. 7-1. *A*, Lateral and, *B*, midsagittal views of the cerebral hemispheres. 1, Superior frontal gyrus; 2, middle frontal gyrus; 3, precentral gyrus; 4, central (Rolandic) sulcus; 5, superior parietal lobule; 6, supramarginal gyrus; 7, postcentral gyrus; 8, sylvian fissure; 9, angular gyrus; 10, occipital gyri; 11, superior temporal gyrus; 12, middle temporal gyrus; 13, inferior temporal gyrus; 14, opercular lobule; 15, triangular gyrus; 16, inferior frontal gyrus (= 14 + 15); 17, orbitofrontal gyrus; 18, superior frontal gyrus; 19, cingulate sulcus; 20, corpus callosum; 21, paracentral lobule; 22, marginal sulcus; 23, precuneus; 24, parieto-occipital fissure; 25, cuneus; 26, calcarine fissure; 27, cingulate gyrus; 28, splenium of corpus callosum; 29, lingual gyrus; 30, parahippocampal gyrus; 31, medial occipitotemporal gyrus; 32, lateral occipitotemporal gyrus; 33, uncus; 34, genu of corpus callosum; 35, subcallosal gyrus; 36, gyrus rectus; 37, olfactory bulb; 38, collateral sulcus. (Modified from Brazis PW, Masdeu JC, Biller J. Localization in clinical neurology. 4th ed. Philadelphia: Lippincott Williams & Wilkins; 2001. p. 453-521. Used with permission.)

2) Long dendritic processes extend toward cortical surface
3) Axons project primarily to thalamus
2. Horizontal cortical organization
  a. Neocortex (primary, unimodal, and heteromodal areas) is organized in six layers
    1) Layers I to IV receive afferents
    2) Layer V projects to spinal cord, brainstem, and basal ganglia
    3) Layer VI projects to thalamus
    4) Corticocortical connections: mainly from layers II and III of primary cortices to layers V and VI of association cortices
  b. Layer I—molecular (plexiform) layer: consists mainly of local interneurons and apical dendrites of pyramidal cells in deeper layer
  c. Layer II—external granular layer
    1) Stellate cells: axons project to deeper cortical layers
    2) Pyramidal cells: axons project to contralateral cortex as commissural fibers
  d. Layer III—external pyramidal layer: pyramidal cells with projections to ipsilateral cortices (association fibers) or contralateral hemisphere (commissural fibers)
  e. Layer IV—internal granular layer
    1) Consists mainly of stellate cells
    2) Receives afferent glutaminergic input from thalamus
    3) Prominent layer in primary sensory cortices
  f. Layer V—internal pyramidal layer
    1) Pyramidal cells: axons project to basal ganglia, brainstem, spinal cord, and contralateral cortex (commissural fibers)
    2) Prominent layer in primary motor cortex, which contains giant pyramidal cells of Betz
  g. Layer VI—multiform layer: pyramidal cells with projections to thalamus and layer IV
3. Vertical (columnar) cortical organization
  a. Each column is a functional unit of cortex
  b. Specificity of connection with target cells is maintained and afferent feedback from the same target is received
  c. Layer IV is the main input layer in each column
  d. Afferents from a specific group of neurons in thalamus project to a designated cortical column (layer IV): the organizational specificity of neuronal columns is mirrored in subcortical modulating nuclei (e.g., thalamus, basal ganglia)
4. Intercortical connections
  a. Association fibers: connection between different cortices in same hemisphere
    1) U-fibers (short association fibers)
    2) Superior longitudinal fasciculus

3) Cingulum (part of the Papez circuit)

4) Inferior longitudinal fasciculus

5) Uncinate fasciculus

b. Commissural fibers: connection between the two cerebral hemispheres

1) Corpus callosum

2) Anterior commissure

3) Posterior commissure

4) Hippocampal commissure

c. Projection fibers: corticosubcortical fibers

C. Cortical Localization

1. Frontal lobe

a. Primary motor cortex (Brodmann area 4, M I)

1) Type: idiotypic primary cortex

2) Voluntary discrete movements involving direct projections to spinal cord anterior horn cells and subsequent direct activation of a motor unit

3) Lesion: contralateral pattern of upper motor neuron weakness

a) Acute lesion: hypotonic and flaccid

b) Chronic lesion: spastic, increased reflexes

4) Stimulation or epileptic activity: partial motor seizures with spread (jacksonian march) reflect somatotopic organization of the area

b. Premotor areas (area 6, M II)

1) Type: homotypic unimodal cortex

2) All areas project to primary motor cortex and spinal cord

3) All receive projections from parietal cortex: parieto-premotor pathways are important in goal-directed movements (reaching and grasping)

4) Divisions

a) Ventral and dorsolateral premotor cortex

i) Located on lateral aspect of frontal lobe anterior to M I

ii) Input from parietal lobe and medial premotor areas

iii) Responsible for initiating motor plans in response to sensory stimuli (e.g., stopping at a red light)

iv) Involved in learning to associate a particular sensory stimulus with a particular motor movement (associative learning)

b) Supplementary motor cortex (medial premotor area, area 6, M II)

i) Located on medial aspect of frontal lobe anterior to M I

ii) Input from ipsilateral parietal lobe and prefrontal "presupplementary area"

iii) Presupplementary area is responsible for learning

sequences of a motor plan and supplementary motor cortex is responsible for producing the motor sequence already learned—does *not* initiate motor plans in response to sensory stimuli as the lateral premotor regions do

iv) Blood flow to supplementary motor cortex increases when one is thinking about or planning a movement

v) Contains complete bilateral somatotopic representation of the body

vi) Responsible for coordinating and advance planning of movements on the two sides of the body

vii) Stimulation/epileptic activity: tonic abduction and external rotation/elevation of the contralateral arm with forced head turn toward elevated arm (fencing posture)

c. Frontal eye fields (homotypic unimodal cortex): voluntary conjugate horizontal eye movements (lesion: transient paralysis of contralateral gaze)

d. Broca's area

1) Receives connections from Wernicke's area via arcuate fasciculus

2) Projects to premotor areas involved in motor programs required for speech production

3) Lesion: nonfluent aphasia, typically involving deficits in both language production and motor speech outputs

2. Prefrontal lobe

a. Type: homotypic heteromodal cortex (all three regions discussed below)

b. Dorsolateral prefrontal cortex

1) Located on convexity of the gyri anterior to areas 8 and 45

2) Interconnects with other heteromodal regions, basal ganglia, and dorsomedial thalamus

3) Important for executive functions, planning, judgment, problem-solving

4) Lesion: poor abstract thought, poor planning, poor judgment and problem solving, psychomotor retardation, motor impersistance and perseveration, poor executive functioning, and dysexecutive syndrome

c. Orbitofrontal cortex

1) Located on inferior surface of frontal lobes and includes the frontal poles

2) Widespread interconnection with limbic system and basal ganglia

3) Responsible for emotional and visceral activities, social behavior, and inhibition of inappropriate behavior in a particular social context as well as judgment

4) Responsible for conscious perception of smell:

> **Lesions of Prefrontal Cortex**
>
> Dorsolateral: poor executive functions, planning, judgment, and problem solving
>
> Orbitofrontal: disinhibition, impulsive behavior, poor judgment and insight
>
> Medial frontal and anterior cingulate
>> Abulia, indifference, poor speech output, impaired initiation of a behavior or motor movement with reduced spontaneous movements
>> Associated with urinary incontinence and gait disturbance

               receives input from piriform cortex via thalamic relay

    5) Impairment: disinhibited, impulsive behavior; poor judgment and insight; emotional lability; euphoria and excessive and inappropriate laughter and jocular affect, especially with right hemispheric lesions; speech apraxia; environmental dependency syndrome with utilization; perseveration; hyperorality; hypersexuality

    6) Impairment also associated with obsessive-compulsive behavior

    7) Lesions of orbitofrontal cortex
       a) Meningioma: commonly involving the sphenoid wing or olfactory groove
       b) Closed head injury: usually affecting orbitofrontal and anterior temporal areas because of the irregular surface of the anterior and middle cranial fossae

    8) Stimulation/epileptic activity
       a) Motor and gestural automatisms that may be complex (bicycling, walking around the room)
       b) Olfactory hallucinations and forced thinking with anterior frontopolar focus

  d. Mesial frontal cortex and anterior cingulate cortex
    1) Interconnections with limbic system (especially amygdala)
    2) Important role in initiation, motivation, and goal-oriented behavior
    3) Impairment: abulia, indifference, poor speech output, impaired initiation of a behavior or motor movement with reduced spontaneous movements; associated with urinary incontinence and gait disturbance
    4) With severe impairment: akinetic mutism (no spontaneous behavior)
    5) Anterior cerebral artery distribution strokes or ruptured anterior communicating artery aneurysms can selectively involve mesial frontal structures
    6) Stimulation/epileptic activity: complex motor and gestural automatisms

  e. Wisconsin Card Sorting Test
    1) Sensitive measure of function of prefrontal cortex
    2) The subject is asked to sort the cards according to a certain perceptual attribute of a visual stimulus (e.g., color, form, number) and, then, challenges the subject to shift cognitive sets without warning
    3) Patients with frontal lobe lesions have difficulty with this task because of poor cognitive flexibility and perseveration)

3. Parietal lobe
  a. Primary somatosensory cortex (S I, postcentral gyrus): idiotypic primary cortex
  b. Secondary somatosensory cortex (S II) on the parietal operculum (on superior lip of sylvian fissure): homotypic unimodal cortex
    1) Direct input from thalamus and postcentral gyrus (S I)
    2) Bilateral receptive fields (mostly contralateral), receives and integrates information from both sides of the body
    3) Provides somatosensory input to motor cortex
    4) Projections to limbic system: important for tactile learning
  c. Dorsal M pathway: occipitoparietal visuospatial pathway responsible for visuomotor tasks (see below)
  d. Impairment
    1) Lesion of primary somatosensory cortex (S I): primary somatosensory deficits (e.g., touch, vibration, joint position, stimulus localization), sparing pain and temperature sensations, which are projected to second somatosensory cortex (S II)
    2) Lesion of S II at parietal operculum: pseudothalamic syndrome
       a) Impairment of pain and temperature (may have complete loss of elementary sensory modalities)
       b) Syndrome of delayed pain and paresthesias, as may occur sometimes with thalamic infarcts
    3) Parietal somatosensory association cortices
       a) Complex somatosensory functions
       b) Lesions produce "cortical sensory deficits" (e.g., two-point discrimination, graphesthesia, stereognosis, and recognition of bilateral simultaneous stimulation)
    4) Impairment of nondominant hemisphere: anosognosia, dressing apraxia, geographic agnosia, constructional apraxia, hemispatial sensory neglect

5) Lesions of dominant hemisphere: finger agnosia, acalculia, agraphia, alexia, aphasia (primarily conduction aphasia and/or transcortical sensory aphasia), right-left disorientation, conduction apraxia

    a) Angular gyrus syndrome (lesion of angular gyrus, heteromodal cortex): anomia, alexia, constructional difficulties, acalculia, dysgraphia, finger anomia, right-left disorientation (aphasia may be present if lesion extends to superior temporal gyrus and Wernicke's area)

    b) Gerstmann's syndrome: acalculia, dysgraphia, finger anomia, right-left disorientation

6) Lower homonymous quadrantanopia from damage to optic radiations (if lesion extends deep enough)

7) Balint's syndrome: optic ataxia, ocular apraxia, simultanagnosia (bilateral lesions)

8) Reduced slow phase of optokinetic nystagmus

4. Temporal lobe

  a. Primary auditory cortex (idiotypic primary cortex)

    1) Located on dorsomedial aspect of superior temporal gyrus

    2) Has a well-defined tonotopic map reflecting cochlear organization

    3) Unilateral lesions do not cause hearing loss, but subject may have difficulty localizing sound stimuli in space, especially from the opposite side

  b. Auditory association cortex (homotypic unimodal cortex): no well-defined tonotopic map

  c. Wernicke's area

  d. Middle and inferior temporal lobes: memory and learning

  e. Limbic area: inferior and medial temporal areas

  f. Uncus receives olfactory and gustatory input

  g. Subcortical occipitotemporal projections and optic radiations (Meyer's loop)

  h. Insular cortex: taste area II (taste area I is on dorsal aspect of lateral sulcus near insular cortex)

  i. Impairment

    1) Superior homonymous quadrantanopia

    2) Cortical hearing loss with bilateral temporal (or subcortical) lesions

    3) Auditory agnosia with lesions of bilateral, more than unilateral, temporal cortex (and/or corresponding subcortical areas): difficulty recognizing different sounds (nonverbal auditory agnosias may also result from right-sided lesions)

    4) Dysacusis: perception of particular sounds as unpleasant

    5) Pure word deafness (often bilateral lesions)

      a) A verbal auditory agnosia (due to auditory-verbal disconnection)

      b) Patients can hear and react to environmental auditory cues and can understand written language, but are unable to understand spoken language

    6) Wernicke's aphasia (dominant lesions)

    7) Klüver-Bucy syndrome: bilateral anterior temporal lobe lesions (see below)

    8) Amnesia

      a) Nondominant hemisphere: amnesia for nonverbal, visuospatial information

      b) Dominant hemisphere: amnesia for verbal information)

    9) Amusia

      a) Example of nonverbal auditory agnosia

      b) Difficulty with recognition of songs, primarily because of disturbance of recognition of different characteristics of music composition (e.g., rhythm, pitch, tone) due to right temporal lobe lesions

      c) Left temporal lobe lesions: not true amusia, patient has difficulty understanding lyrics

      d) Left temporal lobe lesions in musicians who analyze different aspects of music composition may produce some degree of amusia

    10) Ageusia (lack of taste): possibly occurs with bilateral lesions of insular cortex

    11) Semantic dementia: dominant anterior temporal lobe is site of word meaning (object-word associations)

    12) Prosopagnosia (defined below)

      a) Lesion in posteroinferior temporo-occipital region

      b) Usually bilateral lesions, but nondominant hemisphere lesion may be sufficient

  j. Stimulation/epileptic phenomena

    1) Complex visual hallucinations of people, animals, etc. from a posterior temporal lobe epileptic focus

    2) Auditory hallucinations

    3) Olfactory hallucinations (especially unpleasant odor, "uncinate fits"), gustatory hallucinations, epigastric rising sensation, intense fear (or pleasure), usually associated with alteration of consciousness and associated with complex partial seizures arising from medial temporal lobe

    4) Alternation of memory

      a) Déjà vu: sensation of familiarity with a previously unfamiliar experience, place, or event

      b) Déjà entendu: sensation of familiarity with a previously unfamiliar auditory experience (e.g., sound, music, speech, or narrative)

      c) Jamais vu: sensation of unfamiliarity with a previously familiar experience, place, or event

      d) Jamais entendu: sensation of unfamiliarity with a previously familiar auditory experience

5) Palinopsia
   a) Recurrence of an image no longer present in visual field
   b) May occur with posterior temporo-occipital epileptic focus
6) Automatisms are associated with the complex partial seizures arising from, or spreading to, mesial temporal lobe
7) Postictal cough

5. Occipital lobe
   a. Primary visual (striate) cortex (V1)
      1) Type: idiotypic primary cortex (area 17)
      2) Located along the banks of calcarine fissure
      3) Layer IV
         a) Receives the majority of input from lateral geniculate nucleus
         b) Projects primarily to layers II and III, which then project to association cortices
      4) Projections to superficial layer of superior colliculus and pulvinar: responsible for production of saccades and rapid shifting of gaze to another point in the visual field in response to a novel stimulus
         a) Other sensory cortices project to deep layers of superior colliculus
         b) Superior colliculus acts as a sensory integration center
         c) Novel visual stimuli
            i) Retinal ganglion cells and primary visual cortex project to superior colliculus (e.g., moving vehicle entering the far right visual field)
            ii) Other sensory input (e.g., auditory—projections from corresponding primary sensory [auditory] cortex) to deep layers of superior colliculus
            iii) Superior colliculus: integrated sensory response to direct gaze toward novel stimuli
      5) Occipital pole: central (macular) vision
      6) More anterior portions of calcarine cortex: peripheral vision
      7) Impairment
         a) Homonymous hemianopsia: may or may not spare macular area (vascular lesions often spare the macula because of dual blood supply)
         b) Anton's syndrome: bilateral lesions of medial occipital lobe (usually acute onset) cause cortical blindness associated with denial of the deficit, of which the patient is unaware, and confabulation
      8) Stimulation/epileptic phenomena
         a) Simple elementary visual hallucinations, primarily geometric shapes and patterns (usually bright, colorful, positive symptoms, but may be negative

symptoms such as amaurosis, scotoma, or visual field defects)
         b) Eye deviation, nystagmoid eye movements

Important Cortical Syndromes

Angular gyrus syndrome
   Dominant angular gyrus lesion
   Anomia, alexia, constructional difficulties, acalculia, dysgraphia, finger anomia, right-left disorientation ± aphasia

Gerstmann's syndrome
   Dominant angular gyrus lesion
   Acalculia, dysgraphia, finger anomia, right-left disorientation

Anton's syndrome
   Bilateral medial occipital lobe lesion
   Cortical blindness associated with denial of the deficit, for which the patient is unaware, and confabulation

Balint's syndrome
   Lesion involves occipitotemporal pathways bilaterally, often seen with Alzheimer's disease
   Optic ataxia, ocular apraxia, simultanagnosia

Klüver-Bucy syndrome
   Bilateral anterior temporal lobe lesion
   Hyperorality and oral exploratory behavior, altered eating habits, weight gain, emotional blunting, blunting of response to fear and aggression, and altered sexual activity (hyposexuality > hypersexuality)

Fregoli syndrome
   Belief that the strangers are identified by the patient as familiar
   Usually seen in context of dementia

Capgras' syndrome
   Belief that a family member is an imposter
   Usually associated with paranoid delusions in the context of dementia

Ganser syndrome
   "Syndrome of approximate answers"; answers are consistently nearly correct but not correct
   Usually seen in context of psychiatric disease and malingering but may also be seen in degenerative dementias

Charcot-Wilbrand syndrome
   Impaired ability to produce an internal image of a named object

b. Visual association areas (peristriate cortices)
   1) Type: homotypic unimodal cortex
   2) Located in the peristriate occipital areas (areas 18 and 19) and middle and inferior temporal gyri (areas 20, 21, 37)
   3) Synthesis of visual input including perception of different aspects of visual input as well as perception of motion and integration with other sensory modalities
   4) Parallel pathways: projections to parietal and temporal lobes
   5) Dorsal M pathway ("where pathway") (Fig. 7-2)
      a) Originates in M cells of retina that project to magnocellular portion of lateral geniculate nucleus
      b) Follows dorsal pathway to middle temporal (MT) and medial superior temporal (MST) areas to reach the posterior parietal area
         i) MT and MST were originally defined in monkey brains; the anatomic correlate in human brain is primarily the junction of occipital, parietal, and temporal lobes
         ii) Bilateral lesions of MT can cause motion agnosia (akinetopsia), inability to perceive motion
      c) M cells do not respond to change in color contrast, but MT neurons are sensitive to color analyzed primarily in the P pathway
      d) M pathway carries information on perception of depth, analysis of motion, and spatial orientation ("where") of a particular visual input
      e) Important for reaching and grasping (visuomotor tasks, transmits information about the location of an object in space): impairment causes optic ataxia (impaired visually guided reaching and grasping)
      f) Important role in shifting direction of gaze in response to visual stimuli: impairment causes ocular apraxia
      g) Important for understanding the meaning of an image as a whole: impairment results in simultanagnosia while perception of different components of the object remains intact
      h) Balint's syndrome: the combination of optic ataxia, ocular apraxia, and simultanagnosia (usually occurs with bilateral lesions)
      i) Other signs of impairment: abnormal depth perception, unilateral or bilateral inferior quadrantanopia, abnormal slow component of optokinetic nystagmus
   6) Ventral P pathway ("what pathway," Fig. 7-2)
      a) Originates in P cells in retina that project to parvocellular portion of lateral geniculate nucleus

   b) Follows the ventral pathway to inferior temporal cortex
   c) Concerned primarily with perception of form and color; important in recognition of faces and objects and pattern identification
   d) P cells do respond to changes in color contrast
   e) Impairment of ventral P pathway can cause the following:
      i) Aperceptive visual agnosia: cannot recognize objects by visual presentation or draw the objects (cannot perceive the objects); lesions usually involve occipital or bilateral occipitotemporal projections; this is in contrast to associative visual agnosia in which perception is intact and patient can draw the object but is unable to visually recognize the object (the latter disturbance may be seen in lesions involving the posterior parietal area, sparing the cortices responsible for perception)
      ii) Achromatopsia: cortical color blindness occurring with lesions of inferior occipitotemporal

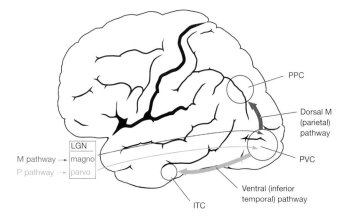

Fig. 7-2. The dorsal M (parietal) pathway, also called the "where pathway," projects from primary visual cortex (PVC) to the posterior parietal cortex (PPC) responsible for visuomotor tasks and perception of depth, analysis of motion, and spatial orientation ("where") of a particular visual input. The M pathway originates in M cells in the retina, which project to the magnocellular portion of the lateral geniculate nucleus (LGN). The ventral P (inferior temporal) pathway, also called the "what pathway," projects from primary visual cortex to the inferior temporal gyrus cortex (ITC) responsible for perception of form and color and important in recognition of faces and objects and pattern identification. The P pathway originates in P cells in the retina, which project to the parvocellular portion of the lateral geniculate nucleus.

projections in the P pathway (nondominant hemisphere or bilateral) and accompanied by a superior quadrantanopia because the lesion involves inferior striate cortex (inferior to the calcarine sulcus) or inferior temporal projections

   iii) Color agnosia: patient can read color plates but cannot name colors; intact knowledge of colors (e.g., patient knows that the color of sky is blue)

   iv) Prosopagnosia: difficulty recognizing familiar faces and objects, lesion involves occipitotemporal areas unilaterally (right-sided) or bilaterally affecting fusiform gyri

   v) Difficulty revisualizing the characteristics and appearance of objects and people

   vi) Unilateral or bilateral superior quadrantanopia

II. Consciousness and Attention

A. Definition: (arousal, attention, and awareness of self and the environment)

B. Basic Anatomy of Consciousness

1. Ascending reticular activating system
   a. Brainstem reticular formation: complex aggregates of medium-sized neurons, most distinctive organization is in medulla and caudal pons
   b. Neurons have long dendrites generally radiating perpendicular to brainstem tegmentum
   c. Receives extensive input from major somatic and sensory pathways, including cerebral cortex, for modulation of activity
   d. Projects to cerebral cortex directly or via thalamic relay to modulate cortical activity
   e. Interconnections between thalamus and cerebral cortex (cortico-thalamo-cortical loops) are important for coordinating cortical activity and processing sensory input
   f. Midbrain reticular formation most important for arousal
      1) Projections to basal forebrain and diencephalon are the anatomic substrate for arousal
      2) Lesion may cause alpha coma
   g. Three functional divisions
      1) Efferents to thalamic reticular nucleus (which then sends inhibitory projections to other thalamic nuclei)
      2) Efferents to hypothalamus and basal forebrain
      3) Diffuse cortical projections, mainly from raphe nuclei (serotonergic) and locus ceruleus (noradrenergic)
   h. Three anatomic divisions
      1) Midline (raphe)
      2) Lateral (mainly receives afferent input)
      3) Medial (mainly responsible for efferent output)
   i. Neurochemically defined divisions
      1) Cholinergic neurons
         a) Basal forebrain cholinergic neurons: important in attention, regulation of behavior, learning, memory
         b) Mesopontine tegmentum cholinergic neurons: projections to thalamus and brainstem; important in regulation of arousal and REM sleep
      2) Serotonergic neurons
         a) Located in raphe nuclei of brainstem midline
         b) Reduced firing rate with transition from awake state to sleep
      3) Noradrenergic neurons
         a) Located in pons and medulla
         b) Largest group is in locus ceruleus (in pons)
         c) Responsible for regulation of arousal

Achromatopsia

Cortical color blindness

Lesions of the occipital lobe inferior to the calcarine sulcus, essentially involving the inferior occipitotemporal projections, produce a superior visual field defect and loss of color vision in the preserved inferior visual field (color perception of both the superior and inferior visual fields are affected, but the superior visual field defect masks the achromatopsia of the superior field)

Prosopagnosia

Patients fail to identify faces and objects (the latter is more difficult when there are many members in a particular category)

Identification of a unique object (e.g., "my car") is particularly difficult

Visual identification of famous individuals and those familiar to the patient is difficult, and patients may use other cues, such as voice or a unique physical characteristic, to identify the person

No difficulty identifying sex, age, and emotional state

Lesion localizes to the right fusiform gyrus or, more commonly, to fusiform gyri bilaterally

d) Responsible for global release of norepinephrine, which modulates and enhances arousal

e) Neurons of locus ceruleus increase firing in response to presentation of stimuli

 i) Selective phasic activation for focused selective attention

 ii) High persistent activation associated with distractibility and increased emotional reactivity

 4) Histaminergic neurons

2. Thalamus

a. Relay neurons: reciprocal connections with cerebral cortex

b. Reticular nucleus: local inhibitory projections to mainly other thalamic nuclei

3. Basal forebrain

a. Includes nucleus basalis (of Meynert) and septal nuclei

b. Cholinergic neurons project diffusely to cerebral cortex

4. Cerebral cortex: diffuse localization

C. Anatomy of Attention

1. Inferior posterior parietal cortex and the primary and association sensory cortices are important for perception of a novel stimulus and initiation of a response to the stimulus

a. Superior colliculus, pulvinar, and parietal lobe have extensive connections with the frontal eye fields: all important for perception of a novel visual stimulus

b. Sensory cortices selectively inhibit the thalamic nucleus reticularis and reduce the inhibitory effect of this nucleus on other thalamic nuclei, promoting thalamic relay of sensory input

2. Prefrontal cortex (especially mesial frontal area), frontal eye fields, and anterior cingulate cortex are responsible for executing spatial attention and selectively focusing attention on the novel stimulus (while inhibiting attention to the other, less important stimuli in the environment) as well as nonspatial attention

a. Lesion can cause nonspatial inattention: motor and verbal impersistence, perseveration, and akinetic mutism with severe involvement of the mesial frontal lobes bilaterally or a diffuse cortical process

3. Striatum (especially caudate)

a. Projects to prefrontal areas and is an important modulator of prefrontal function

b. Lesion of caudate or frontostriatal projections: apathy and disinhibition (unilateral or bilateral)

4. Primary and association sensory cortices

5. Thalamus and ascending reticular activating system promote arousal and are important in maintenance of consciousness

D. Dysfunction of Attention

1. Diffuse inattention

a. Acute confusional state (i.e., delirium)

b. Chronic dysfunction of attention and memory as a confabulatory state (e.g., Korsakoff's syndrome)

c. Depression or other psychiatric disease

d. Subcortical dementia—global inattention associated with a "frontal-dysexecutive syndrome" and possibly other frontal lobe features: may be caused by involvement of striatofrontal projections and other subcortical pathways as in normal-pressure hydrocephalus, Binswanger's disease, or CADASIL (cerebral autosomal dominant arteriopathy with subcortical infarcts and leukoencephalopathy)

2. Unilateral inattention

a. Unilateral signs: spatial sensory neglect (most sensitive exam is with bilateral simultaneous stimuli), hemiakinesia (motor neglect), anosognosia (unawareness of the deficit), allesthesia (stimulation of the affected side of the body is interpreted as stimulation of the unaffected side)

b. May be difficult to determine when there is severe deficit of the primary sensory modality

 1) Visual inattention may be difficult to determine if patient has a dense hemianopia

 2) Examining the patient after directing the eyes toward the unaffected side would help to distinguish hemispatial inattention from hemianopsia (deficit persists regardless of the direction of gaze)

c. Right hemispheric lesions usually cause contralateral spatial neglect (not usually seen with left hemispheric lesions)

 1) Right hemisphere (likely the inferior parietal area) is responsible for attention for both sides of the body, and left hemisphere only for the right (contralateral) side of the body

 2) Anosognosia: patient is unaware of the acquired deficits (e.g., hemiparesis and nonmotor perceptual and cognitive dysfunction), most commonly seen with acquired right hemisphere lesions

 3) Anosodiaphoria: patient is indifferent to his/her condition despite the recognition of hemiparesis or hemisensory deficits, often with right hemisphere lesions

 4) Right hemisphere lesions may also be associated with the following:

 a) Aprosody, i.e., reduced "emotional flow" and misperception of emotional tone in one's speech (right hemisphere involvement, especially right parietotemporal region)

 b) Misperception of facial expressions (right parieto-occipital lesion)

c) Topographagnosia or topographic disorientation, i.e., impaired spatial orientation and navigation in the environment; involvcment of right posterior parahippocampal region, infracalcarine cortex of either hemisphere, or less commonly, right parietal lesions

d. Hemiakinesia or motor neglect: reduction of exploratory motor behavior to the neglected side, primarily a result of sensory inattention and feedback

III. MEMORY AND LEARNING

A. Definitions

1. Learning
   a. Acquisition of new knowledge and experience and alteration of behavior as a result of the experience
   b. In its simplest form, it represents change in response over time to repeated exposure to the same stimulus
2. Memory: storage and retrieval mechanism for learned knowledge
3. Plasticity
   a. Learned behavior can be modified with modulation and alteration of adaptable "plastic" neuronal pathways
   b. Alterations in neuronal excitability and synaptic connectivity are physiologic correlates of plasticity and are responsible for learning and memory
4. Encoding: acquisition or learning of new information
5. Retrieval: recall of knowledge previously encoded and stored as long-term memory
6. Modalities of memory
   a. Explicit (declarative) memory
      1) Knowledge that requires conscious recall and acquisition: example is semantic memory, which is factual knowledge and meaning of people, places, and things; requires fast acquisition and conscious recall (e.g., geography)
      2) First step for acquisition of knowledge (encoding) involves perception of sensory input, executed by association cortices and their connections, e.g., visual association cortices are involved in "understanding" and encoding of specific aspects of a particular visual stimulus before it is stored
      3) Acquisition of explicit knowledge (encoding) is executed by mesial temporal lobe and surrounding structures, including parahippocampal and entorhinal cortices through the excitatory loop of Papez
      4) Long-term storage of explicit memory: distributed network involving association cortices (after encoding by mesial temporal structures)

5) Different aspects of a particular experience are stored in different brain regions, and memory for a certain experience is eventually stored in a distributed network
6) Disease of a particular brain region causes loss of previously acquired knowledge in that brain region and loss of ability to acquire new knowledge in that brain region
7) Types of explicit knowledge
   a) Semantic
      i) Knowledge of facts, objects, and abstract concepts unrelated to events (e.g., geography)
      ii) Semantic memory requires inferotemporal association areas and other regions outside mesial temporal lobe
      iii) Semantic memory loss usually accompanies episodic memory loss
      iv) Isolated semantic memory loss may be seen in a form of frontotemporal dementia (semantic dementia) and can also be seen in Alzheimer's disease in conjunction with memory and other deficits
   b) Episodic
      i) Knowledge of past events that have been encoded and stored with certain associations established in particular time and place
      ii) Short term: limited capacity, requires repetitive recall

---

Types of Memory

Explicit (declarative) memory: knowledge that requires conscious recall and acquisition; requires fast acquisition and conscious recall
    Semantic memory
    Episodic memory

Implicit (nondeclarative) memory: knowledge that does not require conscious recall; acquisition is generally slow
    Procedural memory
    Priming

Verbal vs. nonverbal memory

Anterograde vs. retrograde memory

Short-term vs. long-term memory

Working memory

---

iii) Long term: long-lasting or permanent, relatively more resistant to dementing illness and cerebral insult than short-term memory

iv) Anterograde memory: knowledge for experiences that occur after a certain event (anterograde memory loss refers to inability to acquire new information after a particular insult)

v) Retrograde memory: previously acquired information

b. Implicit (nondeclarative) memory
  1) Knowledge that does not require conscious recall, acquisition is generally slow
  2) Types of implicit knowledge
    a) Procedural memory
      i) Knowledge for performing a motor task is slowly acquired (learned) by repeatedly performing the same task
      ii) Acquisition is slow and incremental, the knowledge is resistant to forgetfulness by degenerative conditions
      iii) Motor skill learning likely occurs with the participation of the pyramidal, extrapyramidal, and cerebellar motor systems and their cortical projections
      iv) Cortical pathways important for skilled motor movements: motor cortex, premotor cortex, supplementary motor cortex, the parietal lobe (lesion of these pathways may produce apraxis [see below])
    b) Priming: perceptual (nonmotor) priming is linked to modality-specific neocortices

7. Division of memory based on the type of knowledge stored
  a. Verbal
    1) Generally stored in left hemisphere (dominant hemisphere)
    2) Anterograde amnesia for verbal memory (i.e., defective acquisition of verbal information) may be seen with left temporal lobe injury
  b. Nonverbal
    1) Generally stored in right hemisphere
    2) Anterograde amnesia for visual memory may be seen with right temporal lobe injury; patient may have difficulty recognizing faces, objects, etc.

8. Working memory
  a. Temporarily held knowledge that is used to execute the operation at hand
  b. Essentially, temporary operational memory that is lost after the operation is executed
  c. Performed mainly by prefrontal cortex, especially dorso-

lateral frontal cortex and its connections with basal ganglia and cerebellum

d. Frontal dysexecutive amnesia: fluctuating difficulty with acquisition of memory mainly because of difficulty with allocating attention for acquisition of information

B. Anatomy
1. Limbic system
  a. Basal forebrain: cholinergic projections to hippocampal formation
    1) Septal area
      a) Connections with hippocampus and hypothalamus
      b) Medial septal nucleus has cholinergic projections to hippocampus
    2) Substantia innominata
      a) Nucleus basalis of Meynert
        i) Cholinergic projections to amygdala and neocortex, commonly affected in Alzheimer's dementia
        ii) Receives projections from subiculum
      b) Connections with paleocortex and olfactory bulb
    3) Amygdala complex: connections with hippocampal formation responsible for attachment and association of an emotion with a particular memory
  b. Hippocampal formation
    1) Dentate gyrus: three cell layers
      a) Granule cell layer: unipolar cells projecting to molecular layer
      b) Molecular layer
      c) Polymorphic layer
    2) Hippocampus proper
      a) Subsections (cornu ammonis [CA]): CA1-4 (CA4 no longer considered a subsection)
      b) Focal damage to CA1 and CA2 is sufficient to cause anterograde amnesia
      c) CA2 is generally resistant to metabolic, vascular (anoxic), and degenerative insults with few exceptions (argyrophilic grain disease [Braak's disease] selectively affects CA2)
    3) Subicular complex
      a) Consists of the subiculum proper, presubiculum, and parasubiculum
      b) Projects to mamillary body
  c. Pathways
    1) Intrinsic hippocampal connections: all excitatory, repetitive, self-exciting circuits involved in long-term potentiation implicated in synaptogenesis, learning, and plasticity
      a) Perforant pathway projects from entorhinal cortex

to granule cells of dentate gyrus (Fig. 7-3)
b) Granule cell axons ("mossy fibers") project to pyramidal cells of CA3 and to less extent to CA1; dentatohippocampal mossy projections are dependent on presynaptic calcium influx and not on NMDA receptors
c) CA3 pyramidal cells have excitatory projections to CA1 pyramidal cells (Schaffer collateral pathway), commissural projections to opposite hippocampus, projections to fimbria of the fornix (minor component of fornix), and adjacent CA3 cells
d) Excitation of CA1 pyramidal cells is dependent on activation of NMDA receptors; this requires adequate depolarization of the postsynaptic cell to relieve blockade of the receptor by magnesium, allowing calcium influx and maintenance of long-term potentiation
e) CA1 pyramidal cells project primarily to the subiculum (and fornix to a much lesser degree)
    i) Subiculum: feedback projections to entorhinal cortex provide reentrant excitatory loops
    ii) Subiculum also projects through fornix (major component of the axons of fornix) to mamillary bodies, septal region, and hypothalamus: this is the main hippocampal output

f) Hippocampal output is primarily via the fornix from the subiculum (much more than the CA3 and CA1 pyramidal cells)
2) Excitatory reentrant circuit involved in learning and long-term potentiation: hippocampus → fornix → mamillary body → mamillothalamic tract → anterior nucleus of thalamus → thalamocingulate radiation → cingulate gyrus → cingulum → entorhinal cortex → hippocampal formation (Fig. 7-4)
3) Subcortical connections
4) Commissural interhemispheric connections between the two hippocampi (projections from CA3 pyramidal cells)
5) Projections from parahippocampal and entorhinal cortices to hippocampal formation
6) Reciprocal connections between parahippocampal and entorhinal cortices with heteromodal association cortices
2. Cerebellum
    a. Participates in learning motor tasks
    b. Learning motor skills entails modulation of certain parallel fiber–Purkinje cell synapses that are activated at the same time as climbing fiber input
    c. Long-term depression
        1) Mossy fibers synapse with cerebellar granule cells, whose axons, parallel fibers, synapse on Purkinje cells to relay information about direction, position, amplitude, and speed of movement (see Fig. 9-5)
        2) Climbing fiber input to Purkinje cells modifies their response to parallel fibers (hence, to mossy fibers) that are activated concurrently
        3) This serves as a feedback and acts to compare expected with actual movement and "correct" the movement; this occurs through weakening of parallel fiber–Purkinje cell synapses and is called "long-term depression"

IV. Emotional Behavior

A. Anatomy
1. Amygdala
    a. Mediator of acquisition of emotional memory; important role in emotional responses, particularly ones involving conditioned fear
    b. Connections with centers concerned with emotional expression: prefrontal cortex, cingulate cortex, and parahippocampal cortex
    c. Bilateral amygdala function is needed to recognize "body language" and cues to emotional attachment of the presented stimuli

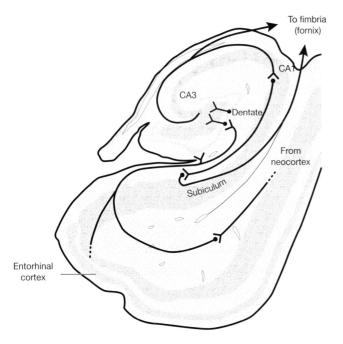

Fig. 7-3. Cross-section of the mesial temporal lobe showing anatomic pathways of the hippocampus proper.

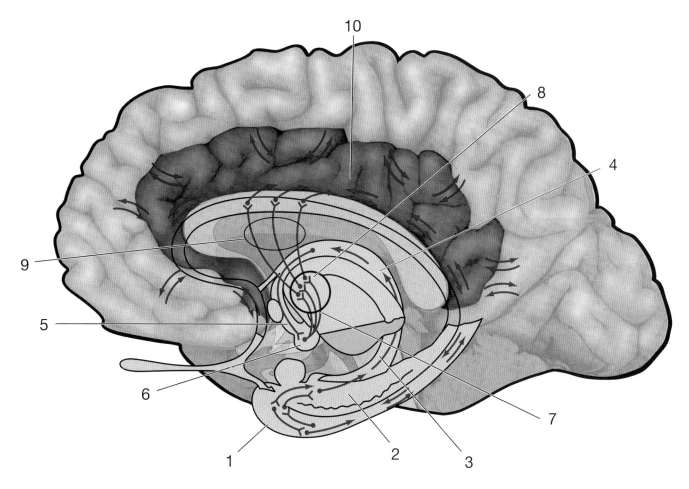

Fig. 7-4. Circuit of Papez. 1, Entorhinal cortex; 2, hippocampus proper; 3, fimbria of fornix; 4, body of fornix; 5, column of fornix; 6, mamillary body; 7, mamillothalamic tract; 8, anterior nucleus of thalamus; 9, thalamocingulate radiation; 10, cingulate gyrus.

d. Klüver-Bucy syndrome (see below): bilateral anterior temporal lobectomies that included the amygdala (first clue that amygdala is involved with emotional experience)

e. Basolateral nuclear group
  1) Receives input from sensory association cortices and projects to central nuclear group
    a) Interprets the emotional significance of a stimulus
    b) Example, amygdala can mediate emotional response to visual stimuli through connections with inferior temporal cortex, which responds to emotionally charged visual input such as faces

f. Central nuclear group
  1) Main output center of amygdala: initiates the emotional response to a stimulus after receiving input from basolateral nuclear group
  2) Connects with centers responsible for primitive emotional responses: hypothalamus and brainstem

    3) Output mediating autonomic emotional response: for mediating autonomic expression and motor and endocrine responses as in "fight-or-flight" response
      a) Via stria terminalis: projections to hypothalamic paraventricular nucleus
      b) Via ventral amygdalofugal pathway: projections to brainstem via medial forebrain bundle
    4) Output mediating conscious perception of emotions: projections via amygdalofugal pathway to basal forebrain (nucleus accumbens), orbitofrontal cortex, and cingulate gyrus

2. Hypothalamus: responsible for coordinating a set of autonomic and somatic responses to emotional stimuli through connections with periaqueductal gray matter and visceral brainstem nuclei (e.g., "fight-or-flight" response)

3. Cerebral cortex
  a. Damage to left hemisphere more likely associated with depression than damage to right hemisphere

b. Right hemisphere lesions may be associated with excessive and inappropriate cheerfulness

c. Prefrontal cortex

  1) Orbitofrontal

    a) Connections with limbic system and reticular formation

    b) Responsible for judgment and social behavior and inhibition of inappropriate behavior in a particular social context

  2) Medial frontal (anterior cingulate cortex): involved mainly with motivation

d. Temporal lobe

  1) Involved in modulation of emotional behavior

  2) Hyperoral, hypersexual, irritable behavior of Klüver-Bucy syndrome (discussed below), with lesions affecting amygdala, uncus, and portions of the hippocampi bilaterally

  3) "Temporal lobe personality" observed in patients with temporal lobe epilepsy: hypergraphia, hyper-religiosity, altered sexual behavior (hyposexuality > hypersexuality), circumstantiality of speech (with excessive detail about minute points), euphoria, sadness, emotionality, and, sometimes, anger and aggressive behavior

V. LANGUAGE AND APHASIAS (TABLE 7-1, FIG. 7-5)

A. Definition of Aphasia
1. Acquired impairment of language processes that may include disturbance in comprehension and/or formulation of language symbols (across all modalities, not only verbal)

B. To Be Distinguished From
1. Disturbance of articulation: dysarthria (disturbance of mechanical articulation) or speech apraxia (usually with buccofacial apraxia that occurs with lesions involving the pathways extending from superior temporal to prefrontal cortex)
2. Mutism
  a. Akinetic mutism: amotivational, akinetic state characterized by poor effort to initiate speech, lesion usually localized to mesial frontal lobes
  b. Aphemia: pure anarthria, no speech output
    1) Usually due to bilateral lesions of the corticobulbar (upper motor neuron) tract, often from bilateral capsular infarcts limited to corticobulbar fibers (written language and verbal comprehension are preserved)

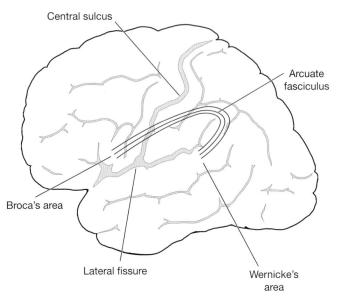

Fig. 7-5. Primary language centers.

  2) Unilateral (left-sided) lesion of precentral gyrus has also been reported
3. Pure word deafness (auditory verbal agnosia) caused by bilateral lesions of superior temporal gyrus, sparing the dominant auditory association cortex (Wernicke's area): difficulty understanding spoken language and with repetition
4. Aphonia
5. Delirium
6. Psychiatric disorder and hysteria

C. Lateralization
1. Left hemisphere is dominant for language in 99% of right-handed persons and 2/3 of left-handed persons

D. Cortical Localization of Language in Bilingual Persons
1. Cortical localization of different languages is same if second language is acquired *before* adolescence
2. Cortical localization of second language is different from first language (organized differently in Broca's area, not Wernicke's) if second language is acquired *after* adolescence

E. Broca's "Motor" Aphasia
1. Nonfluent aphasia with markedly reduced speech output
2. Effortful speech marked by short phrases and sentences with intact meaning ("telegraphic speech")
3. Agrammatic content

Table 7-1. **Classification of Aphasias**

Aphasia type	Fluency of verbal output	Naming	Comprehension	Repetition	Paraphasic errors
Broca's	Nonfluent	Impaired	Intact	Impaired	Rare
Transcortical motor	Nonfluent	Impaired	Intact	Intact	Rare
Wernicke's	Fluent	Impaired	Impaired	Impaired	Common
Transcortical sensory	Fluent	Impaired	Impaired	Intact	Common

4. Abnormal naming and repetition
5. Most patients have some degree of comprehension disturbance, mainly for grammatically complex sentences (in general, comprehension tends to be relatively preserved)
6. Writing is usually abnormal (including copying written material) because of involvement of Exner's area, which is inferior and adjacent to Broca's area (often considered part of Broca's area rather than independent language area)
7. Associated with damage to inferior and middle posterior frontal lobe (Broca's area)
8. Lesions usually extend to involve premotor, primary motor, and subcortical areas
   a. There may be associated disturbance of articulation, prosody, and speech (and orobuccal) apraxia
   b. Dominant (left) premotor cortex projects to opposite premotor cortex as well as to ipsilateral primary motor cortex
      1) Lesion involving the left premotor cortex would cause bilateral apraxia
      2) Most lesions also involve primary motor cortex and cause weakness, which masks the apraxia on the contralateral side, but patients may continue to have left-sided apraxia

F. Transcortical Motor Aphasia
1. Nonfluent speech with preserved ability to repeat words and relatively preserved comprehension
2. May be seen with lesions anterior or superior to Broca's area and in subcortical white matter
3. Aphasia due to thalamic lesions may mimic this
4. Watershed infarcts in distribution between the anterior cerebral artery and middle cerebral artery territories in the dominant hemisphere may cause a transcortical motor aphasia

G. Wernicke's "Sensory" Aphasia
1. Fluent speech with normal or increased verbal output
2. Normal grammar, but empty, meaningless speech with

frequent neologisms; highly learned phrases may be intact but are often used out of context and impart little meaning
3. Impaired comprehension, naming, and repetition as well as reading out loud and writing
4. Paraphasias (both phonemic and semantic) and neologisms
   a. Phonemic (literal) paraphasias: when a portion of the word is misspoken ("sable" for "table")
   b. Global (verbal) paraphasias: when the entire word is misspoken ("table" becomes "orange")
   c. Semantic paraphasia: verbal paraphasia in which the misspoken word is in the same category as the intended word ("apple" for "orange")
5. Associated with damage to posterior 2/3 of superior temporal gyrus (auditory association cortex)
6. Lesions may extend to involve the second temporal gyrus and adjacent parietal lobe, including the angular gyrus

H. Transcortical Sensory Aphasia
1. Preserved ability to repeat words without comprehension of the verbal or written words: patients may repeat the command but be unable to follow it
2. Fluent speech similar to Wernicke's aphasia (except for preserved repetition), with impaired comprehension and naming
3. May be seen with lesions of posterior middle temporal gyrus, angular gyrus, and corresponding deep white matter
4. Aphasia due to thalamic lesions may mimic this
5. Watershed infarcts in the distribution between the middle cerebral artery and posterior cerebral artery territories in dominant hemisphere may cause a transcortical sensory aphasia

I. Global Aphasia
1. Severe limitation of all language functions (fluency, comprehension, repetition, naming); involves all modalities (talking, understanding, reading, writing)

2. Nonfluent speech with severe limitation of naming, repetition, and comprehension (although the latter may be affected less)
3. Lesions usually involve the entire perisylvian area, including inferior frontal and posterior temporal lobes
4. Aphasia typically improves and evolves to mimic either Broca's or Wernicke's aphasia
5. Aphasia due to lesion predominantly affecting the frontal lobe tend to evolve to Broca's aphasia

J. Conduction Aphasia
1. Primary limitations of repetition out of proportion to other aspects of language
2. Fluent speech, with some hesitation and variable amount of phonemic paraphasias
3. Good articulation and intact comprehension
4. Naming may be affected by paraphasic errors
5. Anatomic localization: usually left arcuate fasciculus extending from left superior temporal gyrus (other areas that may be involved include left supramarginal gyrus and left primary auditory cortex, insula, and adjacent subcortical white matter)

K. Subcortical Aphasia
1. Considerable variation
2. Typically acute onset with mutism with evolution and recovery to dysarthric speech
3. Mild-to-moderate anomia
4. Almost always associated with dysarthria
5. Variable impairment of fluency, comprehension, and repetition
6. May sometimes resemble transcortical aphasia
7. Usually striatocapsular or thalamic (especially ventro-lateral and anteroventral nuclei)
8. Associated with other neurologic deficits such as hemiparesis
9. Good prognosis for recovery

L. Anomic Aphasia
1. Fluent, spontaneous speech with disturbance of word retrieval (occasional hesitation for word-finding and circumlocution)
2. Normal comprehension, repetition, reading, and writing
3. Lesions may occur anywhere in left hemisphere and sometimes right hemisphere (most commonly, the dominant inferior parietal and anterior temporal lobes)
4. Anomia may be category-specific (differentially affecting certain semantic category such as living vs. nonliving) with lesions of dominant anterior temporal lobe

5. Anomia often remains the residua of more severe aphasias
6. Typical aphasia in Alzheimer's disease

M. Nonfluent Aphasias: poor verbal output with effortful speech
1. Broca's aphasia
2. Transcortical motor aphasia
3. Global aphasia
4. Anomic aphasia (word finding difficulties produce hesitant speech that can be interpreted incorrectly as a nonfluent aphasia)

N. Fluent Aphasias: generous verbal output but often meaningless
1. Wernicke's aphasia
2. Transcortical sensory aphasia
3. Conduction aphasia

O. Other Cortical Areas Involved in Speech and Language
1. Insular cortex: important for planning or coordinating articulatory movements of speech
2. Right hemisphere: important for prosody, or emotional intonation of language, including gesturing
   a. Anterior (motor) aprosodia
      1) Poor *production* of emotional overtones of language (gestural or spoken)
      2) Associated with lesions of nondominant frontoparietal region
   b. Posterior (sensory) aprosodia
      1) Poor *perception* of emotional overtones of language (gestural or spoken)
      2) Associated with lesions of nondominant posterior temporoparietal region
3. Right hemisphere is also important for the pragmatic aspect of language: using the sentence in appropriate social setting, sarcasm, humor
   a. The true meaning of a particular sentence or phrase can vary depending on context of the conversation or narrative
   b. This is understood and applied by the right hemisphere
4. Mesial frontal regions: important for initiation of speech, as well as attention and emotion (lesions can cause akinetic mutism, not aphasia)

P. Other Language Disturbances
1. Agraphia
   a. Aphasic agraphia: language disturbance, and not a pyramidal, extrapyramidal, ataxic, or apraxic disturbance

1) Almost all patients with aphasia have some degree of agraphia
2) Dominant frontal aphasic agraphia (Exner's area)
   a) Usually accompanies Broca's aphasia
   b) Poor written output with agrammatism
3) Dominant parietotemporal aphasic agraphia
   a) Usually accompanies Wernicke's aphasia
   b) Good written output, but meaningless and with paraphasic errors
   b. Pure agraphia: lesion localized to the posterior frontal and superior parietal areas
   c. Apractic agraphia
   d. Visuospatial agraphia: lesion localized to nondominant temporoparietal junction
2. Alexia with agraphia
   a. With pure angular gyrus lesion: accompanied by acalculia, finger agnosia, right-left disorientation (Gerstmann's syndrome)
   b. With angular gyrus lesion extending to Wernicke's area: Gerstmann's syndrome plus sensory aphasia
   c. Associated also with visual field defects
3. Alexia without agraphia
   a. Usually occurs with lesions involving dominant (left) medial occipital lobe (and medial temporal lobe) and splenium of corpus callosum: affecting the right hemifield and transfer of information about the left hemifield to the angular gyrus
   b. May be accompanied by right visual field defect or hemiachromatopsia (when the lesion involves the occipital cortex inferior to the calcarine fissure)
   c. Patients have word blindness but not letter blindness (patients retain the ability to read letters)

VI. APRAXIA

A. Inability to Perform Learned Tasks in the Absence of Sensory Impairment, Pyramidal Weakness, Extrapyramidal Disturbances, or Poor Comprehension

B. Anatomy of Praxis (Fig. 7-6)
1. Information is transmitted from Wernicke's area (dominant hemisphere) for comprehension of verbal commands
2. Information is then projected to dominant premotor area via the arcuate fasciculus and, subsequently, to left motor cortex and right premotor area via the corpus callosum (which then projects to the right primary motor cortex)

3. Lesions involving Wernicke's area, arcuate fasciculus, or left premotor area cause apraxis on both sides of the body, including buccofacial apraxia and speech apraxia.
   a. Dominant anterior (frontal) lesions: contralateral (right) hemiparesis (masking apraxis) and ipsilateral (left-sided) apraxia because the verbal command is not transmitted to the right premotor area; often associated with imitation behavior and utilization, which are release phenomena that occur because of reduced frontal lobe inhibition
   b. Dominant posterior (parietal) lesions: buccofacial apraxia, bilateral limb apraxia
4. Lesions involving only anterior corpus callosum (potentially may occur with anterior cerebral artery territory infarcts): callosal apraxia

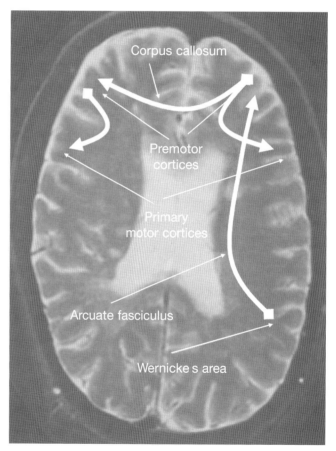

Fig. 7-6. Proposed anatomy of praxis. Wernicke's area is responsible for recognition and decoding of verbal command. This activates the dominant premotor area (via arcuate fasciculus), which in turn communicates directly with the ipsilateral primary motor cortex and indirectly with the contralateral primary motor cortex. The dominant premotor cortex sends projections to the contralateral premotor cortex via corpus callosum. Lesions along these pathways may produce abnormalities of praxis.

a. Selective apraxia of left limb and alien limb phenomenon

b. Anterior callosal lesion disconnects left hand representation (right primary motor and premotor cortices) from verbal left hemisphere, which usually results in apraxia to verbal commands confined to left hand (alien hand phenomenon)

C. Ideomotor Apraxia

1. Inability to execute a motor command

2. Spatial and temporal errors

3. Lesions most commonly involve left inferior parietal lobe (angular or supramarginal gyrus): inability to comprehend command and greater difficulty understanding the quality of a motor performance by patient or others (discrimination of movements), as compared with more anterior lesions

4. Anterior (frontal) lesions often involve mesial frontal lobe, including supplementary motor cortex, which is responsible for bimanual coordination, with relative preservation of comprehension and discrimination of movements

D. Ideational Apraxia

1. Definition: failure to execute a *series* of acts in a particular sequence, although individual movements are correct (as compared with ideomotor apraxia, in which the execution of the individual movements is abnormal)

2. Loss of the perception (idea) behind the skilled movements

3. Example: writing and mailing a letter

4. Poor localization

a. May occur with bilateral frontal and parietal lesions

b. Most commonly, with lesions of left parieto-occipital junction

E. Gait Apraxia

1. Magnetic gait, described as difficulty lifting the feet off the floor

2. Anatomic substrate

a. Pathways originate from medial frontal lobes, loop around lateral ventricles, and project to deep gray matter (most important, frontostriatal pathways)

b. May be affected by hydrocephalus, bilateral subcortical infarcts, or periventricular small vessel disease

F. Conceptual Apraxia

1. Unable to recall the type of action associated with a particular object or tool: content errors

2. Patient cannot demonstrate the use of a tool such as scissors (with pantomiming or when given the tool)

3. Unable to develop tools from available material

4. Impaired mechanical knowledge: demonstrates poor judgment in selecting the appropriate tool for a particular action

G. Conduction Apraxia: impaired imitation of movement, with relatively preserved comprehension and discrimination of movements

Nima Mowzoon, M.D.

I. DELIRIUM

A. **Characterized by Altered Sensorium With Confusion, Inattention, and Disorientation of Acute Onset** (chronic symptoms are usually referred to as encephalopathy)

B. **Acute or Subacute in Onset**

C. **Fluctuating Course** (over minutes or hours)

D. **Altered Consciousness** (including alertness and orientation): patients can be lethargic or combative and agitated

E. **Attentional Deficits**
1. Reduced ability to focus, sustain, or shift attention
2. Patients are usually distractible and unable to maintain attention to a particular task, yet can be more attentive to trivial stimuli than the more important task at hand

F. **Disorganized Thinking, Circumstantiality, Tangentiality, and Disorganized Content of Speech With Poor Comprehension:** attributed mostly to altered consciousness, decreased alertness, working memory deficits, and inattention
1. Hallucinations: often visual, may be release phenomenon
2. Delusions: often persecutory (may be situational, as in agitated patient requiring restraint)
3. Behavioral dyscontrol: inappropriate social conduct, impulsivity, poor judgment, poor insight, confabulation, impersistence, perseveration (together with poor working memory and inattention demonstrate the importance of prefrontal cortex in maintenance of arousal and attention)

G. **Altered Sleep-Wake Cycle:** excessive daytime drowsiness, "sundowning," even complete reversal of sleep-wake cycles

H. **Altered Psychomotor Activity**
1. Psychomotor hypoactivity and retardation with lethargy and decreased arousal
2. Psychomotor hyperactivity (prominent in drug withdrawal): associated with agitation
3. Fluctuation of psychomotor activity (hypoactive-hyperactive)

I. **Differential Diagnosis**
1. Metabolic: hypoxia, endocrinopathies (e.g., thyroid disease, pituitary failure, Cushing's syndrome, hypoglycemia, hyperglycemia); organ failure (e.g., hepatic encephalopathy, uremic encephalopathy, acute intermittent porphyria); electrolyte abnormalities (e.g., hypernatremia, hyponatremia, central pontine myelinolysis, hypercalcemia); nutritional deficiencies (vitamin B_{12} deficiency, Wernicke's encephalopathy)
2. Infectious: systemic (sepsis), meningitis, encephalitis, focal (cerebritis, subdural or epidural abscess)
3. Inflammatory: fulminant multiple sclerosis, acute disseminated encephalomyelitis, primary central nervous system (CNS) angiitis, systemic vasculitis with CNS involvement (as with systemic lupus erythematosus or rheumatoid arthritis), and others
4. Traumatic: subdural hemorrhage, epidural hemorrhage, subarachnoid hemorrhage, contusion, concussion, and others
5. Tumors: primary, metastatic, meningeal carcinomatosis, paraneoplastic limbic encephalopathy
6. Toxic: intoxication, withdrawal (sedatives and anxiolytics, including benzodiazepines, barbiturates, amphetamine, cocaine, alcohol, and other drugs of

abuse), industrial (heavy metals, including mercury, carbon monoxide, and others)

7. Perioperative: especially with heart operations or those with long periods of hypotension and resultant global hypoxia, anesthetic effect

8. Paroxysmal: status epilepticus, status migrainosus, postictal state

9. Vascular: hypertensive encephalopathy, ischemic infarcts (especially brainstem infarcts), hemorrhagic disease, transient ischemic attack (TIA), venous infarcts (especially with thrombosis of the straight sinus and vein of Galen, which can cause venous infarcts of the thalamus bilaterally; this usually produces coma or stupor, not delirium)

J. Treatment

1. Focuses on correcting underlying cause of delirium and symptomatic measures, including treating agitation and behavioral dyscontrol

2. General approach and management is discussed in Chapter 10

II. Mild Cognitive Impairment (MCI)

A. **Definition:** cognitive impairment that does not interfere with activities of daily living and is not severe enough to meet criteria for dementia

B. **It Can Encompass**

1. Impairment in a single cognitive domain: memory, language, attention, executive function, visuospatial *or*

2. Deficits in multiple domains

C. **Patients May or May Not Be Aware of Deficits**

D. **Amnestic MCI**

1. Patients present with predominant memory impairment, with or without other domain involvement

2. These patients are likely to develop Alzheimer's disease (AD)

E. **Single, Nonmemory-Domain MCI**

1. A condition in which a single domain other than memory is affected, such as language, executive function, attention, and visuospatial function

2. These patients may eventually develop non-AD abnormality such as frontotemporal dementia

F. **Multiple-Domain MCI:** may be related to early

presentations of vascular dementia, dementia with Lewy bodies, or AD

G. **About 80% of Patients With MCI Eventually Convert to Dementia by 6 Years**

H. **Risk Factors for Progression After Diagnosis**

1. Apolipoprotein E (APOE) ε4 allele carrier

2. Poor performance on semantic cueing memory test

3. Reduced hippocampal volumes derived from magnetic resonance images (MRIs)

I. **Measurements of the Entorhinal Cortex:** may be equally useful in discriminating between the "worried-well" and MCI likely to progress to AD

J. **Neuropathology**

1. Transitional pathology usually does not meet full criteria for diagnosis of any disease state but is indicative of underlying disease process

2. Patients with amnestic MCI are likely to have medial temporal lobe involvement (e.g., amyloid deposition, neurofibrillary lesions, hippocampal sclerosis)

K. **Treatment**

1. Donepezil
   a. Associated with lower rate of progression to AD during first 12 months of treatment
   b. This effect is not observed after 3 years of treatment

2. Vitamin E: not shown to be of benefit

III. Alzheimer's Disease

A. **Risk Factors**

1. Age

2. Female sex (likely a survival effect based on age)

3. Low level of education

4. Down syndrome
   a. Patients with Down syndrome eventually develop AD lesions, but this is considered a distinct entity
   b. Mothers of children with Down syndrome are considered at greater risk for developing AD than the general population

5. Head trauma, especially repeated or severe trauma, as in dementia pugilistica

6. APOE ε4 as susceptibility gene
   a. Homozygous carrying two genes are at increased risk of developing AD by age 85
   b. Effect is predominantly on age at onset rather than on

development of disease and is seen in both heterozygotes and homozygotes

   c. APOE genotyping should not be used for diagnosis or risk assessment because many APOE ε4 carriers never develop AD (AAN recommendations)

7. Genetic/familial predisposition
   a. There may be family history of dementia in first-degree relatives
   b. Familial AD with genes linked to the following chromosomes:
     1) 21 (amyloid precursor protein [APP]), 14 (presenilin-1 [PS-1]), 1 (PS-2)
     2) Autosomal dominant forms of AD typically present at early age (40-70 years)
     3) Several other candidate genes, including insulin-degrading enzyme (IDE), are being investigated in relation to late-onset AD

B. Clinical Features: memory deficits and subsequent development of multiple cognitive deficits causing significant impairment of daily functioning

1. Established criteria for diagnosis of AD are listed in Table 7-2
2. Early memory deficits, including impaired episodic memory and reduced delayed recall on semantic memory tests
   a. Relative sparing of procedural memory and old remote memory
   b. Preclinical stage may be categorized as "amnestic MCI"
3. Language deficits: anomia, poor comprehension, semantic paraphasias
4. Visuospatial impairment and environmental disorientation; impaired visual processing and visual agnosia; posterior cortical atrophy, with prominent visuospatial dysfunction and relative preservation of memory, is typically related to AD and may present as Balint's syndrome
   a. Oculomotor apraxia: inaccurate shift of voluntary gaze to visual stimuli
   b. Optic ataxia: inaccurate movement of hand when reaching for a target using visual guidance
   c. Simultanagnosia: failure of visual recognition of the whole picture
5. Apraxia: ideational, ideomotor, conceptual
6. Agnosia (mainly visual)
7. Impairment of executive function: usually responsible for functional decline in activities of daily living required for DSM-IV diagnosis of dementia and AD
8. Behavioral and psychiatric symptoms: usually relatively preserved early in the disease except for social withdrawal

   a. Indifference and apathy most common
   b. Behavioral dyscontrol with advanced disease: agitation, aggression, irritability, anxiety, and disinhibition
   c. Psychiatric manifestations
     1) Depression: patients with AD are at higher risk for developing clinical depression (may be due to loss of noradrenergic neurons in locus ceruleus)
     2) Hallucinations: auditory or visual (the latter if prominent posterior cerebral involvement)
     3) Paranoid delusions (especially persecutory): common examples are delusions of theft of property or infidelity and false beliefs that an intruder is living in the house (phantom boarder) or the caretaker or a family member is an imposter (Capgras' syndrome)
   d. Less frequently, strangers may be identified as family members (Fregoli syndrome)
9. Extrapyramidal symptoms: parkinsonian rigidity and myoclonic jerks in *late* stages of AD
10. Sleep disturbance: "sundowning," sleep-wake cycle reversals, REM sleep behavior (usually does not occur unless there are concurrent diffuse Lewy bodies)

C. Imaging (Fig. 7-7)
1. MRI: mesiotemporal and hippocampal atrophy, may be evident in preclinical stage of MCI
   a. Useful in excluding reversible causes of altered sensorium, which may include structural lesions
   b. Focal cortical atrophy with sparing of mesial temporal lobe and hippocampus may indicate alternative disease process such as frontotemporal dementia or corticobasal degeneration
2. Positron emission tomography (PET) and single photon emission computed tomography (SPECT): glucose hypometabolism (on PET) and hypoperfusion (on SPECT) of posterior temporal and parietal structures, followed by changes in frontal association in advanced stages

D. Other Features
1. EEG may show diffuse slowing of the background

Functional Imaging in Alzheimer's Disease
Glucose hypometabolism and hypoperfusion (as measured by PET and SPECT) of the posterior temporal and parietal structures, followed by changes in the frontal association areas in the advanced stages

Table 7-2. **Criteria for Diagnosis of Alzheimer's Disease**

I.   Criteria for clinical diagnosis of *probable* Alzheimer's disease:
  a. Dementia established by clinical examination and documented by mental status examination, and confirmed by neuro-psychologic tests
  b. Deficits in two or more areas of cognition
  c. Progressive worsening of memory and other cognitive functions
  d. No disturbance of consciousness
  e. Onset between ages 40 and 90, most often after age 65 *and*
  f. Absence of systemic disorders or other brain diseases that in and of themselves could account for progressive deficits in memory and cognition

II. Diagnosis of *probable* Alzheimer's disease is supported by:
  a. Progressive deterioration of specific cognitive functions such as language (aphasia), motor skills (apraxia), and perception (agnosia)
  b. Impaired activities of daily living and altered patterns of behavior
  c. Family history of similar disorders, particularly if confirmed with pathology examination *and*
  d. Laboratory results of:
    i.   Normal CSF examination with lumbar puncture
    ii. Normal pattern or nonspecific changes on EEG (an example of the latter may be increased diffuse slow-wave activity or bitemporal slowing)
    iii. Neurodiagnostic evidence of cerebral atrophy with progression documented by serial observation

III. Other clinical features consistent with the diagnosis of *probable* Alzheimer's disease, after *exclusion* of causes of dementia other than Alzheimer's disease, include:
  a. Plateau in the course of progression of the illness
  b. Associated symptoms of depression; insomnia; incontinence; delusions; illusions; hallucinations; catastrophic verbal, emotional, or physical outbursts; sexual disorders; and weight loss
  c. Other neurologic signs and symptoms such as increased muscle tone, gait disorder, and myoclonus
  d. Seizures in advanced age
  e. Normal neuroimaging features for age

IV. Features that make the diagnosis of *probable* Alzheimer's disease *uncertain* or *unlikely* include:
  a. Sudden, apoplectic onset
  b. Focal neurologic findings such as hemiparesis, sensory loss, visual field deficits, and incoordination early in the course of the illness
  c. Seizures or gait disturbances at the onset or very early in the course of the illness

V.   Clinical diagnosis of *possible* Alzheimer's disease:
  a. May be made on the basis of the dementia syndrome, in the absence of other neurologic, psychiatric, or systemic disorders sufficient to cause dementia, and in the presence of variations in the onset, in the presentation, or in the clinical course
  b. May be made in the presence of a second systemic or brain disorder sufficient to produce dementia, which is not considered to be *the* cause of the dementia
  c. Should be used in research studies when a single, gradually progressive severe cognitive deficit is identified in the absence of other identifiable cause

VI. Criteria for diagnosis of *definite* Alzheimer's disease are:
  a. Clinical criteria for probable Alzheimer's disease
  b. Histopathologic evidence obtained from biopsy or autopsy

VII. Classification of Alzheimer's disease for research purposes should specify features that may differentiate subtypes of the disorder, such as:
  a. Familial occurrence
  b. Onset before age 65
  c. Presence of trisomy 21
  d. Coexistence of other relevant conditions such as Parkinson's disease

CSF, *cerebrospinal fluid;* EEG, *electroencephalogram.*
From McKhann G, Drachman D, Folstein M, Katzman R, Price D, Stadlan EM. *Clinical diagnosis of Alzheimer's disease: Report of the NINCDS-ADRDA Work Group under the auspices of Department of Health and Human Services Task Force on Alzheimer's Disease. Neurology. 1984;34:939-44. Used with permission.*

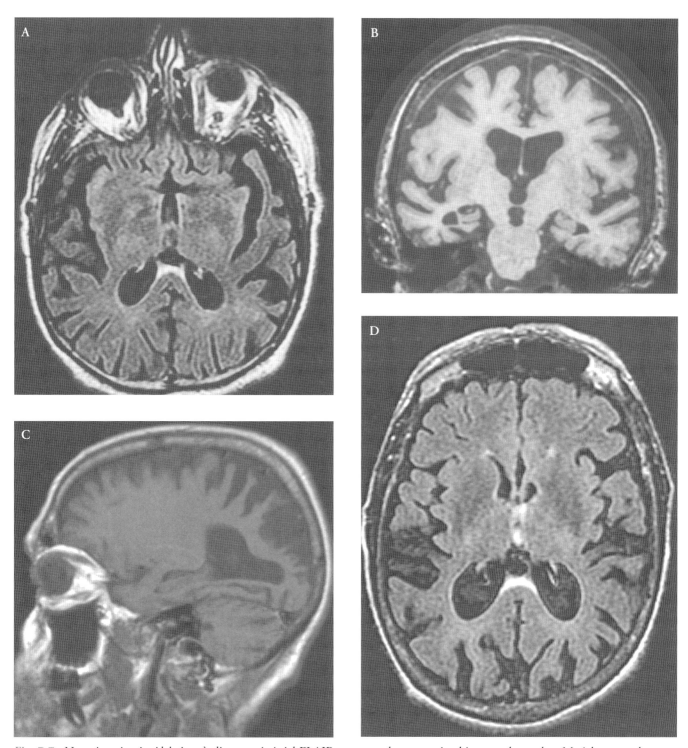

Fig. 7-7. Neuroimaging in Alzheimer's disease. *A,* Axial FLAIR sequence demonstrating bitemporal atrophy. Mesial temporal structures and hippocampi are better seen in coronal sequences (*B*). *B,* Coronal T1-weighted image shows asymmetric, bilateral hippocampal atrophy, which seems more prominent on the right. There is also diffuse cortical atrophy, but the degree of hippocampal atrophy is more pronounced. *C,* Sagittal T1-weighted and, *D,* axial FLAIR images of another patient with Alzheimer's disease who presented with Balint's syndrome. Note the prominent occipitoparietal atrophy in both *C* and *D.*

activity or temporal slowing (usually normal in the early stages)

2. Other potential associations
   a. Increase in cerebrospinal fluid (CSF) tau protein and decrease in CSF $A\beta_{1-42}$ and $A\beta_{1-40}$, but there is extreme variability in test results between subjects and these abnormalities may be seen in other degenerative disease states
   b. Main goal of laboratory testing: rule out reversible causes of altered sensorium (including depression), structural lesions, chronic infections (e.g., neurosyphilis), inflammatory conditions (e.g., steroid-responsive encephalopathy), thyroid disease, vitamin deficiencies, other metabolic conditions, and iatrogenic causes (e.g., medications)

E. Pathologic Features (Fig. 7-8 and 7-9)
1. Nerve cell loss
   a. Early involvement of entorhinal cortex and hippocampus may account for early memory deficits
   b. Early selective involvement of layers II and IV of CA1 and subiculum
   c. Other: frontal, temporal, parietal neocortex; limbic cortex, basal forebrain, brainstem
2. Neurofibrillary tangles
   a. Tangle stages (referring to distribution of tangles): good clinical correlation
   b. Paired helical filaments consisting of hyperphosphorylated tau protein
   c. Early presence in mesiotemporal structures
   d. Pathologic evolution: dispersed and perinuclear tau established aggregates into paired helical filaments late stage of neuronal death and remaining "ghost tangle"
   e. Pathologic differential diagnosis of "tauopathies" (diseases with filamentous tau deposits) is listed in Table 7-3
3. Plaques
   a. Plaque stages: poor clinical correlation
   b. Diffuse plaques: extracellular loose aggregates of amyloid and preamyloid material

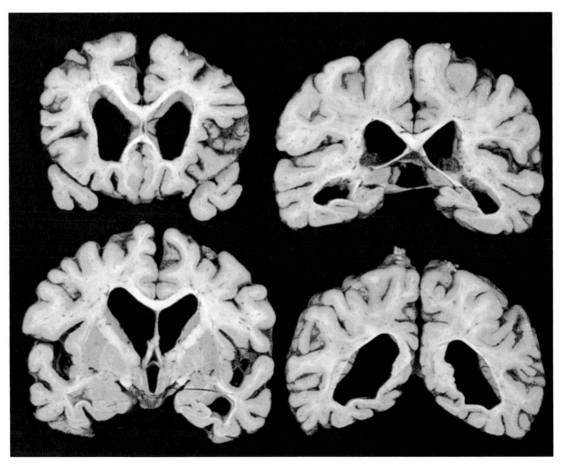

Fig. 7-8. Gross specimen of a brain with Alzheimer's disease. Note profound bilateral hippocampal atrophy disproportionate to diffuse cortical atrophy. (From Okazaki H, Scheithauer BW. Atlas of neuropathology. New York: Gower Medical Publishing; 1988. p. 220. By permission of Mayo Foundation.)

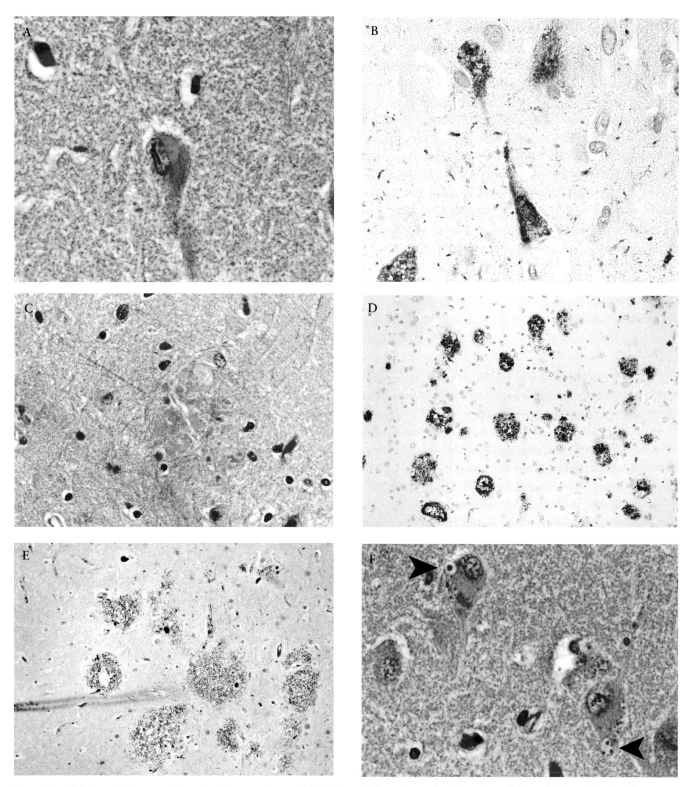

Fig. 7-9. Alzheimer's disease. Neurofibrillary tangles are faintly basophilic and may be flame-shaped (*A* and *B*) or globular filamentous structures. They are neuronal inclusions composed of aggregates of hyperphosphorylated tau protein as paired helical filaments and are usually best demonstrated with tau immunohistochemistry (*B*). *C*, Diffuse plaques: extracellular poorly defined depositions of amyloid protein. They may be detected better with use of β-amyloid immunohistochemistry (*D*) or Bielschowsky's silver stain (*E*). Granulovacuolar degeneration may be seen in some neurons (*F*, *arrowheads*).

Table 7-3. **Diseases With Filamentous Tau Deposits**

Alzheimer's disease
Pick's disease
FTD-17
Corticobasal degeneration
Progressive supranuclear palsy
Down syndrome
ALS/PD/dementia complex
Dementia pugilistica
Multiple system tauopathy

ALS, amyotrophic lateral sclerosis; FTD, frontotemporal dementia; PD, Parkinson's disease.

   c. Primitive plaques: extracellular spherical, well-defined aggregates of amyloid and preamyloid material
   d. Neuritic (mature) plaques: extracellular focal aggregates of amyloid material with dense core and surrounding halo, dystrophic, tau-positive neurites
   e. End-stage (burned-out) plaques: extracellular compact core of amyloid material
   f. Molecular biology: APP cleaved by β- and γ-secretase, producing insoluble Aβ protein (Aβ_{1-42}, Aβ_{1-40})
4. Granulovacuolar degeneration
   a. Neuronal intracytoplasmic vacuoles containing granules
   b. Predominantly affect hippocampal pyramidal cells
   c. May also be seen in Down syndrome and, to a lesser extent, aging brains
5. Amyloid angiopathy
   a. Deposition of amyloid in the wall of small-sized and medium-sized cortical and leptomeningeal arteries in most patients with AD
   b. Abnormal deposition of amyloid may obliterate the vessels, resulting in hemorrhage

F. Treatment Strategies
1. Cholinesterase inhibitors
   a. Should be discontinued before anticholinergic general anesthesia
   b. Should not be given with other cholinesterase inhibitors or anticholinergic medications
   c. Prescribe with caution if patient has cardiac rhythm disturbance or history of gastrointestinal tract bleeding because cholinergic upregulation can exacerbate these problems
   d. Used as monotherapy for MCI or dementia
   e. May be used in combination with vitamin E or memantine (moderate to severe dementia)
   f. Tacrine (Cognex): no longer available

    1) Short-term half-life (4 hours), administered four times daily
    2) Hepatotoxicity in 40% of patients, frequent blood monitoring needed
  g. Donepezil (Aricept)
    1) Pure acetylcholinesterase inhibitor
    2) Time to maximum concentration is 3 to 5 hours
    3) Once-daily regimen
    4) Introduced at 5 mg/d for 1 month, then increased to 10 mg once daily
    5) Major side effects: nausea, vomiting, diarrhea, vivid dreams
    6) Best tolerated of all available cholinesterase inhibitors
    7) Better tolerated if taken in morning on full stomach
  h. Galantamine (Reminyl)
    1) Acetylcholinesterase inhibitor and allosteric nicotinic modulator
    2) Administered twice daily
    3) Initial dose of 4 mg twice daily for at least 1 month, increased to 8 mg twice daily, and then 12 mg twice daily after 1 month
    4) Nausea, vomiting, diarrhea, vivid dreams are more frequent than with donepezil
  i. Rivastigmine (Exelon)
    1) Acetylcholinesterase and butyrylcholinesterase inhibitor
    2) Administered twice daily
    3) Dose escalation preferably in monthly increments because of the relatively higher side effect rate than with other cholinesterase inhibitors: initial starting dose of 1.5 mg twice daily, then 3 mg twice daily, and 4.5 mg (and possibly 6 mg) twice daily
    4) Higher side effect profile than other cholinesterase inhibitors, may need to slow down the titration schedule
    5) Not metabolized by the liver
2. Memantine (Namenda)
   a. Low affinity for NMDA receptor, with rapid onset and offset of action
   b. Goal of therapy is short-term NMDA receptor activation that may promote memory and learning and avoidance of chronic low-grade NMDA activation that may promote excessive calcium influx and resultant apoptosis
   c. Not metabolized by the liver
   d. Reported side effects: confusion, headaches, dizziness
   e. Initial therapy for patients with moderate to severe dementia
   f. May be used as monotherapy or in conjunction with cholinesterase inhibitors and vitamin E (polytherapy well tolerated)

g. Dose escalation, preferably in weekly increments: starting dose of 5 mg once daily in the evening, next 5 mg twice daily, followed by 10 mg every morning and 5 mg in the evening, and then 10 mg twice daily

h. Should not be administered with medications with similar mechanism of action

3. Other symptomatic measures

a. Acute delirium

1) Acute deterioration of cognition may be due to underlying medical problem such as urinary tract infection

2) Treatment: find and treat the cause and treat symptomatically until cause is found and treated

b. Behavioral, nonpharmacologic management (special attention to the environment and surroundings)

c. Depression: use selective serotonin reuptake inhibitors (SSRIs) (least anticholinergic side effects and may also be effective for concurrent anxiety and agitation)

d. Psychosis: atypical antipsychotic agents recommended, including olanzapine and quetiapine

e. Agitation: antipsychotic agents (preferably, atypical agents), sometimes trazodone may be used as first-line agent

f. Apathy: acetylcholinesterase inhibitors may be considered

IV. FRONTOTEMPORAL DEMENTIAS (FTDS)

A. Genetics

1. Only 20% of cases are inherited, the other 80% are considered sporadic

2. Autosomal dominant inheritance in most inherited FTDs (mutations in the tau gene on chromosome 17 account for most of these, up to 50% [FTD-17])

3. More than 30 tau mutations identified (both coding and noncoding regions): most between exons 9 and 13, which code for the microtubule-binding domains of tau

4. Full penetrance, but the onset of disease and spectrum of clinical symptoms varies significantly even within the same kindred

5. Tau mutation is much less likely to be present in the absence of a family history

6. Tau is a soluble microtubule-binding protein

a. Microtubule-binding domains of tau protein are responsible for binding

b. 3R tau contains 3 microtubule-binding repeats (4R tau contains 4), normal ratio 3 tau:4 tau is 1:1

c. Mutations following exon 10 (chromosome 17) cause abnormal ratio of tau isoforms and reduced microtubule

binding leading to aggregation of insoluble tau filaments and interference with axonal transport

7. FTD-17: associated with parkinsonism, linked with chromosome 17q21-22 (missense mutations with alternate splicing of exon 10 yield predominantly 4R tau, also seen with missense mutations outside of exon 10)

8. FTD-MND (motor neuron disease): associated with motor neuron disease, some cases linked to unknown gene on chromosome 9 and have shorter, more malignant course relating to motor neuron disease

9. FTD-ldh (lacking distinctive histopathology): sometimes referred to as "FTD with ubiquitin-positive, tau-negative inclusions"

10. FTD-Pick/Pick's disease: characterized by tau-positive inclusions without known mutations in tau gene; unlike FTD-17, Pick's inclusions are composed of predominantly 3R tau

11. Possible association with APOE ε4 allele: APOE ε4 carriers (larger increase in ventricular size, no effect on age at onset, poorly established)

B. Clinical Features

1. Occur equally in men and women

2. Mean length of disease: 8 years (range, 2-15)

3. Presenting (early) features may be predominantly behavioral and psychiatric or aphasia

4. Insidious onset and gradual progression

5. Behavioral features

a. Gradual personality change

b. Impaired social interactions and interpersonal conduct: disinhibition, inappropriate social and sexual behavior (including criminal activity and other "antisocial" behavior)

c. Emotional blunting

d. Mental rigidity and inflexibility: inability to adapt to new situations

---

Frontotemporal Dementia (FTD) Phenotypes
Only 20% are inherited

FTD-17: associated with parkinsonism, linked to chromosome 17q21-22; predominantly 4R tau

FTD-MND: associated with motor neuron disease; linked to chromosome 9

FTD-ldh: ubiquitin-positive histochemistry

FTD-Pick (Pick's disease): tau-positive inclusions without known mutations; predominantly 3R tau

e. Distractibility, impersistence, failure to complete tasks
f. Loss of insight
g. Frontal "executive dysfunction": poor judgment, planning, organization, task completion, mental flexibility; poor sequencing; distractibility
h. Perseverative and stereotyped behaviors, repetitive acts (may be complex acts and involve rituals); obsessive-compulsive tendencies often precede overt dementia
i. Utilization behavior: behavior of repetitive grasping and reaching for an object in the visual field, driven solely by digression of attention to the object, despite its irrelevance to the situation at hand
j. Decline in personal hygiene
k. Hyperorality: altered food preferences, overeating, oral exploration of the environment
l. Relative preservation of memory, perception, and visuospatial functions, until advanced stages of disease
m. Abnormalities on testing memory mostly due to deficits in working memory and attention rather than true amnesia
n. Klüver-Bucy syndrome
   1) Results from bilateral damage to anterior temporal lobes and amygdala
   2) Other causes may be ischemia, herpes encephalitis, trauma, temporal lobe surgery
   3) Hyperorality and oral exploratory behavior, altered eating habits, weight gain, emotional blunting, blunting of response of fear and aggression, and altered sexual activity (hyposexuality > hypersexuality)
   4) Aggression is not a component of the syndrome
   5) Hypermetamorphosis: patients are hypersensitive and preoccupied with the most subtle environmental stimuli, by touching or otherwise examining the stimuli
o. Eventually lead to apathetic, akinetic mutism with poor motivation and social withdrawal
6. Psychiatric and affective: apathy, depression, anxiety, psychosis, delusions; inability to express different emotions
7. Language and speech
   a. Combination of nonfluent aphasia with phonemic errors and fluent aphasia with semantic errors and empty spontaneous speech, and other features of aphasia
   b. Other features: immediate repetition of patient's own (palilalia, also called palinphrasia) or another's words; stereotypy (repeated perseverative utterance of single words or phrases)
   c. Neary criteria for primary progressive aphasia
      1) Progressive nonfluent aphasia
         a) Decreased speech output to late mutism, agram-

matism, impaired repetition (early preservation of word meaning)
         b) Anomia is mild and marked by phonologic errors (phonemic paraphasias)
         c) Poor fluency with effortful and hesitant speech (semantic fluency is better)
         d) Phonemic paraphasias
         e) Oral apraxia and stuttering
         f) Associated with alexia, agraphia
         g) Aspontaneity and economy of speech, echolalia, stereotypy of speech, press of speech, perseveration
         h) MRI: asymmetric frontotemporal atrophy (best localized to left frontotemporal area according to functional studies)
      2) Progressive fluent aphasia: semantic dementia (and associative agnosia)
         a) Fluent and grammatical but empty spontaneous speech
         b) Loss of word meaning, impaired naming and word comprehension: "loss of memory for words"; usually aware of impaired naming and reduced vocabulary, but unaware of reduced comprehension
         c) Associated with semantic (not phonemic) paraphasias
         d) Relatively preserved repetition, able to read aloud, write words with regular spelling-to-sound correspondence
         e) Unable to write, read (and spell) irregular words: surface dysgraphia and dyslexia
         f) Preserved phonology and syntax
         g) Both temporal lobes contribute to poor naming and comprehension
         h) Asymmetric temporal atrophy (L>R) associated with impaired word meaning
         i) Asymmetric temporal atrophy (R>L) associated with crossmodal perceptual disorder: difficulty recognizing faces (prosopagnosia), names, and voices; object agnosia; and emotional perception
         j) Normal perceptual matching and drawing reproduction
         k) Some patients may have pressured speech
         l) May progress to mutism

C. Other Asymmetric Variants
1. Right hemisphere
   a. Frontal lobe: bizarre behavior with disinhibition (orbitofrontal), socially inappropriate, compulsive, rigid, altered appearance and dress
   b. Temporal lobe: reduced empathy, sociopathic tendencies, reduced recognition of emotions

2. Left hemisphere
   a. Frontal lobe: nonfluent aphasia with flat behavior
   b. Temporal lobe: semantic dementia, decreased emotional control, facilitated artistic or musical skills

D. Other Features
1. MRI: frontal and/or anterior temporal atrophy with corresponding sulcal widening and eventual hippocampal atrophy (Fig. 7-10)
2. SPECT and PET show decreased frontotemporal regional blood flow and metabolism

E. Neuropathology (Fig. 7-11)
1. Frontal and/or temporal atrophy

a. Affecting mainly orbitofrontal cortex and anterior and medial temporal areas
b. Relative sparing of precentral gyrus and posterior one-third of superior temporal gyrus
2. Neuronal loss and gliosis of layers II and III of frontotemporal cortex and anterior hippocampus; superficial spongiosis with microvacuolation of the superficial cortical layers
3. Hyperphosphorlyated, insoluble filamentous inclusions or spheroids, tau-positive and/or ubiquitin-positive, tau-negative inclusions
   a. Tau-positive inclusions (Table 7-2)
   b. Ubiquitin-positive and tau-negative inclusions seen in FTD with and without motor neuron disease
4. Frontotemporal atrophy lacking distinctive histology (FTD-ldh)
   a. No specific histologic or immunohistochemical characteristics
   b. Neuronal loss and gliosis
   c. Almost all cases have positive immunohistochemistry staining for ubiquitin

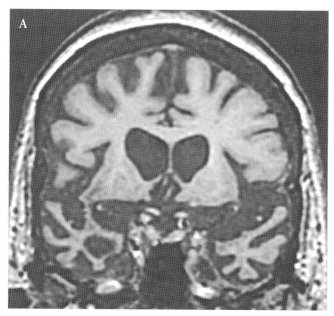

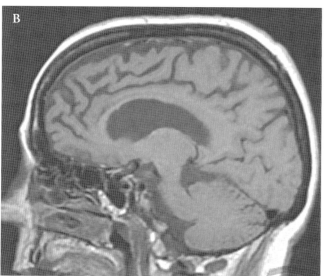

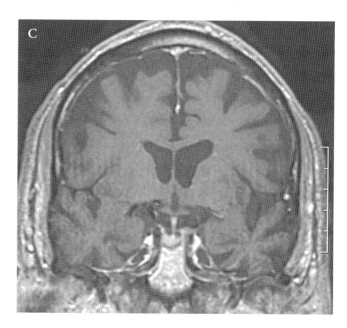

Fig. 7-10. Neuroimaging in frontotemporal dementia (T1-weighted coronal [*A, C*] and sagittal [*B*] images). *A,* Coronal image showing severe atrophy of frontal and anterior temporal cortex. Both the frontal ("knife-like" gyri) and anterior temporal atrophy seem to be more prominent on the right side. *B,* Sagittal image clearly shows prominent mesial frontal atrophy. *C,* Image from patient who presented with primary progressive aphasia shows disproportionate atrophy of left temporal lobe.

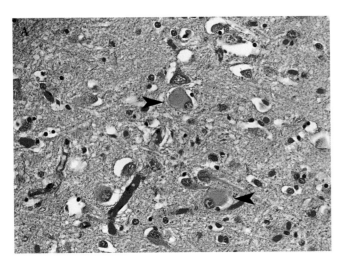

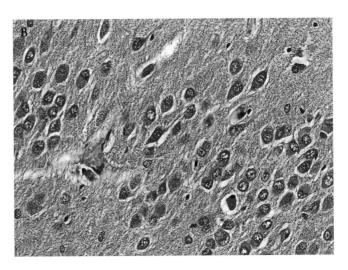

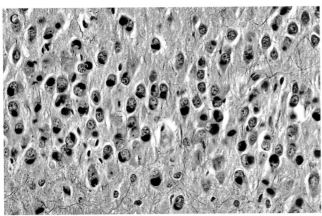

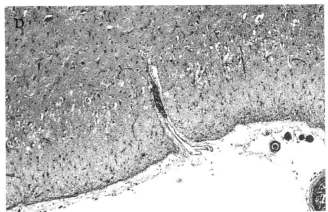

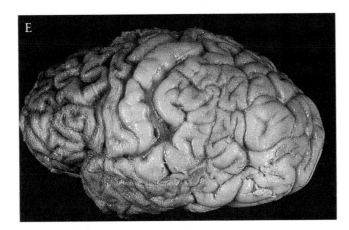

Fig. 7-11. Neuropathology of frontotemporal dementia (FTD). Pick's disease (FTD-Pick): Pick bodies are spherical, well-circumscribed neuronal inclusions that are usually slightly basophilic. *A*, Pick bodies (*arrowheads*) in cortical layers II and III (cortical Pick bodies). *B*, Pick bodies in hippocampus. *C*, Bielschowsky's silver stain demonstrates the neuronal inclusions. *D*, Neocortical microvacuolation, neuronal loss, and gliosis in brain with familial chromosome 17-linked FTD (FTD-17). *E*, Gross specimen of brain with Pick's disease. Note the "knife-like" appearance and marked atrophy of frontal and temporal gyri, with relative sparing of the posterior superior temporal gyrus. (*E* from Okazaki H, Scheithauer BW. Atlas of neuropathology. New York: Gower Medical Publishing; 1988. p. 225. By permission of Mayo Foundation.)

5. Frontotemporal atrophy with motor neuron disease (FTD-MND)
    a. Ubiquitin-immunoreactive, tau-negative inclusion bodies in motor neurons, hippocampus (dentate granule cells), and parahippocampal gyri
    b. Linked to chromosome 9
6. Frontotemporal atrophy with parkinsonism linked to chromosome 17 (FTDP-17): associated with basal

ganglia atrophy and pale substantia nigra in addition to the frontotemporal atrophy described above
7. Pick's disease (FTD-Pick)
    a. Severe frontotemporal atrophy with knife-like gyri, sparing posterior aspect of superior temporal gyrus
    b. Superficial spongiosis: microvacuolation of neocortical layer II with neuronal loss; superficial spongiosis is seen

in all forms of FTD and in most end-stage dementias of other causes
c. Ballooned neurons
d. Pick bodies (tau- and ubiquitin-positive)
   1) Pick bodies are centered in cortical layers II and III (more than layers V and VI) of frontotemporal neocortex, hippocampus (dentate granule cells), parahippocampal gyrus, and amygdala
   2) Pick bodies appear slightly basophilic, argyrophilic, and have a well-defined margin

F. Treatment
1. Behavioral and psychiatric symptoms may respond to SSRIs
2. Marked disinhibition and aggressive behavior may respond to risperidone, olanzapine, or quetiapine
3. In vitro evidence and anecdotal studies suggest that inhibitors of tau phosphorylation (especially glycogen synthase kinase-3 inhibitors, such as lithium and valproic acid) may be beneficial

V. Dementia With Lewy Bodies

A. Risk Factors and Etiology
1. Advanced age
2. Increased frequency of APOE ε4 allele
3. Rare autosomal dominant forms of dementia with Lewy bodies with diffuse Lewy body and neuronal loss in CA2 and CA3 of the hippocampus: may be related to mutation involving the synuclein gene on chromosome 4

B. Clinical Features
1. McKeith criteria (Table 7-4)
   a. Progressive decline in cognition interfering with social and occupational functioning
   b. Prominent or persistent memory impairment in early stages does not typically occur and would be unexpected for this diagnosis
   c. Deficits on tests of attention/concentration, verbal fluency, psychomotor speed, and visuospatial tasks
   d. Two of three core features for clinically probable dementia with Lewy bodies (one for clinically possible dementia with Lewy bodies)
      1) Fluctuating cognition or alertness
      2) Recurrent visual hallucinations
      3) Spontaneous motor symptoms of parkinsonism
2. Cognitive features
   a. Fluctuating cognition, attention, alertness on background of progressive cognitive decline

b. Prominent attentional, executive, and visuospatial deficits
c. Poor working memory
d. "Subcortical" pattern: slowed cognition
e. May not have prominent memory impairment early in disease course
f. Differential diagnosis to include Parkinson's disease with dementia (PDD): illness beginning with parkinsonism syndrome and meeting the criteria for Parkinson's disease with subsequent occurrence of dementia
3. Visual hallucinations
   a. Recurrent, well formed
   b. Typically involve animals, children, or other people
   c. Early on, they tend to occur at night and may be mistaken for hypnogogic hallucinations
4. Parkinsonism
   a. Bilateral, symmetric (most) rigidity, bradykinesia
   b. Tremor less common than in idiopathic Parkinson's disease: postural and symmetric (most)

Table 7-4. McKeith Criteria for Dementia With Lewy Bodies (DLB)

I.   Progressive cognitive decline interfering with social and occupational functioning. Prominent or persistent memory impairment may not necessarily occur in the early stages but is usually evident with progression

II.   Two of three core features for clinically *probable* DLB and one for clinically *possible* DLB:
  a.   Fluctuating cognition with pronounced variations in attention and alertness
  b.   Recurrent visual hallucinations (typically well-formed and detailed)
  c.   Spontaneous motor symptoms of parkinsonism

III.   Deficits on tests of attention/concentration, verbal fluency, psychomotor speed, and visuospatial tasks
IV.   Supportive features (repeated falls, syncope or transient loss of consciousness, delusions, neuroleptic sensitivity, hallucinations of other modalities, REM sleep behavior, depression)

V.   Features suggesting disorder other than DLB
  a.   Focal neurologic deficits or presence of significant cerebrovascular disease on neuroimaging
  b.   Findings on examination or on ancillary testing that another medical, neurologic, or psychiatric disorder sufficiently accounts for the observed clinical features

Modified from McKeith IG, Galasko D, Kosaka K, Perry EK, Dickson DW, Hansen LA, et al. Consensus guidelines for the clinical and pathologic diagnosis of dementia with Lewy bodies (DLB): report of the Consortium on DLB International Workshop. Neurology. 1996;47:1113-24. Used with permission.

c. Shuffling gait

d. Stooped posture

e. Masked facies

f. Not necessarily within 1 year after parkinsonism: the 1-year rule abolished with the new criteria

5. Fluctuation in cognition with variation in attention and alertness

6. Supportive features

a. Neuropsychiatric

1) Systematized delusions (e.g., Capgras' syndrome: patient may believe spouse is replaced by an imposter)

2) Depression, anxiety

3) Tactile or olfactory hallucinations can occur in addition to more typical visual hallucinations

4) Agitation or aggressive behavior

b. Falls: often due to parkinsonism and fluctuating attention

c. Sleep disorders

1) REM sleep behavior disorder: vivid dreams often involving chases or attacks, vocalizations, screaming, and absence of loss of muscle tone; predilection for males

2) Excessive daytime sleepiness

3) Insomnia

4) Periodic limb movements of sleep

d. Neuroleptic sensitivity

e. Syncope: episodes of transient loss of consciousness

f. Autonomic dysfunction: orthostatic hypofunction, urinary incontinence, impotence, constipation (due to Lewy body involvement of peripheral autonomic nervous system and non-nervous system tissues such as gut and cardiac involvement)

C. Imaging

1. Normal vs. whole brain atrophy as seen on MRI, less temporal atrophy than expected in AD

2. PET imaging: bilateral temporoparietal (less prominent than in AD) and occipital hypometabolism (more prominent than in AD)

D. Pathology (Fig. 7-12)

1. Senile plaques and fewer neurofibrillary tangles than AD

2. α-Synuclein–positive Lewy neurites in CA2 and CA3 of hippocampus

3. Lewy bodies: cytoplasmic inclusions found in substantia nigra, limbic regions, and neocortex

a. More densely packed in the center

b. Anti-ubiquitin and anti–α-synuclein immunohistochemistry

c. Diffusely present in cerebral cortex, including limbic and parahippocampal cortices and amygdala, and brainstem; relative sparing of primary neocortex

d. Lewy bodies in parahippocampal and inferior temporal gyri may account for visual hallucinations

E. Treatment

1. Donepezil, galantamine, and rivastigmine: potentially effective for cognitive and behavioral symptoms

2. Dopaminergic therapy: potentially effective for parkinsonism, but increased chance of potential side effects, including hallucinations

3. Atypical neuroleptics for behavioral dyscontrol and agitation, hallucinations: patients at risk for neuroleptic sensitivity

a. Worsening of extrapyramidal or cognitive symptoms; may cause neuroleptic malignant syndrome

b. Quetiapine is the best tolerated antipsychotic agent and has few anticholinergic and antidopaminergic effects

c. Other agents that may be used: clozapine, olanzapine, risperidone

4. SSRIs may be used for depression or emotional lability

5. Sertraline, paroxetine, buspirone for anxiety or obsessive-compulsive behavior

6. Clonazepam and melatonin for REM sleep behavior disorder (minimize use of clonazepam because it can exacerbate dementia, depress level of consciousness, and cause fluctuations in alertness)

7. Fludrocortisone and midodrine for orthostatic hypotension

8. Carbidopa-levodopa, pramipexole, or gabapentin for restless legs syndrome or periodic limb movement disorder

VI. VASCULAR DEMENTIA

A. Heterogeneous Group of Dementing Disorders Resulting From Cerebrovascular Disease (established criteria for diagnosis of vascular dementia are given in Table 7-5)

B. Clinical Spectrum: various vascular disorders can cause dementia

1. Multiple ischemic infarcts due to macrovascular disease

2. Single strategic infarction

a. Caudate nucleus: unilateral or bilateral lesions can produce a behavioral syndrome depending on the location

1) Lesion in dorsolateral caudate: psychomotor depression, apathy, reduced spontaneity

2) Lesion in ventromedial caudate: psychomotor hyper-

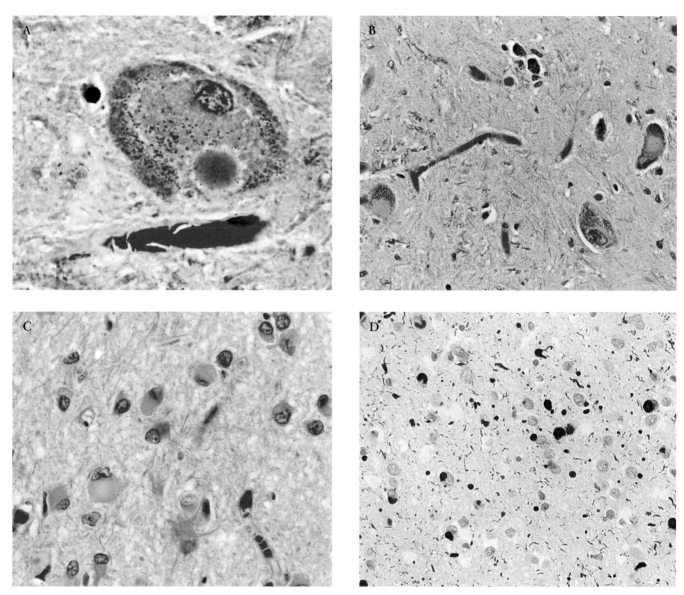

Fig. 7-12. Diffuse Lewy body disease. *A*, Typical classic Lewy body is essentially a neuronal inclusion with a hyaline eosinophilic core and pale halo. (Substantia nigra, hematoxylin-eosin stain.) *B*, Also in the substantia nigra, note the pale bodies that are rounded, granular eosinophilic cytoplasmic inclusions displacing neuromelanin. *C*, Cortical Lewy bodies are rounded, homogeneous eosinophilic structures usually lacking the classic "halo." Cortical Lewy bodies occupy most of the cytoplasm and appear less eosinophilic than brainstem Lewy bodies. *D*, α-Synuclein immunohistochemistry demonstrates the inclusions.

activity, disinhibition, impulsiveness
b. Hippocampi: usually a result of hypoperfusion injury
c. Paramedian thalami
   1) Infarction in territory of Percheron's artery (posterior thalamosubthalamic paramedian artery)
      a) This artery arises at the basilar bifurcation medial to the thalamoperforators and supplies medial thalamus bilaterally and rostral midbrain
      b) Infarction in this arterial distribution can cause

alteration in level of consciousness, lack of spontaneous behavior, and vertical gaze palsy
   d. Right parietal lobe: acute delirium
3. Cerebral hemorrhage(s) due to uncontrolled hypertension, amyloid angiopathy, and others
4. Extensive microvascular disease and arteriosclerosis of deep, penetrating end arterioles: usually "frontal-dysexecutive" syndrome with difficulty performing executive tasks, deficits in attention, psychomotor slowing,

Table 7-5. Criteria for Diagnosis of Vascular Dementia

I.   Criteria for the clinical diagnosis of *probable* vascular dementia include *all* the following:
   a.   Dementia defined by cognitive decline from a previously higher level of functioning and manifested by impairment of memory and of two or more cognitive domains, preferably established by clinical examination and documented by neuropsychologic testing
      i.   Exclusion criteria: cases with disturbances of consciousness, delirium, psychosis, severe aphasia, or major sensorimotor impairment precluding neuropsychologic evaluation. Also excluded are the systemic or primary central nervous system disorders (such as Alzheimer's disease) that can account for the dementia in and of themselves
   b.   Cerebrovascular disease (CVD) defined by presence of focal signs on neurologic examination and evidence of relevant CVD on neuroimaging, including multiple large-vessel infarcts or a single strategically located infarct (angular gyrus, thalamus, basal forebrain, or posterior cerebral artery or anterior cerebral artery territory), as well as multiple basal ganglia and white matter lacunes or extensive periventricular white matter lesions, or combinations thereof
   c.   A relationship between the above two, manifested or inferred by the presence of one or more of the following:
      i.   Onset of dementia within 3 months after a recognized stroke
      ii.   Abrupt deterioration in cognitive function
      iii.   Fluctuating, stepwise progression of cognitive deficits
II.   Clinical features consistent with the diagnosis of *probable* vascular dementia include the following:
   a.   Early presence of gait disturbance
   b.   History of unsteadiness and frequent, unprovoked falls
   c.   Early urinary frequency, urgency, and other urinary symptoms not explained by urologic disease
   d.   Pseudobulbar palsy
   e.   Personality and mood changes, abulia, depression, emotional incontinence, or other subcortical deficits, including psychomotor retardation and abnormal executive function
III.   Features that make the diagnosis of vascular dementia *uncertain* or *unlikely* include:
   a.   Early onset of memory deficit and progressive worsening of memory and other cognitive functions such as language (aphasia), motor skills (apraxia), and perception (agnosia), in the absence of corresponding focal lesions on brain imaging
   b.   Absence of focal neurologic signs other than cognitive disturbance, *and*
   c.   Absence of cerebrovascular lesions on brain computed tomography or magnetic resonance imaging
IV.   Clinical diagnosis of *possible* vascular dementia are:
   a.   Presence of dementia with focal neurologic signs in patients in whom brain imaging fails to confirm definite CVD, *or*
   b.   In the absence of clear temporal relationship between the dementia and the stroke, *or*
   c.   In patients with subtle onset and variable course (plateau or improvement) of cognitive deficits and evidence of relevant CVD
V.   Criteria for diagnosis of *definite* vascular dementia are:
   a.   Clinical criteria for *probable* vascular dementia
   b.   Histopathologic evidence of CVD obtained from biopsy or autopsy
   c.   Absence of neurofibrillary tangles and neuritic plaques exceeding those expected for age, *and*
   d.   Absence of other clinical or pathologic disorder capable of producing dementia
VI.   Classification of vascular dementia for research purposes may be made on the basis of clinical, radiologic, and neuropathologic features, for subcategories or defined conditions such as cortical vascular dementia, subcortical vascular dementia, Binswanger's disease, and thalamic dementia

Data from Román GC, Tatemichi TK, Erkinjuntti T, Cummings JL, Masdeu JC, Garcia JH, et al. Vascular dementia: diagnostic criteria for research studies. Report of the NINDS-AIREN International Workshop. Neurology. 1993;43:250-60.

and apathy (more than other cognitive functions)
   a. Lacunar state (état lacunaire)
      1) Small cavitating lesions in deep gray and white matter that are essentially microinfarcts involving the short, penetrating end arterioles

   2) Frontal white matter tends to be more affected
   b. Binswanger's disease (Fig. 7-13)
      1) Extensive diffuse white matter changes usually associated with hypertension
      2) Onset: usually in sixth to seventh decade

3) Frontal dysexecutive syndrome, poor working memory, inattention, psychomotor retardation with poor apathy and motivation, and other frontal lobe functions may be affected
5. Hereditary vascular disease (e.g., CADASIL [see Chapter 11])
6. Extensive cerebrovascular disease in the setting of Alzheimer's type dementia
   a. Vascular lesions can precipitate dementia in asymptomatic patients with AD
   b. Some have amyloid angiopathy
7. Hypoperfusion injury
   a. May be seen, for example, after cardiopulmonary arrest, carotid endarterectomy, heart surgery
   b. May cause watershed infarcts, which can include deep white matter between distributions of anterior and middle cerebral arteries
   c. May affect neocortex (primarily layers III and V), hippocampi (primarily CA1 and presubiculum), and cerebellar Purkinje cells
   d. Results in neuronal loss and gliosis: "hippocampal sclerosis" and neocortical laminar necrosis
8. Vasculitis and other angiopathy
   a. Primary CNS angiitis
   b. Systemic CNS vasculitis in Wegener's granulomatosis,

rheumatoid arthritis with vasculitis, and others
   c. Sneddon's syndrome: microangiopathic syndrome of small strokes, extensive white matter disease, livedo reticularis, seizures, miscarriages; associated with antiphospholipid antibodies (see Chapter 11)
   d. Spatz-Lindenberg disease
   e. Susac syndrome (see Chapter 11)

C. Clinical Presentation
1. Variable
2. Evidence of cerebrovascular disease with brain imaging
3. Exclusion of extensive white matter lesions from the definition portends a worse prognosis
4. Close temporal relation between onset of cognitive deficits and cerebrovascular disease (onset of dementia abruptly or within 3 months after cerebrovascular insult) may portend a worse prognosis
5. Presence of bilateral cortical and deep gray matter "symptomatic" infarcts
6. Abrupt onset with stepwise progression of deficits is considered typical (slow progression seen less often)
7. Extensive white matter disease as in Binswanger's dis-

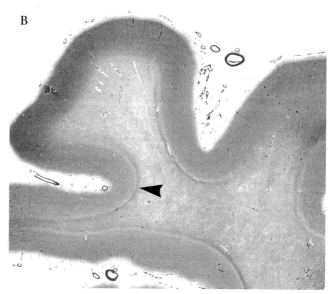

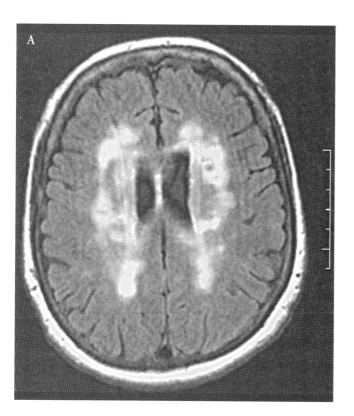

Fig. 7-13. *A*, FLAIR image of a patient with Binswanger's disease. Note the extensive confluent T2 signal abnormality involving white matter (particularly deep and periventricular white matter) and sparing of gray matter and subcortical U-fibers. *B*, Low-power microscopy demonstrates diffuse, confluent myelin pallor in subcortical white matter and sparing of U-fibers (*arrowhead*). These characteristic changes were noted throughout the subcortical white matter.

ease or status lacunaris as well as lacunes involving deep gray matter and frontostriatal and frontothalamic connections can produce a "frontal-subcortical" syndrome

   a. Deficits involve the executive functions ("frontal-dysexecutive" dysfunction) as above: lack of insight, judgment, planning, motivation; patients can have apathy, psychomotor retardation, inattention, and dysfunction of working memory

   b. With status lacunaris, the signs and symptoms corresponding to sustained lacunes would be expected

   c. Akinetic rigid syndrome with pseudobulbar palsy, pseudobulbar palsy, spasticity, and other pyramidal and long tract signs (such as exaggerated deep tendon reflexes and extensor plantar responses) may be seen

8. Anterograde amnesia: may or may not be present (impairment of memory is a requirement for the NINDS-AIREN criteria of probable vascular dementia)

D. Treatment: primarily involves preventive therapy for cerebrovascular disease

1. Antihypertensive treatment, especially calcium channel blockers (which may have a neuroprotective role as well), has been shown to decrease incidence of dementia

2. Anticholinesterase inhibitors may be potentially beneficial (the data may be clouded by concurrent AD lesions in patients studied)

VII. ARGYROPHILIC GRAIN DEMENTIA

A. Pathologic Diagnosis

B. Comorbidity: may coexist with AD or another degenerative dementing illness

C. Presentation: some patients present with behavioral and personality changes, followed by memory deficits, with no other cognitive disturbance

D. Pathology: involves mainly entorhinal cortex, hippocampus (CA2), amygdala, and hypothalamus

1. Spindle-shaped or comma-shaped tau-immunoreactive argyrophilic grains, which are essentially straight filaments

2. Tau protein that accumulates is mostly 4R tau (four-repeat isoform)

3. Ballooned neurons (mostly in amygdala)

4. Neurofibrillary tangles in subthalamic nucleus

5. "Thorny" astrocytes are tau-positive glial inclusions

VIII. NORMAL-PRESSURE HYDROCEPHALUS

A. Also Known as Adult Hydrocephalus Syndrome

B. Clinical Manifestations

1. Chronic history with gradual onset usually comprises patients with true normal pressure hydrocephalus

2. Gait disturbance: characterized by apractic, magnetic gait, described as unsteadiness, wide-based gait with short steps and difficulty picking the feet up off the floor

3. Dementia: characterized by bradyphrenia, disturbance of working memory, "frontal-dysexecutive syndrome" with hydrocephalus impinging on periventricular frontostriatal projections

4. Urinary incontinence: typically with lack of concern for incontinence and associated with urgency at the onset

5. Other akinetic-rigid parkinsonian features are possible

6. Also possible: pyramidal involvement including spasticity, exaggerated reflexes, extensor plantar responses

7. Not really "normal pressure": prolonged monitoring has revealed intermittent, transient elevations of CSF pressure (Lundberg, or B, waves)

C. Ancillary Testing

1. MRI (Fig. 7-14)

   a. Ventriculomegaly out of proportion to cortical atrophy

   b. Periventricular white matter changes assumed to be due to transependymal edema and CSF flow

   c. Decreased aqueductal attenuation (signal-void) presumed to be due to poor compliance of ventricular wall

2. "Large volume" lumbar puncture

Normal-Pressure Hydrocephalus

Triad of gait disturbance (apractic, magnetic gait), urinary incontinence, and dementia (characterized by bradyphrenia, inattention, and frontal-dysexecutive/frontal-subcortical pattern of cognitive impairment)

Intermittent transient elevations of intracranial pressure (Lundberg, or B, waves)

Ancillary testing: MRI, "large-volume" diagnostic spinal tap, and radionuclide cisternography

a. Removal of 20 to 50 mL of CSF with subsequent examination 1 hour and then 24 hours after procedure

b. Positive response (improvement in clinical symptoms) has good predictive value for improvement with a shunt procedure

3. Radionuclide cisternography: rapid diffusion of radioisotope into the ventricles and failure to rise into the sagittal areas

D. Treatment

1. Shunt procedures

a. Treatment of choice for those who are good surgical candidates; gait and urinary function are more likely to improve than cognitive deficits

b. Benign prognostic predictors of response to shunt procedures include young age, relatively recent onset and short duration (<36 months), prominent and early gait disturbance, relatively early or absent cognitive disturbance, improvement after large-volume CSF withdrawal, elevated CSF opening pressures, a known underlying cause (not idiopathic)

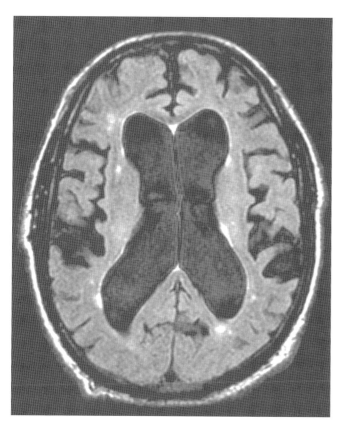

Fig. 7-14. Normal-pressure hydrocephalus. Note marked dilatation of the lateral ventricles that is out of proportion to the atrophy. (Axial FLAIR sequence.)

IX. DEMENTIA RELATED TO TRAUMA

A. Acute Syndrome: acute injury can cause concussion, contusion, intracranial hemorrhagic disorders such as subdural hematoma, deficits ranging from mild attentional deficits to delirium, sometimes accompanied by loss of consciousness

B. There May Be Delayed Deterioration

C. Postconcussive Syndrome

1. Inattention, impaired working memory, executive dysfunction, slowed cognitive speed, headaches, dizziness, and psychiatric symptoms

2. Usually follows most major traumatic concussions (transient or long-lasting)

D. Contusions: usually frontotemporal, can cause any combination of symptoms

1. Frontal lobe symptoms

a. Disturbance of planning, judgment, reasoning, and abstract thought

b. Cause disinhibition and inappropriate social conduct (especially with orbitofrontal and inferior frontal lesions) and anosmia (with damage to olfactory bulbs)

2. Temporal lobe symptoms: disturbance of learning and short-term memory, Klüver-Bucy syndrome with bilateral anterior temporal contusions

E. Permanent Deficits: may be seen with intracranial hemorrhage, including contusions, and diffuse axonal injury

F. Dementia Pugilistica

1. Chronic traumatic encephalopathy of boxing, with progressive cognitive dysfunction

2. Associated with boxing but can occur with soccer and other contact sports (not well studied)

3. 17% of retired professional boxers have the syndrome

4. Rare in amateur boxers

5. Symptoms of chronic encephalopathy associated with dementia pugilistica

a. Extrapyramidal syndrome of akinetic-rigid parkinsonism, associated with tremors, incoordination and ataxia, and pyramidal signs

b. Cognitive deficits: inattention, slowed speech, slowed cognitive speed, poor executive functioning such as judgment, planning, insight, and reasoning

c. Behavioral characteristics: change in personality, apathy, disinhibition, emotional lability

6. MRI: usually nonspecific; can show diffuse atrophy,

subdural hygromas, contusions (frontotemporal, coup-contrecoup)

7. Neuropathology: there may be changes of AD
   a. Tau- and ubiquitin-immunoreactive neurofibrillary tangles in superficial neocortical layers (in contrast to deep location of neurofibrillary tangles of AD)
   b. Amyloid plaques
   c. Neuronal loss involving cerebellar Purkinje cells and frontotemporal neocortical areas
8. Treatment: primarily symptomatic

X. AMYOTROPHIC LATERAL SCLEROSIS/ PARKINSON'S DEMENTIA COMPLEX (OF GUAM)

A. Prominent, Early Dementia
1. Characterized by mental slowness, apathy, irritability, poor abstraction, depression that may progress eventually to akinetic mutism

B. Parkinsonism
1. Characterized by axial rigidity, with eventual development of postural deformities and postural tremor

C. Pyramidal Features
1. Hyperreflexia, spasticity, and bilateral extensor responses

D. Motor Neuron Disease
1. May precede the dementia and parkinsonism, sometimes by several years

E. Associated With Peripheral Neuropathy

F. Pathology
1. Generalized atrophy, with pallor of substantia nigra and locus ceruleus
2. Neuronal loss and gliosis affecting mesial temporal structures, deep gray matter (striatum, thalamus, and substantia nigra), brainstem tegmentum, and anterior horn cells
3. Tau-immunoreactive neurofibrillary tangles in some of the aforementioned structures

XI. PRION DISORDERS (TRANSMISSIBLE SPONGIFORM ENCEPHALOPATHIES)

A. Creutzfeldt-Jakob Disease (CJD)

1. Rapidly progressive dementing prion disease that can be accompanied by ataxia, myoclonus, pyramidal and extrapyramidal tract signs, and other features, usually causing death in less than 1 year
2. 85% of cases are sporadic (few reported cases of accidental inoculation and cannibalism [kuru]); 15% are inherited in autosomal dominant fashion
3. Prions do not self-replicate but act as molecular chaperones, altering the structure and function of normal prion protein (PrP)
4. PrP: a membrane-associated protein (gene located on chromosome 20p) attached to cell membrane by a glycolipid at its C-terminus; role unknown
5. PrP^C: normal isoform of membrane-bound PrP, primarily α-helical structure
6. PrP^{Sc}: abnormal isoform of PrP protein, with a higher β-pleated sheet content; insoluble, more resistant to proteolysis and tendency to polymerize and accumulate intracellularly (causing neuronal loss, gliosis, and vacuolization) and extracellularly (in plaques)
7. Exact mechanism of conversion of PrP^C to PrP^{Sc} is unknown but appears to involve conformational changes independent of other posttranslational modifications
8. PrP^{Sc} has the ability to bind to PrP^C and perpetuate further conversion to the abnormal isoform
9. Polymorphism at codon 129: susceptibility factor
   a. Codon 129 of the prion gene (*PRNP*) codes for either methionine (Met) or valine (Val)
   b. Homozygosity for either Met or Val confers susceptibility
      1) 90% of cases of sporadic CJD (sCJD) are homozygous for either Met or Val
      2) Homozygosity for Met at codon 129 confers susceptibility for iatrogenic CJD (iCJD)
      3) Homozygosity for Met at codon 129 confers susceptibility for variant CJD (vCJD): 100% of patients with vCJD are homozygous for Met
   c. Several other mutations of *PRNP* have been associated with familial CJD (fCJD)
      1) The most common mutation is glutamine → lysine miscoding at codon 200 (E200K)
      2) Second most common mutation is aspartate (D) → asparagine (N) miscoding at codon 178 (D178N mutation); concomitant with this mutation, the residue at codon 129 determines susceptibility
         a) Val at codon 129 → fCJD phenotype
         b) Met at codon 129 → fatal familial insomnia phenotype
10. Highest concentration of abnormal prion protein is in

cell membrane and lysosomes
11. Abnormal aggregation of abnormal prion protein may affect synaptic transmission and induce dendritic swelling, which may be primarily responsible for spongiform pathologic features
12. Extracellular aggregation and polymerization of abnormal prion protein with high β-pleated sheet content may result in formation of plaques in the form of amyloid (amyloidosis is the hallmark of vCJD, kuru, and Gerstmann-Sträussler-Scheinker syndrome much more frequently than fCJD or sCJD)
13. Histopathology (Fig. 7-15)
    a. Macroscopic appearance is quite variable (normal to severe atrophy)
    b. Spongiform change (status spongiosus): intracellular vacuolation of neuropil primarily affecting the gray matter (neocortical and deep gray matter), representing focal areas of swollen axonal and dendritic processes which occur primarily at synapses
    c. Neuronal loss: greatest in neocortical layers III to V
    d. Reactive gliosis: massive reactivation and proliferation of astrocytes
    e. PrP-immunoreactive amyloid fibrils and plaques: variable, extent depends on CJD type (as mentioned above)
14. Ancillary testing
    a. CSF 14-3-3 (marker of neuronal loss, normally present in CNS neuronal cytoplasm)
        1) High sensitivity (94%-97%) and specificity (84%-87%) for sCJD; specificity is higher in the appropriate clinical context
        2) Much lower sensitivity for fCJD and vCJD

3) Level of CSF 14-3-3 tends to increase during course of the illness; it is important to retest if initial result is negative
4) This is a distinguishing feature from other dementing illnesses
5) Elevated CSF 14-3-3 reflects neuronal destruction and may be elevated in any condition causing rapid neuronal death, such as stroke, trauma, Hashimoto's encephalopathy, and viral encephalitis (including human immunodeficiency virus [HIV] encephalopathy)
    b. EEG pattern can change with disease progression
        1) Earliest change may be slow-wave abnormalities
        2) With disease progression, diphasic or triphasic sharp waves may appear
            a) These appear at first to be sporadic
            b) With further disease progression, they evolve into a characteristic pattern of periodic sharp waves, usually occurring at intervals of 0.5 to 1 second
        3) Myoclonic jerks often occur in conjunction with periodic sharp waves
    c. Brain MRI: increased T2 signal in neocortex, thalamus, caudate, and putamen, but not in globus pallidus; most changes are asymmetric (Fig. 7-16)
        1) Classic "cortical ribbon sign" best noted on diffusion-weighted imaging, which is result of neocortical neuronal loss
        2) "Pulvinar sign": characterized by T2 hyperintesity of pulvinar nuclei, often symmetric when bilateral, and reported only with vCJD
15. Sporadic CJD

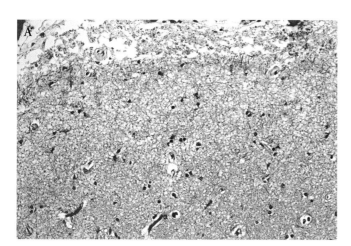
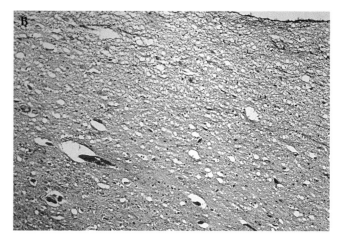

Fig. 7-15. Histopathology of Creutzfeldt-Jakob disease. *A*, Status spongiosus with coarse vacuolation of the cortex and, *B*, the deep gray matter (thalamus) in advanced disease.

a. Age at onset: usually between 50 and 75 years

b. Average duration of symptoms: 7 months

c. Acute or subacute presentation is possible

d. Marked by rapidly progressive dementia, myoclonus, ataxia

e. Early signs may be difficulty with memory and concentration, change in personality, apathy, inappropriate behavior, and psychiatric symptoms (psychosis, aggression, others)

f. Vegetative functions affected relatively early: poor appetite, poor sleep hygiene, others

g. Other symptoms that eventually develop include myoclonus (which may be stimulus-induced [startle] or spontaneous), ataxia, and pyramidal and extrapyramidal (chorea, athetosis) symptoms

h. Final stage: usually marked by akinetic mutism

i. Clinical variants

   1) Heidenhain variant: rapidly progressive cortical blindness; primarily occipital lobes are affected

   2) Amyotrophic variant: prominent, early lower motor neuron signs

   3) Brownell-Oppenheimer (cerebellar) variant: early, prominent, rapidly progressive ataxia

   4) Stern-Garcia (extrapyramidal) variant: early, promi-

nent parkinsonism and other extrapyramidal features, primarily affects deep gray matter, including basal ganglia

j. Criteria

   1) Definite sCJD: diagnosis requires histopathologic examination

   2) Probable sCJD: progressive dementia with duration less than 6 months and two of the following:

      a) Myoclonus

      b) Visual or cerebellar deficits

      c) Pyramidal or extrapyramidal features

      d) Akinetic mutism and ancillary findings of periodic EEG epileptiform activity, CSF 14-3-3, or typical MRI findings

   3) Possible sCJD: progressive dementia with duration less than 2 years and two of aforementioned four features

16. Variant CJD

a. Young age at onset (average age, 27 years)

b. Average duration of illness: about 14 months

c. Restricted to homozygous Met/Met genotype at codon 129 of *PRNP*

d. Early psychiatric and sensory symptoms, with later development of ataxia leading to dementia and myoclonus

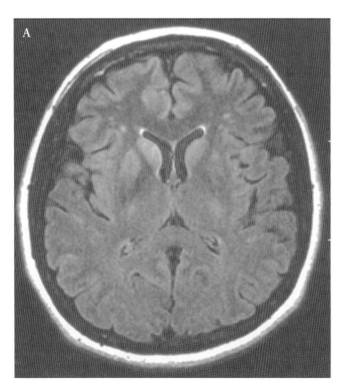
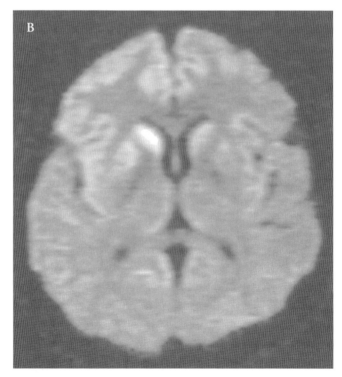

Fig. 7-16. MRI image from a 54-year-old woman with Creutzfeldt-Jakob disease. Note increased signal in the caudate and putamen bilaterally (asymmetric) in the *A,* FLAIR nand, *B,* diffusion-weighted imaging sequences.

e. Sensory symptoms include dysesthesias in the limb(s) more than the face

f. 77% of patients have a high signal in posterior thalamus-pulvinar bilaterally

g. CSF 14-3-3 less useful

h. EEG usually does not show the typical periodic EEG activity

i. Premortem diagnosis by tonsil biopsy is sometimes helpful: may show positive PrP immunohistochemistry

j. Histopathology
1) Numerous prion amyloid plaques consisting of aggregates of the abnormal prion protein
2) Spongiform changes are most prominent in thalamus and basal ganglia

17. Iatrogenic CJD
a. Associated with corneal transplants from contaminated surgical instruments, contaminated pituitary hormones, dural grafts from human cadavers, and pericardial grafts

b. Inoculation of surgical instruments likely from inadequate temperatures of autoclaving (required temperature for steam autoclaving is now 134°C)

c. Direct inoculation of CNS by the causative agent (as with corneal transplants): clinical course identical to that of sCJD

d. Indirect inoculation (as with cadaveric pituitary hormones): prominent early ataxia and late dementia (spongiform changes and neuronal loss most prominent in cerebellum, more often than in deep neocortical layers)

e. Some patients have characteristic periodic activity on EEG (depends on disease stage)

f. Most cases: positive CSF 14-3-3

18. Familial CJD
a. Age at onset: usually earlier and course usually longer than sCJD

b. Except for E200K, most known mutations do not show periodic EEG changes

c. Peripheral neuropathy possibly associated with the E200K mutation

B. Fatal Familial Insomnia

1. Mutation of *PRNP* responsible for fatal familial insomnia is D178N (aspartate to asparagine at codon 178) in addition to Met residue at codon 129, as mentioned above

2. Severe neuronal loss and gliosis affect ventral and mediodorsal thalamic nuclei more than inferior olivary nuclei and cerebellum, with little spongiform change

3. Average age at onset: 48 years (25-61)

4. Disease duration: can range between 6 months and 3 years

5. Syndrome of intractable insomnia with dysautonomia

6. Clinical course: subacute onset, rapidly progressive, intractable insomnia, followed by dysautonomia (primarily sympathetic hyperactivity such as hypertension, tachycardia, hyperhidrosis), ataxia, myoclonus, pyramidal signs, and extrapyramidal features such as tremor

7. Cognitive function tends to be spared until late in the disease: mainly poor attention, disorientation, confusion, hallucinations

8. EEG generally shows diffuse slowing, not periodic sharp waves characteristic of sCJD

C. Sporadic Fatal Insomnia

1. Clinical and pathologic features identical to those of fatal famial insomnia in the absence of a mutation of *PRNP*

D. Gerstmann-Sträussler-Scheinker (GSS) Syndrome

1. Presentation usually in the third to fourth decades

2. Slow clinical course (3-8 years' duration)

3. Histopathology: neuronal loss, gliosis, minimal spongiform change, and abundant PrP-amyloid deposits and plaques (Fig. 7-17)

4. Most cases have prominent and early ataxia, with later involvement of cognition, and pyramidal and extrapyramidal signs

5. Cognitive impairment can be various combinations of inattention, deficits in working memory and short-term memory, psychomotor retardation, disorientation

6. Mutation subtype dictates the clinical manifestations
a. Ataxic GSS (P102L): most common mutation, presenting with ataxia and varying degrees of dementia
b. Telencephalic GSS (A117V): predominantly dementia (± ataxia), variable presentation depending on the residue at codon 129
c. Progressive spastic paraparesis (P105L): early and progressive spastic paraparesis that may originally present with a clumsy hand; with progression, ataxia and cognitive decline may develop
d. Slowly progressive dementia (Y145Stop): disease course may be as long as 20 years

E. Kuru

1. Reported in the Fore tribe of New Guinea

2. Transmission: exposure to infected tissue by cannibalism

3. Incubation period can range from 4.5 months to 40 years (rare cases of kuru in patients with a long incubation period)

4. Average length of disease until death: 12 months

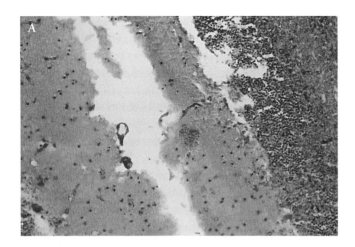

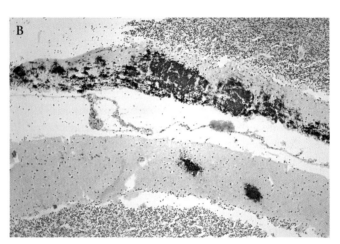

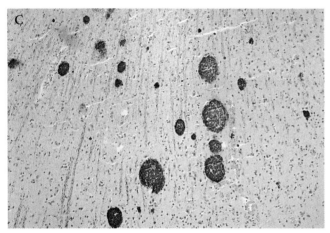

Fig. 7-17. Gerstmann-Straüssler-Scheinker disease. *A,* Eosinophilic floccular plaque in cerebellar molecular layer. These are described as granular clusters of eosinophilic material. Note large number of prion protein immunoreactive floccular plaques in the molecular layer of the cerebellum (*B*) and in cerebral cortex (*C*). Most have a multicentric appearance.

5. Predominant clinical feature: ataxia
6. Early phase is marked by dysarthria, gait ataxia, truncal instability (there may be "clawing" of the toes when standing with feet together), titubation, and postural tremor
7. With progression, there is worsening of ataxia and dysarthria, and patients may develop emotional lability, psychomotor retardation, and uncontrollable laughter
8. Histopathology: neuronal loss highest in cerebellum >> basal ganglion, thalamus, mesial temporal lobe, with prominent amyloid deposits and dense-core plaques
9. Homozygosity for Met at codon 129: susceptibility gene

XII. OTHER INFECTIOUS AND INFLAMMATORY CAUSES OF DEMENTIA

A. Objective
1. Discuss some examples of infectious entities associated with progressive dementias
2. Neurology of infectious disease is described in detail in other chapters

B. HIV-associated Dementia Complex
1. Wide range of severity of cognitive symptoms (from mild cognitive impairment to advanced dementia), associated with motor symptoms
2. Syndrome with symptoms of mild severity is referred to as "HIV1-associated minor cognitive/motor disorder"
3. Cognitive disturbance is a variable combination of the following symptoms (but primarily a "subcortical dementia" pattern of deficits): disturbance of working memory, attention, and concentration, and bradyphrenia (slowness in thinking), in addition to poor initiation, psychomotor slowing, apathy, and psychiatric symptoms such as psychosis, mania, agitation, and obsessive-compulsive behavior
4. Insidious onset and variable progression (may be stable for several years or progressive throughout)
5. Motor symptoms may be a combination of pyramidal and extrapyramidal symptoms: tremors (especially postural tremors), ataxia, myoclonus, exaggerated reflexes and tone, extensor plantar responses; also bowel and bladder symptoms in more advanced stages of disease
6. Diffuse atrophy and periventricular and deep white matter abnormal signal on MRI

C. General Paresis of Neurosyphilis
1. Gradually progressive behavioral syndrome is quite variable in presentation (usually 3-40 years after primary infection with *Treponema pallidum*)

a. Frontal-dysexecutive syndrome: inattention, poor planning, poor judgment, and dysfunction of other executive tasks

b. Psychiatric: psychosis, delusions, hallucinations, depression, mania, aggression, agitation, irritability

c. Juvenile paresis may occur from primary congenital infection presenting in first or second decade of life

d. Brain gummas are extremely rare

e. Concurrent symptoms (e.g., tabes dorsalis, Argyll-Robertson pupils) and serum and CSF serology tests may assist in diagnosis

f. Treatment usually does not reverse the dementing illness

D. Dementia Associated With Late Neuroborreliosis

1. Cognitive impairment associated with third stage of Lyme disease (occurs in <10% of patients)

2. Chronic progressive encephalomyelitis with white matter involvement and cognitive disorder with primary symptoms of inattention and apathy; associated with psychomotor retardation, depression, emotional lability, attention-deficit/hyperactivity disorder, and possibly extrapyramidal symptoms of tremor and bradykinesia

3. This dementia can be treated; is reversible to some degree

E. Whipple's Disease

1. Dementia, supranuclear palsy, and myoclonus (about 1-5 years after onset of systemic symptoms such as the gastrointestinal tract symptoms of malabsorption, abdominal pain, weight loss)

2. The dementia has a "frontal-subcortical pattern": primarily affects attention and working memory

3. 20% of patients have the pathognomonic oculomasticatory myorhythmia

F. Postencephalitic Dementia Associated With Herpes Simplex Infection

1. Postencephalitic cognitive disorder can persist after the acute infection, especially in elderly or immunocompromised patients

2. May also occur in the context of other viral encephalitides

3. Risk factors: delay in administration of acyclovir in acute stage, age, and low level of consciousness in acute presentation

4. Cognitive disorder primarily affecting language and memory, may mimic frontotemporal dementia

5. Varying degree of aphasia

6. Behavioral symptoms: apathy, aggression, agitation, disinhibition, poor executive functions, possibly Klüver-Bucy phenotype

G. Dementia Associated With Multiple Sclerosis

1. Usually less severe than most other dementias

2. 60% of patients with multiple sclerosis have a cognitive complaint at some point during the illness

3. Patients with progressive multiple sclerosis tend to have more cognitive deficits than those with relapsing-remitting multiple sclerosis

4. Degree of cognitive impairment can vary from mild cognitive deficits to advanced dementia

5. Most common complaint is "memory problems"
   a. This may be impaired working memory due to depression or otherwise inattention due to fatigue and other multiple sclerosis–related symptoms
   b. Some patients may have difficulty with retrieval of short-term and remote memories

6. Psychiatric symptoms
   a. Depression and other affective disorder (rarely, psychosis)
   b. Change in personality: may be "frontal-lobe behavior" of disinhibition, apathy

7. Other behavioral manifestations thought to be due to extensive subcortical plaque burden, especially affecting frontostriatal subcortical pathways
   a. Psychomotor retardation and impaired information-processing speed, abnormal set-shifting tasks
   b. Frontal-dysexecutive syndrome with abnormal abstract thought, judgment, planning, organization
   c. Pseudobulbar palsy
   d. Emotional lability: "emotional incontinence," extremes of emotions, inappropriate laughter or crying
   e. Relative preservation of language

8. MRI
   a. Neuroimaging evidence of atrophy and ex-vacuo ventriculomegaly correlates weakly with degree of cognitive impairment
   b. Degree of "plaque burden" correlates better with degree of cognitive impairment
   c. Degree of corpus callosal atrophy correlates with frontal-subcortical dysfunction
   d. Involvement of neocortical gray matter by demyelination: good correlation with degree of cognitive impairment

9. Donepezil: recently reported to improve cognitive function in multiple sclerosis

XIII. Toxic-Metabolic Causes of Dementia

A. Introduction

1. For a more extensive discussion of toxic and metabolic disorders of the nervous system, see Chapter 17

2. Refer to the corresponding chapters for a more complete discussion

3. Metabolic encephalopathies are not discussed here

B. Alcoholic Dementia

1. Debatable topic because most patients also have a nutritional deficiency, Korsakoff's syndrome, or medical complications such as hepatic encephalopathy

2. Occurs with long-term history (≥10 years) of heavy intake of alcohol

3. Possible exacerbating factors believed to predispose to the neurotoxic effect of alcohol: periodic binge drinking and thiamine deficiency

4. Clinical manifestations: very gradual onset and slow progression of cognitive and behavioral deficits
   a. Cognitive dysfunction is primarily a "frontal-dysexecutive" disorder with inattention, poor working memory, poor planning and judgment, impaired abstraction and reasoning, and circumstantiality of speech and thought
   b. Also poor motivation and initiation, disinhibition, socially inappropriate behavior, and paranoid ideation

5. With ongoing exposure to alcohol, syndrome slowly progresses

6. With cessation or reduction of alcohol intake, cognitive deficits may be reversed to some degree

7. MRI
   a. May show diffuse atrophy, which may be more pronounced in prefrontal areas
   b. Changes may be reversible if alcohol intake is discontinued

8. Functional imaging shows reduced metabolism in mesial frontal cortex

C. Wernicke-Korsakoff Syndrome

1. Usually in setting of chronic alcoholism or nonalcohol-related malnutrition

2. Thought to be due to thiamine deficiency

3. Wernicke's encephalopathy
   a. Acute presentation of delirium and global confusional state, ataxia (axial, not appendicular), nystagmus and ophthalmoparesis (especially cranial nerve VI palsy, commonly bilateral ± other cranial nerves), sometimes followed by Korsakoff's syndrome
   b. There may be apathy and inattention in alert patients
   c. Classic triad is not present in up to 90% of cases, so it is important to have a low threshold for treating alcoholics with any *one* of the following symptoms:
      1) Alteration of consciousness (ranging from acute confusion to coma)
      2) Ataxia

      3) Ophthalmoparesis
      4) Nystagmus
      5) Hypothermia
      6) Hypotension
      7) Memory deficits
   d. Untreated Wernicke's encephalopathy: 20% mortality rate
   e. Evidence for use of thiamine (well-established practice) is based on a series of case reports and two small randomized controlled trials
   f. Ophthalmoparesis is likely due to involvement of cranial nerve nuclei III, VI, or vestibular nuclei
   g. Ataxia may be due to involvement of superior cerebellar peduncle (possibly vestibular system, peripheral and central)
   h. Some evidence suggests treatment of Wernicke's encephalopathy with thiamine supplements reverses ophthalmoparesis and ataxia within minutes to hours, with a more gradual recovery of the nystagmus; impairment of memory is slower and often incomplete

4. Korsakoff's syndrome
   a. Chronic amnestic syndrome, both anterograde and retrograde components for events as far back as several years
   b. Is often the "chronic phase" of acute Wernicke's encephalopathy

5. Peripheral neuropathy may be associated with Wernicke-Korsakoff syndrome

6. Polyneuropathy associated with thiamine deficiency without other features of Wernicke-Korsakoff syndrome is sometimes called "dry beriberi"

7. MRI
   a. Abnormal T2 signal in anterior diencephalon, medial thalami, periaqueductal region, mamillary bodies, sometimes with contrast enhancement in acute stage
   b. In chronic stage, mamillary bodies and anterior diencephalon may show atrophy

8. Pathology (Fig. 7-18)
   a. Microscopic appearance: petechial hemorrhage, congestion, atrophy of mamillary bodies and sometimes anterior hypothalamus, thalami, and periaqueductal gray matter
   b. Microscopic appearance
      1) Capillary dilatation, endothelial hyperplasia, hemosiderin-laden macrophages with areas of petechial hemorrhage in acute stage
      2) Chronically, neuronal loss, gliosis, spongiform appearance
      3) Hemosiderin-laden macrophages may persist into chronic stage

9. Treatment
   a. Thiamine and adequate nutritional supplementation

b. Abstinence from alcohol

c. Amnestic syndrome associated with Korsakoff's syndrome is not reversed with thiamine supplementation, but further progression is usually halted

D. Marchiafava-Bignami Disease

1. Described originally in malnourished Italian males who consumed large amounts of red wine; has since been described in association with chronic alcoholism (rarely in nonalcoholics)
2. Hallmark: symmetrical demyelination of corpus callosum, affecting most prominently the central portion (other regions or entire corpus callosum may be involved) (Fig. 7-19)
3. Other structures may be affected: optic chiasm, cerebellar peduncles, pons, anterior or posterior commissures, deep white matter
4. Patients with chronic disease usually also have atrophy of corpus callosum
5. In addition to demyelination, there is usually necrosis, hemorrhage, and cavitation of affected areas
6. Variable presentation
   a. Acute presentation: various degrees of altered mentation and consciousness (patients are often stuporous or comatose), seizures, death
   b. Subacute presentation: various degrees of altered mentation, gait disturbance, behavioral abnormalities
   c. Chronic presentation: mild, progressive dementia
   d. Subacute and chronic presentations may have "disconnection syndrome" of left-sided apraxia and alien hand phenomenon, hemialexia without agraphia, "mirror image" movements, and others
7. MRI
   a. Contrast enhancement of acute lesion
   b. T2 hyperintensity of affected region, with hypointensity on T1-weighted images
   c. Atrophy of corpus callosum of chronic lesion, most prominent in anterior part of corpus callosum

E. Hepatic Encephalopathy (see Chapter 17)

F. Uremic Encephalopathy (see Chapter 17)

G. Industrial Agents

1. Lead, mercury, manganese, aluminum (see Chapter 17)
2. Aluminum toxicity has been associated with dialysis dementia

H. Hypothyroidism

1. Associated with lethargy, psychomotor retardation, apathy, depression, poor attention
2. May be associated with encephalopathy ("encephalopathy associated with autoimmune thyroiditis," and known previously as "Hashimoto's encephalopathy")

I. Hashimoto's Encephalopathy

1. Rare
2. Diagnosis of exclusion
3. Proposed to be a nonvasculitic, autoimmune meningo-encephalitis, but some cases with this diagnosis may be vasculitic because adequate angiographic and histopathologic data are lacking
4. Characterized by subacute onset of delirium, headaches, seizures, ataxia, myoclonus, psychosis, and possibly stroke-like events

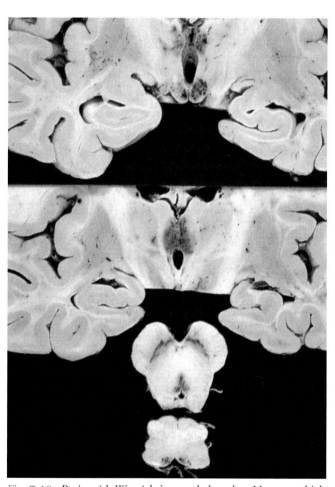

Fig. 7-18. Brain with Wernicke's encephalopathy. Note petechial hemorrhages in hypothalamus (especially mamillary bodies), periaqueductal gray matter, and medulla. (From Okazaki H, Scheithauer BW. Atlas of neuropathology. New York: Gower Medical Publishing; 1988. p. 253. By permission of Mayo Foundation.)

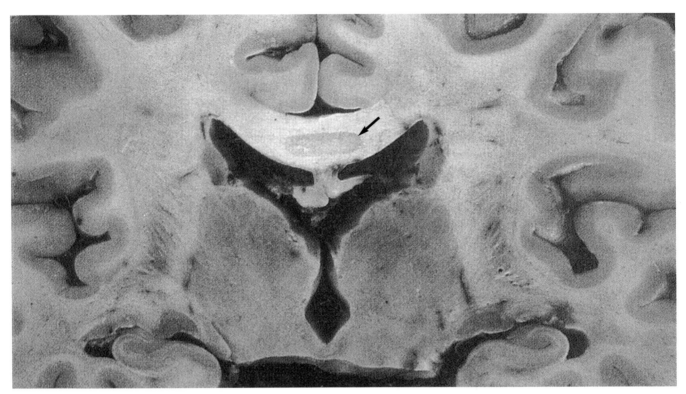

Fig. 7-19. Brain with Marchiafava-Bignami disease. Note discoloration of the central portion of corpus callosum (*arrow*). Microscopic examination would show demyelination and necrosis. (From Ellison D, Love S, Chimelli L, Harding B, Lowe J, Roberts GW, et al. Neuropathology: a reference text of CNS pathology. London: Mosby; 1998. p. 25.20. Used with permission.)

5. Classic description
   a. Autoimmunity against thyroid peroxisomes and increase in anti-thyroid peroxisomal antibodies
      1) No evidence that the antibodies cause the encephalopathy
      2) Thus more appropriate name is "encephalopathy associated with autoimmune thyroiditis"
   b. Typically presents when patient is euthyroid (hypothyroidism has also been observed at presentation) or with subclinical hypothyroidism (normal T3 [triiodothyronine] and T4 [thyroxine], with elevated sTSH [sensitive thyrotropin test])
6. Likely to be a spectrum of autoimmune disorders
   a. May be associated with systemic autoimmune disorders such as Sjögren's syndrome and systemic lupus erythematosus
   b. This spectrum of nonvasculitic autoimmune meningoencephalitis is also known as "nonvasculitic autoimmune inflammatory meningoencephalitis"
7. MRI: normal in most cases, but may show multifocal changes

8. CSF: may be completely normal or have increased protein levels (mostly mild increase)
9. EEG abnormalities: variable and reversible (normalize with corticosteroid treatment)
   a. Primarily, generalized slow-wave abnormalities
   b. Lateralized slowing is possible
   c. Triphasic and atypical triphasic waves are possible
   d. Rarely, epileptiform discharges
   e. Rarely, photomyogenic response
10. Often quick recovery when treated with corticosteroids (also called "steroid-responsive encephalopathy associated with autoimmune thyroiditis")

J. Adult Polyglucosan Body Disease
1. Rare, slowly progressive syndrome
2. Late onset: commonly presents between fifth and seventh decades
3. Ashkenazi Jewish patients: deficiency of glycogen branching enzyme (GBE) due to mutation of *GBE* gene (mutation not present in other populations)
4. Accumulation of cytoplasmic periodic acid-Schiff–posi-

tive polyglucosan bodies in CNS and peripheral nervous system (most abundant in myelinated fibers)

5. Manifestations
   a. Peripheral neuropathy (80% of patients)
   b. Dementia (64%)
   c. Neurogenic bladder (72%)
   d. Upper motor neuron signs (80%)
6. Combination of upper and lower motor neuron involvement mimics amyotrophic lateral sclerosis
7. Polyglucosan bodies
   a. Nonspecific pathologic finding (in the absence of corresponding clinical features) and may be seen in nerve biopsy specimens from normal subjects and occasionally from patients with axonal neuropathies and amyotrophic lateral sclerosis
   b. Pathologic equivalent in normal aged brains is corpora amylacea that are typically in superficial cortical layers but are scattered throughout the parenchyma in adult polyglucosan body disease

XIV. RELATED TOPICS

A. Depression-Associated Dementia: pseudodementia

1. Patients usually are aware of their problem and have good insight
2. May also have an underlying dementia: demented patients who become depressed have more severe symptoms than nondemented patients with depression
3. Psychiatric symptoms (depression plus psychosis) may represent prodrome of a neurodegenerative dementia
4. Cognitive deficits: primarily involve attention, set-shifting tasks, and working memory much more frequently than short-term memory (not immediate recall) and remote memory deficits
5. Poor motivation, impairment in cognitive tasks that require effort
6. Psychomotor retardation
7. Ganser syndrome: "syndrome of approximate answers"
   a. Answers are consistently nearly correct but not correct
   b. Usually seen in context of psychiatric disease and malingering, but may also occur in degenerative dementias
8. Vegetative functions affected, such as poor sleep hygiene and appetite
9. Involvement of noradrenergic pathways can explain anhedonia, apathy, anorexia: this can occur with involvement of locus ceruleus
10. Involvement of serotonergic and cholinergic pathways may explain guilt, depressed mood, and suicidal ideations

11. First-line agents are SSRIs: have the least anti-cholinergic effect and are better tolerated

B. Transient Global Amnesia

1. Paroxysmal and transient loss of memory that may last up to 24 hours but usually less than 12 hours
2. Acutely, both anterograde and retrograde amnesia
3. Predominant form of memory affected: anterograde episodic memory (the period of amnesia is usually limited to the time during the episode)
4. Intact remote memory, immediate recall, and personal identity
5. No other neurologic deficits
6. Recovery
   a. Retrograde amnesia resolves to a brief period immediately before the episode
   b. Typically, permanent loss of memory for the time immediately before the episode and the entire time during the episode (no learning)
7. Etiology: unknown
8. Incidence: 5.2 per 100,000 in Rochester, MN (higher for population older than 50 years)
9. Differential diagnosis
   a. Complex partial seizures, TIA (rare, transient ischemia of hippocampus bilaterally), migraine, toxic (alcohol, drug intoxication)
   b. Symptoms must be differentiated from aphasia (language function is normal) or delirium
   c. Neurologic examination is often normal, other than memory deficits
10. Differential diagnosis also includes psychogenic amnesia: most commonly suppression of unpleasant memories as well as psychogenic "fugue" state, in which patients awaken from the amnesia and find themselves in an unfamiliar or strange place, without knowledge of how they got there; these psychogenic "fugue" states may be due to malingering or a dissociative state
11. Benign prognosis; up to 24% of patients have recurrent episodes, none are at greater risk for subsequent stroke

XV. CHILD AND ADOLESCENT BEHAVIORAL NEUROLOGY

A. Pervasive Developmental Disorders

1. Autism
   a. 90% to 100% concordance rate in monozygotic twins
   b. Most frequent associated chromosomal abnormality: fragile X
   c. The risk of recurrence of autism in families is about 5%

after the birth of a first affected child

   d. Autistic regression generally begins between 18 and 24 months of life; by school-age, symptoms may resolve, but children may continue to have impaired social skills

   e. Impaired communication skills (verbal and nonverbal) and social skills

     1) Apathetic, do not seek social interactions and may or may not accept approaches by others

     2) Some children may be interactive and talk to people in a persistent way

     3) The children usually do not spontaneously seek interaction with people and do not wish to share interests and achievements with others

   f. Restricted range of behaviors and stereotypies: stereotypic and repetitive (motor) mannerisms, such as repetitive rocking

   g. Inflexible adherence to routines and rituals

   h. Language abnormalities

     1) Echolalia (repetition of phrases said by others)

     2) Palilalia (repetition of phrases said by the patient)

     3) Aprosodia (speech is monotonic, a mechanical quality)

   i. Up to 85% are mentally retarded (excluding Asperger's syndrome)

   j. IQ is the most important predictor of long-term outcome

   k. Up to 25% of patients develop seizures

   l. Asperger's syndrome: this term is reserved for a milder phenotype of the spectrum of autism in which the early language development is normal and IQ is often normal

     1) The children are often socially inept and unable to form peer relations, often most apparent in late childhood

     2) They often have considerable difficulty interpreting emotional attachment of gestures and body language of others

     3) They have difficulty understanding abstract concepts such as the punch line of a joke

2. Developmental dyslexia

   a. Unexpected difficulty learning to read, despite normal intelligence

   b. Diagnosis is usually delayed until third grade

   c. Early identification and intervention important for preventing long-term reading difficulties

3. Attention-deficit/hyperactivity disorder

   a. Prevalence reported at 1% to 20%; prevalence in childhood is 6% to 10% and in adulthood 2% to 7%

   b. Characterized by inattention, impulsivity, distractibility, hyperactivity

   c. Generally complete recovery by adulthood but up to

70% of adults with the disorder report that it has persisted since childhood

   d. Few patients (10%) develop antisocial personality disorder or other psychiatric illness

   e. Some patients have concurrent tics (more common in boys)

   f. Neurologic examination is normal, other than inattention and frontal-executive dysfunction

   g. Treatment

     1) Mainstay is psychostimulants such as methylphenidate, dextromethorphan, and pemoline (tics are not a contraindication)

     2) α-Agonists may also be used (especially with concurrent tics): clonidine, guanfacine; clonidine is a central agonist of α_2-adrenoreceptors and effective in reducing impulsivity and hyperactivity

     3) Antidepressants: tricyclic agents, SSRIs, bupropion, venlafaxine

     4) Mood stabilizers: carbamazepine, valproic acid

B. Mental Retardation

1. Definition: controversial

2. Has been defined loosely as below average intelligence with deficits in adaptive behavior

   a. Below-average intelligence

     1) Defined as 2 SD below mean on accepted standardized developmental and psychometric testing (defined by most authorities as IQ <70)

     2) Some authorities grade this as mild (55-70), moderate (40-55), severe (25-40), and profound (<25)

   b. The need for support in areas of adaptive functions

     1) Communication, self-care, social skills, home living, community use, self-direction, health and safety, functional academics, leisure, work

     2) The degree of support required has been graded as intermittent, limited, extensive, and pervasive

3. 1% to 3% of the population in developed countries (3/4 have been classified as "mild")

4. M>F (1.4:1): male excess has been attributed to X-linked genetic disorders and prevalence of boys with autism

5. Mild mental retardation is more prevalent in lower socioeconomic groups: this may be due partly to poor prenatal care and increased incidence of maternal smoking and drug use (including alcohol), all of which have been associated with a higher prevalence of mental retardation

6. Severe mental retardation is equal in prevalence among different socioeconomic groups: prenatal factors (chromosomal abnormalities and other genetic disorders) are probably more important in this group than other potential factors

7. Higher risk of mental retardation with lower birth weight, malnutrition, autism
8. Prenatal causes of mental retardation: congenital developmental malformations (see Chapter 1), chromosomal abnormalities (discussed below), abnormal synaptic connections and dendritic spine anomalies, endogenous or exogenous toxic causes (e.g., maternal smoking, alcohol use, or use of cocaine during pregnancy), infectious causes (e.g., toxoplasmosis, cytomegalovirus)
9. Perinatal causes: perinatal trauma or birth asphyxia, toxic or metabolic (e.g., hyperbilirubinemia)
10. Postnatal causes: inborn errors of metabolism, trauma, CNS infections, toxic, metabolic, or systemic conditions (subclinical lead poisoning, iron deficiency anemia) (approximately 1/3 of children with sickle cell disease have IQ of 50-70)
11. Chromosomal abnormalities
    a. Chromosomal abnormalities that commonly appear on examination questions are discussed here (noteworthy is the long list of genetic disorders associated with mental retardation, most of which are outside the scope of this chapter and not discussed further)
    b. Down syndrome
        1) Most common chromosomal aneusomy
        2) Trisomy 21 is usually (more than 90% of cases) a triplicate copy of the chromosome
            a) Presence of the extra chromosome 21 results from abnormal separation of chromosomes during meiosis
            b) The risk of occurrence of this triplicate copy of the chromosome increases proportionally with maternal age
        3) Trisomy 21 may also occur (<10%) from translocation of a portion of the long arm of chromosome 21 to another chromosome: this mechanism is *not* dependent on maternal age
        4) Most patients develop pathologic features of AD by late 30s and early 40s (progressive dementia and deterioration in cognitive function [resembling AD patients] usually develop much later)
            a) The gene encoding APP is located on chromosome 21
            b) Trisomy 21 yields an elevation of APP and more β-amyloid deposition
        5) Clinical features
            a) Hypotonic at birth: tone improves with age
            b) Brachycephaly
            c) Narrowed palpebral fissures
            d) Prominent epicanthal folds

e) Brushfield's spots (small white spots in the iris)
f) High-arched hard palate
g) Cardiac anomalies
h) Duodenal atresia
i) Short, broad hands, with clinodactyly of the fifth finger due to hypoplastic middle phalanx
j) Variable degrees of mental retardation
k) Social skills may be relatively preserved in some (not all) patients
l) More than 50% will have seizures by age 50 years (80% in patients with dementia)
c. Trisomy 18 (Edwards' syndrome)
    1) Full trisomy of chromosome 18 in more than 90% of patients, other 10% have translocation of a portion of the chromosome or mosaicism
    2) Congenital malformations, most commonly cardiac malformations (e.g., ventricular or atrial septal defects)
    3) Developmental disability and global psychomotor retardation
    4) Hypotonic infants (later become hypertonic)
    5) Hearing loss
    6) Cleft lip (5%-10% of patients)
d. Cri du chat syndrome
    1) Most cases caused by deletion of a portion of short arm of chromosome 5
    2) Weak, "meowing" cry in newborn infants
    3) Round face, microcephaly, hypertelorism, prominent epicanthal folds, low-set ears, and micrognathia (abnormally small jaw)
    4) Severe psychomotor and mental retardation
e. Fragile X syndrome
    1) Most common maternally inherited cause of mental retardation (1/1,500 boys)
    2) Most frequent chromosomal abnormality associated with autism
    3) The fragile-X gene has been named "fragile X mental retardation-1" (*FMR1*); located on the long arm of X chromosome (Xq27.3)
        a) Fragile X permutation tremor/ataxia phenotype
            i) Trinucleotide repeat expansion between 50-200
            ii) It is a syndrome of "permutation" that has been associated with normal intelligence, ataxia, and essential tremor
            iii) A family history of mental retardation in subsequent generations (due to anticipation, described below) in the appropriate clinical context should prompt clinicians to consider this diagnosis
        b) Fragile X phenotype

i) Trinucleotide repeat expansion more than 200 CGG repeats ("full mutation") has been associated with mental retardation in almost all males and about half of females

ii) Hypermethylation of the trinucleotides occurs at high repeat rates (proportional to the number of the repeats) and is believed to cause transcriptional inactivation and, consequently, loss of FMR1 protein expression

c) Anticipation: large repeats (>50) transmitted from parent to offspring are unstable ("fragile") and tend to expand from generation to generation

4) Clinical features

a) Mental retardation, as defined above

b) Hyperkinetic or autistic behavior

c) Macro-orchidism in mature males (develops during or after puberty)

d) Characteristic facial features: long face and palpebral fissures, prominent ears, relatively large head, high-arched palate

e) Hyperexpansile metacarpophalangeal joints and "double-jointed" thumbs

f) Pes planus

g) Less common features: hand calluses, single palmar creases, seizures (20% of patients)

f. Prader-Willi syndrome

1) Caused by deletion of paternal 15q11-q13 chromosomal region; deletion of maternal 15q11-q13 causes Angelman's syndrome (genetic imprinting and uniparental disomy)

2) Mild to moderate mental retardation

3) Neonatal hypotonia

4) Hyperphagia, food seeking, morbid obesity

5) Short stature

6) Hypogonadotropic hypogonadism: boys with hypoplastic scrotum and small penis; girls with hypoplastic or absent labia minora, amenorrhea, infertility

7) Hypopigmentation relative to the family in 75% of patients

8) Small hands and feet

g. Angelman's syndrome ("happy puppet syndrome")

1) Caused by deletion of maternal 15q11-q13 chromosomal region

2) Usually severe psychomotor retardation

3) Hyperactivity

4) Ataxia

5) Hypotonia, "floppy infants"

6) Seizures: usually manifest before age 2 years, often intractable

7) Usually absence of intelligible speech

8) Facies: large mandible and open mouth expression with constant tongue protrusion, macrostomia (excessively large mouth); excessive laughing and smiling with bursts of laughter, happy disposition

h. Rett syndrome

1) Sporadic or familial (X-linked dominant); 80% to 85% of patients have classic Rett syndrome, 50% of patients with atypical syndrome have a mutation in *MECP* gene on X chromosome

2) Occurs in girls, lethal in boys

3) "Acquired" microcephaly (deceleration of head growth)

4) Usually severe mental retardation: generally normal development by 7 to 18 months of age, followed by developmental arrest, then rapid regression and progressive encephalopathy

5) Disease progression reaches a plateau before adolescence

6) Intractable seizures; after childhood, seizures may be better controlled

7) Striking deterioration in growth

8) Hyperventilation and apnea

9) Loss of purposeful use of the hands and stereotypic hand movements

10) Loss of communication skills

11) Hypoactivity

12) Truncal ataxia

13) Relatively high incidence of sudden death

14) Prolonged QT interval

i. Williams syndrome

1) Rare cause of mental retardation: patients have difficulty especially with visuospatial skills and visuo-

---

Rett Syndrome

X-linked dominant disorder predominantly in young girls

Associated with mutation of the *MECP* gene

Developmental arrest and regression

Stereotypic hand movements and loss of purposeful use of the hands

Loss of communication skills

Deceleration of head growth and "acquired" microcephaly

Seizures

motor integration skills

   2) Supravalvular aortic stenosis

   3) Short stature

   4) Infantile hypercalcemia

   5) Facial dysgenesis: "elfin-like" facies and micrognathia (abnormally small jaw)

C. Cerebral Palsy

1. McKeith's definition: "a persisting qualitative motor disorder due to nonprogressive interference with development of the brain occurring before the growth of the central nervous system is complete"

2. Terminology refers to syndrome-symptom complex, not a particular etiology

3. Nonprogressive, persistent motor disorders and/or static encephalopathy (highly variable between patients)

4. The insult may occur during the prenatal (most cases), perinatal, or first few years postnatal period; phenotype and clinical manifestations often transform with time

5. Physiologic classification: spastic, dyskinetic (includes choreoathetoid and dystonic, ataxic, hypotonic, and mixed types)

6. Topographic classification: quadriplegia, diplegia, hemiplegia

7. Physiologic and topographic classifications may have poor reliability

8. Functional classification focuses on degree of severity, and therapeutic classification consists of nontreatment, modest interventions, need for a cerebral palsy treatment team, and pervasive supports

9. Spastic cerebral palsy

   a. The most common type (75% of patients)

   b. These patients often have early hypotonia, followed by spasticity; motor development is often delayed

   c. Early fetal or neonatal diffuse hypoperfusion injury can produce ischemia in bilateral watershed distribution affecting the deep white matter and causing spastic diplegia

10. Associated with attention-deficit/hyperactivity disorder, mental retardation, developmental learning disabilities, and seizures (depending to some degree on cause)

11. Cerebral palsy is better predicted by recurrent seizures in perinatal and neonatal periods than other perinatal abnormalities

12. Most patients have normal to above-average intelligence

13. Treatment: limited to symptomatic management

REFERENCES

Caselli RJ, Boeve BF, Scheithauer BW, O'Duffy JD, Hunder GG. Nonvasculitic autoimmune inflammatory meningoencephalitis (NAIM): a reversible form of encephalopathy. Neurology. 1999;53:1579-81.

Colombo R. Age and origin of the *PRNP* E200K mutation causing familial Creutzfeldt-Jacob disease in Libyan Jews. Am J Hum Genet. 2000;67:528-31.

Cummings J. Treatment of Alzheimer's disease: current and future therapeutic approaches. Rev Neurol. 2004;1:60-9.

Fox RJ, Kasner SE, Chatterjee A, Chalela JA. Aphemia: an isolated disorder of articulation. Clin Neurol Neurosurg. 2001;103:123-6.

Gambini A, Falini A, Moiola L, Comi G, Scotti G. Marchiafava-Bignami disease: longitudinal MR imaging and MR spectroscopy study. AJNR Am J Neuroradiol. 2003;24:249-53.

Goldman JS, Farmer JM, Van Deerlin VM, Wilhelmsen KC, Miller BL, Grossman M. Frontotemporal dementia: genetics and genetic counseling dilemmas. Neurologist. 2004;10:227-34.

Harper C. Wernicke's encephalopathy: a more common disease than realised: a neuropathological study of 51 cases. J Neurol Neurosurg Psychiatry. 1979;42:226-31.

Harper C, Fornes P, Duyckaerts C, Lecomte D, Hauw JJ. An international perspective on the prevalence of the Wernicke-Korsakoff syndrome. Metab Brain Dis. 1995;10:17-24.

Harper CG, Giles M, Finlay-Jones R. Clinical signs in the Wernicke-Korsakoff complex: a retrospective analysis of 131 cases diagnosed at necropsy. J Neurol Neurosurg Psychiatry. 1986;49:341-5.

Harris JC. Developmental neuropsychiatry. Vol 2. New York: Oxford; 1998.

Hodges JR. Frontotemporal dementia (Pick's disease): clinical features and assessment. Neurology. 2001;56 Suppl 4:S6-10.

Jordan BD. Chronic traumatic brain injury associated with boxing. Semin Neurol. 2000;20:179-85.

Jordan BD, Relkin NR, Ravdin LD, Jacobs AR, Bennett A, Gandy S. Apolipoprotein E ε4 associated with chronic traumatic brain injury in boxing. JAMA. 1997;278:136-40.

King BH, State MW, Shah B, Davanzo P, Dykens E. Mental retardation: a review of the past 10 years: part I. J Am Acad Child Adolesc Psychiatry. 1997;36:1656-63.

Knopman DS, DeKosky ST, Cummings JL, Chui H, Corey-Bloom J, Relkin N, et al. Practice parameter: diagnosis of dementia (an evidence-based review): report of the Quality Standards Subcommittee of the American Academy of Neurology. Neurology. 2001;56:1143-53.

Kuban KC, Leviton A. Cerebral palsy. N Engl J Med. 1994;330:188-95.

MacKeith RC, Mackenzie ICK, Polani PE. Memorandum on terminology and classification of "cerebral palsy." Cerebral Palsy Bull. 1959;5:27-35.

McKhann G, Drachman D, Folstein M, Katzman R, Price D, Stadlan EM. Clinical diagnosis of Alzheimer's disease: report of the NINCDS-ADRDA Work Group under the auspices of Department of Health and Human Services Task Force on Alzheimer's Disease. Neurology. 1984;34:939-44.

Miller JW, Petersen RC, Metter EJ, Millikan CH, Yanagihara T. Transient global amnesia: clinical characteristics and prognosis. Neurology. 1987;37:733-7.

Neary D, Snowden JS, Gustafson L, Passant U, Stuss D, Black S, et al. Frontotemporal lobar degeneration: a consensus on clinical diagnostic criteria. Neurology. 1988;51:1546-54.

Oostra BA, Willems PJ. A fragile gene. Bioessays. 1995;17;941-7.

Rabadi MH, Jordan BD. The cumulative effect of repetitive concussion in sports. Clin J Sport Med. 2001;11:194-8.

Robertson NP, Wharton S, Anderson J, Scolding NJ. Adult polyglucosan body disease associated with an extrapyramidal syndrome. J Neurol Neurosurg Psychiatry. 1998;65:788-90.

Román GC, Tatemichi TK, Erkinjuntti T, Cummings JL, Masdeu JC, Garcia JH, et al. Vascular dementia: diagnostic criteria for research studies. Report of the NINDS-AIREN International Workshop. Neurology. 1993;43:250-60.

Sawka AM, Fatourechi V, Boeve BF, Mokri B. Rarity of encephalopathy associated with autoimmune thyroiditis: a case series from Mayo Clinic from 1950 to 1996. Thyroid. 2002;12:393-8.

Schauble B, Castillo PR, Boeve BF, Westmoreland BF. EEG findings in steroid-responsive encephalopathy associated with autoimmune thyroiditis. Clin Neurophysiol. 2003;114:32-7.

Shapiro BK. Cerebral palsy: a reconceptualization of the spectrum. J Pediatr. 2004;145 Suppl:S3-7.

Sindern E, Ziemssen F, Ziemssen T, Podskarbi T, Shin Y, Braasch F, et al. Adult polyglucosan body disease: a postmortem correlation study. Neurology. 2003;61:263-5.

Singhi PD. Cerebral palsy-management. Indian J Pediatr. 2004;71:635-9.

State MY, King BH, Dykens E. Mental retardation: a review of the past 10 years: part II. J Am Acad Child Adolesc Psychiatry. 1997;36:1664-71.

Trivedi JR, Wolfe GI, Nations SP, Burns DK, Bryan WW, Dewey RB Jr. Adult polyglucosan body disease associated with Lewy bodies and tremor. Arch Neurol. 2003;60:764-6.

QUESTIONS

1. Which of the following is *not* a histologic feature of Alzheimer's disease?
   a. Hirano bodies
   b. Neuritic plaques and neurofibrillary tangles
   c. Granulovacuolar degeneration of neurons
   d. Alzheimer type II astrocytes
   e. Deposition of amyloid in walls of leptomeningeal and cortical blood bessels

2. Damage to which of the following structures results in loss of the ability to form new memories?
   a. Fornix
   b. Orbitofrontal gyrus
   c. Calcarine cortex
   d. Hypothalamus
   e. None of the above

3. Which of the following are *not* a common feature of dementia with Lewy bodies?
   a. Early visual hallucinations
   b. Parkinsonism, with poor response to levodopa
   c. Fluctuating mental status
   d. "Alien hand" phenomenon
   e. Sensitivity to neuroleptics
   f. All the above are common characteristics of dementia with Lewy bodies

4. Which of the following is *not* a feature of subcortical dementia?
   a. Psychomotor slowing
   b. Cognitive decline
   c. Bradyphrenia (slowness in mental processing)
   d. Change in mood and personality
   e. All the above are features of subcortical dementia

5-9. Match the following cortical functions with the appropriate cortex. An answer may be used once, more than once, or not at all.

5. Executive functions

6. Elemental sensory perception

7. Processing of sensory information

8. Emotional properties of information processing

9. Processing of motor information

10. Which of the following is *not* a feature of frontotemporal dementia?
    a. Nascent artistic ability
    b. Semantic aphasia
    c. Achromatopsia
    d. Klüver-Bucy syndrome
    e. All the above are features of frontotemporal dementia

11. In which of the following aphasias is written language preserved?
    a. Broca's aphasia
    b. Transcortical mixed aphasia
    c. Aphemia
    d. Transcortical motor aphasia
    e. None of the above

12. Digit span (immediate recall) is spared in all the following disorders *except*:
    a. Transient global amnesia
    b. Korsakoff's psychosis
    c. Alzheimer's disease
    d. Major depression
    e. Digit span is spared in *none* of the above

a. Unimodal cortex

b. Idiotypic primary cortex

c. Heteromodal cortex

d. Paralimbic cortex

Answers

1. Answer: d.
Neuritic plaques and neurofibrillary tangles are the most important histologic features of Alzheimer's disease. Hirano bodies, granulovacuolar degeneration, and amyloid deposition in blood vessels are commonly seen as well. Alzheimer type II astrocytes are reactive astrocytes that occur in conditions associated with hyperammonemia and liver failure.

2. Answer: a.
The fornix is an important part of the circuit of Papez, and lesions of the fornix can result in the loss of ability to form new memories.

3. Answer: d.
All the choices are common characteristics of dementia with Lewy bodies except for the "alien hand" phenomenon, which is characteristic of corticobasal degeneration.

4. Answer: e.
All the choices listed are common in subcortical dementia. The most common feature is bradyphrenia.

5. Answer: c.

6. Answer: b.

7. Answer: a.

8. Answer: d.

9. Answer: a.

10. Answer: c.
Achromatopsia is generally not a feature of frontotemporal dementia.

11. Answer: c.
Aphemia is distinguished from the other aphasias listed by preserved written language.

12. Answer: d.
Major depression is the only disorder listed associated with poor attention and abnormal immediate recall, with relatively preserved short-term memory. A diagnostic characteristic of the amnestic syndromes, including Alzheimer's disease and Korsakoff's psychosis, is relatively preserved immediate recall and more prominent difficulty with learning and remembering new information. Transient global amnesia is also associated with retrograde and anterograde amnesia, with relatively preserved immediate recall.

MOVEMENT DISORDERS 8

Nima Mowzoon, M.D.

I. BASAL GANGLIA NEUROBIOLOGY (FIG. 8-1)

A. Introduction

1. Components
   a. Basal ganglia (large subcortical nuclei)
   b. Basal ganglia consist of caudate nucleus, putamen, globus pallidus, amygdaloid complex
   c. Caudate nucleus, putamen, and nucleus accumbens together are called the striatum
   d. Globus pallidus with the putamen is called the lenticular nucleus
   e. Basal ganglia have connections with substantia nigra and subthalamic nucleus
2. Function
   a. Major role in control of motor movements and cognitive and affective functions

B. Striatum and Pallidostriatal Connections

1. Main input to the basal ganglion: cerebral cortex (mainly frontal lobe)
2. Other sources of input to the striatum are from
   a. Thalamus: excitatory input
   b. Dopaminergic neurons of substantia nigra pars compacta
      1) Dopaminergic input to spiny striatal neurons with dopamine$_1$ (D$_1$) receptors: dopamine acts on D$_1$ receptors on striatal output neurons projecting to substantia nigra pars reticulata and globus pallidus interna (direct pathway); these output neurons are γ-aminobutyric acid (GABA)ergic, with substance P and dynorphin as cotransmitters
      2) Dopaminergic input to spiny striatal neurons with D$_2$ receptors: dopamine acts on D$_2$ receptors on striatal output neurons projecting to globus pallidus externa (indirect pathway); these output neurons are GABAergic, with enkephalin as cotransmitter
      3) The substantia nigra pars compacta input facilitates the direct pathway via D$_1$ receptors and inhibits the indirect pathway via D$_2$ receptors

   4) Degeneration of dopaminergic substantia nigra pars compacta input (which occurs with idiopathic Parkinson's disease) leads to relative activation of the indirect pathway and resultant hypokinetic movement disorder (Fig. 8-1 *B*)
   5) Dopaminergic input to both pathways acts to enhance excitatory cortical input
   c. Large aspiny striatal interneurons: excitatory (cholinergic) and influenced by cortical input
   d. Neighboring medium spiny neurons: collateral inhibition
3. The majority of the neurons are medium spiny projection neurons, which are GABAergic inhibitory cells projecting to globus pallidus and subtantia nigra
4. Main cortical input: excitatory glutaminergic synapses on dendritic spines of GABAergic neurons
5. Output (primarily GABAergic, inhibitory)
   a. Globus pallidus interna and substantia nigra pars reticulata as a functional unit
      1) Receive inhibitory GABAergic input from striatal projection neurons with substance P and dynorphin as cotransmitters
      2) GABAergic cells with projections to ventrolateral and ventroanterior thalamus (excitatory relay to cerebral cortex)
   b. Globus pallidus externa
      1) Receives inhibitory GABAergic input from striatal neurons with enkephalin as cotransmitter
      2) GABAergic cells with projections to subthalamic nucleus

C. Subthalamic Nucleus

1. Receives inhibitory GABAergic input from globus pallidus externa
2. Receives excitatory glutaminergic input from cerebral cortex
3. Contains excitatory neurons with glutamate as the primary neurotransmitter

A

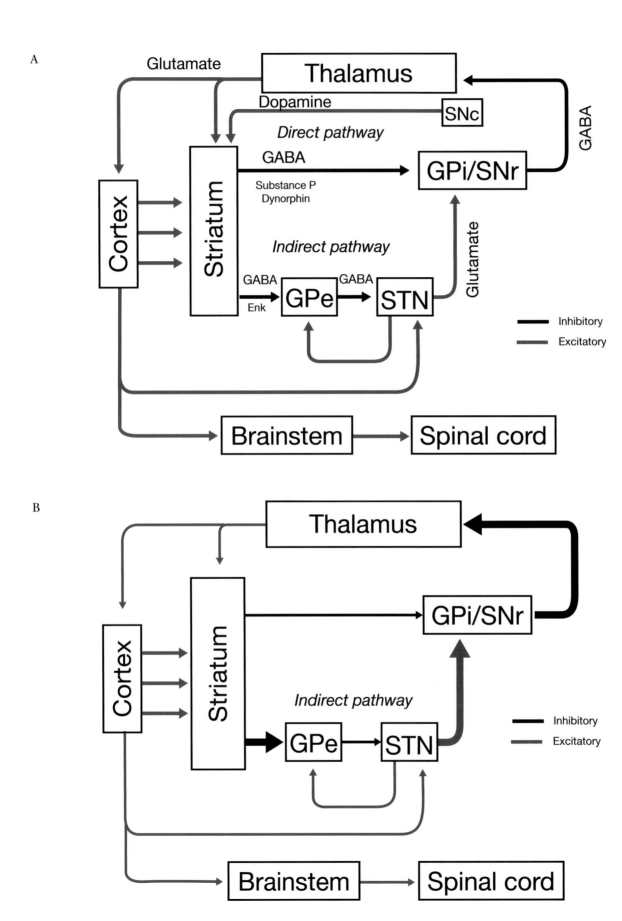

C

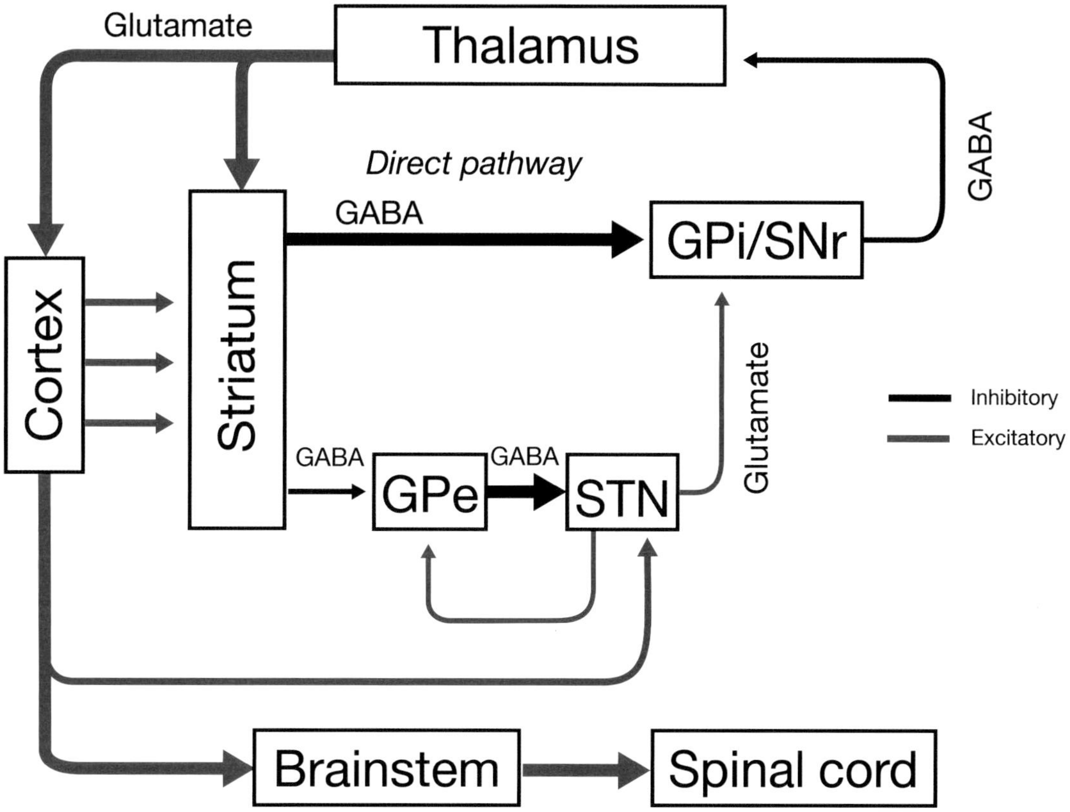

Fig. 8-1. *A*, Basal ganglia pathways. *B*, Pathophysiology of hypokinetic movement disorders such as idiopathic Parkinson's disease. *C*, Pathophysiology of hyperkinetic movement disorders such as Huntington's disease. Enk, enkephalins; GABA, γ-aminobutyric acid; GPe, globus pallidus externa; GPi, globus pallidus interna; SNc, substantia nigra pars compacta; SNr, substantia nigra pars reticulata; STN, subthalamic nucleus.

4. Output: excitatory and mainly to globus pallidus interna and substantia nigra pars reticulata, some projections to globus pallidus externa as excitatory feedback

D. Intrinsic Circuits
1. Direct pathway (Fig. 8-1 *C*)
   a. Dopaminergic activation of D_1 receptors
   b. Direct phasic inhibition of globus pallidus interna and substantia nigra pars reticulata (transmitter, GABA; cotransmitters, substance P and dynorphin) by striatal projection neurons, which in turn, reduce inhibition of the thalamus by globus pallidus interna and substantia nigra pars reticulata
   c. Activates thalamocortical excitatory pathways and promotes movement
   d. Net result: augmentation of movement
   e. Hyperactive in hyperkinetic disorders
2. Indirect pathway (Fig. 8-1 *B*)
   a. Dopaminergic activation of D_2 receptors

b. GABAergic inhibition of globus pallidus externa (cotransmitter, enkephalin), causing reduced inhibition of the subthalamic nucleus and subsequent activation of subthalamic nucleus excitatory projections to globus pallidus interna and substantia nigra pars reticulata
   c. Indirect excitatory stimulation of the globus pallidus interna and substantia nigra pars reticulata, increasing inhibition of the thalamus and subsequent reduction of excitatory thalamocortical projections
   d. Net result: reduction of movement
   e. Hyperactive in hypokinetic disorders

E. Physiology
1. At rest
   a. Low-frequency spontaneous discharge of medium spiny striatal neurons (relatively hyperpolarized because of an inward rectifying potassium current)
   b. High-frequency spontaneous discharge of globus pallidus interna and substantia nigra pars reticulata

2. With movement
    a. Corticostriatal pathway activates a desired motor program: excitatory corticostriatal input overcomes the inward rectifying potassium current (requires temporal and spatial summation of excitatory input to multiple dendritic spines simultaneously) → activation of striatum → stimulates striatal phasic inhibition to globus pallidus interna and substantia nigra pars reticulata (overcoming excitation from subthalamic nucleus), decreasing the frequency of spontaneous discharges of globus pallidus interna and substantia nigra pars reticulata and promoting excitatory thalamocortical input for the desired movement (Fig. 8-1 *C*)
    b. Corticosubthalamic pathway inhibits undesired motor programs: excitatory cortical input to the subthalamus increases subthalamic glutaminergic excitation of inhibitory globus pallidus interna and substantia nigra pars reticulata cells, increasing inhibition of the thalamocortical input for the undesired movement
    c. End result:
        1) Reduction of undesired movements (excitation of globus pallidus interna and substantia nigra pars reticulata by cortical stimulation of subthalamic nucleus and release of inhibition of subthalamic nucleus via the indirect pathway)
        2) Promotion of the desired motor programs (striatal inhibition of globus pallidus interna and substantia nigra pars reticulata via the direct pathway)

F. **Parallel Circuits** (Table 8-1)
1. Five parallel circuits have different corticostriatal input from specific cerebral cortical areas and project back to the same cortical areas via a thalamic relay
2. Responsible for the role of basal ganglia in cognition and affective functions in addition to motor and oculomotor functions

II. HYPOKINETIC MOVEMENT DISORDERS

A. **Idiopathic Parkinson's Disease**
1. Risk factors
    a. Age
    b. Sex (M > F)
    c. Family history
    d. History of exposure to toxins: higher risk with exposure to pesticides, herbicides, welding (manganese poisoning), or for agricultural workers
    e. History of head trauma
2. Inherited parkinsonism (Table 8-2)
    a. *PARK1* gene
        1) Autosomal dominant
        2) Missense mutation or triplication of the α-synuclein gene on chromosome 4q
        3) α-Synuclein: role in synaptic function and transmitter release
        4) L-dopa–responsive parkinsonism with young age at

Table 8-1. Basal Ganglia Parallel Circuits

Circuit	Cortical origin of circuit	Striatum	Output (GPi/SNr)	Thalamic nucleus	Function
Motor	Primary motor, supplementary motor, premotor, posterior parietal	Putamen	GPi SNr	VL, VA, CM	Motor planning & execution
Oculomotor	Frontal eye fields, supplementary eye fields, posterior parietal	Caudate	SNr	VA, DM	Saccades
Behavior (dorsolateral prefrontal)	Dorsolateral prefrontal	Dorsal caudate	GPi	VA, DM	Executive tasks
Behavior (orbitofrontal)	Orbitofrontal	Ventral caudate	GPi	VA, DM	Social behavior
Limbic	Anterior cingulate	Nucleus accumbens	Ventral pallidum	DM	Motivation

CM, centromedian nucleus; DM, dorsomedial nucleus; GPi, globus pallidus interna; SNr, substantia nigra pars reticulata; VA, ventral anterior nucleus; VL, ventral lateral nucleus.

onset, associated with dystonia, and more prominent dementia than sporadic Parkinson's disease

b. *PARK2* gene

1) May be responsible for up to half of inherited cases with early-onset parkinsonism

2) Autosomal recessive

3) Early-onset parkinsonism with early dystonia

4) Mutation of parkin protein (gene on chromosome 6)

5) Parkin protein is required for protein degradation via the proteasome complex

a) Ubiquitination of a protein (no longer needed by the cell) is the key step in marking that protein for subsequent degradation by the proteasome

b) Ubiquitination requires the action of ubiquitin-activating enzyme (E1), ubiquitin-conjugating enzyme (E2), and ubiquitin ligase (E3); Parkin is an E3 ubiquitin ligase

---

Genetics of Idiopathic Parkinson's Disease

PARK1: autosomal dominant (α-synuclein gene on chromosome 4)

PARK2: Autosomal recessive (parkin gene on chromosome 6)

Both: early parkinsonism and dystonia

Table 8-2. Inherited Forms of Parkinson's Disease

Gene	Pattern of inheritance	Chromosome of gene locus	Key clinical feature
PARK1 (α-synuclein)	AD	4	Dementia*
PARK2 (Parkin)	AR	6	Dystonia*
PARK3	AD	4, 2p	
PARK4	AD	4p	Dementia
PARK5	AD	4p	
PARK6	AR	1p	*
PARK7	AR	1p, loss of DJ-1	Dystonia*
PARK8	AR	12	*
PARK9	AR	1p	
PARK10	Unkown	1p	Late-onset parkinsonism

AD, autosomal dominant; AR, autosomal recessive.
Early-onset parkinsonism.

c) Abnormal accumulation of the substrate protein eventually causes selective cell death of dopaminergic neurons

d) Lewy bodies do not form in the absence of ubiquitinated protein inclusions

3. Clinical features

a. Tremor

1) Characterized as rest tremor

2) May also be a postural or kinetic tremor (rest tremor typically dampens with posture or action)

3) Usually unilateral onset in an extremity

4) Tremor may spread to involve contiguous extremities

b. Rigidity

1) Not velocity-dependent or direction-dependent

2) "Cogwheeling": usually indicative of superimposed tremor

c. Bradykinesia

1) Reduced arm swing

2) Generalized slowness in movements

3) Slowness and difficulty with manual dexterity (Fig. 8-2)

4) Micrographia

5) Masked facies (hypomimia)

6) Sialorrhea because of bulbar bradykinesia

d. Postural instability

1) Loss of postural reflexes

2) Retropulsion as may be found on the "pull test"

e. Gait disturbance

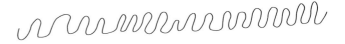

Fig. 8-2. "Sine wave" in a patient with parkinsonism. Note the repetitive dampening of the amplitude and subsequent attempts to correct it.

Cardinal Features of Parkinson's Disease

Tremor

Rigidity

Bradykinesia

Postural instability and gait disturbance

---

1) Stooped posture: characteristic "shuffling" festinating gait with short stride, with tendency to lean forward

2) Propulsion: involuntary and unwanted forward acceleration when patient wants to stop

3) Difficulty initiating gait and gait "freezing" after gait already initiated (sudden inability to take another step)

4) Difficulty with turns

f. Associated features

1) Hypokinetic speech: characterized by reduced amplitude and sometimes acceleration of rate

2) Autonomic features

a) Most commonly, orthostatism, usually not a presenting feature

b) Other less common features: urinary symptoms (hesitancy, nocturia, incontinence), sexual dysfunction, intermittent increased sweating

3) Behavioral and cognitive features

a) Bradyphrenia (mental slowing), with difficulty with attention, and poor initiation and working memory

b) Depression in up to 2/3 of patients and anxiety (especially associated with akinetic "off" state)

c) Dementia may develop after many years

i) Difficulty with frontal lobe executive and visuospatial functions, with some language deficits

ii) Difficulty with attentional tasks and those involving timed responses

4. Neuroimaging

a. Magnetic resonance imaging (MRI): generally not helpful

b. Fluorodopa positron emission tomography (PET): reduced uptake in dopaminergic striatal and nigrostriatal pathways, proportional to severity of disease and pathology

5. Histopathology (Fig. 8-3)

a. Macroscopic pigmentary loss and microscopic neuronal loss of substantia nigra pars compacta, with microglial activation and cytoplasmic pigmentation of macrophages

b. Locus ceruleus, intermediolateral cell column, and dorsal motor nucleus of the vagus nerve may be affected

c. Lewy bodies in surviving neurons in areas affected (sparing neocortex): cytoplasmic inclusions with dense eosinophilic core containing hyperphosphorylated neurofilament proteins, lipids, iron, ubiquitin, and α-synuclein

6. Treatment (Table 8-3)

a. Levodopa

1) Precursor of dopamine

2) Should be taken on empty stomach because it competes with amino acids in crossing the blood-brain barrier by a transporter

3) Formulations

a) Immediate release (IR) carbidopa-levodopa

i) More predictable response than controlled release

ii) Start at 1 tablet of 25/100 IR 3 times daily and increase to ceiling dose of 3 1/2 tablets 3 times daily

iii) If not tolerated, may start at 1/4 of 25/100 IR tablet

iv) Should be taken 1 hour before meals

b) Controlled-release (CR) carbidopa-levodopa

i) Twice daily regimen: start at 1 tablet of 25/100 CR twice daily and increase to ceiling dose of 4 to 6 tablets twice daily

ii) Should be taken 2 hours before meals

iii) Onset of action: usually about 2 hours

iv) May be used as initial therapy in absence of clinical fluctuations

v) Disadvantage: delayed and unpredictable absorption and response, may cause severe dyskinesias

4) Increments in dose should be made weekly because a week is required to determine cumulative effect of drug

5) Inconclusive evidence about potential levodopa toxicity as initial agent

6) Simpler to use and initiate than the agonists

7) Most efficacious and potent medical treatment

8) Greater incidence of motor fluctuations and dyskinesias than with dopamine agonists

9) Adverse effects

a) Nausea

i) Due to premature conversion of levodopa to dopamine in the circulation by the peripheral dopa decarboxylase enzyme (L-aromatic amino acid decarboxylase)

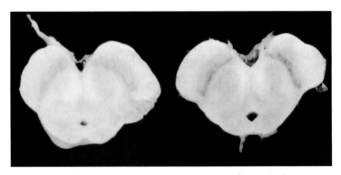

Fig. 8-3. Pallor of the substantia nigra in Parkinson's disease (*left*) compared with normal (*right*). (From Okazaki H, Scheithauer BW. Atlas of neuropathology. New York: Gower Medical Publishing; 1988. p. 227. By permission of Mayo Foundation.)

Table 8-3. **Medical Treatment for Parkinson's Disease**

Drug	Usual starting dose	Maximal dose (usual target dose)	Adverse effects
Amantadine (Symmetrel)	100 mg bid-tid	100 mg tid	Anticholinergic-like (dry mouth, urinary retention, constipation), hallucinations, livedo reticularis, insomnia
Carbidopa-levodopa	25/100 mg tid IR, bid CR	1,500 mg/day (300-1,200 mg/day)	Nausea, orthostatic hypotension, dyskinesias, hallucinations & psychosis
Entacapone (Comtan)	200-mg tablets, 1 tablet taken with each levodopa dose	Up to 8 doses daily	Nausea, diarrhea, prolongation of all levodopa-induced dyskinesias & other side effects
Pergolide (Permax)	0.05 mg	6.0 mg/day (1.5-3.0 mg/day)	Nausea, orthostatic hypotension, dyskinesias, vivid dreams, hallucinations & psychosis, somnolence, headaches, dyspepsia, valvular heart disease (rare), pleuropulmonary fibrosis (rare)
Pramipexole (Mirapex)	0.125 mg tid	1.5 mg tid (3.0-4.5 mg/day)	Nausea, orthostatic hypotension, dyskinesias, vivid dreams, hallucinations & psychosis, somnolence, sleep attacks (rare)
Ropinirole (Requip)	0.25 mg tid	5 mg 5 times daily (3-25 mg/day)	
Selegiline (Eldepryl)	5 mg bid—given in early part of day because of insomnia	Same as starting dose	Insomnia, vivid dreams & nightmares, potentiation of dopaminergic effects
Trihexyphenidyl	1 mg daily-bid	6 mg tid (2 mg tid)	Anticholinergic (dry mouth, urinary retention, constipation, visual blurriness, memory impairment)

bid, twice daily; CR, controlled release; IR, immediate release; tid, three times daily.

ii) Dopamine in the circulation does not penetrate blood-brain barrier but can penetrate into brain-stem chemoreceptor trigger zone that lacks blood-brain barrier, and this is responsible for nausea

iii) Common cause of nausea at initiation of levo-dopa therapy is inadequate doses of carbidopa; this drug does not cross blood-brain barrier and acts to inhibit peripheral dopa decarboxylase enzyme; approximately 100 to 150 mg of carbidopa per day is required to saturate this peripheral enzyme

iv) May be treated with dry bread or cracker (low protein), adding carbidopa to each dose, domperidone (Motilium), or trimethobenzamide (Tigan) 250 mg 1 to 3 times daily as needed

  b) Dyskinesias
    i) Dystonia (parkinsonian)
    ii) Choreiform (levodopa-induced): reduce dose of levodopa for peak-dose dyskinesias

  c) Orthostatic hypotension (management discussed in another chapter)
  d) Visual hallucinations and psychosis
  e) Insomnia and vivid dreams (discussed below)

b. Dopamine agonists (Table 8-3)
  1) Directly activate dopamine receptors
  2) Activation of both D_1 and D_2 receptors needed for optimal physiologic response
  3) All have high affinity for D_3 receptors
  4) More likely than levodopa to produce psychosis, hallucinations, and orthostatic hypotention
  5) Less likely than levodopa to produce dyskinesias
  6) Synergistic effect with concomitant use of levodopa to exacerbate dyskinesias while reducing the "off" state, necessitating a lower levodopa dose
  7) Pergolide and bromocriptine
    a) Ergot derivatives, higher chance of ergot side effects such as potential for vasoconstriction (e.g.,

Reynaud's phenomenon), erythromelalgia, pulmonary and retroperitoneal fibrosis (rare)

b) Pergolide: recently reported cases of noninflammatory fibrotic degeneration of cardiac valves is believed to involve serotonin-mediated abnormal fibrogenesis via $5-HT_{2B}$ receptors in fibroblasts of heart valves

8) Pramipexole and ropinirole: nonergolines, have lower rate of adverse effects than traditional dopamine agonists above; may rarely cause sleep attacks and leg edema

c. COMT inhibitors

1) They inhibit catechol *O*-methyltransferase (COMT) and increase plasma level of levodopa

2) Formulations

a) Tolcapone (Tasmar)

i) Rarely used because of reported cases of acute fulminant liver failure, requiring frequent monitoring of liver function enzymes

ii) Reversible central- and peripheral-acting COMT inhibitor

b) Entacapone (Comtan)

i) Reversible peripheral-acting (including gastrointestinal tract, erythrocytes, and liver)

ii) Shorter duration of action than tolcapone

iii) Given as 200-mg dose with each dose of levodopa

3) They do not delay time to reach peak plasma level of levodopa

4) They do not delay absorption of levodopa

5) They act to prolong "on" time

6) Have predisposition to levodopa-induced dyskinesias and other adverse effects (e.g., nausea), sometimes requiring decrease in levodopa dose

7) Other adverse effects: abdominal cramps, abdominal pain, severe diarrhea (1.3% of patients) related to allergic hypersensitivity—otherwise, well tolerated

---

COMT Inhibitors

Tolcapone
A reversible central and peripheral-acting COMT inhibitor

Entacapone
A reversible peripheral-acting COMT inhibitor; shorter half-life than tolcapone (usually given with each levodopa-carbidopa [Sinemet] dose)

---

d. Anticholinergic agents

1) Usually less effective than levodopa or dopamine agonists

2) May be selectively more effective for tremor and dystonia poorly responsive to levodopa or dopamine agonist when added

3) Dose-related therapeutic effect

4) Most commonly used formulations: trihexyphenidyl (Artane) and benztropine mesylate (Cogentin)

5) Adverse effects: dry mouth, blurred vision, urinary retention, forgetfulness, hallucinations, psychosis

e. Adjunctive therapy

1) Amantadine

a) Used in early stages: may delay need for levodopa

b) Used as adjunctive therapy: reduce the required doses of dopaminergic treatment

c) May be effective in reducing levodopa-induced dyskinesias

d) Excreted unchanged in the urine: dose needs to be reduced in patients with renal impairment and in elderly

e) Can cause cognitive impairment

2) Selegiline

a) Selectively inhibits monoamine oxidase (MAO)-B and not MAO-A at doses below 10 mg daily

b) Daily dose above 10 mg can inhibit MAO-A and may induce hypertensive crisis with ingestion of tyramine-containing food

c) Delays the need for levodopa if started early, but no long-term benefit

d) Unclear if it has neuroprotective effect

e) Metabolized to amphetamine and methamphetamine

f) May have a synergistic effect with levodopa

f. Sleep disturbance and treatment

1) Parkinsonism-related akathisia (restlessness) or other motor symptoms: fourth dose of carbidopa-levodopa IR

2) Insomnia and fragmented sleep

a) Parkinsonian symptoms: nocturnal awakenings from rigidity and difficulty turning in bed, nocturnal akathisia, nocturnal leg cramps and dystonias (including early morning dystonias)

i) Initial insomnia: use carbidopa-levodopa IR at bedtime

ii) Awakening 2 to 3 hours after sleep onset: use CR formulation or dopamine agonist before sleep

iii) Awakening after 3 to 5 hours or early morning hours: use carbidopa-levodopa IR on awakening

b) Medication effect: alerting effect, insomnia, hallucinations, vivid dreams, nightmares, or dyskinesias—reduce dopaminergic medications, add hypnotics, or reduce or discontinue causative drug if possible

c) Primary sleep disturbance: restless legs syndrome associated with Parkinson's disease (treat with dopamine agonist or gabapentin)

d) Depression (may afflict up to 40% of patients with Parkinson's disease): treat with selective serotonin reuptake inhibitor (SSRI) or a bedtime tricyclic antidepressant

e) Circadian rhythm disturbance: treat with melatonin

3) Hypersomnia and excessive daytime sleepiness

a) Secondary to insomnia and fragmented sleep

b) Obstructive sleep apnea (primary sleep disorder): associated with idiopathic Parkinson's disease

c) Depression

d) Narcolepsy-like disorder with hallucinations and sleep attacks

4) Excessive nocturnal motor activity

a) Rapid eye movement (REM) sleep behavior disorder (RBD)

i) Up to 30% of patients with Parkinson's disease develop RBD at some time

ii) Up to 40% of patients with idiopathic RBD eventually develop Parkinson's disease at mean of 12.7 years after RBD onset

iii) Loss of skeletal muscle atonia during REM sleep

iv) Excessive chin muscle tone and limb motor activity noted on polysomnography

v) Usually associated with dreams of being chased or threatened, may involve violent and aggressive motor activity

vi) Sporadic in frequency and severity

vii) Must distinguish from "sundowning," (patient appears awake and confused)

viii) Treatment: small doses of clonazepam (Klonopin) or melatonin at bedtime

b) Periodic limb movements of sleep: occurs more frequently in patients with Parkinson's disease

5) Hallucinations

a) Medication-induced: levodopa (vivid dreams, nightmares), anxiolytics, anticholinergics, antidepressants

b) Associated with sundowning and dementia

c) Associated with RBD

d) Treatment

i) Discontinue the weaker antiparkinsonian medi-cine believed to exacerbate hallucinations (e.g., amantadine)

ii) If continued, treatment options may include clozapine, quetiapine (Seroquel), or olanzapine (Zyprexa)

g. General approach to initial symptomatic treatment in mild to moderate parkinsonism

1) Consider treatment with levodopa or dopamine agonist if symptoms interfere with daily activity

2) If minimal interference with daily activity: may start with selegiline, amantadine, or anticholinergic agent

3) Onset of symptoms at young age (<40-50 years): many prefer to start with dopamine agonist (no motor fluctuations or dyskinesias in absence of levodopa, much less potent than levodopa) or combination therapy (levodopa and dopamine agonist)

a) Patients with early onset parkinsonism are more prone to dyskinesias and fluctuating motor responses and response to levodopa is less predictable

4) Onset of symptoms at older age: start with levodopa IR 25/100 3 times daily 1 hour before meals and titrate weekly or consider an agonist; initial dose may be smaller and titration slower if nausea or other prominent adverse effects

h. General approach to advancing Parkinson's disease (Fig. 8-4)

1) "Wearing off" effect

a) Most common type of motor fluctuation in advancing disease

b) Recurrence of parkinsonian symptoms and clinical deterioration before next dose

c) If response to levodopa during the "on" phase is adequate, move next dose to an earlier time and shorten the time between doses

d) If response to levodopa during the "on" phase is inadequate, increase individual levodopa dose before making any adjustment in timing of next dose

e) Addition of dopamine agonist after adjustments to levodopa regimen has been made reduces motor fluctuations

f) Addition of COMT inhibitors may also increase the "on" phase but predispose to levodopa-induced adverse effects (e.g., dyskinesias)

2) Dyskinesias

a) Dystonic in absence of chorea: usually parkinsonian (most commonly, early morning or nocturnal dystonia such as painful foot cramps)

b) Choreiform with or without dystonia: usually levodopa-induced

c) Usually peak-dose (Off-On-Dyskinesia-On-Off)

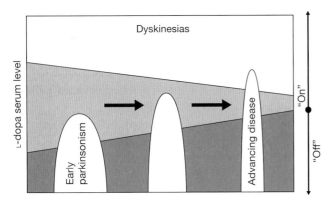

Fig. 8-4. Development of dyskinesias with advancing disease and narrowing of the "therapeutic window." Each curve represents serum levels of levodopa-carbidopa combination (Sinemet). Dark gray area is "off" phase without dyskinesias; light gray area is "on" phase *without* dyskinesias; white area is "on" phase *with* peak-dose dyskinesias. With advancing Parkinson's disease (*arrows*) and degeneration of dopamine storage, the predisposition to dyskinesias and motor fluctuations increases. Furthermore, the pharmacokinetics of levodopa-carbidopa combination is less "smooth," with a sharper rise and fall, and serum levels attain higher peak levels.

and rarely biphasic (Off-Dyskinesia-On-Dyskinesia-Off)
d) Mechanism thought to involve overactivity of direct striatum—globus pallidus interna pathway
e) Peak-dose dyskinesias: reduce amount of levodopa IR and consider discontinuing adjunctive selegiline or COMT inhibitors
f) Consider addition of amantadine
g) Rapid motor fluctuations with alternating dyskinesias and "off" states, consider addition of an agonist (use adequate dose and avoid rapid titration of dose)
h) Biphasic dykinesias (true biphasic dyskinesias are rare): shortening the time between doses
3) "On-Off" phenomenon
a) Unpredictable, abrupt episodes of parkinsonism
b) Usually treated with increasing levodopa dose or addition of dopamine agonists
4) Freezing
a) Usually occurs because of rigidity and bradykinesia, represents difficulty with initiating movements (walking, getting up from a seated position, etc.)
b) "Off" phase, end-dose freezing responds to short-

ening the time between levodopa doses and taking the next dose at earlier time, addition of a COMT inhibitor or agonist
c) If clinical response to levodopa is inadequate, treatment is to increase the respective levodopa dose
d) Liquid levodopa as "rescue therapy" can be effective given relatively short onset of symptoms
e) Rarely, occur as a peak-dose effect (may respond to a slight decrease in the respective levodopa dose)
i. Surgical treatment of Parkinson's disease
1) Thalamotomy
a) Now obsolete
b) Alleviates or abolishes contralateral rest tremor or rigidity in 80% to 90% of patients
c) Also effective for contralateral dyskinesias
d) No effect on bradykinesia, postural instability, or other axial symptoms
e) Complications: weakness, numbness, paresthesias, dysarthria, delayed-onset dystonia (more common with bilateral procedures previously done)
2) Unilateral pallidotomy
a) Improves rigidity, postural instability, and bradykinesia (as opposed to thalamotomy), although not much greater benefit over L-dopa treatment.
b) Most important benefit: dyskinesias (both levodopa-induced chorea type and parkinsonian dystonic type)
c) Complications: hemiparesis, aphasia, facial weakness (more common with bilateral procedures)
3) Deep brain stimulation
a) Electrodes implanted in ventralis intermedius nucleus of thalamus, subthalamic nucleus, globus pallidus interna, and other subcortical nuclei
b) Components: lead, power source (implantable pulse generator), and extension wire connecting the two
c) Implantable pulse generator is usually subcutaneous in infraclavicular area
d) Stimulator implanted in thalamus, usually unilaterally
e) Stimulator implanted in subthalamic nucleus and globus pallidus interna, usually bilaterally
f) Mechanism of action thought to involve
i) Depolarization inhibition and block
ii) Activation of inhibitory pathways
iii) Desynchronization of tremor-causing intrinsic pacemaker activity of excitatory neurons
g) Deep brain stimulation of thalamus
i) Most effective for parkinsonian tremor (and essential tremor)

ii) Minimal benefit for other parkinsonian features such as rigidity, bradykinesia, dyskinesias

iii) Best used in patients with tremor-predominant disease, when tremor is not effectively treated medically

h) Deep brain stimulation of globus pallidus interna

i) Improves all symptoms including dyskinesias

ii) Does not reduce need for antiparkinsonian agents

iii) Ideal candidate: patient with levodopa-responsive idiopathic Parkinson's disease who has unrelenting dyskinesias and motor fluctuations

i) Deep brain stimulation of subthalamic nucleus

i) Reduces all cardinal features of idiopathic Parkinson's disease, including postural instability and gait disorder

ii) Does reduce the need for antiparkinsonian agents significantly

iii) Ideal candidate: patient with levodopa-responsive idiopathic Parkinson's disease who has unrelenting dyskinesias and motor fluctuations

4) Generally, good surgical candidates: younger than 75; multiple antiparkinsonian agents, including combinations, have been tried; no dementia, behavioral problems, or mood disorders

B. Multiple System Atrophy (MSA)

1. Often multiple overlapping clinical features (see below)
2. Autonomic features: Shy-Drager syndrome
   a. Presenting complaints in half of the patients; will be present in most patients during the clinical course
   b. Most common presenting symptoms: orthostatism and urinary incontinence
   c. Postural hypotension
   d. Postprandial hypotension
   e. Anhidrosis
   f. Urinary incontinence
      1) Detrusor hypofunction and denervation: loss of parasympathetic innervation and retention
      2) Detrusor hyperreflexia
      3) Sphincter weakness from involvement of Onuf's nucleus (sacral cord)
   g. Male impotence
   h. Iris atrophy
   i. Constipation
3. Extrapyramidal features: striatonigral degeneration (MSA-P)
   a. These are presenting features in less than half of patients but occur in most patients during course of the disorder
   b. Most often bradykinesia and rigidity, less often tremor
   c. Severe hypophonia

d. Postural myoclonus: jerking of outstretched hands
e. Up to 30% of patients may respond to levodopa: response is usually brief and limited, exacerbated by orthostatism
f. Levodopa-induced dyskinesias are usually dystonic
g. Prominent and early antecollis with gait instability and possibly early falls

4. Cerebellar features: olivopontocerebellar atrophy (MSA-C)
   a. Presenting feature in only about 5% of patients
   b. Eventually develops in up to half of patients
   c. Appendicular and axial dysmetria are more common than oculomotor dysmetria
5. Other features
   a. Stridor (as well as sleep apnea and other sleep-related breathing disorders)
      1) Due to abductor weakness of vocal cords
      2) May cause sudden nocturnal death
   b. Pyramidal features: long-tract signs include spasticity, extensor plantar responses, hyperreflexia
   c. Rare and unexpected features

Important Pathologic Features of Parkinsonian Syndromes

Idiopathic Parkinson's disease
Substantia nigra pallor and neuronal loss, Lewy bodies in surviving neurons in substantia nigra

Multiple system atrophy
Glial and neuronal cytoplasmic and nuclear inclusions positive for α-synuclein; neuronal loss and gliosis involving inferior olivary nucleus, pons, cerebellum, and intermediolateral cell column of thoracic cord

Progressive supranuclear palsy
Tau-immunoreactive deposition—neuropil threads, tufted astrocytes, globose neurofibrillary tangles; neuronal loss and gliosis in upper brainstem, locus ceruleus, substantia nigra, periaqueductal gray matter, superior colliculus

Corticobasal degeneration
Superficial cortical neuronal loss and gliosis of frontoparietal cortex, ballooned neurons, intraneuronal "corticobasal" inclusions, tau-positive astrocytic plaques

1) Dementia
   a) Includes focal cortical symptoms such as apraxia
   b) Cognitive dysfunction described in a small proportion of patients: abnormalities in attentional tasks, working memory, and speed of thinking
2) Slowing of saccades and supranuclear gaze palsy

6. Histopathology (Fig. 8-5)
   a. Neuronal loss and gliosis in inferior olivary nucleus, pons, cerebellum, intermediolateral cell column of thoracic cord, putamen, and substantia nigra
   b. Glial and neuronal inclusions
      1) Oligodendrocyte nucleus and cytoplasm
      2) Neuronal nucleus and cytoplasm
      3) May be the primary pathologic change and precede neuronal loss
      4) Found primarily in motor cortex, basal ganglia, pons, and intermediolateral cell column
      5) Major component of inclusions is α-synuclein ("synucleinopathy")

6) Other constituents: ubiquitin, β-crystallin, tubulins
7. Investigations
   a. MRI (Fig. 8-6)
      1) Rule out other disorders
      2) T2 imaging: putaminal hypointensity and atrophy and nigral atrophy—not specific
      3) Atrophy of cerebellum, cerebellar peduncles, pons (may see "hot-cross-bun sign" with pontine atrophy)
   b. Functional imaging
      1) Fluorodopa PET: decreased uptake in striatonigral projections, reduced metabolism in putamen and caudate
   c. Thermoregulatory sweat test and autonomic testing
   d. Sleep study for evaluation of stridor

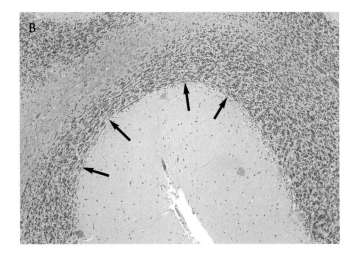

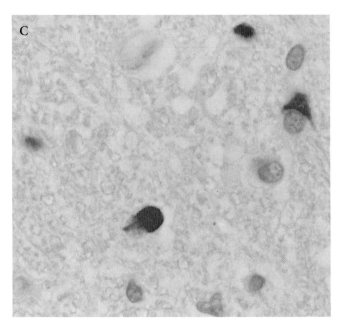

Fig. 8-5. Histopathology of multiple system atrophy. *A*, Macroscopically, there is often atrophy and discoloration of the putamen and pallor of the substantia nigra and locus ceruleus in striatonigral-type multiple system atrophy. Microscopically, the disease is characterized by cerebellar Purkinje cell loss (*arrows* in *B*) and α-synuclein–positive cytoplasmic inclusions (*C*).

e. Electromyography (EMG) of the external urethra or anal sphincter: long duration, high-amplitude neurogenic potentials indicating denervation and involvement of Onuf's nucleus (segments S2 and S3)

8. Treatment
   a. Orthostatism
      1) Discontinuation of agents exacerbating orthostatic hypotension
      2) Increase fluid and salt intake in diet
      3) Elevate head of bed at 30 degrees (to increase renin secretion)
      4) Compressive elastic stockings
      5) Medications
         a) Fludrocortisone
         b) Midodrine
   b. Urinary incontinence
      1) Bedside urinal or condom catheter (males) for simple urge incontinence
      2) Intermittent self-catheterization for urinary retention
      3) Anticholinergic agents (oxybutynin 2.5-5 mg 2-3 times daily) or propantheline bromide (15-60 mg daily) for detrusor hyperreflexia
      4) Indwelling catheters
      5) Surgery (last resort)
   c. Anhidrosis: patients warned against extreme heat (environmental or during exercise)

d. Other measures
   1) Physical therapy
   2) Stridor: continuous positive pressure or tracheostomy for refractory vocal cord paresis
e. Parkinsonism: carbidopa-levodopa (may worsen orthostatic hypotension)

C. Progressive Supranuclear Palsy

1. Clinical features
   a. Supranuclear ophthalmoplegia
      1) Vertical saccades (especially downward) > horizontal saccades affected earlier than pursuit movements
      2) Slow and hypometric saccades
      3) Limitation of convergence and "wide-eyed stare" due to bilateral exophoria and bilateral lid retraction
      4) Apraxia of eyelid movements (especially opening)
      5) Saccadic intrusions on primary gaze and square wave jerks
      6) Reduced vestibulo-ocular reflex suppression
      7) Reduced fast component of optokinetic nystagmus

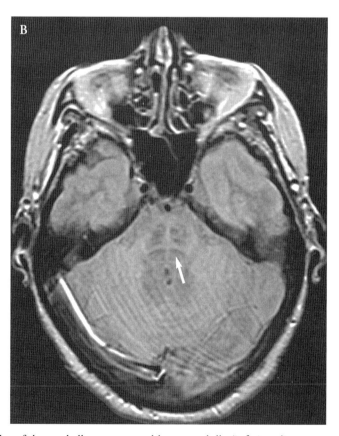

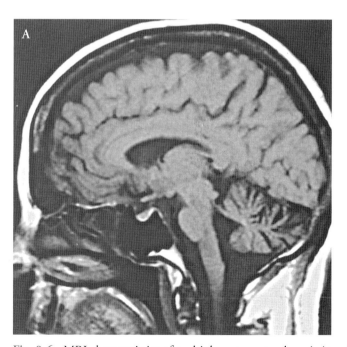

Fig. 8-6. MRI characteristics of multiple system atrophy. *A*, Atrophy of the cerebellum, pons, and lower medulla (inferior olivary nuclei) are seen best in sagittal T1-weighted images. *B*, The "hot-cross-bun sign" (*arrow*) may result from pontine atrophy; it is seen best in axial T2-weighted and proton density images.

8) Eventually, complete bilateral ophthalmoplegia
b. Parkinsonism and early falls
  1) Prominent, early axial rigidity and early impairment of axial and postural reflexes with retropulsion
  2) Prominent hyperextended posture during walking (as compared with antecollis in patients with multiple system atrophy)
  3) Symmetric bradykinesia
  4) Rest tremor is uncommon
  5) Unresponsive or poor response to levodopa
c. Pseudobulbar palsy
  1) "Emotional incontinence": crying or laughter inappropriate to context of conversation
  2) Dysarthria: spastic and sometimes hypernasal speech
  3) Dysphagia
  4) Drooling
  5) Increased jaw jerk
d. Cognitive disturbance
  1) Impaired attention and mental slowing
  2) Frontal-executive dysfunction
  3) Frontal release signs
  4) Possibly ideomotor apraxia (uncommon)
  5) Personality change: apathy, irritability, disinhibition
e. Other: hypertension (presumably from degeneration of brainstem adrenergic nuclei)

2. Investigations
a. MRI
  1) Localized midbrain atrophy (reduced anteroposterior diameter)
  2) Enlarged third ventricle
  3) Atrophy of red nucleus
  4) Possibly frontal or temporal atrophy
b. Functional imaging
  1) Global metabolic reduction, including bilateral frontal lobes (especially anterior cingulate cortex), basal ganglia, thalamus, upper brainstem
  2) Fluorodopa PET: reduction of ^{18}F-dopa influx into caudate and putamen
c. Polysomnography: diminished total sleep time and REM sleep

3. Histopathology (Fig. 8-7)
a. Atrophy (with neuronal loss and gliosis) of upper brainstem structures, pallor of substantia nigra and locus ceruleus
b. Other areas may be affected: periaqueductal gray matter, superior colliculus, substantia nigra, subthalamic nucleus, red nucleus, dentate nucleus, basal ganglia (globus pallidus > putamen), hippocampal structures
c. Abnormal tau deposition, including neuropil threads (tau-positive fibers) and tau-positive tufted astrocytes

(abnormal "tufted" fibers)
d. Iron pigmentation of globus pallidus
e. Hallmark: unusual globose neurofibrillary tangles (prominent in brainstem)
  1) Pretangles: neurons with nonfilamentous cytoplasmic tau deposits
  2) Bundles of straight filaments (as opposed to paired helical filaments in Alzheimer's disease)

4. Treatment
a. Few patients have response to dopaminergic agents: minimal response may be appreciated with bradykinesia and rigidity
b. Trials of NMDA receptor antagonists (e.g., amantadine) and acetylcholinesterase inhibitors have been disappointing

D. Corticobasal Degeneration

1. PARA syndrome (**p**rogressive **a**symmetric **r**igidity and **a**praxia) asymmetric or focal presentation of following symptoms:
a. Affected limb may be both rigid (extrapyramidal) and spastic (pyramidal)
b. There may be dystonic posturing of limb and myoclonus (which may be action-induced or stimulus-sensitive)
c. Cortical sensory loss
d. Ideomotor apraxia (sometimes ideational apraxia)—usually unilateral or classic "alien limb phenomenon" (spontaneous involuntary movements more noticed with eyes closed)
  1) Limb may become useless when severe
  2) Usually occurs with nondominant hand
  3) Usually due to involvement of parietal lobe or supplementary motor cortex but also to subcortical interconnections with frontal lobe, premotor cortex, cingulate gyrus, and corpus callosum
e. Mirror movements: likely signify parietal and, sometimes, corpus callosal damage
f. Progressive rigidity or dystonia may mask alien limb phenomenon

2. Other features
a. Apraxia of speech
b. Oculomotor apraxia
c. Apraxia of eyelid movements (also in progressive supranuclear palsy)
d. Asymmetric long-tract and pyramidal findings: extensor plantar response, hyperreflexia, spasticity
e. Dementia: psychomotor slowing, impaired attention and concentration, frontal-executive dysfunction, and possibly visuospatial involvement (may have oculomotor apraxia or other features of Balint's syndrome)

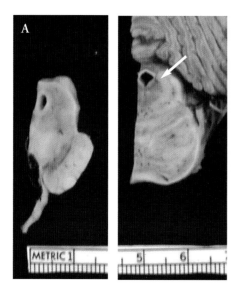

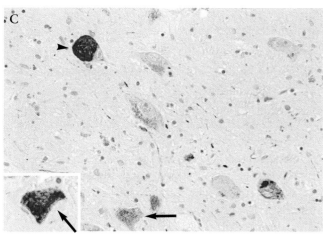

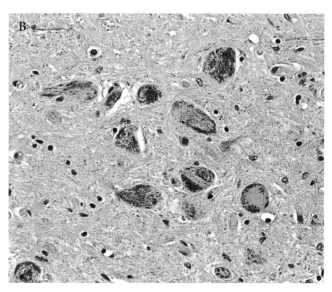

Fig. 8-7. Histopathologic features of progressive supranuclear palsy. *A,* Macroscopically, atrophy of upper brainstem structures and pallor of the substantia nigra and locus ceruleus (*white arrow*) are apparent. *B,* The most important microscopic feature is the globose tangles, which are basophilic, tau-immunoreactive, argyrophilic structures in the gray matter. *C,* Tau immunohistochemistry in a section from thalamus demonstrates neuronal accumulation of tau protein, some aggregating into tau-immunoreactive "globose" neurofibrillary tangles (*arrowhead*) and "pretangles" (*arrows*).

3. Histopathology (Fig. 8-8)
   a. Frontoparietal and perirolandic cortical atrophy, with neuronal loss and gliosis involving superficial layers and subcortical white matter (Fig. 8-8 *A*)
      1) "Status spongiosus" in more severely affected areas: spongiform change due to neuronal dropout
   b. Ballooned neurons: swollen, achromatic (loss of cytoplasmic staining), immunoreactive to phosphorylated neurofilament epitopes and αβ-crystallin, and sometimes tau- and ubiquitin-positive
   c. Substantia nigra: severe depigmentation, neuronal loss, gliosis
   d. Intraneuronal "corticobasal" inclusions in substantia nigra (and cortical layer II): inclusions have positive tau and negative ubiquitin immuoreactivity
   e. Astrocytic plaques: tau-positive thick glial inclusions deposited in distal processes of cortical astrocytes, specific for corticobasal degeneration

   f. Tau filaments are double-stranded paired helical filaments that are more polymorphic than those in Alzheimer's disease
4. Neuroimaging (Fig. 8-9)
   a. MRI: asymmetric frontoparietal and midcallosal atrophy
   b. MRI T2-weighted: mild putaminal and pallidal hypointensity
   c. PET: hypometabolism of frontoparietal cortex, lenticular nucleus, and thalamus bilaterally
5. Upper limb somatosensory evoked potentials may be abnormal
6. Treatment strategies
   a. One-fourth of patients may have some benefit from levodopa (far less than expected with idiopathic Parkinson's disease)
   b. Amantadine may benefit 13% of patients (rigidity and gait)
   c. Dopamine agonists produce little improvement, if any
   d. Clonazepam may be helpful in treating myoclonus and dystonia

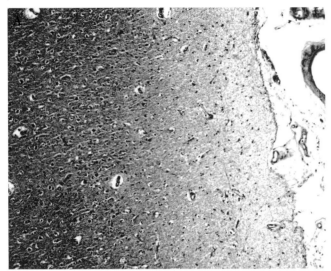

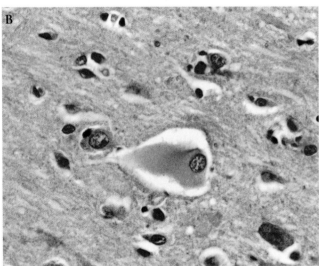

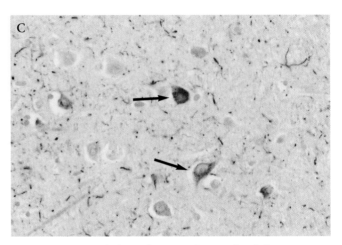

Fig. 8-8. Histopathologic features of corticobasal degeneration. *A*, Neuronal loss and microvacuolation of superficial layers of cerebral cortex. *B*, Characteristic swollen cortical neurons. *C*, Tau-positive intraneuronal inclusions, appearing as globular or angular inclusions (*arrows*).

    2) Ages between 40 and 60: dementia and parkinsonism
  d. May also have pyramidal tract signs, choreoathetosis, or ataxia
  e. Dementia: primarily "subcortical," with poor attention and concentration and poor working memory
  f. Imaging may show calcification of basal ganglia, dentate nucleus, and periventricular region (Table 8-4)
    1) Most apparent on computed tomography (CT) (Fig. 8-10)
    2) Hyperintense areas noted on MRI T2-weighted images
  g. No effective treatment
2. Neurodegeneration with brain iron accumulation type I (now called pantothenate kinase-associated neurodegeneration [PKAN] and formerly known as Hallervorden-Spatz disease)
  a. Rare autosomal recessive disorder (linkage analysis: pantothenate kinase gene on chromosome 20p12.3-p13)
  b. Histopathology
    1) Excessive iron deposition, with rusty brown discoloration of medial globus pallidus (more than substantia nigra pars reticulata)
    2) Iron deposition both intracellular and extracellular: neurons, glia, microglia
    3) Spheroids: dystrophic axonal swellings and degenerating myelinated axons (primary neuroaxonal dystrophy)
    4) Neuronal loss, gliosis, and demyelination
    5) Tau-immunoreactive neurofibrillary tangles with paired helical filaments (phosphorylated tau)

  e. SSRIs may help treat depression (if ineffective, try tricyclic agents)
  f. Speech therapy and percutaneous endoscopic gastrostomy tube placement for dysphagia if needed
  g. Rehabilitation for limb apraxia

E. Heredodegenerative Parkinsonian Disorders
1. Idiopathic calcification of the basal ganglion (Fahr's disease)
  a. Syndrome of progressive dementia and parkinsonism, extensive calcification of basal ganglia
  b. Usually sporadic but may be inherited as autosomal dominant disorder (locus on chromosome 14)
  c. Presentation
    1) Ages between 20 and 40: schizophrenia-like psychosis and other psychiatric manifestations

6) Widespread accumulation of α-synuclein

c. Clinical presentation

1) Variants

a) Late infantile: onset between ages 1 and 3

b) Juvenile (classic): onset between ages 7 and 12

c) Adult (rare)

2) Childhood onset: predominant features are dystonia, rigidity, and postural and gait imbalance

3) Adulthood onset (rare): parkinsonism may be predominant presentation, with asymmetric rigidity

4) Neurocognitive deficits

a) Depression, personality changes

b) Deficits in attention, concentration, working memory, visuospatial tasks

5) Other features may include dysarthria, choreoathetosis, retinitis pigmentosa and optic nerve degeneration, seizures, and few patients with pyramidal signs (spasticity, hyperreflexia, and extensor plantar responses)

6) Tics and myoclonus in latter stages of disease

d. Neuroimaging

1) MRI

a) Characteristic low signal changes in basal ganglia

b) "Eye of the tiger" sign: small area of anteromedial high signal on T2-weighted images, with surrounding low signal

2) Nonenhanced CT: bilateral low-density basal ganglia

e. Treatment

1) Iron chelation not effective

2) Levodopa for parkinsonism (some may respond)

3) Benzodiazepines for choreoathetosis

4) Antiepileptic drugs for seizure control

3. Wilson's disease (progressive hepatolenticular degeneration)

a. Autosomal recessive (chromosome 13q14.3): mutation in *ATP7B* (encoding a copper-transporting P-type ATPase), involved in vesicular transport of copper

Table 8-4.   **Differential Diagnosis of Symmetric Basal Ganglia Calcification**

Idiopathic
Fahr's disease
Wilson's disease
Amyloid angiopathy
Hypercalcemia
Hypoparathyroidism
Postinfectious: tuberculosis, congenital HIV, toxoplasmosis, cysticercosis
Toxic: lead, chemotherapy agents (methotrexate), radiotherapy
Perinatal anoxia
Carbon monoxide intoxication
Cockayne's syndrome

HIV, human immunodeficiency virus.

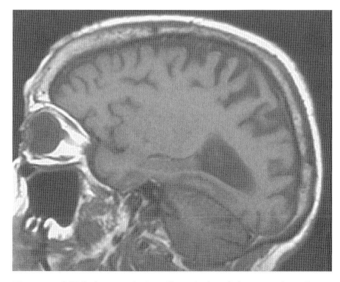

Fig. 8-9. MRI characteristics of corticobasal degeneration showing selective frontoparietal atrophy. (Sagittal T1-weighted image.)

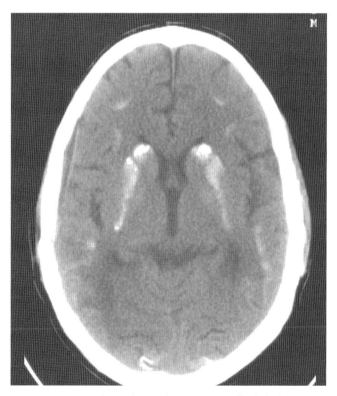

Fig. 8-10. Nonenhanced CT characteristics of Fahr's disease showing intense calcification in basal ganglia.

b. Pathophysiology
   1) After absorption, copper binds to albumin; most albumin-copper complex is transported to liver, most of which is excreted via the biliary tract.
   2) A proportion of this copper binds to ceruloplasmin and is secreted into circulation; this binding depends on action of P-type ATPase, which is affected with Wilson's disease
   3) Abnormal copper accumulation with affinity for brain and liver occurs in absence of adequate binding of copper to ceruloplasmin
   4) Low ceruloplasmin levels in the patients may be attributed to rapid liver degradation of unbound protein
c. Clinical features (clinical and phenotypic heterogeneity)
   1) Juvenile onset: presentation is most commonly liver disease
   2) Adult onset: presentation is most commonly neurologic disease
   3) Liver manifestations
      a) Most commonly, progressive cirrhosis
      b) Clinical heterogeneity: asymptomatic elevation of liver enzymes to fulminant liver failure
      c) Chronic hepatitis
         i) May originally present as acute hepatitis episode
         ii) May be associated with renal tubular dysfunction
      d) Fulminant liver failure
         i) Associated with intravascular hemolysis from massive release of copper into circulation from hepatocytes (>75 μg/dL)
         ii) Definitive treatment is liver transplantation (otherwise, 100% mortality)
   4) Neurologic manifestations
      a) Cranial motor (common)
         i) Dysarthria
         ii) Sialorrhea
         iii) Dysphagia
         iv) Cranial dystonia
         v) Risus sardonicus: fixed grimace from dystonic posturing of selected facial muscles
      b) Tremor (most common neurologic symptom)
         i) Most common: postural and mixed type tremors
         ii) Classic: irregular proximal kinetic or postural described as "wing-beating" with flexed elbows
         iii) May be paroxysmal rest, action/kinetic, or postural (or a combination)
      c) Other
         i) Parkinsonism

      ii) Generalized dystonia
      iii) Ataxia: gait, appendicular, scanning dysarthria
      iv) Below average memory function
      v) Seizures: rare (6%), more likely to occur after initiation of chelation therapy
   5) Psychiatric manifestations
      a) Commonly noted at onset of other presenting symptoms (may precede other features)
      b) Emotional lability, psychosis, depression, disinhibition, impulsive behavior, loss of insight, change in personality, aggressiveness, irritability, sexual preoccupation
   6) Ophthalmologic manifestations
      a) Kayser-Fleischer rings (Fig. 8-11)
         i) Uniformly concentric and present in periphery of cornea
         ii) Copper-containing granules in Descemet's membrane
         iii) Almost always present with neurologic or psychiatric symptoms
      b) "Sunflower cataracts": copper deposition in the lens
      c) Also possible: difficulty with smooth pursuits, nystagmus, impaired convergence, and, less commonly, apraxia of eyelid opening
   7) Renal manifestations: hypercalciuria, hyperphosphaturia, nephrocalcinosis, and aminoaciduria
d. Diagnostic testing
   1) Liver function tests
   2) Serum ceruloplasmin (normal 20-40 mg/dL)

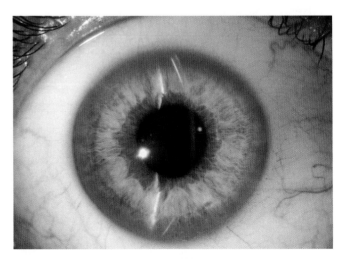

Fig. 8-11. Slit-lamp examination of patient with Wilson's disease, demonstrating Kayser-Fleischer ring. (Courtesy of Brian R. Younge, MD.)

a) Usually low in Wilson's disease (75% of patients have liver symptoms at onset and 90% have neurologic symptoms)

b) May be reduced in 10% to 20% of asymptomatic carriers

c) False-negative results (elevated levels) with oral contraceptives, hormone replacement therapy, systemic illness (acute phase reactant)

d) False-positive results (low levels) with liver failure, nephrotic syndrome, protein-losing enteropathy, Menkes syndrome

3) 24-Hour urine copper

a) Symptomatic patients: usually in excess of 100 μg/day

b) False-positive results (elevated levels) with liver failure or nephrotic syndrome, biliary or obstructive liver disease, increased dietary copper

c) Copper-free diet for 24 hours preceding test and copper-free collection jars needed for accurate measurement

4) Slit-lamp examination to look for Kayser-Fleischer rings

5) Serum copper

a) Total serum copper: not reliable, reduced with low ceruloplasmin level

b) Free serum copper: level increases as liver storage is saturated

6) Liver biopsy—measurement of liver copper level

a) Normal, below 15 μg/g

b) Heterozygotes, 55-200 μg/g

c) Wilson's disease, above 200 μg/g

7) Imaging characteristics

a) Normal or generalized atrophy

b) CT: bilateral putaminal hypodensity

c) MRI: T2 hyperintensity signals in thalami, putamen, dentate nuclei, brainstem

    i) Occasionally central core of decreased signal intensity

    ii) Rarely "face of the panda" sign in midbrain

d) Fluorodeoxyglucose (FDG)-PET: abnormal glucose metabolism in cerebellum and striatum

8) Genetic testing

a) Not widely available

b) Difficult because of diversity of mutations in *ATP7B* gene

e. Histopathology (Fig. 8-12)

1) Red brownish discoloration of putamen, with symmetric atrophy and cavitation in advanced cases

2) Neuronal loss and reactive gliosis in involved regions

3) Alzheimer type II cells

a) Often seen in globus pallidus, thalamus, brainstem (nonspecific and may be seen in other hepatic encephalopathies)

b) Are characterized by enlarged vesicular nucleus and sparse cytoplasm

4) Opalski cells

a) Seen in small number of cases

b) Round cells with densely eosinophilic cytoplasm, small central nucleus

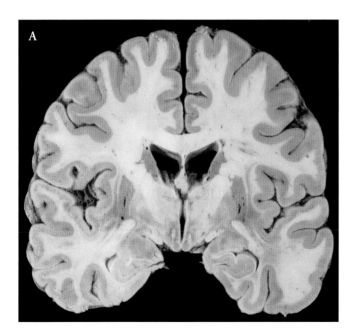

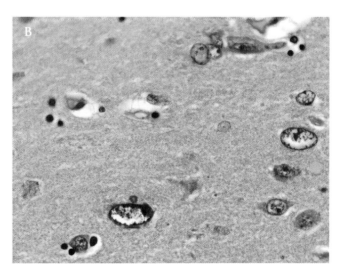

Fig. 8-12. Wilson's disease. *A*, There is often atrophy and cavitation of the putamen. *B*, Alzheimer type II cells are characterized by enlarged vesicular nuclei and sparse cytoplasm.

c) Not entirely specific to Wilson's disease, also occur in non-wilsonian chronic hepatic encephalopathy

f. Treatment

1) Reversal of liver and neurologic damage is optimal with early intervention

2) Reduction of copper intake: avoidance of food rich in copper, especially liver and shellfish

3) Inhibition of copper absorption and increased copper elimination

   a) Zinc

      i) Induced synthesis of metallothionein by enterocytes, which binds copper and zinc

      ii) Dietary copper stored temporarily in enterocytes bound to metallothionein, excreted when the enterocyte is excreted

      iii) Well-tolerated

      iv) Onset of action: up to 2 weeks (induction of metallothionein synthesis)

      v) Used for chronic management of copper overload or maintenance therapy, also for patients who do not tolerate chelating agents

      vi) Formulation: acetate or sulfate, 50 mg 3 times daily

      vii) Does not promote excretion of copper in urine

      viii) Urine copper levels should diminish with time: measure 24-hour urine copper before therapy, first month after the therapy, then every 3 months

   b) Ammonium tetrathiomolybdate

      i) Works in the enteric lumen to form a complex with albumin and copper (both in the enteric lumen and bloodstream), and acts to limit copper transport to the target tissues

      ii) The complex is then excreted

      iii) Liver storage is slowly depleted

      iv) Usual starting dose: 20 mg 3 times daily with meals, with slow titration and addition of three doses of 20 to 60 mg in between doses

      v) Small potential chance of bone marrow suppression, but usually well tolerated

      vi) May be appropriate induction agent with the relatively fast onset of action

      vii) Not approved by U.S. FDA

4) Copper chelation and increased copper elimination

   a) Penicillamine

      i) Copper chelator and inducer of metallothionein, resulting in excretion of copper in urine up to 10 to 15 mg in 24 hours (goal 2-5 mg/24 hours)

      ii) 24-Hour urine copper measured monthly

      iii) Administered on an empty stomach at 250 mg 4 times daily (initial dose is 250 mg once daily, and titrated by 250 mg every 3-5 days until desired copper excretion is obtained)

      iv) 30% to 50% of patients initially have worsening of neurologic function (possibly caused by mobilization of copper from liver storage and deposition in brain)

      v) Improvement in neurologic function occurs as early as 2 weeks, may be delayed for several months

      vi) Tremor usually responds better than dystonia or psychiatric symptoms

      vii) Adverse effects—acute (sensitivity): rash, fever, eosinophilia, thrombocytopenia, leukopenia, lymphadenopathy

      viii) Adverse effects—chronic reactions: bone marrow suppression, lupus-like syndrome, Goodpasture's syndrome, myasthenic syndrome, loss of taste, skin discoloration, aphthous stomatitis

   b) Trientine

      i) Not as potent as penicillamine, may avoid the initial clinical worsening

      ii) Used when penicillamine is not tolerated

5) Liver transplantation

   a) Indicated for fulminant liver failure (100% fatality) or progressive liver failure not responding to medical therapy

   b) Results in reduction of neurologic and psychiatric symptoms

4. Spinocerebellar ataxia 3 (SCA3, Machado-Joseph disease) (see Chapter 9)

a. Ataxia, ophthalmoplegia, pyramidal and extrapyramidal features, polyneuropathy

b. Extrapyramidal features are usually akinetic parkinsonism and dystonia

F. Secondary Parkinsonism

1. Drug-induced parkinsonism (see Section IV below)

2. Toxic parkinsonism

a. Manganese: most common cause of environmental toxin

   1) Miners and industrial workers at risk (welders)

   2) Primarily affects globus pallidus and subthalamic nucleus more than striatum (sparing substantia nigra)

   3) Symmetric parkinsonism with prominent rigidity, "cock-walk" gait characterized by prominent foot action dystonia and flexed arm posture, and oculogyric crisis

   4) Behavioral symptoms including dementia may precede or accompany parkinsonian features

   5) May progress for some time after cessation of exposure

6) MRI: striatal T1 symmetric bilateral high signal in pallidum (due to accumulation of manganese)

b. MPTP (1-methyl-4-phenyl-1,2,3,6-tetrahydropyridine)

1) Highly toxic to substantia nigra, may promote active nigrostriatal degenerative process

2) MPTP is converted to MPP+, a mitochondrial toxin that concentrates in mitochondria, interfering with energy production and metabolism

3) Symptoms mimic idiopathic Parkinson's disease and are responsive to levodopa, with early dyskinesias and motor fluctuations

4) Concentration and visuospatial impairments possible

5) Pathology: nigrostriatal degeneration similar to idiopathic Parkinson's disease (without Lewy bodies) with cytoplasmic inclusion bodies (chronic exposure) or mitochondrial inclusion bodies (acute exposure)

c. Cyanide

1) Mitochondrial toxin

2) Acute intoxication with inhalation is often fatal within minutes

3) Oral intake may cause hyperventilation, cardiopulmonary distress, agitation, gastrointestinal distress with nausea and vomiting, followed by worsening pulmonary distress, seizures, coma, possibly death

4) If patient survives the acute stage, delayed-onset parkinsonism and dystonia with prominent rigidity may develop

5) Optic atrophy, polyneuropathy, cerebellar ataxia, myelopathy with chronic low-grade exposure

6) MRI: bilateral hyperintense T2 and hypointense T1 symmetric pallidal signals

7) Histopathology: white matter and pallidal necrosis with loss of Purkinje cells may be seen at autopsy of survivors of acute or chronic exposure

d. Methanol

1) Acute intoxication

a) Manifestations usually delayed for several hours (until methanol is metabolized to formaldehyde and formic acid)

Toxic causes of parkinsonism affecting the globus pallidus include carbon monoxide, cyanide, and manganese

Methanol affects primarily the putamen

---

b) Includes gastrointestinal upset, headache, retinal toxicity, respiratory failure, metabolic acidosis, delirium, coma, death

2) Delayed-onset parkinsonism develops in survivors of acute stage or those with chronic low-grade exposure

3) Bilateral symmetric putaminal atrophy, gliosis, and MRI signal change

e. Carbon monoxide

1) Acute intoxication: headache, nausea, impaired vision, dizziness with mild exposure, seizures, coma, and possibly death when more severe

2) Survivors may develop parkinsonism

3) Chronic exposure can cause blindness, parkinsonism, pyramidal and extrapyramidal features, and a neurobehavioral syndrome of poor attention and concentration and psychiatric manifestations

4) Pathology: pallidal hemorrhagic discoloration (acute) and atrophy, gliosis, and cavitation (chronic)

3. Metabolic parkinsonism

a. Hepatic encephalopathy: parkinsonism associated with asterixis, myoclonus, chorea, encephalopathy

b. Postanoxic parkinsonism: associated with pallidal lesions (as in carbon monoxide poisoning)

c. Hypoparathyroidism: associated with basal ganglia calcifications

d. Hypothyroidism (not true parkinsonism): slowing of activity may mimic parkinsonism

e. Central pontine myelinolysis: associated with extrapontine lesions that occur with rapid correction of hyponatremia

4. Vascular parkinsonism

a. Multiple small lacunes in deep gray matter

b. Parkinsonism primarily affecting gait and presenting as loss of postural stability and falls (primarily lower body involvement); apractic gait with difficulty initiating each step

c. Pseudobulbar affect, urinary incontinence with subcortical dementia

d. Associated with vascular dementia

e. Pyramidal involvement is common: hyperreflexia and extensor plantar responses are more common than upper motor neuron distribution weakness

f. Poor response to dopaminergic agents

5. Normal-pressure hydrocephalus (see Chapter 7)

a. Gait characterized by parkinsonian and ataxic features, may result from involvement of frontostriatal periventricular pathways

b. Other cardinal parkinsonian features (bradykinesia, rigidity, tremor) may be present

6. Posttraumatic parkinsonism

a. Akinetic rigid syndrome after a single traumatic event *or*

b. Dementia pugilistica: constellation of dementia primarily affecting frontal-executive functions, psychiatric manifestations, and parkinsonism

7. Infectious and postencephalitic parkinsonism

a. Occurred in the early 1900s with the worldwide epidemic of encephalitis lethargica (von Economo's encephalitis)

1) Often fatal, but over half of survivors developed parkinsonism, dementia, and psychiatric manifestations after encephalitis

2) Onset of symptoms was immediate or delayed (up to 1-2 decades) after the insult

3) Subcortical dementia with neuropsychiatric manifestations and personality changes

4) Other features: catatonia, cataplexy, chorea, tremor, tics, dystonias including blepharospasm, torticollis (all less common than akinetic-rigid parkinsonian features)

5) Histopathology: neuronal loss and gliosis in substantia nigra, globus pallidus, locus ceruleus; neurofibrillary tangles

6) Some respond to treatment with levodopa and other dopaminergic agents

b. Acquired immunodeficiency syndrome (AIDS): currently the most common infectious cause

1) Akinetic-rigid parkinsonism with primary infection, especially with AIDS dementia complex

2) Opportunistic infections such as toxoplasmosis

c. Neurosyphilis

d. Viral: coxsackievirus, western equine, poliomyelitis, subacute sclerosing panencephalitis, varicella-zoster

e. Creutzfeldt-Jakob disease

f. Whipple's disease: supranuclear ophthalmoplegia and oculomasticatory myorhythmia

8. Guam parkinsonism-dementia complex

a. Dementia and parkinsonism with/without amyotrophic lateral sclerosis (ALS)-like illness

b. Onset in middle-age

c. High incidence of ALS-like illness in same population, sometimes associated with parkinsonism and dementia

d. Neuronal loss and gliosis associated with neurofibrillary tangles in cerebral cortex, anterior horn cells, deep gray matter, substantia nigra, brainstem tegmentum, hippocampus, amygdala

9. Parkinsonism associated with FTD-17

a. Associated with frontotemporal dementia

b. Linked to chromosome 17, many with mutation of tau gene

c. Tau-positive inclusions, neuronal loss, and gliosis in substantia nigra

III. HYPERKINETIC SYNDROMES

A. Tremor Disorders

1. Phenomenology of tremors

a. Tremor frequency may vary and should not be used to characterize tremor clinically

b. Rest tremor

1) Activation of contralateral limb can exacerbate tremor and increase its amplitude

2) Classic appearance of pill-rolling movement of thumb and fingers or alternating supination-pronation

3) Associated with parkinsonian syndromes, including idiopathic Parkinson's disease; may be seen with severe essential tremor when action-postural component is severe

c. Action tremor

1) Tremor occurring with voluntary muscle contraction

2) Subtypes

a) Postural: observed with sustained posture

b) Isometric: muscle contraction against a rigid object

c) Kinetic: goal-oriented or nongoal-oriented, may be task-specific

d) Intention: occurrence and exacerbation during visually guided targeted movements; if isolated and low frequency (<5 Hz), then usually cerebellar sign

2. Specific tremor disorders

a. Physiologic tremor

1) Fine, low-amplitude, high-frequency (7-12 Hz) tremor

2) May be exaggerated and clinically apparent with stress, anxiety, fear, metabolic condition (hyperthyroidism, hypocalcemia) drug-induced (stimulants [e.g., cocaine], nicotine, corticosteroids, thyroxine, alcohol withdrawal, caffeine)

Tremor Frequencies	
Tremor	Frequency, Hz
Physiologic	7-12
Essential	4-12
"Rubral" and cerebellar outflow	4.5-5 (variable)
Parkinsonian	4-5
Orthostatic	13-18

b. Essential tremor
  1) Etiology
     a) Sporadic
     b) Familial
        i) Genetic heterogeneity
        ii) Some families follow autosomal dominant pattern of inheritance
        iii) Possible genetic loci on chromosomes 2, 3, 4
  2) Mechanism
     a) Unknown
     b) Speculation: central oscillatory generator may be in Guillain-Mollaret triangle, especially inferior olive and cerebellum
  3) Clinical features
     a) Postural and kinetic tremor (4-12 Hz) involving upper extremities: starts unilaterally or bilaterally, but eventually involves both upper extremities
     b) May be asymmetric: more prominent in initially affected limb
     c) Tremor usually noticed with handwriting, holding objects, or other fine motor movements (Fig. 8-13)
     d) When severe, it may persist at rest, although dampened
     e) Tremor reduced with alcohol intake, usually remits with sleep, exacerbated with stress
     f) Tremor frequency and amplitude may dampen with age
     g) May be associated with head, voice, or tongue tremor (tremor of chin or lips more likely to be seen with Parkinson's disease)
  4) Variants
     a) Isolated chin tremor
        i) Rare
        ii) Autosomal dominant pattern of inheritance
        iii) Tremor of the mentalis muscle
        iv) More often seen in Parkinson's disease, when not isolated
     b) Isolated voice tremor: may be associated with classic essential tremor or cerebellar disease
     c) Task-specific tremor (e.g., primary writing tremor): 4 to 7-Hz tremor occurring with only certain tasks or positions associated with those tasks (e.g., writing)
  5) Treatment
     a) β-Blockers: propranolol (Inderal) studied most extensively
        i) Inderal LA (long-acting) may be started at 40 mg daily, and increased in small increments to optimal doses 240-320 mg/day, as tolerated and if needed
        ii) Tremor reduction up to 60%
        iii) Contraindicated if asthma, diabetes mellitus, marked bradycardia, second- or third-degree atrioventricular block, heart failure
     b) Primidone (Mysoline)
        i) As effective as propranolol but more adverse effects
        ii) Converted to phenylethylmalonamide and phenobarbital, the latter with longer half-life
        iii) To minimize the adverse effects, start with small doses of 50 mg/day and with subsequent titration, may be divided as 3-times-daily regimen
        iv) May be titrated up to maximum of 750 mg/day (250 mg 3 times daily)
     c) Second-line agents: carbonic anhydrase inhibitors (e.g., methazolamide), gabapentin, benzodiazepines
     d) Surgical treatment
        i) Thalamotomy
        ii) Thalamic stimulation: high success rate (tremor reduced in up to 90% and abolished in 50% of cases); bilateral procedures have lower complication rates than thalamotomy
c. Parkinsonian tremor
  1) Usual onset in one limb
  2) Usually a pure resting tremor
  3) Sometimes isolated finding with no other cardinal features

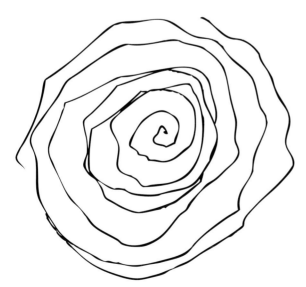

Fig. 8-13. Hand drawing of spiral figure by a patient with essential tremor. The action-kinetic tremor is easily demonstrated with this maneuver.

4) May be associated with action-postural tremor, which may or may not be of same frequency
   a) Seen as "re-emergent" tremor: tremor at first suppressed with posture but reemerges after a few seconds
   b) Rarely, parkinsonism may present with a pre-dominantly action-postural tremor
d. Primary orthostatic tremor
   1) In patients older than 40 years
   2) Symptoms
      a) Sensation of unsteadiness, fear of falling
      b) Discomfort in legs when standing
      c) Difficulty initiating walking
      d) Symptoms attenuate by walking
      e) Symptoms disappear by sitting
   3) Usually a 13 to 18-Hz tremor involving weight-bearing muscles of legs, trunk, and possibly arms bilaterally, suggesting a possible central generator
   4) Considered a task-specific tremor by some authorities
   5) PET shows increase in cerebellar activity: possible cerebellar generator but mechanism unknown
   6) Treated with low dose of clonazepam
   7) Second-line agents: primidone, valproate, gabapentin with variable success
e. Dystonic tremor
   1) Focal irregular tremors that are kinetic and postural, do not occur with complete rest
   2) True dystonic tremor—tremor is essentially phasic dystonia and may respond to sensory tricks (e.g., phasic cervical dystonia presenting as head tremor): treat with botulinum toxin type A (Botox)
   3) Tremor associated with dystonia: usually a focal dystonia associated with kinetic and postural tremor in another distribution (e.g., hand tremor in patients with spasmodic torticollis)
   4) Dystonia-gene associated with tremor: isolated action tremor with an inherited dystonia
f. Holmes' tremor (formerly, rubral tremor)
   1) Mechanism thought to involve nigrostriatal pathway (dopaminergic denervation), midbrain tegmentum, and cerebellar output (including but not limited to cerebellorubral pathways)
   2) Usually occurs with interruption of these pathways by a focal lesion (e.g., hemorrhage, infarction), may also be seen in Wilson's disease
   3) Irregular, proximal > distal, usually low-frequency (<5 Hz) tremor present at rest and with action and posture
   4) May be more noticeable with action and posture
   5) Medical treatment usually not efficacious; may be treated with stereotactic thalamotomy or thalamic stimulation

g. Palatal tremor (formerly, palatal myoclonus) (Fig. 8-14)
   1) Most symptomatic cases due to pontine hemorrhage or infarct
   2) Generated within Guillain-Mollaret triangle, specifically, pathway between dentate nucleus, red nucleus, and inferior olivary nucleus
   3) Olivocerebellar projection is *spared* and may be *necessary* for development of palatal tremor
   4) Histopathology: hypertophic degeneration of inferior olivary nucleus (cytoplasmic vacuolation and astrocytic proliferation, with argyrophilic fibers made of fibrous astrocytes and neurites)
   5) Symptomatic cases: palatal movements caused by *levator* veli palatini muscle, associated with ocular oscillopsia (which may be symmetric or nonconjugate)
   6) Essential (1/4 of cases): palatal movements by *tensor* veli palatini muscle, not associated with ocular oscillopsia
h. Hereditary geniospasm (chin tremor)
   1) Genetic heterogeneity with linkage to chromosome 9q13-21 in some families
   2) Episodes of involuntary tremor of tip of chin, tongue, and lower lip, may last seconds to hours
   3) Typical age at presentation: infancy or early childhood
   4) Movements precipitated by stress, concentration, emotion
   5) Frequency of episodes tends to decrease with age
   6) Benign prognosis
   7) No associated abnormalities
i. Fragile X premutation
   1) "Premutation" carriers with 50 to 200 repeats of CGG trinucleotide repeat expansion in 5'-untranslated region of *FMR1* gene (normal, 6-40, full mutation >200)
   2) Full mutation (fragile X syndrome) associated with phenotypic heterogeneity: mental retardation, autism, hyperactivity, learning disabilities, and physical stigmata (e.g., long face, large ears, macroorchidism) (see Chapter 7)
   3) "Premutation" recently noted to be associated with a neurodegenerative disorder characterized by the following:
      a) Intension tremor in men older than 50 years
      b) Most common complaint: gait instability
      c) Progressive neurologic syndrome characterized by cerebellar gait ataxia, executive cognitive deficits, mild parkinsonism, erectile dysfunction, peripheral

neuropathy, behavioral problems such as outbursts, anxiety
- d) Penetrance increases with age
- e) MRI: generalized atrophy and T2 hyperintensities of middle cerebellar peduncles in most reported cases
- f) Histopathology: neuronal and astrocytic intranuclear inclusions throughout cerebrum and cerebellum, most numerous in hippocampus, also involve ependymal and subependymal cells, epithelial lining cells of choroid plexus; Purkinje cell loss and dystrophic cerebellar white matter changes
- j. Titubation
  1) Low-frequency oscillation, primarily involving the axial musculature and appearance of a tremor involving entire body
  2) Usually a cerebellar tremor, associated with cerebellar disorders

B. Chorea
1. Definitions
   a. Unsustained, nonstereotypic movements with variable speed and direction, may be rapid or brief, may flow from one extremity to the next
   b. Tardive chorea may be more stereotypic
   c. Choreoathetosis: chorea occurring concurrently with athetosis or dystonic movements
   d. Ballismus (ballism): large-amplitude random movements, most prominent at the proximal limbs
   e. Hemichorea or hemiballismus: refers to hemibody distribution of the movement disorder
2. Clinical features
   a. Mild chorea may appear as restlessness or uneasy movements
   b. Parakinesia: chorea that may seem semipurposeful and may "blend into" purposeful movements
   c. Inability to maintain tone: maintaining handgrip ("milkmaid's grip") or maintaining protrusion of tongue ("flycatcher's tongue")
   d. Hyperkinetic gait and posture: characterized by intrusions of random, nonstereotypic limb and trunk movements and lurching
   e. Dysarthria
      1) Characterized by poor coordination of phonation,

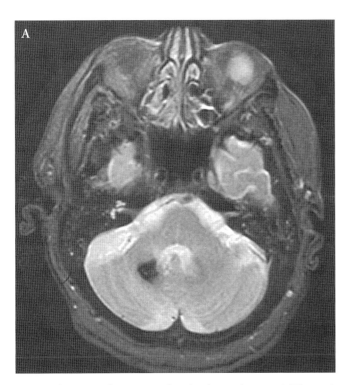 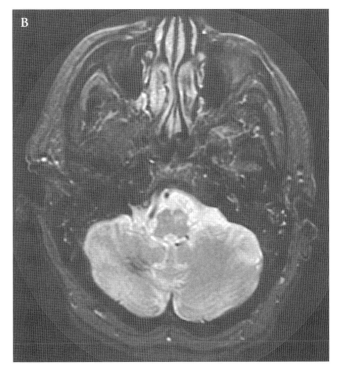

Fig. 8-14. MRI of patient with palatal myoclonus. *A*, The patient sustained a hemorrhage in the right dentate nucleus (area of low T2 signal, hemosiderin deposition of old hemorrhage). *B*, The lesion affected predominantly dentatorubroolivary outflow, leading to hypertrophic olivary degeneration (abnormal signal in ventral left medulla), with sparing of olivocerebellar projections. (Axial T2-weighted images.)

resonance, articulation, and respiration, producing irregular variation in the articulatory tone and rate

2) Choreiform movements of mouth, tongue, lips as well as diaphragmatic movements may interfere with pronunciation, articulation, and rate and volume of speech output

3. Primary chorea: benign nonprogressive causes
   a. Benign familial chorea
      1) Many early reports may have referred to other disorders
      2) Nonprogressive chorea at young age of onset, expected to improve by young adulthood
      3) May be associated with mild cognitive deficits and delayed motor milestones
      4) Genetically heterogeneous (recently, autosomal dominant inheritance linked to chromosome 14 [*TITF1*] reported)
   b. Senile chorea
      1) Gradual onset of orolingual chorea in elderly
      2) Mouthing, tongue protrusion, others

4. Primary chorea: neurodegenerative causes
   a. Huntington's disease
      1) Autosomal dominant inherited movement disorder characterized by neuropsychiatric manifestations and chorea
      2) Equally common in men and women
      3) Usual age at onset: fourth to fifth decade
      4) Mean survival: 17 years
      5) Genetics
         a) Huntington's disease gene near the tip of short arm of chromosome 4 (4p16.3): unstable expansion of CAG repeat sequence on exon 1
         b) Everyone with 40 or more repeats develops disease (high penetrance)
         c) Gene product, huntingtin protein, is overexpressed and may play role in endocytosis and intracellular trafficking (it is a component of microtubules and vesicle membranes)
         d) Anticipation: intergenerational expansion of the mutation from instability of the gene
            i) Age at onset inversely proportional to the length of the repeat, but length of the repeat is not an accurate predictor of age at onset
            ii) Inherent instability of the trinucleotide repeat is exaggerated in spermatogenesis (more than oogenesis), thus greater repeat lengths and earlier age at onset in affected offspring if inherited from the affected father
         e) Progression of disease not clearly affected by length of the repeat

6) Pathogenesis and possible mechanisms of neuronal death
   a) NMDA–mediated excitotoxicity
   b) Defective mitochondrial energy metabolism (reduced oxidative phosphorylation) causing reduced ATP production and ATPase activity and intracellular influx of calcium (because normal resting membrane potential is not maintained)
   c) Defective mitochondrial energy metabolism potentiates excitotoxic injury
   d) Free radical formation
   e) Mutant huntingtin protein may be resistant to ubiquitin-dependent proteasomal protein degradation, leading to formation of cytoplasmic and intraneuronal protein aggregates, triggering apoptosis and interfering with gene transcription

7) Clinical features
   a) Presenting symptoms may be motor (67% of cases), behavioral (15%-20%), or both (25%)
   b) Motor symptoms
      i) Chorea usually begins as uneasy, fidgety movements, clumsiness, "nervous" twitching or mannerisms evolving into semi-intentional movements
      ii) With progression, chorea becomes more noticeable; combined with smooth, writhing movements (athetosis), it may consist of grimacing, head bobbing, alternating extension-pronation and nonstereotypic flexion-supination postures of fingers
      iii) With evolution, choreoathetosis may become constant; gait and posture may be interrupted by intrusions of hyperkinetic movements as irregular lurching, or "dancing," plus features of parkinsonism and ataxia
      iv) With evolution, there is a trend of decrease in hyperkinetic motor activity, while athetosis, dystonia, bradykinesia, and other parkinsonian features become more noticeable
      v) Progressive dysphagia and dysarthria (as above)
   c) Cognitive features
      i) Deficits in frontal executive functions (poor judgment, planning, and organization and poor executive functioning), poor attention and concentration, reduced verbal fluency
      ii) Memory deficits: procedural learning, recent and remote memory (as opposed to Alzheimer's disease)
   d) Psychiatric manifestations
      i) Change in personality and frontal lobe dysfunc-

tion: apathy, disinhibition, loss of interest, altered sexual behavior, increased antisocial behavior
   ii) Irritability, explosive behavior, agitation
   iii) Depression
   iv) Anxiety
   v) Psychosis (schizophrenia-like illness)
   e) Juvenile Huntington's disease (Westphal variant): early dementia, parkinsonism, dystonia, possibly myoclonus and seizures
8) Neuropathology (Fig. 8-15)
   a) Caudate and putamen mainly involved (pallidum is much less affected): neuronal loss and gliosis with macroscopic atrophy
   b) Neuronal intranuclear and intracytoplasmic inclusions (protein aggregates)
   c) Loss of small spiny nigrostriatal GABAergic projection neurons
   d) Decreased levels of GABA and glutamic acid decarboxylase in striatum and substantia nigra
9) Neuroimaging
   a) MRI: selective caudate (and possibly putaminal) atrophy
   b) PET: bilateral caudate hypometabolism may be an earlier, more sensitive marker
10) Genetic testing
   a) Most useful and cost-effective if typical clinical presentation and questionable family history
   b) Informed consent and genetic counseling recommended
11) Treatment and management
   a) Dopamine receptor blockers and dopamine-depleting agents for chorea, psychosis, and behavioral symptoms
      i) Typical antipsychotics are not well tolerated and can induce tardive dyskinesias
      ii) Atypical antipsychotics better tolerated and do not induce tardive dyskinesias
      iii) Atypical antipsychotic—clozapine: effective for psychosis but not for chorea; disadvantage is high cost and risk of agranulocytosis
      iv) Atypical antipsychotic—olanzapine: effective for both chorea and psychiatric symptoms (may increase stroke risk in elderly)
   b) Riluzole: corticostriatal glutamate release inhibitor; may potentially improve chorea
   c) Remacemide: glutamate/NMDA receptor antagonist, may marginally improve chorea (no evidence of neuroprotection)
   d) Coenzyme Q10: mitochondrial complex I enhancer, possible decline in measure of disability (not statistically significant), possible benefit on behavioral symptoms
   e) Anticonvulsants (e.g., valproate): may be helpful for chorea and psychiatric and behavioral symptoms, including aggression and irritability

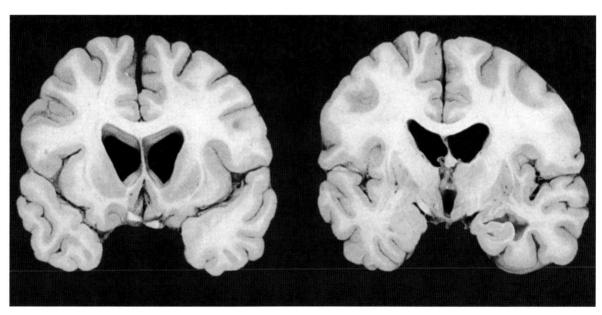

Fig. 8-15. Huntington's disease. The head of the caudate nucleus is often concave because of selective atrophy of the nucleus. (From Okazaki H, Scheithauer BW. Atlas of neuropathology. New York: Gower Medical Publishing; 1988. p. 226. By permission of Mayo Foundation.)

f) Monoamine-depleting drugs (e.g., reserpine, tetrabenazine): effective for both chorea and psychiatric manifestations (Note: tetrabenazine may be most effective for chorea but has not been approved in U.S.)

g) Lithium: for aggressive behavior, mood disorder

h) Propranolol may help treat aggression, irritability

i) SSRIs: help manage depression, chronic anxiety, aggression, obsessive-compulsive behavior

j) Physical, speech, occupational therapy

k) Prevention of medical complications

l) Surgical treatments (pallidotomies or porcine striatal transplantations) have been disappointing

b. Huntington's disease-like illnesses

1) Phenotype and clinical presentation identical to Huntington's disease, different genotype

2) Huntington's disease-like (HDL)-1: dominant inheritance (chromosome 20)

3) HDL-2: chromosome 16 (trinucleotide repeat)

4) HDL-3: autosomal recessive (chromosome 4)

5) HDL-4: autosomal dominant

c. Dentatorubro-pallidoluysian atrophy (DRPLA, Haw River syndrome)

1) Due to unstable trinucleotide repeat at chromosome 12p13.31

2) Autosomal dominant with high penetrance

3) Described in Japan and in African-American family

4) Age at onset: inversely correlated with size of CAG repeats

5) Anticipation: earlier age at onset and larger size of CAG repeat in succeeding generations

6) Paternal inheritance: larger number of repeats and younger age at onset (exaggerated anticipation with spermatogenesis)

7) Usual age at onset: third decade

8) Progressive myoclonic epilepsy, with ataxia, cognitive decline, dystonia, chorea, and possibly parkinsonism

9) Seizures less prominent after age 20 years

10) Degeneration of dentate nucleus, pallidum, red nucleus, subthalamic nucleus, with neuronal loss and intranuclear neuronal inclusions

d. Neuroacanthocytosis

1) Broad category of neurologic disease associated with acanthocytes (erythrocytes with irregular spines)

2) Associated with abnormal lipid metabolism

a) Abetalipoproteinemia (Bassen-Kornzweig syndrome): associated with progressive ataxia, pigmentary retinopathy, severe malabsorption of fat-soluble vitamins (e.g., vitamins A, E)

b) HARP (**h**ypoprebetalipoproteinemia, **a**cantho-cytosis, **r**etinitis pigmentosa, **p**allidal degeneration) syndrome

3) Associated with normal lipid metabolism

a) Amyotrophic choreoathetosis with acanthocytosis (see below)

b) McLeod's syndrome (see below)

c) MELAS (syndrome of mitochondrial myopathy, lactic acidosis, and strokes) (see Chapter 24)

d) Neurodegeneration with brain iron accumulation type I

4) Amyotrophic choreoathetosis with acanthocytosis

a) Mean age at onset: between second and third decade

b) Usual symptoms at onset: chorea, orofacial dyskinesias

c) May develop other hyperkinetic involuntary movements such as tics, dystonia, parkinsonism

d) Cognitive impairment

e) Psychiatric manifestations, personality change

f) Muscular weakness and wasting predominantly in lower extremities

g) Seizures

h) Histopathology: neuronal loss and gliosis in striatum (caudate > putamen)

i) Investigations and laboratory data

i) Acanthocytosis on peripheral blood smear

ii) Normal lipid profile

iii) Increased creatine kinase levels

iv) EMG evidence of diffuse neurogenic process with denervation potentials mimicking ALS

v) MRI: caudate and putaminal atrophy, some with cortical atrophy and ventricular enlargement

vi) PET: marked caudate and putaminal hypo-metabolism

j) Management

i) Physical therapy, speech therapy, occupational therapy as needed

ii) Antiepileptics for seizures

iii) Usually poor response of parkinsonism to levodopa or dopamine agonists

iv) Treatment of chorea

5) McLeod's syndrome

a) X-linked recessive: caused by a mutation in gene for Kell group of erythrocyte antigens

b) Change in erythrocyte cytoskeletal structure possibly responsible for formation of acanthocytes

c) Age at onset: later than other types of neuro-acanthocytosis

d) Associated with axonal neuropathy, myopathy, chorea, seizures, cognitive impairment

e) Oral dyskinesias and lip and tongue biting less common than with other types of neuro-acanthocytosis

f) Systemic manifestations more common in McLeod's syndrome than in other types of neuro-acanthocytosis: hemolytic anemia, cardiomyopathy, splenomegaly

g) MRI: caudate and cortical atrophy, striatal T2 hyperintensity

6) Hereditary choreoacanthocytosis

a) Autosomal recessive (genetic linkage to chromosome 9q21)

b) Age at symptom onset: usually between 25 and 45 years

c) Predominant symptom: chorea, with acanthocytosis

d) Other neurologic manifestations: dystonia, parkinsonism, progressive supranuclear palsy, apraxia of eye opening

e) Psychiatric manifestations: dementia, pychosis, personality change

f) Axonal neuropathy, similar to that in McLeod's syndrome

g) Atrophy of putamen and caudate

5. Secondary chorea

a. Immune-mediated: Sydenham's chorea

1) Epidemiology

a) Autoimmune-mediated

b) Female predominance (F:M ratio 2:1)

c) Age at onset: 3 to 17 years (mean 9-10 years)

d) Associated with group A β-hemolytic streptococcal infection: chorea usually occurs about 4 to 8 weeks after streptococcal pharyngitis, not skin infection

2) Clinical features

a) Usual symptom at onset: insidious development of chorea

b) Chorea rapidly spreads, becoming generalized (20% hemichorea)

c) Duration of chorea: 1 week to 2 years (mean 8-9 months)

d) Chorea may recur (20%-30% of cases)

e) Chorea may be replaced by weakness

f) Other motor manifestations: motor and vocal tics, hypometric saccades, and, rarely, oculogyric crisis

g) Behavioral changes: irritability, restlessness, obsessive-compulsive symptoms, emotional lability, depression, anxiety, personality changes, attention-deficit/hyperactivity disorder

3) Diagnosis

a) Laboratory evidence of recent streptococcal infec-tion: increased erythrocyte sedimentation rate, ASO titers, throat cultures, and 46% of patients have anti-neuronal antibodies reacting to sub-thalamic nucleus and caudate antigens

b) MRI evidence of basal ganglia T2 hyperintense lesions

c) Correlation of persistent MRI lesions with persist-ent chorea

d) Striatal hypermetabolism on PET and single photon emission computed tomography (SPECT) imaging

4) Treatment

a) Valproate (first choice), dopamine receptor block-ers (e.g., pimozide), carbamazepine, gabapentin

b) Possible role of immunosuppression (e.g., cortico-steroids) or immunomodulatory agents (e.g., intra-venous immunoglobulin, plasmapheresis) for disabling chorea refractory to conventional antichorea agents

5) Outcome

a) May develop chorea later during pregnancy or with oral contraceptives or other drugs

b) Self-limiting condition, often remits after 8 to 9 months (up to half of patients may have "persistent chorea")

b. Immune-mediated: systemic lupus erythematosus

1) 1% to 4% of systemic lupus erythematosus patients develop chorea

2) May be generalized chorea or hemichorea

3) Usual age at onset: second to third decade, with female predominance

4) Chorea may respond to dopamine receptor blockers or corticosteroids

5) If associated with antiphospholipid antibody syn-drome, chorea may respond to aspirin or warfarin

c. Other immune-mediated chorea

1) Paraneoplastic

a) Anti-Hu and CRMP antibodies

b) Small cell carcinoma of the lung, non-Hodgkin's lymphoma, CNS lymphoma, renal cell carcinoma, thymoma

c) MRI: abnormal T2 signal in basal ganglia

2) CNS vasculitis: primary CNS angiitis or systemic vasculitis with CNS involvement (e.g., Behçet's syn-drome, polyarteritis nodosa, Henoch-Schönlein purpura)

3) Associated with anticardiolipin antibodies

d. Infectious chorea

1) Acute manifestation of bacterial meningitis, aseptic meningitis

2) Tuberculous meningitis with basal ganglia infarcts

3) Toxoplasmosis (usually with AIDS)
e. Systemic metabolic (examples below)
   1) Hyperthyroidism and thyrotoxicosis
   2) Nonketotic hyperglycemia
   3) Toxins: toluene, manganese, carbon monoxide
f. Drug-induced
   1) Most common: levodopa-induced
   2) Others: anticonvulsants (lamotrigine), estrogens, lithium, dopaminergic agonists, methadone
   3) Oral contraceptive-induced chorea may be seen in patients with history of Sydenham's chorea
   4) Tardive dyskinesia: after prolonged use of dopamine receptor blocking agents
   5) Cocaine and amphetamines
g. Vascular
   1) Strokes (ischemic and hemorrhagic), intracerebral hemorrhage, vascular malformations reportedly involving the subthalamic nucleus, thalamus, and striatum: unusual complication of acute vascular lesions (less than 1% with acute stroke)
   2) Spontaneous improvement over time; few are persistent
   3) Other uncommon vascular causes: moyamoya disease and "post-pump chorea" (latter is complication of extracorporeal circulation)
   4) Treatment: dopamine receptor blocking agents or depleters, anticonvulsants
   5) Stereotactic surgery: considered for persistent cases
h. Female hormone-mediated
   1) Generalized or unilateral
   2) Associated with pregnancy or hormones
   3) Previous history of Sydenham's chorea or cyanotic heart disease as a predisposition
   4) Chorea associated with pregnancy (chorea gravidarum)
      a) Occurs in the first half of first pregnancy
      b) Often hemilateral distribution
      c) Usually persists until after delivery
      d) May recur in later pregnancies
      e) Resolves spontaneously
i. Ballism
   1) Large-amplitude ballistic proximal limb movements with wild flailing appearance; classically, a hemilateral distribution
   2) Classically associated with subthalamic lesions (e.g., ischemic or hemorrhagic lesions): contralateral to the lesion, often with hypotonia of involved limb
   3) Lesions outside the subthalamic nucleus (e.g., striatum) may also produce ballism
   4) Differential diagnosis: similar to chorea, with emphasis on vascular and neoplastic or structural causes

C. Dystonias
1. Definition: syndrome of sustained muscle contractions producing abnormal postures or repetitive movements involving different distributions
  a. Slow or rapid
  b. Usually more stereotyped than chorea
  c. Action dystonia is more prominent during voluntary movement, may be task-specific
  d. Dystonia is often exacerbated by stress, anxiety, fatigue; alleviated with rest or sensory tricks (*geste antagoniste*)
  e. Primary dystonias usually start with a focal distribution
    1) Young-onset dystonias (age ≤26): onset of symptoms in lower extremity and evolving into generalized dystonia
    2) Adult-onset dystonias (age >26): onset of symptoms in upper extremity and rarely evolving into a more generalized dystonia
  f. Classification according to distribution:
    1) Focal: one body region
    2) Multifocal: at least two noncontiguous body regions
    3) Hemidystonia: at least two ipsilateral body regions
    4) Segmental: adjacent body regions
    5) Generalized: involvement of both lower extremities *or* one lower extremity and trunk *and* another body region
  g. Classification according to etiology: primary vs. secondary
2. Primary dystonias (childhood onset in 10%-15% of cases, adult onset in 85%-90%)
  a. Primary generalized dystonias
    1) Onset: usually in childhood or young adulthood as focal dystonia with later generalization
    2) May begin as focal lower extremity action dystonia that may be noticeable during walking and less apparent with rest, sitting, walking backward, running
    3) Later, dystonia may become apparent at rest and generalize to contiguous body regions, interfering with gait
    4) With more constant dystonic postures at rest, patient becomes confined to bed or wheelchair
    5) Absence of involvement of other neurologic systems, including cognition
    6) Inherited dystonias (Table 8-5)
      a) Autosomal dominant early-onset dystonia (*DYT1* gene)
        i) GAG deletion in gene causes abnormality in ATP-binding protein, torsin A (function not fully understood)
        ii) Most common form of inherited dystonias (90% of primary generalized dystonia in Jewish

Ashkenazi families and 50% in the non-Jewish population)

b) Myoclonus-dystonia (*DYT11*)

  i) Autosomal dominant: chromosome 7q21 (gene product, ε-sarcoglycan); another locus may be on chromosome 18

  ii) Age at onset: usually in first decade

  iii) Alcohol-responsive myoclonus and variable dystonia (both involving axial and limb muscles)

  iv) May have tremor

  v) Head, arms, upper body primarily affected

  vi) Hyperkinetic movements sensitive and responsive to alcohol

  vii) Psychiatric features: mood disorder, obsessive-compulsive disorder, substance abuse

viii) Generally poor response to medication, but valproate and trihexyphenidyl may be effective

c) Dopa-responsive dystonia (DRD, *DYT5*)

  i) Autosomal dominant with incomplete penetrance: chromosome 14

  ii) Females preferentially affected

  iii) Mutation of gene coding for guanosine triphosphate cyclohydrolase-1, which is rate-limiting step for synthesis of tetrahydrobiopterin (cofactor for tyrosine hydrolase, rate-limiting step in synthesis of dopamine), thus decreasing dopamine synthesis

  iv) Multiple point mutations of the gene have been identified

  v) Usually childhood onset (first decade), but may

Table 8-5. Classification of Primary Inherited Dystonias

Syndrome (gene)	Inheritance	Comments
Early-onset dystonia (*DYT1*)	AD (chr 9q24: GAG deletion of gene for torsin A [ATP-binding protein])	Childhood onset
Autosomal recessive dystonia in Gypsies (*DYT2*)	AR (not mapped)	Childhood onset; Spanish Gypsies
Dystonia-parkinsonism/"Lubag" syndrome (*DYT3*)	X-linked recessive	Filipino men; segmental or generalized dystonia, parkinsonism, myoclonus, chorea
Whispering dysphonia (*DYT4*)	AD	Described in Australian families
Dopa-responsive dystonia (*DYT5*)	AD (chr 14q22: GTP cyclohydrolase I gene)	Dystonia with or without parkinsonism; Diurnal variation
Segawa syndrome (*DYT5*)	AR (chr 11p15.5: tyrosine hydrolase gene)	Marked response to levodopa
Adolescent-onset dystonia (*DYT6*)	AD (chr 8p)	Mennonite families; Adolescent or adult onset; Cranial or cervical segmental
Adult-onset focal dystonia (*DYT7*)	AD (chr 18p)	Adult-onset focal dystonia: cervical, cranial; German families
Paroxysmal nonkinesigenic dyskinesia (*DYT8*)	AD (chr 2q)	Paroxysmal choreoathetosis
Paroxysmal choreoathetosis with ataxia and spasticity (*DYT9*)	AD (chr 1p)	Paroxysmal, episodic choreoathetosis associated with ataxia & spasticity; Childhood onset
Paroxysmal kinesigenic dyskinesia (*DYT10*)	AD (chr 16p)	Childhood onset; Episodic choreoathetosis induced by startle
Myoclonus-dystonia (*DYT11*)	AD (chr 7: gene for ε-sarcoglycan)	Childhood onset; Alcohol-sensitive myoclonic jerks & dystonia
Rapid-onset dystonia-parkinsonism (*DYT12*)	AD (chr 19q)	Subacute onset of parkinsonism & dystonia
Multifocal and segmental dystonia (*DYT13*)	AD (chr 1p)	Primarily described in Italian families; Childhood or adult onset; Cranial, cervical, upper limb dystonia

AD, autosomal dominant; AR, autosomal recessive; chr, chromosome.

occur at any age

    vi) Usually starts as foot focal-action dystonia, later evolves to focal or generalized dystonia

    vii) Parkinsonian symptoms over time: may be only manifestation in rare adult-onset cases

    viii) Diurnal fluctuations: may be normal in early morning, with increasing severity of symptoms by end of day

    ix) Marked response to levodopa

    x) Both dystonia and parkinsonian symptoms respond to levodopa, motor fluctuations and dyskinesias do not develop

d) Paroxysmal kinesigenic dyskinesia (*DYT10*)

    i) Autosomal dominant: chromosome 16p

    ii) Mean age at onset: 12 years, male predominance

    iii) Episodic paroxysmal unilateral or bilateral choreoathetosis and dystonia, lasts from few seconds to 5 minutes

    iv) Attacks may be precipitated by sudden movements, startle, or hyperventilation

    v) Treatment: phenytoin, phenobarbital, carbamazepine, valproate

e) Paroxysmal nonkinesigenic dyskinesia (*DYT8*)

    i) Autosomal dominant: chromosome 2q

    ii) Episodic paroxysmal, unilateral or bilateral choreoathetosis, dystonia, ballism of longer duration (less frequency) than paroxysmal kinesigenic dyskinesia (minutes to several hours)

    iii) Attacks may be precipitated by alcohol, caffeine, fatigue, psychologic stressors

    iv) Treatment: anticonvulsants (less responsive than paroxysmal kinesigenic dyskinesia), benzodiazepines, dopamine receptor antagonists

    v) Inherited type must be differentiated from secondary causes such as multiple sclerosis or psychogenic

f) Paroxysmal exertional dyskinesia

    i) Autosomal dominant

Autosomal Dominant Paroxysmal Dyskinesias

Paroxysmal kinesigenic dyskinesia: episodes of unilateral or bilateral choreoathetosis and dystonia lasting few seconds to 5 minutes; precipitated by sudden movements, startle, or hyperventilation

Paroxysmal nonkinesigenic dyskinesia: episodes of unilateral or bilateral choreoathetosis, dystonia, and ballism lasting several minutes to hours; precipitated by alcohol, caffeine, fatigue, psychologic stressors

---

    ii) Paroxysmal episodes lasting 5 to 30 minutes, induced by exercise

    iii) Unilateral or bilateral dystonia or choreoathetosis primarily affecting legs

    iv) Treatment: acetazolamide, antimuscarinic agents, benzodiazepines

g) X-linked dystonia-parkinsonism (*DYT3*, Lubag syndrome)

    i) Heterogeneous disorder of parkinsonism, dystonia, tremor, chorea, myoclonus affecting Filipino adult men

    ii) Onset: usually fourth to fifth decade

    iii) Duration: usually 10 to 12 years

    iv) Poor response to medical treatment, but some may respond to levodopa

    v) Pathology: caudate and putaminal atrophy

h) Rapid-onset dystonia-parkinsonism (*DYT12*)

    i) Sporadic or inherited (gene locus on chromosome 19q13)

    ii) Subacute onset of upper body dystonia and parkinsonism in childhood or adulthood: primarily bulbar dystonia

    iii) Poor response to levodopa or dopaminergic agents

i) Niemann-Pick disease type C

    i) Inherited disorder of cholesterol metabolism resulting in lysosomal accumulation of low-density-lipoprotein–derived cholesterol

    ii) *NPC1* gene on chromosome 18q11

    iii) Syndrome of progressive CNS degeneration marked by dementia, cataplexy, dysarthria, dystonia, dysphagia, vertical supranuclear gaze palsy, seizures

    iv) Patients usually present at preschool age with gait ataxia and "clumsiness" and/or hepatosplenomegaly

b. Primary focal dystonias

    1) Usually sporadic, may be genetically determined

    2) More common in women, except for writer's cramp

    3) Cervical dystonia: spasmodic torticollis

        a) Most common form of primary focal dystonia

        b) Onset: between ages 30 and 50

        c) Usually rotational torticollis or laterocollis (retrocollis less common, anterocollis almost never seen)

        d) Symptoms often absent in early morning, exacerbated throughout day

        e) Sensory tricks usually effective in the early stages of disease

        f) Spontaneous remission in 20% of patients, high recurrence rate

    4) Cranial dystonias

a) Blepharospasm
  i) Bilateral repetitive contractions of orbicularis oculi: may be as brief as repetitive blinking or prolonged and forceful closure of the eyelids
  ii) May be associated with dystonic movement of face, jaw, tongue, and oral and pharyngeal muscles
  iii) Essential blepharospasm: isolated focal dystonia involving the lids
  iv) Meige's syndrome (craniocervical dystonia): dystonic involvement of cervical and cranial musculature, more extensive than the lids
  v) May be induced or aggravated by exposure to bright lights, wind, watching television, reading, stress
  vi) May be alleviated with sensory tricks (e.g., touching upper lids or voluntary facial movements, pinching the neck, talking, singing)
b) Oromandibular dystonia
  i) Primarily involves jaw muscles bilaterally or unilaterally (e.g., trismus, jaw deviation, bruxism, involuntary jaw opening)
  ii) May include tongue protrusion, platysma contraction, pursing lip movements
c) Spasmodic dysphonia
  i) Often begins as task-specific dystonia affecting talking or singing
  ii) Some with voice tremor (may be presenting symptom)
  iii) Adductor variety: 90% of cases, excessive contraction of thyroarytenoid causes strained voice
  iv) Abductor variety: separation of vocal cords by excessive contraction of posterior cricoarytenoid muscles causes breathy voice
5) Limb dystonia
  a) Least common form of focal dystonia
  b) May be part of a segmental dystonia
  c) Upper extremity focal dystonia is usually action dystonia and task-specific (e.g., writer's cramp)
    i) Patients with writer's cramp are able to write larger on a blackboard using proximal muscles but writing is slow and effortful
6) Trunk dystonia
  a) Repetitive and stereotyped movements of exaggerated lordosis, kyphosis, scoliosis, or opisthotonic posturing
  b) Improvement with sensory tricks, running, or walking backward
c. Treatment
  1) Botulinum toxin (BTX)
    a) Most potent known neurotoxin
    b) First-line treatment for adult-onset focal dystonias (BTX type A)
    c) Weakens targeted muscle by inhibiting neuromuscular transmission: specifically, it is incorporated into motor nerve endings and prevents release of acetylcholine from presynaptic membrane into neuromuscular junction
    d) Mechanism of action: BTX type A cleaves SNAP-25 (synaptosome-associated protein), and BTX type C cleaves syntaxin
      i) Both SNAP-25 and syntaxin are cytoplasmic presynaptic membrane-associated proteins
    e) BTX types B and F cleave synaptobrevin (or vesicle-associated membrane protein [VAMP])
    f) All these compounds inhibit acetylcholine release from presynaptic membrane
    g) May be effective in up to 95% of cases
    h) Resistance may develop in 5% to 20% of patients, BTX type B may be tried
  2) Medical treatment
    a) Dopaminergic (Sinemet)
    b) Dopaminergic antagonists
    c) Dopamine-depleting agents
    d) Anticholinergic (e.g., trihexyphenidyl, benztropine): may be effective in up to 40% of patients
    e) Baclofen: may be effective in up to 20%
    f) Clonazepam: may be effective in up to 15%
    g) Anticonvulsants (e.g., carbamazepine, gabapentin)
  3) Surgical treatment
    a) Peripheral denervation procedures: bilateral anterior cervical rhizotomy, microvascular decompression, ramisectomy, peripheral nerve lysis, myectomy
    b) Deep brain stimulation
    c) Unilateral thalamotomy
3. Secondary dystonias
  a. Usually sudden onset, rapid progression
  b. Onset may be as early as infancy
  c. Abnormal imaging features
  d. Usually caused by structural or metabolic factor
  e. Differential diagnosis: traumatic, iatrogenic (drugs), toxic, perinatal complications, basal ganglia structural lesions, encephalitis, psychogenic
  1) Posttraumatic
    a) Dystonia may emerge as posttraumatic hemiparesis resolves
    b) Latent period from trauma to dystonia development: may be from 1 day to 6 years
    c) Poor prognosis, tends to be medically refractory but may respond to BTX type A and surgical options

D. Tic Disorders

1. Tics: repetitive, rapid, brief, stereotypic jerklike movements (motor) and localizations (vocal); simple or complex
2. Waxing and waning course, asymptomatic interictally
3. Tics worsen with stress, alleviated with rest
4. Premonition and some degree of volitional suppression and voluntary control
5. Vocal tics: may interrupt normal prosody of speech
   a. Simple vocal tics (e.g., sniffing, coughing)
   b. Complex vocal tics: coprolalia (vocalizing obscenities), palilalia (repeating one's own words), echolalia (repeating another person's words)
6. Motor tics
   a. Simple motor tics: rapid (clonic-type), slower (dystonic), examples are twitches and jerks involving different parts of body
   b. Complex motor tics: coordinated sequence of motor activity such as a head shake and kicking
7. Gilles de la Tourette's syndrome (criteria of Tourette Syndrome Classification Study Group)
   a. Onset: usually before age 21
   b. Volitional suppression of tics and immense sense of distress when tics are suppressed
   c. Criteria
      1) Presence of multiple motor tics and one or more vocal tics at some time during course of the illness
      2) Tics occurring many times daily intermittently for at least 1 year, without a period of absence for 3 months or more
      3) Onset before age 21
      4) Tics changing over time
      5) No other condition to explain the tics
   d. Associated features (may precede the tics)
      1) Associated with obsessive-compulsive disorder or trait in half of patients
      2) Attention-deficit/hyperactivity disorder (50%-75% of patients): inattention, distractibility, impulsive behavior, hyperactivity, difficulty with school performance
      3) Major depression
      4) Oppositional defiant disorder
   e. Pathophysiology
      1) Exact mechanisms largely unknown
      2) Abnormal dopaminergic transmission
         a) Striatal dopamine receptor hypersensitivity possibly responsible for negative feedback and reduced release of dopamine by acting on presynaptic dopaminergic receptors
         b) Therapeutic response to dopamine receptor antagonists (blocking presynaptic dopaminergic receptors) and worsening of symptoms with dopaminergic agonists
         c) Decreased level of cerebrospinal fluid (CSF) dopamine metabolite, homovanillic acid
      3) Cholinergic, GABAergic, noradrenergic systems may also be involved
      4) Functional MRI: reduced basal ganglia and thalamic activation with tic suppression, while increased activity in right caudate, right frontal cortex, and other cortices involved in inhibition (prefrontal, parietal, temporal, and cingulate cortices)
      5) Widespread cortical activation with tics
      6) Immunologic mechanisms: post-streptococcal autoimmunity
         a) Post-streptococcal autoimmunity suggested by exacerbation of Tourette's syndrome symptoms by group A β-hemolytic streptococcus infection
         b) Pediatric autoimmune neuropsychiatric disorders associated with streptococcal infections (PANDAS), also called pediatric infection-triggered autoimmune neuropsychiatric disorders (PITANDS)
      7) Genetic heterogeneity: likely polygenic influence
8. Treatment
   a. Tic suppression
      1) Alpha agonists
         a) Clonidine
            i) May need several weeks to take effect
            ii) Side effects: sedation, insomnia, irritability, dry mouth
            iii) Acute withdrawal may cause hypertension, tachycardia, increased agitation
         b) Guanfacine
            i) Single daily dose, less sedating than clonidine
            ii) Initiated at 0.5 mg daily, may be titrated to 4-mg daily dose
      2) Neuroleptics
         a) Typical neuroleptics: haloperidol (0.5-20–mg daily dose), pimozide (0.5-10–mg daily dose)
            i) Higher binding to D_2 receptors, higher incidence of parkinsonism and tardive dyskinesias

---

Major obsessions and compulsions are observed in half of the patients with Tourette's syndrome

The presence of both motor and vocal tics are required for diagnosis of Tourette's syndrome

ii) Prolonged QT interval with pimozide
   b) Atypical neuroleptics: decrease vocal and motor tics (seen in controlled trials)
      i) Risperidone (Risperdal): starting dose 0.5 mg at night, gradual titration to maximal daily dose 16 mg (single or twice daily divided dose)
      ii) Olanzapine (Zyprexa): may start at 2.5-mg daily dose (maximal daily dose 15 mg), may increase stroke risk in elderly
  3) Monoamine depletors
   a) Tetrabenazine: depletes presynaptic dopaminergic storage, not available in the U.S.
   b) Reserpine: initial nighttime dose of 0.25 mg (maximal daily dose 1-3 mg)
   c) Not associated with tardive dyskinesias
   d) Associated with nausea, parkinsonism, akathisia, depression, anxiety
  4) Other:
   a) Clonazepam
   b) Baclofen
   c) BTX for motor tics affecting stereotypic muscle groups
 b. Treatment of associated conditions
  1) Obsessive-compulsive behavior: SSRIs
  2) Attention-deficit/hyperactivity disorder: stimulants (methylphenidate, dextroamphetamine, atomoxetine, pemoline)

E. Myoclonus

1. Definition: sudden, brief involuntary movements caused by contraction (positive) or inhibition of contraction (negative) of certain muscle groups
  a. Negative (asterixis): toxic-metabolic vs. structural, poor response to treatment
  b. Positive: cortical (often stimulus-sensitive), brainstem, spinal/segmental
2. May be classified by localization (Table 8-6)
  a. Cortical myoclonus: cortical reflex myoclonus is usually focal myoclonus activated by active or passive movements
  b. Subcortical myoclonus: often generalized
  c. Spinal myoclonus: confined to a specific dermatome or spreads along propriospinal pathways and involves multiple segments, may be rhythmic
  d. Peripheral myoclonus: remains in the distribution of irritated peripheral nerves or roots
3. Treatment
  a. Clonazepam: hyperekplexia, postanoxic myoclonus, essential myoclonus, palatal myoclonus, spinal myoclonus
  b. Valproate: cortical, posthypoxic, epileptic, hiccups
  c. Levetiracetam

  d. Piracetam
  e. Acetazolamide (second-line for cortical or epileptic myoclonus)
  f. Zonisamide
  g. Primidone
4. Nonepileptic
  a. Physiologic myoclonus
   1) Hypnic jerks and nocturnal myoclonus: stereotyped, repetitive dorsiflexion and occasionally hip and knee flexion; associated with restless legs syndrome
   2) Hiccups
   3) Benign infantile myoclonus
   4) Anxiety- or exercise-induced
  b. Myoclonus in neurodegenerative disease
   1) Inherited metabolic encephalopathies (progressive myoclonic epilepsies): focal or multifocal action- and stimulus-sensitive reflex myoclonus
   2) Cerebellar degenerative conditions: spinocerebellar degeneration, celiac disease
   3) Alzheimer's disease
    a) Usually observed during late stages, but may be seen as prominent and early feature in inherited forms of Alzheimer's disease
    b) Both cortical and subcortical origin, may be stimulus-sensitive
   4) Creutzfeldt-Jakob disease

Table 8-6. Classification of Myoclonus Based on Localization

Cortical (focal, multifocal, or generalized)	Subcortical	Spinal	Peripheral
Cortical reflex myoclonus	Reticular reflex myoclonus	Segmental or "propriospinal" (rhythmic jerks affecting 1 segment of cord)	May originate from peripheral nerve, plexus, or nerve roots
Spontaneous cortical myoclonus	Hyperekplexia (exaggerated startle)		
Epilepsia partialis continua	Drug-induced myoclonus	Causes: tumor, trauma, ischemia, viral infections	
	Essential myoclonus		
	Dystonic myoclonus		
	Periodic myoclonus		
	Palatal myoclonus		

a) Characteristic generalized stimulus-sensitive cortical myoclonus
b) Associated with periodic bilateral synchronized discharges

5) Parkinsonism (usually cortical myoclonus)
  a) Parkinson's disease
    i) Myoclonus rare, most often reported in relation to levodopa intake (when it occurs)
    ii) Peak-dose, action-induced multifocal myoclonus possible but uncommon
  b) Postencephalitic parkinsonism
  c) Encephalitis lethargica (1917-1928 epidemic)
    i) Hyperkinetic/myoclonic form: encephalitis algo-myoclonica
    ii) Focal and generalized myoclonus: abdominal myoclonus producing distinct umbilical movements
  d) Drug-induced parkinsonism
  e) MSA
    i) Myoclonus may be described as "irregular jerky tremor"; electrophysiologic evidence of action and postural myoclonus ("minipolymyoclonus")
    ii) Usually stimulus-sensitive focal reflex myoclonus, cortical or brainstem origin
    iii) Photic reflex myoclonus: markedly responsive to levodopa
  f) Corticobasal degeneration
    i) Usually focal and predominantly distal cortical myoclonus
  g) Diffuse Lewy body disease
    i) Small-amplitude distal limb "minipolymyoclonus"
    ii) Cortical origin
    iii) May be stimulus-sensitive and exaggerated with systemic insults

6) Other neurodegenerative disorders: neurodegeneration with iron accumulation type I, Wilson's disease

c. Essential myoclonus
1) General features
  a) Only abnormality is myoclonus; no dementia, ataxia, seizures, or EEG abnormalities
  b) Normal somatosensory evoked potentials
  c) Generalized, multifocal, unilateral, or segmental
  d) Reflex myoclonus not described
2) Sporadic essential myoclonus
  a) Variable age at onset (2-64 years)
  b) Generally does not have marked progression or disability
3) Hereditary essential myoclonus
  a) Autosomal dominant with phenotypic heterogeneity
  b) Male = female
  c) Onset: first or second decade
  d) Benign course, normal life span
  e) Higher incidence of essential tremor (myoclonus may be sensitive to alcohol in these patients)
  f) Myoclonus is usually prominent in upper body
  g) Myoclonus may be induced with action and dampened with alcohol (rebound effect with withdrawal of alcohol)
  h) Myoclonus may respond to clonazepam and 5-hydroxytryptophan
4) Inherited myoclonus-dystonia
  a) Autosomal dominant inheritance (gene locus on chromosome 7q21) with incomplete penetrance: mutations of ε-sarcoglycan gene at this locus
  b) Age at onset of myoclonus: usually before 20 (range 6 months-38 years)
  c) Benign course; no ataxia, seizures, or dementia
  d) Normal life span
  e) Myoclonus usually distributed in upper body, involving neck and arms, followed by trunk and bulbar muscles
  f) Dystonia may be seen, usually in same distribution as the myoclonus; is rarely the sole feature
  g) Myoclonus usually at rest; exaggerated with stress, startle, caffeine, action; sometimes dramatically alleviated by alcohol (response to alcohol is not consistent within and between families)
  h) Some families have psychiatric manifestations (obsessive-compulsive disorder, major affective disorder)
  i) Treatment
    i) Marked improvement reported with γ-hydroxybutyric acid
    ii) Moderate improvement reported with clonazepam and valproate
    iii) Stereotactic thalamotomy or deep brain stimulation for refractory cases

d. Posthypoxic (Lance-Adams syndrome)
1) Generalized cortical myoclonus, usually occurs with recovery from an anoxic insult (e.g., cardiorespiratory arrest, drug overdose)
2) Usually preceded by a period of coma
3) Associated with protracted seizures, usually before myoclonus, attributed to major neocortical injury
4) Synchronized olivary discharge: possible "pacemaker"
5) May respond to oral administration of serotonin (CSF serotonin metabolites are decreased)

e. Posttraumatic
f. Drug-induced

1) Psychotropic medications: tricyclic antidepressants, SSRIs, monoamine oxidase inhibitors, lithium, buspirone, clozapine
2) Antimicrobial agents: penicillin, cephalosporins, quinolones, imipenem, isoniazid, acyclovir, vidarabine: nonrhythmic, asymmetric myoclonus
3) Antihistamines: multifocal, asymmetric, stimulus-sensitive myoclonus
4) Narcotics: morphine, hydromorphine, meperidine, fentanyl: intoxication or withdrawal
5) Anticonvulsants: phenytoin, carbamazepine, valproate, vigabatrin
6) Anesthetics: isoflurane, midazolam
7) Contrast media: ascending myoclonic spasms, segmental myoclonus
8) Calcium channel blockers: irregular, symmetric, dystonic myoclonus
9) Levodopa
10) Physostigmine
11) Metoclopramide
g. Toxin-induced: aluminum, bismuth, mercury, tetanus toxin, strychnine, toluene (gases, metals, organic solvents, pesticides)
h. Metabolic-induced (e.g., uremia, hepatic encephalopathy, hypercarbia, hypoglycemia)
   1) Often multifocal, arrhythmic myoclonic jerks affecting face and axial and proximal extremity muscle groups
   2) Patients may develop a negative myoclonus that may affect any part of the body (asterixis), with involvement of the hands (essentially flapping motion of the hand as a result of the negative myoclonus)
   3) Negative myoclonus may also be seen with post-hypoxic encephalopathy or structural lesion (especially if unilateral)
   4) Most common localization for unilateral asterixis: thalamus (often from thalamic hemorrhage)
i. Viral infections
5. Epileptic myoclonus
   a. Features
      1) Usually cortical origin
      2) Myoclonus associated with generalized seizures, including myoclonic seizures
      3) Myoclonus may accompany generalized seizures
      4) Seizures are the predominant feature, encephalopathy may or may not follow
   b. Associated epileptic syndromes: Lennox-Gastaut, infantile spasm, juvenile myoclonic epilepsy
   c. Other examples: photosensitive myoclonus, isolated epileptic myoclonic jerks, epilepsia partialis continua

d. Progressive myoclonic epilepsies
   1) Neuronal ceroid-lipofuscinosis
      a) Core features
         i) Autosomal recessive inheritance, except for adult form
         ii) Developmental regression
         iii) Hypotonia
         iv) Extrapyramidal symptoms
         v) Seizures
         vi) Myoclonus
         vii) Involvement of visual pathways, blindness
         viii) Granular osmophilic deposits: storage bodies with saposins as major storage material
      b) Infantile form: *CLN1* (Haltia-Santavuori disease)
         i) Chromosome 1p32 (gene product is palmitoyl protein thioesterase)
         ii) Normal development in early infancy
         iii) Developmental "plateau," then regression
         iv) Early and progressive blindness
         v) Ages 2 to 3: rapid neurologic deterioration marked by: hypotonia, ataxia, microcephaly, myoclonus, seizures, dystonia, choreoathetosis
         vi) Repetitive hand movements reminiscent of Rett syndrome
         vii) Nonreactive EEG by age 3
         viii) Thalamic involvement: MRI may show increased T2 signal bilaterally
         ix) Death by age 8 to 11 years
      c) Late infantile form: *CLN2*
         i) Chromosome 11p15 (tripeptidyl peptidase 1)
         ii) Age at onset: between 2 and 3 years, usually with seizures, followed by myoclonus, ataxia, cognitive decline
         iii) Visual symptoms apparent later
         iv) Generalized atrophy may be seen on neuroimaging
      d) Late infantile form: *CLN5* (Finnish)
         i) Chromosome 13q21-32
         ii) Age at onset: about 5 years, with clumsiness and hypotonia, followed by visual impairment, ataxia, myoclonus
      e) Juvenile onset: *CLN3* (Batten disease)
         i) Chromosome 16
         ii) Age at onset: between 5 and 10 years, usually with visual failure, followed by epilepsy, cognitive decline
         iii) Most patients are blind by second decade of life
         iv) Electroretinogram usually very low or unrecordable at diagnosis
         v) Myoclonus usually subtle, not a prominent feature

vi) Other features: ataxia, parkinsonism, or psychiatric manifestations

vii) Ultrastructural appearance of curvilinear and fingerprint bodies; vacuolated lymphocytes

viii) Cerebral and cerebellar atrophy

f) Northern epilepsy: *CLN8*

    i) Childhood-onset, progressive epilepsy with mental retardation

    ii) Age at onset: about 5 to 10 years, with seizures (all generalized tonic-clonic, some complex partial)

    iii) Progressive cognitive decline into adulthood

    iv) Visual involvement not a key feature, no myoclonus

    v) Neuroimaging consistent with brainstem and cerebellar atrophy

g) Adult-onset neuronal ceroid-lipofuscinosis (Kufs' disease)

    i) Onset in the fourth decade, but may occur earlier

    ii) Dementia, psychosis, pyramidal or extra-pyramidal symptoms, and seizures

    iii) No visual symptoms

2) Unverricht-Lundborg disease: autosomal recessive

    a) Chromosome 21q (crystatin B)

    b) Myoclonus or tonic-clonic seizures at onset, between ages 8 and 13 years

    c) Severe myoclonus: may be evoked by stimuli

    d) Repetitive morning myoclonus

    e) Seizures may be difficult to control

    f) Progression of ataxia and dementia is mild and later in the course

    g) Clinical course variable

    h) Electroencephalogram: background slowing, frontal beta activity, marked photosensitivity

3) DRPLA (dentatorubro-pallidoluysian atrophy): autosomal dominant (chromosome 12, atrophin)

4) Juvenile neuroaxonal dystrophy: autosomal recessive (chromosome 20p)

5) Juvenile Huntington's disease

6) Myoclonic epilepsy with ragged red fibers (MERRF)

    a) Broad spectrum, with variability within families

    b) Symptoms may begin at any age

    c) Myoclonus, ataxia, tonic-clonic seizures, dementia; less commonly, myopathy, neuropathy, deafness, optic atrophy

7) Sialidosis types I and II: autosomal recessive (chromosome 6p, lysosomal sialidase)

8) Gaucher's disease type 3: autosomal recessive (chromosome 1q, lysosomal glucocerebrosidase)

9) GM_2 gangliosidoses: autosomal recessive (chromosome 5q, β-hexosaminidase)

10) Lafora's disease: autosomal recessive (chromosome 6q, laforin)

    a) Characterized by Lafora bodies (polyglucosan inclusions in neurons and other tissues) (Fig. 8-16)

    b) Onset: in second decade

    c) Dementia, myoclonus, seizures

    d) Diagnosis may be made by examining eccrine sweat gland ducts on skin biopsy

6. Hyperekplexia and startle syndromes

a. Exaggerated motor response to unexpected auditory (and visual) stimuli

b. Startle response may be of cortical or brainstem origin

c. Hereditary or sporadic

d. Genetic heterogeneity

    1) Almost always autosomal dominant

    2) Autosomal dominant inheritance described in patients with mutations in gene encoding alpha$_1$ sub-unit of the glycine receptor on chromosome 5q

e. Clinical heterogeneity

    1) Severe form

        a) Patient may have continuous stiffness and flexed posture during awake state (possibly since infancy)

        b) Apnea and cardiorespiratory arrest possible

        c) Apneic attacks possible

        d) Episodes of repetitive myoclonic jerks

        e) Exaggerated startle may interfere with walking and cause falls: exacerbated during adolescence, may be variably alleviated in adult life

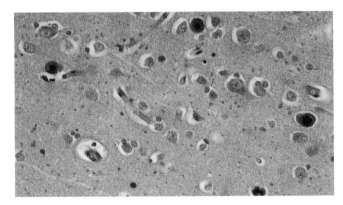

Fig. 8-16. Lafora bodies are neuronal and glial inclusions occupying most of the cytoplasm, typically with a deeply stained core and less dense periphery. (From Ellison D, Love S, Chimelli L, Harding B, Lowe J, Roberts GW, et al. Neuropathology: a reference text of CNS pathology. London: Mosby; 1998. p. 1.7. Used with permission.)

f) Exaggerated tone and stiffness tends to improve in first year of life, but exaggerated startle persists

g) Other associations: seizures, low intelligence

2) Mild form

a) Only excessive startle without other features described above

f. Symptomatic hyperekplexia from ischemic or hemorrhagic strokes, perinatal anoxia, and other similar insults to CNS

g. Treatment: clonazepam and other benzodiazepines, valproate, 5-hydroxytryptophan, piracetam

IV. DRUG-INDUCED MOVEMENT DISORDERS

A. Drug-Induced Parkinsonism

1. Symmetric or asymmetric parkinsonism clinically indistinguishable from idiopathic Parkinson's disease

2. May be seen with most neuroleptics with D_2 receptor blockade and presynaptic dopamine depletors (D_2 receptors most closely associated with parkinsonian effects)

a. Phenothiazines (e.g., chlorpromazine [Thorazine], prochlorperazine [Compazine], fluphenazine [Prolixin])

b. Thioxanthenes (e.g., thiothixene [Navane])

c. Butyrophenones (e.g., haloperidol [Haldol], droperidol)

d. Diphenylbutylpiperidine (e.g. pimozide)

e. Thienobenzodiazepine (e.g., olanzapine [Zyprexa])

f. Benzamides (e.g., metoclopramide [Reglan])

g. Presynaptic monoamine depletors (inhibit reuptake)

1) Reserpine

2) Tetrabenazine (action shorter than reserpine, also may block dopamine receptors)

3. Clozapine and quetiapine: least propensity to cause parkinsonism

4. Other drugs that may potentially cause parkinsonism: valproate, flunarizine, verapamil (a calcium channel blocker, mechanism of action is thought to be mitochondrial chain dysfunction), lithium

5. Treatment: discontinuation of causative drug

6. If parkinsonism persists, consider subclinical parkinsonism (debatable) and treat accordingly (amantadine, levodopa)

B. Acute Dystonic Reactions

1. Abrupt onset of dystonic posturing and movements primarily involving cervicocranial musculature and sometimes as oculogyric crisis

2. Typically occurs within 2 to 24 hours after first dose of offending drug (90% in first 5 days)

3. May be painful, distribution may vary during a single episode

4. Usually occur as a reaction to medications that block dopamine D_2 receptors (e.g., neuroleptics)

5. Other possible offending agents: tetrabenazine, methamphetamine, calcium channel blockers

6. Usually resolves spontaneously after drug withdrawal; may treat with benztropine mesylate (Cogentin) or diphenhydramine (Benadryl)

C. Akathisia

1. Sensation of inner restlessness and tension and urge to move

2. Usually seen as an acute (possibly very early) phenomenon, but may also be tardive

3. Result of ingestion of typical and atypical neuroleptics, dopamine depletors such as reserpine, and SSRI antidepressants

4. Treatment: decrease the dose or discontinue offending agent if possible

5. If persists, may treat with small doses of propranolol, amantadine, anticholinergics, or clonidine (acts to stimulate central α_2-receptors and reduce noradrenergic activity)

D. Tardive Dyskinesia

1. Usually occurs after 3 months to several years of treatment with a neuroleptic

2. Pathophysiology

a. Unclear but thought to involve supersensitivity of the dopamine receptors by chronic blockade of dopamine receptors

b. Possibly decreased GABA and glutamic acid decarboxylase (GAD) activity in pallidum, subthalamic nucleus, and substantia nigra

3. Possible genetic susceptibility genes: polymorphism in the $5\text{-}HT_{2A}$ receptor gene as a risk factor

4. Stereotypic, repetitive involuntary movements involving mainly oral, buccal, lingual, perioral muscles

5. Movements may be characterized as athetosis (slow, writhing) or chorea (rapid and irregular jerking)

6. If mild, movements may "blend into" normal movements or be masked by them

7. Mouth may have a stereotypic pattern of chewing, smacking, or repetitive tongue protrusion ("flycatcher tongue")

8. Stereotypic pattern differentiates this from most other choreas, as in Huntington's disease

9. Distal limbs may be affected

10. May be associated with irregular respiratory patterns and intermittent hyperventilation

11. May be transient (but more than 3 months' duration) or persistent

12. Masked by increases in neuroleptic; increased by anxiety, stress, or rapid alternating movements of hands
13. Clozapine and quetiapine: lowest incidence of tardive dyskinesias and other tardive syndromes, including tardive parkinsonism
14. Drugs known to induce tardive dyskinesia (Table 8-7): usually dopamine receptor antagonists
15. Treatment: pharmacologic treatment often indicated when movements are not abolished with elimination of the causative agent
    a. Atypical antipsychotic agents: clozapine and quetiapine
    b. Presynaptic dopamine depleters: reserpine, tetrabenazine
    c. Clonazepam
    d. Vitamin E

E. Tardive Dystonia

1. Usually involves repetitive axial twisting, retrocollis, opisthotonos with elbow extension and wrist flexion
2. May occur within 4 days to 23 years after exposure to offending agent (usually a dopamine antagonist)
3. Treatment: as for tardive dyskinesias

F. Neuroleptic Withdrawal Syndrome (see Chapter 6)

1. Usually a complication of dopamine antagonists blocking D_2 receptors
2. Hyperthermia, extrapyramidal syndrome usually consisting of rigidity and dystonia, altered mental status, autonomic features (tachycardia, diaphoresis, labile blood pressure)
3. May develop after first dose or after prolonged treatment
4. Treatment: primarily supportive, discontinuation of offending agent; consider bromocriptine, dantrolene, or levodopa

Table 8-7. Drugs Associated With Tardive Syndromes

Phenothiazines: chlorpromazine (Thorazine), prochlorperazine (Compazine), thioridazine (Mellaril), perphenazine, fluphenazine (Prolixin)
Thioxanthenes: chlorprothixene, thiothixene (Navane)
Butyrophenones: haloperidol (Haldol), droperidol
Diphenylbutylpiperidine: pimozide
Thienobenzodiazepine: olanzapine (Zyprexa)
Benzamides: metoclopramide (Reglan)
Loxapine
Risperidone
Ziprasidone
Calcium channel blockers: flunarizine, cinnarizine
Tricyclic antidepressants: amoxapine

5. Residual catatonia possible, some respond to electroconvulsive therapy

G. Withdrawal Emergent Syndrome

1. Caused by abrupt withdrawal of neuroleptics
2. Usual manifestation: nonstereotypic choreic hyperkinetic movements involving different muscle groups randomly
3. May also manifest as parkinsonism (mechanism is poorly understood)
4. Treatment: reintroduction of the neuroleptic and subsequent tapering of the agent slowly

V. MISCELLANEOUS

A. Hemifacial Spasms

1. Involuntary, episodic synchronous contraction of the muscles supplied by the ipsilateral facial nerve
2. Usually caused by compression of facial nerve by an aberrant blood vessel; less commonly, by other compressive lesions (aneurysms, tumors, arteriovenous malformations, which may compress the nerve as it exits from the brainstem)
3. Other causes may include intraparenchymal brainstem abnormalities (as in multiple sclerosis)
4. The generator usually localizes to the peripheral facial nerve (considered a peripheral, segmental myoclonus)
5. Main component is contraction of orbicularis oris muscles, eventually may spread to involve other facial muscles supplied by facial nerve
6. Contractions can range from individual muscle twitches to sustained muscle contraction caused by series of muscle twitches, producing sustained eye closure or tonic facial contraction.
7. Treatment
   a. Usually poor response to agents such as baclofen or anticonvulsants
   b. BTX injections usually effective (at least moderate improvement in up to 92% of cases)
   c. Surgery considered for refractory cases: craniectomy, microvascular decompression

B. Stiff-Man Syndrome

1. CNS disorder manifested as progressive, fluctuating signs of motor neuron hyperexcitability (including spasms)
2. Pathophysiology thought to involve cerebellar and alpha motor neuron loss of inhibitory GABAergic neurons

3. Association with anti-GAD immunoreactivity and diabetes mellitus type 1: thought to possibly be an autoimmune disorder

4. May occur as a paraneoplastic syndrome; reported to be associated with breast cancer (association with anti-amphiphysin antibodies and sometimes a syndrome of progressive encephalomyelitis), possibly thymoma, small cell lung cancer, lymphoma

5. Presentation: typically begins with axial hypertonicity and spasms with exaggerated lumbar lordosis, back pain

6. Subsequent involvement of proximal limb muscles (legs > arms), eventual impairment of gait from the rigidity

7. Deep tendon reflexes usually brisk, no weakness, no sensory loss

8. Cortical and cranial-bulbar functions usually spared

9. Occasional autonomic involvement

10. Diagnostic testing
    a. EMG: continuous motor unit activity in paraspinal and abdominal muscles
    b. Anti-GAD antibodies positive in up to 70% of cases
    c. Anti-amphiphysin antibodies positive in up to 5% of cases
    d. CSF may have oligoclonal bands

11. Treatment
    a. First-line agent: diazepam
       1) Promotes GABA transmission
       2) Usually high dose (up to 100 mg/day) is required
    b. Alternative: another benzodiazepine (e.g., clonazepam)

c. Other agents that may be effective: valproate, vigabatrin
d. Potential role for plasma exchange, intravenous immunoglobulin, prednisone, other immunosuppressants such as azathioprine and cyclosporine

C. Restless Legs Syndrome and Periodic Limb Movements (see Chapter 19)

D. Painful Legs and Moving Toes Syndrome

1. Etiology: usually peripheral nerve trauma, peripheral neuropathy, radiculopathy, idiopathic

2. Mechanism undetermined; EMG suggests both peripheral and central generators

3. Pain usually precedes the movement disorder by days to years, may be exacerbated with walking or putting pressure on the affected limb

4. Pain is not always present

5. Movements vary, may be difficult to explain

6. Movements usually involve the toes (may spread proximally) and include clawing, fanning, and circular movements as well as different combinations of flexion, extension, and other movements

7. Stress can exacerbate both pain and movements

8. Symptoms: usually mild at onset, intensify with time

9. Treatment: usually disappointing; anticonvulsants (gabapentin, progabide), tricyclic antidepressants, dopaminergic agents (levodopa, pramipexole), sympathetic ganglionic blockade

REFERENCES

Adler CH, Ahlskog E, editors. Parkinson's disease and movement disorders: diagnosis and treatment guidelines for the practicing physician. Totowa (NJ): Humana Press; 2000.

Andermann F, Keene DL, Andermann E, Quesney LF. Startle disease or hyperekplexia: further delineation of the syndrome. Brain. 1980;103:985-97.

Artieda J, Obeso JA. The pathophysiology and pharmacology of photic cortical reflex myoclonus. Ann Neurol. 1993;34:175-84.

Bonifati V, Rizzu P, van Baren MJ, Schaap O, Breedveld GJ, Krieger E, et al. Mutations in the DJ-1 gene associated with autosomal recessive early-onset parkinsonism. Science. 2003 Jan 10;299:256-9. Epub 2002 Nov 21.

Fahn S, Frucht SJ, Hallett M, Truong D, editors. Advances in neurology: myoclonus and paroxysmal dyskinesias. Vol 89. Philadelphia: Lippincott Williams & Wilkins; 2002.

Grimes DA, Han F, Bulman D, Nicolson ML, Suchowersky O. Hereditary chin trembling: a new family with exclusion of the chromosome 9q13-q21 locus. Mov Disord. 2002;17:1390-2.

Hallett JJ, Harling-Berg CJ, Knopf PM, Stopa EG, Kiessling LS. Anti-striatal antibodies in Tourette syndrome cause neuronal dysfunction. J Neuroimmunol. 2000;111:195-202.

Hallett JJ, Kiessling LS. Neuroimmunology of tics and other childhood hyperkinesias. Neurol Clin. 1997;15:333-44.

Horvath J, Fross RD, Kleiner-Fisman G, Lerch R, Stalder H, Liaudat S, et al. Severe multivalvular heart disease: a new complication of the ergot derivative dopamine agonists. Mov Disord. 2004;19:656-62.

Jacquemont S, Hagerman RJ, Leehey MA, Hall DA, Levine RA, Brunberg JA, et al. Penetrance of the fragile X-associated tremor/ataxia syndrome in a permutation carrier population. JAMA. 2004;291:460-9.

Jarman PR, Wood NW, Davis MT, Davis PV, Bhatia KP, Marsden CD, et al. Hereditary geniospasm: linkage to chromosome 9q13-q21 and evidence for genetic heterogeneity. Am J Hum Genet. 1997;61:928-33.

Jellinger KA. Recent developments in the pathology of Parkinson's disease. J Neural Transm Suppl. 2002;62:347-76.

Krusz JC, Koller WC, Ziegler DK. Historical review: abnormal movements associated with epidemic encephalitis lethargica. Mov Disord. 1987;2:137-41.

Le WD, Xu P, Jankovic J, Jiang H, Appel SH, Smith RG, et al. Mutations in NR4A2 associated with familial Parkinson disease. Nat Genet. 2003 Jan;33:85-9. Epub 2002 Dec 23. Erratum in: Nat Genet. 2003;33:214.

Leehey MA, Munhoz RP, Lang AE, Brunberg JA, Grigsby J, Greco C, et al. The fragile X premutation presenting as essential tremor. Arch Neurol. 2003;60:117-21.

Liscum L, Klansek JJ. Niemann-Pick disease type C. Curr Opin Lipidol. 1998;9:131-5.

Luquin MR, Scipioni O, Vaamonde J, Gershanik O, Obeso JA. Levodopa-induced dyskinesias in Parkinson's disease: clinical and pharmacological classification. Mov Disord. 1992;7:117-24.

Peterson BS. Neuroimaging studies of Tourette syndrome: a decade of progress. Adv Neurol. 2001;85:179-96.

Quinn NP. Essential myoclonus and myoclonic dystonia. Mov Disord. 1996;11:119-24.

Quinn NP, Marsden CD. The motor disorder of multiple system atrophy. J Neurol Neurosurg Psychiatry. 1993;56:1239-42. Erratum in: J Neurol Neurosurg Psychiatry 1994;57:666.

Rubio JP, Danek A, Stone C, Chalmers R, Wood N, Verellen C, et al. Chorea-acanthocytosis: genetic linkage to chromosome 9q21. Am J Hum Genet. 1997;61:899-908.

Schenck CH, Bundlie SR, Mahowald MW. Delayed emergence of a parkinsonian disorder in 38% of 29 older men initially diagnosed with idiopathic rapid eye movement sleep behaviour disorder. Neurology. 1996;46:388-93. Erratum in: Neurology. 1996;46:1787.

Shiang R, Ryan SG, Zhu YZ, Hahn AF, O'Connell P, Wasmuth JJ. Mutations in the alpha 1 subunit of the inhibitory glycine receptor cause the dominant neurologic disorder, hyperekplexia. Nat Genet. 1993;5:351-8.

Singer HS. Neurobiology of Tourette syndrome. Neurol Clin. 1997;15:357-79.

Stern E, Silbersweig DA, Chee KY, Holmes A, Robertson MM, Trimble M, et al. A functional neuroanatomy of tics in Tourette syndrome. Arch Gen Psychiatry. 2000;57:741-8.

Suhren O, Bruyn GW, Tuynman JA. Hyperexkplexia: a hereditary startle syndrome. J Neurol Sci. 1966;3:577-605.

Tassone F, Hagerman RJ, Garcia-Arocena D, Khandjian EW, Greco CM, Hagerman PJ. Intranuclear inclusions in neural cells with premutation alleles in fragile X associated tremor/ataxia syndrome. J Med Genet. 2004;41:e43.

The Tourette Syndrome Classification Study Group. Definitions and classification of tic disorders. Arch Neurol. 1993;50:1013-6.

von Economo C. Encephalitis lethargica: its sequelae and treatment. (Translated and adapted by KO Newman.) London: Oxford University Press; 1931.

QUESTIONS

1. A 60-year-old man presents with a several-month history of unexplained falls. On neurologic examination, you notice hypometric vertical saccades, hyperextended posture, prominent axial rigidity, and abnormal postural reflexes. This disorder is also likely to comprise all the following *except*:
   a. Limitations of convergence
   b. Asymmetric rest tremor
   c. Impaired attention
   d. Pseudobulbar palsy and "emotional incontinence"

2. Which of the following is not an "α-synucleinopathy"?
   a. Multiple system atrophy
   b. Idiopathic Parkinson's disease
   c. Progressive supranuclear palsy
   d. Neurodegeneration with brain iron accumulation type I (formerly, Hallervorden-Spatz disease)
   e. Diffuse Lewy body disease

3. All the following conditions are associated with bilateral basal ganglia calcification except:
   a. Wilson's disease
   b. Fahr's disease
   c. Hypoparathyroidism
   d. Leigh's disease
   e. History of perinatal anoxia

4-12. Match the disorder (4-12) with the appropriate pathologic features (a-i). Choices a-i may be used once, more than once, or not at all.

4. Huntington's disease

5. Multiple system atrophy

6. Wilson's disease

7. Progressive supranuclear palsy

8. Amyotrophic choreoathetosis with acanthocytosis

9. Neuronal ceroid-lipofuscinoses

10. Idiopathic Parkinson's disease

11. Corticobasal degeneration

12. Neurodegeneration with brain iron accumulation type I (formerly, Hallervorden-Spatz disease)

13. A 65-year-old man presents with a several-month history of right hand weakness and gait imbalance. Neurologic examination demonstrates mild rest tremor of the right hand, mild "cogwheel" rigidity, and gait marked by mildly stooped posture (antecollis), short stride, reduced arm swing on the right, and difficulty on turns. There is no sign or symptom indicative of autonomic dysfunction, dementia, or pyramidal tract and cerebellar involvement. What is the most likely diagnosis and what is the next most appropriate step?
   a. Idiopathic Parkinson's disease, obtain MRI of the brain and neuropsychometric evaluation.
   b. Idiopathic Parkinson's disease, start carbidopa-levodopa
   c. Multiple system atrophy, start carbidopa-levodopa
   d. Multiple system atrophy, obtain MRI to rule out a structural cause of parkinsonism, no need to treat with levodopa given the generally poor response
   e. Idiopathic Parkinson's disease, observe and follow the patient and consider treatment when there is progression of disease

a. Neuronal loss and gliosis involving the caudate

b. Glial and neuronal inclusions, α-synuclein-positive immunohistochemistry

c. Curvilinear and "fingerprint" bodies

d. Lewy bodies limited to substantia nigra and degeneration of nigrostriatal projections

e. Tau-positive neuropil threads and tufted astrocytes; globose neurofibrillary tangles

f. Alzheimer type II cells and Opalski cells

g. Excessive intracellular and extracellular iron deposition and spheroids

h. Ballooned neurons and tau-positive astrocytic plaques

i. Bunina bodies

ANSWERS

1. Answer: b.
This patient likely has progressive supranuclear palsy. Axial
rigidity and falls are commonly the first signs. The supranuclear
vertical ophthalmoplegia may not be obvious at onset. Usually
before frank ophthalmoparesis develops, the saccades become
hypometric and slow and the fast component of optokinetic
nystagmus may be reduced. Patients characteristically have a
"wide-eyed star," with poor convergence. With more advanced
disease, there is often cognitive involvement and a pseudobulbar affect with "emotional incontinence." However, asymmetric rest tremor would be atypical for this entity, and
symmetric rigidity-parkinsonism (especially axial) is more
typical.

2. Answer: c.
Progressive supranuclear palsy is a tauopathy, with abnormal
tau deposition. Histopathologic study of the other disorders
listed usually demonstrates positive immunoreactivity for
α-synuclein.

3. Answer: d.
All the listed possibilities are associated with bilateral basal
ganglia calcification except Leigh's disease, which usually causes
necrosis of the basal ganglia (especially the putamen).

4. Answer: a.

5. Answer: b.

6. Answer: f.

7. Answer: e.

8. Answer: a.

9. Answer: c.

10. Answer: d.

11. Answer: h.

12. Answer: g.

13. Answer: b.
The presentation and neurologic examination findings are highly suggestive of idiopathic Parkinson's disease. The next most
appropriate step is to start treatment because of the patient's
disability. The asymmetry of symptoms and lack of cerebellar
or autonomic features make this less likely to be multiple system atrophy.

THE CEREBELLUM AND CEREBELLAR DISORDERS

Nima Mowzoon, M.D.

I. ANATOMY

A. Anatomic Divisions

1. Anterior lobe: anterior to primary fissure, receives majority of input from spinocerebellar tracts
2. Posterior lobe: between primary and dorsolateral fissures; receives majority of input from neocortex
3. Flocculonodular lobe: receives input from vestibular nuclei

B. Functional Subdivisions

1. Vestibulocerebellum
   a. Function
      1) Orienting eyes during movement
      2) Coordinating position of head and limbs in response to position and motion through connections with medial and lateral vestibulospinal tracts
      3) Has a role in smooth pursuit
   b. Cerebellar component: flocculonodular lobe
   c. Afferents: information from vestibular nuclei (mossy fibers) enters via inferior cerebellar peduncle to synapse in the flocculonodular lobe
   d. Efferents: information from flocculonodular lobe returns to vestibular nuclei; this includes inhibitory Purkinje cell input to medial and lateral vestibular nuclei
   e. Vestibular nuclei project to contralateral abducens nucleus and their axons also form the origins of vestibulospinal tracts
   f. Note: Some output from the nodulus is transmitted to fastigial nucleus; from here, fastigial nucleus axons influence vestibular nuclei (bilaterally), the reticular formation, and contralateral ventrolateral thalamus
   g. Dysfunction: vertigo, nystagmus, truncal ataxia, deficits in visual pursuit
2. Spinocerebellum—vermis (Fig. 9-1)
   a. Function
      1) Monitors ongoing execution of movement (especially proximal limbs and axial musculature)

2) Role in maintenance of muscle tone
   b. Cerebellar component: vermis
   c. Afferents (mossy fiber): primary somatosensory input via inferior cerebellar peduncle (from dorsal spinocerebellar and cuneocerebellar tracts, mostly muscle spindle input) and superior cerebellar peduncle (from ventral and rostral spinocerebellar tracts)
   d. Efferents: information from vermis projects to fastigial nucleus
   e. Efferents from fastigial nucleus

Functional Subdivisions of the Cerebellum

Vestibulocerebellum

   Involves the flocculonodular lobe

   Connections with the vestibular system

Spinocerebellum

   Vermis—responsible for axial and proximal limb motor control (synaptic relay in fastigial nucleus)

   Paravermis (intermediate zone)—responsible for distal limb motor control (synaptic relay in nucleus interpositus [globose and emboliform nuclei])

Cerebrocerebellum

   Involves the lateral cerebellar hemispheres and dentate nucleus

   Responsible for planning and initiation of movement, precision in control of rapid movements, and conscious assessment of errors in movement

---

1) Descending fibers to ipsilateral and contralateral reticular formation, origin of reticulospinal tracts
2) Descending fibers to ipsilateral and contralateral vestibular nuclei, origin of vestibulospinal tracts
3) Ascending fibers via superior cerebellar peduncle to primary motor cortex through synaptic relay in ventrolateral thalamic and red nuclei, influencing descending motor pathways

  f. Dysfunction: syndromes may overlap with paravermal syndromes; truncal ataxia

3. Spinocerebellum—paravermis (intermediate lobe) (Fig. 9-2)
  a. Function
    1) Monitors ongoing execution of limb movement
    2) Postural tone
    3) Modulates descending motor systems
  b. Cerebellar component: paravermal region and anterior lobe
  c. Afferents to paravermis: somatosensory information from dorsal spinocerebellar and cuneocerebellar tracts (via inferior cerebellar peduncle) ventral and rostral spinocerebellar tracts (via superior cerebellar peduncle)
  d. Efferents: information from anterior lobe projects to nucleus interpositus (globose and emboliform nuclei)
  e. Efferents from nucleus interpositus (ascends via decussating superior cerebellar peduncle) to
    1) Contralateral red nucleus (its axons descend in rubrospinal tract, which decussates immediately after it originates)
    2) Contralateral ventrolateral thalamic nucleus, which projects to cerebral cortex
  f. Dysfunction: limb dysmetria

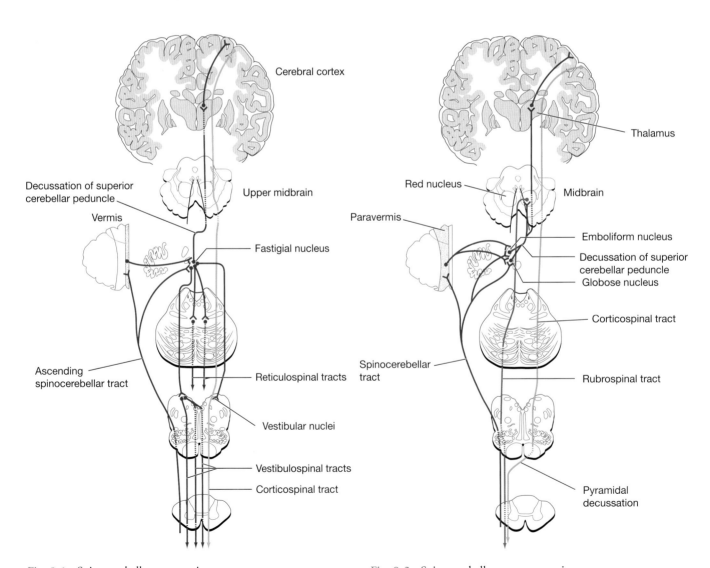

Fig. 9-1. Spinocerebellum—vermis.

Fig. 9-2. Spinocerebellum—paravermis.

4. Cerebrocerebellum (Fig. 9-3)
   a. Function: initiation, planning, and timing of movement; precision in control of rapid movements and conscious assessment of errors in movement (fine dexterity)
   b. Cerebellar component: lateral cerebellar hemispheres (posterior lobes)
   c. Afferents (mossy fiber): corticopontocerebellar fibers via middle cerebellar peduncle
   d. Efferents from dentate nucleus (ascends via decussating superior cerebellar peduncle) to
      1) Contralateral red nucleus (dentatorubral tract)
      2) Contralateral ventrolateral thalamic nucleus (dentatothalamic tract), which projects to cerebral cortex
   e. Dysfunction: delay in initiation and termination of movement and limb ataxia, limb dysmetria, dysarthria, intention tremor, kinetic tremor, nystagmus

C. Cytoarchitecture of Cerebellar Cortex (Fig. 9-4 and 9-5)
1. Granular layer: contains mainly granule cells, which receive most input from the mossy fibers, and Golgi cells, which modify granule cell output
2. Purkinje cell layer: contains Purkinje cells, the major source of output of cerebellar cortex
3. Molecular layer: contains mainly axons from granule cells (forming parallel fibers), Purkinje cell dendrites, basket cells, stellate cells

II. PHYSIOLOGY

A. Purkinje Cells
1. Purkinje cells are large γ-aminobutyric acid (GABA)ergic neurons
2. They send inhibitory projections to deep cerebellar nuclei
3. Purkinje cell axons form the primary (inhibitory) output of the cerebellar cortex
4. Contain three synaptic domains
   a. Distal dendritic spines: each Purkinje cell synapses with as many as 200,000 parallel fibers
   b. Proximal dendritic processes: innervated by multiple synapses from a single climbing fiber
   c. Cell body and axon hillock: inhibitory input from local interneurons (basket and stellate cells)

B. Climbing Fiber Input to Purkinje Cells (Fig. 9-5)
1. Climbing fibers arise primarily from neurons of the inferior olivary nucleus; the axons form the

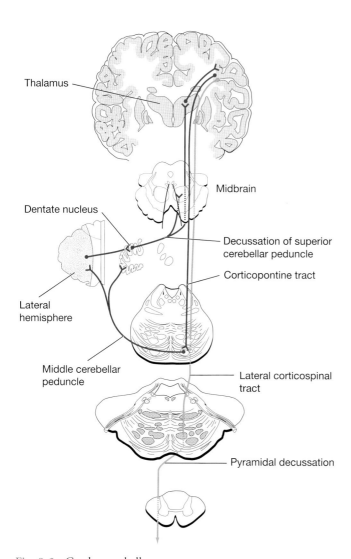

Fig. 9-3. Cerebrocerebellum.

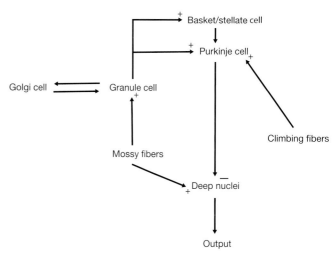

Fig. 9-4. Circuitry of cerebellar neurons. +, excitatory synapse; −, inhibitory synapse.

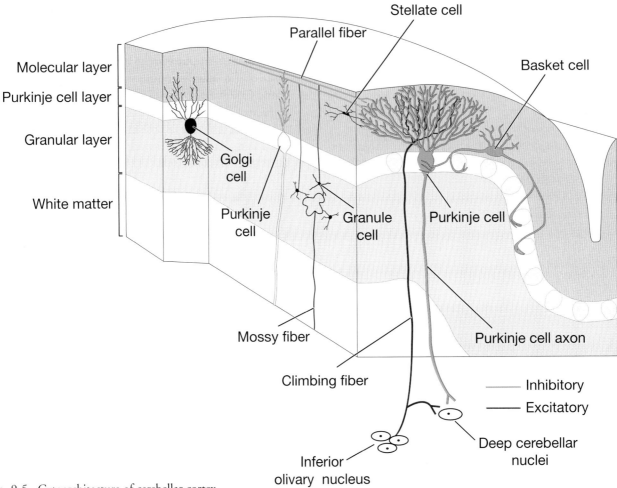

Fig. 9-5. Cytoarchitecture of cerebellar cortex.

olivocerebellar pathway (essentially carries motor error signals to the cerebellum)

2. Each climbing fiber may contact up to 10 Purkinje cells, but each Purkinje cell has contact with only one climbing fiber

3. Climbing fibers modify responses of Purkinje cells to mossy fiber input

4. Complex spikes: powerful phasic excitation generated by Purkinje cell, which is activated by climbing fiber input

   a. Each action potential in the climbing fiber generates a large depolarization in the Purkinje cell

   b. Bursts of small-amplitude action potentials following a large-amplitude spike produced by voltage-dependent Ca^{2+} conductance

   c. Synchronized, rhythmic firing produced by the electronic coupling of dendritic spines of neurons of the inferior olivary nucleus via gap junctions (may be responsible for the oscillatory properties of the inferior olivary nucleus

neurons and may partly explain palatal myoclonus)

   d. "Error detection and correction" function

      1) Produced as a consequence of a transient change in ongoing limb movements

      2) Complex spikes act to correct mismatches between the intended and actual movement

C. Mossy Fiber Input to Purkinje Cells (Fig. 9-5)

1. Mossy fibers arise from the vestibular nuclei, reticular formation, spinal cord, pontine nuclei (i.e., vestibulocerebellar, spinocerebellar, cuneocerebellar, reticulocerebellar, and pontocerebellar pathways)

   a. Mossy fibers arising in the spinal cord relay sensory information from the periphery via spinocerebellar tracts

   b. Mossy fibers arising in the pontine nuclei relay cortical inputs via the corticopontocerebellar pathway

2. Mossy fibers form excitatory synapses on granule cells (L-glutamate, via AMPA and metabotropic glutamate receptors)

a. Terminals (rosettes) contact the short dendrites of several granule cells, forming a complex called the glomerulus
b. Granule cells give rise to the parallel fibers in the molecular layer, which provide input to Purkinje cells
c. One mossy fiber contacts many granule cells
d. Each granule cell receives input from many mossy fibers
3. Simple spikes: discharge by Purkinje cell activated by parallel fibers (temporal and spatial summation of input from several parallel fibers is needed to trigger a Purkinje cell)
4. High discharge rates (50-300 Hz) provide information continuously to Purkinje cells about movement and allow continuous modulation of movement

D. Basket Cells and Stellate Cells: spatial modulation of Purkinje cell output
1. Basket and stellate cells reside in the molecular cell layer
2. They are activated by the parallel fibers
3. They provide GABAergic inhibitory input to surrounding "off-beam" Purkinje cells, while each mossy fiber provides excitatory input to a cluster of granule cells that in turn stimulate via parallel fibers a central array of "on-beam" Purkinje cells
4. This arrangement of lateral inhibition around the central array of facilitatory Purkinje cells resembles center-surround antagonism and provides spatial modulation of cerebellar cortex output

E. Golgi Cells: temporal modulation of Purkinje cell output
1. Dendrites of Golgi cells are in both the granular layer (contacted by mossy fibers) and molecular layer (contacted by excitatory parallel fiber synapses)
2. Golgi cells provide feedback inhibition (GABAergic) to the glomeruli, control the "gain" of the granule cell, and shorten the duration of bursts in the parallel fibers

F. Cerebellar Nuclei
1. Dentate nucleus: receives input primarily from the cerebellar hemispheres and projects primarily to the thalamus
2. Neurons in the cerebellar nuclei are tonically active and provide powerful excitatory postsynaptic potentials to their targets, including the motor relay nuclei of the thalamus, the red nucleus, vestibular nuclei, and reticular formation—via these projections, the cerebellum controls oculomotor, postural, and limb movements
3. Excitatory input to the deep cerebellar nuclei is via collaterals of mossy and climbing fibers, and inhibitory input is from Purkinje cells; the function of deep cerebellar nuclei depends on summation of the excitatory and inhibitory inputs
4. Purkinje cell output is influenced by modulatory influence of climbing fiber and mossy fiber inputs to the same Purkinje cell
5. The response of cerebellar nuclear neurons consists of an initial excitation, Purkinje cell–mediated inhibition, and then rebound bursts of excitation; the inhibitory "pulse" is important for cortical and subcortical feedback for prompt initiation and termination of a particular movement
6. Olivary-cerebellar nucleus-olivary loop
   a. Direct excitatory input from the inferior olivary nucleus to the cerebellar nuclei via climbing fiber collaterals
   b. Cerebellar nuclei, in turn, provide inhibitory GABAergic projections to the inferior olivary nucleus
7. Olivomesodiencephalic loop
   a. An excitatory loop involving projections from dentate nucleus to the mesodiencephalic junction and contralateral red nucleus and excitatory projections from these nuclei to the inferior olivary nucleus, and finally, the projection from the inferior olivary nucleus to dentate nucleus (Mollaret's triangle)
   b. This loop represents an excitatory, reverberating circuit that may be important in the pathophysiology of palatal myoclonus and essential tremor

III. CONGENITAL, FAMILIAL, AND ACQUIRED DISORDERS OF THE CEREBELLUM (TABLE 9-1)

A. Congenital Ataxias
1. Behr syndrome
   a. Autosomal recessive inheritance
   b. Optic atrophy and cerebellar ataxia beginning in early childhood; other features include nystagmus, scotoma, and bilateral retrobulbar neuritis
   c. Spasticity, spastic ataxic gait, mental retardation, and posterior column sensory loss
   d. Nerve biopsy findings consistent with chronic neuropathy with axonal degeneration and regeneration
2. Dandy-Walker syndrome (Fig. 9-6 A)
   a. Autosomal recessive or sporadic (Dandy-Walker variant with hydrocephalus and facial dysmorphism has been associated with deletion involving chromosome 3q25)
   b. Cystic dilatation of the fourth ventricle
   c. Dysplasia of the cerebellar vermis
   d. Heterogeneous clinical syndrome

Table 9-1. **Differential Diagnosis for Cerebellar Disorders**

Disease category	Acute or recurrent ataxia	Chronic progressive ataxia
Vascular	Cerebellar hemorrhage Cerebellar infarction Cerebellar ischemic attacks	
Infectious	Acute postinfectious cerebellitis (e.g., varicella) Brainstem encephalitis	CJD and Gerstmann-Sträussler-Scheinker syndrome Chronic panencephalitis of congenital rubella
Inflammatory and demyelinating	Miller Fisher syndrome Bickerstaff's brainstem encephalitis Multiple sclerosis Disseminated encephalomyelitis	Multiple sclerosis
Neoplastic	Paraneoplastic cerebellar degeneration Paraneoplastic opsoclonus Posterior fossa tumor	Cerebellar astrocytoma Cerebellar hemangioblastoma Ependymoma Medulloblastoma Paraneoplastic syndromes
Trauma	Hematoma Postconcussion syndrome Vertebrobasilar occlusion or dissection	
Toxic and metabolic	Drug ingestion Alcoholic cerebellar degeneration (acute exacerbation)	Alcoholic cerebellar degeneration Vitamin E deficiency Thiamine deficiency Hypothyroidism

Familial/congenital	Episodic ataxia type 1
	Episodic ataxia type 2
	Hyperammonemia (usually deficient urea
	  cycle enzymes, expecially OTC deficiency)
	Hartnup disease
	Maple syrup urine disease
	Pyruvate dehydrogenase deficiency
	Biotin-dependent carboxylase deficiency
		Cerebellar dysplasia/aplasia
		Dandy-Walker syndrome
		Congenital ataxia (see text)
		Basilar impression
		Hexosaminidase deficiency
		Niemann-Pick disease type C
		Autosomal dominant ataxias (see text)
		Autosomal recessive ataxias (see text)
		Ataxias with X-linked recessive inheritance
		  Adrenoleukodystrophy
		  Leber's optic neuropathy

Paroxysmal	Migraine (basilar) Benign paroxysmal vertigo Epilepsy	
Sporadic degenerative		Sporadic cerebellar degeneration Multiple system atrophy (OPCA)
Other	Foramen magnum compression Intermittent hydrocephalus Idiopathic, sporadic	Foramen magnum compression Hydrocephalus Idiopathic, sporadic

CJD, Creutzfeldt-Jakob disease; OPCA, olivopontocerebellar atrophy; OTC, ornithine transcarbamoylase.

1) Presenting symptoms usually within the first year of life: generally related to hydrocephalus and posterior fossa symptoms such as apneic spells, cranial nerve palsies, nystagmus, papilledema, bulging of anterior fontanelle
2) Infants may have poor head control and spasticity, poor feeding, and hyperirritability

3) Older children often have delayed motor and intellectual development, seizures in 20% to 30%
   e. Associated with
   1) Agenesis of the corpus callosum
   2) Cortical heterotopias
   3) Cerebral gyral abnormalities
   4) Occipital encephalocele
   5) Syringomyelia
   6) Aqueductal stenosis
   7) Hemimegalencephaly
   f. Differential diagnosis for posterior fossa collection of cerebrospinal fluid should include
   1) Familial vermian agenesis (e.g., Joubert syndrome, see below)
   2) Trapped fourth ventricle
   3) Enlarged cisterna magna (because of cerebellar

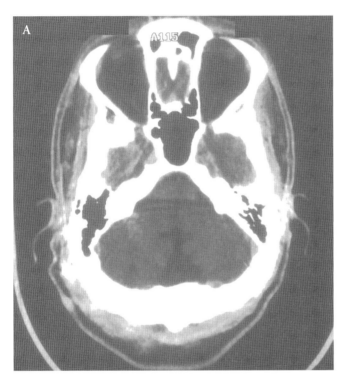

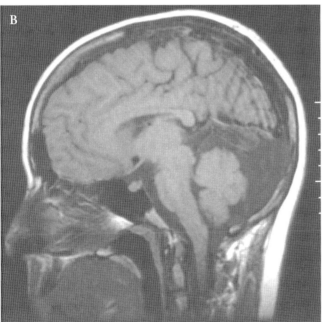

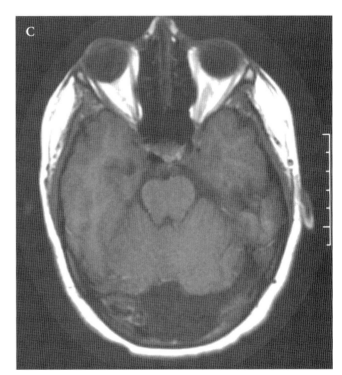

Fig. 9-6. Dandy-Walker malformation and arachnoid cyst. *A*, Dandy-Walker nonenhanced computed tomogram shows the characteristic features of vermian hypoplasia and cystic dilatation of the fourth ventricle without enlargement of the posterior fossa. *B* and *C*, Magnetic resonance images (T1 weighted) show a true retrocerebellar arachnoid cyst of developmental origin associated with a pronounced mass effect. Note displacement of the transverse sinuses and remodeling of the underlying occipital bone from the arachnoid cyst. The bone remodeling is the result of a chronic mass effect.

atrophy or agenesis or associated with benign infantile macrocephaly)

    4) Arachnoid cyst (may present as posterior fossa mass in infancy or childhood or may cause hydrocephalus or may be asymptomatic) (Fig. 9-6 *B* and *C*)

3. Classic Joubert syndrome (Joubert syndrome type 1)
   a. Autosomal recessive inheritance, linked to chromosome 9
   b. Hypotonia in infancy
   c. Developmental delay, ataxia, abnormal breathing pattern, including episodic apnea and tachypnea, and later development of mental retardation
   d. Oculomotor apraxia, nystagmus, ptosis
   e. Other features: renal disease, ocular colobomas, liver fibrosis, polydactyly, pigmentary retinopathy
   f. Hypoplastic or dysplastic cerebellar vermis with enlargement of the fourth ventricle
   g. "Molar tooth sign" (brainstem abnormalities that resemble a tooth): elongated superior cerebellar peduncle, deep interpeduncular fossa, dysplasia of the superior cerebellar vermis

4. Cerebello-oculorenal syndrome (Joubert syndrome type 2)
   a. Autosomal recessive inheritance, linked to chromosome 11
   b. Phenotypic presentation similar to classic Joubert syndrome
   c. Infantile onset of ataxia, hypotonia, psychomotor developmental delay, oculomotor disorders (oculomotor apraxia and nystagmus)
   d. Ocular manifestations: retinal dystrophy (sometimes called "Leber's congenital amaurosis")
   e. Renal abnormalities: cystic dysplastic kidneys or juvenile nephronophthisis
   f. Polydactyly, high-arched palate, hypertelorism
   g. Molar tooth sign (as above), cerebellar vermian dysplasia, kinked corpus callosum

5. COACH syndrome (**c**erebellar vermis hypoplasia, **o**ligophrenia, congenital **a**taxia ocular **c**oloboma, and **h**epatic fibrosis)
   a. Early-onset ataxia, cerebellar vermis hypoplasia (molar tooth sign)
   b. Moderate mental retardation
   c. Ocular coloboma
   d. Liver fibrosis
   e. Hypertelorism
   f. Progressive renal insufficiency has been reported

6. Gillespie syndrome
   a. Autosomal recessive inheritance
   b. Partial or complete aniridia: aplasia involving only the pupillary zone of the iris, giving the appearance of fixed dilated pupils in a hypotonic infant; congenital cataracts; and corneal opacities

    c. Nonprogressive cerebellar ataxia, associated with cerebellar hypoplasia
    d. Mental deficiency

7. Gomez-Lopez-Hernandez syndrome (cerebellotrigeminal dermal dysplasia)
   a. Craniosynostosis
   b. Gait and truncal ataxia, cerebellar anomaly
   c. Trigeminal anesthesia, absence of corneal reflexes, corneal opacities, scalp alopecia
   d. Midface hypoplasia, apparently low-set ears, mental retardation, and short stature

8. Marinesco-Sjögren syndrome
   a. Rare autosomal recessive disorder
   b. Cerebellar ataxia, developmental delay, and mental retardation
   c. Additional features: congenital cataracts, short stature, skeletal deformities, hypogonadism
   d. Variable neuromuscular manifestations such as chronic myopathy and demyelinating sensorimotor neuropathy
   e. Major clinical overlap with congenital cataracts facial dysmorphism neuropathy (CCFDN) syndrome
   f. Features that distinguish Marinesco-Sjögren syndrome from CCFDN include more severe mental retardation; marked cerebellar atrophy; chronic myopathy, with specific ultrastructural features seen on muscle biopsy; absence of facial dysmorphism; and microcornea
   g. Muscle histopathology
      1) Dystrophic-like changes: variation in fiber size, fibrosis, adipose tissue replacement, necrosis, proliferation of internal nuclei, rimmed vacuoles
      2) Autophagocytosis: autophagic vacuoles

9. Congenital disorder of glycosylation, type Ia (carbohydrate-deficient glycoprotein syndrome type 1a)
   a. Psychomotor retardation
   b. Generalized hypotonia, hyporeflexia, truncal ataxia, cerebellar hypoplasia
   c. Demyelinating peripheral neuropathy
   d. Decreased serum glycoproteins (total serum glycoproteins deficient in sialic acid and in galactose and *N*-acetylglucosamine)
   e. Reduced serum activity of *N*-acetylglucosaminyltransferase
   f. Type Ia: Phosphomannomutase affected, an enzyme necessary for the synthesis of guanosine diphosphate-mannose, mapped to chromosome 16p

10. Cerebellar ataxia 1
   a. Other names include cerebelloparenchymal disorder III, cerebellar hypoplasia, nonprogressive Norman type
   b. Autosomal recessive inheritance, chromosome 9q
   c. Nonprogressive autosomal recessive congenital cerebellar ataxia and mental insufficiency

d. Short stature

e. Severe loss of granule cells; heterotopic Purkinje cells

11. Cerebellar ataxia 3
    a. Infantile-onset nonprogressive cerebellar ataxia
    b. Normal intellectual function
    c. Brisk deep tendon reflexes and, occasionally, spasticity
    d. Short stature, pes planus
    e. Magnetic resonance imaging (MRI): cerebellar vermian atrophy

12. Dysplastic gangliocytoma of the cerebellum (Lhermitte-Duclos disease)
    a. Typical presentation in young adults with symptoms of increased intracranial pressure due to obstructive hydrocephalus
    b. Cowden disease (multiple hamartomas syndrome): predisposing and associated condition
    c. MRI: laminated increased T2 signal
    d. Pathology: cellular disorganization, hypertrophied granule cells, and axonal hypermyelination in the molecular layer of the cerebellum, with global hypertrophy of the cerebellum and coarse gyri macroscopically

B. **Familial Ataxias—Autosomal Recessive**

1. Friedreich's ataxia
    a. Genetics and pathogenesis
        1) In more than 90% of persons affected, a mutation involves expansion of GAA triplet repeats within the first intron of the *FRDA* gene (chromosome 9q13-q21.1), impairing exon splicing and decreased production of frataxin protein
        2) Point mutation (about 6%)
        3) Frataxin protein is likely located in mitochondria and is possibly a mitochondrial iron transporter
        4) Deficiency of frataxin may cause excess intramitochondrial iron and subsequent oxidative stress
        5) Reduced frataxin levels in skeletal muscle, heart, pancreas, liver, kidney, central nervous system (spinal cord > cerebellum > cerebral cortex)
        6) The length of the repeat correlates directly with the severity of disease and the presence of cardiomyopathy and inversely with age at onset
    b. Typically develops around the time of puberty, with gait disorder and clumsiness
    c. Mixed sensory and cerebellar ataxia
    d. Cerebellar dysfunction
        1) Progressive limb and gait ataxia, cerebellar dysarthria
        2) Early ataxia of the lower limbs and axial control; subsequent appendicular ataxia of the upper limbs and cranial musculature
        3) Results from the loss of Purkinje cells, degeneration of

the dentate nucleus, axonal loss and demyelination of the superior cerebellar peduncles, and degeneration of the spinocerebellar tracts

e. Sensory symptoms
    1) Mainly large-fiber sensory loss (vibratory and proprioceptive), areflexia
    2) Axonal sensory neuropathy
    3) Likely secondary to involvement of large myelinated fibers (scanty paranodal and segmental demyelination), with wallerian degeneration of the posterior columns, nuclei gracilis and cuneatus, and medial lemniscus (Fig. 9-7)
    4) Degeneration of the dorsal root ganglia (Fig. 9-8)

f. Pyramidal involvement
    1) Initially, may be mild; mainly extensor plantar responses
    2) Eventually, may cause weakness in lower extremities, spasticity, and flexor spasms
    3) Distal wasting and amyotrophy, mainly in the lower extremities
    4) Degeneration of the corticospinal tracts is most severe in lumbar segments and least apparent in cervical segments (Fig. 9-7)

g. Progressive bulbar deficits (dysarthria, dysphagia)

h. Skeletal abnormalities
    1) Kyphoscoliosis (Fig. 9-9 *A* and *B*)
    2) Pes cavus, pes planus, and equivarus

i. Other manifestations that may be involved
    1) Cardiac involvement: widespread T-wave inversions, hypertrophied cardiomyopathy (50% of cases), asymmetrical septal hypertrophy, symmetrical concentric ventricular hypertrophy, or subaortic stenosis
    2) Diabetes mellitus
    3) Optic atrophy
    4) Sensorineural hearing loss
    5) Sphincter disturbance, usually mild

j. Nerve conduction studies: normal compound muscle action potentials and reduced or absent sensory nerve action potentials

k. Prognosis
    1) Slow, variable progression
    2) Age at death varies, usually late 30s (range, 21-69 years)
    3) Wheelchair-dependent usually in second decade

l. Treatment
    1) Possible benefit of idebenone on heart wall thickness
    2) Combination of coenzyme Q and vitamin E may improve cardiac and skeletal muscle bioenergetics
    3) Possible role of iron chelation therapy
    4) Close monitoring for cardiac abnormalities, diabetes, scoliosis, hearing loss, etc.

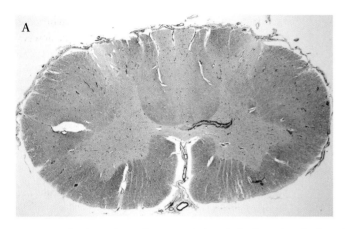
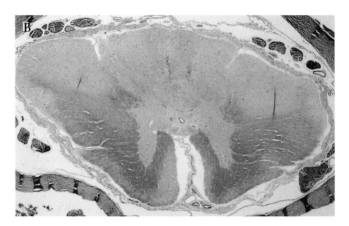

Fig. 9-7. Sections through, *A*, cervical and, *B*, thoracic spinal cord from a patient with Friedreich's ataxia. Degeneration is more prominent in the gracile fasciculus than the cuneate fasciculus. The thoracic section shows degeneration of the spinocerebellar tracts and the lateral and anterior funiculi, the location of the corticospinal tracts. The corticospinal tracts are often spared at the cervical level, as is here. (Luxon fast blue.)

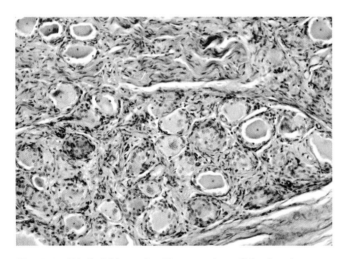

Fig. 9-8. Friedreich's ataxia. Degeneration of the dorsal root ganglion is indicated by dense clusters of cells called the nodules of Nageotte.

2. Friedreich's ataxia 2—autosomal recessive inheritance, chromosome 9p23-p11
3. Ataxia with isolated vitamin E deficiency
   a. Mutation of α-tocopherol transfer protein gene, located on chromosome 8q13.1-q13.3 (most commonly frameshift deletions)
   b. Phenotypically resembles Friedreich's ataxia, with low or undetectable vitamin E levels without malabsorption
   c. Large-fiber sensory loss with areflexia
   d. Ataxia and dysarthria
   e. Onset is usually in childhood (frameshift mutations), middle-age onset (usually point mutations)

   f. Head titubation and dystonia are more frequent than in Friedreich's ataxia
   g. Cardiac involvement is less frequent than in Friedreich's ataxia
   h. Other findings: xanthelasma, tendon xanthomas, retinitis pigmentosa, deafness, sphincter involvement
   i. Laboratory findings: very low vitamin E levels; cholesterol and triglyceride levels may be high
   j. Treatment: vitamin E supplements and high fat diet
4. Abetalipoproteinemia (Bassen-Kornzweig syndrome)
   a. Rare, gene localized to chromosone 4q24 (microsomal triglyceride transfer protein)
   b. Absence of apolipoprotein B-containing proteins (such as very-low-density lipoprotein, chylomicrons, low-density lipoprotein)
   c. Neonatal and infantile onset of diarrhea, followed by slow onset and progression of the neurologic syndrome
   d. Early-onset ataxia resembles Friedreich's ataxia, with ataxia, areflexia, proprioceptive sensory loss, and extensor plantar responses
   e. Gait disturbances usually develop by age 10 years
   f. Low levels of lipids, including serum cholesterol, and severe malabsorption of fat-soluble vitamins A, D, E, and K
   g. Peripheral blood acanthocytosis
   h. Pigmentary retinopathy
   i. Pes cavus and scoliosis
   j. Laboratory findings: acanthocytosis, decreased serum level of cholesterol, low levels of low-density lipoprotein, very-low-density lipoprotein, and triglycerides
   k. Electrodiagnostic evaluation
      1) EMG and nerve conduction studies: predominantly

axonal peripheral neuropathy
2) Abnormal sensory evoked potentials (implying involvement of posterior columns)
3) Abnormal visual evoked resonses and electro-retinography (implying retinal degeneration and optic neuropathy)
l. Treatment: reduced fat intake and high doses of vitamin E and administration of vitamins A, D, and K
5. Ataxia-telangiectasia
a. Genetics and pathogenesis
1) Mutation of the AT mutant (*ATM*) gene located on chromosome 11q22-q23
2) ATM protein is located predominantly in the nucleus, has a main role in cell cycle control and mitogenic signal transduction
b. Clinical features
1) Phenotypic variation in age at onset and severity of symptoms

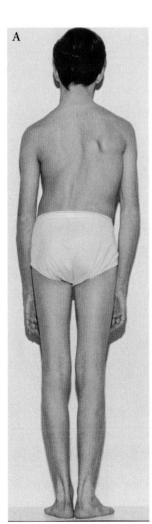
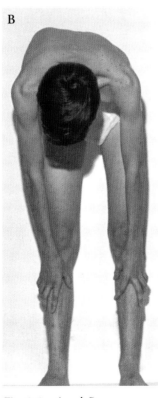

Fig. 9-9. *A* and *B*, Kyphoscoliosis in a patient with Friedreich's ataxia.

2) Usual age at onset is between 1 and 2 years, when the patient learns to walk; later onset may predict slower progression
3) Most patients are wheelchair-bound by age 10
4) Ataxia (predominantly truncal) is usually the first symptom (later, appendicular ataxia), ataxic dysarthria
5) Oculomotor apraxia, jerky pursuit movements with loss of optokinetic nystagmus and limitation of upgaze, slow saccades with long latency
6) Choreoathetosis and dystonia
7) Large-fiber sensory neuropathy may occur late in the disease
8) Reduced or absent deep tendon reflexes, sometimes with extensor plantar responses
9) Oculocutaneous telangiectasias usually occur after onset of ataxia, about 4 to 6 years of age (Fig. 9-10)
10) Progressive distal muscle atrophy may occur late in the disease
11) Predisposition to neoplasia, mainly leukemia or B-cell lymphoma
12) Before age 20 years, malignancies are mostly lymphoid
13) In older adults, malignancies are commonly solid
14) Immunodeficiency (60%) and frequent sinopulmonary infections, T-cell deficiency, and absent or small thymus gland
c. Laboratory features
1) Increased level of alpha fetoprotein
2) Decreased serum levels of IgA, IgE, IgG, especially IgG2
3) IgM level may be increased
d. Pathology
1) Cerebellar atrophy, especially affecting vermis
2) Cell loss involving the inferior olivary nucleus, dentate nucleus, Purkinje cells, and granule cells (abnormal arborization and ectopic localization)
3) Degenerative changes in the spinal cord affect the posterior and lateral columns and anterior horn cells (Fig. 9-11)
4) Demyelinating peripheral neuropathy
5) Hypoplastic or absent thymus gland
6. Autosomal recessive ataxia with oculomotor apraxia
a. Autosomal recessive, chromosome 9: *aprataxin* or *senataxin*
b. Childhood onset, more common in Japanese and Portuguese populations
c. Ataxia (gait and appendicular arm > leg), cerebellar atrophy
d. Oculomotor apraxia and possibly optic atrophy
e. No immunodeficiency or chromosomal instability

f. Peripheral neuropathy (distal symmetrical motor or sensory mainly involving large fibers)

g. Mental retardation may occur

h. Hypoalbuminemia

7. Cockayne syndrome

  a. Autosomal recessive inheritance (chromosome 5)

  b. Autosomal dominant inheritance (chromosome 10)

  c. Mental retardation, microcephaly, hydrocephalus, seizures

  d. Pyramidal and extrapyramidal features are possible

  e. Ataxia

  f. Retinal degeneration, optic atrophy, cataracts, blindness

  g. Short stature, contractures, progeric features, brittle hair

  h. Photosensitivity, abnormal UV sensitivity has been noted in cultured skin fibroblasts

  i. Computed tomography (CT): calcification of the basal ganglia

8. Xeroderma pigmentosum

  a. Defect in DNA excision repair after exposure to UV light

  b. Ataxia, dementia/mental retardation and microcephaly, seizures, choreoathetosis, spasticity, sensorineural hearing loss, large-fiber sensory peripheral neuropathy

  c. Photosensitivity and skin malignancies

  d. Phenotypic differences with Cockayne syndrome: presence of skin tumors and absence of intracranial calcification

9. Refsum's disease

  a. Rare, autosomal recessive inheritance

  b. Deficiency in peroxisomal enzyme phytanoyl-CoA hydroxylase prevents α-oxidation of phytanic acid

  c. Accumulation of phytanic acid produces neurotoxicity

  d. Onset: second to third decade of life

  e. Relapsing-remitting course

  f. Early pigmentary retinal degeneration and night blindness

  g. Demyelinating sensorimotor polyneuropathy

  h. Sensorineural deafness

  i. Ataxia

  j. Skin manifestation (ichthyosis)

  k. Cardiac arrhythmias

  l. Laboratory features

    1) Increased phytanic acid levels in plasma and urine

    2) Cultured fibroblasts have reduced ability to oxidize phytanic acid

  m. Treatment: dietary reduction in phytanic acid may help the neuropathy

10. Cerebrotendinous xanthomatosis

  a. Autosomal recessive

  b. Defect in liver bile acid synthesis (27-hydroxylase): impaired formation of cholic acid

  c. Abnormal high-density lipoprotein: reduced cholesterol content suggesting decreased capacity to remove excess cholesterol from peripheral tissues

  d. Accumulation of cholesterol and related products in various tissues

  e. Tendon xanthomas, xanthelasma, and cataracts

  f. Deposits found in the cerebellar white matter

  g. Slowly progressive neurologic manifestations include ataxia, pyramidal signs, peripheral neuropathy, cognitive decline

  h. Other features: seizures, palatal myoclonus, pseudobulbar palsy

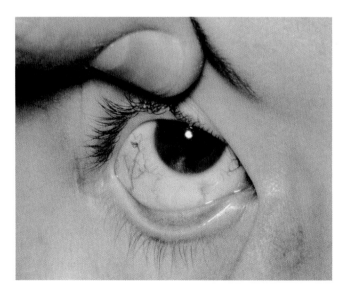

Fig. 9-10. Ocular telangiectasia in patient with ataxia-telangiectasia.

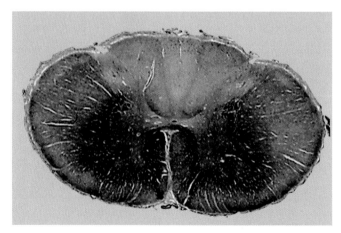

Fig. 9-11. Ataxia-telangiectasia. Section through cervical spinal cord from patient with ataxia-telangiectasia demonstrating marked degeneration of the posterior columns (more prominent in gracile fasciculus) and less severe degeneration in lateral funiculi. (Luxol fast blue stain.)

i. Neuroimaging may show cerebral and cerebellar atrophy
j. Treatment
   1) Cholic acid and chenodeoxycholic acid: compensate for the deficient bile acids in the intrahepatic pool and decrease cholestanol synthesis and levels
   2) Simvastatin or lovastatin: decrease cholesterol synthesis and cholestanol levels
11. Childhood ataxia with central nervous system hypomyelination
   a. Also called vanishing white matter leukoencephalopathy
   b. Autosomal recessive inheritance
   c. Associated with mutations in any of the five genes coding for translation initiation factor 2B (eIF2B)
   d. Childhood onset of chronic progressive ataxia, seizures, possibly cognitive deficits, spasticity, optic atrophy, episodes of coma
   e. Episodic deterioration, may follow minor trauma, fever, or stress
   f. Pathology confined to the white matter: diffuse leukoencephalopathy with astrocytic dropout and "foamy" oligodendrocytes (Fig. 9-12)
   g. Cerebellar atrophy, primarily involving the vermis
   h. Increased glycine in cerebrospinal fluid
12. Spinocerebellar ataxia with axonal neuropathy (SCAN 1)
   a. Mutation in the gene encoding tyrosyl-DNA phosphodiesterase 1 (DNA repair enzyme)
   b. Gradual onset of gait ataxia in the second decade, with sensorimotor neuropathy, areflexia, and normal intelligence
13. Cayman ataxia
   a. Mutation in the gene encoding caytaxin on the short arm of chromosome 19
   b. Early childhood onset of cerebellar dysarthria and gait ataxia and mental retardation
14. Early-onset cerebellar ataxia with retained tendon reflexes
   a. Age at onset: first two decades of life
   b. Ataxia and large-fiber polyneuropathy with preserved deep tendon reflexes

Autosomal Recessive Ataxias Related to DNA Repair Defects

Ataxia-telangiectasia

Spinocerebellar ataxia with axonal neuropathy (SCAN 1)

Cockayne syndrome

c. Pancerebellar syndrome affecting different cerebellar functions (appendicular, gait, speech, and oculomotor control)
d. Pyramidal involvement, cardiomyopathy, and skeletal deformities are absent or rare
e. Cerebellar atrophy may be evident
15. Baltic myoclonus (Unverricht-Lundborg disease)
   a. See Chapter 8
   b. Mutation in the gene encoding for cystatin B, chromosome 21q
   c. Myoclonic or generalized epilepsy, mental deterioration, ataxia, pyramidal symptoms
16. Charlevoix-Saguenay spastic ataxia
   a. Point mutation in the SACS gene on chromosome 13, resulting in loss of expression of sacsin
   b. Early childhood onset of spastic ataxia with amyotrophy, described in Quebec
   c. Ataxic gait, dysarthria, nystagmus
   d. Pyramidal tract involvement: progressive spastic paraparesis with extensor plantar responses
   e. Sensorimotor peripheral neuropathy
   f. Associated with mitral valve prolapse, pes cavus, and pes planus, prominent retinal myelinated nerve fibers (striations)
   g. Loss of myelinated axons, onion bulb formation, cerebellar atrophy with Purkinje cell loss, denervation atrophy noted on muscle biopsy
   h. Absence of somatosensory evoked potentials in the lower extremities and delayed visual evoked responses
17. Infantile-onset spinocerebellar ataxia
   a. Autosomal recessive inheritance, chromosome 10q
   b. Infantile onset: clumsiness and athetosis in the hands and face, hypotonia, hyporeflexia
   c. By school age: sensorineural hearing loss, ophthalmoplegia
   d. By age 10 to 15: sensorimotor polyneuropathy, optic atrophy, female hypogonadism, seizures
   e. Progressive ataxia and dementia
   f. Wheelchair-bound by late teens

C. Familial Ataxias—Autosomal Dominant (Table 9-2)
1. General features
   a. Features of all spinocerebellar ataxias (SCAs): cerebellar syndrome including ataxia and dysarthria
   b. Features of most SCAs
      1) Upper motor neuron signs (SCAs 1, 3, 7, 12, and, less commonly, 6 and 8)
      2) Parkinsonism (SCA 3)
      3) Axonal polyneuropathy (SCAs 1, 2, 3, 4, 8, 18, 25)
      4) Anticipation (most prominent in SCA 7, dentatorubral-pallidoluysian atrophy [DRPLA], and SCA 1)

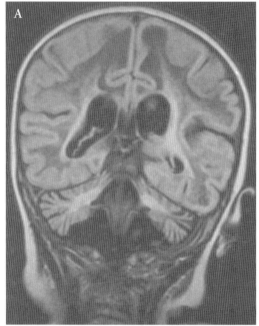

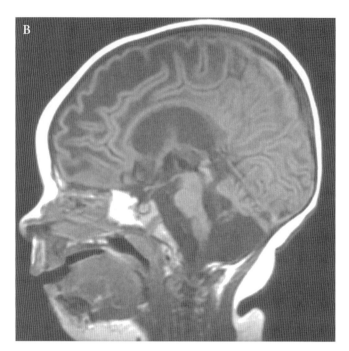

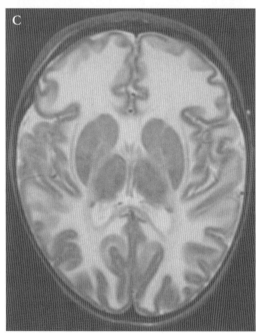

Fig. 9-12. Childhood ataxia with central nervous system hypomyelination. Conventional magnetic resonance images from patient with developmental regression, seizures, and spasticity. *A* and *B*, T1-weighted images; *C*, T2-weighted image. Almost the entire subcortical white matter appears homogeneously hyperintense on the T2-weighted image and severely hypointense on the T1-weighted images. Note pronounced atrophy of posterior fossa structures, including brainstem and cerebellum. The images also show a septum cavum, ex-vacuo dilatation of all the ventricles, and prominent cisterns, as a result of the atrophy.

     b) SCA 2, SCA 7: hypometric saccades (reduced velocity)
     c) Hypometric saccades are also noted in the later stages of SCA 1, SCA 3, never in SCA 6
     d) SCA 3: gaze-evoked nystagmus, parkinsonism, spasticity
     e) SCA 6 (and episodic ataxia 2): downbeat nystagmus, benign course
     f) SCA 7: macular dystrophy and pigmentary retinal degeneration, blindness
  3) Seizures: SCA 7, SCA 10, DRPLA
  4) Genetic features
     a) Length of repeats usually are inversely correlated with age at onset
     b) Anticipation, particularly paternal
  5) Pathologic features
     a) SCAs 1, 2, 3: severe degeneration of the nuclei

  c. Age at onset
    1) Childhood: SCAs 2, 7, 13, DRPLA
    2) Young adulthood: SCAs 1, 2, 3, 21
    3) Older adult: SCA 6
  d. Selective features
    1) Cognitive impairment: SCAs 1, 2, 3, 7, DRPLA
    2) Ophthalmologic findings
      a) SCA 1: hypermetric saccades (increased amplitude)

Table 9-2. **Classification of Autosomal Dominant Cerebellar Ataxias (ADCAs)**

Phenotypic classification	Genotypic classification	Mutation (protein)	Predictive clinical phenotype*	Major sites of pathologic change†
ADCA I	SCA 1	CAG repeat expansion in chr 6p23 (ataxin-1)	Pyramidal signs, EP (rare), hypermetric saccades	Purkinje cells, inferior olivary nuclei, pons, dentate nucleus, cerebellar peduncles, spinal cord
ADCA I	SCA 2	CAG repeat expansion in chr 12q (ataxin-2)	Dementia, myoclonus, tremor, hypometric saccades, hyporeflexia	Purkinje cells, inferior olivary nuclei, pons, middle and inferior cerebellar peduncles, spinal cord
ADCA I	SCA 3	CAG repeat expansion in chr 14q (ataxin-3)	Pyramidal signs, EP, ophthalmo-plegia	Basal ganglia,‡ pontine nuclei, dentate nucleus, red nucleus, cranial nerve nuclei, spinal cord (spinocerebellar tracts, Clarke's columns, posterior columns, anterior horn cells) Inferior olivary nuclei and Purkinje cells are spared
ADCA I	SCA4	Chr 16q	Cerebellar signs ± pyramidal signs or polyneuropathy	Lack of adequate data
ADCA II	SCA 7	CAG repeat expansion in chr 3p (ataxin-7)	Pigmentary retinal degeneration and macular dystrophy, blindness	Degeneration of the cerebellum, retinal ganglion cells, basal pons, inferior olivary nuclei Neuronal intranuclear inclusions, predominantly in the inferior olivary nuclei
ADCA III	SCA 5	Chr 11	Pure cerebellar syndrome	
ADCA III	SCA 6	CAG repeat expansion in chr 19q (CACNA1)	Benign course Pure cerebellar syndrome—slowly progressive ataxia (pyramidal signs and EP unusual)	Neuronal loss and gliosis limited to Purkinje cells and inferior olivary nuclei
DRPLA		CAG repeat expansion in chr 12p	Dementia Ataxia, seizures, myoclonus, chorea	Globus pallidus, red nucleus, subthalamic nucleus, dentate nucleus

Chr, chromosome; DRPLA, dentatorubral-pallidoluysian atrophy; EP, extrapyramidal signs; SCA, spinocerebellar ataxia.
*Features with some predictive value for specific gene defects; all patients will have ataxia and dysarthria and most will have polyneuropathy.
†Pathologic changes usually consist of degenerative processes, i.e., neuronal loss and gliosis.
‡Including the globus pallidus, subthalamic nucleus, substantia nigra.

pontis and spinocerebellar tracts, sparing of the optic nerve (pontocerebellar atrophy)
b) SCA 1, SCA 2 (not SCA 3): severe neuronal loss and degeneration involving Purkinje cells, inferior olivary nuclei, and olivocerebellar pathways
c) SCA 3: sparing of Purkinje cells and inferior olivary nuclei
d) SCA 6: pure cerebellar atrophy, isolated involve-

ment of Purkinje cells and inferior olivary nucleus neurons
e. Symptomatic classification
1) Autosomal dominant cerebellar ataxia (ADCA) I: cerebellar syndrome with pyramidal and extrapyramidal features, ophthalmoplegia, and dementia (SCAs 1, 2, 3, 4, 8, 12, 17)
2) ADCA II: cerebellar syndrome and pigmentary

macular degeneration and macular dystrophy (SCA 7)

    3) ADCA III: limited to cerebellar syndrome, possibly mild pyramidal signs (SCAs 5, 6, 10, 11, 14, 15)

2. SCA 1 (ADCA I)

  a. CAG repeat leads to unstable, polymorphic expansion (higher number of repeats correlates with disease severity and earlier age at onset) in chromosome 6p, with coding of a novel protein (ataxin-1)

  b. Anticipation (especially paternal)

  c. Onset: about third or fourth decade of life

  d. Cerebellar signs and symptoms (ataxic gait, dysarthria), pyramidal signs (spasticity, hyperreflexia, clonus, extensor plantar responses), and extrapyramidal signs (dystonia, chorea, parkinsonism)

  e. Initial symptoms: usually slowness of limb movements, slow and infrequent eye blinking, saccadic pursuit eye movements, hypermetric saccades, and end-gaze nystagmus on lateral gaze

  f. With disease progression, saccades become progressively slowed, leading to complete ophthalmoplegia

  g. Axonal polyneuropathy, sensory ± motor

  h. Cognitive impairment in some patients

  i. Motor evoked potentials: markedly prolonged peripheral and central motor conduction times

  j. MRI shows cerebellar and pontine atrophy

  k. Pathology

    1) Severe loss of Purkinje cells, worse in the vermis

    2) Neuronal loss in the dentate nucleus, substantia nigra, red nucleus, pontine nuclei, and inferior olivary nucleus; also degeneration in superior, middle, and inferior cerebellar peduncles, including olivocerebellar pathways

    3) Degenerative changes in the spinal cord affect anterior horn cells, corticospinal tracts, posterior columns, spinocerebellar tracts, and Clarke's columns

3. SCA 2 (ADCA I)

  a. CAG repeat expansion in chromosome 12q, with coding of a novel protein (ataxin-2)

  b. Paternal anticipation

  c. Longer repeats correlate with earlier onset, incidence of myoclonus, and more rapid progression

  d. Mean age at clinical onset: second to fourth decades

  e. Earlier age at onset is associated with faster progression and development of dementia

  f. Progressive ataxia, hyporeflexia, slow saccades with progression to supranuclear ophthalmoplegia and complete ophthalmoparesis

  g. Extrapyramidal signs are less common

  h. More likely than SCA 1 or 3 to cause kinetic and postural tremor, myoclonus, early dementia, slow saccades, and hyporeflexia

  i. Pathology

    1) Macroscopic: pontine and cerebellar atrophy (Fig. 9-13)

    2) Microscopic: neuronal loss and gliosis involving Purkinje cells, inferior olivary nuclei, middle and inferior cerebellar peduncles, pontine nuclei, substantia nigra, and spinal cord (posterior columns, spinocerebellar tracts, Clarke's columns, anterior horn cells, corticospinal tracts, ventral and dorsal roots)

4. SCA 3 (ADCA I): Machado-Joseph disease

  a. CAG repeat expansion in chromosome 14q

  b. Gene product is ataxin-3 (cytoplasmic protein, nuclear inclusions only with disease)

  c. The length of repeats is inversely proportional with age at onset

  d. Ataxia, ophthalmoplegia, pyramidal and extrapyramidal features, polyneuropathy

  e. Three clinical phenotypes

    1) Type I: onset in adolescents—ataxia, ophthalmoparesis, pyramidal (spasticity and hyperreflexia) and extrapyramidal (rigidity, dystonia) features, facial and lingual fasciculations

    2) Type II: early to middle adulthood onset (mean, 36 years)—ataxia, pyramidal features, dystonia, polyneuropathy

    3) Type III: later onset (mean, 40 years)—ataxia, ophthalmoparesis, peripheral neuropathy, lower motor neuron symptoms of weakness, atrophy, and fasciculations

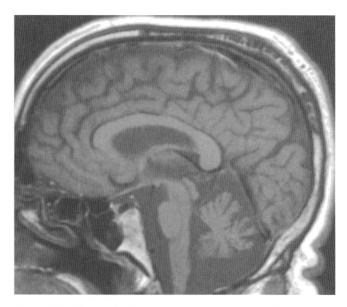

Fig. 9-13. T1-weighted magnetic resonance image from patient with spinocerebellar ataxia type 2 demonstrating marked pontocerebellar atrophy.

4) Type IV: oldest onset, adult (usually in the 40s)—parkinsonism, oral and facial fasciculations, sensory neuropathy, bulging eyes

  f. Pathology
  1) Neuronal loss and gliosis affecting the basal ganglia (globus pallidus, subthalamic nucleus, substantia nigra), red nucleus, pontine nuclei, dentate nucleus (Fig. 9-14), spinocerebellar tracts and Clarke's columns, cranial nerve nuclei, posterior columns, anterior horn cells
  2) Nucleus ambiguus and dorsal nucleus of the vagus may be affected
  3) Inferior olivary nuclei and Purkinje cells tend to be spared

5. SCA 7 (ADCA II)
  a. CAG repeat expansion in chromosome 3p
  b. Age at onset may vary from birth to 65 years
  c. Onset usually occurs with progressive visual loss, with macular degeneration
  d. With progression, ataxia of gait is followed by ataxic dysarthria and appendicular ataxia
  e. Early onset cases: deep tendon reflexes may be decreased
  f. Dementia, pyramidal signs, and peripheral neuropathy may be present
  g. Degenerative changes may be present in the cerebellum, retinal ganglion cells, basal pons, inferior olivary nucleus, with neuronal intranuclear inclusions

6. SCA 6 (ADCA III)
  a. Polymorphic CAG repeat in chromosome 19p

  b. *CACNA1A* gene coding for the α_{1A} voltage-dependent P/Q type calcium channel subunit (highest expression is in Purkinje cells)
  c. Age at onset is usually later than for most other autosomal dominant ataxias (fourth to fifth decades)
  d. Indolent benign course
  e. Ataxia (slow onset and progression)
  f. Horizontal gaze-evoked nystagmus and downbeat nystagmus
  g. Large-fiber peripheral neuropathy
  h. Other features may include pyramidal signs, possibly episodic ataxia
  i. Pathology
  1) Confined to the cerebellum and inferior olivary nuclei
  2) Severe loss of Purkinje cells, with proliferation of Bergmann glia, neuronal loss and gliosis in the inferior olivary nuclei (Fig. 9-15)

7. Episodic ataxia type 1
  a. Point mutation in the *KCNA1* gene, encoding the α subunit of voltage-gated potassium channels Kv1.1 responsible for the delayed rectifier potassium currents
  b. Early-childhood onset with brief attacks of ataxia and dysarthria (± dystonic or choreic features) 1 to 2 minutes in duration; attacks may occur several times daily
  c. Provoked by abrupt postural change, emotional stimulus, and caloric stimulation of the vestibular apparatus
  d. Interictal myokymia of the face and limbs
  e. Electromyography (EMG) at rest may show continuous spontaneous activity (neuromyotonia)
  f. Good prognosis: begins in early childhood and becomes milder with age

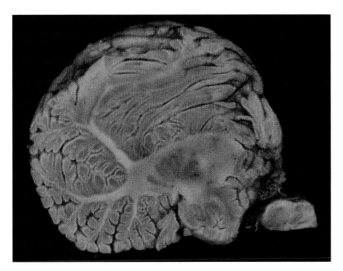

Fig. 9-14. Atrophy and discoloration of the dentate nucleus in spinocerebellar ataxia type 3 (Machado-Joseph disease). Note relative sparing of cerebellar folia (location of Purkinje cells) compared with the prominent atrophy seen in spinocerebellar ataxia type 2 (Fig. 9-13).

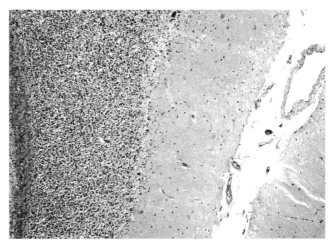

Fig. 9-15. Spinocerebellar ataxia type 6 is marked by severe loss of Purkinje cells and gliosis. There is relative sparing of the granule cells. (Hematoxylin-eosin.)

g. Diagnosis is based on clinical impression and interictal EMG findings

h. Management
   1) Avoidance of sudden movements
   2) Acetazolamide: may be less effective than for episodic ataxia type 2 in reducing attacks in some, not all, patients
   3) Phenytoin, carbamazepine

8. Episodic ataxia type 2
   a. Nonsense mutation causing truncation of the *CACNA1A* gene coding for α_{1A} voltage-dependent calcium channel subunit
      1) Missense mutations of the same gene are associated with familial hemiplegic migraines
      2) CAG expansion in the 3' end of the gene causes SCA 6
   b. Attacks last longer than those of episodic ataxia type 1 (>10 minutes) and are precipitated by emotional stress and physical exertion, not startle
   c. Attacks consist of ataxia (± vertigo, nausea, vomiting, headaches)
   d. Weakness is also possible during an attack (neuromuscular junction dysfunction?), 10% of patients have hemiplegic episodes
   e. Interictal gaze-evoked nystagmus
   f. With progression, chronic progressive gait ataxia may develop
   g. Cerebellar atrophy is possible
   h. Jitter and blocking may be seen on single-fiber EMG
   i. Treatment of choice: acetazolamide (500-700 mg daily); daily acetazolamide therapy often completely eliminates the attacks (better and more predictable response than episodic ataxia type 1)

9. DRPLA
   a. Autosomal dominant inheritance; due to unstable CAG trinucleotide repeat expansion (usually 49 to 75) on chromosome 12p13.31, with high penetrance
   b. Anticipation: paternal transmission tends to increase the repeat length more than maternal transmission
   c. Onset before age 20: usually progressive myoclonic epilepsy with seizures, dementia, ataxia, and myoclonus
   d. Onset after age 20: ataxia, dementia, choreoathetosis
   e. Most cases have been reported from Japan
   f. Homozygotes may have a more severe syndrome and spastic paraplegia or posterior column involvement
   g. MRI may show cerebellar and brainstem atrophy and hyperintense T2 lesions in the white matter in adults
   h. Pathology: neuronal loss and gliosis of the dentate nucleus and globus pallidus (posterior columns may be involved in severe cases)

D. Selected Acquired Ataxia
1. See Table 9-1 for differential diagnosis of cerebellar disorders
2. Toxic causes (see Chapter 17)
   a. Alcoholic cerebellar degeneration
      1) Due to both nutritional deficiency (such as thiamine deficiency) and alcohol neurotoxicity
      2) Gradually occurs only after 10 years or more of excessive alcohol intake
      3) Chronic midline cerebellar syndrome with truncal ataxia and titubation
      4) Atrophy of the superior and anterior parts of the vermis occurs with chronic alcoholism
      5) Loss of Purkinje cells, thinning of the molecular layer, and proliferation of Bergmann glia
   b. Chemotherapy agents: 5-fluorouracil, cytosine arabinoside, piperazine
   c. Metals (see Chapter 17)
      1) Organic mercury
         a) Paresthesias, ataxias, deafness, visual field constriction, and cortical blindness
         b) Causes neuronal degeneration, edema, gliosis in cerebellar granular layer, calcarine cortex, insular cortex, and dorsal root ganglia
      2) Thallium
      3) Bismuth
   d. Anticonvulsants (e.g., phenytoin)
      1) Transient cerebellar signs with supratherapeutic levels
      2) Purkinje cell loss in patients receiving long-term phenytoin treatment
3. Infectious causes (refer to the corresponding section for more detail)
   a. Acute or subacute onset
      1) Cryptogenic is most common
      2) Second most common is varicella (peak incidence 5-6 years of age)
      3) Coxsackievirus groups A and B, echovirus, Epstein-Barr virus, poliovirus
      4) *Borrelia burgdorferi* infection (Lyme disease), *Mycoplasma* infection, *Plasmodium falciparum*, cysticercosis, tuberculosis, Whipple's disease
      5) Human immunodeficiency virus and complications, including progressive multifocal leukoencephalopathy and toxoplasmosis
   b. Chronic: chronic panencephalitis of congenital rubella
4. Prion disease
   a. Creutzfeldt-Jakob disease (especially new variant Creutzfeldt-Jakob disease)
   b. Gerstmann-Sträussler-Scheinker syndrome
5. Autoimmune causes

a. Paraneoplastic cerebellar degeneration (see Chapter 16)
   1) Subacute or acute onset with initial rapid progression and subsequent stabilization of the neurologic course
   2) Usually a pancerebellar syndrome
   3) Other systems that may be slightly affected include pyramidal and extrapyramidal systems, cognition, and peripheral nerves
   4) Most common associated tumors: ovarian cancer, lung cancer, lymphoma
   5) "Pure paraneoplastic cerebellar degeneration"
      a) Anti-Purkinje cell antibodies (anti-Yo and anti-Tr antibodies) and anti-mGluR1 antibodies are associated with a pancerebellar syndrome
      b) Associated tumors: gynecologic and breast tumors usually with anti-Yo (PCA-1) antibodies, adenocarcinoma of lung, Hodgkin's lymphoma
   6) Paraneoplastic encephalomyelitis with or without paraneoplastic cerebellar degeneration
      a) Associated with anti-Hu (antineuronal antibody [ANNA]-1) antibodies: usually associated with small cell lung carcinoma and breast cancer
   7) Paraneoplastic opsoclonus with or without paraneoplastic cerebellar degeneration
      a) Associated with anti-Ri (ANNA-2) antibodies
      b) Ovarian and breast cancers, small cell lung carcinoma
      c) Female preponderance
   8) Paraneoplastic cerebellar degeneration with Lambert-Eaton myasthenic syndrome: more than half of the patients with paraneoplastic cerebellar degeneration and anti–voltage-gated calcium channel antibodies may also have Lambert-Eaton myasthenic syndrome
b. Ataxia with gluten sensitivity
   1) Gluten sensitivity observed in 41% of idiopathic sporadic ataxias as defined by presence of circulating antigliadin antibodies (IgG with or without IgA) (Hadjivassiliou et al.)
   2) Malabsorption is not a cause of the ataxia
   3) Slowly progressive ataxia (may be rapid with development of cerebellar atrophy within a year after onset)
   4) Antibodies bind to Purkinje cells
   5) Sensorimotor peripheral neuropathy, mononeuritis multiplex, pure motor neuropathy, small-fiber neuropathy
   6) Mild cognitive changes
   7) Association with HLA-DQ2, HLA-DQ8, HLA-DQ1
   8) Jejunal biopsy specimens may appear normal because bowel involvement is patchy

   9) Response of the neurologic symptoms to a gluten-free diet is unclear
c. Ataxia with anti-GAD antibodies
   1) Onset: usually middle-aged women, but age at onset varies
   2) Slowly progressive ataxia with dysarthria, associated with peripheral neuropathy, slow saccades, and stiffness (15% of patients)
   3) Associated with thyroiditis and diabetes mellitus (organ-specific antibodies, including anti-parietal cell antibodies)
d. Bickerstaff's brainstem encephalitis
   1) Most frequent preceding symptoms are related to an upper respiratory tract infection
   2) Most frequent initial symptoms are diplopia and gait disturbance
   3) Clinical features: disturbance of consciousness, ophthalmoplegia, hyperreflexia, ataxia
   4) Frequent symptoms: pupillary abnormalities, facial weakness, bulbar palsy, pyramidal involvement with extensor plantar responses
   5) Flaccid limb weakness (likely close association and overlap with Guillain-Barré syndrome in a continuous spectrum)
   6) Serum antibodies to GQ1b ganglioside
   7) MRI may show high T2 signal involving brainstem, thalamus, cerebellum (may regress with clinical course)
   8) Cerebrospinal fluid findings vary: may be normal or show albuminocytologic dissociation or pleocytosis
   9) Electrodiagnostic evaluation may mimic acute motor axonal neuropathy and show low distal compound muscle action potentials
   10) No definitive pathologic features
   11) Treatment: intravenous immune globulin or plasma exchange may be tried
e. Sporadic degenerative ataxias
   1) Sporadic cerebellar degeneration
      a) Age at onset is usually after 50 years
      b) Clinical presentation is limited to cerebellar signs and symptoms
      c) Clinicians must exclude inherited causes of ataxia even in the absence of a family history
      d) Cerebellar atrophy may be found with disease progression
      e) Pathology findings may be nonspecific or consistent with multiple system atrophy
   2) Multiple system atrophy (see Chapter 8 for details)

References

Aicardi J, Barbosa C, Andermann E, Andermann F, Morcos R, Ghanem Q, et al. Ataxia-ocular motor apraxia: a syndrome mimicking ataxia-telangiectasia. Ann Neurol. 1988;24:497-502.

Albin RL. Dominant ataxias and Friedreich ataxia: an update. Curr Opin Neurol. 2003;16:507-14.

Bolla L, Palmer RM. Paraneoplastic cerebellar degeneration: case report and literature review. Arch Intern Med. 1997;147:157-62.

Dotti MT, Federico A, Signorini E, Caputo N, Venturi C, Filosomi G, et al. Cerebrotendinous xanthomatosis (Van Bogaert-Scherer-Epstein disease): CT and MR findings. AJNR Am J Neuroradiol. 1994;15:1721-6.

Fogli A, Wong K, Eymard-Pierre E, Wenger J, Bouffard JP, Goldin E, et al. Cree leukoencephalopathy and CACH/VWM disease are allelic at the EIF2B5 locus. Ann Neurol. 2002;52:506-10.

Gomez MR. Cerebellotrigeminal and focal dermal dysplasia: a newly recognized neurocutaneous syndrome. Brain Dev. 1979;1:253-6.

Hadjivassiliou M, Grunewald RA, Davies-Jones GA. Gluten sensitivity as a neurological illness. J Neurol Neurosurg Psychiatry. 2002;72:560-3.

Hannan MA, Sigut D, Waghray M, Gascon GG. Ataxia-ocular motor apraxia syndrome: an investigation of cellular radiosensitivity of patients and their families. J Med Genet. 1994;31:953-6.

Horoupian DS, Zucker DK, Moshe S, Peterson HD. Behr syndrome: a clinicopathologic report. Neurology. 1979;29:323-7.

Jaeken J, Eggermont E, Stibler H. An apparent homozygous X-linked disorder with carbohydrate-deficient serum glycoproteins. Lancet. 1987;2:1398.

Jaeken J, Stibler H. A newly recognized inherited neurological disease with carbohydrate deficient secretory glycoproteins. In: Wetterberg L, editor. Genetics of neuropsychiatric diseases. Proceedings of an international symposium held at the Wenner-Gren Center; 1989 May 26-28; Stockholm, Sweden. Wenner-Gren Center International Symposium Series. Vol 51. London: Macmillan Press; 1989. p. 69-80.

Johnson WG, Murphy M, Murphy WI, Bloom AD. Recessive congenital cerebellar disorder in a genetic isolate: CPD type VII? [Abstract.] Neurology. 1978;28:352-3.

Klockgether T. Hereditary ataxias. In: Jankovic JJ, Tolosa E, editors. Parkinson's disease and movement disorders. 4th ed. Philadelphia: Lippincott Williams & Wilkins; 2002. p. 553-65.

Koskinen T, Santavuori P, Sainio K, Lappi M, Kallio AK, Pihko H. Infantile onset spinocerebellar ataxia with sensory neuropathy: a new inherited disease. J Neurol Sci. 1994;121:50-6.

Kumar S, Rankin R. Renal insufficiency is a component of COACH syndrome. Am J Med Genet. 1996;61:122-6.

Kvistad PH, Dahl A, Skre H. Autosomal recessive non-progressive ataxia with an early childhood debut. Acta Neurol Scand. 1985;71:295-302.

Lagier-Tourenne C, Chaigne D, Gong J, Flori J, Mohr M, Ruh D, et al. Linkage to 18qter differentiates two clinically overlapping syndromes: congenital cataracts-facial dysmorphism-neuropathy (CCFDN) syndrome and Marinesco-Sjögren syndrome. J Med Genet. 2002;39:838-43.

Lynch DR, Farmer J. Practical approaches to neurogenetic disease. J Neuroophthalmol. 2002;22:297-304.

Margolis G, Kilham L. Virus-induced cerebellar hypoplasia. Res Publ Assoc Res Nerv Ment Dis. 1968;44:113-46.

McHale DP, Jackson AP, Campbell DA, Levene MI, Corry P, Woods CG, et al. A gene for ataxic cerebral palsy maps to chromosome 9p12-q12. Eur J Hum Genet. 2000;8:267-72.

Merlini L, Gooding R, Lochmuller H, Muller-Felber W, Walter MC, Angelicheva D, et al. Genetic identity of Marinesco-Sjögren/myoglobinuria and CCFDN syndromes. Neurology. 2002;58:231-6.

Montermini L, Rodius F, Pianese L, Molto MD, Cossee M, Campuzano V, et al. The Friedreich ataxia critical region spans a 150-kb interval on chromosome 9q13. Am J Hum Genet. 1995;57:1061-7.

Moreira MC, Barbot C, Tachi N, Kozuka N, Mendonca P, Barros J, et al. Homozygosity mapping of Portuguese and Japanese forms of ataxia-oculomotor apraxia to 9p13, and evidence for genetic heterogeneity. Am J Hum Genet. 2001;68:501-8.

Murray C, Shipman P, Khangure M, Chakera T, Robbins P, McAuliffe W, et al. Lhermitte-Doclos disease associated with Cowden's syndrome: case report and literature review. Australas Radiol. 2001;45:343-6.

Nelson J, Flaherty M, Grattan-Smith P. Gillespie syndrome: a report of two further cases. Am J Med Genet. 1997;71:134-8.

Nystuen A, Benke PJ, Merren J, Stone EM, Sheffield VC. A cerebellar ataxia locus identified by DNA pooling to search for linkage disequilibrium in an isolated population from the Cayman Islands. Hum Mol Genet. 1996;5:525-31.

Odaka M, Yuki N, Yamada M, Koga M, Takemi T, Hirata K, et al. Bickerstaff's brainstem encephalitis: clinical features of 62 cases and a subgroup associated with Guillain-Barré syndrome. Brain. 2003;126:2279-90.

Parisi MA, Dobyns WB. Human malformations of the midbrain and hindbrain: review and proposed classification scheme. Mol Genet Metab. 2003;80:36-53.

Richardson JP, Mohammad SS, Pavitt GD. Mutations causing childhood ataxia with central nervous system hypomyelination reduce eukaryotic initiation factor 2B complex formation and activity. Mol Cell Biol. 2004;24:2352-63.

Sasaki K, Suga K, Tsugawa S, Sakuma K, Tachi N, Chiba S, et al. Muscle pathology in Marinesco-Sjögren syndrome: a unique ultrastructural feature. Brain Dev. 1996;18:64-7.

Sudha T, Dawson AJ, Prasad AN, Konkin D, de Groot GW, Prasad C. De novo interstitial long arm deletion of chromosome 3 with facial dysmorphism, Dandy-Walker variant malformation and hydrocephalus. Clin Dysmorphol. 2001;10:193-6.

Sztriha L, Al-Gazalli LI, Aithala GR, Nork M. Joubert's syndrome: new cases and review of clinicopathologic correlation. Pediatr Neurol. 1999;20:274-81.

Valente EM, Salpietro DC, Brancati F, Bertini E, Galluccio T, Tortorella G, et al. Description, nomenclature, and mapping of a novel cerebello-renal syndrome with the molar tooth malformation. Am J Hum Genet. 2003;73:663-70.

Van Dyke DH, Griggs RC, Murphy MJ, Goldstein MN. Hereditary myokymia and periodic ataxia. J Neurol Sci 1975;25:109-18.

Verloes A, Lambotte C. Further delineation of a syndrome of cerebellar vermis hypo/aplasia, oligophrenia, congenital ataxia, coloboma, and hepatic fibrosis. Am J Med Genet. 1989;32:227-32.

Wiesner GL, Snover DC, Rank J, Tuchman M. Familial cerebellar ataxia and hepatic fibrosis: a variant of COACH syndrome with biliary ductal proliferation [abstract]. Am J Hum Genet. 1992 Suppl:A110.

QUESTIONS

1-5. Match the following conditions (1-5) with the associated gene mutation (a-e):

1. Childhood ataxia with central hypomyelination   a. *ATM*

2. Ataxia telangiectasia   b. *Ataxin*

3. Spinocerebellar ataxia (SCA) 1   c. *Frataxin*

4. Megencephalic leukoencephalopathy with subcortical cysts   d. *MLC1*

5. Friedreich's ataxia   e. *eIF2B*

6. Which of the following is *not* a feature of classic Joubert syndrome (Joubert syndrome type 1)?
   a. Infantile hypotonia
   b. Ataxia and developmental delay
   c. Abnormal breathing pattern
   d. Retinal dystrophy
   e. "Molar tooth sign"

7-10. Match the following disorders (7-10) with the corresponding treatments (a-d):

7. Bassen-Kornzweig syndrome   a. Reduced fat intake and high dose vitamin E

8. Refsum's disease   b. Cholic acid, chenodeoxycholic acid, and simvastatin

9. Cerebrotendinous xanthomatosis   c. Dietary restriction of phytanic acid

10. Ataxia with isolated vitamin E deficiency   d. High fat intake and vitamine E supplements

ANSWERS

1. Answer: e.

2. Answer: a.

3. Answer: b.

4. Answer: d.

5. Answer: c.

6. Answer: d.
All the features listed are typical of classic Joubert syndrome except for retinal dystrophy, which is a feature of cerebello-oculorenal syndrome (Joubert syndrome type 2).

7. Answer: a.

8. Answer: c.

9. Answer: b.

10. Answer: d.

Kelly D. Flemming, M.D.

I. PRINCIPLES OF COMA AND DELIRIUM
(SEE CHAPTER 7, PART A)

A. Consciousness: definition and anatomy

1. Consciousness
   a. Consists of arousal (ability to interact with external environment, wakefulness) and awareness of content (ability to perceive and understand content)
   b. States of consciousness are defined in Table 10-1
2. Anatomical structures involved in consciousness
   a. As noted above, consciousness is defined by arousal and awareness of content, thus certain parts of the brain are involved in these activities
   b. Arousal is predominantly a function of the ascending reticular activating system (ARAS)
      1) ARAS cell bodies are in pons and midbrain and the axons ascend in the central tegmental tract
      2) ARAS receives collaterals from somatic and special sensory systems
      3) ARAS projects to the reticular nucleus of thalamus and to hypothalamus (which projects to limbic cortex and basal forebrain)
      4) In addition, the midline raphe nuclei and locus ceruleus project diffusely to cerebral cortex
   c. Awareness of content is a direct function of the cerebral hemispheres and the projections to them from thalamus, hypothalamus, brainstem
   d. The anatomical structures of the ARAS and their connections are noted in Figure 10-1 and Table 10-2 (for additional details on anatomical structures involved in consciousness and attention, see Chapter 7)
   e. Change in consciousness may be due to diffuse, multifocal, or strategic lesions

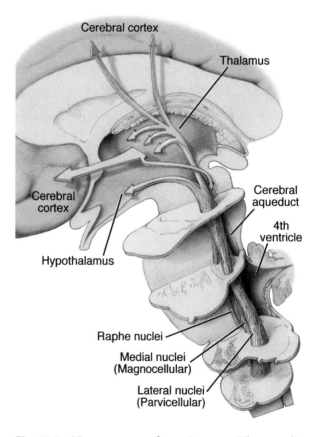

Fig. 10-1. Neuroanatomy of consciousness. The ascending reticular activating system is responsible for arousal and projects to the thalamus, hypothalamus, raphe nuclei, and locus ceruleus. The cerebral hemispheres interpret content of awareness. (From Wijdicks EFM. Neurologic catastrophes in the emergency department. Boston: Butterworth-Heinemann; 2000. p. 3-39. By permission of Mayo Foundation.)

Three Anatomical Areas to Alter Level of Consciousness
Reticular formation (upper midbrain)
Bilateral diencephalon (thalamus)
Bilateral cerebral hemisphere

Table 10-1. Levels of Consciousness

State	Description
Obtundation	Mild-to-moderate decreased level of alertness and interest in environment
	Appears to be in sleep state
	May have avoidance reactions to noxious stimuli
Stupor	Decreased level of alertness
	Aroused by vigorous stimuli
Coma	Decreased level of alertness
	Eyes closed
	No response to noxious stimuli
	No understanding of external stimuli—utters no understandable words and unable to localize noxious stimuli
	Extensor or flexor posturing may be present
Persistent vegetative state	May occur after a period of coma
	Arousal present, but no awareness
	Not able to understand content of sensory stimuli
	Eyes open and appear to be tracking
Delirium	Fluctuating change in cognition and consciousness not attributable to dementia
	Common findings include disorientation, misperception of sensory stimuli, visual hallucinations
	Commonly due to medical condition, medications, withdrawal or toxic syndromes or combination
Akinetic mutism	Alert appearing, but unable to recognize content
	Spontaneous motor activity is lacking
Locked-in syndrome	Paralysis of extremities and lower cranial nerves
	No impairment of consciousness
	May be able to communicate with eye movements
	Often due to large pontine lesions sparing ascending reticular activating system

Table 10-2. Structures Involved in Consciousness and Their Connections

Structure	Description	Input	Output
Reticular formation	Ascending reticular activating system originates in upper pons and midbrain	Motor paths Sensory paths	Thalamus (reticular nucleus) Hypothalamus, projects to limbic system Brainstem (raphe nuclei, locus ceruleus), projects to cerebral cortex
Diencephalon	Reticular nucleus of thalamus, serves as gating mechanism for information reaching cortex (consciousness)	All other thalamic nuclei except non-specific nuclei of thalamus and anterior nucleus of thalamus Ascending reticular activating system	Cerebral cortex
Cerebral cortex	Widespread cerebral cortex	Reticular nucleus of thalamus Raphe nuclei and locus ceruleus	Reticular nucleus of thalamus Corticocortical connections

1) Toxic-metabolic causes affect cerebral hemispheres and brainstem in diffuse manner
2) Unilateral supratentorial lesions with mass effect toward opposite hemisphere or with central herniation may result in reduced level of consciousness, as may multifocal supratentorial lesions
3) Diencephalic lesions (usually bilateral) may result in reduced levels of consciousness
4) Infratentorial lesions involving ARAS may result in reduced levels of consciousness

B. Clinical Approach to Coma

1. Differential diagnosis is listed in Table 10-3
2. Clinical history
   a. Obtain information from witnesses about onset and course, medical history, and medications
   b. Specifically obtain information about recent injury or trauma, seizure-like activity, recent symptoms (including fever, previous medical problems)
3. Examination: used to localize the problem and determine prognosis (Fig. 10-2)
   a. General examination
      1) Look for signs of trauma (Battle's sign, i.e., bruising of

Table 10-3.   **Differential Diagnosis of Coma**

Vascular	Ischemic stroke—bihemispheric, diencephalic, upper brainstem			Hyper- or hypoglycemia
	Cerebral venous thrombosis			Hypercapnia
	Hemorrhage—subarachnoid, intraparenchymal, subdural, epidural			Hyper- or hyponatremia
				Hypothyroid
	Pituitary apoplexy			Hyper- or hypothermia
	Diffuse hypoxia			Lactic acidosis and mitochondrial disease
	Hypertensive encephalopathy			Porphyria
Infectious	Cerebral abscess			Uremia
	Subdural empyema			Wernicke's encephalopathy
	Viral encephalitis	Toxins	Carbon monoxide
	Malaria		Cyanide
	Typhoid fever		Ethylene glycol
	Sepsis		Lead
	Syphilis		Methanol
	Postinfectious encephalomyelitis	Medications, drugs	Alcohol
Inflammatory	Acute demyelinating encephalomyelitis		Anticholinergics
	Multiple sclerosis (fulminant)		Barbiturates
	Multifocal leukoencephalopathy		Lithium
Neoplastic	Any neoplasm—bihemispheric, unilateral hemisphere with midline shift and herniation, diencephalic, upper brainstem, associated with hydrocephalus		Opiates
			Psychotropics
			Benzodiazepines
		Other	Status epilepticus
			Hydrocephalus
Paraneoplastic	Limbic encephalitis		Trauma
Metabolic	Addisonian crisis		Reye's syndrome
	Diabetic ketoacidosis	Mimics	Locked-in syndrome
	Dialysis encephalopathy		Catatonia
	Hepatic encephalopathy		Conversion reaction
	Hyper- or hypocalcemia		Neuromuscular weakness—Guillain-Barré syndrome, myasthenia gravis
	Hypermagnesemia		

mastoid), cerebrospinal fluid (CSF) leak
   2) Evidence of seizure activity: tongue biting, urinary incontinence
   b. Level of consciousness
      1) See Table 10-1
      2) Glasgow Coma Scale (GCS) score is commonly used
   c. Respiratory
      1) Respiratory pattern should be observed, may provide localization information (Fig. 10-2)
      2) Many patients require mechanical ventilation, obscuring ability to observe these patterns
   d. Eyes
      1) Oculocephalic (doll's eyes)
         a) Remember to rule out cervical spine injury before performing this maneuver
         b) Rotate head from side to side or vertically
            i) In normal functioning brainstem, eyes move opposite the head movement and are conjugate

      ii) Normal function implies that cranial nerves (CNs) III and VI (horizontal) or CNs III and IV (vertical) are intact in pons and midbrain, also the medial longitudinal fasciculus that connects CNs III and VI
   2) Caloric testing
      a) Be sure tympanic membrane is intact and head of bed is at 30 degrees
      b) Instill cold water in ear
      c) If brainstem is intact, tonic deviation of eyes toward cold ear (this also assesses CNs III and VI, medial longitudinal fasciculus, and vestibular input [CN VIII])
   3) Pupils: observe size and reactivity (for pupillary pathways, see Chapter 3)
      a) Midposition, fixed pupils: rule out trauma, eye drops, medications (atropine) or poisoning as cause of fixed pupils

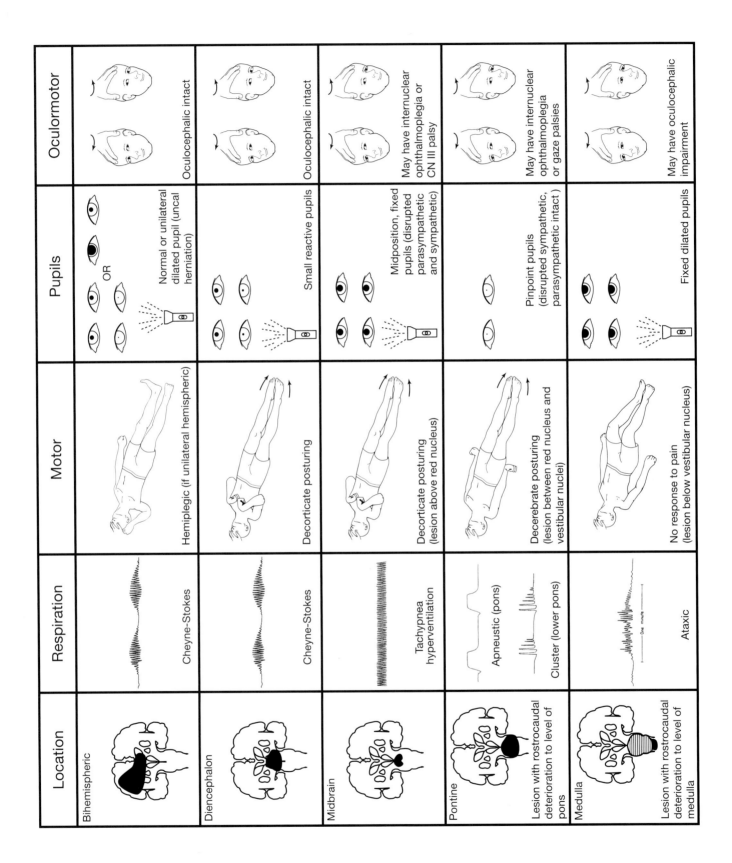

Location	Respiration	Motor	Pupils	Oculomotor
Bihemispheric	Cheyne-Stokes	Hemiplegic (if unilateral hemispheric)	Normal or unilateral dilated pupil (uncal herniation)	Oculocephalic intact
Diencephalon	Cheyne-Stokes	Decorticate posturing	Small reactive pupils	Oculocephalic intact
Midbrain	Tachypnea hyperventilation	Decorticate posturing (lesion above red nucleus)	Midposition, fixed pupils (disrupted parasympathetic and sympathetic)	May have internuclear ophthalmoplegia or CN III palsy
Pontine Lesion with rostrocaudal deterioration to level of pons	Apneustic (pons) Cluster (lower pons)	Decerebrate posturing (lesion between red nucleus and vestibular nuclei)	Pinpoint pupils (disrupted sympathetic, parasympathetic intact)	May have internuclear ophthalmoplegia or gaze palsies
Medulla Lesion with rostrocaudal deterioration to level of medulla	Ataxic One minute	No response to pain (lesion below vestibular nucleus)	Fixed dilated pupils	May have oculocephalic impairment

Fig. 10-2. Examination findings in coma.

Glasgow Coma Scale

Points	Best eye	Best verbal	Best motor
6	---	---	Obeys commands
5	---	Oriented	Localizes pain
4	Sponta-neous	Confused	Withdraws in response to pain
3	To speech	Inappropriate	Flexion (decorticate)
2	To pain	Incompre-hensible	Extension (decerebrate)
1	None	None	None

    i) Often a result of diffuse midbrain lesion or midbrain damage from transtentorial herniation
    ii) Sympathetic tone and parasympathetic tone are impaired, causing midposition pupils
    iii) Efferent path of light reflex is impaired, so pupils are unreactive
  b) Pinpoint pupils: rule out toxins and medications (narcotics) as cause
    i) Typically found with pontine lesion
    ii) Bilateral impairment of sympathetic nerves produces pinpoint pupils because of unopposed tonic parasympathetics (CN III)
    iii) May also have small pupils from lesions in upper brainstem (above red nucleus) and diencephalic region because of impaired sympathetic outflow from hypothalamus
  c) Fixed, dilated pupils: rule out toxins and metabolic dysfunction (e.g., hypothermia, barbiturates); can be related also to extensive medullary lesion
  d) Unequal pupil size: consider Horner's syndrome (sympathetic dysfunction) vs. CN III nerve palsy (see Chapter 3)
  e) Poor pupil reactivity: consider if the lesion is afferent (CN II), efferent (CN III), or in midbrain tectum
 4) Gaze preference
  a) Horizontal gaze preference may occur at level of frontal cortex or in pons
  b) Gaze preference at level of pons can affect medial longitudinal fasciculus and CN VI or nucleus of CN VI

    i) Patients look *toward* the side of hemiparesis if there is concomitant corticospinal tract damage
    ii) Oculocephalic maneuver will *not* overcome gaze preference
  c) Gaze preference at the level of the frontal cortex is result of frontal eye field being affected
    i) Patients look *away* from side of hemiparesis if the corticospinal tract is also involved
    ii) Oculocephalic maneuver will overcome gaze preference (i.e., patient's eyes will cross midline with oculocephalic maneuver)
 5) Spontaneous eye movements
  a) Skew deviation: may localize to midbrain (CNs III and IV)
  b) Periodic alternating gaze: eyes deviate side to side; may be related to bilateral cerebral hemisphere dysfunction
  c) Ocular bobbing: may localize to pons
e. Motor response to stimulus
 1) Rubrospinal tracts beginning in midbrain project to ventral horn cells of contralateral flexors of upper extremities
 2) Pontine reticulospinal tracts and medullary vestibulospinal tracts (both excitatory) project to ventral horn cells of extensors of extremities
 3) Corticospinal tract projects to extremities to control fine motor movements, and varying influences of corticospinal and extrapyramidal tracts result in normal tone
 4) Decorticate posturing, i.e., flexion of upper extremities, extension of lower extremities: the lesion is *above* the red nucleus and cortical influence is impaired (Fig. 10-2)
 5) Decerebrate posturing, i.e., extension of all four extremities: the lesion is *below* the red nucleus and *above* the vestibular nuclei (Fig. 10-2)
 6) Lesions *below* the vestibular nuclei may result in absent movement of the extremities because of disruption of projections from vestibular and pontine reticular nuclei that provide extensor tone; the medullary reticulospinal tract remains intact and is inhibitory to motor neurons controlling extensors of the extremities

C. Clinical Management of Comatose Patients (Table 10-4)

D. Brain Death
1. Definition: cessation of all brain and brainstem function

Table 10-4. **Clinical Management of Comatose Patients**

Airway, breathing, circulation	Assess airway
	Intubate if necessary
	Check oxygen saturation, administer oxygen as needed
	Assess blood pressure and pulse
	Place cardiac monitor
Stat lab tests	Check glucose finger stick
	Arterial blood gas
	Electrolytes, complete blood count, calcium, magnesium, ammonia, drug levels, PT, PTT
	Consider toxin screen
Supportive measures	Thiamine 50-100 mg IV
	Naloxone (Narcan) 1 ampule IV
	Glucose D-50 IV (at least 25 mL)
History	Gather basic clinical history
Examination	If signs or symptoms suggestive of meningitis (altered mental status, fever, meningismus), consider empiric antibiotics and perform lumbar puncture if safe
	If signs or symptoms suggest herniation (progressive obtundation, decorticate or decerebrate posturing, unilateral CN III palsy), initiate measures to lower ICP
	If clinical evidence of seizures, load with antiepileptic medication
CT	CT of head without contrast
	Check and clear cervical spine
Lumbar puncture	Consider lumbar puncture to rule out subarachnoid hemorrhage or infection if no evidence on CT of herniation and no other cause for coma found
Other	Treat specific metabolic, CT, or lumbar puncture results
	Obtain further clinical history

CN, cranial nerve; CT, computed tomography; D-50, 50% dextrose in distilled water; ICP, intracranial pressure; IV, intravenous; PT, prothrombin time; PTT, partial thromboplastin time.

2. Criteria for brain death vary among countries
3. Only consider applying the following criteria after ruling out possible confounding conditions: severe metabolic disturbances, drug intoxication (sedatives, barbiturates, etc.), poisoning, neuromuscular blocking agents, severe hypothermia (temperature <32°C), hypotension
4. Criteria include
   a. Coma
   b. Absence of motor responses
      1) These include absence of response to deep central

pain and absence of decorticate or decerebrate posturing
   2) Spinal cord–mediated reflexes are compatible with brain death, including flexor plantar response, rapid flexion of arms, raising one or all limbs off the bed and sitting up ("Lazarus sign"), or jerking of one limb or multifocal spinal myoclonus
c. Absence of pupillary responses to light; pupils at midposition
d. Absence of corneal reflexes
e. Absence of gag reflex
f. Absence of cough with tracheal suctioning
g. Absence of sucking and rooting reflexes
h. Absence of respiratory drive (apnea) at $PaCO_2$ 60 mm Hg or at 20 mm Hg above normal baseline pressure
   1) Apnea test is important component of evaluation of patient for brain death
   2) Subject should fulfill all above criteria before apnea test is considered
   3) Additional prerequisites for the test: positive fluid balance, absence of hypothermia (core temperature >32.2°C), systolic blood pressure >90 mm Hg, arterial $PaCO_2 \geq 40$ mm Hg, arterial $PaO_2 \geq 200$ mm Hg
   4) Apnea: the lack of any spontaneous respirations after discontinuation of the ventilator
   5) Positive apnea test (apnea related to brain death): $PaCO_2$ level is more than 60 mm Hg without respirations
   6) Patients with chronic hypercapnea (CO_2 retainers, e.g., patients with chronic obstructive pulmonary disease) have higher $PaCO_2$ levels at baseline: apnea test may be unreliable and a confirmatory test should be considered
   7) $PaCO_2$ level increases 3 to 6 mm Hg per minute and 6 to 8 minutes may be needed to reach target level of 60 mm Hg; this may be facilitated if apnea test is started at baseline of 40 mm Hg
   8) Because severe hypoxemia predisposes patient to cardiac arrhythmias and must be avoided, ventilate for 15 minutes with 100% oxygen before the test and through a catheter placed at the level of the carina during testing
   9) Baseline arterial blood gases should be measured and repeated at regular intervals until the criterion for positive apnea test is met
i. Interval between two evaluations according to age
   1) Term to 2 months old: 48 hours
   2) >2 months to 1 year old: 24 hours
   3) >1 year but <18 years old: 12 hours
   4) ≥18 years old: first exam may be used (according to

some authorities) with overwhelming clinical evidence of brain death

   j. Confirmatory test

     1) Term to 2 months old: 2 confirmatory tests

     2) >2 months to 1 year old: 1 confirmatory test

     3) >1 year but <18 years old: optional

     4) ≥18 years old: optional

   k. Optional confirmatory tests: electroencephalography (EEG), cerebral angiography, transcranial Doppler, nuclear studies

E. Clinical Approach to Delirium

1. Definition: fluctuating alteration of consciousness and cognition due to general medical condition
2. Predisposing factors
   a. Elderly
   b. Dementia
   c. Metabolic disturbances
   d. Visual or auditory impairment
3. Causes
   a. Many of same factors that result in coma may result in delirium, but delirium more commonly is due to toxic-metabolic mechanisms
   b. Other common causes: medications, withdrawal syndromes, systemic infections, surgery, electrolyte fluctuations, hypoxemia (see Chapter 7)
4. Management
   a. Identify precipitating factors
   b. Adjust environment to improve sleep-wake cycle, reduce noxious stimuli, reduce noise
   c. Medications if needed may include neuroleptics

II. INTRAPARENCHYMAL CEREBRAL HEMORRHAGE (ICH)

A. Pathophysiology

1. ICH results in shear force through brain parenchyma
2. Imaging studies show rebleeding may occur within first 12 hours after onset of symptoms
3. Edema (both vasogenic and cytotoxic) occurs and may cause clinical deterioration, generally between 24 and 72 hours

B. Differential Diagnosis: varies according to site (Table 10-5)

1. Hypertensive hemorrhages usually occur in deep locations, in following order of decreasing prevalence:
   a. Basal ganglia (Fig. 10-3)
   b. Subcortical white matter

   c. Cerebellum

   d. Thalamus

   e. Pons

2. Amyloid angiopathy
   a. Common cause of lobar intraparenchymal hemorrhages in elderly (generally >65 years)
   b. Congophilic (amyloid) material is deposited in small blood vessels of brain and meninges and may result in hemorrhage
   c. This amyloid is similar to that deposited in Alzheimer-type plaques (Fig. 10-4)
   d. High risk of hemorrhage recurrence, especially if the patient carries APOE ε2 or ε4 allele

C. Clinical Presentation

1. Focal neurologic deficits
2. Headache
3. Nausea, vomiting
4. Alteration in level of consciousness

D. Diagnostic Evaluation

1. Computed tomography (CT) of head: hyperdensity consistent with blood
2. Magnetic resonance imaging (MRI)
   a. May be useful to rule out underlying structural abnormality such as arteriovenous malformation or tumor
   b. Gradient echo sequences may demonstrate silent micro-hemorrhages in patients with amyloid angiopathy or those with cavernous malformations
   c. Can be used to determine approximate timing of hemorrhage (Fig. 10-5, Table 10-6)
3. Angiography: may be required to rule out aneurysm or arteriovenous malformation, especially in lobar-related hemorrhages

E. Management

1. Supportive measures
2. Blood pressure: should maintain mean arterial pressure less than 120 to 130 mm Hg
3. Mechanical ventilation: may be required, especially in comatose patients
4. Corticosteroids (methylprednisolone, dexamethasone): clinical trials have not shown benefit
5. Surgical options: several randomized clinical trials evaluated surgical evacuation of hemorrhage vs. supportive care—mixed results but majority showed no difference in surgery vs. supportive care; one trial showed that surgery could improve mortality but not morbidity; ongoing studies are evaluating whether early surgery may help

6. Recombinant factor VIIa
   a. Early treatment with recombinant factor VIIa after onset of ICH limits growth of the hematoma, reduces mortality, and improves functional outcomes
   b. Increased risk of thromboembolic complications

F. Outcome
1. Most consistent and sensitive predictors of outcome: size (volume) of hemorrhage and initial GCS score
2. Possible additional predictors: deep location, intraventricular extension, time to presentation
3. Volume more than 60 mL or GCS score less than 8 (or both) predicts poor outcome

III. Subarachnoid Hemorrhage (SAH)

A. Pathophysiology
1. SAH: extravasated blood in subarachnoid space
   a. Dural innervation is the substrate for pain
   b. Patients may have altered levels of consciousness, nausea, and vomiting with hydrocephalus
2. Most common cause of all SAHs: trauma
3. Most common cause of nontraumatic SAHs: aneurysm rupture

Table 10-5.   **Differential Diagnosis of Intraparenchymal Cerebral Hemorrhage**

Hypertensive—most commonly basal ganglia, internal capsule, pons, cerebellum
Hypertensive vasculopathy, eclampsia
Cerebral amyloid angiopathy—commonly lobar, older patients
Arteriovenous malformation
Cavernous malformation
Aneurysm rupture—can result in both subarachnoid hemorrhage and intraparenchymal cerebral hemorrhage
Moyamoya disease—typically basal ganglia
Vasculitis
Primary central nervous system tumor
Metastatic tumor—renal cell carcinoma, melanoma, lung cancer, choriocarcinoma
Bleeding diathesis—low platelet count, disseminated intravascular coagulation
Hemorrhagic conversion of ischemic stroke
Venous hypertension and infarction—typically cortical
Traumatic contusion—usually frontal pole and tip of temporal lobe
Medications—sympathomimetics, thrombolytic medication, warfarin

B. Presentation
1. Thunderclap headache or "the worst headache of my life"
2. Nausea, vomiting
3. Meningismus
4. Patient may have altered level of consciousness
5. May have focal neurologic symptoms if ICH present in addition to SAH
6. Ocular hemorrhage
   a. Subhyaloid hemorrhage
   b. Retinal hemorrhage
   c. Vitreal hemorrhage (Terson's syndrome)

C. Diagnosis
1. Complaint of a thunderclap headache should alert clinician to diagnosis of SAH
2. Head CT without contrast
   a. 92% of patients scanned within 24 hours after symptom

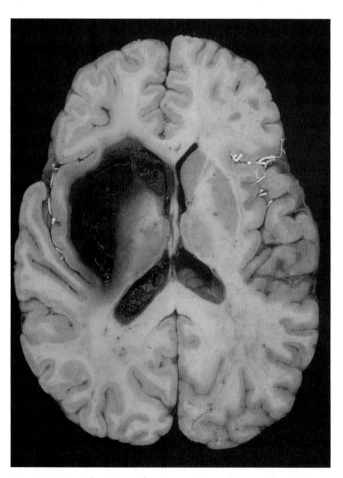

Fig. 10-3. Axial section of gross specimen showing hemorrhage in the basal ganglia, with intraventricular extension. Patient was hypertensive.

Table 10-6.   Magnetic Resonance Imaging Characteristics of Intraparenchymal Cerebral Hemorrhage

		T1 signal		T2 signal	
Stage	Timing	Central*	Peripheral†	Central*	Peripheral†
Hyperacute	<12 h	↔	↔	↑	↑
Acute	12-72 h	↔	↔	↓	↑
Early subacute	4-7 d	↔	↑	↓/↔	↓↓
Late subacute	1-4 wk	↑↑	↑↑	↑↑	↑↑
Chronic	Months	↑	↓	↑	↓
Late chronic	Months-years	↓↓	↓↓	↑	↓↓

↓, *decreased;* ↓↓, *markedly decreased;* ↑, *increased;* ↑↑, *markedly increased;* ↔, *isodense.*
Central part of the hemorrhage.
†*Peripheral part of the hemorrhage.*

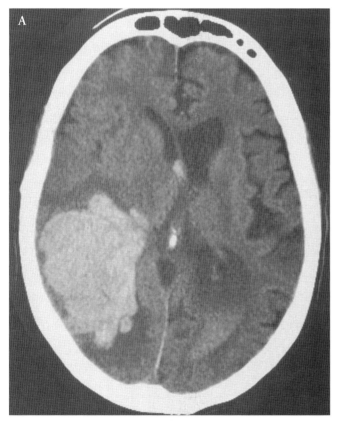

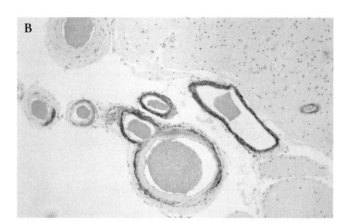

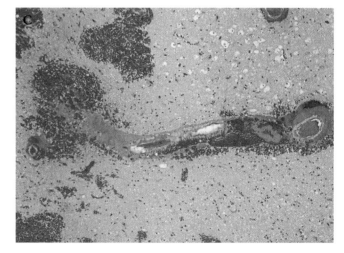

Fig. 10-4. *A,* CT, without contrast, of head showing intraparenchymal hemorrhage due to amyloid angiopathy. *B,* Cortical and leptomeningeal amyloid deposits are best demonstrated with β-amyloid immunohistochemistry. Note extensive β-amyloid deposition in the media and adventitia of the leptomeningeal arteries and arterioles. *C,* Micrograph of intraparenchymal hemorrhage due to amyloid angiopathy showing patchy, confluent microhemorrhagic areas around an arteriole. Note the surrounding ischemic brain parenchyma. (Hematoxylin-eosin.)

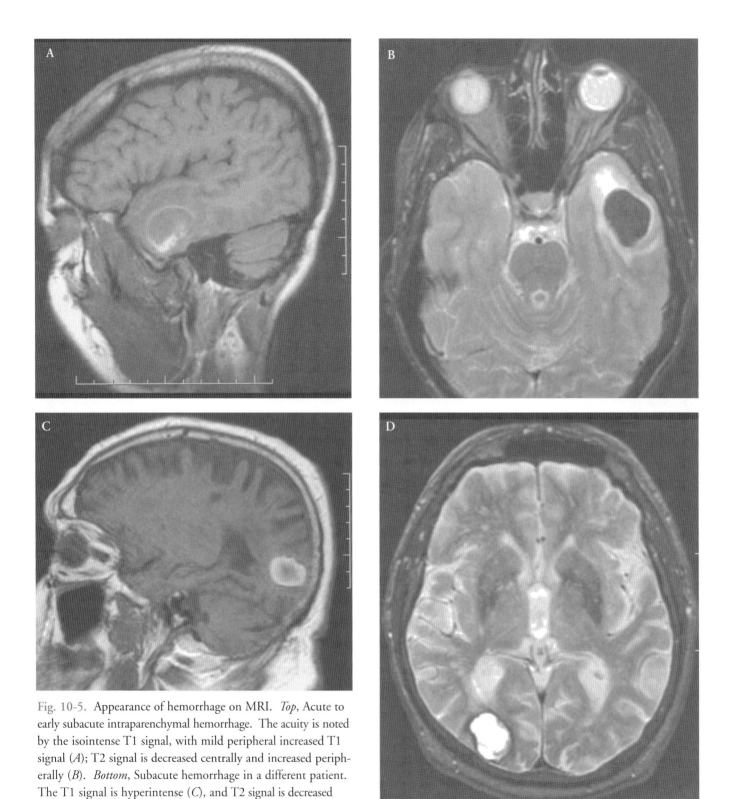

Fig. 10-5. Appearance of hemorrhage on MRI. *Top*, Acute to early subacute intraparenchymal hemorrhage. The acuity is noted by the isointense T1 signal, with mild peripheral increased T1 signal (*A*); T2 signal is decreased centrally and increased peripherally (*B*). *Bottom*, Subacute hemorrhage in a different patient. The T1 signal is hyperintense (*C*), and T2 signal is decreased peripherally and hyperintense centrally (*D*).

onset show blood (hyperdensity) in subarachnoid spaces (Fig. 10-6 *A*)

b. CT findings "normalize" in up to 10% of patients by day 3 and in 50% by day 7

c. Note: if CT is negative but SAH is strongly suspected clinically, perform lumbar puncture if not otherwise contraindicated

d. Note: look closely in interpeduncular region for subtle

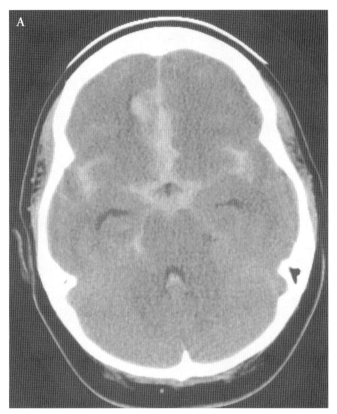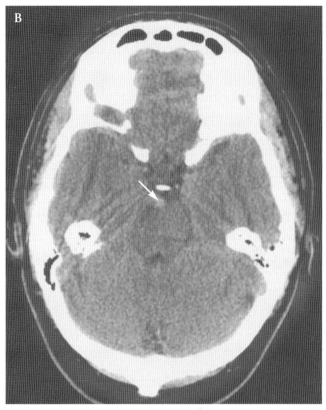

Fig. 10-6. Subarachnoid hemorrhage in different patients. *A*, Subarachnoid blood is distributed diffusely in the cisterns and fissures, including sylvian fissure. *B*, Note small amount of perimesencephalic (pretruncal) (*arrow*) subarachnoid blood. This patient has a benign form of subarachnoid hemorrhage with a good prognosis. *A* and *B*, CT without contrast.

blood that may represent perimesencephalic SAH (Fig. 10-6 *B*), which has a more benign prognosis and is not usually associated with aneurysm rupture
3. Lumbar puncture
   a. Perform following tests on CSF: opening pressure, leukocyte count, erythrocyte count in tubes 1 and 4, protein, glucose, Gram's stain, xanthochromia
   b. Distinguishing traumatic tap from SAH
      1) If traumatic tap: erythrocyte count should decrease from tube 1 to tube 4
      2) Xanthochromia: should be evident with SAH but not traumatic tap if symptoms started at least 6 hours earlier
         a) Xanthochromia: yellow tinge to CSF noted after CSF is centrifuged
         b) It results from breakdown products of erythrocytes and may be present if ictus was at least 6 hours before CSF examination
         c) Thus, CSF examination performed less than 6 hours after onset may yield false-negative results because insufficient time has lapsed for erythrocytes to break down and form xanthochromia
         d) For the same reason, xanthochromia is usually not

observed in traumatic tap
      e) Positive xanthochromia may also be seen when CSF protein is very high or patient has hyperbilirubinemia
   c. Note on CSF
      1) For every 750 to 1,000 erythrocytes, 1 leukocyte
      2) For every 1,000 erythrocytes, 1 mg/dL of protein
4. Angiography is necessary if nontraumatic SAH is expected
   a. Angiography can help detect the presence and morphology of aneurysm and related abnormality
   b. Conventional angiography is superior to magnetic resonance angiography (MRA) or CT angiography in this situation
   c. Most common cause of nontraumatic SAH: saccular or berry aneurysms
   d. Ruptured aneurysms are commonly smaller than 10 mm in diameter
   e. Giant aneurysm, saccular aneurysm more than 25 mm in diameter may also rupture (Fig. 10-7); angiography is helpful in determining size, morphology, and relation of aneurysm to other blood vessels

D. **Differential Diagnosis**
1. Differential diagnosis of thunderclap headache (see Chapter 18)
2. Differential diagnosis of SAH is listed in Table 10-7

E. **Management of SAH**
1. Aims: to support patient and prevent complications
2. Complications
   a. Rebleeding
      1) Timing: early
      2) Risk: 4% in first 24 hours, 1% daily thereafter for first 2 weeks
      3) Treatment: endovascular coiling vs. surgical clipping
   b. Hydrocephalus
      1) Timing: early
      2) Risk: 20% to 25% of patients develop hydrocephalus
      3) Treatment: external ventricular drain or ventriculo-peritoneal shunt
   c. Vasospasm
      1) Timing: 4 to 14 days
      2) Risk: up to 50% of patients have asymptomatic vasospasm, 15% to 20% develop infarctions
      3) Monitor: can be detected with transcranial Doppler ultrasonography, angiography
      4) Medical treatment
         a) Augment blood pressure
         b) Increase volume status
         c) Nimodipine: reduces cerebral infarction rate due

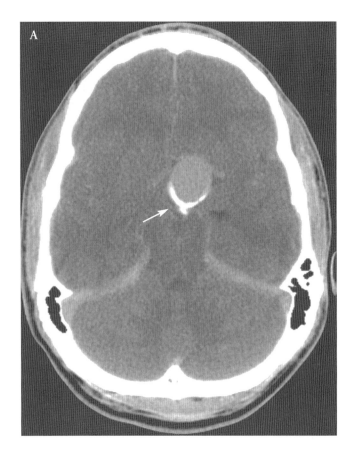

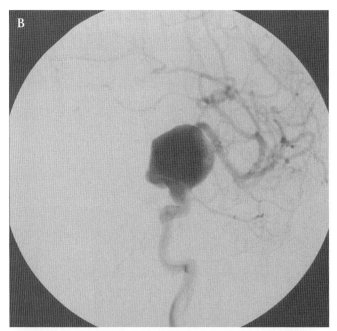

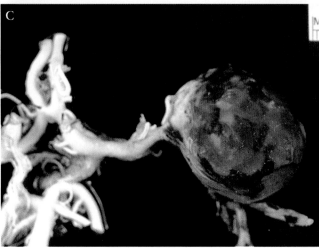

Fig. 10-7. *A* and *B*, Giant aneurysm of left internal carotid artery. *A*, CT without contrast showing subarachnoid blood and aneurysm (*arrow*) with mild mural calcification. The aneurysm is slightly hyperdense, suggesting partial thrombosis. *B*, Conventional angiogram showing the giant aneurysm, approximately 2.5 cm in diameter, at the supraclinoid segment of left internal carotid artery. *C*, Gross specimen of giant middle cerebral artery aneurysm from another patient.

to vasospasm but does not affect incidence of vasospasm

      d) Endovascular treatment: angioplasty or intra-arterial papaverine

  d. Cardiovascular complications

    1) Electrocardiographic changes (U waves)

    2) Arrhythmia

    3) Myocardial stunning (possibly due to catecholamine surge)

  e. Seizures

    1) Occur in 10% to 20% of patients

    2) More common if associated intracerebral hemorrhage

    3) Controversy about need for prophylactic antiepileptic use, but treatment definitely indicated when seizure occurs

  f. Pulmonary edema: neurogenic pulmonary edema may occur but is rare

  g. Hyponatremia

    1) Occurs in 10% to 30% of patients typically 2 to 10 days after symptom onset

    2) May be secondary to cerebral salt-wasting syndrome

F. Outcome of SAH

1. Mortality rate: approximately 30%
2. For patients who arrive at hospital with SAH, initial World Federation of Neurosurgeons (WFNS) grade and GCS score are used to determine outcome
3. Other factors that may contribute: age, amount of blood by CT (Fisher grade), seizures
4. Poor-grade SAH (WFNS grade 4-5): poor outcome if patient does not improve any grade within first 48 hours despite supportive treatment and ventriculostomy when needed

Table 10-7.   **Etiologies of Subarachnoid Hemorrhage**

Trauma

Aneurysm

Angiographically negative subarachnoid hemorrhage (pretruncal or perimesencephalic hemorrhage)

Arteriovenous malformation

Cavernous malformation

Vasculitis

Bleeding diathesis

IV. UNRUPTURED INTRACRANIAL ANEURYSM

A. Epidemiology

1. Approximately 3% to 5% of U.S. general population harbors an unruptured intracranial aneurysm
2. U.S. annual incidence of SAH: 30,000
3. This statistic suggests not all unruptured intracranial aneurysms found incidentally will rupture
4. Location
  a. More than 90% of aneurysms: anterior circulation (anterior communicating and posterior communicating arteries are most common)
  b. 5% to 10%: posterior circulation
  c. Multiple aneurysms: 20% to 30% of patients

B. Causes

1. Risk factors for aneurysm formation
  a. Female sex
  b. Hypertension
  c. Smoking
  d. Cocaine and/or methamphetamine use
  e. Certain connective tissue diseases (see below)
  f. Family history of two or more first-degree relatives
2. Good population-based data indicate polycystic kidney disease is associated with intracranial aneurysm formation
3. Case report and case series data suggest the following may predispose to intracranial aneurysm formation:
  a. Aortic coarctation

World Federation of Neurosurgeons Grading Scale for Subarachnoid Hemorrhage

Grade	Focal deficit	Glasgow Coma Scale score
1	Absent	15
2	Absent	13-14
3	Present	13-14
4	May/may not be present	7-12
5	May/may not be present	3-6

b. Pseudoxanthoma elasticum

c. Ehlers-Danlos syndrome type IV

d. Marfan syndrome

e. Neurofibromatosis

C. Clinical Presentation

1. Unruptured intracranial aneurysms may present with symptoms that are related to the aneurysm or the aneurysm may be noted incidentally when cerebral imaging study is performed for symptoms unrelated to aneurysm

2. Symptoms may include

  a. Compression

    1) Unruptured intracranial aneurysms may compress nearby structures

    2) Posterior communicating artery aneurysms often produce ipsilateral CN III palsy

  b. Ischemic stroke: unruptured intracranial aneurysms may thrombose, producing thromboembolic stroke

3. Diagnosis

  a. Occasionally large aneurysms may be detected on unenhanced CT

    1) Aneurysm often appears as slightly hyperdense well-circumscribed structure

    2) Occasionally, aneurysm wall may appear calcified

  b. Diagnosis can be made with noninvasive studies such as MRA or CT angiography

  c. Further characterization of the aneurysm may require conventional angiography, especially if endovascular coiling or surgical intervention is considered

4. Natural history

  a. Debated

  b. International Study of Unruptured Intracranial Aneurysms (ISUIA) provides data from selected population on the natural history of these aneurysms

    1) Predictors of future rupture: posterior circulation aneurysm (including posterior communicating artery aneurysm), increasing size, and previous SAH from separate aneurysm (Table 10-8)

    2) Patients with an anterior circulation aneurysm smaller than 7 mm and no previous history of SAH: very low risk of future rupture

5. Treatment

  a. Options: observation, surgical clipping, endovascular coiling

  b. Treatment is based on

    1) Patient age

    2) Natural history of aneurysm in individual patient

    3) Risk of coiling vs. open surgery based on angioarchitecture of aneurysm

V. OTHER ANEURYSMS

A. Infectious Aneurysms

1. Epidemiology

  a. 3% of all intracranial aneurysms

  b. 2% to 12% of all patients with infectious endocarditis

2. Pathogenesis

  a. Aneurysm dilatation may result from

    1) Direct infection of intima and inflammation of muscularis from septic emboli

    2) Septic emboli to vasa vasorum, causing destruction of adventitia and muscularis

  b. May occur within 7 to 10 days after initial infection

  c. Etiology

    1) Majority of infectious intracranial aneurysms due to bacterial sources

    2) Infectious endocarditis is most common source for septic emboli, but contiguous spread from parameningeal infection or seeding from remote site may also produce arteritis and aneurysm

    3) Fungal intracranial aneurysms are more commonly due to contiguous spread but are exceedingly rare and

Table 10-8.   **Five-Year Cumulative Rupture Rates of Unruptured Intracranial Aneurysms**

| | Diameter, mm | | | | |
| | <7 | | | | |
Location	Group 1*	Group 2†	7-12	13-24	≥25
Cavernous carotid artery	0	0	0	3%	6.4%
MCA, ACA, ICA	0	1.5%	2.6%	14.5%	40%
Posterior circulation or PCoA	2.5%	3.4%	14.5%	18.4%	50%

ACA, anterior cerebral artery; ICA, internal carotid artery; MCA, middle cerebral artery; PCoA, posterior communicating artery.
*Patients without a previous history of subarachnoid hemorrhage.
†Patients with a previous subarachnoid hemorrhage from a separate aneurysm.
From International Study of Unruptured Intracranial Aneurysms Investigators. Unruptured intracranial aneurysms: natural history, clinical outcome, and risks of surgical and endovascular treatment. Lancet. 2003;362:103-10. Used with permission.

usually in immunocompromised patients

    4) Organisms

      a) *Streptococcus* (most common)

      b) *Staphylococcus aureus*

      c) *Enterococcus*

      d) *Aspergillus* (rare)

      e) Phycomycetes (rare)

3. Clinical presentation

  a. Incidental

  b. Headache

    1) Neurologic deficit in setting of endocarditis or fever

    2) Seizures

4. Natural history

  a. Exact risk of rupture of infectious aneurysms: not known because of their rarity

  b. Rupture usually occurs early after disease onset; may be the clue leading to diagnosis of endocarditis

5. Diagnosis

  a. MRI of head may suggest aneurysm, but conventional angiography is best to make the diagnosis

  b. Aneurysms often are distal in arterial tree, so currently MRA is sometimes unreliable in making the diagnosis (Fig. 10-8)

6. Treatment

  a. Targeted antibiotic treatment and surgery in selected patients

  b. Surgery is considered for

    1) Ruptured aneurysm

    2) Life-threatening mass effect of aneurysm

    3) Evidence of enlargement

    4) Easily accessible single aneurysms

B. Fusiform Aneurysms

1. Epidemiology

  a. Uncommon

  b. Estimated prevalence by autopsy studies: 0.05%

2. Pathogenesis

  a. Risk factors for development of this aneurysm type: smoking, hypertension, male sex, age

  b. Concomitant pathology in other vessels is common, with high incidence of abdominal aortic aneurysms

  c. More common in posterior than anterior circulation

3. Radiographic diagnosis

  a. Dilatation of arterial segment(s) 1.5 times normal size without a definable neck; may also be tortuous and/or elongated

  b. Best defined by both cross-sectional imaging and angiography (Fig. 10-9)

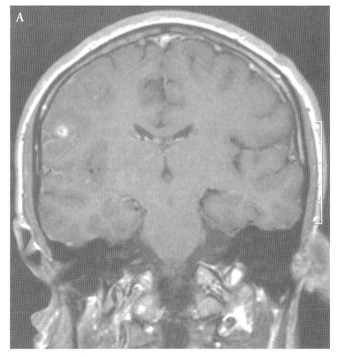 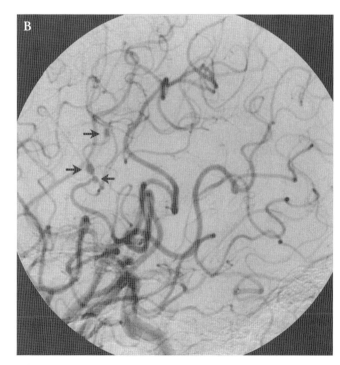

Fig. 10-8. Infectious ("mycotic") aneurysm. *A*, Coronal MRI, T1-weighted with gadolinium, showing area of enhancement in right frontal lobe. *B*, Conventional angiogram demonstrating three small fusiform aneurysms (*arrows*) of opercular branch of right middle cerebral artery.

4. Clinical presentation
   a. Typically in patients older than 60 years
   b. Asymptomatic
   c. SAH
   d. Mass effect (compression)
   e. Ischemia (thrombosed aneurysm with thromboemboli)
5. Natural history
   a. Risk of hemorrhage: reportedly rare, but may be as high as 2.3% annually in posterior circulation if there is enlargement of entire basilar artery with a superimposed aneurysmal segment
   b. Risk of ischemia: may be as high as 5% to 6% annually for posterior circulation aneurysms
   c. Mortality: median survival with posterior circulation fusiform aneurysms is approximately 7 to 8 years
   d. Most common cause of death: cerebral ischemia
6. Treatment
   a. Treatment options are limited
   b. In selected patients, vessel may be sacrificed or feeding vessel may be occluded to reduce flow to the parent vessel; this may reduce chance of aneurysm enlarging (but this has not been proved definitively)

C. **Dissecting Aneurysms**
1. Pathogenesis
   a. False aneurysms resulting from intimal tear and intramural hemorrhage
   b. Most commonly are extracranial; may be saccular or fusiform
   c. Angiography or MRA may help distinguish between dissecting and typical acquired aneurysms
      1) This distinction is not always possible
      2) Suggestive features: evidence of false lumen, intimal flap, retention of contrast in lumen or tapering of artery at proximal end of the aneurysm
2. Etiology
   a. Trauma
   b. Atherosclerosis
   c. Fibromuscular dysplasia
   d. Infection
   e. Arteritis
3. Clinical presentation
   a. Cerebral infarction or transient ischemic attack
   b. Extracranial dissecting aneurysms rarely rupture; because their extradural location eliminates concern about SAH, treatment is typically aimed at preventing further ischemia
   c. Intracranial dissecting aneurysms
      1) May present with ischemia
      2) Are intradural, thus substantial risk of SAH
      3) Over half of patients experience rebleeding after initial hemorrhage, with substantial increase in morbidity
4. Treatment: surgical vs. endovascular repair depending on location and size

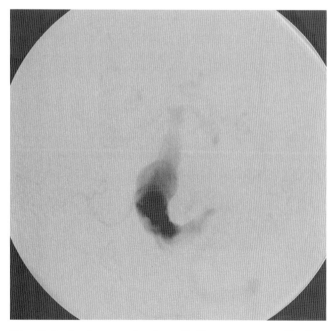 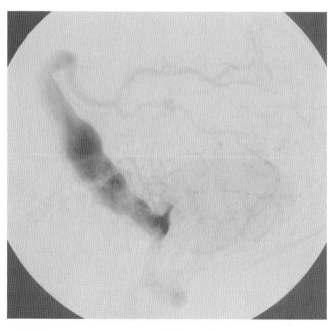

Fig. 10-9. Angiograms showing a fusiform aneurysm of basilar artery. *Left,* Anteroposterior view; *right,* lateral view. (From Flemming KD, Wiebers DO, Brown RD Jr, Link MJ, Nakatomi H, Huston J III, et al. Prospective risk of hemorrhage in patients with vertebrobasilar nonsaccular intracranial aneurysm. J Neurosurg. 2004;101:82-7. Used with permission.)

D. Neoplastic Aneurysms

1. Exceedingly rare
2. Have been described in association with many types of primary and metastatic brain tumors
3. Tumor emboli infiltrate and weaken vessel wall and may result in aneurysm formation
4. Typically located distally; may be saccular or fusiform in shape

VI. NEUROLOGIC INTENSIVE CARE PRINCIPLES

A. Intracranial Pressure (ICP)

1. Physiology
   a. The skull is a fixed structure not allowing expansion
   b. Intracranial volume (~1,900 cm³) consists of three compartments: brain (80%), blood (10%), CSF (10%)
   c. Monroe-Kellie doctrine: if the volume of one of these compartments increases, the volume of another must decrease to maintain normal ICP (0-20 mm Hg)
   d. First measures in preventing increasing ICP: generally CSF is shifted to spinal subarachnoid space and arterial and venous structures collapse, reducing blood volume
   e. If these measures are not effective, the brain may begin to herniate because of increasing ICP, or if ICP increases above mean arterial pressure, then cerebral perfusion pressure will drop and ischemia result
   f. Autoregulation
      1) Changes in cerebral perfusion pressure between 60 and 160 mm Hg do not alter cerebral blood flow because of autoregulation
         a) Above or below these pressures, flow is related to pressure (Fig. 10-10)
         b) In patients with long-standing hypertension, the entire curve is shifted to the right; therefore, it is important not to aggressively treat blood pressure to levels that can decrease cerebral blood flow
         c) The shift in autoregulation is an important adaptive mechanism against large increases in blood pressure that may otherwise cause hypertensive encephalopathy
      2) Autoregulation may become impaired, resulting in pressure-dependent flow if brain injury occurs, with the brain becoming more susceptible to ischemia

2. Causes of raised ICP (Table 10-9)
   a. Space-occupying mass, for example, brain tumor, abscess
   b. Brain edema
      1) Cytotoxic: fluid accumulation within cells
      2) Vasogenic: proteinaceous fluid leaks into extracellular space from capillaries

Relation Between Cerebral Perfusion Pressure and Intracranial Pressure

Formula	Normal
ICP	0-20 mm Hg (adult)
CPP = MAP – ICP	70-100 mm Hg (adult)
$CBF = \dfrac{CPP}{CVR}$	20-70 mL/100 g tissue/min
MAP = DBP + 1/3 (SBP – DBP)	70-110 mm Hg (adult)

CBF, cerebral blood flow; CPP, cerebral perfusion pressure; CVR, cerebral vascular resistance; DBP, diastolic blood pressure; MAP, mean arterial pressure; SBP, systolic blood pressure.

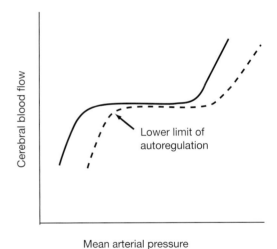

Fig. 10-10. Cerebral autoregulation. When cerebral autoregulation is intact, cerebral blood flow remains constant if the mean arterial pressure is between 60 and 160 mm Hg. However, with long-standing hypertension, the entire curve shifts to the right (*dashed line*). (From Wijdicks EFM. The clinical practice of critical care neurology. 2nd ed. New York: Oxford University Press; 2003. p. 107-25. By permission of Mayo Foundation.)

3) Interstitial: CSF pushed into extracellular space in periventricular white matter in hydrocephalus
   c. Hydrocephalus: increased CSF from
      1) Overproduction: rare, choroid plexus papilloma
      2) Ventricular obstruction: obstructive hydrocephalus

3) Arachnoid granule obstruction: nonobstructive, communicating hydrocephalus
d. Venous thrombosis: impairs CSF reabsorption
3. Diagnosis: clinical signs
   a. Headache
   b. Vomiting
   c. Papilledema
   d. Herniation syndromes (see below)
   e. Hypertension and bradycardia
   f. Transient visual obscurations
   g. False localizing CN VI palsy
4. Indications for ICP monitoring
   a. GCS score less than 8
   b. Severe head trauma
   c. ICP waveforms
      1) Plateau (A) waves
         a) Sudden surges in ICP to 50 to 80 mm Hg lasting 5 to 20 minutes

   b) Presence of A waves suggests failing compliance of the brain to ICP and risk for ischemia
   2) B waves: smaller surges in ICP to 20 mm Hg for 1 to 2 minutes
5. Management (Table 10-10)
   a. Measures to reduce intracranial pressure are aimed at reducing volume of CSF, brain, or blood (or combination)
   b. Specific measure for reducing intracranial pressure: depends on the abnormality
6. Herniation syndromes: supratentorial (Fig. 10-11)
   a. Subfalcine
      1) Herniation of brain tissue under falx cerebri
      2) Generally occurs with unilateral space-occupying mass in a cerebral hemisphere
   b. Central (diencephalic)
      1) Diencephalon is displaced downward through tentorium cerebelli, resulting in rostrocaudal

Table 10-9. Etiologies of Increased Intracranial Pressure

Vascular	Intracerebral hemorrhage with mass effect
	Epidural hemorrhage with mass effect
	Subarachnoid hemorrhage
	Large hemispheric ischemic stroke with mass effect
	Venous thrombosis
	Jugular vein ligation (radical neck dissection)
	Superior vena cava syndrome
Infectious	Abscess or empyema with mass effect
	Any meningitis or encephalitis (especially brucellosis, Lyme disease, cryptococcosis)
Inflammatory	Behçet's syndrome
	Systemic lupus erythematosus
	Sarcoidosis
Neoplastic	Mass lesion
	Carcinomatous meningitis
Toxic/ metabolic	Vitamin A intoxication
	Endocrine disturbances—adrenal insufficiency, hyper- or hypoparathyroidism, hyperthyroidism
	Hepatic encephalopathy
	Certain medications—anabolic steroids, tetracycline, cyclosporine
Trauma	Brain trauma with edema
Other	Hydrocephalus
	Pseudotumor cerebri
	Reye's syndrome
	Eclampsia

Table 10-10. Management of Increased Intracranial Pressure

Measure	Compartment	Recommended
General	Several	Head of bed at 30 degrees Normothermic Pain control
CSF drainage	↓ CSF	External ventricular drain Lumbar drain
Hyperventilation	↓ Blood (vasoconstriction)	Hyperventilate to P_{CO_2} of 30 mm Hg
Osmotic diuresis	↓ Brain volume*	Mannitol 0.25-1 g/kg bolus, then consider repeat every 8 h; titrate to serum osmolality <310
Barbiturates	↓ Metabolic activity of brain and thus blood flow	Pentobarbital
Hypothermia	↓ Metabolic activity of brain and thus blood flow	Cooling blankets
Surgery	↓ Brain	If intracranial pressure not controlled by medical management and surgical lesion present

CSF, cerebrospinal fluid.
*Cells shrink from osmotic diuresis.

A

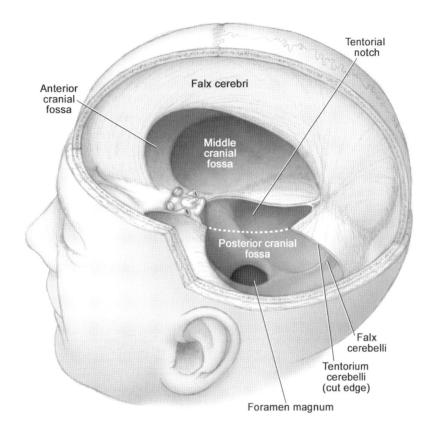

B

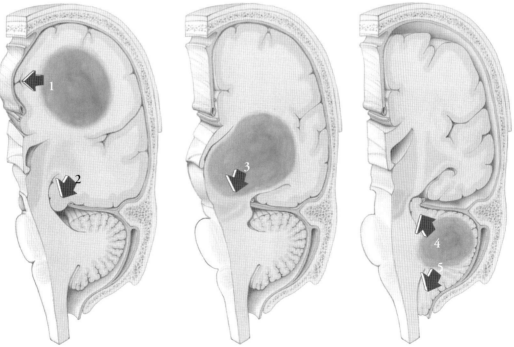

Fig. 10-11. *A,* Dura mater and its folds divide the intracranial contents into compartments (cranial fossae). The free edges of the tentorium cerebelli form the tentorial notch (Kernohan's notch). *B,* Herniation syndromes. *1,* Subfalcine herniation; *2,* uncal herniation; *3,* central or diencephalic herniation; and, *4,* cerebellar upward and, *5,* tonsillar herniation. (From Wijdicks EFM. The clinical practice of critical care neurology. 2nd ed. New York: Oxford University Press; 2003. p. 107-25. By permission of Mayo Foundation.)

deterioration of sequential brainstem structures
2) May result in Duret's hemorrhages of brainstem (Fig. 10-12), pituitary stalk shearing (diabetes insipidus), and bilateral occipital infarctions from compression of posterior cerebral artery
3) Duret's hemorrhages result from shearing and traction on the basilar perforators and compression of their intramedullary portions
4) Reduced level of consciousness appears early in this herniation syndrome
   c. Tentorial (uncal)
   1) Uncus is displaced over edge of tentorium cerebelli, trapping ipsilateral CN III (dilation of pupil) and compressing midbrain
   2) If herniation continues, both central and tonsillar herniation may occur
   3) Ipsilateral CN III palsy usually is first sign, followed by loss of consciousness and brainstem findings
   4) Uncal herniation may also compress posterior cerebral artery, resulting in infarction (Fig. 10-13)
7. Herniation syndromes: infratentorial (Fig. 10-11)
   a. Upward cerebellar: cerebellar vermis ascends rostral to tentorium cerebelli, compressing the midbrain, may compress the cerebral aqueduct
   b. Tonsillar
   1) Cerebellar tonsils herniate through foramen magnum, compressing the medulla

2) Can occur with supratentorial or infratentorial lesions or with increased ICP

B. Respiratory Parameters
1. Critically ill patients in neurologic intensive care unit may have respiratory difficulties related to brain or brainstem dysfunction, neuromuscular weakness, or primary pulmonary disease
2. Indications for intubation
   a. Inability to protect airway in patient with frequent hypoxic episodes
   b. Comatose (GCS score <8): controversial
   c. Impending neuromuscular failure: "20/30/40" rule
   1) Tachypnea, tachycardia, paradoxical breathing
   2) Vital capacity: <20 mL/kg (normal adult, 40-70 mL/kg)
   3) Maximum inspiratory pressure: −30 cm H_2O (normal, −70 to −100 cm H_2O)
   4) Maximum expiratory pressure: 40 cm H_2O (normal, 140-200 cm H_2O)
   d. Refractory Hypoxemia
   e. Need for therapeutic hyperventilation (to reduce ICP)

VII.   OTHER NEUROLOGIC EMERGENCIES

A. Status Epilepticus
1. Incidence: 6.8-41/100,000 population annually
2. Definition

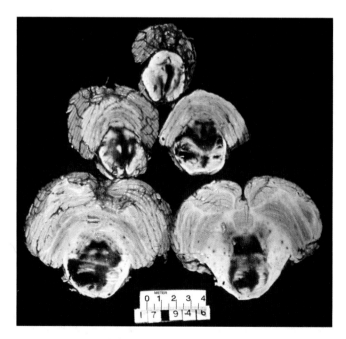

Fig. 10-12. Duret's hemorrhages produced by severe downward herniation. (See the text for explanation.)

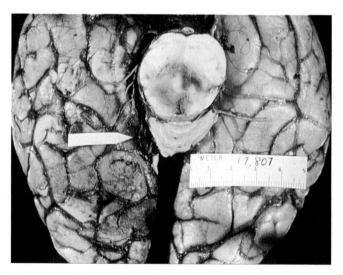

Fig. 10-13. Compression of the posterior cerebral artery (*white arrow*) by uncal herniation produces ipsilateral occipital infarction. Note midline Duret's hemorrhage in brainstem.

a. Older definitions characterize status epilepticus as seizure duration longer than 30 minutes or two seizures or more with incomplete recovery between the two (the reason being brain injury is known to occur by 30 minutes)

b. Newer definition suggested to prevent brain injury and promote early treatment: seizure duration longer than 5 minutes or two seizures or more with incomplete recovery

c. Diagnosis is based on neurologic examination consistent with seizure activity and confirmed by EEG (Fig. 10-14)

3. Types of status epilepticus

a. Generalized: generalized tonic-clonic, absence, myoclonic, tonic, and clonic

b. Partial: simple partial (motor, sensory, visual, auditory, or language) and complex partial

4. Causes

a. Any acute or chronic brain lesion or toxic-metabolic disturbance can produce seizures and status epilepticus

b. Most common cause of status epilepticus: acute insult (most commonly vascular event [stroke]; next most common, withdrawal or low levels of antiepileptic drugs; also tumors, meningitis, encephalitis, metabolic derangements, trauma)

c. Remote symptomatic lesions comprise approximately 30% of cases of status epilepticus and 5% are idiopathic or unknown

d. In children, prolonged febrile convulsions and low antiepileptic drug levels are common

5. Management

a. An algorithmic approach to treatment is given in Figure 10-15 and details about medications are listed in Table 10-11 (see also Chapter 12)

b. ABCs: assess airway, breathing, and circulation (intubate if necessary, assess vital signs and oxygen saturation)

c. Check blood glucose level

d. Establish intravenous access: administer thiamine and D5 saline

e. Draw blood for laboratory studies: blood gas, electrolytes, magnesium, calcium, glucose, toxicology screen, blood count, and drug levels if patient takes antiepileptic medications

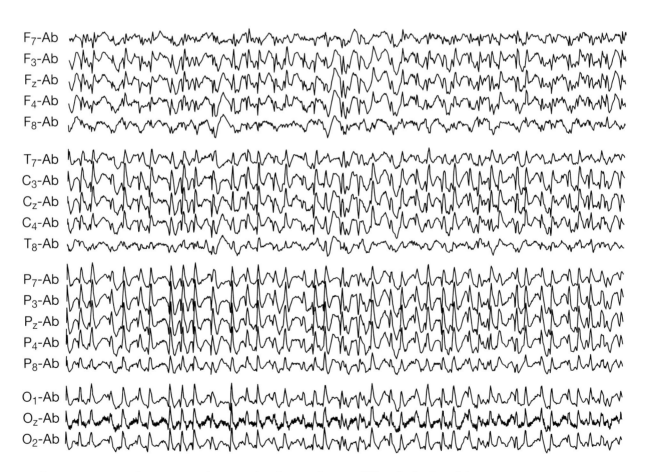

Fig. 10-14. EEG, nonconvulsive status epilepticus, showing continuous, diffuse rhythmic activity.

f. Consider benzodiazepine: lorazepam or diazepam used most commonly
   1) Advantage: rapid onset of action, can be given intravenously (IV), intramuscularly (IM), or rectally (diazepam)
   2) Midazolam also can be considered, but because of short half-life and sedation, is usually favored as infusion after consideration of fosphenytoin
g. If seizures persist, fosphenytoin should be considered
   1) Is effective within 10 to 30 minutes after IV administration
   2) Also available IM, but takes longer to be absorbed
   3) Loading dose: 15 to 20 mg/kg phenytoin equivalents
   4) Additional 5 to 10 mg/kg can be considered if seizures persist
h. At this point, consider intubation, head CT, and moving patient to EEG-monitored intensive care unit
i. Typical reasons why seizures persist after load of fosphenytoin: inadequate fosphenytoin loading dose, structural brain lesion, or metabolic derangement
j. Phenobarbital load, propofol infusion, or midazolam infusion could be considered
k. If seizures persist despite all the above, consider pentobarbital coma or general anesthesia
l. Treat to "burst suppression" for 12 to 48 hours, then withdraw sedation with constant EEG monitoring
m. Intravenous valproate sodium may be considered an alternative to fosphenytoin especially if patient has allergy to phenytoin (dilantin), patient takes valproic acid and valproic acid levels are low or patient is hemodynamically unstable

6. Outcome: depends on cause in generalized tonic-clonic status epilepticus
   a. Short-term complications
      1) Death: 10% to 20% of patients
      2) Rhabdomyolysis

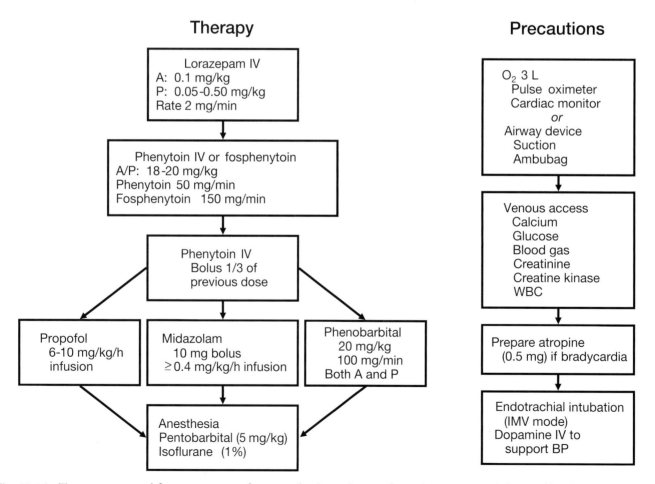

Therapy

Lorazepam IV
A: 0.1 mg/kg
P: 0.05-0.50 mg/kg
Rate 2 mg/min

↓

Phenytoin IV or fosphenytoin
A/P: 18-20 mg/kg
Phenytoin 50 mg/min
Fosphenytoin 150 mg/min

↓

Phenytoin IV
Bolus 1/3 of
previous dose

Propofol
6-10 mg/kg/h
infusion

Midazolam
10 mg bolus
≥0.4 mg/kg/h infusion

Phenobarbital
20 mg/kg
100 mg/min
Both A and P

↓

Anesthesia
Pentobarbital (5 mg/kg)
Isoflurane (1%)

Precautions

O₂ 3 L
Pulse oximeter
Cardiac monitor
or
Airway device
Suction
Ambubag

↓

Venous access
Calcium
Glucose
Blood gas
Creatinine
Creatine kinase
WBC

↓

Prepare atropine
(0.5 mg) if bradycardia

↓

Endotracheal intubation
(IMV mode)
Dopamine IV to
support BP

Fig. 10-15. Treatment protocol for management of status epilepticus. See text for explanation. A, adults; BP, blood pressure; IMV, intermittent mechanical ventilation; IV, intravenous; P, pediatriac patient; WBC, white blood cells. (From Wijdicks EFM. Neurologic catastrophes in the emergency department. Boston: Butterworth-Heinemann; 2000. p. 3-39. By permission of Mayo Foundation.)

3) Aspiration
4) Cardiac dysrhythmias
b. Long-term complications
  1) Development of epilepsy (mesial temporal sclerosis): 20% to 40% of patients
  2) Encephalopathy: cortical atrophy, anoxia

B. Guillain-Barré Syndrome

1. Description: also referred to as "acute inflammatory demyelinating polyradiculoneuropathy" (AIDP), which reflects its localization, pathology, and pathogenesis
2. Epidemiology: incidence is 1/100,000 population
3. Pathogenesis
   a. Immune response with myelin damage
   b. Two-thirds of patients have antecedent respiratory tract infection (Epstein-Barr virus, cytomegalovirus, *Mycoplasma*) or gastrointestinal tract infection (especially *Campylobacter jejuni*, cytomegalovirus)

c. Other possible precipitating events: vaccinations, trauma, surgery, cancer
4. Clinical presentation
   a. Presentation: approximately 2 to 4 weeks after viral illness
   b. "Ascending paralysis": patients may develop distal paresthesias in extremities, followed within hours to days by lower extremity weakness that may ascend to involve upper extremities and cranial nerves (facial weakness, dysphagia, ptosis)
   c. Aspiration pneumonia may occur if dysphagia is severe
   d. Radicular pain or cramps may occur
   e. Respiratory failure may not be presenting symptom, but can occur early after other symptoms requiring frequent monitoring (see below)
5. Physical examination findings
   a. Symmetric weakness
   b. Hyporeflexia or areflexia
   c. Minimal loss of sensation despite paresthesias
   d. Autonomic symptoms: cardiac conduction arrhythmias, orthostatic hypotension, hypertension, paralytic ileus, bladder dysfunction, abnormal sweating
6. Variant forms
   a. Miller Fisher variant
      1) Patient presents with ophthalmoplegia, ptosis, ataxia, and hyporeflexia
      2) Associated with the GQ1b ganglioside
   b. Pharyngeal-cervical-brachial variant
7. Differential diagnosis (see Chapter 21)
8. Diagnostic evaluation
   a. Head or spine imaging: may be important to rule out alternative lesion
   b. Electromyography
      1) Demyelinating polyradiculopathy, but can also have features of axonal degeneration
      2) Demyelinating: slowed motor conduction velocities and distal latencies, motor conduction block, temporal dispersion, slowed or absent F waves
      3) H-reflex may be helpful
   c. CSF
      1) Protein is usually more than 50 mg/dL (usually within first week)
      2) Few cells: if high leukocyte count, consider alternative diagnosis such as Lyme disease, human immunodeficiency virus infection, or other meningeal processes
   d. GM1b ganglioside: found in some cases of *Campylobacter*-associated AIDP
   e. GQ1b ganglioside: found in some cases of Miller Fisher variant

Table 10-11. **Medications Used to Manage Status Epilepticus**

Medication	Loading dose, mg/kg, intravenous	Maintenance dose	Therapeutic level, µg/mL
Lorazepam	0.1		---
Diazepam	0.15		---
Phenytoin	18-20	300 mg/d (adults) 4-6 mg/kg daily (children)	10-20
Fosphenytoin	18-20 mg/kg phenytoin equivalents	Same as phenytoin	10-20
Valproate (Depacon)	15-20		50-100
Phenobarbital	20	200-320 mg/d (adult) 3-6 mg/kg daily (children)	10-40
Propofol	1-3	6-10 mg/kg per hour	---
Midazolam	0.2	1-10 µg/kg per minute	---
Pentobarbital	5	1-5 mg/kg per hour	---

9. Specific therapy
   a. Intravenous immunoglobulin (IVIG) or plasma exchange can be considered depending on cost and availability
   b. Treatments can improve strength outcome earlier than placebo and decrease time of ventilator
   c. Generally not considered for mild cases when patients are ambulatory
   d. If clinical symptoms progress after reaching a plateau with treatment, additional therapy or alternate therapy can be considered
   e. IVIG (immune globulin)
      1) Utility: can improve strength earlier than natural history
      2) Regimen: 0.4 g/kg daily for 5 days
      3) Side effects: aseptic meningitis, acute renal failure, anaphylaxis, pseudohyponatremia
      4) Contraindications
         a) Hypersensitivity to IVIG, human albumin, or thimerosal
         b) Isolated immunoglobulin A deficiency with antibodies to IgA
   f. Plasma exchange
      1) Utility: improve strength earlier than natural history
      2) Regimen: five exchanges on alternate days with 5% albumin
      3) Side effects: hypovolemia, allergy, catheter-related problems (infection, access), hypocalcemia, thrombocytopenia, hypokalemia
      4) Contraindications: septic shock, recent myocardial infarction, marked dysautonomia, active bleeding
10. Supportive therapy
   a. Intensive care unit warranted for following:
      1) Patients with rapid progression of symptoms
      2) Bulbar and/or facial dysfunction
      3) Severe autonomic dysfunction (arrhthymia, hypotension)
      4) Respiratory compromise
         a) Occurs in about one-third of patients
         b) Prediction of respiratory compromise in Guillain-Barré syndrome (the 20/30/40 rule): if vital capacity is less than 20 mL/kg, maximum inspiratory pressure less than −30 cm H_2O, maximum expiratory pressure less than 40 cm H_2O
   b. Other supportive measures
      1) Monitor for respiratory changes
      2) Deep venous thrombosis prevention
      3) Decubitus ulcer prevention
      4) Gastritis prevention
      5) Pain control

6) Enteral feeding if necessary
7) Stool softener
8) Recognition and treatment of ileus
9) Monitoring for arrhythmia
10) Consider tracheostomy if prolonged course
11) Recognition and treatment of bladder paralysis
12) Recognition and treatment of depression
11. Clinical course and outcome
   a. Clinical course: most patients reach plateau at 2 weeks and slowly improve over months
   b. Serial respiratory monitoring is required because patient's condition may deteriorate rapidly, requiring mechanical ventilation (occurs in about one-third of patients)
   c. Majority of patients have good long-term outcome

C. Hemicraniectomy for Malignant Ischemic Stroke

1. Background and indications
   a. Large-distribution hemispheric ischemic stroke patients often deteriorate because of formation of cytotoxic and vasogenic edema
   b. Transtentorial herniation may develop in some patients about 48 to 96 hours after ictus
   c. Despite medical treatments (hyperventilation, mannitol, hypothermia) to reduce ICP, mortality rate may be as high as 50% to 80%
   d. Decompressive surgery: removal of frontotemporoparietal bone ipsilateral to ischemic stroke, then opening of dura mater to allow outward herniation of the brain, potentially preventing downward herniation (Fig. 10-16)
   e. No randomized clinical trials to guide clinical management
   f. Determining which patients go on to herniation and die may improve selection for surgery; this has been debated and may include the following:
      1) Hypodensity in more than 50% of middle cerebral artery territory
      2) Early nausea and vomiting
      3) National Institutes of Health Stroke Scale score more than 20 for left hemisphere or more than 15 for right hemisphere
      4) Involvement of anterior cerebral artery or posterior cerebral artery territories in addition to middle cerebral artery territory
2. Outcome
   a. Overall mortality rate from case series is lower than natural progression of large middle cerebral artery territory strokes
   b. Patients older than 50 years undergoing hemicraniectomy for ischemic stroke had increased mortality and morbidity compared with those younger than 50 (80% severely

disabled or dead in "older than 50" group vs. 32% in "younger than 50" group)

   c. Timing of surgery, side of infarct, herniation before surgery, and number of vascular territories involved did not significantly affect outcome according to one meta-analysis of case series and reports

3. Indication

   a. Debated, awaiting clinical trial evidence to become available

   b. Generally, patients who are young (<50 years) and have signs and symptoms of malignant hemispheric infarction (noted above) could be considered for the procedure

D. Acute Spinal Cord Compression

1. Etiology

   a. Differential diagnosis for acute myelopathy is discussed in Chapter 20

   b. Consider cauda equina syndrome and acute polyradiculoneuropathies in differential diagnosis of patient presenting with acute paraparesis

   c. Conus medullaris syndrome and cauda equina lesion are compared in Table 10-12

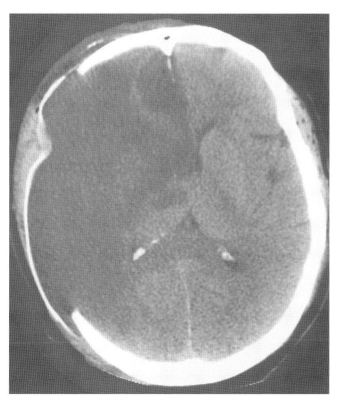

Fig. 10-16. CT showing a large right hemispheric stroke and hemicraniectomy.

2. Clinical history and physical examination

   a. Weakness in both lower extremities (can be asymmetric)

   b. Reflexes likely diminished early after compression; Babinski's sign may be present

   c. Sensory loss in myelopathic pattern (i.e., sensory level to pin)

   d. Urinary retention (check postvoid residual)

   e. Decreased rectal tone

   f. May or may not be associated with pain, depending on cause

   g. Respiratory compromise with high cervical lesions

   h. Dysautonomia (hypotension, bradycardia)

3. Diagnostic evaluation

   a. Imaging

     1) MRI of region presumedly affected is the test of choice

     2) CT myelography can be performed in patients who cannot undergo MRI

   b. CSF: if no obvious structural cause for myelopathy, lumbar puncture is often done to look for inflammatory or infectious cause

4. Treatment

   a. Corticosteroids

     1) Indications: tumor, demyelination, trauma

     2) Dose for cord compression: 100 mg dexamethasone, then 6 mg every 4 hours for 3 to 5 days

     3) Dose for trauma

       a) Within 3 hours: 30 mg/kg methylprednisolone IV, then 5.4 mg/kg per hour continuous infusion for 23 hours

Table 10-12. Cauda Equina Syndrome Versus Conus Medullaris Lesion

	Cauda equina	Conus medullaris
Pain	Often present	Uncommon
Motor weakness	Often asymmetric	Often symmetric weakness in distal > proximal muscles
Sensory distribution	Often asymmetric, dermatomal, saddle region	Often symmetric, saddle region
Reflexes	Absent	Achilles reflex absent, patellar reflex may be preserved
Bladder symptoms	May be present	Often present early on

b) Within 3 to 8 hours, 30 mg/kg methylprednisolone, then 5.4 mg/kg per hour continuous
infusion for 48 hours

4) Radiation consultation

a) Indications: radiation-responsive tumor

b) EMERGENT!

b. Neurosurgical consultation

1) Indications: if evidence of structural compression
(e.g., tumor, disk, epidural hematoma)

2) EMERGENT!

c. Supportive management

1) Place Foley catheter to avoid overdistension of bladder

2) Consider abdominal binder if hypotension is due to
dysautonomia

3) Have atropine at bedside if bradycardia is due to
dysautonomia

4) Monitor respiratory status, especially if cervical or
thoracic lesion

5. Outcome

a. Early diagnosis and treatment are important

b. 80% to 100% of patients improve if still ambulatory
when treatment begins

c. 30% improve if mild weakness when treatment begins

d. 2% to 6% improve if paraplegic before treatment begins

VIII. Trauma

A. Subdural Hematoma (Fig. 10-17 and 10-18)

1. Etiology: trauma causing tearing of bridging veins
traversing subdural space

2. Clinical presentation

a. Usually recent history of trauma

b. May present with subacute confusion or focal neurologic
symptoms

c. May have headache

3. Diagnostic evaluation

a. CT may show acute (increased attenuation), subacute
(isodense), or chronic blood (similar to fluid attenuation)
over cerebral convexity or, less often, interhemispheric or
posterior fossa along tentorium cerebelli; crescentic or
concave shape

b. Can be associated with midline shift or edema

4. Management

a. Check prothrombin time (PT) (international normalized
ratio [INR]), partial thromboplastin time (PTT), complete
blood count

b. Reverse anticoagulation if applicable

c. Surgical indications: symptomatic, blood more than
1 cm

d. Observation: may be indicated if small, asymptomatic
hemorrhage

B. Epidural Hematoma (Fig. 10-19)

1. Etiology

a. Usually due to blunt skull trauma and injury to the
middle meningeal artery (less common, venous sinus)

b. Most commonly occur laterally over cerebral hemisphere
(temporal or temporoparietal)

2. Clinical presentation

a. Blunt head injury, often with loss of consciousness

b. Patient may improve briefly, then deteriorate rapidly to
somnolence, contralateral hemiparesis and "blown" pupil
on ipsilateral side (CN III compressed at the tentorial
edge because of herniation—Kernohan's notch)

3. Diagnostic evaluation: CT shows lenticular-shaped
acute blood (hyperdensity) against the skull with mass
effect and midline shift; often with ipsilateral soft tissue
injury (Fig. 10-17 *B*)

4. Treatment

a. Check PT (INR), PTT, complete blood count

b. Reverse anticoagulation if applicable

c. Surgery

C. Head Injury

1. Classification

a. Impact damage occurs immediately; treatment is aimed
at preventing subsequent swelling, infection, or ischemia

b. Head injury may result in focal or diffuse damage

1) Focal damage

a) Contusion (Fig. 10-20)

i) Most common in frontotemporal regions
(frontal pole, orbitofrontal cortex, and temporal
pole)

ii) Can also occur opposite head impact (i.e.,
contracoup)

b) Intraparenchymal hemorrhage: can occur alone or
in conjunction with subdural bleeding

c) Subdural hemorrhage (see above)

d) Epidural hemorrhage (see above)

2) Diffuse damage: diffuse axonal injury

a) Shear force causes immediate axonal damage

b) Subsequent release of neurotransmitters results in
calcium influx into cells, contributing to further
damage

c) Typical locations where axonal damage may be
visible are at gray matter–white matter junction or
along white matter fiber tracts: centrum semiovale, corpus callosum, fornix, superior and
middle cerebellar peduncles, brainstem

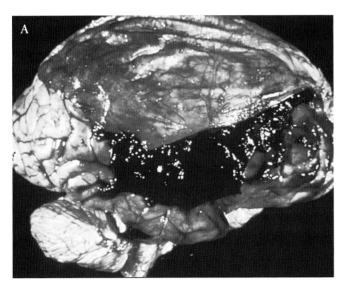

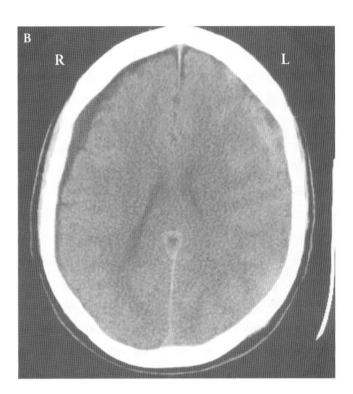

Fig. 10-17. Subdural hematoma. *A*, Gross specimen. *B*, CT showing appearance of chronic (*right*) and subacute (*left*) subdural hematoma. The chronic hematoma appears hypodense to the brain, whereas the subacute hematoma is modestly hyperdense.

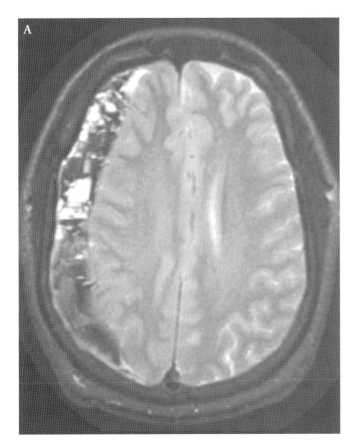

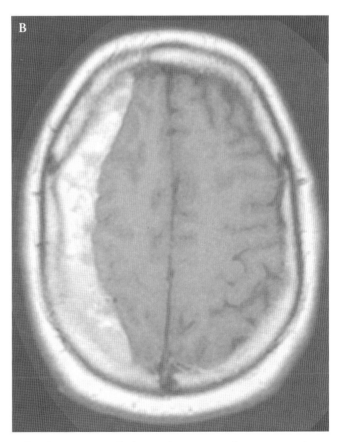

Fig. 10-18. MRI characteristics of subacute subdural hematoma. In early subacute stage, the hemorrhage appears heterogeneously hypointense on T2-weighted images (*A*) and hyperintense on T1-weighted images (*B*).

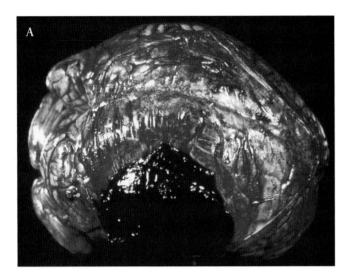

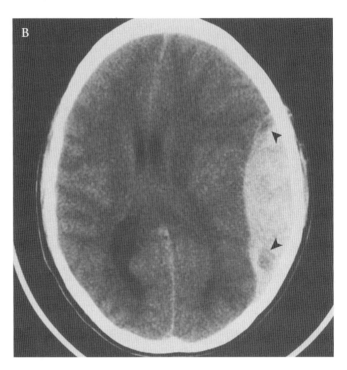

Fig. 10-19. Epidural hematoma. *A*, Gross specimen. *B*, On CT, epidural hematoma appears as a biconvex hyperdense lesion, often with substantial mass effect (as shown here). Small low-density areas within the hemorrhage (*arrowheads*) are likely hyperacute, unretracted, semiliquid blood building up rapidly.

2. Diagnostic evaluation and approach to management
   a. If multiple injuries, the following priorities should be kept in order:
      1) Airway
      2) Breathing
      3) Circulation
      4) Assess for chest and abdominal injury
      5) Assess for head and spinal injury
      6) Assess for limb injury
   b. Specific components of assessment of head injury
      1) History of event: circumstances surrounding event
      2) Persistent headache or vomiting
      3) Lacerations or bruising
      4) Assess for signs of skull fracture
      5) Level of consciousness: eye, verbal, motor responses (GCS score)
      6) Pupil response
      7) Eye movements
      8) Other cranial nerve lesions
3. Deterioration and complications
   a. Herniation syndrome: increased ICP may result in herniation (following principles of Monroe-Kellie doctrine) (see above)
   b. Infection
      1) Dural tears occurring with compound depressed skull fracture or basilar skull fracture may be potential route for infection

      2) Meningitis or abscess formation can occur
   c. Cerebral edema
   d. Cerebral ischemia
      1) May be focal or diffuse
      2) Impaired autoregulation makes brain vulnerable to small shifts in blood pressure

D. Spinal Cord Trauma
1. General
   a. Majority of injuries involve cervical spine, followed by thoracic, then lumbar spine
   b. One in five patients may have more than one spinal cord segment involved
2. Mechanism and types of injury
   a. Burst fracture: generally result of vertical compression; fracture of vertebral body
   b. Ligamentous injury: involves either anterior longitudinal ligament (generally with hyperextension injury) or posterior interspinous ligament (with anterior flexion injury)
   c. Rotational force can result in dislocation and/or fracture
3. Clinical history and examination
   a. Determine mechanism of injury if possible (e.g., hyperextension, axial loading, forced flexion)
   b. Clinical symptoms: pain, weakness, sensory loss, bowel and bladder function
   c. Assess for tenderness over spinous processes, swelling, or sudden "step-off" of vertebral processes

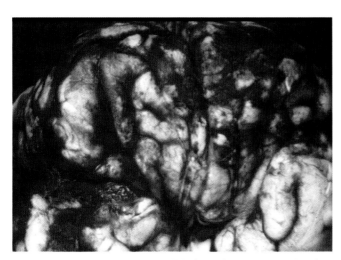

Fig. 10-20. Gross specimen with bifrontal contusions related to trauma.

d. Determine spinal cord involvement: level and whether lesion is complete or incomplete (preservation of long tract function)
1) Paradoxical breathing: abdominal breathing due to loss of thoracic musculature
2) Autonomic instability: bradycardia, hypotension
3) Flaccid limbs with reduced reflexes
4) Sensory level
5) Urinary retention
6) Priapism
e. Remember: cervical spine injury may also result in arterial dissection
4. Diagnostic evaluation
a. Important to evaluate if
1) Spinal cord is injured in addition to ligament or bone
2) If no spinal cord injury, assess stability of ligamentous or bone injuries to prevent spinal cord damage
b. Important to be cautious with patients who are comatose until such injuries can be ruled out
c. Cervical spine plain X-rays
1) Lateral and anterior-posterior views
2) May need additional views: open mouth (view odontoid), oblique, flexion-extension, swimmer's view)
3) Indications in recent trauma
a) Unconscious
b) Cervical pain, neck injury by history
c) Neurologic deficit suggesting cervical spine injury
d. Thoracolumbar spine plain X-rays
1) Lateral and anterior-posterior views
2) Indications in recent trauma
a) Unconscious

b) Complaints of thoracic or lumbar level pain and/or swelling
c) Fall from distance or thrown from vehicle
d) Neurologic deficit suggesting spine injury
e. Spinal CT: indications
1) Provide additional information about fractures
2) Patient has neurologic deficit and unable to undergo MRI
f. MRI: indications
1) Bony injury level different from examination level
2) No bony injury noted on plain films, but myelopathic by examination
5. Treatment
a. Unstable lesion requires operative intervention or immobilization
b. Corticosteroids: dose for trauma depends on time of injury
1) Within 3 hours: 30 mg/kg methylprednisolone IV, then 5.4 mg/kg per hour continuous infusion for 23 hours
2) Within 3 to 8 hours: 30 mg/kg methylprednisolone, then 5.4 mg/kg per hour continuous infusion for 48 hours
c. Supportive management
1) Place Foley catheter to avoid overdistension of bladder
2) Consider abdominal binder if hypotension is due to dysautonomia
3) Have atropine at bedside if bradycardia is due to dysautonomia
4) Monitor respiratory status, especially if cervical or thoracic lesion
5) Spine board for transfers until injury is ruled out
6. Outcome
a. If spinal cord involvement is complete below level of injury on initial examination, 3% of patients gain some function within 24 hours
b. If spinal cord involvement is complete and no change in function after 24 hours, further recovery is unlikely

IX. PERIVENTRICULAR-INTRAVENTRICULAR HEMORRHAGE OF PREMATURE NEONATES

A. Occurrence: in 20% to 40% of premature neonates with birth weight less than 1,500 g (may occur occasionally in full-term infants, different cause)

B. Time of Occurrence
1. 50% of cases occur in first 24 hours, with a large portion occurring in the first 6 hours of life

2. More than 90% of cases occur within first 72 hours postpartum

C. Origin of Hemorrhage

1. In subependymal germinal matrix, often in region of caudate, near foramen of Monro (Fig. 10-21)
2. May be result of rupture of thin-walled vessels in germinal vascular plate

D. Hemorrhage Grades

1. Grade I: confined to caudate head and subependymal layer (usually asymptomatic)
2. Grade II: extension into lateral ventricle, without ventriculomegaly
3. Grade III: extension into lateral ventricle, with ventriculomegaly (some may be clinically silent)
4. Grade IV: extension into parenchyma

E. Presentation

1. May be asymptomatic (especially grade I hemorrhage)
2. Acute neurologic deterioration with rapid development of coma, stupor, tense fontanelle, apnea, bradycardia, hypotension, metabolic acidosis, unreactive and midposition pupils, changes in muscle tone with decerebrate or decorticate posturing, and clonic limb movements (are not usually true focal seizures)

F. Diagnostic Testing

1. Bloody or xanthochromic CSF with elevated protein levels
2. Ultrasound through open fontanelles (noninvasive and highly accurate, with 90% sensitivity), may be used to follow progression of ventriculomegaly
3. CT if ultrasound not available

G. Management

1. Surgical evacuation is not indicated because of generally poor operative outcome
2. No treatment is usually indicated for grades I and II hemorrhage (good prognosis)
3. Daily lumbar punctures tend to reduce immediate harmful effects of the hemorrhage (this approach has not been shown to prevent long-term complications such as progressive hydrocephalus, which may eventually require a shunt)
4. If long-term lumbar punctures are necessary, alternative options may include placement of external ventricular drainage or ventricular catheter with a subcutaneous reservoir
5. In 50% of patients, progression of hydrocephalus stops and sometimes resolves spontaneously
6. If there is evidence of continued progression of hydrocephalus despite these temporary measures, placement of a ventriculoperitoneal shunt (or conversion of a subcutaneous reservoir to ventriculoperitoneal shunt) may eventually be indicated

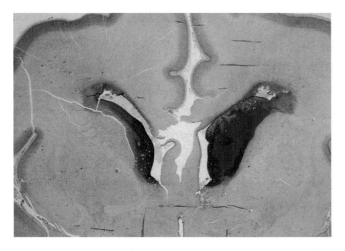 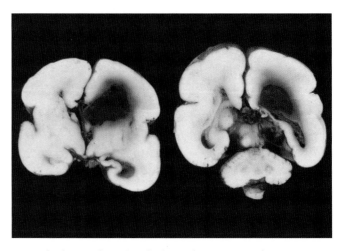

Fig. 10-21. *A,* Coronal section showing typical periventricular-intraventricular hemorrhage (grade I) involving germinal matrix overlying the caudate head, rostral to foramen of Monro. *B,* Postmortem specien from different neonate showing a larger hemorrhage (grade IV) extending into the brain parenchyma and lateral ventricle. (From Okazaki H, Scheithauer BW. Atlas of neuropathology. New York: Gower Medical Publishing; 1988. p. 279. By permission of Mayo Foundation.)

REFERENCES

Bradley WG, Daroff RB, Fenichel GM, Jankovic J. Neurology in clinical practice: principles of diagnosis and management. Vol 2. 4th ed. Philadelphia: Butterworth-Heinemann (Elsevier); 2004.

Chin RF, Neville BG, Scott RC. A systematic review of the epidemiology of status epilepticus. Eur J Neurol. 2004;11:800-10.

Flemming KD, Brown RD Jr. Natural history of intracranial vascular malformations. In: Winn HR, editor. Youmans neurological surgery. Vol 2. 5th ed. Philadelphia: Saunders; 2004. p. 2159-83.

Flemming KD, Brown RD Jr, Wiebers DO. Subarachnoid hemorrhage. Curr Treat Options Neurol. 1999;1:97-112.

Flemming KD, Wiebers DO. Unruptured intracranial aneurysms. In: Noseworthy JH, editor. Neurologic therapeutics: principles and practice. London: Martin Dunitz; 2003. p. 518-23.

Gupta R, Connolly ES, Mayer S, Elkind MS. Hemicraniectomy for massive middle cerebral artery territory infarction: a systematic review. Stroke. 2004 Feb;35:539-43. Epub 2004 Jan 5.

Manno EM. New management strategies in the treatment of status epilepticus. Mayo Clin Proc. 2003;78:508-18.

Rowland LP. Merritt's neurology. 10th ed. New York: Lippincott Williams & Wilkins; 2000.

Wijdicks EFM. Neurologic catastrophes in the emergency department. Boston: Butterworth-Heinemann; 2000.

Wijdicks EFM. The clinical practice of critical care neurology. 2nd ed. New York: Oxford University Press; 2003.

QUESTIONS

1. A patient presents with the acute onset of severe headache, nausea, and vomiting. This is the worst headache she has ever had. The patient comes to the emergency department, where you examine her within 30 minutes after headache onset. Initial CT study of the head is normal. What do you do next?
   a. Lumbar puncture immediately
   b. MRI of the brain
   c. Conventional angiography
   d. Observe patient and perform lumbar puncture 6 to 12 hours after symptom onset

2. If the patient in question 1 does have subarachnoid hemorrhage, at what time intervals are secondary complications such as rebleeding, hydrocephalus, and vasospasm likely to occur?
   a. Rebleeding, early (1-3 days); hydrocephalus, early; vasospasm, early
   b. Rebleeding, early; hydrocephalus, early; vasospasm, late (4-14 days)
   c. Rebleeding, late; hydrocephalus, late; vasospasm, late

3. Which of the following is *true* about the location and differential diagnosis of intracerebral hemorrhage?
   a. A basal ganglia hemorrhage is most commonly due to an arteriovenous malformation
   b. Hypertensive hemorrhages occur most commonly in the deep hemispheres or brainstem as opposed to a lobar location
   c. Multiple intracranial hemorrhages are common in hypertensive hemorrhage
   d. Cavernous malformation hemorrhage occurs most commonly in the cerebellum

4. Despite treatment with benzodiazepines and phenytoin, a patient continues in status epilepticus. What is your next step?
   a. Consider intubating patient and starting a propofol drip
   b. Consider intubating patient and giving intravenous valproic acid
   c. Intubate patient and place under general anesthesia with pentobarbital
   d. Monitor patient with continuous electroencephalography for 1 hour and observe whether phenytoin is effective

5. A patient presents with numbness in his toes and bilateral footdrop, which developed over the past 12

hours. You admit the patient, and over the next 12 hours, the weakness ascends to involve the proximal and distal legs and his hands start to become weak. Because you recognize this as possible Guillain-Barré syndrome, what respiratory parameters would require intubation?
   a. Vital capacity, <40 mL/kg; maximum inspiratory pressure (PImax), < (−)40 cm H_2O; maximum expiratory pressure (PEmax), <40 cm H_2O
   b. Vital capacity, <40 mL/kg; PImax, < (−)30 cm H_2O; PEmax, <20 cm H_2O
   c. Vital capacity, <20 mL/kg; PImax, < (−)30 cm H_2O; PEmax, <40 cm H_2O

6. On examination of an unresponsive male patient, you note that he has Cheyne-Stokes respirations. The patient is moaning, but no clear words come out. He briefly opens his eyes to sternal rub. The left pupil is dilated to 7 mm and unreactive and the right pupil is 3 mm. The patient localizes pain with his left arm and leg movement, but displays decorticate posturing on the right. What is the patient's Glasgow Coma Score (GCS)?
   a. 7
   b. 8
   c. 9
   d. 10

7. In the patient in question 6, CT showed an epidural hematoma. While the patient is in the emergency department before going to the operating room, which of the following can be used to lower his intracranial pressure?
   a. Warming blankets
   b. Trendelenberg position
   c. Keep stimulating the patient to assure examination findings are not changing
   d. Pain control

8. A young woman 8 weeks' pregnant is admitted for intractable nausea and vomiting of several days' duration. You are called several days after admission to evaluate the patient because of acute onset of ataxia and confusion. What is the most likely consideration?
   a. Guillain-Barré syndrome—Miller Fischer variant
   b. Wernicke's encephalopathy
   c. Ischemic stroke
   d. Vitamin B_{12} deficiency

9. A 50-year-old patient presents with a single seizure. MRI shows a cavernous malformation with intra-lesional, but not extralesional, hemorrhage in the left temporal lobe. What is the best management at this time?
    a. Treat medically with antiepileptic medication
    b. Stereotactic radiosurgery
    c. Endovascular coiling
    d. Surgical resection

10. A patient presents with a 1-week history of progressive leg weakness. Examination shows complete paraplegia with no movement of the lower extremities and a sensory level at T-10. MRI of the thoracic spine shows a large disk at the appropriate level. One day postoperatively, the examination findings are the same. What do you tell the patient regarding prognosis?
    a. There is a 50% chance that over 1 year the patient will become ambulatory
    b. There is a 25% chance that over 1 year the patient will become ambulatory
    c. There is a 10% chance that over 1 year the patient will become ambulatory
    d. It is unlikely that the patient will become ambulatory

ANSWERS

1. Answer: d.
The concern is possible subarachnoid hemorrhage. CT of the head can be falsely negative for subarachnoid hemorrhage within the first 24 to 48 hours. Lumbar puncture is definitely required if suspicion is high for subarachnoid hemorrhage. The red blood cell count over several tubes and presence of xanthochromia can help distinguish between a subarachnoid hemorrhage and a traumatic tap. However, xanthochromia (yellow tinge to cerebrospinal fluid) will only be seen after blood products have time to break down, approximately 6 to 12 hours after onset of symptoms. One should wait 6 hours before performing lumbar puncture and observe patient closely. Xanthochromia can also be seen with high cerebrospinal fluid levels of protein and increased bilirubin level.

2. Answer: b.
The highest risk for rebleeding is within the first 24 hours. Hydrocephalus may also present early within the first several days. Vasospasm generally occurs between 4 and 14 days.

3. Answer: b.
Hypertensive hemorrhages generally occur in the basal ganglia, thalamus, pons, cerebellum, and brainstem. This location and the appropriate history of long-standing hypertension can help make the diagnosis. Lobar hemorrhages may be due to amyloid angiopathy in older patients, arteriovenous malformations, aneurysmal rupture, venous thrombosis, or be drug- or toxin-related. Multiple intracranial hemorrhages may be due to metastases, multiple cavernous malformations, bleeding diathesis, vasculitis, venous thrombosis, a cardiac source (endocarditis, myxoma, angiosarcoma) or be drug- or toxin-related.

4. Answer: a.
At this point and while continuing to treat patient, laboratory studies and head imaging should be performed to determine the possible cause. Intubation should be considered because additional medical management may result in sedation and inability to protect the airway. (Review Figure 10-15 for additional medical management options.)

5. Answer: c.
Remember the "20/30/40" rule for consideration of intubation in neuromuscular failure: vital capacity <20 mL/kg, PImax < (–)30 cm H_2O, PEmax <40 cm H_2O.

6. Answer: c.
GCS = E2V2M5 = 9 (remember, it is *best* motor). Examination findings suggest a left supratentorial mass causing transtentorial herniation and trapping ipsilateral cranial nerve III at Kernohan's notch (along the tentorial edge where the midbrain and diencephalon meet).

7. Answer: d.
Consider mannitol, pain control, and normothermia before sending the patient to the operating room. Intubation with hyperventilation could also be considered.

8. Answer: b.
Hyperemesis gravidarum is a risk factor for Wernicke's encephalopathy, which may present with ataxia, amnestic state, and extraocular motility abnormalities. It is treatable with thiamine. Another consideration in a pregnant woman is increased risk of certain cerebrovascular complications, including ischemic arterial stroke, venous thrombosis, and rupture of an arteriovenous malformation, which generally occur in the third trimester or postpartum.

9. Answer: a.
Many patients with cavernous malformations and seizures respond well to medical management alone (antiseizure medication). However, if there is mass effect, marked extralesional hemorrhage, or recurrent hemorrhage, surgery could be considered. It is often curative. If the cavernous malformation is located in noneloquent tissue, some may advocate early surgical intervention. Radiotherapy generally is not recommended for cavernous malformations.

10. Answer: d.
If examination shows complete loss below the affected spinal cord level 24 hours after presentation, recovery is unlikely.

CEREBROVASCULAR DISEASE **11**

Kelly D. Flemming, M.D.

I. ANATOMY OF THE CEREBRAL AND SPINAL VASCULATURE

A. The Aortic Arch and Its Three Major Vessels (Fig. 11-1)

1. The aortic arch gives rise to 3 major branches: the brachiocephalic, left common carotid, and left subclavian arteries
2. The brachiocephalic artery gives rise to the right common carotid and right subclavian arteries
3. The vertebral arteries branch off the subclavian artery

B. The Carotid Artery (Fig. 11-2)

1. The common carotid artery bifurcates into the internal

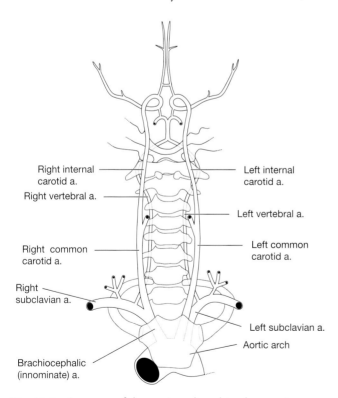

Fig. 11-1. Anatomy of the aortic arch and its three major branches. a, artery.

and external carotid arteries at approximately the cervical vertebral level 3-4

2. The main branches of the internal carotid artery are listed in Table 11-1
3. The internal carotid artery is composed of several segments
   a. Cervical: no branches arise from this segment
   b. Petrous: internal carotid artery enters the carotid canal of the temporal bone; a few minor branches (vidian, caroticotympanic) arise from this segment
   c. Cavernous: traverses the cavernous sinus along with cranial nerves III, IV, VI, and V_1 and V_2; a few minor branches (meningohypophyseal trunk, inferolateral trunk, capsular arteries) arise from this segment
   d. Clinoid: small segment; no branches
   e. Ophthalmic: most commonly intradural; gives rise to ophthalmic artery (supplies the retina) and superior hypophyseal artery
   f. Communicating segment: begins proximal to the origin of the posterior communicating artery and ends where the carotid terminates; the two major branches are the

Table 11-1. **Main Branches of Internal Carotid Artery System**

Branch	Supplies
Ophthalmic	Eye (retina)
Anterior choroidal	Optic tract, posterior limb of internal capsule, cerebral peduncle, choroid plexus, medial temporal lobe, globus pallidus, lateral geniculate body
Posterior communicating	Anastomoses with posterior cerebral artery
	Anterior thalamoperforate branches from posterior communicating artery extend to anterior portions of thalamus

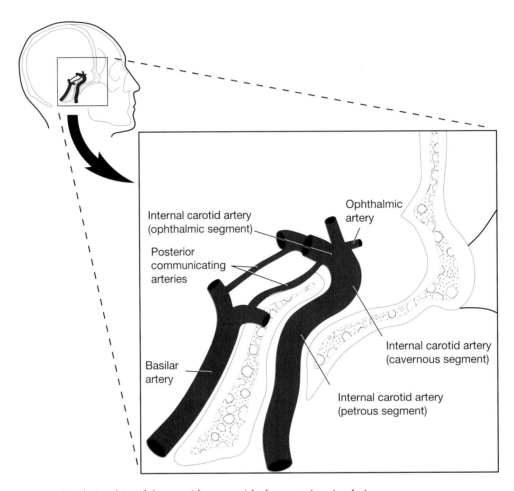

Fig. 11-2. Neuroanatomic relationship of the carotid artery with the posterior circulation.

posterior communicating artery and anterior choroidal artery

  g. At the carotid terminus, the artery bifurcates into the anterior and middle cerebral arteries

C. Anterior Cerebral Artery (ACA) (Fig. 11-3)
1. Composed of perforating vessels and cortical vessels
  a. Perforating or penetrating arteries (including recurrent artery of Heubner) supply deep structures: head of caudate nucleus, corpus callosum, part of fornix
  b. Cortical branches supply the medial aspect of the cerebral hemisphere

D. Middle Cerebral Artery (MCA) (Fig. 11-4)
1. Has both perforating branches and cortical branches
2. Perforating branches
  a. Arise from segment M_1 (extends from carotid terminus to MCA bifurcation) and
  b. Are called the lateral lenticulostriate arteries

  c. Supply the basal ganglia and internal capsule
3. Cortical branches: supply lateral aspect of cerebral hemisphere and anterior temporal lobe

E. Anastomoses
1. Collateral circulation: refers to alternative paths of blood supply (should one artery be impaired or occluded)
2. Several anastomoses supply collateral circulation to the brain
  a. Circle of Willis (Fig. 11-5)
    1) An anastomotic ring connecting the anterior circulation (carotid artery system) and posterior circulation (vertebrobasilar system)
    2) Less than 35% of people have a complete circle of Willis
    3) Components of the circle of Willis are shown in Figure 11-5
  b. Leptomeningeal collaterals: refers to anastomoses of distal cortical arteries

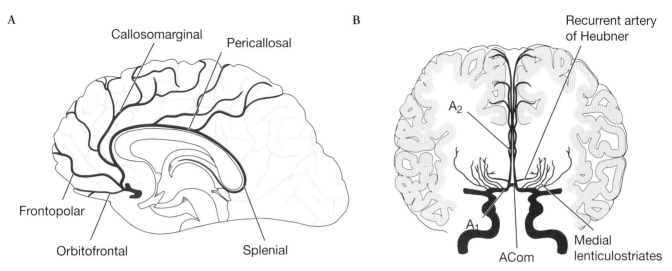

Fig. 11-3. Anterior cerebral artery (ACA). *A*, Medial aspect of cerebral hemisphere with cortical branches of ACA. *B*, Coronal section of cerebral hemispheres with cortical and penetrating branches of ACA. A_1, A_2, segments of ACA; *ACom*, anterior communicating artery.

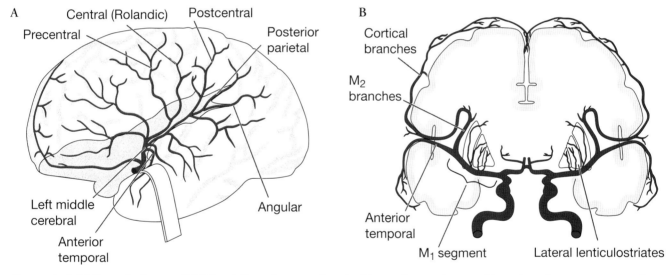

Fig. 11-4. Middle cerebral artery (MCA). *A*, Lateral aspect of cerebral hemisphere with cortical branches of MCA. *B*, Coronal section of cerebral hemispheres with cortical and penetrating branches of MCA. M_1, M_2, segments of MCA.

c. External carotid or extracranial vertebral artery-to-intracranial artery anastomoses
   1) External carotid artery commonly anastomoses with ophthalmic artery, serving as collateral circulation for distal internal carotid artery

F. **Vertebral Artery** (Fig. 11-6)
1. The right and left vertebral arteries arise from the respective subclavian arteries
2. The vertebral arteries ascend through the transverse foramina of vertebral bodies C6 to the axis; minor meningeal branches arise from these segments
3. Vertebral arteries enter the foramen magnum and pierce the dura mater
4. Intracranial vertebral arteries extend the length of the medulla and join at the pontomedullary junction to form the basilar artery
5. Important branches of the intracranial vertebral arteries include the following:
   a. Anterior spinal artery—supplies midline medulla,

including the pyramids, and extends caudally to supply ventrolateral spinal cord

b. Posterior spinal artery—supplies a portion of lateral medulla and extends caudally to supply posterior funiculus of spinal cord

c. Paramedian perforating arteries—supply the paramedian aspect of the medulla

d. Posterior inferior cerebellar artery (PICA)—supplies lateral medulla and inferior aspect of the cerebellum (Fig. 11-7 *A*)

G. Basilar Artery (Fig. 11-6)

1. Formed by union of left and right vertebral arteries at pontomedullary junction
2. Extends to the interpeduncular fossa where it ends by branching into the posterior cerebral arteries (PCAs)
3. Median and paramedian perforating branches supply their respective areas (Fig. 11-7 *B*)
4. Two long circumferential branches, anterior inferior cerebellar artery (AICA) and superior cerebellar artery (SCA), supply lateral pons inferiorly and superiorly, respectively, and a portion of the cerebellum
5. SCA also supplies part of midbrain

H. Posterior Cerebral Artery (PCA) (Fig. 11-6)

1. Basilar artery bifurcates into right and left PCAs at the interpeduncular fossa
2. Each PCA gives rise to both perforating and cortical arteries
3. Perforating branches arise from segments P₁ and P₂ of PCA
   a. Supply the thalamus
   b. Supply portions of the midbrain (Fig. 11-7 *C*)
4. Cortical branches
   a. Medial occipital artery gives rise to parieto-occipital and calcarine branches (supply visual cortex)
   b. Lateral occipital artery gives rise to temporal artery (supplies inferior temporal lobe)

I. Blood Supply to Deep Structures and Cerebellum (Tables 11-2 and 11-3)

J. Arterial Vascular Supply: borders of the arterial vascular supply are shown in Figure 11-8

K. Cerebral Venous System (Fig. 11-9)

1. Venous drainage occurs from pial venous plexuses that

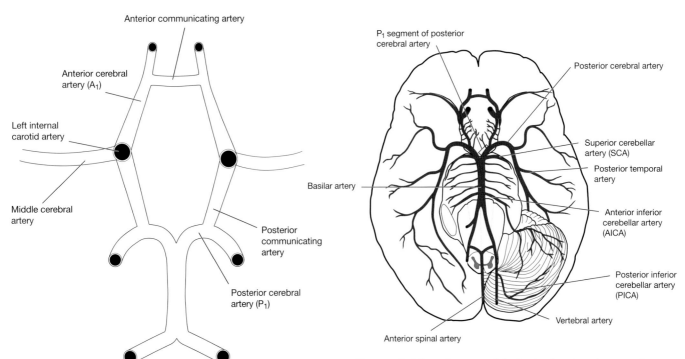

Fig. 11-5. Components of circle of Willis.

Fig. 11-6. Ventral aspect of the brain showing the posterior circulation.

> The middle meningeal artery enters the skull via the foramen spinosum

form within the substance of brain and drain into larger cerebral veins that, in turn, pass through subarachnoid space to empty into dural venous sinuses; small veins of the scalp communicate with dural venous sinuses via emissary veins

2. Dural venous sinuses are formed where periosteal and meningeal layers separate; these venous structures have no valves
3. Important dural venous sinuses: superior sagittal, inferior sagittal, straight (rectus), transverse, and sigmoid sinuses
4. Cavernous sinus: important venous structure composed of network of venous channels; situated on either side of sella turcica, with some interconnecting channels
5. Ophthalmic veins drain into the cavernous sinus, from which blood drains to superior and inferior petrosal veins to transverse and jugular veins, respectively
6. Deep cerebral veins
   a. Drain deep structures (e.g., basal ganglia, deep white matter, diencephalon) into the internal cerebral vein and great cerebral vein
   b. Internal cerebral veins
   c. Basal vein of Rosenthal
   d. Great cerebral vein of Galen
7. Superficial cerebral veins
   a. Superficial veins drain cerebral cortex and superficial subcortical white matter into venous sinuses
   b. Superior cerebral veins
   c. Inferior cerebral veins
   d. Superficial middle cerebral vein
   e. Superior anastomotic vein (Trolard)
   f. Inferior anastomotic vein (Labbé)

L. **Spinal Cord Vasculature**
1. Blood supply to the spinal cord emerges from anterior and posterior spinal arteries (branches of vertebral arteries) and from spinal branches of segmental arteries
2. Anterior spinal artery
   a. Paired anterior spinal arteries branch from vertebral arteries and join to form a single artery that descends along the anterior (ventral) aspect of the medulla and spinal cord

Table 11-2. Blood Supply to Basal Ganglia and Thalamus

Structure	Supply
Striatum	Lateral striate branches (MCA)
Head of caudate	Recurrent artery of Heubner (ACA)
Head of caudate, anteromedial portion	Anterior choroidal
Lateral globus pallidus	Lateral striate branches (MCA) and anterior choroidal
Medial globus pallidus	Anterior choroidal and perforating branches (PCOM)
Internal capsule	
Anterior limb	Lateral striate branches (MCA) and medial striates (ACA)
Genu	Internal carotid artery branches and lateral striate branches (MCA)
Posterior limb	Lateral striate branches (MCA) and anterior choroidal
Anterior thalamus	Anterior thalamoperforating branches (PCOM)
Medial thalamus	Posterior thalamoperforating branches from P_1 segment PCA and tip of basilar + posterior choroidal
Lateral thalamus	Thalamogeniculate from P_2 segment PCA

ACA, anterior cerebral artery; MCA, middle cerebral artery; PCA, posterior cerebral artery; PCOM, posterior communicating artery.

Table 11-3. Blood Supply to Cerebellum

Artery	Supplies
Posterior interior cerebellar arery (PICA)	Inferolateral surface of cerebellum, inferior vermis (uvula and nodulus), cerebellar tonsil Lateral medulla
Anterior inferior cerebellar artery (AICA)	Inferior surface of cerebellum, flocculus, dentate nucleus Caudal pontine tegmentum
Superior cerebellar artery (SCA)	Medial portion supplies superior cerebellar vermis Lateral portion supplies superior hemispheres and also supplies deep nuclei, superior medullary velum, and lateral portion of upper pontine tegmentum

A

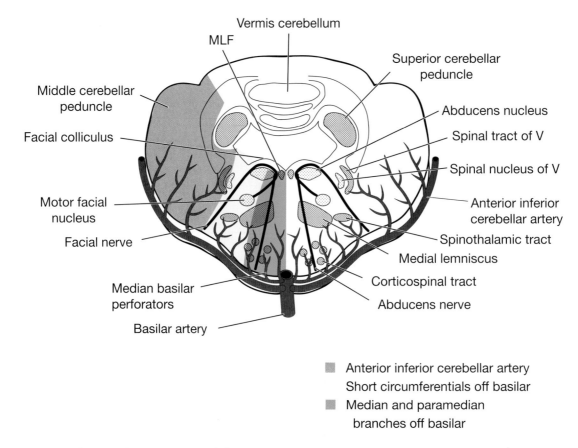

Fig. 11-7. Arterial supply to the brainstem. *A,* Medulla. *B,* Pons.

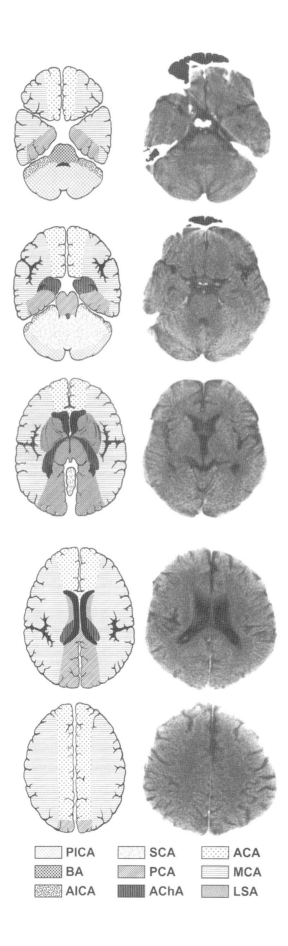

b. As anterior spinal artery descends along spinal cord, anastomotic branches from the anterior radicular arteries contribute to the vessel's continuity

c. Supplies midline medulla (including pyramids) and provides sulcal branches that enter anterior median fissure of the spinal cord to supply anterior and lateral funiculi (Fig. 11-10 *A*)

3. Posterior spinal artery

a. Paired posterior spinal arteries arise from vertebral arteries (and occasionally PICA) and descend on posterior surface of spinal cord, medial to dorsal roots

b. Like the anterior spinal artery, these arteries receive contributions from radicular arteries as they descend

c. These arteries supply posterior third of spinal cord, including the posterior columns

4. Segmental arteries and radicular arteries

a. Maintain continuity of anterior and posterior spinal arteries at each level of spinal cord

b. Include ascending cervical, intercostal, and lumbar arteries

c. Contribute branches that further divide into anterior and posterior radicular arteries

d. May be up to 31 pairs of radicular arteries: not every radicular artery contributes to spinal cord vascularization

e. Cervical cord has the most contributions; thoracic and lumbar segments have fewer (perhaps 2-4) arteries that contribute to spinal cord blood supply, making the region more vulnerable to ischemia

f. Blood supply to mid-thoracic (T4-T6) cord is relatively tenuous: the vascular watershed zone of spinal cord, most vulnerable to ischemic insults

---

The blood supply to the mid-thoracic (T4-T6) spinal cord is relatively tenuous: the vascular watershed zone of the spinal cord, most vulnerable to ischemic insults

---

Fig. 11-8. Arterial vascular distributions. ACA, anterior cerebral artery; AChA, anterior choroidal artery; AICA, anterior inferior cerebellar artery; BA, basilar artery; LSA, lenticulostriate artery; MCA, middle cerebral artery; PCA, posterior cerebral artery; PICA, posterior inferior cerebellar artery; SCA, superior cerebellar artery. (From Wijdicks EFM. Catastrophic neurologic disorders in the emergency department. 2nd ed. New York: Oxford University Press; 2004. p. 191-222. By permission of Mayo Foundation.)

A

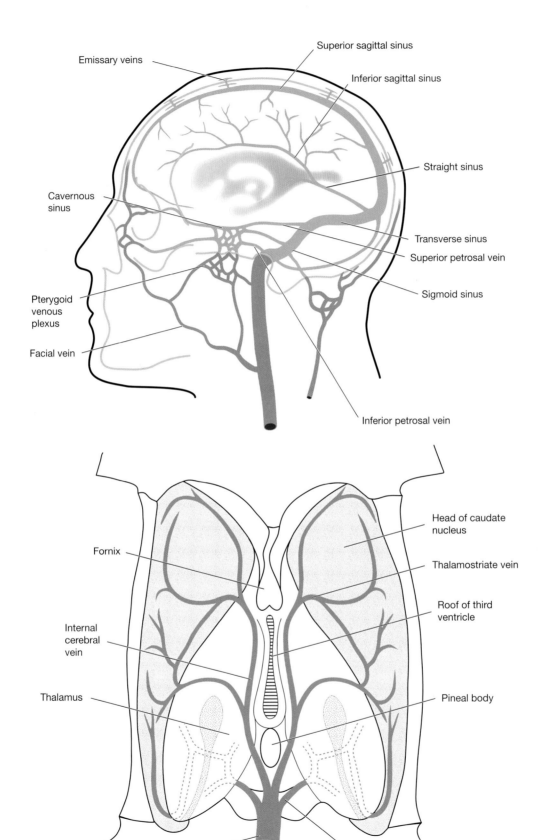

Fig. 11-9. *A*, Venous sinuses. *B*, Deep, subependymal venous system depicted from above.

A

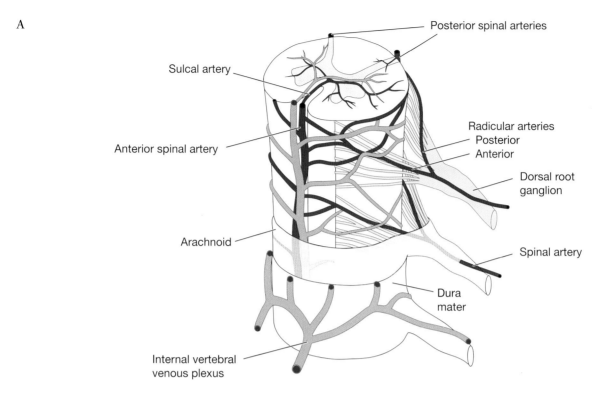

B

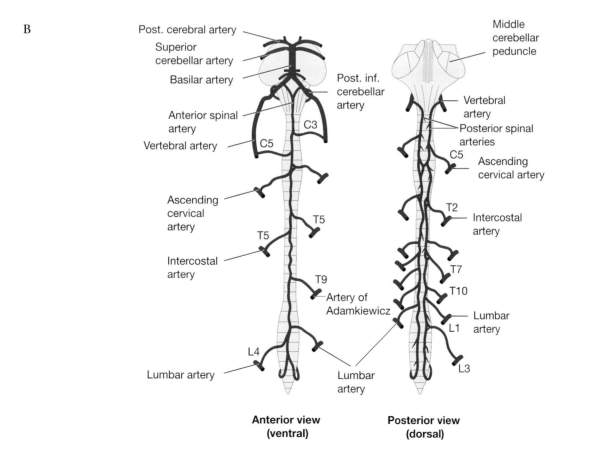

Fig. 11-10. *A* and *B*, Vascular supply of the spinal cord.

g. Artery of Adamkiewicz: large anterior radicular artery at level T12, L1, or L2; major source of blood to lower thoracic and upper lumbar cord (Fig. 11-10 *B*)

5. Veins of spinal cord
   a. Anterolateral and anteromedian veins drain anterior cord
   b. Posterolateral and posteromedian veins drain posterior cord
   c. These veins drain into radicular veins, which empty into the epidural venous plexus
   d. The epidural venous plexus has longitudinal connections with other veins of central nervous system (extending all the way to the brainstem region) and can drain into segmental veins and systemic venous system

II. ISCHEMIC STROKE PATHOPHYSIOLOGY

A. Principles of Cellular Injury and Vascular Biology

1. Cellular injury and ischemia
   a. Normal cerebral blood flow in humans is approximately 50 to 60 mL/100 g of brain tissue per minute to supply oxygen and glucose to tissues and remove lactic acid
   b. When flow decreases to 20 to 40 mL/100 g per minute, neuronal dysfunction occurs
   c. When flow is less than 10 to 15 mL/100 g per minute, irreversible tissue damage occurs
   d. Because of extensive collateral circulation, there is variability in perfusion changes within an ischemic lesion
   e. In the central core of the infarction, severity of hypoperfusion results in irreversible cellular damage
   f. Around this core is a region of decreased flow in which either the critical flow threshold for cell death has not been reached or the duration of ischemia has been insufficient to cause irreversible damage, the so-called ischemic penumbra
   g. If flow is not restored, this penumbra may result in permanent and irreversible damage
   h. Secondary effects of ischemia
      1) In addition to lack of energy supply to the tissue, other mechanisms contribute to cell death
      2) Excess glutamate release and impaired glutamate reuptake during ischemia results in prolonged elevations of calcium in the cytosol; this elevated calcium in turn triggers proteases, lipases, endonucleases, and cytokines, which result in neuronal cell death

2. Pathology (Fig. 11-11 and 11-12)
   a. Acute (1 day–1 week)
      1) Gross: affected area is edematous
      2) Microscopic

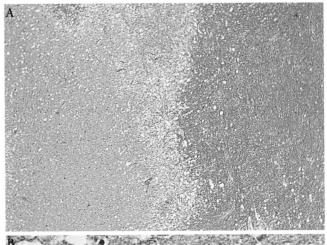
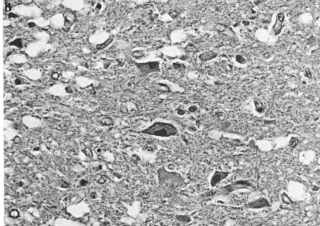
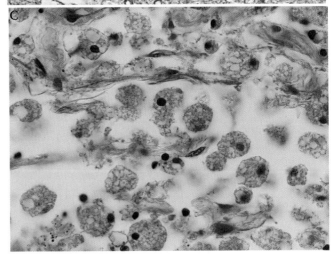

Fig. 11-11. Acute and subacute ischemic infarct. In the acute stage of infarction, there is often a clear interface between the pale zone of ischemia and richly stained normal tissue. *A*, The edge of the infarct is marked by vacuolation of the neuropil. *B*, Neurons in the region of the acute ischemic event often appear pyknotic and intensely eosinophilic, appearing as "little red cells." *C*, Foamy macrophages usually appear in the subacute stage and can persist for several months after the insult.

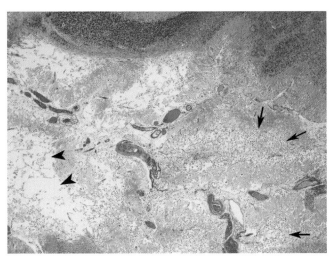

Fig. 11-12. Old ischemic infarct. In the chronic stage (after several weeks), liquefactive necrosis leads to cystic cavitation (*arrowheads*). This is the result of resorptive action of macrophages on damaged tissue (*arrows*).

       a) Acutely, there are eosinophilic pyknotic neurons; there is neuropil vacuolation, often most prominent at the edge of the infarct
       b) Within 1 to 3 days, an inflammatory response is seen, followed by mononuclear cell influx by days 3 to 5; the latter phagocytize dying cells
    b. Subacute (1 week–1 month)
      1) Gross: tissue destruction, liquefactive necrosis
      2) Microscopic: reactive astrocytes and prominent macrophage infiltration and phagocytosis are often seen
    c. Chronic (>1 month)
      1) Gross: cavitation of affected area with surrounding gliosis
      2) Microscopic: cystic cavity forms, surrounded by gliosis; there may be residual macrophage infiltration (Fig. 11-12)

B. Atherogenesis
1. Is an important pathologic lesion responsible for cerebral infarction
2. Atherosclerotic plaque formation requires several sequential steps that are set into motion by certain triggers: hypertension, diabetes mellitus, obesity, chronic inflammation or infection, oxidized lipoproteins
3. Triggers result in activation of endothelial cells and expression of white blood cell adhesion protein
4. Certain adhesion molecules allow migration of white blood cells into the intima, and these monocytes transform into macrophages
5. Subsequently, macrophages engulf specific lipoproteins and become "foam" cells, which can secrete mediators that allow continued accumulation of other monocytes, promote smooth muscle cell proliferation in the vessel, and change the extracellular matrix, degrading the collagen protective structure
6. The plaque is dynamic and may change over time because of continued triggers and risk factors: increased lipid content, intramural hemorrhage, calcification
7. The artery may show progressive narrowing of the lumen to occlusion or endothelial integrity may become vulnerable from proliferation of metalloproteinases degrading stability of the plaque
8. If the plaque become unstable and ruptures, the subendothelium is exposed, and platelets can adhere and aggregate, resulting in thrombus formation
9. Atherosclerosis is most common at arterial bifurcations (Fig. 11-13)

III. Clinical Ischemic Syndromes

A. **Large-Artery Disease:** clinical syndromes (Table 11-4)

B. **Small-Vessel Disease** (lacunar stroke): clinical syndromes
1. Lacunar stroke refers to a 1.5-cm (greatest diameter) or smaller ischemic stroke within the distribution of a penetrating end artery (Additional information is given below, but the clinical-anatomic descriptions are provided here)
2. More than 20 lacunar syndromes have been described; the most common syndromes are listed in Table 11-5

IV. Overview of Ischemic Stroke Mechanisms and Etiologies

A. **Mechanisms and Causes of Ischemia**
1. Definitions
    a. Ischemic stroke: a fixed focal neurologic deficit attributable to an arterial or venous territory and lasting longer than 24 hours
    b. Transient ischemic attack (TIA): a transient focal neurologic deficit attributable to an arterial territory and lasting less than 24 hours (by definition), most last less than 20 minutes

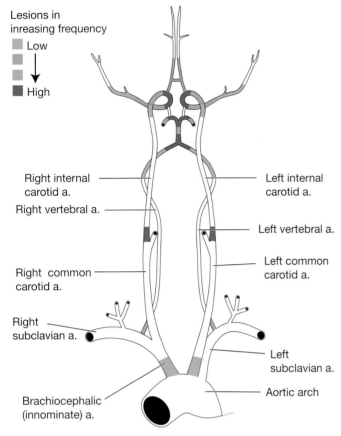

Lesions in
inreasing frequency

■ Low

↓

■ High

Right internal
carotid a.

Right vertebral a.

Right common
carotid a.

Right
subclavian a.

Brachiocephalic
(innominate) a.

Left internal
carotid a.

Left vertebral a.

Left common
carotid a.

Left
subclavian a.

Aortic arch

Fig. 11-13. Distribution and frequency of atherosclerotic
lesions in extracranial and intracranial arteries. a, artery.

c. Reversible ischemic neurologic deficit (RIND): a focal
neurologic deficit that lasts longer than 24 hours, but
resolves by 3 weeks
2. Mechanisms
   a. Hypoperfusion: may be global or focal, the latter in the
   setting of a single-vessel fixed stenosis
   b. Thrombosis (e.g., thrombus at site of atherosclerotic
   plaque rupture)
   c. Embolism
      1) Cardiac: thrombus, myxomatous emboli, vegetation
      2) Artery to artery: cholesterol, platelet, thrombotic emboli
      3) Rare: air, fat, or amniotic fluid emboli
3. Causes
   a. Etiology of thrombosis or emboli can be divided into
   several categories (from proximal to distal)
      1) Cardioembolic source
      2) Large-vessel disease of extracranial vessels (aorta,
      carotid arteries, vertebral arteries)
      3) Large-vessel disease of intracranial vessels
      4) Small-vessel disease (lacunar)

5) Abnormalities intrinsic to blood itself, i.e.,
coagulation defects
6) Venous infarction
7) Other
   b. Desite thorough diagnostic evaluation, 15% to 35% of
   cerebral infarctions remain cryptogenic, i.e., no definable
   source
4. Prevalence: overall prevalence of selected cerebral
infarction causes in a general population of patients is
approximately
   a. Cardioembolic in 30%
   b. Large-vessel disease in 20%
   c. Small-vessel disease in 20%
   d. Other in 3%
   e. Cryptogenic in 27%
5. Differential diagnosis of ischemic stroke is listed in
Table 11-6
6. General approach to ischemic stroke evaluation
   a. First goal: determine if patient is a candidate for acute
   therapy, such as thrombolytic agents
   b. Second goal: prevent recurrent ischemic stroke
      1) This involves diagnostic investigations to determine
      cause of ischemic stroke, specifically a cause that
      would require treatment other than an antiplatelet
      agent, such as surgery or anticoagulation
      2) Identify risk factors such as hyperlipidemia, hyperten-
      sion, others
   c. Third goal: prevent early and late complications of
   ischemic stroke
      1) Poststroke depression
      2) Myocardial infarction (MI)
      3) Pulmonary emboli/deep venous thrombosis
      4) Aspiration pneumonia
7. General approach to ischemic stroke evaluation is
shown in Fig. 11-14
   a. Localizing a stroke requires knowledge of neuroanatomy
   and typical clinical presentations (Tables 11-4 and 11-5)
   b. Localization can be aided by cross-sectional imaging
   studies such as computed tomography (CT) and magnetic resonance imaging (MRI)
   c. CT
      1) May be negative early in ischemic stroke
      2) Cortical ischemia may take 24 hours to evolve
      3) Early signs of cortical ischemia may include
         a) Sulcal effacement (most apparent with side-to-side
         comparison)
         b) Loss of distinction between gray and white matter
         c) Dense MCA sign or hyperdense basilar artery may
         also be seen, suggesting clot within the arteries
   d. MRI (Fig. 11-15)

Table 11-4.   Large-Vessel Clinical Syndromes*

Vessel	Clinical presentation
Internal carotid artery	Ipsilateral retinal ischemia (amaurosis)
	Sensorimotor dysfunction similar to involvement of middle and anterior cerebral artery territories
Middle cerebral artery (M1)	Contralateral face and arm > leg weakness
	Aphasia (dominant hemisphere)
	Contralateral sensory loss
	Cortical sensory loss (nondominant hemisphere)
	Contralateral visual field defect
	Gaze deviation ipsilateral to lesion
Middle cerebral artery, anterior division	Contralateral face and arm > leg weakness
	Broca's aphasia (dominant hemisphere)
Middle cerebral artery, posterior division	Contralateral sensory loss
	Wernicke's aphasia (dominant hemisphere)
	Gerstmann's syndrome (dominant hemisphere)
	Cortical sensory loss/neglect (nondominant hemisphere)
	Contralateral visual field defect
Anterior cerebral artery	Contralateral leg weakness
	Contralateral leg sensory loss
	Apraxia
	Abulia (bilateral)
Anterior choroidal artery	Contralateral homonymous hemianopia (lateral geniculate body)
	Contralateral face, arm, leg weakness (posterior limb internal capsule)
	Contralateral face, arm, leg sensory loss (thalamus)
Posterior cerebral artery (precommunicating)	Contralateral sensory loss (thalamus)
	Cognitive dysfunction (thalamus)
	Thalamic aphasia (rarely)
	Visual dysfunction as for postcommunicating segment
Posterior cerebral artery (postcommunicating segment)	Contralateral homonymous hemianopia
	Visual agnosias
Posterior inferior cerebellar artery	Horner's syndrome
	Ipsilateral hemiataxia
	Ipsilateral palatal weakness
	Hoarse voice
	Decreased pain and temperature on ipsilateral face and contralateral limbs
Anterior inferior cerebellar artery	Ipsilateral deafness
	Ipsilaeral facial weakness (lower motor neuron)
	Ipsilateral hemiataxia
	Contralateral sensory loss in limbs
Superior cerebellar artery	Ipsilateral ataxia
	Decreased sensation contralaterally
	Diplopia
Basilar perforators, median and paramedian pontine perforators	Contralateral limb weakness if unilateral or quadriparesis if bilateral
	Hemiataxia may develop (crossing pontocerebellar fibers)
	Cranial nerve/nuclear VI and VII palsies
	Internuclear ophthalmoplegia
Midbrain basilar, posterior cerebral artery perforators	Ipsilateral nuclear or fascicular cranial nerve III palsy
	Contralateral face, arm, leg weaknes (corticospinal tracts)
	Rubral tremor (red nucleus) may develop
	Ataxia (decussation of superior cerebellar peduncle) may occur
Anterior spinal and vertebral perforators to median and paramedian medulla	Ipsilateral tongue weakness (cranial nerve/nucleus XII)
	Contralateral arm and leg have reduced vibration sensation and proprioception (medial lemniscus)
	Contralateral arm and leg weakness (medullary pyramids)

*For brainstem syndromes, see Chapter 4.

Table 11-5. Lacunar Syndromes

Syndrome	Typical clinical presentation	Typical localization
Pure motor hemiparesis	Contralateral face, arm, leg weakness	Internal capsule Corona radiata
Pure sensory stroke	Contralateral face, arm, leg sensory loss	Thalamus (ventral posterolateral and postero-medial nuclei)
Sensorimotor stroke	Contralateral face, arm, leg weakness Contralateral face, arm, leg sensory loss	Thalamocapsular
Ataxic-hemiparesis	Hemiataxia and hemiparesis on same side of body	Basis pontis Thalamocapsular Corona radiata
Clumsy hand dysarthria	Facial weakness Dysarthria Slight hemiparesis Cerebellar dysmetria	Basis pontis

1) Random diffusion of water molecules: relatively free in extracellular space and restricted in intracellular space in normal state; best measured by diffusion-weighted imaging (DWI)
2) Rapid dysfunction of cellular metabolism and ion exchange pumps cause massive shift of water from extracellular to intracellular compartment: cytotoxic edema
3) Cytotoxic edema forming early in ischemic stroke restricts diffusion of water molecules, resulting in increased signal on DWI and decreased signal on apparent diffusion coefficient (ADC) map
4) Diffusion signal increases very early (within minutes-hours) and remains positive for about 2 weeks, then normalizes so that acute to subacute infarcts can be distinguished from old infarcts and background ischemic white matter changes
5) Patients with transient symptoms may also have abnormalities on DWI
6) FLAIR and T2-weighted images are also helpful for ischemic stroke
7) Caution: not all diffusion hyperintensity is an ischemic stroke; positive diffusion abnormalities have been described in neoplastic, infectious, and demyelinating processes
8. Special situation: stroke in the young—atherosclerosis is a common cause in younger patients, but nonathero-

sclerotic arteriopathies such as dissection and cardioembolic sources are frequent
9. Special situation: stroke during pregnancy
   a. Ischemic stroke and hemorrhage may occur during pregnancy
   b. Pregnancy represents a special situation in which the body is preparing for an event that requires rapid coagulation at the time of birth
   c. Coagulation changes during pregnancy and postpartum period
      1) When the placenta separates, maternal blood flows at 700 mL/min and is reduced by myometrial compression and thrombotic occlusion of the vessels
      2) Coagulation is activated and fibrinogen is increased and coagulation inhibitors are decreased; coagulation system and fibrinolytic systems are important in controlling fibrin deposition in uteroplacental circulation while simultaneously preventing fibrin deposition in rest of vascular system
      3) Changes typically begin in first trimester and increase maximally by late pregnancy
      4) Erythrocyte mass increases at about 10 weeks and increases progressively until term
      5) Plasma volume increases at about 10 weeks' gestation and increases progressively until 30 to 34 weeks, after which it plateaus
      6) Mean increase in plasma volume by 30 to 34 weeks is 50%
      7) Because volume increases by 50% and erythrocyte mass increases only by 18% to 30%, the hematocrit decreases: anemia (30-34–week nadir)
      8) Changes of the specific coagulation factors in pregnancy are noted in Table 11-7
   d. Pregnancy and postpartum–associated cerebrovascular complications can include
      1) Subarachnoid hemorrhage
         a) Incidence: 20 per 100,000 pregnancies
         b) Etiology: aneurysmal rupture, arteriovenous malformation (AVM) rupture, trauma
         c) More common to occur during pregnancy than postpartum period
      2) Intraparenchymal hemorrhage
         a) Incidence: 4 per 100,000
         b) Etiology: AVM rupture, cavernous malformation rupture, eclampsia, venous thrombosis
         c) More common during postpartum period than during pregnancy
      3) Venous thrombosis (with ischemia and/or hemorrhage)
         a) Incidence: 10 to 20 per 100,000 (higher in underdeveloped countries)

Table 11-6.   Differential Diagnosis of Ischemic Stroke

Cardiac disorder
  Atrial fibrillation
  Mitral stenosis
  Left ventricular thrombus
  Atrial myoma
  Dilated cardiomyopathy
  Anterior wall myocardial infarction
  Prosthetic valves
  Endocarditis (bacterial, nonbacterial, marantic)
  Patent foramen ovale
  Atrial septal aneurysm
  Mitral valve calcification
  Fibroelastoma
  Pulmonary fistula (Osler-Weber-Rendu disease)
  Air or fat emboli (rare)
Large-vessel extracranial disorder
  Atherosclerosis
  Dissection
  Radiation vasculopathy
  Fibromuscular dysplasia
  Vasculitis
    Takayasu's vasculitis
    Giant cell arteritis
Large-vessel intracranial disorder
  Atherosclerosis
  Dissection
  Inflammatory vasculitis
    Isolated CNS angiitis
    Necrotizing vasculitides (Wegener's granulomatosis,
      polyarteritis nodosa, Churg-Strauss syndrome,
      lymphomatoid granulomatosis)
    Hypersensitivity angiitis with connective tissue
      disease (sarcoidosis, systemic lupus erythematosus,
      Sjögren's syndrome, rheumatoid arthritis)
    Susac syndrome (retinocochleocerebral arteriopathy)
    Kohlmeier-Degos disease
    Behçet's syndrome
  Infectious vasculitis
    Varicella-zoster virus
    Human immunodeficiency virus
    Hepatitis B and C
    Epstein-Barr virus
    Cytomegalovirus
  Noninflammatory vasculopathies
    Moyamoya disease
    Drug-induced (cocaine, methamphetamine, phenyl-
      propanolamine, ergotamines)
    Postpartum cerebral angiopathy

  Radiation-induced
  Eales disease
  Arterial dolichoectasia
  Endovascular lymphoma
  Thrombosed aneurysm with emboli
Small-vessel disease
  Lipohyalinosis/atherosclerosis
  Vasculitis
    Varicella-zoster vasculitis
    Cryoglobulin-related angiitis
    Angiitis related to lymphomatoid malignancies
    Henoch-Schönlein purpura
Hematologic and coagulation disorders
  Disorders of coagulation factors
    Protein C or S deficiency
    Antithrombin III deficiency
    Activated protein C resistance/factor V Leiden
      mutation
    Prothrombin 20210 mutation
  Disorders of red blood cells
    Sickle cell anemia
    Polycythemia (primary or secondary)
    Paroxysmal nocturnal hemoglobinuria
  Disorders of white blood cells
    Lymphoma
    Leukemia
  Disorders of platelets
    Disseminated intravascular coagulation
    Thrombotic thrombocytopenic purpura
    Idiopathic thrombocytopenic purpura
    Essential thrombocythemia
    Thrombocytosis
    Paraproteinemia
    Uremia
  Disorders of plasma cells
    Myeloma
    Cryoglobulinemia
  Other
    Antiphospholipid antibody syndrome
    Hyperhomocystinemia
  Malignancy-associated coagulopathy
Other
  CADASIL
  Sneddon's syndrome
  Fabry's disease
  MELAS
  Homocystinuria
  Organic acidemias

CADASIL, cerebral autosomal dominant arteriopathy with subcortical infarcts and leukoencephalopathy; CNS, central nervous system; MELAS, myopathy, encephalopathy, lactic acidosis, and stroke-like episodes.

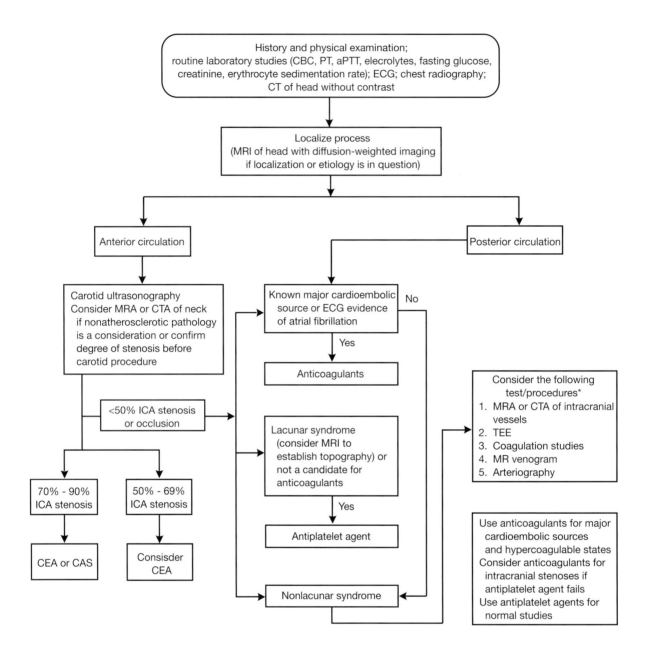

Fig. 11-14. Evaluation of ischemic stroke. aPTT, activated partial thromboplastin time; CAS, carotid artery stenting; CBC, complete blood cell count; CEA, carotid endarterectomy; CT, computed tomography; CTA, computed tomographic angiography; ECG, electrocardiography; ICA, internal carotid artery; MR, magnetic resonance; MRA, magnetic resonance angiography; MRI, magnetic resonance imaging; PT, prothrombin time; TEE, transesophageal echocardiography. *Indications for diagnostic testing (factors increasing the pretest probability of disease): 1) intracranial arterial evaluation (MRA or CTA): stereotyped transient ischemic attacks in single vascular territory or cortical ischemic event; female; Asian, Hispanic, or African Americans; and patient younger than 50 years, 2) TEE: personal history of cardiac disease, physical examination consistent with heart murmur or congestive heart failure, abnormal ECG, patient younger than 50 years with no other source found, and ischemic events in multiple territories or cortical ischemic event, 3) coagulation studies: patient younger than 45 years and personal or family history of thrombotic events, 4) MR venogram: if clinical suspicion (headache, thrombotic risk factors, young age) or radiographically stroke overlaps arterial territories, and 5) arteriography: clinical suspicion for inflammatory or infectious vasculitis. (From Flemming KD, Brown RD Jr, Petty GW, Huston J III, Kallmes DF, Piepgras DG. Evaluation and management of transient ischemic attack and minor cerebral infarction. Mayo Clin Proc. 2004;79:1071-86. By permission of Mayo Foundation.)

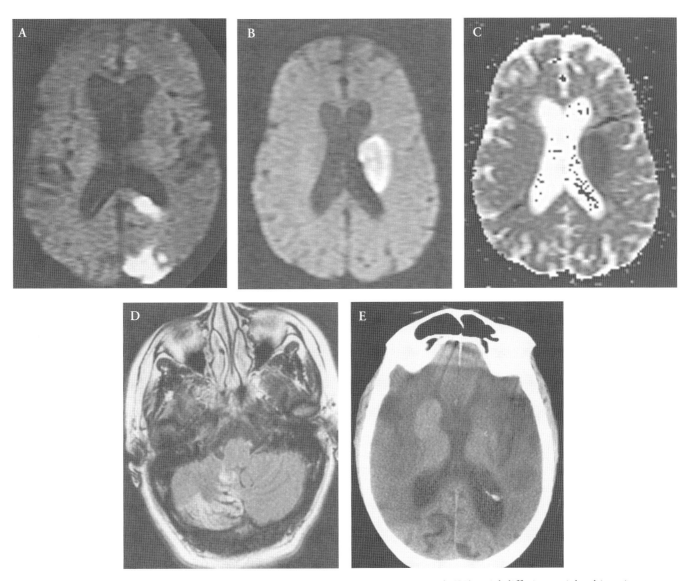

Fig. 11-15. Neuroimaging of acute ischemic strokes. *A*, Magnetic resonance imaging (MRI), axial diffusion-weighted imaging (DWI) showing area of restricted diffusion involving left occipital lobe and splenium of corpus callosum (posterior cerebral artery distribution infarct due to cardioembolism). Patient presented with alexia without agraphia. *B* and *C*, MRI of 79-year-old patient with acute infarct involving left corona radiata. Acute infarct appears hyperintense on DWI (*B*) and low signal on ADC (apparent diffusion coefficient) mapping (*C*). Distribution is that of lateral lenticulostriate branches of left middle cerebral artery. *D*, MRI FLAIR sequences of patient with right cerebellar infarct in distribution of right posterior inferior cerebellar artery—vertebral artery. *E*, Computed tomogram of patient with old infarct in distribution of left middle cerebral artery (MCA) who now presents with right MCA stroke, showing very prominent area of low attenuation involving most of right MCA territory, complete effacement of the sulci of the right cerebral hemisphere, and mild mass effect.

b) Most common in postpartum period (80%)
c) Often associated with predisposing factor for thrombosis such as factor V Leiden mutation, dehydration, concurrent infection, sickle cell anemia
4) Pituitary apoplexy (Sheehan's syndrome)
5) Arterial stroke
   a) Incidence: 3.5 to 5 per 100,000

b) Highest risk in postpartum period
c) Causes vary, with some pregnancy-specific and some not pregnancy-specific
d) Pregnancy-specific causes: eclampsia (common), choriocarcinoma (rare), amniotic fluid embolism (rare), postpartum cerebral angiopathy (rare), peripartum cardiomyopathy (rare)

Table 11-7.   Changes in Specific Coagulation Factors in Pregnancy

Increased	Decreased	No change
Fibrinogen (doubles)	Factors XI, XIII	Factors II, V, IX
Factors VII, VIII, X, XII	Platelets (±)	Angiotensin III
Plasminogen (50%)	Fibrinolytic systems (highest in 3rd trimester)	Total protein S
PAI-1 and PAI-2		Protein C
Blood volume	Tissue plasminogen activator	
D-dimer		
β-Thromboglobulin (platelet)	Free protein S	
Fibrinopeptide A (first peptide cleaved from fibrinogen)		

PAI, plasminogen activator inhibitor.

V. Ischemic Stroke by Etiology

A. Cardioembolic Ischemic Stroke

1. Approximately 20% to 30% of cerebral infarctions in a general population are result of a cardioembolic source
2. "Major cardiac risk sources" are established as causative risk factors for TIA and cerebral infarction
3. "Minor risk sources" are established as potential sources and carry an uncertain risk of recurrent stroke because of inconclusive data in epidemiologic literature (Table 11-8)
4. Nonvalvular atrial fibrillation
   a. Prevalence: 1% of general population, 10% of population older than 75 years
   b. Risk factors for thromboembolism in patients with atrial fibrillation include
      1) Previous stroke or TIA
      2) History of hypertension
      3) Congestive heart failure or impaired left ventricular dysfunction
      4) Advanced age
      5) Diabetes mellitus
      6) Coronary artery disease
      7) Left atrial thrombus or spontaneous echo contrast
   c. Risk of stroke: may be as high as 10% to 12% per year with associated risk factors
   d. Treatment
      1) Anticoagulation with warfarin is superior to aspirin in secondary prevention of stroke in patients with atrial fibrillation

Table 11-8.   Major and Minor Cardiac Risk Sources

Major risk sources	Minor risk sources
Atrial fibrillation	Mitral valve prolapse
Mitral valve stenosis	Severe mitral annular calcification
Prosthetic cardiac valve	Patent foramen ovale
Recent myocardial infarction	Atrial septal aneurysm
Left ventricular or atrial thrombus	Calcific aortic stenosis
	Left ventricular regional wall motion abnormalities
Atrial myxoma	Mitral valve strands
Infectious endocarditis	
Dilated cardiomyopathy	
Marantic endocarditis	

2) Practice guidelines recommend adjusted dose anticoagulation in high-risk patients
   a) High-risk patients: those older than 75 years, patients older than 60 with diabetes or coronary artery disease, all patients with risk factors for thromboembolism
   b) Risk factors for thromboembolism: heart failure, left ventricular ejection fraction less than 0.35, history of hypertension, previous thromboembolism, rheumatic heart disease, prosthetic heart valves, thrombus detected on echocardiography
   c) Goal international normalized ratio (INR) is 2.0 to 3.0 except for patients with rheumatic heart disease or prosthetic valves who may require a higher INR
   d) Low-risk patients without risk factors for thromboembolism younger than 75 years can be treated with aspirin alone if they have not had a previous ischemic stroke or TIA
5. Impaired myocardial function and cardiomyopathy
   a. Can result in cardioembolic ischemic stroke
   b. Cardiomyopathy with left ventricular ejection fraction less than 30% increases risk of ischemic stroke
   c. Anticoagulation is recommended for patients with thromboembolic events related to cardiomyopathy
6. Myocardial infarction
   a. Risk factors for ischemic stroke after MI: older age, apical or anterior wall MI, coexistence of left ventricular dysfunction or atrial fibrillation, echocardiographic evidence of mural thrombi or severe wall motion abnormalities, previous history of stroke, history of hypertension before MI, history of systemic or pulmonary embolism
   b. Most cardioembolic events occur within first 2 weeks after acute MI, and one-third occur within the first

month; stroke risk is greatest in the first week and persists for 4 to 6 months

   c. In absence of aforementioned risk factors, old MI is not usually responsible for acute cerebrovascular ischemic event

   d. Treatment: short-term anticoagulation in addition to aspirin may be recommended for high-risk patients with recent MI

7. Left atrial spontaneous echo contrast

   a. Echocardiographic finding

   b. May represent local blood stasis; often seen with atrial fibrillation or left atrial thrombus

   c. Unclear whether patients with this finding (by itself) benefit from antiplatelet or anticoagulation therapy

   d. This finding should lead to further evaluation with Holter monitor or telemetry for paroxysmal atrial fibrillation

8. Infectious endocarditis

   a. Typical sources

     1) *Staphylococcus aureus*

     2) *Streptococcus viridans*

   b. Risk factors

     1) Intravenous drug use (generally involving the right-sided heart valves)

     2) Prosthetic heart valves

     3) Structural heart valve or other cardiac disease

   c. Neurologic complications

     1) Ischemic stroke due to emboli

     2) Mycotic aneurysm formation with potential rupture

     3) Intracranial abscesses

   d. Diagnosis

     1) Transesophageal echocardiography (TEE)

     2) Blood cultures

   e. Clinical picture: new cardiac murmur, fever, Janeway lesions, Osler's nodes, Roth's spots

   f. Treatment

     1) Appropriate antibiotics depending on culture results

     2) Surgery may be needed for ruptured mycotic aneurysm or asymptomatic large or enlarging mycotic aneurysm

9. Nonbacterial thrombotic endocarditis (NBTE)

   a. Libman-Sacks endocarditis

     1) May be associated with systemic lupus erythematosus

     2) Valvular vegetations consist of immune complexes, white blood cells, fibrin and platelet thrombi, fibrosis

     3) Mitral, aortic, and tricuspid valves are usually affected

   b. Marantic endocarditis

     1) This term usually refers to NBTE in patients with malignancy

     2) The pathology is very similar to that of Libman-Sacks endocarditis

     3) Often, platelet and fibrin thrombi, usually of aortic and mitral valves

   c. Sources

     1) Systemic lupus erythematosus

     2) Human immunodeficiency virus (HIV) infection

     3) Antiphospholipid antibody syndrome

     4) Malignancies (usually adenocarinomas)

   d. Neurologic complications

     1) Ischemic stroke

     2) Systemic emboli are also common

   e. Diagnosis

     1) TEE

     2) Blood cultures to rule out infection

     3) Other systemic findings to suggest specific source (e.g., known malignancy, HIV infection, lupus)

   f. Treatment

     1) Anticoagulation is generally considered

     2) If heart valve is damaged, surgery or valvuloplasty may be considered

10. Osler-Weber-Rendu disease (see also Chapter 13)

   a. Autosomal dominant condition characterized by numerous telangiectasias in multiple organs, including lung, liver, kidney, skin, brain

   b. Neurologic manifestations due most commonly to cerebral ischemia from pulmonary fistulae

   c. Treatment: treat pulmonary fistulae

11. Valvular heart disease and prosthetic (mechanical) heart valves

   a. Valvular heart disease and mechanical, prosthetic valves increase risk for ischemic stroke

   b. Risk factors for ischemic stroke with prosthetic valves: advanced age, previous thromboembolic event, left ventricular dysfunction, associated atrial fibrillation, left atrial thrombus, mitral position of valve, tilting disk valve, and caged-ball valves

   c. Risk of thromboembolism is also higher with multiple (rather than single) prosthetic valves

   d. Anticoagulation is preferred over antiplatelet agents for prosthetic valves; level of anticoagulation depends on type of prosthetic valve

12. Patent foramen ovale (PFO)

   a. Association between PFO and cerebral infarction has been controversial, with varying results from epidemiologic studies; population-based echocardiographic study suggests prevalence of 25% in general population

   b. Risk factors thought to increase probability that PFO is associated with cerebral infarction: size, shunting characteristics (right to left), associated atrial septal aneurysm, known deep venous thrombosis, cortical stroke

   c. Treatment is controversial

d. Treatment options for secondary prevention: antiplatelet drugs, anticoagulation, closure of PFO with endovascular device, or open heart surgery and PFO repair

e. No definitive data on which treatment is better than aspirin and each has its own associated risks

f. Studies on both device closure and surgery suggest recurrent stroke risk is 3% to 4% per year; this suggests other mechanisms may have a role and appropriate selection needs to be refined

13. Diagnostic testing for cardioembolic ischemic mechanisms

a. Electrocardiography (ECG) (electrocardiogram)—all patients should have ECG to evaluate for dysrhythmia, MI, or suggestion of ventricular dysfunction

b. Echocardiography
   1) May be used to confirm major sources and to detect minor sources of cardioembolism
   2) TEE vs. transthoracic echocardiography (TTE)
      a) Sensitivity and specificity for left ventricular thrombi similar for TEE and TTE
      b) Advantages of TTE: noninvasive, provides a better estimate of left ventricular function than TEE
      c) Disadvantage of TTE: difficulty in achieving adequate window in larger patients
      d) Advantages of TEE
         i) Far superior to TTE for left atrial thrombus
         ii) More sensitive than TTE for detecting other potential sources of cardioembolism: aortic atheromatous disease or dissection, spontaneous echo contrast, PFO, atrial septal aneurysm

c. Blood cultures: if endocarditis is suspected

d. Laboratory tests: consider additional tests such as antinuclear antibody (ANA), ds-DNA, erythrocyte sedimentation rate, HIV, malignancy screen if NBTE is discovered

B. Extracranial Large-Artery Disease

1. Differential diagnosis of extracranial large-vessel disease is listed in Table 11-6

2. Prevalence: approximately 15% to 20% of strokes are secondary to large-vessel disease

3. Aortic atherosclerosis
   a. Epidemiologic data suggest that aortic plaque 4 mm or larger is independent risk factor for ischemic stroke
   b. Stroke risk is greater for complex, mobile plaques larger than 5 mm
   c. Diagnosis: TEE is preferred test for diagnosis of aortic atherosclerosis; however, because optimal treatment is unclear, it may not be necessary to perform TEE only to look for aortic disease

d. Treatment
   1) Currently, best antithrombotic management is not defined, with conflicting data on anticoagulation vs. antiplatelet agents
   2) The only randomized clinical trial suggests anticoagulation is not superior to antiplatelet agents

4. Aortic dissection
   a. Pathology and pathophysiology
      1) Result of spontaneous medial hemorrhage and cleavage creating a false lumen that communicates with true lumen via an intimal tear
      2) Two-thirds of aortic dissections involve the ascending aorta
   b. Clinical
      1) Clues to diagnosis on history: chest and/or back pain (although may not be elicited in patients with aphasia or altered mental status)
      2) Clues to diagnosis on examination: aortic regurgitation murmur, hypotension, reduced peripheral pulses, different blood pressure recordings between upper limbs
      3) Neurologic complications of aortic dissection: TIA, cerebral infarction, spinal artery syndrome, syncope, ischemic peripheral neuropathy
   c. Diagnosis
      1) Chest X-ray may show widened mediastinum, but sensitivity is only moderate
      2) Definitive diagnosis can be made by TEE or chest CT
   d. Treatment
      1) Management of aortic dissection complicated by stroke is controversial
      2) Many series suggest poor prognosis for patients with aortic dissection and stroke whether treated medically or surgically

5. Internal carotid artery stenosis: atherosclerosis (Fig. 11-16)
   a. Epidemiology: extracranial atherosclerosis of carotid bifurcation is more common than intracranial stenosis
   b. Clinical (see section above on large-vessel syndromes involving internal carotid artery)
   c. Diagnosis (discussed below)
   d. Treatment of symptomatic internal carotid artery stenosis and occlusion
      1) Term "symptomatic stenosis or occlusion" refers to cerebral infarction or TIA symptoms in anterior circulation ipsilateral to atheromatous diseased internal carotid artery
      2) Symptomatic internal carotid artery stenosis 70% to 99%
         a) Northern American Symptomatic Carotid

Symptomatic Internal Carotid Disease Ipsilateral to
Anterior Circulation Symptoms

0%-<50%: no clear treatment superior to aspirin
daily

50%-69%: carotid endarterectomy plus aspirin
daily superior to aspirin daily in selected patients
(absolute risk reduction, 6.3%)

70%-99%: carotid endarterectomy plus aspirin daily
superior to aspirin daily (absolute risk reduction, 17%)

100% occluded: no clear treatment superior to
aspirin daily

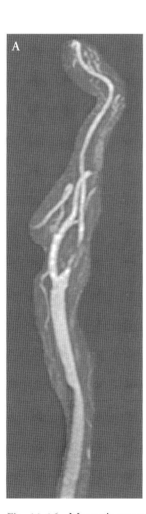 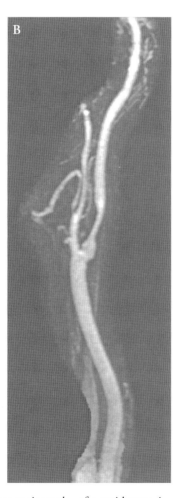

Fig. 11-16. Magnetic resonance angiography of carotid stenosis.
A, Very high-grade stenosis (near occlusion) of proximal left
internal carotid artery with reduced caliber of the distal internal
carotid artery. *B*, Moderately severe stenosis (50%-70%) in
area of right carotid bulb.

Endarterectomy Trial (NASCET): the 2-year ipsilateral stroke rate was 26% in medically treated vs.
9% in carotid endarterectomy (CEA) group

3) Symptomatic internal carotid artery stenosis 50% to
69%
  a) 5-Year risk of fatal or nonfatal ipsilateral stroke was
22% in medically treated group and 15.7% in the
surgically treated group
  b) Greater benefit of surgery for
    i) Men than for women
    ii) Patients who have had stroke than for those with
TIAs
    iii) Patients with hemispheric symptoms than for
those with retinal symptoms
  c) Increased risk of perioperative stroke or death in
patients with diabetes, increased blood pressure,
contralateral occlusion, or left-sided carotid disease
4) Internal carotid artery stenosis <50%: no data suggest
CEA is beneficial over medical management
5) Symptomatic internal carotid artery occlusion (100%
blockage)
  a) Best medical management (anticoagulation vs.
antiplatelet therapy) and best surgical management
have not been defined
  b) Ongoing studies are aimed at defining best medical
management
6) Alternative to CEA is carotid angioplasty and stenting
(CAS)
  a) CAVATAS trial—carotid angioplasty with or without stent vs. CEA had no major difference in 30-
day and 3-year vascular end points
  b) SAPPHIRE trial—randomized trial of CAS (using
distal protection device) vs. CEA in both asymptomatic and symptomatic "high-risk" patients; study
concluded CAS was not inferior to CEA
  c) Recommendations
    i) More data needed to determine when CAS vs.
CEA should be considered
    ii) Currently, CAS should be reserved for patients
at high risk for CEA
  d) "High risk" for CEA includes clinically significant
cardiac disease (congestive heart failure, abnormal
stress test, need for heart surgery), severe pulmonary disease, contralateral internal carotid artery
occlusion, contralateral laryngeal nerve palsy, previous radical neck surgery or radiotherapy to the
neck, recurrent stenosis after endarterectomy, age
older than 80 years
7) Medically, antiplatelet agents are recommended after
CEA or CAS

8) Evidence that HMG-CoA reductase inhibitors ("statins") are beneficial as secondary prevention for vascular events in these patients
6. Extracranial cerebral artery vasculitides
   a. Takayasu's arteritis presents in younger patients; giant cell arteritis presents in older patients
   b. Takayasu's arteritis (pulseless disease)
      1) Epidemiology
         a) More common in young, females
         b) Pathology
            i) Granulomatous arteritis
            ii) Vessels affected: aorta and carotid, vertebral, and subclavian arteries
      2) Clinical presentation
         a) TIA or stroke
         b) Upper extremity claudication
         c) May have fevers, fatigue, weight loss
         d) Asymmetric pulses and blood pressures in upper extremities
         e) Increased erythrocyte sedimentation rate
      3) Diagnosis
         a) Clinical symptoms and signs
         b) Increased erythrocyte sedimentation rate
         c) Magnetic resonance angiographic, CT angiographic, or conventional angiographic evidence that extracranial large arteries affected
      4) Treatment
         a) Immunosuppressants
         b) Reconstructive surgery or endovascular surgery
   c. Giant cell arteritis
      1) Epidemiology: more common after age 50
      2) Pathology
         a) Inflammatory vasculitis affecting medium and large extracranial branches of aortic arch
         b) Pathologic picture: intimal thickening; inflammation within the media, with fragmented internal elastic lamina; T-cell lymphocytes, macrophages, and multinucleated macrophages may be seen
      3) Clinical presentation
         a) Systemic symptoms: fever, weight loss, malaise
         b) Jaw claudication
         c) Temporal headaches with scalp tenderness
         d) Ischemic stroke is uncommon but may occur in anterior or posterior circulation
      4) Diagnosis
         a) Increased erythrocyte sedimentation rate (in most patients)
         b) Irregularities may be found on angiography of extracranial blood vessels
         c) Temporal artery biopsy (biopsy on one side and if negative, consider contralateral biopsy; preferable to biopsy before corticosteroid treatment, but can perform biopsy up to 2 weeks after initiation of corticosteroid treatment)
      5) Treatment: high-dose prednisone
7. Arterial dissection: carotid (Fig. 11-17), vertebral arteries
   a. Epidemiology
      1) Common cause of stroke in patients younger than 45 years (2% of strokes in general population, but 10%-25% of strokes in young)
      2) About half of cases are associated with some identifiable trauma (including catheter procedures) and half have no predisposing event
      3) Conditions that may predispose to dissection: fibromuscular dysplasia, Ehlers-Danlos syndrome type IV, Marfan's syndrome, polycystic kidney disease, pseudoxanthoma elasticum, osteogenesis imperfecta

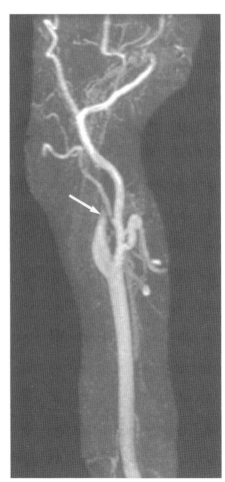

Fig. 11-17. Magnetic resonance angiography of carotid dissection. The flame-like tapering (*arrow*) of internal carotid artery is suggestive of dissection.

b. Pathology
   1) Intimal tear with resultant false lumen
   2) Occurs most commonly at extracranial sites
      a) Internal carotid arteries: usually 2 to 3 cm distal to bifurcation
      b) Vertebral arteries: at point of curving around the atlas immediately before penetrating dura mater (usually around C1-2 junction)
   3) Intimal direction of the dissection may cause arterial occlusion, whereas the adventitial direction may cause pseudoaneurysm or subarachnoid hemorrhage (if intracranial)
c. Clinical presentation
   1) May have anterolateral cervical and/or retro-orbital pain associated with carotid dissection, or posterior head pain with vertebral dissection
   2) Horner's syndrome and rarely lower cranial nerve palsies may be present with carotid dissection (due to involvement of contents of the carotid sheath)
   3) Vertebral dissection most commonly presents with posterior inferior cerebellar artery (first branch off vertebral artery) ischemia, thus lateral medullary syndrome
   4) Carotid dissection may present with any anterior circulation symptomatology
d. Diagnosis
   1) Carotid ultrasonography has low sensitivity for carotid dissection if vessel is nonstenotic
   2) Magnetic resonance or CT angiography of neck is noninvasive test of choice and typically demonstrates tapered narrowing of the vessel, with a "flame-like" appearance; other findings are double lumen (true and false lumens) and intimal flap
   3) Conventional cerebral angiography is more sensitive than magnetic resonance or CT angiography but is invasive and used when noninvasive studies are inconclusive
e. Treatment
   1) No randomized clinical trial data about whether anticoagulation is better than antiplatelet agents for cerebral arterial dissection
   2) Because most strokes are due to thromboembolism, many clinicians treat extracranial arterial dissection with anticoagulation for 3 to 6 months, then switch to an antiplatelet agent
   3) Angioplasty and stenting can be considered in cases refractory to medical therapy but there is risk of further dissection of the vessel
8. Fibromuscular dysplasia (Fig. 11-18)
   a. Epidemiology: more common in young females and Caucasians

b. Pathology
   1) Nonatherosclerotic, noninflammatory arteriopathy: tunica media with disorganized smooth muscle cells and loss of smooth muscle cells (sometimes hyperplasia) and general disorganization of arterial wall
   2) Disruption of internal elastic lamina
   3) Vessels affected: renal (most common, 60%-75%), extracranial carotid or vertebral arteries (second most common, 20%-30%), intracranial vessels, iliac artery, femoral artery, subclavian artery, visceral arteries, others
c. Clinical presentation
   1) May be asymptomatic
   2) May present with focal cerebral ischemia (TIA or ischemic stroke) or rarely global hypoperfusion
   3) Patients can be predisposed to arterial dissection (Fig. 11-18 C and D)
   4) Hypertension due to involvement of renal arteries
d. Diagnosis
   1) Fibromuscular dysplasia: best demonstrated by arteriography, but advanced magnetic resonance angiography may be helpful
   2) Angiographic appearance of "string of beads," i.e., constricted arterial segments alternating with normal or dilated segments
   3) Less common angiographic appearance: smooth concentric tubular lesions
   4) Rarely, diverticular outpouchings may lead to aneurysm formation
e. Treatment
   1) Management of concomitant renal disease in hypertension
   2) Antiplatelet agent for ischemic symptoms
   3) Endovascular angioplasty considered for symptomatic arteries
9. Diagnostic evaluation of extracranial large-vessel disease
   a. Goals of evaluating extracranial arterial circulation
      1) Define degree of arterial stenosis
      2) Determine location and nature of pathology (atherosclerosis, dissection, or arteritis)
      3) Identify concomitant vascular lesions
   b. Choice of diagnostic study depends on the clinical suspicion of pathologic process
   c. Carotid ultrasonography
      1) Sensitivity and specificity of color-flow duplex carotid ultrasonography for internal carotid artery stenosis of more than 70% are 87% to 95% and 86% to 97%, respectively
      2) False-positive carotid ultrasonographic readings of total carotid occlusion (when there is near total

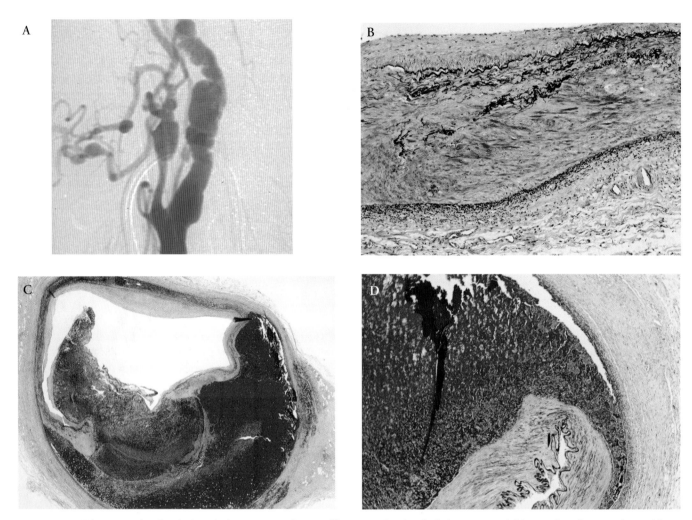

Fig. 11-18. Fibromuscular dysplasia. *A*, Appearance of severe fibromuscular dysplasia in extracranial internal and external carotid arteries on conventional angiography. Note "string of beads" with characteristic luminal narrowing alternating with aneurysmal dilatations. *B*, Histopathologic features include thin tunica media and disorganized smooth muscle cells, disarranged laminae, and disrupted internal elastic lamina. This disruption of the structure of the thin media predisposes the artery to dissection. *C*, Arterial dissection secondary to fibromuscular dysplasia in the same patient as in Panel *A*. The intimal tear in the center allows entrance of hematoma into the media, with more acute blood tearing through and expanding the media. *D*, Higher magnification of a different arterial dissection in the same patient, showing the plane of dissection between the adventitia and tunica media.

occlusion by arteriography) can occur in 2% to 7.5% of cases, necessitating a confirmatory test

3) Advantages: inexpensive, noninvasive, high sensitivity and specificity for detecting stenosis

4) Disadvantages: operator-dependent, not as sensitive or specific for nonatherosclerotic lesions

  d. CT angiography

1) Sensitivity and specificity of CT angiography to determine internal carotid artery stenosis greater than 70% are 74% to 100% and 83% to 100%, respectively; sensitivity for detecting carotid artery occlusion is 100%

2) Advantages: noninvasive

3) Disadvantages: availability, contrast dye load (contraindications are allergy, severe renal insufficiency)

  e. Magnetic resonance angiography

1) Sensitivity of 83% to 95% and specificity of 89% to 94% for detection of extracranial internal carotid artery stenosis of more than 70% (magnetic resonance angiographic technique influences sensitivity and specificity markedly)

2) Advantage: noninvasive

3) Disadvantages: cost, availability, contraindicated for patients with ferromagnetic devices (including pacemakers)

f. Arteriography
   1) Advantages
      a) Considered "gold standard" for assessment of degree of internal carotid artery stenosis
      b) Superior to magnetic resonance angiography for detection of plaque morphology, evidence of dissection, and fibromuscular dysplasia
   2) Disadvantages
      a) Cost, availability, technical skill
      b) 0.5% to 1% risk of cerebral infarction, TIA, or hematoma formation during procedure
      c) Renal failure and contrast allergies are contraindications
g. Currently, TEE is superior to magnetic resonance angiography of aortic arch for detection and quantification of aortic plaque

C. Intracranial Large-Artery Disease

1. Differential diagnosis of intracranial large-artery disease is listed in Table 11-4
2. Atherosclerosis
   a. Epidemiology
      1) Intracranial stenosis may account for up to 5% to 10% of all ischemic strokes
      2) Pretest probability (prevalence) increases in women, Asian, African or Hispanic Americans, diabetics, patients with cortical symptoms or recurrent stereotyped TIAs in a single vascular territory, and posterior circulation events
      3) Most common intracranial sites for atherosclerosis: internal carotid artery (petrous, cavernous, and clinoid segments), main trunk of MCA, vertebral artery (segments V3 and V4) and basilar artery
   b. Clinical presentation
      1) Patients may present with stroke, TIA, and rarely presyncope due to intracranial atherosclerosis
      2) Mechanism of stroke related to intracranial disease may be hemodynamic, result from artery-to-artery emboli, or be related to sudden occlusion or thrombosis of vessel
   c. Natural history
      1) Suggested overall annual risk of stroke in setting of symptomatic intracranial stenosis is 3% to 15%
      2) Anterior circulation: 7% to 10% annually
      3) Posterior circulation: 3% to 15% annually
   d. Diagnosis: conventional angiography, magnetic resonance angiography, CT angiography, transcranial Doppler sonography
   e. Treatment
      1) Controversy about current approach and treatment of intracranial atherosclerotic stenosis
      2) Decision-making should take into account location and accessibility of the intracranial artery, level of severity (length of segment involved, degree of stenosis, tortuosity of the vessel), patterns of collateral flow, response to previous therapy, and expertise of interventionalists and surgeons
      3) Medical management: generally, antiplatelet agents are indicated (this is based on one retrospective study and two prospective clinical trials)
      4) Warfarin and Aspirin Study of Intracranial Disease (WASID)
         a) Retrospective, multicenter study evaluating patients with symptomatic intracranial stenosis defined as 50% to 99% narrowed by angiography; authors concluded a probable role for warfarin and proposed an ongoing prospective trial
         b) Prospective WASID: warfarin was not superior to aspirin in preventing recurrent vascular events in patients with symptomatic intracranial stenosis
      5) Warfarin Aspirin Recurrent Stroke Study (WARSS)
         a) Randomized 2,206 patients with mild-to-moderate ischemic stroke to either aspirin (325 mg/d) or warfarin with a goal INR of 1.4-2.8; a total of 259 were included in the study who had "large-artery disease" as the mechanism of initial stroke
         b) Aspirin was equal to warfarin in efficacy
      6) Endovascular intervention
         a) Intracranial angioplasty and stenting are feasible, but large clinical trials do not exist to identify when this therapy is superior to medical or surgical therapy
         b) Generally, if medical management fails, angioplasty and stenting can be considered
         c) Risk of angioplasty and stenting in the intracranial circulation is higher than extracranial disease and depends on the symptomatic vessel; basilar artery is the highest risk because of many perforating vessels
      7) Surgical management: bypass procedures available for anterior and posterior circulations, but no proven benefit for intracranial stenosis
3. Inflammatory arteritis
   a. Vasculitis may be isolated to central nervous system (CNS) or be a manifestation of systemic vasculitis
   b. Systemic vasculitides that may be associated with CNS (intracranial) involvement: polyarteritis nodosa, Wegener's granulomatosis, systemic lupus erythematosus, Churg-Strauss syndrome (rare in CNS), essential cryoglobulinemic vasculitis

4. Isolated CNS (granulomatous) angiitis (Fig. 11-19)
   a. Pathology
      1) May involve small arteries and veins of brain and spinal cord
      2) Inflammation of vessels consists of granulomas with multinucleated giant cells and lymphocytes predominantly
   b. Clinical presentation
      1) Usually subacute onset and course with some combination of symptoms listed below
      2) Focal neurologic deficit due to ischemic stroke (rarely hemorrhage)
      3) Seizures
      4) Encephalopathy
      5) Headache
      6) May have systemic symptomatology
   c. Diagnosis
      1) Systemic markers of inflammation: generally normal
      2) Cerebrospinal fluid (CSF) examination: may be normal or show elevated protein; white blood cells may or may not be present
      3) MRI: may show areas of ischemia (white and gray matter involvement); enhancement of the meninges may or may not be present
      4) Magnetic resonance angiography: may show irregularities of vessels; not sensitive for the small vessels that generally are involved
      5) Arteriography
         a) May show "beading" of vessels with alternating stenosis and dilatation
         b) This angiographic finding itself is not diagnostic and differential diagnosis of the angiographic findings include vasospasm (due to migraine, sympathomimetics, hypertensive crisis), sarcoid angiopathy, infectious arteritis, radiation vasculopathy, atherosclerosis, fibromuscular dysplasia, intravascular lymphoma, and leptomeningitis
         6) Brain parenchymal and leptomeningeal biopsy
            a) Gold standard for diagnosis
            b) Because of frequently patchy involvement, negative biopsy findings do not exclude the diagnosis
   d. Treatment: immunosuppression, generally with cyclophosphamide and corticosteroids
5. Infectious arteritis
   a. Rare
   b. Causes: herpes zoster ophthalmicus, hepatitis B and C, HIV, cytomegalovirus, Epstein-Barr virus, bacterial aortitis, syphilis
   c. Herpes zoster ophthalmicus associated with ipsilateral M₁ segment MCA stenosis resulting in contralateral

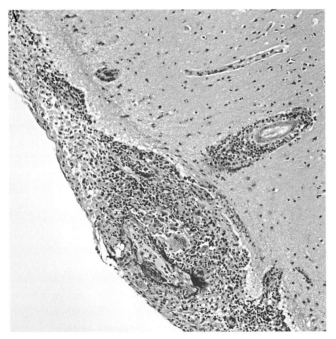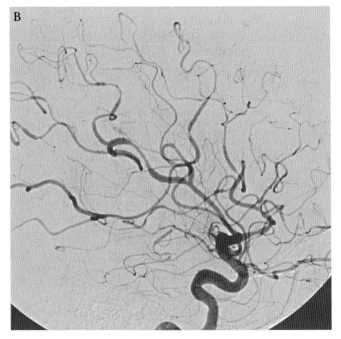

Fig. 11-19. Primary central nervous system vasculitis. *A*, Extensive leptomeningeal acute and chronic cellular infiltrates and necrotizing vasculitis of small-sized leptomeningeal and parenchymal arteries. *B*, Classic angiographic appearance of primary central nervous system vasculitis, with characteristic "beading" of vessels with alternating stenosis and dilatation, although this is not diagnostic by itself.

symptoms; CSF studies may confirm presence of virus
and treatment may be a combination of acyclovir with or
without corticosteroids and antiplatelet agents

6. Intracranial dissection
   a. Rare cause of ischemic stroke, more typical in young
      than old patients
   b. Because pseudoaneurysms may form, subarachnoid
      hemorrhage is possible
   c. Treatment unclear; pseudoaneurysms may require
      intervention

7. Moyamoya disease
   a. Epidemiology: rare; most prevalent in Japan and Asia
   b. Male:female ratio is 1:1.8
   c. Nonatherosclerotic occlusive arteriopathy
   d. Pathology
      1) Endothelial hyperplasia and fibrosis, intimal thicken-
         ing, and abnormal elastic laminae
      2) This leads to severe progressive occlusion of distal
         intracranial internal carotid arteries and collateral
         circulation from perforating arteries that may show
         lipohyalinosis and microaneurysm formation due to
         increased blood flow
   e. Radiographically characterized by bilateral stenosis or
      occlusion of distal intracranial internal carotid arteries or
      vessels of circle of Willis, prominent moyamoya collateral
      vessels; the latter often arise from enlarged penetrating,
      perforating branches of internal carotid arteries, ACAs,
      and MCAs (Fig. 11-20)
   f. Cases with typical radiographic features of moyamoya
      disease on one side should be labeled "possible" moya-
      moya disease because many eventually develop bilateral
      radiographic findings on follow-up scans
   g. Radiographic pattern may be seen in true moyamoya dis-
      ease or in association with various entities, including
      Down syndrome, dissection, sickle cell anemia, antiphos-
      pholipid antibody syndrome, radiotherapy
   h. Clinical presentation
      1) Most commonly present in childhood (mean age, 5
         years); less common peak age at onset, between 30
         and 40 years
      2) Children: commonly present with TIAs (usually
         motor deficits) and/or seizures; TIAs may be precipi-
         tated by hyperventilation or exercise
      3) Adults: may present with ischemia or hemorrhage
         (due to abnormal collateral development or
         aneurysms); the latter is intracerebral (often involving
         deep white matter, thalamus, or basal ganglia) or
         intraventricular and occurs more frequently in women
         with this condition
   i. Diagnosis

A

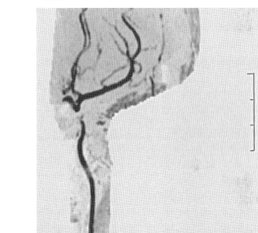

B

C

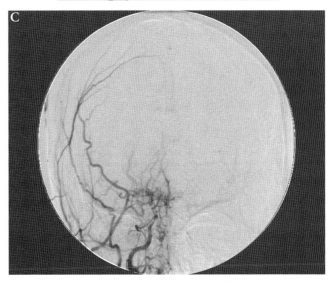

Fig. 11-20. Moyamoya disease. *A* and *B*, Magnetic resonance
angiography shows bilateral distal internal carotid artery
stenosis and stenosis of right M_1 and A_1. *C*, Conventional
angiography demonstrates the typical multiple small lenticulostriate collaterals.

1) MRI may show areas of ischemia or hemorrhage, generally in anterior circulation

2) Magnetic resonance angiography may show intracranial stenoses of circle of Willis

3) Arteriography (conventional angiography) is gold standard for diagnosis and allows better visualization of collateral circulation than magnetic resonance angiography does

4) SPECT or positron emission tomography (PET) may be used to assess cerebrovascular reserve

  j. Treatment

1) Antiplatelet agents commonly used

2) If patients present with ischemia or have poor cerebrovascular reserve, superficial temporal artery–to–middle cerebral artery bypass is considered with or without encephalomyoarteriosynangiosis or encephaloduroarteriosynangiosis

3) Role of bypass in patients who present with hemorrhage is less clear

8. Drug-related ischemic strokes

  a. Can occur with use of any sympathomimetic or vasospastic medication

  b. Due to either vasospasm or drug-induced vasculopathy

  c. Examples: methamphetamines, cocaine

  d. Clinical presentation

1) Patients present with ischemia and sometimes hemorrhage

2) In severe cases, diffuse vasospasm can increase intracranial pressure, resulting in reduced level of consciousness, seizures, severe headache

9. Diagnosis of intracranial large-vessel vascular disease

  a. Options for evaluation of intracranial disease: transcranial Doppler ultrasonography, CT angiography, magnetic resonance angiography, conventional arteriography

  b. Transcranial Doppler ultrasonography

1) Noninvasive technique to assess proximal intracranial internal carotid artery, M_1 segment of MCA, A_1 segment of ACA, vertebral arteries, and proximal aspect of basilar artery

2) Sensitivity and specificity: for all vessels, sensitivity of 89% to 98%, specificity of 87% to 96% for detecting stenosis greater than 50%

3) Advantages: noninvasive, portable

4) Disadvantages: operator-dependent; the transcranial window may not allow insonation in up to 20% of patients

  c. CT angiography

1) Sensitivity: approximately 78% to 80% for detection of 70% to 99% stenosis and 100% for occluded segments

2) Advantage: noninvasive

3) Disadvantage: use of contrast dye

  d. Magnetic resonance angiography

1) Sensitivity and specificity: sensitivity and specificity of 3D time-of-flight angiography to detect stenoses greater than 50% are 85% to 88% and 96% to 97%, respectively

2) Advantage: noninvasive

3) Disadvantage: contraindicated for patients with ferromagnetic devices

  e. Conventional cerebral arteriography

1) Advantages

   a) Superior to noninvasive studies for evaluating arteries distal to circle of Willis, such as those involved in vasculitis

   b) Superior for detecting AVMs or dural arteriovenous fistulas that may present with transient neurologic deficits

   c) Superior for defining plaque and vessel pathology

2) Other indications may include equivocal or conflicting noninvasive studies

3) Disadvantages: as noted above

D. Lacunar Small-Vessel Disease

1. Epidemiology: 20% of all cerebral ischemic events

2. Pathology

  a. Small subcortical infarction generally less than 1.5 cm resulting from occlusion of a penetrating end artery

  b. Lacunes predominate in basal ganglia, thalamus, centrum semiovale, brainstem, internal capsule

  c. Autopsy studies: pathology underlying lacunar infarctions is most commonly microatheroma, lipohyalinosis, and fibrinoid necrosis, but approximately 5% to 10% of autopsy cases do not have these findings, implying that lacunar infarctions possibly could result from embolic source

3. Risk factors: typical atherosclerotic risk factors, most notably hypertension, smoking, diabetes mellitus

4. Clinical lacunar syndromes are outlined in Table 11-5

5. Diagnosis

  a. Because lipohyalinosis and microatheroma are not visible by any diagnostic technique, clinical onset, patient risk factors, examination, and topography of infarction become important

  b. Patients presenting with a typical lacunar syndrome with typical risk factors and location of the cerebral infarction most likely have small-vessel disease or a true lacunar infarction

  c. For patients without typical risk factors or with an atypical syndromic presentation or unusual location of radiographic infarct, other mechanisms of stroke are considered

   d. Carotid artery disease should be considered in patients with lacunar infarcts in anterior circulation

6. Treatment: unless other mechanisms are found, antiplatelet agents and aggressive risk factor management are warranted for lacunar infarction

E. Hypercoagulability

1. Epidemiology

   a. Prevalence of specific coagulation disorders in the general population is listed in Table 11-9

   b. Coagulation disorders account for 1% to 4.8% of all ischemic strokes in a general population

   c. Pretest probability (prevalence) of coagulation disorders increases in younger patients (younger than 45 years), patients with previous history of clotting dysfunction, and patients with cryptogenic stroke

2. Etiologies—differential diagnosis of coagulation defect disorders and hematologic disorders associated with ischemic stroke are listed in Table 11-6

3. Diagnosis

   a. All patients: complete blood count, activated partial thromboplastin time, INR, erythrocyte sedimentation rate

   b. Additional testing in selected patients: homocysteine, coagulation factors, disseminated intravascular coagulation panel, factor V and prothrombin 20210 mutations, antiphospholipid antibodies and lupus anticoagulant, and hemoglobin electrophoresis

4. Treatment

   a. Anticoagulation with warfarin is recommended for patients with ischemic stroke related to antiphospholipid antibody syndrome

Table 11-9. **Prevalence of Coagulation Defects in General Population**

Factor	Prevalence in population
Antiphospholipid antibody	2-5%
Factor V Leiden mutation/APC resistance	1-9%
Congenital protein C deficiency	1/36,000
Congenital protein S deficiency	1/15,000-20,000
Congenital antithrombin III deficiency	1/2,000-5,000
Homocysteine (moderate)	30% of stroke population

APC, activated protein C.

   1) This recommendation is based mainly on retrospective studies

   2) No current consensus about whether intermediate-intensity warfarin (INR 2.0-2.9) or high-intensity warfarin (INR $\geq$3.0 or more) is better

   3) Recent subgroup analysis of WARSS trial suggested no difference in outcome with aspirin vs. warfarin (INR 1.4-2.8)

   b. Increased homocysteine level can be treated with supplemental vitamin B_{12}, B_6, and folate (response of homocysteine levels to treatment has been reported, but no studies have demonstrated benefit of this treatment in secondary prevention of recurrent strokes)

   c. High-risk sickle cell anemia patients may be treated successfully with transfusion therapy

F. Cerebral Venous Thrombosis

1. Epidemiology: rare

2. Superior sagittal sinus is most common site of thrombosis (associated with trauma, parasagittal meningiomas, meningeal infiltrative process, pregnancy-related, or hypercoagulable state)

3. Differential diagnoses and predisposing conditions: malignancy, pregnancy and postpartum period, oral contraception, factor V Leiden (common), hyperhomocysteinemia, prothrombin 20210 mutation (common), proteins C and S deficiencies, contiguous infectious extension (ear or mastoid), dehydration, dural arteriovenous fistula

4. Clinical symptoms

   a. Headache: due to increased intracranial pressure and involvement of pain-sensitive structures

   b. Other symptoms of increased intracranial pressure: papilledema, false localizing CN VI palsy

   c. Focal neurologic deficits (if cerebral venous infarct or hemorrhage)

   d. Seizures

   e. In children with deep venous thrombosis, coma often develops, sometimes death occurs

   f. Adults with deep venous thrombosis may have altered consciousness or psychiatric symptoms

5. Diagnosis (Fig. 11-21): made by magnetic resonance venography, CT venography, or conventional angiography

6. Treatment

   a. Anticoagulation is recommended treatment

   b. Mechanical clot disruption or endovascular administration of thrombolytics considered if increased intracranial pressure, altered mentation and somnolence, and poor response to anticoagulation

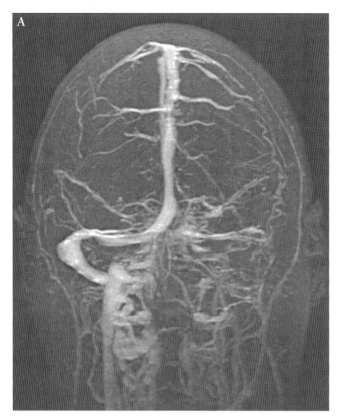
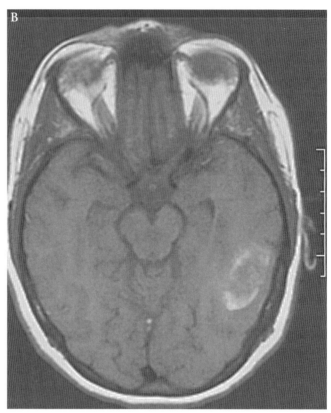

Fig. 11-21. A 47-year-old woman taking oral contraceptives had veno-occlusive disease and venous infarction. *A*, Magnetic resonance venogram demonstrates extensive thrombosis of left transverse and sigmoid sinuses that extends to involve left internal jugular vein. *B*, Nonenhanced T1-weighted magnetic resonance image shows hemorrhagic venous infarction in left temporal lobe.

G. Other Ischemic Syndromes
1. Cerebral autosomal dominant arteriopathy with subcortical infarcts and leukoencephalopathy (CADASIL)
   a. Pathology (Fig. 11-22)
      1) Ischemic subcortical strokes, demyelination
      2) Osmophilic granules seen with electron microscopy
      3) Widespread myelin pallor in white matter; multiple small infarcts in white matter and basal ganglia
      4) Thickened vessels of white matter and meninges, smudgy granular media and loss of muscle cell nuclei (the osmophilic granules are visible with electron microscopy and are of uncertain significance)
   b. Genetics
      1) Chromosone 19 (19q13.1) (missense mutation of *Notch3* gene)
      2) *Notch3* gene encodes a transmembrane protein thought to be involved in cell signaling during embryonic development (the ligand binding domain contains 34 epidermal growth factor-like repeats; the intracellular domain is involved in cell signaling)
      3) Of 33 coding exons of *Notch3* gene, exons 3 and 4 are commonly involved
   c. Clinical syndrome
      1) Migraine headaches with aura: earliest symptom; mean age at onset, 30 years
      2) Stroke or stroke-like episodes (often recurrent): most frequent manifestation of the disease; mean age at onset, 49 years
      3) Progressive dementia: reported in one-third of patients; mean age at onset, 60 years
      4) Some cognitive impairment may be secondary to multiple ischemic events
      5) Pseudobulbar affect
      6) Urinary incontinence
      7) Gait disturbance
      8) Pyramidal tract signs
   d. Diagnosis
      1) Genetic testing
      2) Skin biopsy: electron microscopy may identify osmophilic granules in arterial smooth muscle

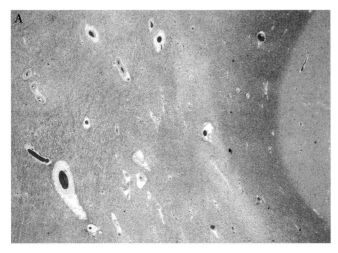

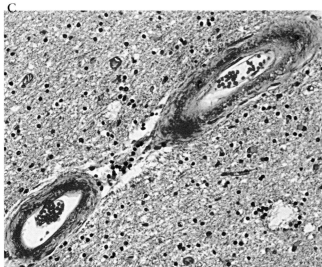

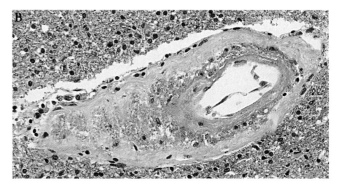

Fig. 11-22. CADASIL. *A*, Subcortical microcavitation and pallor and neuronal loss and gliosis, with relative preservation of cerebral cortex (on right) and U fibers beneath the cortex. (Movat stain.) *B*, Small-sized artery with deposition of granular material in media, degeneration of arterial wall, and destruction of media (Movat stain.) *C*, Subcortical small-sized arteries with eosinophilic granular material in media of vessel wall. (Hematoxylin-eosin.)

3) MRI of brain: generally shows confluent deep white matter changes often affecting anterior temporal lobe
  e. Treatment
    1) No treatment known to delay disease progression
    2) Antithrombotics typically used for general ischemic stroke prevention
2. Vascular cognitive impairment and dementia (see Chapter 7)
  a. Vascular dementia (encompasses dementia associated with multiple types of cerebrovascular pathology)
    1) Multi-infarct dementia
      a) Sudden focal neurologic dysfunction in addition to cortical cognitive impairment (aphasia, agnosia, apraxia)
      b) Neuroimaging shows multiple infarctions
    2) Single infarct dementia
      a) Strategically located single cerebral infarction can impair memory and cognitive function

b) Typical locations: thalamus, basal forebrain, caudate nucleus
    3) Subcortical ischemic vascular dementia (Binswanger's disease) (see Fig. 7-13)
      a) Unlike single and multi-infarct dementias, onset may be gradual and progressive
      b) Lacunar disease and incomplete white matter ischemia are underlying pathology
      c) Typical cognitive features: executive dysfunction, poor planning and abstraction, memory loss, psychomotor retardation, emotional lability
    4) Mixed vascular and Alzheimer's dementias
  b. Vascular cognitive impairment: patients with cognitive and functional impairment without dementia in setting of vascular disease
  c. Treatment
    1) Risk factor management
    2) Acetylcholinesterase inhibitors may show some benefit
3. Heritable disorders of connective tissue
  a. Marfan's syndrome
    1) Autosomal dominant
    2) Clinical phenotype: long limbs and digits, joint laxity, pectus deformity, subluxation of lens, arachnodactyly
    3) Ischemic infarcts may occur and may be related to enlargement of aortic root and associated mitral or aortic valve disease (e.g., mitral valve prolapse or aortic regurgitation) or aortic dissection

4) Predisposes to cerebral aneurysm formation

b. Pseudoxanthoma elasticum (see Chapter 13)
  1) Autosomal recessive hereditary disease of connective tissue characterized by progressive dystrophic mineralization of elastic fibers
  2) Clinical phenotype: skin lesions, loss of visual acuity, cardiovascular and cerebrovascular complications
  3) Few data about mechanism of the disorder and stroke
  4) Ischemic stroke may occur and be related to arterial dissection
  5) Clinical presentation resembling Binswanger's disease has been described
  6) Patients may be at increased risk for cerebral aneurysm formation

c. Ehlers-Danlos syndrome type IV (see also Chapter 13)
  1) Autosomal dominant disorder: mutation of gene encoding type III procollagen
  2) Patients are predisposed to rupture of arteries, bowel, and uterus
  3) Cerebrovascular complications: predisposition of intracranial aneurysm formation, arterial dissection, possible cavernous-carotid fistula

4. Cogan's syndrome
  a. Autoimmune arteritis involving small- or medium-sized vessels
  b. Clinical phenotype
    1) Interstitial keratitis, scleritis, or uveitis: patients often present with symptoms of visual blurring, photophobia or ciliary injection; may lead to bilateral blindness
    2) Vestibuloauditory dysfunction: vertigo, tinnitus, hearing loss; may present with abrupt onset and resemble Meniere's disease
    3) Systemic vasculitis observed in 10%; there may be aortitis; aortic aneurysm formation possible
  c. Diagnosis
    1) History, examination (neurologic and ophthalmologic)
    2) Laboratory studies to rule out other systemic vasculitides
  d. Treatment: consider immunosuppressants

5. Eales' disease
  a. Clinical manifestations
    1) Young adults
    2) Visual loss (monocular or binocular) with evidence of retinal vasculitis and periphlebitis (vasculitis of retinal arteries and veins), recurrent vitreous hemorrhage, microaneurysms of retinal vessels
    3) CNS vasculitis: focal infarcts, aseptic meningitis
  b. Diagnosis
    1) Clinical presentation

2) Fluorescein angiography
3) Laboratory tests to rule out other systemic vasculitides
  c. Treatment: immunosuppressants may be considered
  d. Late complications: neovascularization, retinal detachment, glaucoma

6. Susac syndrome (retinocochleocerebral vasculopathy)
  a. Pathology
    1) Microangiopathy affecting arterioles of the brain, retina, cochlea
    2) Some perivascular lymphocytic infiltration, but not definitively vasculitic
  b. Clinical characteristics
    1) Acute to subacute encephalopathy, visual loss, sensorineural hearing loss
    2) Cerebral symptoms: behavioral, affective, and cognitive dysfunction; ataxia, corticospinal tract involvement
    3) Ophthalmologic findings: visual field losses; retinal arteriolar stenosis or occlusions
    4) Otologic findings: low-to-mid–frequency sensorineural hearing loss
  c. Diagnosis
    1) Clinical manifestations
    2) MRI: multiple, small, punctate areas of increased T2 signal and contrast enhancement seen in both cerebral gray matter and white matter
    3) Rule out other vasculitides
  d. Treatment: controversial
    1) Immunosuppressants
    2) Plasma exchange

7. Sneddon's syndrome
  a. Pathology
    1) Vasculopathy without vasculitis has been found on brain biopsy
    2) Skin biopsy may show noninflammatory vasculopathy of medium-sized arteries with intimal hyperplasia
  b. Clinical manifestations
    1) Livedo reticularis (reticulated skin pattern caused by impaired superficial venous drainage of skin)
    2) Ischemic stroke
    3) Seizures
    4) Dementia
    5) Antiphospholipid syndrome may coexist and should be considered in all cases
  c. Diagnosis
    1) Clinical picture
    2) Livedo reticularis may be associated with other entities
    3) Rule out systemic vasculitides
  d. Treatment: antithrombotics (antiplatelet agents or

warfarin have been used)

8. Kohlmeier-Degos disease (malignant atrophic papulosis)
   a. Extremely rare
   b. Pathology
      1) Vasculopathy of skin, cerebral circulation, other organs
      2) A fibrous intimal proliferation can be accompanied by thrombosis
   c. Clinical manifestations
      1) Skin manifestations: raised papules with white center (due to progressive fibrosis of the small- and medium-sized arteries of skin causing infarcts of skin)
      2) Gastrointestinal tract manifestations: ulcers, bowel dysmotility, dilatation, possibly perforation
      3) Neurologic manifestations: ischemic stroke, TIA
   d. Treatment: not clear

9. Acute posterior multifocal placoid pigment epitheliopathy (APMPPE)
   a. Acute chorioretinal vasculitis in young adults
   b. Prodrome of flu-like illness with fever, lymphadenopathy, myalgias
   c. Both eyes are usually affected simultaneously; less commonly, unilateral involvement with involvement of other eye shortly thereafter
   d. Multiple well-circumscribed "placoid" white-gray lesions of retinal pigment epithelium
   e. Papilledema and optic neuritis may occur
   f. Cerebral vasculitis reported (in association with ocular findings): TIAs, ischemic strokes, aseptic meningitis
   g. Systemic vasculitic manifestations: erythema nodosum, microvascular nephropathy, immune-mediated thyroiditis
   h. Treatment: immunosuppressants; prednisone used for isolated ocular involvement

10. Mitochondrial myopathy, encephalopathy, lactic acidosis, and stroke-like episodes syndrome (MELAS)
    a. Rare disorder of mitochondrial DNA (most cases are an A to G point mutation in the dihydrouridine loop of transfer RNA gene at mt3243)
    b. Clinical manifestations
       1) Progressive encephalopathy
       2) Seizures
       3) Ischemic stroke (generally does not follow arterial borders)
       4) Deafness
       5) Myopathy
    c. Diagnosis
       1) Increased blood lactic acid and lactate-to-pyruvate ratio
       2) CSF lactate and pyruvate
       3) Muscle biopsy: may show ragged red fibers in skeletal muscle
       4) Molecular genetic analysis
       5) MRI: ischemic areas crossing arterial boundaries; basal ganglia may show calcification
       6) Magnetic resonance SPECT
    d. Treatment
       1) Coenzyme Q10 is tried
       2) Supportive
       3) Disease is progressive

H. Hypoxic-Ischemic Encephalopathy

1. Pathophysiology
   a. Anoxia: absence of oxygen in the tissue from pulmonary failure and resulting decrease in partial pressure of oxygen (e.g., pulmonary embolism, neuromuscular respiratory failure, strangulation, status epilepticus), cardiac arrest (inability to circulate oxygenated blood), or anemia and lack of oxygen-carrying capacity (e.g., carbon monoxide inhalation)
   b. Severe hypoglycemia can mimic clinical and pathologic features of hypoxic encephalopathy
   c. CNS structures most sensitive to anoxia: cerebellar Purkinje cells, dentate nucleus, globus pallidus, hippocampus (CA1 pyramidal cells), cerebral cortex layers III and V

2. Clinical manifestations are heterogeneous
   a. Usually result of *global* ischemia preferentially affecting structures most sensitive to anoxia, but *focal* ischemia may occur from underlying focal cerebrovascular disease
   b. Severity of symptoms: depends on duration of hypoxic event
   c. Syncope: brief episode of hypoxia causing brief loss of consciousness, followed by complete restoration of neurologic function; if episode is long enough, may be associated with clonic movements and, rarely, tonic-clonic seizures
   d. More prolonged global hypoxia can cause one or more of following: altered consciousness (obtundation, stupor, coma), neuropsychiatric and behavioral syndrome, predominantly anterograde amnestic syndrome
   e. Acute mountain sickness: syndrome of headache, nausea, vomiting, and altered consciousness due to diffuse cerebral edema
   f. Agitation and combativeness may occur as patient awakens from anoxic coma
   g. Postanoxic amnestic syndrome is believed to be due to selective hippocampal ischemic injury (usually from cardiopulmonary arrest)
   h. Movement disorder
      1) Stimulus-sensitive and action myoclonus (usually result of cortical damage)

2) Delayed-onset myoclonus may occur days to weeks after cognitive recovery from anoxic coma

3) Dystonic and akinetic-rigid parkinsonism (usually result of damage to basal ganglia)

i. Seizures

   1) Simple, complex partial, generalized tonic-clonic, or myoclonic seizures

   2) Myoclonus status epilepticus portends extremely poor prognosis; other seizure types have no prognostic value

   3) Myoclonus often involves facial, appendicular, and axial musculature; is often resistant to treatment

   4) Usual electroencephalographic (EEG) pattern of myoclonus status epilepticus: burst suppression

   5) Focal or generalized myoclonus may occur during cardiac resuscitation and needs to be differentiated from myoclonus status epilepticus

j. Watershed infarcts as result of prolonged arterial hypotension

   1) Arterial border zones between bilateral ACAs and MCAs (preservation of facial and distal lower limb motor function): bibrachial palsy with relatively less severe lower limb motor involvement (*man-in-a-barrel syndrome*), transcortical motor aphasia, or more extensive subcortical white matter damage and leukoencephalopathy

   2) Arterial border zones between bilateral MCAs and PCAs: Balint's syndrome (asimultanagnosia, optic ataxia, ocular apraxia, see Chapter 7, part A) and transcortical sensory aphasia

   3) Anoxic myelopathy often affecting mid-thoracic level

k. Delayed postanoxic encephalopathy (leukoencephalopathy)

   1) Most often reported after carbon monoxide inhalation

   2) Occurs in comatose patients who awaken within 24 to 48 hours after hypoxic insult and resume neurologic function for 4 to 14 days or longer

   3) Subsequently, patients abruptly develop "confusion" and behavioral symptoms (apathy, irritability, agitation, mania) and pyramidal and/or extrapyramidal symptoms (spasticity, rigidity, dystonia, quadraparesis)

   4) The syndrome may progress, halt, or, less commonly, the patient may recover partially or completely

   5) Pathology: extensive damage to bilateral subcortical white matter (leukoencephalopathy), ranging from demyelination to hemorrhagic necrosis

   6) Reduction of arylsulfatase A activity (a lysosomal enzyme important for lipid metabolism of myelin) may predispose to leukoencephalopathy

l. Cranial nerves

   1) Early loss of corneal reflex and ophthalmoplegia are poor prognostic indicators

   2) Dilated, fixed pupils result from asystole

     a) Persistence through resuscitation portends poor prognosis

     b) If resuscitation is successful, pupillary function is usually restored in 6 hours

3. Pathology (Fig. 11-23)

a. Macroscopic

   1) Acute or subacute: diffuse cerebral edema with loss of gray-white matter differentiation

   2) Chronic: watershed infarcts, cortical laminar necrosis, hippocampal sclerosis

b. Neuronal loss and gliosis of vulnerable areas: CA1 (Sommers' sector) of hippocampus, frontoparietal cortex, basal ganglia, cerebellar Purkinje cells, spinal cord (mid-thoracic segments, particularly anterior horn cells and Clarke's column)

c. Earliest observations in ischemic neurons: pyknotic nuclei and eosinophilic cytoplasm

d. Later, nuclei become eosinophilic and blend into cytoplasmic background

4. Diagnostic testing (Fig. 11-24)

a. CT: watershed infarcts, loss of gray-white matter differentiation may or may not be seen (usually seen after a few days)

b. MRI: widespread increased T2/FLAIR signal may be seen in neocortex, hippocampus, cerebellum, thalamus; watershed infarcts and sulcal edema can also be seen

c. EEG patterns

   1) Electrocerebral inactivity is usually present for up to an hour after cardiac arrest, but portends a poor prognosis if persistent

   2) Periodic patterns (generally poor prognosis): generalized periodic sharp waves, spikes or spike-and-wave discharges (may be associated with clinical myoclonus); bilateral periodic lateralized epileptiform discharges (PLEDs); burst-suppression pattern

   3) Invariant monorhythmic patterns: alpha coma pattern portends poor prognosis (most patients die or remain in a persistent vegetative state)

d. Somatosensory evoked potentials (SSEPs)

5. Poor prognostic factors (Tables 11-10 and 11-11)

a. No pupillary reaction (admission to day 3)

b. No motor response to pain (admission to day 3)

c. Sustained upward or downward gaze

d. Myoclonic status eplilepticus

e. Unwitnessed cardiac arrest

f. Elderly (>75 years old)

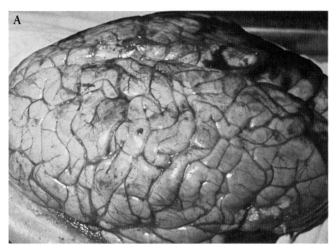

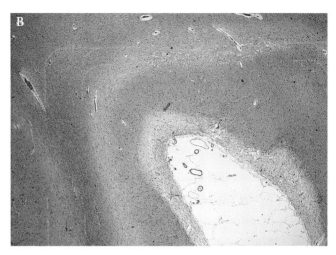

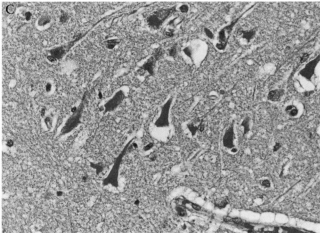

Fig. 11-23. Anoxic brain injury. *A,* Gross autopsy specimen demonstrating diffuse global edema of the brain (patient had cardiac arrest). Microscopic examination showed laminar necrosis of cerebral cortex, *B,* and ischemic neurons in CA1 sector (Sommer's sector) of hippocampus, *C.* Ischemic hippocampal neurons have pyknotic nuclei and densely eosinophilic cytoplasm; most of these neurons have nuclei that have become more eosinophilic and appear to be assimilated into the background of eosinophilic cytoplasm.

g. Organ failure or other medical comorbidities

h. Absence of cortical SSEPs bilaterally in first week

i. EEG: alpha coma pattern, burst-suppression pattern, or isoelectric EEGs in first week

6. Treatment

  a. Supportive measures

  b. Therapeutic mild hypothermia in adults after cardiac arrest due to ventricular fibrillation may improve neurologic outcome

I. Spinal Cord Ischemia and Infarction

1. Unknown incidence

2. Pathophysiology

  a. Mid-thoracic segments are in vascular watershed zones, most vulnerable to hypoperfusion and ischemic insult

  b. Mechanisms may include hypoperfusion, emboli, or thrombosis

  c. Because spinal cord is contained in spinal canal with fixed dimensions, any change in contents occurs at expense of CSF, blood, or spinal tissue; thus, if intraspinal canal pressure increases, blood flow to spinal

cord slows and hypoxia results

3. Differential diagnosis (Table 11-12)

4. Clinical presentation

  a. Anterior spinal artery syndrome

  b. Pain and temperature loss below level of lesion, with sparing of posterior columns

  c. Upper motor neuron loss below level of lesion

  d. Lower motor neuron lesion loss at segment of injury

5. Diagnostic tests

  a. MRI of spine (or alternatively CT myelography) may help rule out other causes of myelopathy; MRI may show increased T2 signal in spinal cord

  b. Evaluation for potential causes may depend on history and recent procedures and could include search for aortic disease, cardioembolic disease, coagulopathies, or vasculitides, depending on pretest probability of likelihood

6. Treatment

  a. No randomized trials

  b. Primary prevention

    1) Prevention in iatrogenic cases

    2) Intraoperative monitoring with SSEPs during aortic surgery

    3) Avoiding hypotension

  c. Acute treatment

    1) Methylprednisolone can be tried

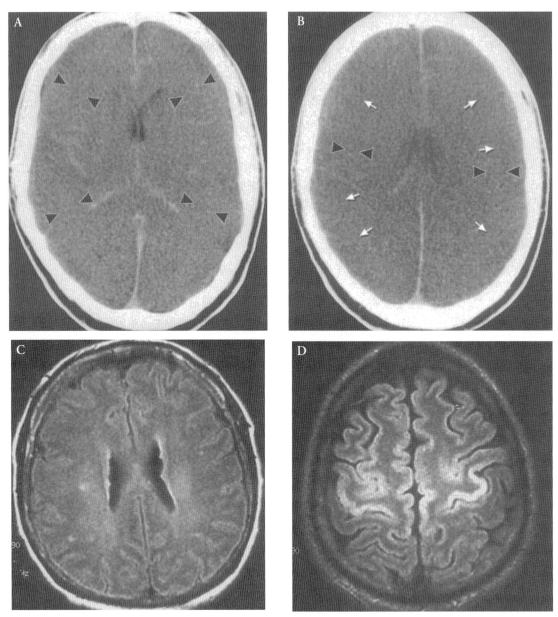

Fig. 11-24. Neuroimaging in hypoxic-ischemic encephalopathy. *A* and *B*, Unenhanced CT demonstrating diffuse cerebral edema with loss of gray-white matter differentiation (*arrowheads*) in a patient who had cardiac arrest. Note absence of sulci (*arrows* in *B*). *C*, Sulcal effacement due to diffuse cerebral edema is noted in this axial FLAIR MRI. *D*, Neocortical anoxic injury shown by widespread T2 signal abnormalities, predominantly affecting the cortical ribbon (axial FLAIR MRI). (*A* and *B*, from Wijdicks EFM. Catastrophic neurologic disorders in the emergency department. 2nd ed. New York: Oxford University Press; 2004. p. 94-105. Used with permission. *C* and *D*, from Wijdicks EFM. Neurologic complications of critical illness. 2nd ed. New York: Oxford University Press; 2002. p. 123-42. By permission of Mayo Foundation.)

      2) Lumbar drain to reduce intrathecal pressure has been tried with varying success
  d. Secondary prevention
      1) Consider antiplatelet agents or anticoagulation if embolic source
      2) Supportive treatment: bowel and bladder function

7. Prognosis
  a. Varies depending on degree of damage and etiology
  b. 20% to 25% of patients have no improvement, 20% have good recovery with minimal disability, rest have poor prognosis
  c. Chronic pain can be disabling feature

Table 11-10. **Factors Predicting Poor Prognosis After Hypoxic-Ischemic Injury in Adults**

Factor	Sensitivity, %	Specificity, %	95% CI of false-positive test rates, %
Pupillary reaction absent at admission	30-50	69-100	
Pupillary reaction absent at day 3	22-55	100	0-11.9
Motor response 1-3 on GCS on day 1	63-95	30-79	
Motor response 1-2 on GCS on day 3	56-92	93-100	
Motor response 1 on GCS on day 3	11-58	100	0-6.7
GCS 3-5 in first 24 hours	63-82	54-100	
Alpha coma pattern	15-43	71-100	
Burst-suppression pattern or isoelectric EEG first week	31-84	71-100	0.2-5.9
Bilateral absence of N20 on SSEPs first week	28-73	100	0-2

EEG, electroencephalography; GCS, Glasgow Coma Scale; SSEP, somatosensory evoked potential.
Modified from Zandbergen EGJ, de Haan RJ, Stoutenbeek CP, Koelman JHTM, Hijdra A. Systematic review of early prediction of poor outcome in anoxic-ischaemic coma. Lancet. 1998;352:1808-12. Used with permission.

Table 11-11. **Guidelines to Identify Patients With Poor or Good Prognosis After Cardiopulmonary Arrest**

Time after cardiac arrest	Clinical signs: patients with virtually no chance of regaining independence	Clinical signs: patients with best chance of regaining independence
Initial examination	No pupillary light reflex, in absence of another cause	Pupillary light reflexes present Motor response: flexor or extensor Spontaneous eye movements roving or orienting conjugate
1 day	Motor response: no better than decorticate posturing Spontaneous eye movements disconjugate or nonorienting	Motor response: withdrawal or better Eye opening improved at least 2 grades
3 days	Motor response: no better than decorticate posturing	Motor response: withdrawal or better Spontaneous eye movements normal
1 week	Motor response: not obeying commands Spontaneous eye movements disconjugate or nonorienting (no spontaneous eye opening at 3 days)	Motor response: obeying commands
2 weeks	Abnormal oculocephalic reflexes (no spontaneous eye opening at 3 days; not obeying commands at 3 days)	Normal oculocephalic reflexes

Modified from Levy DE, Caronna JJ, Singer BH, Lapinski RH, Frydman H. Predicting outcome from hypoxic-ischemic coma. JAMA. 1985;253:1420-1. Used with permission.

VI. PRINCIPLES OF TREATMENT: ISCHEMIC STROKE

A. Primary Prevention

1. Asymptomatic carotid artery stenosis
   a. Asymptomatic carotid artery stenosis greater than 60% by ultrasonography carries risk of ipsilateral ischemic stroke of 11% over 5 years (roughly, 2% annually)
   b. Some data suggest certain patients may have slightly higher annual risk (i.e., 3%-4%): ulcerative plaque,

stenosis greater than 80% (controversial), progression of disease over time
   c. Medical options for treatment: antiplatelet agents, statins, other atherosclerotic risk factor management
   d. Surgical options for treatment: information based on two randomized studies (Asymptomatic Carotid Artery Study [ACAS] and Asymptomatic Carotid Stenosis Trial [ACST]; three other negative trials were performed before ACAS)
   e. ACAS: patients undergoing CEA for asymptomatic

Table 11-12. **Differential Diagnosis of Spinal Cord Infarction**

Etiology	Specific
Vasculitis	Polyarteritis nodosa, Behçet's syndrome, giant cell arteritis (vertebral arteries)
Embolic	Atrial myxoma, mitral valve disease, endocarditis, patent foramen ovale, fibrocartilaginous emboli from herniated disks
Systemic hypoperfusion	Cardiorespiratory arrest, aortic rupture or dissection, coarctation of aorta
Iatrogenic	Thoracolumbar sympathectomy, scoliosis surgery, cardiac catheterization, aortography, renal artery embolization, umbilical artery catheterization, vertebral angiography, aortic surgery, surgical repair of coarctation, retroperitoneal lymph node dissection
Infectious	Syphilis, mucormycosis, meningitis
Miscellaneous	Sickle cell anemia, cocaine, decompression sickness, antiphospholipid antibody syndrome, Crohn's disease, cervical subluxation, atherosclerosis of aorta

---

Intravenous Tissue Plasminogen Activator (IV-tPA) for Ischemic Stroke

Must be given within 3 hours after clear onset of ischemic symptoms

Patients receiving IV-tPA are 30% more likely to have minimal or no disability at 3 months

All subgroups of stroke benefit (large vessel, cardioembolic, lacunar disease)

No change in mortality at 3 months

6.4% symptomatic hemorrhage rate (3% fatal hemorrhage)

---

carotid stenosis (60%-99%), followed by daily aspirin, had ipsilateral stroke or any perioperative stroke or death risk of 5.1% at 5 years, compared with 11% at 5 years in medical arm (aspirin daily). Patients were younger than 80 years and had no notable medical comorbidities

   f. Angioplasty/stent options for treatment: limited clinical trial data mixing both symptomatic and asymptomatic patients; more data needed for definitive recommendations

2. Antithrombotics in primary prevention
   a. Aspirin: beneficial in preventing first MI in men and ischemic stroke in women
   b. No primary prevention studies for other antithrombotics

B. Treatment of Acute Stroke

1. Intravenous tissue plasminogen activator (tPA)
   a. National Institute of Neurological Disorders and Stroke (NINDS) trial published in *New England Journal of Medicine* in 1995
   b. Randomized, placebo-controlled double-blind clinical trial: patients treated with 0.9 mg/kg tPA intravenously were 30% more likely to have minimal or no disability at 3 months (absolute reduction of 11%-13% over placebo)
   c. No difference in mortality

   d. Positive results were seen across all subgroups of stroke subtypes
   e. Hemorrhagic risk: 6.4% risk of symptomatic hemorrhage (50% mortality); overall early mortality, 3%
   f. Who is a candidate? (Table 11-13)
   g. Administration
     1) tPA 0.9 mg/kg intravenously (10% bolus; 90% drip over 60 minutes)
     2) No aspirin, heparin, or warfarin within 24 hours after tPA administration
   h. Management after thrombolysis
     1) Blood pressure checks
     2) Neurologic checks
     3) Frequency: every 15 minutes for 1 hour, then every 30 minutes for 6 hours, then every hour until 24 hours after initial infusion
     4) Treatment goals
       a) Maintain blood pressure less than 185/110 mm Hg
       b) Use small doses of agents with short half-life to avoid hypotension

2. Intra-arterial tPA
   a. Experimental: phase 2 and phase 3 clinical trials have shown improved recanalization and outcome in small numbers of patients
   b. Indications
     1) Precise criteria are evolving because this treatment is still considered experimental
     2) Patients with anterior circulation event up to 6 hours after ictus with persistent thrombus by imaging
     3) Patients with basilar artery occlusion up to 12 hours after ictus have been considered

Table 11-13. **Candidates for Intravenous Tissue Plasminogen Activator (tPA)**

	Consider tPA	No tPA
Clinical	≤3 hours* from focal anterior or posterior circulation ischemic symptom onset†	>3 hours from focal anterior or posterior circulation ischemic symptom onset†
	Fixed major or progressive deficit	Rapidly resolving or minor deficit
	Alert or somnolent patient	Obtunded or comatose patient
	No seizure(s) in association with stroke	Seizure(s) at onset of stroke
	No history of intracranial hemorrhage or bleeding diathesis	History of intracranial hemorrhage or bleeding diathesis
	No history of ischemic stroke or serious head injury within 3 months	Ischemic stroke or serious head injury within 3 months‡
	Blood pressure elevations rapidly responsive to use of labetalol and similar agents and maintained at ≤185 mm Hg systolic, ≤110 mm Hg diastolic pretreatment	Blood pressure elevations persistently >185 mm Hg systolic, >110 mm Hg diastolic despite antihypertensive therapy Patients requiring aggressive therapy to maintain above levels (e.g., sodium nitroprusside) excluded
	Absence of gastrointestinal or urinary tract hemorrhage within 21 days	Gastrointestinal or urinary tract hemorrhage within 21 days
	No major surgery within 14 days	Major surgery within 14 days
	No recent myocardial infarction	Recent myocardial infarction
	No recent arterial puncture at a noncompressible site	Recent arterial puncture at a noncompressible site§
	No recent lumbar puncture	Recent lumbar puncture§
	Female patient who is not pregnant	Pregnant female patient
	Normal aPTT, INR ≤1.5; not on warfarin or heparin	On heparin with elevated aPTT *or* Not on anticoagulation and INR >1.5 *or* On warfarin with any INR‖
	Platelet count ≥100,000/mm³	Platelet count <100,000/mm³
	Glucose 50-400 mg/dL	Glucose <50 or >400 mg/dL
Computed tomography	No evidence for significant early infarction,¶ hemispheric swelling, or hemorrhage	Evidence for significant early infarction¶ with focal mass effect, hemispheric swelling, or hemorrhage
	Absence of intracranial tumor	Intracranial tumor

aPTT, activated partial thromboplastin time; INR, international normalized ratio.

*There is no evidence that intravenous tPA given 3-6 hours after onset of symptoms is efficacious, and it is typically not used after 3 hours following symptom onset. Intra-arterial thrombolysis may still be considered in selected patients who have had symptoms for longer than 3 hours.

†For patients who wake up with stroke symptoms, the time they went to sleep defines the time of symptom onset.

‡Selected patients with minor cerebral infarction within the last 3 months may be considered for intravenous tPA depending on clinical circumstances.

§The risk of hemorrhagic complication in the setting of a recent lumbar puncture or arterial puncture at a noncompressible site is uncertain. Treatment in these situations should be considered cautiously for selected patients after review of the findings of the lumbar puncture or arterial puncture, the clinical circumstances, and review with the consulting neurologist.

‖The safety of use of tPA in patients on warfarin, at any INR, has not been documented. Treatment in patients on warfarin should be considered cautiously for selected patients after review with the consulting neurologist.

¶The safety and efficacy of tPA in patients with computed tomography showing early infarct changes (EICs) is still controversial, and its use in these patients should be decided by the consulting neurologist. However, intravenous tPA generally is not contraindicated for patients with EICs. In most patients with early findings suggesting a pronounced cerebral infarction (i.e., >1/3 of middle cerebral artery distribution) tPA is typically not used because of hemorrhage risk and low likelihood of efficacy.

Modified from Fulgham JR, Ingall TJ, Stead LG, Cloft H, Wijdicks EFM, Flemming KD. Management of acute ischemic stroke. Mayo Clin Proc. 2004;79:1459-69. By permission of Mayo Foundation.

c. Risks
1) Similar to intravenous tPA
2) Hemorrhage rate may be slightly higher
3. Aspirin: data combined from Chinese Acute Stroke Trial (CAST) and Internal Stroke Trial (IST) suggest that nine deaths or nonfatal strokes could be prevented per 1,000 patients treated acutely
4. Heparin
a. Many randomized clinical trials have shown no benefit (outcome) in use of heparin acutely for ischemic stroke
b. No data about use of heparin in setting of acute TIA
c. Heparin may be considered in setting of cerebral venous thrombosis
5. MERCI retrieval device
a. Approved for endovascular clot removal
b. Use and indications: data are evolving
c. Risk of stroke and arterial rupture

C. **Supportive Therapy and Management in Treatment of Acute Stroke**
1. Blood pressure
a. Avoid hypotension in immediate postischemic stroke period
b. Goal mean arterial pressure in patients treated with thrombolytics is 120 mm Hg or less
c. Goal mean arterial pressure in patients not treated with thrombolytics is 130 mm Hg or less
d. Treat with short-acting agents to avoid sustained hypotension
2. Blood glucose
a. Hyperglycemia after ischemic stroke may reflect stress response
b. Hyperglycemia is risk factor for poor outcome and infarction in the ischemic penumbra
c. Consider treatment with insulin if blood glucose is more than 200 mg/dL
3. Other supportive measures
a. Aspiration precautions if bulbar involvement
b. Deep venous thrombosis prophylaxis in bed-bound patients
4. Hemicraniectomy (see Chapter 10)

D. **Secondary Prevention**
1. Antiplatelet agents are indicated for most ischemic strokes
2. Certain coagulopathies, major cardioembolic sources, or vasculitis may require alternative treatments
3. Antithrombotics
a. Choices
1) Aspirin

2) Clopidogrel (Plavix)
3) Combination aspirin and extended-release dipyridamole (Aggrenox)
b. Choice of antiplatelet agent often depends on
1) What patient was taking at time of ischemic event
2) Allergies or intolerances
3) Other comorbidities (e.g., gastrointestinal ulcers)
4) Cost and compliance
c. Antiplatelet agents and efficacy studies are reviewed in Tables 11-14 and 11-15
4. Anticoagulation
a. Warfarin (Coumadin)
1) Mechanism of action
a) Vitamin K antagonist
b) Vitamin K is essential cofactor for factors II, VII, IX, and X for converting precursor proteins to active proteins
c) Half-life of each factor varies (e.g., factor IV = 5 hours; factor II = 60 hours), thus a therapeutic response may take several days
2) Monitoring: prothrombin time, INR
3) Risks: bleeding, purple toe syndrome, many drug interactions, teratogenic
4) Indications
a) Common indications for anticoagulation in the setting of ischemic stroke or TIA: atrial fibrillation, mechanical (prosthetic) heart valves, recent anterior wall MI, cardiomyopathy with left ventricular ejection fraction less than 30%, certain coagulopathies, cerebral venous thrombosis
b) Possible indications (but less adequate trial data): arterial dissection, acute carotid artery occlusion
5. Other secondary prevention
a. Secondary prevention of atherothrombotic mechanisms of stroke requires further evaluation for atherosclerosis risk factors (Table 11-16)
b. Hypertension
1) Independent risk factor for ischemic stroke
2) Incidence of stroke increases in proportion to both diastolic and systolic blood pressures
3) For each increment of 20 mm Hg in systolic blood pressure or 10 mm Hg in diastolic blood pressure, risk of cardiovascular disease doubles over entire range from 115/75 mm Hg to 185/115 mm Hg in patients 40 to 70 years old
4) Several clinical trials have shown treatment of hypertension reduces relative risk of initial stroke and recurrent stroke
5) Recommendations from Joint National Committee on the Prevention, Detection, Evaluation, and

Table 11-14.   **Overview of Antiplatelet Agents**

Drug	Dose	Mechanism of action	Side effects
Aspirin	50-325 mg/day	Inhibits cyclooxygenase, thereby reducing platelet thromboxane A_2, potent platelet aggregator Partially impedes platelet aggregation induced by ADP, collagen, and thrombin	Gastrointestinal irritation Bleeding
Ticlopidine (Ticlid)	250 mg bid	Selective antagonists of ADP-induced platelet aggregation	Neutropenia Diarrhea Bleeding Rash TTP
Clopidogrel (Plavix)	75 mg/day	Similar to ticlopidine	Gastrointestinal upset Diarrhea Bleeding TTP (rare)
Aspirin (25 mg)–extended-release dipyridamole (200 mg) (Aggrenox)	1 tablet bid	Inhibits cellular uptake of adenosine (an antiaggregant), increases platelet intracellular levels of cGMP through inhibition of cGMP phosphodiesterase; elevated cGMP inhibits several processes involved in platelet aggregation	Headache Dizziness Gastrointestinal upset Bleeding

ADP, adenosine diphosphate; bid, twice daily; cGMP, cyclic guanosine monophosphate; TTP, thrombotic thrombocytopenic purpura.
From Flemming KD, Wiebers DO. Optimizing antiplatelet therapy to prevent ischemic stroke. Emerg Med. 2002;34:28-37. Used with permission.

Treatment of High Blood Pressure
  a) Goal blood pressure less than 140/90 mm Hg in most patients
  b) Goal blood pressure less than 130/80 mm Hg in patients with diabetes or chronic kidney disease
  c) Prehypertension: 120-139/80-89 mm Hg
6) Treatment
  a) Lifestyle modification such as weight control, physical activity, moderation of sodium intake
  b) Selected medications depend on patients' comorbidities
  c) Clinical trials have evaluated diuretics, β-blockers, angiotensin-converting enzyme (ACE) inhibitors, angiotensin receptor blockers, others
  d) ACE inhibitors, angiotensin receptor blockers, or diuretics may be preferred
c. Hyperlipidemia
  1) Strongest association of hypercholesterolemia and stroke is with carotid artery distribution ischemic strokes
  2) Data from studies in patients with known coronary artery disease show relative risk reductions of stroke between 20% and 31% over 4 to 5 years with HMG-CoA reductase inhibitors or statin lipid-lowering agent
  3) Treatment goals: guidelines from National Cholesterol Education Program (Adult Treatment Panel III - 2001)
    a) Low-density lipoprotein (LDL) less than 100 mg/dL
    b) High-density lipoprotein more than 40 mg/dL
    c) Triglycerides less than 150 mg/dL
    d) This LDL goal applies to patients with previous MI, known diabetes, or patients in whom 10-year risk of coronary artery disease is more than 20%; this goal would apply to most atherothrombotic ischemic stroke patients and those with known carotid artery disease or any patients with ischemic stroke and previous history of coronary artery disease
  4) Coordinating Committee of the National Cholesterol Education Program update (2004)
    a) Optional LDL goal of less than 70 mg/dL in high-

Table 11-15. **Comparison of Major Antiplatelet Trials**

	Patient selection	Medication	Primary end point	Results
TASS	Recent TIA or stroke	Ticlopidine 250 mg bid Aspirin 1,300 mg/day	Nonfatal stroke or death	Event rate: 17% for ticlopidine, 19% for aspirin (12% relative risk reduction) over 3 years
CAPRIE	Recent ischemic stroke or recent MI or symptomatic peripheral vascular disease	Clopidogrel 75 mg/day Aspirin 325 mg/day	Ischemic stroke, MI, or vascular death	Clopidogrel group had annual 5.32% risk of primary end point compared with 5.83% for aspirin group Relative risk reduction of 8.7% in favor of clopidogrel
ESPS-2	Recent ischemic stroke or TIA	Placebo Aspirin 25 mg bid Dipyridamole 200 mg bid Aspirin/dipyridamole combination	Stroke, death, and stroke or death	Stroke risk compared with placebo was reduced by 18% with aspirin alone, 16% with dipyridamole alone, and 37% with combination therapy Risk of stroke or death was reduced by 24% with the combination
MATCH	Recent ischemic stroke or TIA	Clopidogrel 75 mg/day Clopidogrel 75 mg/day plus aspirin 75 mg/day	Composite of ischemic stroke, MI, vascular death, or rehospitalization for acute ischemia	15.7% in combination group reached primary end point compared with 16.7% in clopidogrel alone group Relative risk reduction, 6.4%; absolute risk reduction, 1% (nonsignificant)

bid, twice daily; CAPRIE, Clopidogrel versus Aspirin in Patients at Risk of Ischemic Events; ESPS, European Stroke Prevention Study; MI, myocardial infarction; TASS, Ticlopidine Aspirin Stroke Study; TIA, transient ischemic attack.

    risk patients

  b) High-risk patients: established coronary artery disease *plus* multiple major risk factors (especially diabetes), severe and poorly controlled risk factors, multiple risk factors of the metabolic syndrome, and acute coronary artery syndromes

5) Overall recommendations

  a) Ischemic stroke or TIA patients with elevated cholesterol, coronary artery disease, or evidence of an atherosclerotic origin should be treated according to NCEP III guidelines

  d. Tobacco smoking

    1) Smoking is an important, independent risk factor for ischemic stroke

    2) Smoking increases risk of stroke nearly 2 to 4-fold and increases risk of carotid disease 5-fold

    3) Based on data from observational studies, stroke risk in cigarette smokers apparently is reduced by 60% with smoking cessation

    4) By 5 years after smoking cessation, the level can be reduced to that of a "never smoker"

  e. Diabetes mellitus

Table 11-16. **Atherosclerotic Risk Factors**

Well documented	Less Well Documented
Hypertension	Obesity
Hyperlipidemia	Physical inactivity
Tobacco smoking	Impaired fasting glucose level
Diabetes mellitus	Metabolic syndrome
Asymptomatic carotid artery disease	Poor diet/nutrition
	Alcohol abuse
	Hyperhomocystinemia
	Hormone replacement therapy/oral contraceptive use
	Inflammatory processes
	Sleep apnea

1) Diabetic patients have both increased susceptibility to atherosclerosis and increased prevalence of atherogenic risk factors, notably hypertension, hyperlipidemia, obesity
2) Presence of diabetes increases risk of stroke by 2 to 6-fold
3) Careful attention should be given to glucose control, but also other associated atherosclerotic risk factors such as hypertension and hyperlipidemia
  f. Hormone replacement
    1) Not recommended for patients who have had ischemic stroke; recent data suggest it may actually increase risk of ischemic stroke, myocardial infarction, and deep venous thrombosis
    2) Studies reviewing timing and doses of hormone replacement therapy in relation to vascular disease are ongoing

VII. VASCULAR MALFORMATIONS

A. **AVM, Cavernous Malformations, Venous Angiomas, and Dural Arteriovenous Malformations:** the most common types of cerebrovascular malformations

B. **Clinical Presentation, Natural History, and Treatments of Vascular Malformations:** compared in Table 11-17

C. **Radiographic Findings of Selected Vascular Malformations** (Fig. 11-25 and 11-26)

D. **Capillary Telangiectasia**

1. Small, dilated capillaries without smooth muscle or elastic fibers
2. Most commonly occurs in pons, also in dentate nucleus and middle cerebellar peduncle
3. Usually an incidental finding, rarely symptomatic
4. MRI: increased T2 signal and contrast enhancement

E. **Sturge-Weber Syndrome** (see also Chapter 13)
1. Pathogenesis: unknown, sporadic
2. Clinical features
  a. Port-wine stain of face (facial angioma), typically in distribution of ophthalmic or maxillary division of CN V
  b. Leptomeningeal angioma of brain, typically on same side as port-wine stain
  c. Leptomeningeal angioma may result in
    1) Seizures
    2) Static or progressive focal neurologic deficits
    3) Developmental delay
    4) Visual field deficits
  d. Ocular abnormalities: glaucoma, choroid angioma, heterochromia of iris
3. Diagnosis
  a. Typical clinical features
  b. MRI with and without contrast: leptomeninges are thickened, large leptomeningeal angioma, atrophic brain beneath angioma

F. **Wyburn-Mason's Syndrome** (Bonnet-Dechaume-Blanc syndrome)
1. Congenital, *not* inherited
2. Rare syndrome with unilateral AVM involving retina, brain, and sometimes skin

G. **Osler-Weber-Rendu Disease** (hereditary hemorrhagic telangiectasia) (see also Chapter 13)
1. Autosomal dominant (chromosones 9q and 12q)
2. Telangiectasias occur in multiple organs, including lung, liver, kidney, skin, brain
3. Epistaxis is most common presentation, followed by gastrointestinal tract bleeding
4. Neurologic manifestations usually due to cerebral ischemia from pulmonary fistulas
5. In one series, only 3.7% of patients had intracranial vascular formation; intracranial vascular malformations associated with syndrome are varied

H. **Spinal Vascular Malformations**
1. Classification
  a. Dural arteriovenous fistula
  b. Intradural spinal cord AVMs

Table 11-17. **Comparison of Common Vascular Malformations**

Type	Description	Clinical presentation	Bleeding risk	Treatment
AVM	Fistulous connections of arteries and veins without normal intervening capillary beds Thought to be congenital Majority are supratentorial	Generally present between 20 and 40 years Equal male:female ratio Hemorrhage (most common) Seizures Asymptomatic Headache Focal neurologic deficit Steal phenomenon	2%-3% annually Risk factor: previous hemorrhage Potential risk factors: small (<3 cm), deep venous drainage	May include observation, surgical removal, endovascular embolization, gamma knife surgery May depend on location of AVM (superficial vs. deep), associated aneurysms, patient's age, Spetzler-Martin grade Gamma knife surgery generally reserved for small (<3 cm) deep AVM Surgical removal generally recommended when patient is at risk for hemorrhage, has had hemorrhge, or AVM is surgically accessible with low morbidity
Cavernous malforma-tion	Circumscribed, multilobulated angiographically occult vascular malformations Consists of sinusoidal vascular channels (caverns) lined by a single layer of endothelium Lack of intervening brain parenchyma is characteristic pathologic marker Some are familial: chromosome 7q (*CCM1* gene), usually Hispanic Americans Majority are supratentorial	Present in 2nd and 4th decades Equal male:female ratio Asymptomatic Seizures (most common presenting symptom) Hemorrhage Focal neurologic deficit	0.7%-4.2% annually Risk factor: previous hemorrhage Possible risk factors: female sex, posterior fossa	Observation is recommended for asymptomatic patients with low risk of hemorrhage Surgical removal may be indicated if 1) lesion has hemorrhaged and is surgically accessible, 2) lesion has resulted in intractable seizure disorder and is surgically accessible, 3) patient has progressive neurologic deficit due to lesion and it is surgically accessible Gamma knife therapy for these lesions is controversial and generally not implemented

Dural arterio-venous malfor-mation	Arteriovenous shunts from dural arterial supply to dural venous drainage channel, dural arteries are thickened and veins dilated in an abnormal	Typically present between ages 40 and 60 with:
		  Pulsatile tinnitus (most common presenting symptom)
		  Unilateral headache
		  Hemorrhage
			1.8% annually
			Risk factors: cortical, venous drainage, aneurysmal venous structure
				Management may include observation, endovascular embolization, surgery, gamma knife therapy
				Indications for treatment:
				  Hemorrhage
				  Progressive neurologic deficit
				  High risk DAVF

Table 11-17 (continued)

Type	Description	Clinical presentation	Bleeding risk	Treatment
	vascular network within the wall of venous sinus Cause can be idiopathic, trauma, venous thrombosis, surgery, tumor Transverse/sigmoid sinus most common location May be missed on both CT and MRI/MRA Angiography, including external carotid injections, is necessary for diagnosis	Note: carotid-cavernous fistulas will also produce chemosis and proptosis		Intractable symptoms
Venous angioma	Congenital Pathologically characterized by anomalous veins separated by normal brain tissue Drain normal cerebral tissue May be associated with cavernous malformations	Usually found incidentally for other reasons, rarely symptomatic Hemorrhage, venous thrombosis, focal deficit, seizures, and headaches have been rarely reported	0.2%-0.6% annually	Treatment generally not necessary because venous angiomas are rarely symptomatic Removal of lesion would cause venous infarction because venous angioma drains normal brain

AVM, arteriovenous malformation; CT, computed tomography; MRA, magnetic resonance angiography; MRI, magnetic resonance imaging.

c. Pial (perimedullary) arteriovenous fistulas
d. Cavernous malformations of spinal cord
2. Dural arteriovenous fistulas of spinal cord
  a. Acquired lesions generally occur in older (>40 years) men
  b. Gradual progressive myelopathy likely due to venous hypertension and subsequent spinal cord ischemia
  c. Radicular pain may precede onset of myelopathic symptoms
  d. Rarely can be acute decline in course (Foix-Alajouanine syndrome)
  e. Lower cord segments more commonly involved than cervical segments
  f. Low-flow fistula
  g. Diagnosis can be made by spinal cord MRI assessing for

flow voids
  h. CT myelography or spinal angiography may be necessary if MRI is negative and clinical suspicion is strong
3. Intramedullary AVMs
  a. Male/female incidence is similar; present earlier than dural arteriovenous fistulas of spinal cord
  b. May be associated with vascular malformations elsewhere
  c. Uniform distribution over each spinal segment
  d. High-flow shunting
  e. Acute presentation with back pain, meningismus, and occasionally loss of consciousness with myelopathy
  f. Occasionally may be gradual progressive myelopathic syndrome
  g. Diagnosis by MRI and confirmed by spinal angiograph

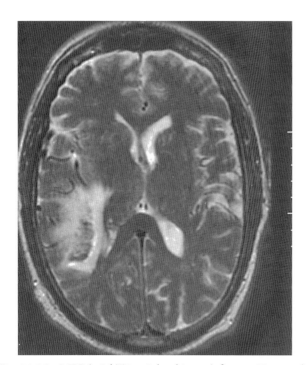

Fig. 11-25. MRI (axial T2-weighted image) from a 50-year-old with subacute right temporal intraparenchymal hemorrhage due to arteriovenous malformation, extending into most anterior aspect of right parietal lobe. The malformation is apparent as multiple enlarged vessels (flow voids), mostly situated in the sylvian fissure.

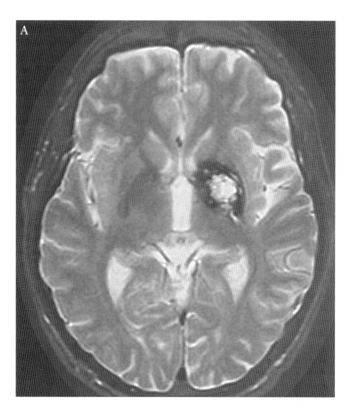

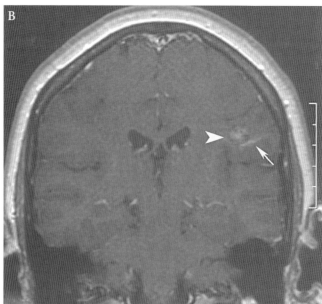

Fig. 11-26. MRI of cavernous malformation (cavernous angioma) A, Axial T2-weighted image demonstrates characteristic appearance of cavernous malformation in deep gray matter. Note heterogeneous reticulated "mulberry" or "popcorn-like" appearance of the lesion core, surrounded by hypointense rim suggestive of hemosiderin deposition. B, Coronal T1-weighted image with contrast demonstrates cavernous malformation in another patient (*arrowhead*) and adjacent venous angioma (*arrow*).

REFERENCES

Albers GW, Amarenco P, Easton JD, Sacco RL, Teal P. Antithrombotic and thrombolytic therapy for ischemic stroke: the Seventh ACCP Conference on Antithrombotic and Thrombolytic Therapy. Chest. 2004;126 Suppl:483S-512S.

Barnett HJ, Taylor DW, Eliasziw M, Fox AJ, Ferguson GG, Haynes RB, et al, North American Symptomatic Carotid Endarterectomy Trial Collaborators. Benefit of carotid endarterectomy in patients with symptomatic moderate or severe stenosis. N Engl J Med. 1998;339:1415-25.

CAVATAS Investigators. Endovascular versus surgical treatment in patients with carotid stenosis in the Carotid and Vertebral Artery Transluminal Angioplasty Study (CAVATAS): a randomised trial. Lancet. 2001;357:1729-37.

Chimowitz MI, Kokkinos J, Strong J, Brown MB, Levine SR, Silliman S, et al. The Warfarin-Aspirin Symptomatic Intracranial Disease Study. Neurology. 1995;45:1488-93.

Erkinjuntti T, Roman G, Gauthier S, Feldman H, Rockwood K. Emerging therapies for vascular dementia and vascular cognitive impairment. Stroke. 2004 Apr;35:1010-7. Epub 2004 Mar 4.

Executive Committee for the Asymptomatic Carotid Atherosclerosis Study. Endarterectomy for asymptomatic carotid artery stenosis. JAMA. 1995;273:1421-8.

Flemming KD, Brown RD Jr. Secondary prevention strategies in ischemic stroke: identification and optimal management of modifiable risk factors. Mayo Clin Proc. 2004;79:1330-40.

Flemming KD, Brown RD Jr, Petty GW, Huston J III, Kallmes DF, Piepgras DG. Evaluation and management of transient ischemic attack and minor cerebral infarction. Mayo Clin Proc. 2004;79:1071-86.

Flemming KD, Wiebers DO. Optimizing antiplatelet therapy to prevent ischemic stroke. Emerg Med. 2002;34:28-37.

Fulgham JR, Ingall TJ, Stead LG, Cloft HJ, Wijdicks EFM, Flemming KD. Management of acute ischemic stroke. Mayo Clin Proc. 2004;79:1459-69.

Halliday A, Mansfield A, Marro J, Peto C, Peto R, Potter J, et al, MRC Asymptomatic Carotid Surgery Trial (ACST) Collaborative Group. Prevention of disabling and fatal strokes by successful carotid endarterectomy in patients without recent neurological symptoms: randomised controlled trial. Lancet. 2004;363:1491-502. Erratum in: Lancet. 2004;364:416.

Heart Protection Study Collaborative Group. MRC/BHF Heart Protection Study of cholesterol lowering with simvastatin in 20,536 high-risk individuals: a randomised placebo-controlled trial. Lancet 2002;360:7-22; summary for patients in: Curr Cardiol Rep. 2002;4:486-7.

Levy DE, Caronna JJ, Singer BH, Lapinski RH, Frydman H, Plum F. Predicting outcome from hypoxic-ischemic coma. JAMA. 1985;253:1420-6.

Mohr JP, Thompson JLP, Lazar RM, Levin B, Sacco RL, Furie KL, et al, Warfarin-Aspirin Recurrent Stroke Study Group. A comparison of warfarin and aspirin for the prevention of recurrent ischemic stroke. N Engl J Med. 2001;345:1444-51.

North American Symptomatic Carotid Endarterectomy Trial Collaborators. Beneficial effect of carotid endarterectomy in symptomatic patients with high-grade carotid stenosis. N Engl J Med. 1991;325:445-53.

Yadav JS, Wholey MH, Kuntz RE, Fayad P, Katzen BT, Mishkel GJ, et al, Stenting and Angioplasty With Protection in Patients at High Risk for Endarterectomy Investigators. Protected carotid-artery stenting versus endarterectomy in high-risk patients. N Engl J Med. 2004;351:1493-501.

Zandbergen EG, de Haan RJ, Stoutenbeek CP, Koelman JH, Hijdra A. Systematic review of early prediction of poor outcome in anoxic-ischaemic coma. Lancet. 1998;352:1808-12.

Questions

1. A patient presents with right face, arm, and leg hemisensory loss and no other findings. Where does this localize?
   a. Left primary sensory cortex
   b. Left internal capsule
   c. Left thalamus (ventral posterolateral and ventral posteromedial nuclei)
   d. Left lateral midbrain (medial lemniscus)

2. For the patient in question 1, what arterial territory supplies the area involved?
   a. Middle cerebral artery, lenticulostriate branches
   b. Thalamogeniculate arteries of posterior cerebral artery
   c. Superior cerebellar artery
   d. Recurrent artery of Huebner

3. A patient presents with ptosis of the right eye. When the right eyelid is opened, the eye deviates down and out. Abduction and downgaze are intact, but other extraocular movements are impaired. The patient has normal strength and sensation throughout, but does have left hemiataxia. Where does this process localize?
   a. Midbrain, medial (Nothnagel's syndrome)
   b. Pons, medial (Foville's syndrome)
   c. Medulla, lateral (Wallenberg syndrome)
   d. Thalamus (ventral lateral nucleus)

4. A patient has a 20-minute episode of aphasia and weakness of the right hand. Carotid ultrasonography shows a left internal carotid artery occlusion. What is the next appropriate step in the management of this patient?
   a. Superficial temporal artery–to–middle cerebral artery bypass
   b. Carotid endarterectomy
   c. Consider a confirmatory carotid artery test such as magnetic resonance angiography
   d. Clopidogrel

5. The patient in question 4 is found to have a total cholesterol of 193 mg/dL, triglycerides of 91 mg/dL, high-density lipoprotein of 64 mg/dL, and low-density lipoprotein of 111 mg/dL. What would you recommend?
   a. Treatment with a fibrate
   b. Treatment with a statin
   c. Treatment with niacin
   d. No treatment necessary

6. For a patient with asymptomatic carotid artery stenosis of more than 60% to benefit from intervention (endarterectomy or angioplasty/stenting), what is the highest risk one could undertake for treatment to outweigh risk?
   a. 1%
   b. 2%
   c. 3%
   d. 5%

7. A 75-year-old woman presented with weakness of the left face and hand and hemineglect. Electrocardiography demonstrates atrial fibrillation. She has not been receiving antithrombotics and has no contraindications to antithrombotics. Which of the following tests would be helpful (i.e., change management) in further diagnostic evaluation?
   a. Magnetic resonance imaging of the head
   b. Transesophageal echocardiography
   c. Carotid ultrasonography
   d. Antiphospholipid antibodies

8. In the NINDS intravenous tissue plasminogen activator (tPA) study for acute ischemic stroke, what was the outcome effect of intravenous tPA when used for acute ischemic stroke?
   a. tPA group was more likely to have minimal or no disability at 3 months
   b. tPA group had lower mortality rate at 3 months
   c. tPA group achieved higher recanalization rates noted on angiography than non-tPA group

9. In the NINDS intravenous tissue plasminogen activator study for acute ischemic stroke, what was the symptomatic hemorrhage rate?
   a. 20%
   b. 8.8%
   c. 3%
   d. 6.4%

10. A young woman presents with a 2-week history of progressively severe headaches and transient visual obscurations. She has papilledema. Computed tomography shows two small hemorrhages in the left and right parasagittal region. What diagnostic tests may be helpful?
   a. Magnetic resonance imaging of the head
   b. Magnetic resonance angiography of the head

c. Carotid ultrasonography

d. Magnetic resonance venography of the head

11. You are consulted to see a patient who had a cardiac arrest 3 days earlier. The patient can trigger the ventilator. The pupils are 4 mm and equal but minimally reactive to light. There is evidence of decerebrate posturing. There is no verbal output (patient intubated) and no eye opening to pain. You are asked to prognosticate.

a. Patient has a 90% chance of good recovery (able to ambulate and speak) at 1 year

b. Patient has a 50% chance of good recovery (able to ambulate and speak) at 1 year

c. Patient has poor chance of good recovery (able to ambulate and speak) at 1 year

12. Which antiplatelet agent or combination of antiplatelet agents has been shown to be superior to aspirin alone in ischemic stroke prevention in patients with strokes not related to a cardiac source?

a. Clopidogrel plus aspirin

b. Aspirin–extended release dipyridamole combination

c. Pentoxifylline plus aspirin

d. Vitamin E plus aspirin

Answers

1. c.
2. b.
3. a.
4. c.
Because ultrasonography can show occlusion that is falsely positive, a confirmatory test is often helpful. This could be magnetic resonance or computed tomographic angiography or conventional angiography.

5. b.
Data from the National Cholesterol Education Program – Adult Treatment Panel would recommend a goal low-density lipoprotein of less than 100 mg/dL in this patient. Also, data from the Heart Protection Study noted benefit of simvastatin in high-risk patients regardless of the initial level of low-density lipoprotein.

6. c.

7. c.
Patient has a fixed focal deficit in an arterial territory suggestive of stroke. Localization is right middle cerebral artery territory. Clinically, one can localize the process as long as computed tomography of the head has been performed; magnetic resonance imaging may not be necessary. Most likely cause is atrial fibrillation, although 10% to 15 % of patients with atrial fibrillation have concomitant carotid artery stenosis. Both atrial fibrillation and significant carotid artery stenosis would change management. Atrial fibrillation will require anticoagulation regardless of what transesophageal echocardiography shows, so it would not be necessary unless there were possibilities of cardioversion. In this age group, antiphospholipid antibody syndrome would be a low yield test, especially given you have already found one of the most common causes of ischemic stroke. Therefore, the only diagnostic test that may change management would be carotid ultrasonography.

8. a.
Patients receiving intravenous tPA were 30% more likely to have minimal or no disability at 3 months (absolute reduction of 11%-13% over placebo). Note that there was no difference in mortality at 3 months.

9. d.
The symptomatic hemorrhage rate was 6.4%, with half of them fatal.

10. d.
Headaches and symptoms of increased intracranial pressure, with or without focal neurologic deficits, should make one think about cerebral venous thrombosis. Computed tomography of the head can be completely normal in this condition; however, in this case, there are two areas of hemorrhage near the sagittal sinus. Magnetic resonance or comuted tomographic venography or conventional angiography would be the diagnostic test of choice. If confirmed, pregnancy testing, medication review, family history, and special coagulation testing should be pursued.

11. c.
This patient has a Glasgow Coma Scale of 4 on day 3 after cardiac arrest. A motor response of 1 or 2 on the Glasgow Coma Scale on day 3 is highly suggestive of poor neurologic recovery.

12. b.
The combination of extended-release dipyridamole (200 mg) and aspirin (25 mg) twice daily is superior to aspirin (25 mg) twice daily in prevention of stroke or death. Clopidogrel (75 mg) daily is superior to aspirin (325 mg) daily in patients with atherosclerosis, although no statistical significance was seen in the cerebrovascular subgroup. The combination of clopidogrel and aspirin has not been shown to be superior to clopidogrel alone for cerebrovascular patients.

Michael L. Bell, M.D.

I. SEIZURE CLASSIFICATION (TABLES 12-1 AND 12-2)

A. Seizure

1. Abnormal focal or generalized neuronal discharge, often with physical manifestations

B. Epilepsy

1. Refers to a condition in which a person experiences two or more seizures

Table 12-1. **Terms Used to Describe Seizures and Their Definitions**

Term	Definition
Simple	Focal seizure with no change in consciousness
Complex	Focal seizure with altered consciousness
Aura	Subjective symptoms attributable to a seizure (patient experiences but not seen by an observer), e.g., sensory symptoms, psychic symptoms such as déjà vu, abdominal sensations; essentially a simple partial seizure
Prodrome or premonition	Vague sense, agitation preceding seizure
Reflex epilepsy	Precipitated by stimulus (visual, eating, contemplating music, reading, startle)
Postictal	Following a seizure
Automatism	Coordinated, involuntary movement during altered consciousness or postictal
Idiopathic	Unknown cause, often used to describe genetic-related epilepsies, e.g., benign rolandic epilepsy
Cryptogenic	Suspected to be symptomatic, but no symptomatic cause identified on imaging (e.g., infantile spasms with normal MRI)
Symptomatic	Seizures with an identifiable cause (e.g., brain lesion, metabolic)
Semiology	Clinical seizure manifestations

C. Partial (focal) Seizures

1. Simple partial seizures
   a. A spontaneous, uncontrolled neuronal discharge from a focal area of the brain *without* loss of consciousness
   b. Motor seizures: clonic, tonic (asymmetrical, e.g., supplementary motor seizures), automatisms, focal negative myoclonus
   c. Sensory seizures
      1) Elementary sensory symptoms: a simple sensation involving one sensory modality, e.g., tingling, a visual sensation, odor, or taste

Table 12-2. **Simplified Outline of the International Classification of Epileptic Seizures**

Partial (focal) seizures
    Simple partial seizures
    Complex partial seizures
    Partial seizures evolving into secondarily generalized seizures
    Partial status epilepticus
Generalized seizures
    Absence seizures
    Atypical absence seizures
    Myoclonic seizures
    Clonic seizures
    Tonic seizures
    Tonic-clonic seizures
    Atonic seizures
    Infantile spasms
    Variations
    Generalized status epilepticus
Unclassified epileptic seizures (e.g., neonatal seizures)

Modified from International League Against Epilepsy. Seizure types: epileptic seizure types and precipitating stimuli for reflex seizures. 2004 [cited 2005 Apr 19]. Available from: http://www.ilae-epilepsy.org/Visitors/Centre/ctf/seizure_types.cfm. Used with permission.

2) Experiential sensory symptoms
   a) Temporoparieto-occipital junction
   b) Complex perceptions ± affective experience, similar to experiences in life but recognized by the subject as occurring out of context, e.g., déjà vu, jamais vu, flashbacks, feelings of depersonalization
d. Autonomic seizures: involve autonomic functions, e.g., unpleasant abdominal sensation, bradycardia, tachycardia, asystole, drooling, piloerection
e. Psychic seizures: disturbance of higher cerebral functions
f. Gelastic seizures
   1) Bursts of laughter
   2) Related to hypothalamic lesions (usually hamartoma)

2. Complex partial seizures
   a. Spontaneous, uncontrolled neuronal discharge from a focal area of the brain *with* loss of consciousness
   b. Temporal >> frontal > parietal or occipital lobe
   c. May begin as a simple partial seizure
   d. May have automatisms: involuntary complex motor activity during impaired consciousness
      1) Examples are gum chewing, nose wiping, drinking from cup, lip smacking
      2) Usually occur with complex seizures, occasionally with absence seizures
      3) Usually occur ipsilateral to the epileptic focus
      4) May be de novo automatisms, in which the complex motor activity begins after the onset of seizure; reactive automatisms, in which the activity also begins after the onset of seizure but is a reaction to an external stimulus; or perseverative automatisms, which are a continuation of the motor activity that was initiated before seizure onset

3. Partial seizures evolving into secondarily generalized seizures

4. Partial status epilepticus
   a. Epilepsia partialis continua
   b. Aura continua
   c. Limbic status epilepticus (psychomotor status)
   d. Hemiconvulsive status with hemiparesis

D. Generalized Seizures

1. Generalized tonic-clonic seizures

---

a. With or without premonition (rare, hours-days)
b. Tonic phase: eyes open and roll up, pupils dilate, elbows flex, arms pronate, incontinence, moaning, cyanosis and apnea
c. Clonic phase: generalized clonic movements, frequency gradually decreases, amplitude gradually increases, atonic between jerks, tongue biting, cyanosis and apnea
d. Postictal state: drowsy, confused, lethargy, regular respiration resumes, headache, muscle soreness

2. Generalized tonic seizures
   a. Axial, proximal limbs, or axial + proximal + distal limbs involved
   b. Less common than tonic-clonic seizures
   c. Typically lasts seconds, can persist (status)

3. Generalized clonic seizures: same clinical significance as generalized tonic-clonic seizures

4. Absence seizures
   a. Usually occur in children with normal intelligence
   b. Generalized 3-Hz spike-and-wave electroencephalogram (EEG)
   c. Brief duration, usually a few seconds
   d. Abrupt recovery
   e. No postictal phase
   f. Absence with atonic components: primarily affects axial musculature, causing head drop or slumping of the trunk (falls are rare)
   g. Absence with tonic components: asymmetric or symmetric contraction of the flexure or extensor muscles
   h. Absence with automatisms: purposeful or semipurposeful movements occurring without awareness (patient is amnestic for the movements)
   i. Absence with mild clonic movements: clonic movements may sometimes occur with prolonged spells
      1) Are of variable duration and severity
      2) Often involve the eyelids or corner of the mouth
   j. Absence with impairment of consciousness only: no other features

5. Atypical absence seizures
   a. Longer duration than typical absence seizures: may last several minutes
   b. Less abrupt onset and offset
   c. Often loss of postural tone (more pronounced than mild head drop)

Automatisms are involuntary complex motor activity during impaired consciousness

They can occur with complex partial or absence seizures

Atypical absence seizures differ from absence seizures in that duration is often longer, onset and offset can be less abrupt, and loss of postural tone may be more prominent

d. Associated with other seizure types and mental retardation

e. Slow generalized spike-and-wave (<2.5 Hz) when seen in the context of Lennox-Gastaut syndrome (see EPILEPSY SYNDROMES)

f. May have mild clonic, atonic, tonic, or autonomic activity or automatisms

6. Myoclonic seizures
   a. Shocklike jerk
      1) Cortical reflex myoclonus: discharge from sensorimotor cortex
      2) Reticular reflex myoclonus: discharge from brainstem reticular formation
      3) Primary generalized epileptic myoclonus: diffuse bursts of polyspike and wave or spike and wave
      4) Nonepileptic myoclonus: most common

7. Atonic seizures
   a. Drop attacks
   b. Duration: seconds
   c. Spectrum: from head drop to complete loss of tone in entire body

8. Akinetic seizures
   a. Similar to atonic seizures, but tone is preserved
   b. Brief loss of consciousness, motionless

9. Infantile spasms (see description under EPILEPSY SYNDROMES)

10. Variations of generalized seizures (examples are myoclonic atonic, massive myoclonic, tonic-clonic beginning with clonic phase)

11. Generalized status epilepticus
    a. Generalized tonic-clonic seizure
    b. Clonic seizure
    c. Absence seizure
    d. Tonic seizure
    e. Myoclonic seizure

II. EPILEPSY SYNDROMES (TABLE 12-3)

A. Localization-related (focal, local, partial) Cryptogenic or Symptomatic (secondary) Epilepsy (otherwise unclassified)

1. Temporal lobe seizures

> Epileptic myoclonus includes cortical reflex myoclonus (sensorimotor cortex), reticular reflex myoclonus (reticular formation of brainstem), and primary generalized epileptic myoclonus (diffuse epileptic discharge)

a. Initial behavioral arrest and automatisms (usually with complex partial temporal lobe seizures); initial speech arrest and aphasia (usually with dominant temporal lobe seizures)

b. Associated with epigastric rising sensation, nausea, olfactory hallucinations (usually unpleasant smell, "uncinate fits"), sensation of fear and terror and other changes of affect (intense pleasure or intense depression), gustatory hallucinations (with deep opercular focus), and autonomic symptoms

Table 12-3. International Classification of Epilepsy Syndromes

Neonates
  Benign familial neonatal seizures
  Early myoclonic encephalopathy
  Ohtahara syndrome
  Migrating partial seizures of infancy
Infants
  West's syndrome
  Aicardi's syndrome
  Benign myoclonic epilepsy of infancy
  Benign infantile seizures
  Severe myoclonic epilepsy in infancy (Dravet syndrome)
Children
  Benign childhood epilepsy with centrotemporal spikes
  Early-onset benign childhood occipital epilepsy
  Late-onset childhood occipital epilepsy
  Epilepsy with myoclonic absences
  Myoclonic-astatic epilepsy of childhood
  Lennox-Gastaut syndrome
  Landau-Kleffner syndrome
  Epilepsy with continuous spike and waves during slow wave sleep
  Childhood absence epilepsy
  Progressive myoclonic epilepsies
Juveniles/adults
  Idiopathic generalized epilepsies
    Juvenile absence epilepsy
    Juvenile myoclonic epilepsy
    Epilepsy with generalized tonic-clonic seizures only
  Reflex epilepsies
    Idiopathic photosensitive occipital lobe epilepsy
    Primary reading epilepsy
    Startle epilepsy
  Familial temporal lobe epilepsies
  Other symptomatic epilepsies (e.g., Rasmussen's syndrome)

Modified from International League Against Epilepsy. Seizure types: epileptic seizure types and precipitating stimuli for reflex seizures. 2004 [cited 2005 Apr 19]. Available from: http://www.ilae-epilepsy.org/Visitors/Centre/ctf/syndromes.cfm. Used with permission.

c. May arise from mesial temporal lobe (amygdala, hippocampus, associated with mesial temporal sclerosis) or lateral neocortical temporal lobe

d. Auditory hallucinations (superior temporal gyrus)

e. Vertigo and perception of motion

f. Memory misperceptions: dreamy state, déjà vu (perception of familiarity with previously unfamiliar people or events), déjà entendu (perception of unfamiliarity with previously familiar people), jamais vu (perception of familiarity with previously unfamiliar auditory experience), and jamais entendu (perception of unfamiliarity with previously familiar auditory experience)

g. Associated with postictal confusion

h. Interictal personality: emotionality, hypermorality and hyperreligiosity, increased philosophical interest, humorlessness, hypergraphia, circumstantiality of speech, altered libido (hyposexuality more than hypersexuality)

2. Frontal lobe seizures

a. Characterized by abrupt onset, brief duration spells occurring with high frequency (tendency to occur during sleep) with minimal or no postictal confusion

b. Associated with frequent falls during the seizure

c. More frequently associated with secondary generalization and status epilepticus than temporal lobe seizures

d. Prominent motor movements such as clonic jerking of one body part that spreads to involve other body parts, termed "jacksonian march," because of spread of epileptic activity in motor cortex

   1) Head or eyes may turn opposite to side of epileptic focus

   2) Tonic posturing of one limb or "fencer's posturing" (see below) is often seen with seizures arising from supplementary motor cortex

   3) There may be motor or gestural automatisms, such as bicycling or pedaling movements of the lower limbs, sexual gesturing

e. Most common extratemporal partial epilepsy

f. Postictal paralysis (Todd's paralysis): transient paralysis that may follow a partial motor seizure

3. Parietal lobe seizures

a. Associated with positive or negative sensory phenomena

b. There may be tingling (positive), which often starts in body parts with larger cortical representation such as the face or the tongue

c. There may be negative phenomena such as asomatognosia (loss of awareness for a body part or whole side of the body) or metamorphopsia (both usually representing a nondominant parietal focus)

4. Occipital lobe seizures

a. Elementary visual hallucinations, often bright lines, flashes of light, geometric objects (positive or negative visual symptoms)

b. Versive eye movements

B. Neonates

1. Benign neonatal seizures

a. Can be idiopathic with no family history or familial (benign familial neonatal seizures)

b. Also called "fifth-day fits"

c. Clinical presentation

   1) Clonic or myoclonic seizures and apneic events during first few weeks after birth

   2) Seizures usually stop by 6 weeks after birth, no long-term sequelae

   3) Normal development

   4) Later, some of the children have epilepsy (10%-15%) or febrile seizures (33%)

   5) Treatment is often unnecessary, may prescribe phenobarbital for 1 month, then taper

d. Generalized epilepsy

e. EEG

   1) Normal interictally

   2) EEG findings are variable

      a) There may be focal, multifocal, or bilateral sharp waves, spikes, spike-and-waves

      b) There may be a pattern of unreactive, asynchronous theta activity with interspersed spikes (theta point alternant)

f. Benign familial neonatal convulsions is an autosomal dominant channelopathy (Table 12-4)

g. Voltage-dependent potassium channel mutations

   1) Mutations in two genes have been identified: *KCNQ2* on chromosome 20 and *KCNQ3* on chromosome 8

   2) These impair potassium-dependent repolarization, thus causing hyperexcitability

   3) Mutation of the *KCNQ1* gene causes the long QT syndrome (which also is related to impaired repolarization)

Benign familial neonatal convulsions is an autosomal dominant disorder caused by mutation of *KCNQ2* or *KCNQ3*, both genes encoding for potassium channel proteins

These mutations impair potassium-dependent repolarization, resulting in hyperexcitability

2. Early myoclonic encephalopathy
   a. Also called "early-onset progressive encephalopathy with migrant, continuous myoclonus"
   b. Clinical presentation
      1) Erratic, focal myoclonus: migrates randomly to different body parts
      2) Occurs in early infancy (occasionally within first few hours after birth)
      3) The infant may have other seizure types (partial, widespread myoclonus, tonic spasms), but these usually occur later in the course of the disorder
   c. Generalized, symptomatic, or cryptogenic
      1) Multiple causes, a nonspecific diagnosis
         a) Metabolic (nonketotic hyperglycemia)
         b) Inherited (autosomal recessive)
         c) Various developmental malformations
   d. Often cryptogenic
   e. EEG
      1) Generalized or focal epileptiform discharges
      2) EEG often shows burst suppression (as in Ohtahara syndrome)

Early myoclonic encephalopathy is characterized by newborn infants with migrant focal myoclonic epilepsy and progressive psychomotor abnormalities

---

Table 12-4. **Epilepsy Syndromes With Simple Genetic Inheritance**

Generalized epilepsy with febrile seizures plus
    Autosomal dominant
        Sodium channel *SCN1B* (chromosome 19)
        Sodium channel *SCN1A* (chromosome 2)
        Sodium channel *SCN2A*
        GABA$_A$ (chromosome 5)
Benign familial neonatal convulsions
    Autosomal dominant
        Voltage-dependent potassium channel *KCNQ2* (chromosome 20)
        Voltage-dependent potassium channel *KCNQ3* (chromosome 8)
Autosomal dominant partial epilepsy with auditory features
    Autosomal dominant
        LGI1, leucine-rich, glioma-inactivated 1 gene (chromosome 10)

GABA, γ-aminobutyric acid.

---

      3) Myoclonus often does not have an EEG counterpart and EEG may be normal initially
   f. Similar to severe myoclonic epilepsy and Ohtahara, Lennox-Gastaut, and West's syndromes (described below)
      1) In all the epileptiform abnormalities thought to contribute to decline in cerebral function
      2) Severe psychomotor delay
      3) Burst suppression pattern may evolve into hypsarrhythmia later in life
   g. Poor prognosis
      1) More than 50% die, others have profound psychomotor delay
3. Ohtahara syndrome
   a. Also called "early infantile epileptic encephalopathy with suppression bursts"
   b. Clinical presentation
      1) Frequent tonic spasms ± partial seizures
      2) Onset is usually within first 10 days after birth (otherwise, <3 months)
      3) Difficult-to-control seizures
      4) Clinical course is marked by neurologic deterioration
   c. Symptomatic or cryptogenic: usually structural brain abnormality, multiple causes
   d. EEG: burst-suppression pattern
   e. The EEG is the same in Ohtahara syndrome and early myoclonic encephalopathy, causing the two to be confused
   f. Difference: no myoclonic seizures in Ohtahara syndrome
   g. Seizures are difficult to control, vigabatrin may be beneficial in early stages
   h. Poor prognosis, 50% die within first few months
   i. Often progresses to West's syndrome or Lennox-Gastaut syndrome phenotypes
4. Migrating partial seizures of infancy
   a. Clinical presentation
      1) Onset less than 6 months after birth (average, first seizure at 3 months)
      2) Progresses over weeks
      3) Multifocal seizures, shift from hemisphere to hemisphere
      4) Seizures are nearly continuous at times, occur in clusters
      5) Progressive microcephaly and severe psychomotor deterioration
      6) Poor response to anticonvulsants

Ohtahara syndrome is early infantile epileptic encephalopathy with tonic spasms and focal seizures associated with a burst-suppression pattern on EEG

b. Idiopathic: no identifiable cause

5. Pyridoxine (vitamin B_6)-dependent seizures (congenital dependency on pyridoxine)

a. Autosomal recessive disorder

b. Some data suggest this condition results from diminished activity of glutamic acid decarboxylase (GAD); diminished action of GAD leads to increased cerebral concentrations of glutamic acid, which may not normalize after initiation of treatment with doses necessary to stop seizures

c. Age at onset: usually neonatal period but may appear up to 1 year of age

d. Diagnosis: established by response (remission of seizures) to treatment with parenteral pyridoxine and relapse without ongoing treatment

e. Treatment: life-long administration of pyridoxine oral supplements daily

  1) If left untreated, the disease is fatal within days to months

  2) If treatment is delayed, patients develop psychomotor retardation, progressive deterioration of neurologic function, chronic encephalopathy

f. This condition needs to be differentiated from

  1) Pyridoxine deficiency-related seizures: often result from breastfeeding by malnutritioned mothers and may be recurrent, of abrupt onset, and responsive to vitamin B_6 supplementation; in comparison, pyridoxine-dependent seizures occur in setting of normal dietary pyridoxine supplementation, require larger doses of pyridoxine to control seizures, and usually occur earlier than pyridoxine deficiency-related seizures

  2) Pyridoxine-responsive epilepsy (usually infantile spasms): seizure frequency may decrease with pyridoxine supplementation (in addition to other anticonvulsants)

C. Infants

1. Infantile spasms

a. This is not an epilepsy syndrome but a seizure type

---

b. May be symptomatic or idiopathic: poor developmental outcome when symptomatic, mild to no mental retardation in 40% when idiopathic

c. Associated with West's syndrome

d. Clinical presentation

  1) Occurs within first year after birth

  2) Sudden tonic extension or flexion of limbs and axial body

    a) Flexion spasms: flexion of neck, trunk, and limbs, followed by several seconds of tonic activity, or may be mild head droop or waist flexion

    b) Extensor spasm: like the Moro reflex

  3) Spasms occur in clusters, often after awakening

e. EEG

  1) Interictal: hypsarrhythmia (high-amplitude, chaotic slow waves with multifocal spikes and sharp waves), which diminishes during REM sleep

  2) Seizure: electrodecrement (low-amplitude fast activity)

f. Treatment: ACTH, vigabatrin (not currently available in U.S., because of high incidence of retinal toxicity) more effective than other epileptic drugs

g. Benign myoclonus of infancy (described below) can mimic infantile spasms; compared with infantile spasms, benign myoclonus

  1) Identical to infantile spasms by semiology but normal EEG

  2) Clusters occur for weeks or months

  3) Usually much less frequent by 3 months, none by 2 years

  4) Developmentally normal infant

  5) Treatment not needed

2. West's syndrome

a. Triad: infantile spasms, hypsarrhythmia, developmental arrest

b. Symptomatic or cryptogenic

c. Etiology: several prenatal, perinatal, or postnatal insults, such as congenital in utero or acquired infections (e.g., meningitis, encephalitis), hydrocephalus, metabolic

---

Infantile spasms may be idiopathic or symptomatic. When idiopathic, sometimes there is mild or no mental retardation (40%)

Symptomatic infantile spasms are generally associated with poor development

---

Benign myoclonus of infancy appears identical to infantile spasms by semiology, but EEG is normal

---

West's syndrome is a nonspecific diagnosis referring to the triad of infantile spasms, hypsarrhythmia, and developmental arrest

disturbance (postnatal), developmental anomalies (prenatal), tuberous sclerosis, among others (40% cryptogenic)

  d. Developmental arrest or regression may occur before seizures develop

  e. Treatment: as mentioned, ACTH, corticosteroids, and vigabatrin; the latter is drug of choice for infantile spasms associated with tuberous sclerosis

3. Aicardi's syndrome

  a. Triad: Infantile spasms, agenesis of the corpus callosum, retinal malformations

  b. X-linked: occurs predominantly in girls, lethal in boys

4. Benign myoclonic epilepsy of infancy

  a. Clinical presentation

    1) Normal infant or toddler (4 months-3 years)

    2) Spectrum: from subtle head drop to massive widespread generalized myoclonus (less intense than infantile spasm)

    3) Some seizures provoked by intermittent photic stimulation

  b. Idiopathic, generalized

  c. EEG

    1) Normal interictally

    2) Generalized spike and polyspike with jerks

  d. If treated, excellent developmental outcome; some patients have photosensitivity, and some may eventually develop generalized tonic-clonic seizures

  e. Easily controlled with valproate

  f. Similar to a younger version of juvenile myoclonic epilepsy

  g. One-third of infants have a family history (as expected because it is idiopathic, often genetic)

5. Benign infantile seizures

  a. Can be subdivided into "benign familial infantile seizures" and "benign nonfamilial infantile seizures"

  b. Clinical presentation

    1) Partial seizures in first 1 to 2 years after birth

    2) Often occur in clusters × 1 to 3 days, <10/day

    3) Seizures last a maximum of a few minutes

    4) No postictal stupor or status

    5) Normal psychomotor development

  c. Idiopathic

    1) Benign epilepsies typically are idiopathic (e.g., benign

myoclonic epilepsy of infancy), but idiopathic epilepsies are not always benign (e.g., severe myoclonic epilepsy of infancy below)

  d. Usually autosomal dominant inheritance (when familial)

    1) Genetic homogeneity

    2) Associated with familial choreoathetosis during infancy or childhood

  e. EEG

    1) Focal epileptiform discharges

    2) May secondarily generalize

  f. Treatment: responds well to anticonvulsants

6. Severe myoclonic epilepsy in infancy

  a. Also called "Dravet syndrome"

  b. Clinical presentation

    1) Begins within 1 year after birth

    2) No previous brain abnormality except occasionally diffuse atrophy

    3) Myoclonic seizures (begin mild, worsen over time)

    4) Partial seizures develop later

    5) Often, the first seizure occurs with fever, can have prolonged febrile seizures (i.e., can evolve from febrile seizures)

    6) One-fourth of the infants have a family history of seizures

    7) Developmental delay with psychomotor regression due to severe, progressive neurologic deterioration that may be secondary to recurrent seizures

  c. Idiopathic, generalized or focal

  d. EEG

    1) General, focal, and multifocal abnormalities

    2) May be normal interictally (early in disease course)

    3) Photosensitivity is common

  e. Treatment

    1) Seizures are often medically refractory

    2) Valproate and benzodiazepines may be tried

D. Children

1. Benign childhood epilepsy with centrotemporal spikes

  a. Also called "benign rolandic epilepsy of childhood"

  b. Common: accounts for one-fourth of childhood seizures

  c. Clinical presentation

Aicardi's syndrome is the X-linked triad of infantile spasms, agenesis of corpus callosum, and retinal malformations

---

Benign epilepsy syndromes are generally idiopathic

But not all idiopathic epilepsies are benign, e.g., idiopathic Dravet syndrome (severe myoclonic epilepsy in infancy) causes progressive brain damage

1) Onset in childhood, age 4 to 12 years
2) Resolves by middle teens
3) Motor, sensory simple seizures: tonic-clonic movements of face or hand, paresthesias of face or hand, drooling, tingling in mouth, speech arrest
4) Can have secondary generalization, usually nocturnal
5) Seizures increase with sleep: 70% of patients have seizures only during sleep (15% awake only, 15% awake and sleep)
6) Normal development and neurologic examination
d. Idiopathic, focal
e. EEG
1) Centrotemporal spikes: between central and mid temporal leads (Fig. 12-1)
2) Normal background
f. Autosomal dominant inheritance, variable penetrance: although half of the close relatives of the patient may demonstrate the EEG abnormality during childhood, only 12% of them have clinical seizures
g. Treatment
1) Easily controlled with anticonvulsants

2) Often not necessary to treat (physicians often wait until the second seizure)
3) Treatment can be stopped after adolescence (only 10% of patients continue to have seizures 5 years after onset)
2. Early-onset benign childhood occipital epilepsy

Benign childhood epilepsy with centrotemporal spikes is an example of focal idiopathic epilepsy

---

Early-onset benign childhood occipital epilepsy involves *infrequent* seizures (autonomic, hemiconvulsive, and generalized)

Late-onset childhood occipital epilepsy is characterized by *frequent* visual seizures

---

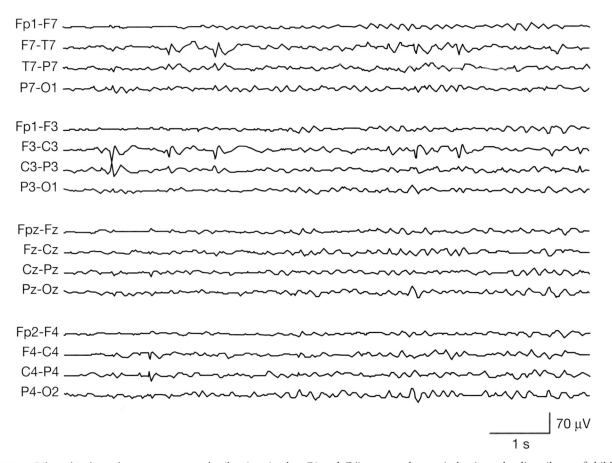

Fig. 12-1. Bilateral independent centrotemporal spikes (maximal at C3 and C4) commonly seen in benign rolandic epilepsy of childhood.

a. Also called "Panayiotopoulos syndrome," "epilepsy associated with ictal vomiting," "childhood epilepsy with occipital paroxysms"
b. Clinical presentation
   1) Most common in children 3 to 6 years old
   2) Autonomic seizures and status epilepticus: commonly, ictal vomiting, eye deviation; often progress to partial clonic or generalized tonic-clonic seizures (often nocturnal)
   3) Visual seizures: elementary or complex visual hallucinations, amaurosis, illusions (such as metamorphopsia), which are often experienced during wakefulness
   4) Infrequent seizures: most patients, 1 to 3 seizures total
   5) Autonomic status epilepticus in almost half of the seizures
c. Overlap with benign childhood epilepsy with centrotemporal spikes (also an idiopathic, benign partial epilepsy)
   1) Excellent response to anticonvulsants
   2) Variable localization of seizures: frequently extra-occipital, the clinical presentation defines the syndrome rather than occipital spikes
d. EEG
   1) Interictal EEG: frequent or nearly continuous bursts or trains of high-voltage rhythmic occipital spikes and spike-wave complexes at a frequency of 1 to 3 Hz, localized to unilateral or bilateral occipital regions, with normal background activity, increases during non-REM sleep, and disappears with eye opening
   2) Ictal EEG: low-voltage fast activity (unilateral or bilateral)
e. Treatment
   1) Not needed if only one seizure or a few brief seizures
   2) Carbamazepine is usually the first-line treatment
3. Late-onset childhood occipital epilepsy (Gastaut type)
   a. Clinical presentation
      1) Children 4 to 8 years old
      2) Visual seizures
         a) Hallucinations, blindness: weekly to several per day
         b) May generalize (rarely)
         c) Often followed by migraine headache
         d) Often induced by photic stimulation
      3) The children commonly have a family history of benign childhood epilepsy with centrotemporal spikes
      4) Both late-onset childhood occipital epilepsy and benign childhood epilepsy with centrotemporal spikes may be benign childhood seizure-susceptibility syndromes with overlapping causes
   b. Idiopathic, benign partial epilepsy
   c. EEG: same as in early-onset benign childhood occipital epilepsy

d. Treatment is recommended because seizures are frequent
4. Epilepsy with myoclonic absences
   a. Rare, with unknown cause
   b. Clinical presentation
      1) Children, average age at onset is 7 years
      2) One-half of the children have developmental delay at time of onset
      3) Prolonged (10-60 seconds) absence seizures are accompanied by bilateral, severe limb myoclonus (may progress to tonic activity)
         a) Myoclonus is rhythmic, corresponds to the spikes of the 3-Hz spike-and-wave EEG pattern
         b) Unlike other absence syndromes, no eye twitching
      4) Most children develop other seizure types
         a) Generalized tonic-clonic seizures
         b) Typical absence seizures
         c) Falls
   c. Significance
      1) Mental impairment is more common than in other childhood absence syndromes
      2) Mental deterioration is thought to be due to seizures
      3) One-half of the patients continue to have seizures as adults
   d. High-dose ethosuximide and valproate usually control the seizures
   e. EEG
      1) Ictal: 3-Hz spike-and-wave pattern
      2) Interictal: intermittent bursts of generalized spike-and-waves on a normal background
5. Myoclonic-astatic epilepsy of childhood
   a. Clinical presentation
      1) The first seizure (often a generalized tonic-clonic seizure) usually occurs in a developmentally normal child 2 to 5 years old
      2) Repeated, sometimes prolonged generalized tonic-clonic seizures
      3) After months of repeated generalized tonic-clonic seizures, other seizure types (myoclonic, absence, and drop-attacks) appear
         a) Drop attacks are myoclonic or atonic seizures
         b) Tonic seizures are uncommon (in contrast to

Epilepsy with myoclonic absences is characterized by long absence seizures with bilateral limb myoclonus

However, unlike atypical absence seizures, EEG shows 3-Hz spike-and-wave activity

Lennox-Gastaut syndrome, in which tonic seizures are a prominent seizure type)
   b. Idiopathic, likely polygenic
   c. EEG: 2 to 3–Hz spike waves (often faster than in Lennox-Gastaut syndrome)
   d. Treatment: valproate, ethosuximide, benzodiazepine, lamotrigine
   e. Some authorities suspect this is a mild or early form of Lennox-Gastaut syndrome

6. Lennox-Gastaut syndrome
   a. Clinical triad: mental retardation, characteristic slow spike-and-wave (2 Hz) EEG, multiple seizure types
   b. Clinical presentation
     1) Children, age at onset is 2 to 8 years
     2) Boys affected more often than girls
     3) The first seizure type is usually drop attacks
     4) Many patients have severe mental retardation preceding onset of seizures
     5) Later, multiple seizure types evolve, often in association with status epilepticus, progressive psychomotor deterioration
       a) Tonic seizures (last a few seconds)
         i) Head/neck flexion or
         ii) Neck extension/arm abduction or
         iii) Generalized tonic stiffening → sudden fall
       b) Atypical absence seizure
         i) Gradual onset and offset (unlike typical absence)
         ii) Longer duration than a typical absence seizure
         iii) May be brief postictal decrease in alertness (unlike typical absence seizure)
       c) Atonic seizure: neck only or whole body
       d) Generalized tonic-clonic seizure
       e) Less common seizure types: partial tonic-clonic, myoclonic
       f) Consider myoclonic-astatic epilepsy if prominent myoclonic seizures
   c. Cryptogenic or symptomatic
   d. Prognosis is usually poor, especially if symptomatic
   e. Progressive deterioration is thought to be related to frequent subclinical epileptic discharges (epileptic encephalopathy)
   f. EEG
     1) Interictal "slow spike-and-wave": double meaning of name (Table 12-5)
       a) Spikes are slow (150 ms, longer than a true spike, which should be <70 ms)
       b) Spike-and-wave rate is also slow (1.5-2.5 Hz) compared with typical absence seizures (3 Hz)
     2) Ictal
       a) Tonic seizure: rhythmic fast activity followed by

Table 12-5. **Syndromes Associated With Characteristic EEG Patterns**

Syndrome	EEG pattern
Childhood and juvenile absence seizures	3-Hz spike-and-wave
Lennox-Gastaut syndrome	Slow spike-and-wave
Generalized seizures	Atypical spike-and-wave Polyspike-and-wave Paroxysmal fast activity Fast repetitive spikes
Infantile spasms, West's syndrome	Hypsarrhythmia

       high-amplitude slow activity
       b) Absence seizure: slow spike-and-wave discharge
   g. Treatment
     1) Valproate: all seizure types
     2) Lamotrigine, felbamate: especially for drop attacks
     3) Carbamazepine and phenytoin: may help generalized tonic-clonic seizures but may worsen atypical absence seizures

7. Landau-Kleffner syndrome
   a. Clinical presentation
     1) Acquired aphasia (word deafness): the main feature of the syndrome
     2) Seizures, may be multiple types: 20% of patients do not have seizures
       a) Generalized tonic-clonic seizures
       b) Partial seizures

The "slow spike-and-wave" pattern characterizes Lennox-Gastaut syndrome, occurring during atypical absence seizures and interictally

"Slow" refers to both the prolonged duration of "spikes" (150 ms) and the slow rate of spike-and-wave activity (1.5-2.5 Hz)

Carbamazepine and phenytoin can worsen atypical absence seizures

---

Landau-Kleffner syndrome refers to acquired epileptic aphasia in children

c) Myoclonic seizures
3) Children, age at onset: 3 to 8 years old
b. Symptomatic, nonspecific (variety of lesions)
c. Magnetic resonance imaging (MRI): usually normal; functional imaging shows temporal abnormalities
d. EEG: variable, multifocal spikes, most commonly temporal
e. Outcome is variable
1) Seizures usually are controlled with medication, seizure disorder resolves with time
2) Persistent language problems in about half the children
f. Treatment
1) Antiepileptic drugs (valproate and lamotrigine) may help decrease seizure frequency and improve cognitive function
2) Corticosteroids have been tried with some success in small series, but data are inadequate
8. Epilepsy with continuous spike-and-wave pattern during slow wave sleep, also referred to as "electrical status epilepticus during sleep"
a. Clinical presentation
1) First seizure occurs in childhood (peak age at onset: 5 years)
2) Multiple seizure types, partial or generalized
3) Seizures occur infrequently, often during sleep
4) Then, seizures accelerate and EEG changes to characteristic pattern (electrical status during slow wave sleep)
5) Psychomotor deterioration (language and motor): thought to be due to seizures
6) Seizures usually resolve by teen years but various degrees of psychomotor abnormalities remain
b. EEG
1) Diffuse or focal interictal discharges (awake)
2) Continuous spike-and-wave pattern during NREM sleep
c. Landau-Kleffner syndrome could be a form of this syndrome (affecting language area) because the two syndromes often have a similar sleep EEG
d. Treatment: same as for Landau-Kleffner syndrome
9. Childhood absence epilepsy
a. Clinical presentation
1) Children (girls, 70%), peak age at onset: 6 years
2) Neurologically and developmentally normal
3) Multiple daily spells usually lasting a few seconds
a) Seizures begin and end abruptly
b) They completely interrupt activity
c) Often, a blank stare
d) May have automatisms
e) Spells often can be provoked, especially hypoglycemia and hyperventilation (which are some-

times used clinically to provoke a spell)
4) Other seizure types
a) About one-third of the children have generalized tonic-clonic seizures later in adolescence (this does not change the diagnosis), but generalized tonic-clonic seizures or myoclonic seizures during treatment do not fit the syndrome definition of childhood absence seizures and carry a worse prognosis
b) Mild ictal jerks of lids, eyes, or eyebrows may occur during the first few seconds of a spell, but any more prominent myoclonus such as perioral myoclonus suggests another syndrome, often with a worse prognosis (e.g., epilepsy with myoclonic absence)
b. Idiopathic
1) Unknown genetic cause, but strong genetic predisposition: family may have history of absence or generalized tonic-clonic seizures
2) Atypical absence seizures suggest symptomatic epilepsies such as Lennox-Gastaut syndrome
3) Typical absence seizures can occur in other types of idiopathic and cryptogenic generalized epilepsy syndromes (e.g., juvenile absence seizures)
4) 80% have remission by adulthood
c. EEG
1) 3-Hz generalized spike-and-wave pattern: may begin faster (up to 4 Hz) and slow at the end to 2.5 Hz
2) Symmetrical, bilateral, synchronous
3) May be frontal predominant
4) Normal background activity
5) Activated by hyperventilation and hypoglycemia (but photic stimulation induces spike-and-wave pattern in only 10%-30% of patients)
6) Discharge generator: thalamus
7) Low-threshold (T-type) calcium channels drive the discharges

---

Hypoglycemia and hyperventilation can often provoke absence seizures

---

Generalized tonic-clonic seizures can occur in childhood absence epilepsy, but this occurs later in adolescence

Early tonic-clonic seizures suggest another diagnosis

a) Ethosuximide acts via T-type calcium channel inhibition

b) γ-Aminobutyric acid (GABA)$_B$ receptors promote T-type calcium channels

c) Thus, GABAergic drugs (vigabatrin, tiagabine) promote absence seizures

8) Differentiating childhood absence epilepsy from

a) Juvenile absence epilepsy

i) Age at onset of childhood absence epilepsy is usually <10 years old and for onset of juvenile absence, 10 to 16 years, but some overlap

ii) More often generalized tonic-clonic seizures in juvenile absence epilepsy, although common also in childhood absence epilepsy

iii) Sometimes myoclonic jerks occur in juvenile absence epilepsy

iv) EEG: 3-Hz spike-and-wave activity, but it may have more polyspikes in juvenile absence epilepsy

v) Juvenile form: somewhat worse prognosis, the child is less likely to outgrow the disease

b) Juvenile myoclonic epilepsy

i) Some of the children have absence seizures, but this is a very different syndrome clinically

ii) Myoclonic jerks on awakening

iii) No 3-Hz spike-and-wave pattern

d. Prognosis

1) More than 90% of the children outgrow the seizures

2) About one-third have generalized tonic-clonic seizures later

e. Treatment

1) First-line treatment: ethosuximide, valproate, lamotrigine

a) Treatment with ethosuximide only prevents absence seizures, it does not prevent generalized tonic-clonic seizures in children with childhood absence epilepsy

b) Valproate and lamotrigine are effective for both generalized tonic-clonic seizures and absence seizures and are considered the drugs of choice in this situation

2) If monotherapy fails, combination therapy with valproate and ethosuximide

3) Anticonvulsant therapy should be stopped if the EEG is normal and the child has not had seizures for 1 to 2 years

10. Progressive myoclonic epilepsies (Table 12-6)

a. Encompasses several progressive disorders, most are lysosomal and mitochondrial disorders

b. Clinical presentation

Absence seizures are driven by T-type calcium channels of the thalamus, which are blocked by ethosuximide and promoted by GABAergic drugs

Therefore, GABAergic anticonvulsants may promote absence seizures

---

Ethosuximide is effective only for absence seizures

---

1) Progressive cognitive deterioration

2) Myoclonus (nonepileptic)

3) Seizures: tonic-clonic, tonic, or myoclonic

4) With or without ataxia, movement disorders

c. Treatment of seizures

1) First-line treatment: valproate

2) Clonazepam and lamotrigine are also used

11. Generalized epilepsy with febrile seizures plus (GEFS+)

a. Clinical presentation

1) Febrile seizures

2) "Plus": this indicates that GEFS+ occurs *after* age 6 years (unlike typical febrile seizures) or is associated with *afebrile* generalized tonic-clonic seizures (unlike typical febrile seizures)

3) One-third of patients have other seizure types: absence, myoclonic, atonic, partial seizures

b. Autosomal dominant channelopathy (Table 12-4)

1) Sodium channel (SCN) or GABA$_A$ receptor: increased inward sodium current or decreased GABA-mediated inhibition both lead to neuronal hyper-excitability

a) SCN1B (chromosome 19)

b) SCN1A (chromosome 2)

c) SCN2A

d) GABA$_A$ receptor

Table 12-6.   Progressive Myoclonic Epilepsies

Lafora body disease

Unverricht-Lundborg syndrome (initally described as "Baltic myoclonus")

Neuronal ceroid lipofuscinosis

Myoclonic epilepsy with ragged-red fibers

Sialidoses

2) Most febrile seizures, unlike GEFS+, show complex inheritance

c. EEG
1) Generalized spike-and-wave or polyspike-and-wave pattern

12. Rasmussen's encephalitis
a. Syndrome of chronic encephalitis with epilepsy in children
b. Intractable, progressive focal seizures; progressive hemiparesis; and cognitive deterioration
c. Radiographic characteristics of slowly progressive cortical atrophy (unilateral more common than bilateral)
d. Antibodies to GLUR3 (glutamate receptor-3) have been implicated in pathogenesis of this disorder

E. Juveniles and Adults

1. Idiopathic generalized epilepsies
a. General category in ILAE classification scheme encompassing
1) Juvenile absence epilepsy
2) Juvenile myoclonic epilepsy
3) Epilepsy with generalized tonic-clonic seizures only

2. Juvenile absence epilepsy
a. Clinical presentation
1) Onset at age 10 to 17 years
2) Developmentally normal children
3) Boys and girls affected equally
4) Initially, infrequent absence seizures: usually not daily (unlike childhood absence epilepsy)
5) Later, tonic-clonic seizures in 75% of patients upon awakening: more common than in childhood absence epilepsy
b. Idiopathic
1) Genetic mechanism is not known
2) One-third of patients have a family history that may include childhood absence epilepsy, juvenile absence epilepsy, juvenile myoclonic epilepsy, or epilepsy with grand mal seizures on awakening
c. EEG
1) Same as childhood absence epilepsy, except spike-and-wave pattern may be slightly faster (3.5-4.5 Hz) and polyspikes are more frequent
d. Prognosis

Juvenile absence epilepsy is characterized by less frequent absence seizures than childhood absence epilepsy and more frequent (75%) development later of tonic-clonic seizures

---

1) Good: most patients are seizure-free with valproate (controls both absence and generalized seizures), ethosuximide, lamotrigine
2) Patients are less likely to outgrow seizures than those with childhood absence epilepsy
a) Patients typically require lifelong anticonvulsant therapy, and to prevent seizures as adults, patients need to avoid sleep deprivation and alcohol (as with juvenile myoclonic epilepsy)
b) Occurrence of myoclonic seizures and generalized tonic-clonic seizures make seizure remission less likely (overlaps with juvenile myoclonic epilepsy)

3. Juvenile myoclonic epilepsy
a. Clinical presentation
1) Age at onset is 8 to 24 years (peak, in teens)
2) Developmentally normal
3) Boys and girls affected equally
4) Myoclonic seizures: the most frequent seizure type
a) Usually predominantly on awakening (early morning or nap)
b) Large-amplitude, bilateral, simultaneous
i) Involves both arms or both legs (can cause falls)
ii) Unlike nonepileptic myoclonus, it is usually focal
c) May be repetitive
d) No loss of awareness
e) Often, reflex seizures, including perioral reflex myoclonia (triggered by reading, talking)
5) Most patients have less frequent generalized tonic-clonic seizures
a) Also, usually occur on awakening
b) Often lead to diagnosis in patients with undiagnosed history of myoclonus on awakening
6) Some patients have typical absence seizures
7) Seizures are provoked by sleep deprivation, alcohol, photic stimulation
b. Idiopathic
1) One-half of patients have a family history of seizures
2) None are symptomatic (MRI is always normal)
3) No consistent genetic cause has been identified

Like juvenile myoclonic epilepsy, juvenile absence epilepsy usually requires lifelong anticonvulsant therapy and avoidance of triggers (sleep deprivation, alcohol)

Childhood absence epilepsy, in contrast, is usually outgrown

4) Overlap in the same family with other generalized epilepsy syndromes: juvenile absence epilepsy, childhood absence epilepsy, and epilepsy with grand mal seizures on awakening

c. EEG
 1) Interictal
   a) Three-fourths of patients have generalized 4 to 6–Hz polyspike-and-wave discharges
   b) If absence seizures, EEG also has 3-Hz spike-and-wave pattern
   c) Often photosensitivity
 2) Ictal: trains of spikes

d. Treatment
 1) First-line: valproate (three-fourths of patients are seizure-free), it controls all seizure types
 2) Second-line: lamotrigine, levetiracetam, topiramate, and zonisamide
 3) Avoid carbamazepine and phenytoin, which are useful in focal seizures but may worsen some primary generalized seizures (myoclonic and absence seizures)

e. Prognosis: it is a lifelong seizure disorder typically requiring lifelong treatment and avoidance of triggers

4. Epilepsy with grand mal seizures on awakening
 a. Clinical presentation
   1) Onset is in second decade
   2) Overlaps clinically with juvenile myoclonic epilepsy and juvenile absence epilepsy
   3) Primary seizure type is generalized tonic-clonic, usually on awakening
   4) Myoclonic or absence seizures may occur but are not predominant
 b. Idiopathic/familial
 c. EEG, treatment, and prognosis: similar to those of juvenile myoclonic epilepsy

5. Idiopathic photosensitive occipital lobe epilepsy
 a. Clinical presentation
   1) Reflex epilepsy, begins about the time of puberty
   2) Occipital lobe seizures provoked by visual stimuli, usually television or video games
   3) Positive visual symptoms (occipital seizures)
     a) The likely origin is the calcarine cortex
     b) Often, colorful rings or spots

   c) May be followed by postictal negative visual symptoms
   d) Head turns may occur toward the visual phenomena
 4) Often spreads to cause autonomic symptoms
   a) Epigastric discomfort, vomiting
   b) Can mimic migraine
 5) Occasional secondarily generalized seizures
b. Idiopathic
c. EEG
 1) Normal background
 2) Interictal epileptiform activity: unilateral or bilateral occipital ± generalized spike-and-wave, enhanced with eye closure
 3) Photoparoxysmal response (epileptiform abnormalities with strobe light) is common
d. Management
 1) Avoid triggers
 2) First-line treatment: often valproate (as for other primary generalized epilepsies)

6. Other types of reflex seizures
 a. Generalized (tonic-clonic and absence) seizures can be triggered by a flash or visual pattern
   1) The most common reflex epilepsy
   2) Multiple idiopathic or symptomatic generalized epilepsy syndromes can have visually evoked seizures, these are not specific to one syndrome
 b. Primary reading epilepsy: seizures occur only when patient is reading
 c. Startle epilepsy
   1) Seizures with unexpected sensory stimuli
   2) Usually frequent seizures (tonic or clonic)
   3) Often associated with developmental delay

7. Temporal lobe epilepsies
 a. Traditional view: temporal lobe epilepsy is usually an acquired, symptomatic epilepsy
   1) Most commonly associated with mesial temporal sclerosis
   2) One-third of patients have a history of febrile seizures
   3) Patients often have a familial predisposition to epilepsy, but it is usually polygenic and/or multifactorial
 b. Familial forms (monogenic) of temporal lobe epilepsy also occur
   1) Onset is usually in teens or adults
   2) Typically less resistant to treatment
   3) A specific gene has been identified: autosomal

Valproate is usually effective in juvenile myoclonic epilepsy

Carbamazepine and phenytoin can worsen some types of primary generalized seizures (myoclonic, absence)

Focal occipital seizures of the calcarine cortex usually consist of colorful rings or spots, sometimes with head turns toward the visual phenomena

Autosomal dominant partial epilepsy with auditory features is an example of a monogenic temporal lobe epilepsy, caused by a mutation of the *LGI1* (leucine-rich, glioma-inactivated 1) gene

Head turns may be *ipsilateral* to seizure onset (early non-forced head turn) or *contralateral* to seizure onset (forced head turn)

dominant partial epilepsy with auditory features (Table 12-4)
   a) *LGI1* mutation (leucine-rich, glioma-inactivated 1 gene) in some families
   b) Clinical presentation: auditory auras precede complex partial and secondarily generalized seizures
8. Autosomal dominant nocturnal frontal lobe epilepsy
   a. Mutations in *CHRNA4* gene on chromosome 20q and *CHRNB2* gene on chromosome 1p, encoding proteins in M2 transmembrane segment of nicotinic acetylcholine receptors: mutations believed to cause increased acetylcholine sensitivity and channel opening ("gain-of-function" mutations)
   b. Most patients have onset of seizures in first two decades (anytime between infancy to adulthood; mean age, 10 years)
   c. Clusters of brief, stereotypic, nocturnal seizures, which may consist of hyperkinetic bizarre movements with clonic, tonic, or dystonic features, and sometimes, secondary generalization: clinical features similar to non-familial frontal lobe epilepsy
   d. Seizures typically occur in non-REM sleep
   e. Few patients also experience stereotypic seizures during daytime
   f. Not associated with cognitive deficits
   g. Decreased frequency and duration of seizures with time

III. Seizure Semiology

A. Head Turn (Fig. 12-2)
1. Early nonforced head turn: ipsilateral temporal lobe
   a. Voluntary-like, often with dystonic posturing of the contralateral extremity
   b. May be due to neglect and/or weakness contralateral to the seizure
2. Forced head turn: contralateral hemisphere (except if it occurs *after* a generalized seizure)
   a. Prominent contraction of neck muscles, forcing the chin to point toward the shoulder
   b. Tends to occur early in frontal lobe seizures, explosive onset with other motor seizure activity
   c. Tends to occur later in temporal lobe seizures, as the

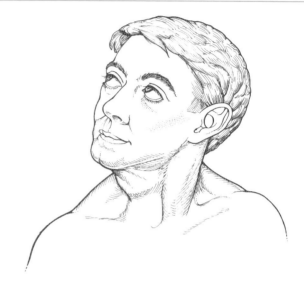

Fig. 12-2. A forced head turn and eye deviation.

   seizure secondarily generalizes ("late forced head turn")
   d. If a forced head turn occurs after a secondarily generalized tonic-clonic seizure, it is usually ipsilateral to seizure onset ("late ipsiversion"), probably because of the spread of seizure activity to the hemisphere contralateral to seizure onset

B. Eye Deviation
1. Accompanies forced head turns (same direction and upward)
2. Eye deviation in isolation at seizure onset suggests seizure activity in the occipital lobe, contralateral to the direction of gaze

C. Focal Clonic
1. Frontal and perirolandic area, contralateral hemisphere
2. Can also occur in temporal lobe complex partial seizures—because of spread of seizure to the surrounding extratemporal cortex

D. Focal Tonic
1. Extended limb
2. Contralateral hemisphere

E. Figure 4 Sign (Fig. 12-3)
1. A tonic limb posture with one arm extended and the

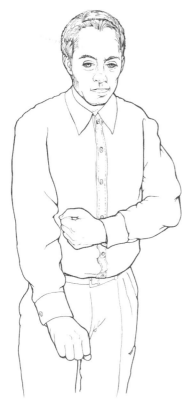

Fig. 12-3. A "figure 4."

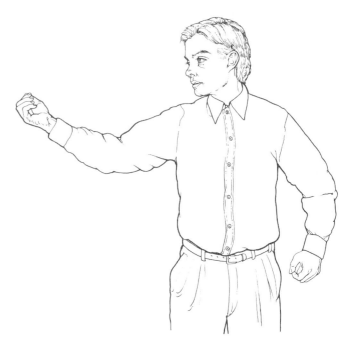

Fig. 12-4. Fencing posture.

Seizures localize to the hemisphere contralateral to the
extended arm in both the figure 4 sign and fencing posture

other flexed at the elbow (forming a "figure 4")
2. The seizure is lateralized to the hemisphere contralateral
   to the extended arm (as with a focal tonic seizure)
3. Figure 4 sign usually occurs as the seizure generalizes
4. A forced head turn may occur (toward the extended arm)

F. Focal Dystonic
1. Sustained contorted posturing of a limb
2. Contralateral hemisphere, possibly due to spread of the
   seizure to the basal ganglia

G. Fencing Posture (Fig. 12-4)
1. Seizures localize to hemisphere contralateral to the
   extended arm, frontal lobe more than temporal lobe
   (supplementary motor area)
2. Lateral abduction and external rotation of the arm at
   the shoulder ± forced head turn to the side of abducted arm
3. Elbow may also flex so the hand is raised to the face

H. Ictal Paresis and Unilateral Immobile Limb
1. Seizures lateralize to contralateral hemisphere

I. Todd's Paralysis
1. Seizures lateralize to contralateral hemisphere
2. Extratemporal lobe > temporal lobe

J. Unilateral Blinking
1. Seizures lateralize to ipsilateral hemisphere
2. Appears like winks (not forceful like a clonic facial seizure)

K. Unilateral Limb Automatism
1. Seizures lateralize to ipsilateral hemisphere
2. Simple or complex automatic behavior
   a. Examples include using a pen, pulling up blanket
   b. The contralateral side does not take part, possibly
      because of neglect

L. Postictal Nose Rubbing
1. Seizures lateralize to hemisphere ipsilateral to hand used
2. Temporal lobe more than frontal lobe

M. Postictal Cough
1. Seizures localize to temporal lobe

N. Bipedal Automatism
1. Frontal lobe more than temporal lobe

2. Bicycling or kicking

O. Hypermotor

1. Violent, restless thrashing of extremities ("hypermotor seizures") suggestive of frontal lobe seizures (supplementary motor area)
2. In contrast, head-and-neck thrashing suggests nonepileptic behavioral event ("pseudoseizure")

P. Gelastic (laughter)

1. Seizures localize to the hypothalamus or mesial temporal lobe

Q. Ictal Spitting

1. Seizures localize to the right temporal lobe

R. Ictal Vomiting or Retching

1. Seizures localize to the right temporal lobe

S. Loud Vocalization

1. Frontal lobe more than temporal lobe
2. Often, nonspeech vocalization (grunting, screaming, moaning) with frontal lobe seizures

T. Speech Arrest

1. Temporal lobe, poorly lateralizing to language-dominant hemisphere
2. Speech preservation during a temporal lobe seizure suggests localization in the nondominant hemisphere, but it can also occur with a dominant hemisphere seizure sparing speech areas—so speech preservation can be misleading

U. Postictal Aphasia

1. Seizures lateralize to the dominant hemisphere

V. Ictal Drooling

1. Seizures lateralize to the nondominant hemisphere

W. Postictal Confusion

1. Is usually more prominent, and persists longer after temporal lobe seizures
2. Is not present or is brief and less prominent after frontal lobe seizures

X. Visual Symptoms

1. Elementary: occipital lobe
   a. Positive visual symptoms > negative ones but either is possible
      1) Circles, spots, shapes, flashes, hemianopsia, scotoma

---

> Unilateral limb automatisms, including nose rubbing, correspond to a seizure focus ipsilateral to the limb used

> Postictal confusion is most prominent after temporal lobe seizures and may be absent after frontal lobe seizures

      2) Often in color
   b. Pattern and progression may be stereotyped for an individual patient
   c. Brief (seconds), with movement and changing shape and size
   d. There may be a postictal headache, can be misdiagnosed as migraine
      1) Migraine aura has more colorful, rounded forms or shapes rather than linear or zigzag lines
      2) Migraine aura is usually briefer (seconds)
2. Complex visual hallucinations or illusions: occipito-temporoparietal junction of nondominant parietal lobe
   a. Relatively rare
   b. Are usually complex and colorful, are often previously experienced images
   c. Can include micropsia (images appear smaller), metamorphopsia (objects appear distorted)

IV. ANTICONVULSANT THERAPY

A. Phenytoin

1. Seizure types
   a. Partial or generalized tonic-clonic seizures (primary or secondary)
   b. Rarely, phenytoin can *worsen* other types of generalized seizures (myoclonic, absence)
2. Mechanism of action: inhibits sodium channels, especially at high rates of firing
3. Metabolism

> Elementary visual symptoms suggest occipital lobe localization, whereas complex visual hallucinations or illusions localize to the nondominant parietal lobe or occipito-temporoparietal junction

> Phenytoin and carbamazepine act by inhibiting sodium channels, especially at high rates of firing

a. Liver (minimal renal excretion)
b. Monitor for toxicity, especially if liver disease
c. May need to follow free plasma concentrations in renal disease because of less protein binding (total may underestimate free level)
d. Nonlinear kinetics: saturable, and concentration-dependent, nonlinear (zero-order) elimination kinetics
   1) As plasma concentration of the drug increases, the elimination mechanism is progressively saturated in a nonlinear fashion, resulting in a disproportionate and logarithmic increase in plasma drug concentrations
   2) Thus, small additional doses may cause a large increment in plasma concentrations when the elimination mechanism is saturated
4. Side effects
   a. Idiosyncratic: dyscrasias, morbilliform rash, Stevens-Johnson syndrome, hepatitis
   b. Cosmetic
      1) Gingival hyperplasia: lessened by good oral hygiene
      2) Probably causes acne, coarse features, and hirsutism
   c. Toxic to tissues (because it is highly alkaline)
      1) Muscle breakdown if phenytoin is injected intramuscularly (therefore, only fosphenytoin is given intramuscularly)
      2) Purple glove syndrome
         a) Severe tissue injury from constriction of blood vessels, can lead to amputation or sepsis
         b) This occurs with intravenous administration, occurs much less frequently with fosphenytoin
   d. Neurotoxicity: because of narrow therapeutic window, blood levels are useful for monitoring for neurotoxicity (unlike newer anticonvulsants) ("narrow therapeutic window" refers to nonlinear, saturable, and concentration-dependent elimination kinetics of phenytoin, discussed above)
      1) Dose-dependent, typically minimal at therapeutic levels
      2) Nystagmus → (at higher blood concentrations) ataxia, dysarthria, diplopia, nausea, dizziness → drowsiness, cognitive difficulties → coma
      3) At high levels, may rarely increase seizure frequency
      4) Movement disorders
   e. Vitamin-related
      1) Folate deficiency/anemia
      2) Increased vitamin D metabolism: causes premature osteoporosis
   f. Chronic
      1) Cerebellar atrophy
      2) Mild peripheral neuropathy
   g. Acute (with intravenous formulation)
      1) Phlebitis, pain, burning sensation (with too rapid infusion)
         a) This occurs because undiluted administration is required (injectable phenytoin is insoluble in standard intravenous fluids)
         b) In comparison, fosphenytoin is freely soluble in all standard intravenous fluids and thus asssociated with fewer local adverse effects such as irritation and superficial phlebitis and systemic adverse effects such as hypotension
      2) Hypotension, conduction abnormalities (need to monitor blood pressure during infusion), especially if cardiac disease
      3) Hypotension and conduction abnormalities are less severe with fosphenytoin
5. Drug interactions
   a. Variable effect in plasma concentration of warfarin
   b. Decreases plasma concentration of
      1) Most anticonvulsants (except for gabapentin and levetiracetam): carbamazepine, oxcarbazepine, topiramate, tiagabine, lamotrigine, zonisamide, valproate, felbamate
      2) Other: benzodiazepines, haloperidol, tricyclic antidepressants, oral contraceptives, digoxin, cyclosporine
   c. The following increase the plasma concentration of phenytoin: cimetidine, carbamazepine, felbamate, fluconazole, fluoxetine, valproate
   d. The following lower the concentration of phenytoin: valproate (decreases total, but increases free levels) and rifampin
6. Monitor: liver function tests
7. Calculating the loading dose if levels are subtherapeutic (estimate only)
   a. If phenytoin level is <10 μg/mL, first-order kinetics
   b. Approaches zero-order kinetics above 10 μg/mL, so small dose increments produce large increases in blood levels
   c. For phenytoin level <10 μg/mL, additional dose to achieve a desired concentration can be estimated as follows:
      1) Additional oral dose (mg/kg) = [volume of distribution (0.7) × desired increment (μg/mL) (desired concentration − measured concentration)]/0.92
      2) Additional intravenous dose (mg/kg) = 0.7 × (desired concentration − measured concentration)
      3) Example: if the total phenytoin concentration is 5 μg/mL and the concentration desired is 10 μg/mL,

the additional intravenous dose will be

$$0.7 \times (10\ \mu g/mL - 5\ \mu g/mL) = 3.5\ mg/kg$$

B. Fosphenytoin
1. Intravenous prodrug of phenytoin
   a. Useful for intravenous load in status epilepticus or if patient is unable to take medication orally
   b. Converted to phenytoin by erythrocytes (using alkaline phosphatase)
   c. Fosphenytoin is a phosphate ester that is water soluble and less alkaline than phenytoin
   d. In contrast, phenytoin is administered in a highly alkaline mixture of propylene glycol (antifreeze) and ethanol and can precipitate if administered too rapidly
      1) Thus, fosphenytoin is less toxic to tissue, and no purple glove syndrome develops
      2) Fosphenytoin can be administered more rapidly than phenytoin and with less hypotension
         a) Maximal fosphenytoin dose: 150 mg of phenytoin equivalents per minute
         b) Maximal phenytoin dose: 50 mg per minute
      3) Because it takes 8 to 15 minutes for fosphenytoin to convert to phenytoin, the more rapid administration of fosphenytoin is offset by the time for conversion
      4) Both drugs take the same time to achieve equivalent phenytoin concentration
   e. Fosphenytoin also can be administered intramuscularly for a loading dose in patient who cannot take medication orally
   f. Otherwise, the side effects are identical to those of phenytoin

---

Liver enzyme-inducing anticonvulsants, like phenytoin, can reduce the effectiveness of low-dose oral contraceptives

Valproate, a liver enzyme inhibitor, also can reduce the effectiveness of low-dose oral contraceptives

---

Fosphenytoin is less toxic to tissue than phenytoin because fosphenytoin is water soluble

Phenytoin, in contrast, is administered in a highly alkaline mixture of propylene glycol and ethanol and can precipitate if administered too rapidly

---

C. Phenobarbital
1. Seizure types
   a. Partial or generalized tonic-clonic seizures (primary or secondary)
   b. Phenobarbital is less effective than phenytoin or carbamazepine for partial seizures
2. Mechanisms of action
   a. GABA$_A$ agonist
   b. Sodium channel antagonist
   c. T-type calcium channel antagonist
   d. Glutamate antagonist
3. Metabolism
   a. Liver with renal excretion of metabolites
   b. Increased risk of toxicity if patient has kidney or liver disease
4. Side effects
   a. Cognitive (dose-dependent)
      1) Sedation, irritability, cognitive difficulties, ataxia
      2) Hyperactivity (children)
      3) Narrow therapeutic window, so plasma levels are useful in monitoring for toxicity (unlike newer anticonvulsants)
   b. Idiosyncratic: rash, aplastic anemia, agranulocytosis, thrombocytopenia, hepatitis
   c. Vitamin deficiencies
      1) Vitamin D deficiency and bone marrow density
      2) Folate, vitamin K deficiencies
   d. Cardiac and respiratory depression
5. Drug interactions
   a. Decreases the plasma concentration of
      1) Most anticonvulsants (except for gabapentin and levetiracetam): valproate, carbamazepine, oxcarbazepine, lamotrigine, topiramate, tiagabine, zonisamide
      2) Other: benzodiazepines, haloperidol, theophylline, cimetidine, warfarin, oral contraceptives
   b. The following increase the plasma concentration of phenobarbital: tricyclic antidepressants and valproate
   c. Cardiac and respiratory depression
6. Monitor: liver function tests

Liver enzyme-inducing anticonvulsants include phenytoin, phenobarbital, and carbamazepine

Oxcarbazepine has less liver enzyme-induction than carbamazepine

D. Primidone

1. Seizure types
   a. Partial or generalized tonic-clonic seizures (primary or secondary)
   b. Primidone is less effective than phenytoin or carbamazepine for partial seizures
2. Mechanisms of action
   a. Multiple: sodium channel antagonist, GABA$_A$ agonist, glutamate antagonist
   b. Primidone is antiepileptic, but so are its metabolites
      1) Metabolized to phenobarbital and phenylethylmalonamide
      2) Therefore, avoid using primidone with phenobarbital
3. Metabolism
   a. Liver with renal excretion of metabolites
   b. Increased risk of toxicity, especially if patient has kidney disease
4. Side effects
   a. Cognitive (dose-dependent)
      1) Common and prominent side effect of primidone, may improve with time
      2) Sedation, irritability, cognitive difficulties, ataxia
   b. Idiosyncratic: rash, aplastic anemia, agranulocytosis, thrombocytopenia, hepatitis, lymphadenopathy
   c. Vitamin deficiencies
      1) Vitamin D deficiency and bone marrow density
      2) Folate, vitamin K deficiencies
5. Monitor: liver function tests

E. Valproate (valproic acid and divalproex sodium)

1. Seizure types: broad spectrum
   a. Partial, generalized tonic-clonic, absence, myoclonic, and tonic seizures and infantile spasms
   b. Is often the drug of first choice for treating primary generalized epilepsy
2. Mechanisms of action
   a. Multiple: sodium channel antagonist, GABA$_A$ agonist, T-type calcium channel antagonist
   b. Note: drugs with multiple mechanisms tend to have a broad spectrum of action (compared with ethosuximide, which blocks only T-type calcium channels and has a narrow spectrum of action, i.e., only absence seizures)
3. Metabolism
   a. Liver (glucuronide) with renal excretion of metabolites
   b. Thus, valproate generally is not used if the patient has liver dysfunction
   c. Can be mixed with food for near-complete absorption
   d. Short half-life
      1) Valproic acid form must be given 3 times daily
      2) Divalproex sodium can be given twice daily

4. Side effects
   a. Cognitive: usually minimal compared with other anticonvulsants (sedation, irritability, cognitive difficulties, ataxia)
   b. Liver
      1) Encephalopathy/hyperammonemia (may occur without other evidence of liver dysfunction)
      2) Mildly increased transaminase levels are common: is dose-related and reversible
      3) Idiosyncratic fatal hepatitis (rare, unpredictable)
         a) Most common in patients younger than 2 years, decreases with age (none in adults)
         b) More common if patient receives anticonvulsant polytherapy
         c) Treated with L-carnitine
   c. Gastrointestinal effects
      1) Nausea, vomiting, gastrointestinal upset
      2) Reduced if valproate is taken with food
      3) Also reduced if the divalproex sodium form is used
   d. Chronic effects: weight gain and thinning of hair
   e. Other effects
      1) Menstrual irregularity, polycystic ovarian syndrome
      2) Tremor (action-like essential tremor)
      3) Pancreatitis: more common in children, can be fatal
      4) Thrombocytopenia, platelet dysfunction: surgical consideration
      5) Teratogenic: spina bifida
   f. Extensive drug interactions
      1) Liver enzyme inhibitor
         a) May increase the concentrations of most anticonvulsants: phenytoin, carbamazepine, phenobarbital, felbamate, lamotrigine, topiramate, tiagabine, ethosuximide
         b) May decrease the concentrations of some anticonvulsants: phenytoin (total plasma concentration), oxcarbazepine
         c) Unaffected: gabapentin and levetiracetam, which are also unaffected by other liver enzyme inducers or inhibitors

---

Valproic acid, a liver enzyme inhibitor, increases the concentrations of most anticonvulsants

---

Gabapentin and levetiracetam are not affected by liver enzyme inducers or inhibitors

---

2) Felbamate increases the valproate level

3) Liver enzyme inducers (carbamazepine, phenytoin, phenobarbital, primidone) decrease the valproate level

4) Valproate reduces the effectiveness of low-dose oral contraceptives

5) Interaction with phenytoin: valproate increases free fraction of phenytoin and decreases total concentration; central nervous system levels determined by the free fraction, so the end result is increased tendency for phenytoin toxicity

5. Monitor: liver function tests

F. Carbamazepine

1. Seizure types
   a. Partial or generalized tonic-clonic seizures (primary or secondary)
   b. Carbamazepine can rarely *worsen* other types of generalized seizures (myoclonic, absence), as phenytoin does

2. Mechanism of action
   a. Inhibits sodium channels (like phenytoin)
   b. The molecule is related to that of tricyclic antidepressants

3. Metabolism
   a. Liver, with renal excretion of metabolites
   b. Use caution if patient has kidney or liver failure

4. Side effects
   a. Generally similar to those of phenytoin, except without cosmetic side effects
      1) Like phenytoin, carbamazepine is usually minimally sedating
      2) A loading dose cannot be given, unlike phenytoin: the dose must be titrated up gradually to avoid toxicity
      3) Like phenytoin, carbamazepine has a narrow therapeutic window
      4) Plasma levels are useful for monitoring for toxicity
   b. Autoinduction
      1) The half-life decreases from *30* hours to 10 to 20 hours after the first few days to weeks of use
      2) Plasma concentrations decrease in first 1 to 2 months;

it may not be necessary to increase the maintenance dose, because the epoxide metabolite also has antiepileptic action and contributes to side effects

   c. Cognitive
      1) Dizziness, fatigue, drowsiness, diplopia, nystagmus, dizziness, headache, ataxia
      2) Often due to starting the drug too rapidly (before autoinduction): dose-dependent
   d. Idiosyncratic
      1) Rash: common (10% of patients) but severe rash (Stevens-Johnson syndrome) is rare
      2) Leukopenia is common: mild, clinically insignificant
      3) Aplastic anemia, agranulocytosis, and thrombocytopenia are rare
      4) Hypersensitivity syndrome is rare: rash, eosinophilia, lymphadenopathy, splenomegaly
   e. Other
      1) Nausea, gastrointestinal upset (reduced if medication is taken with meals)
      2) Dystonia and chorea are rare
      3) Increased transaminase levels: mild, usually insignificant
      4) Hyponatremia: consider if cognitive difficulties
      5) Congestive heart failure
      6) If taken during pregnancy, risk of spina bifida in infant

5. Drug interactions
   a. Decrease the plasma concentration of (liver enzyme induction)
      1) Most anticonvulsants (except gabapentin and levetiracetam): valproate, lamotrigine, tiagabine, topiramate, zonisamide, felbamate, oxcarbazepine
      2) Benzodiazepines, haloperidol, theophylline, warfarin, and oral contraceptives (reduces the effectiveness of oral contraceptives)
   b. Increase the plasma concentration of fluoxetine, tricyclic antidepressants, phenytoin
   c. The following increase the plasma concentration of carbamazepine: erythromycin, clarithromycin, chloramphenicol, propoxyphene, verapamil
   d. The following decrease the plasma concentration of carbamazepine: phenytoin, phenobarbital, primidone, and felbamate
   e. Valproate increases the free fraction of both carbamazepine and its epoxide (inhibits the breakdown of the epoxide); when the level is high enough, the epoxide may also contribute to its toxicity
   f. Isoniazid and carbamazepine increase the plasma concentrations of each other

6. Monitor: liver function tests, complete blood count, and sodium level

Autoinduction of carbamazepine results in reduced plasma concentrations after the first 1 to 2 months of use

The corollary is that dose-related toxicity occurs if the carbamazepine dose is escalated rapidly before autoinduction occurs

G. Oxcarbazepine

1. Chemical cousin of carbamazepine
   a. Differences
      1) Less liver enzyme induction
         a) Thus, fewer drug interactions
         b) No autoinduction, thus can be titrated more rapidly
      2) Metabolites have anticonvulsant effects with less toxicity
         a) Carbamazepine has an epoxide metabolite that is responsible for much of its toxicity
         b) Oxcarbazepine has a 10-monohydroxyl metabolite that is less toxic; anticonvulsant effect is similar to that of carbamazepine
   b. Similarities: both drugs are used for the same seizure types, have the same mechanism (sodium channel antagonist), also have liver metabolism and renal excretion
2. Side effects
   a. Profile similar (except fewer drug interactions and less liver enzyme induction) to that of carbamazepine, less experience
   b. Interferes with contraceptives
   c. If patients have a carbamazepine rash, one-third will also have an oxcarbazepine rash
3. Monitor: complete blood count, sodium levels

H. Benzodiazepines

1. Seizure types
   a. Broad spectrum: partial, generalized tonic-clonic, absence, and myoclonic seizures
   b. Benzodiazepines are particularly useful in status epilepticus (including absence status)
2. Mechanism of action
   a. Potentiates $GABA_A$
   b. Enhances chloride channels, thus hyperpolarizing the neuronal membrane and decreasing neuronal excitability
3. Metabolism

The primary metabolite of oxcarbazepine (10-monohydroxyl metabolite) is less toxic than the primary metabolite of carbamazepine (an epoxide)

No liver autoinduction occurs with oxcarbazepine

Benzodiazepines potentiate $GABA_A$, thus enhancing chloride channels and hyperpolarizing neurons, rendering them less excitable

---

a. Liver, with renal excretion of metabolites
b. Decrease dose in liver disease
c. Dose is usually unchanged in kidney disease

4. Side effects
   a. Cognitive
      1) Somnolence, drowsiness, irritability, psychosis, dysarthria, ataxia, diplopia (as with alcohol)
      2) Tolerance: often used for status epilepticus or infrequent use (e.g., Diastat [rectal diazepam], is used for infrequent or severe seizures)
   b. Hypoventilation: reversed with flumazenil (competitive inhibition)
   c. Cardiovascular collapse
   d. Withdrawal syndrome (mirrors alcohol withdrawal)
   e. Hepatotoxicity
   f. Neutropenia, pancytopenia, thrombocytopenia
5. Specific benzodiazepines
   a. Clonazepam (long half-life): useful (but not first-line agent) for myoclonic, absence, and partial seizures and infantile spasms
   b. Lorazepam, diazepam (medium half-life): useful in status epilepticus
   c. Midazolam (short half-life): anesthetic, can be used for status epilepticus

I. Ethosuximide

1. Seizure type: absence seizures *only*
2. Mechanism of action: antagonist of T-type calcium channels in the thalamus
3. Metabolism: liver, with renal excretion of metabolites
4. Side effects
   a. Usually well tolerated
   b. Cognitive
      1) Drowsiness, dizziness, headache, irritability
      2) Improve with tolerance
   c. Gastrointestinal
      1) Gastrointestinal upset, nausea, vomiting, diarrhea
      2) Dose-related
   d. Idiosyncratic
      1) Rash, leukopenia common
      2) Stevens-Johnson syndrome
      3) Pancytopenia, agranulocytosis, aplastic anemia
5. Monitor: liver function tests, complete blood count

J. Felbamate

1. Seizure types: partial, generalized tonic-clonic, absence, myoclonic, tonic, and atonic seizures
2. Metabolism: liver and kidney (half is excreted unchanged in the urine)
3. Side effects

a. High rates of aplastic anemia and severe, potentially fatal hepatotoxicity compared with other antiepileptic drugs
   1) Required: frequent liver function tests and complete blood count
   2) Felbamate is used in only severe, refractory cases as a last resort (often Lennox-Gastaut syndrome)
   b. Otherwise, mild side effects: nausea, weight loss, insomnia
4. Drug interactions
   a. Increases phenytoin, phenobarbital, and valproate concentrations and carbamazepine epoxide
   b. Decreases carbamazepine level—Note: because carbamazepine epoxide (the active metabolite) increases, the carbamazepine level does not reflect activity and toxicity but underestimates them
5. Monitor: complete blood count, liver function tests, reticulocyte count

K. Tiagabine
1. Seizure types: partial or generalized tonic-clonic seizures (primary or secondary)
2. Mechanism of action: GABA reuptake inhibitor
3. Metabolism
   a. Liver
   b. May be used in renal failure
4. Side effects
   a. Cognitive: somnolence, dizziness, cognitive difficulties, ataxia
   b. Gastrointestinal upset: reduced if tiagabine is taken with meals
   c. Tremor
   d. Few drug interactions
5. Disadvantages
   a. Poor responder rate
   b. Frequent dosing (2-4 times daily)
6. No monitoring is required

L. Gabapentin
1. Seizure types
   a. Partial or secondarily generalized tonic-clonic seizures
   b. Can worsen generalized seizures, especially myoclonic seizures

---

Although felbamate is effective for a broad spectrum of seizure types, it is typically reserved for refractory epilepsy because of high rates of aplastic anemia and severe hepatotoxicity

---

2. Mechanism of action
   a. Increases postsynaptic GABA
   b. Dose-dependent absorption: smaller percentage of agent is absorbed at higher doses
3. Metabolism
   a. Renal excretion, essentially no metabolism before excretion
   b. Longer half-life in the elderly and with renal failure
4. Side effects
   a. Well tolerated
   b. Mild, dose-dependent toxicity
   c. Fatigue, somnolence, headache, ataxia, nausea
   d. No drug interactions
   e. No idiosyncratic reactions
   f. Excellent drug if patient is elderly or has liver failure
5. No monitoring is required

M. Lamotrigine
1. Seizure types
   a. Broad spectrum: partial, generalized tonic-clonic, absence, myoclonic, tonic, and atonic seizures
   b. FDA approved for Lennox-Gastaut syndrome monotherapy and for partial seizures
2. Mechanism of action
   a. Inhibits sodium channels, especially at high rates of firing (like phenytoin and carbamazepine)
   b. Also inhibits glutamate release (unlike phenytoin and carbamazepine, hence the broad spectrum)
3. Metabolism
   a. Liver, with renal excretion of metabolites
   b. Liver enzyme inducers (phenytoin, carbamazepine, phenobarbital) decrease the half-life of lamotrigine
   c. Liver enzyme inhibitor valproate increases the half-life of lamotrigine
   d. Lamotrigine does not affect the metabolism of other drugs
4. Side effects
   a. Typically well tolerated if drug is titrated slowly

Gabapentin is absorbed in a dose-dependent fashion so that a smaller proportion is absorbed at higher doses

---

Gabapentin and levetiracetam are predominantly excreted unchanged in the urine

Both have a longer half-life in the elderly and with renal failure

b. Dizziness, ataxia, blurred vision, diplopia

c. Rash

  1) Tends to be common and more severe than with other anticonvulsants, can cause Stevens-Johnson syndrome

  2) Increased risk with the following:

    a) Rapid titration

    b) Use of valproate

    c) Use in children

d. Can exacerbate carbamazepine toxicity (resolves with decreasing carbamazepine dose)

e. No known chronic toxicity

5. No monitoring is required

N. Levetiracetam

1. Seizure types

  a. Is definitely useful for partial or generalized tonic-clonic seizures (primary or secondary)

  b. May have a broad spectrum, but there is less experience with levetiracetam than with standard broad-spectrum drugs like valproate

2. Mechanism of action

  a. Not known precisely

  b. Inhibits burst firing of neurons without affecting normal neuronal activity

3. Metabolism

  a. Mostly renal (decrease dose in patients who are elderly or have renal failure)

  b. Two-thirds of the drug is excreted unchanged (like gabapentin, topiramate)

  c. One-third is metabolized first (acetamide hydrolysis) but no cytochrome P-450 metabolism

4. Side effects

  a. Well tolerated

  b. Rapid titration

  c. Cognitive

    1) Usually mild

    2) Drowsiness, dizziness, ataxia

  d. Psychiatric

> Lamotrigine has a broad spectrum and can be used for monotherapy in Lennox-Gastaut syndrome

> Lamotrigine is associated with a particularly high risk of Stevens-Johnson syndrome, especially if used in children, titrated rapidly, and used in combination with valproate

  1) Only a small proportion of patients

  2) Agitation, emotional lability, behavioral abnormalities

e. No important drug interactions (including oral contraceptives)

5. No monitoring is required

O. Topiramate

1. Seizure types

  a. Broad spectrum

  b. Partial or generalized tonic-clonic seizures (primary or secondary)

  c. Absence and atonic seizures: used in Lennox-Gastaut syndrome

2. Mechanism of action

  a. Multiple mechanisms like most broad-spectrum drugs

  b. Sodium channel inhibition, $GABA_A$ agonist, NMDA antagonist

3. Metabolism

  a. 80% is eliminated unchanged in the urine (like gabapentin, levetiracetam), some liver metabolism

  b. Liver enzyme inducers increase the proportion of topiramate metabolized by the liver

    1) Decreased half-life with liver enzyme inducers (phenytoin, phenobarbital, carbamazepine)

    2) Valproate has no important effect

4. Side effects

  a. Carbonic anhydrase inhibitor

    1) Renal stone formation (as with acetazolamide and zonisamide): avoid topiramate if patient has personal or family history of stones, advise hydration, do not use with ketogenic diet

    2) Paresthesias (most common adverse effect with monotherapy)

    3) Angle-closure glaucoma

  b. Cognitive

    1) Fatigue, somnolence, dizziness

    2) Word-finding difficulties and mental blunting (dose-dependent)

    3) Most common adverse effects with polytherapy

  c. Weight loss

  d. Few drug interactions

  e. Decreased effectiveness of oral contraceptives

5. No monitoring is required

> Topiramate is a carbonic anhydrase inhibitor, like acetazolamide, and can cause renal stones, paresthesias, and angle-closure glaucoma

P. Zonisamide

1. Seizure types
   a. Broad spectrum
   b. Approved for partial seizures in adults
   c. Used also for generalized seizures in children
2. Mechanism of action
   a. Inhibits sodium channels, T-type calcium channel antagonist
   b. $GABA_A$ agonist
3. Metabolism
   a. Liver with renal excretion of metabolites
   b. One-third of zonisamide is excreted unchanged in the urine
   c. Decrease the dose if the patient is elderly or has renal failure
4. Side effects
   a. Carbonic anhydrase activity: renal stone formation
   b. Cognitive
      1) Somnolence, dizziness, headache, diplopia
      2) Slurred speech, mental blunting, emotional lability
   c. Gastrointestinal: nausea, diarrhea, weight gain
   d. Rash: sulfonamide—zonisamide is contraindicated if patient has sulfonamide allergy
   e. No effect on other anticonvulsant levels
   f. Liver enzyme inducers (carbamazepine, phenytoin, phenobarbital) decrease the plasma concentration of zonisamide
5. No monitoring is required

Q. Vigabatrin

1. Seizure types
   a. Partial and secondarily generalized seizures
   b. Infantile spasms
2. Mechanism of action: decreases breakdown of GABA (inhibitory neurotransmitter)
3. Not currently marketed in the United States: 30% risk of irreversible visual field constriction

R. Pregabalin

1. Approved for adjunctive therapy in partial epilepsy
2. No drug interactions
3. Low protein binding
4. Most of the drug undergoes renal clearance (as with levetiracetam, gabapentin, and topiramate)
5. Adverse effects: drowsiness, ataxia, dizziness, weight gain, euphoria

V. OTHER THERAPIES FOR EPILEPSY

A. Ketogenic Diet

1. Can provide seizure relief when anticonvulsants fail
   a. Typically used for children with refractory seizures,

> Vigabatrin is useful for controlling infantile spasms, but it is not marketed in the U.S. because of a high risk of irreversible visual field constriction

> A ketogenic diet is effective for a broad range of seizure types

especially myoclonic, atonic, tonic, and atypical absence seizures
   b. Is effective across broad range of seizure types
2. Technique
   a. Hospitalize patient for observed starvation for 4 days (until ketotic)
      1) Monitor to avoid hypoglycemia
      2) Goal: 4+ urine ketosis
   b. The ketogenic diet is then introduced—3-4 g fat: 1 g carbohydrate + protein
3. Adverse effects
   a. During diet initiation: hypoglycemia, vomiting, dehydration
   b. Renal stone formation: avoid carbonic anhydrase inhibitors such as topiramate
   c. Vitamin, mineral, and carnitine deficiencies: supplement and, before starting the diet, rule out inborn error of metabolism
   d. Others: hypoproteinemia, renal tubular acidosis, hyperlipidemia, increased liver transaminase levels, pancreatitis, sepsis, long QT syndrome

B. Vagus Nerve Stimulation

1. Rationale
   a. In 30% to 40% of patients, epilepsy is refractory to anticonvulsant therapy
   b. Some patients are not candidates for epilepsy surgery
2. Efficacy
   a. Two large randomized controlled trials showed a modest but statistically significant decrease in seizure frequency
   b. The largest trial showed that high-intensity stimulation decreased seizure frequency by 28% compared with 15% for the low-intensity stimulation "active control" (presumably the placebo effect)
   c. Thus, the treatment effect is only a 13% average decrease in seizure frequency
   d. A smaller proportion had a 75% or greater decrease in seizure frequency

> Vagus nerve stimulation typically produces a modest reduction in seizure frequency
>
> Seizure freedom is an unrealistic goal

    e. No patients were seizure-free

3. Side effects

    a. Hoarseness, dyspnea, cough, and paresthesias

    b. Rare, device infection

    c. Case reports of asystole

    d. None of the typical central nervous system side effects of anticonvulsants

C. Epilepsy Surgery

1. Background

    a. In one-third of patients, epilepsy is refractory to anticonvulsants

    b. If the epilepsy in these patients results from a focal abnormality, resective surgery may be indicated

    c. Resection should be considered if adequate trials of two or three appropriate anticonvulsants prove ineffective, because additional medications are unlikely to stop the seizures

    d. Early surgical consideration is recommended to avoid damaging effects of chronic seizures (central nervous system damage, psychiatric impact, socioeconomic impact)

    e. Other surgical techniques can reduce seizure propagation: corpus callosotomy, multiple subpial resections

2. Surgical options (Table 12-7)

    a. Focal cortical resection: lesional or nonlesional

    b. Temporal lobectomy

        1) Anterior temporal lobectomy: standard approach

        2) Amygdalohippocampectomy: mesial temporal resection

          a) More selective than anterior temporal lobectomy

          b) Useful for mesial temporal lobe epilepsy, including mesial temporal sclerosis

        3) Neocortical temporal resection

    c. Multiple subpial resection

        1) Used for epileptogenic focus in "critical real estate"

        2) Horizontal fibers are severed to curtail spread of synchronous epileptogenic activity while vertical connections are maintained so that cortical function is minimally disrupted

        3) Can be used in combination with resective surgery

        4) Efficacy depends on the size of the lesion, usually does not render patients seizure-free but can reduce the intensity of the seizures

Table 12-7. Types of Surgical Procedures for Epilepsy

Focal cortical resection
Temporal lobectomy
    Anterior temporal lobectomy
    Amygdalohippocampectomy (mesial temporal resection)
    Neocortical temporal resection
Multiple subpial resection
Hemispherectomy
Corpus callosotomy
Deep brain stimulation
Radiotherapy

> Multiple subpial resection can be used in eloquent cortex because vertical connections subserving most cortical function are minimally disrupted

    d. Hemispherectomy

        1) Used if seizure activity is confined to only one poorly functioning hemisphere (e.g., Rasmussen's encephalopathy, Sturge-Weber disease, cerebral dysgenesis)

        2) "Functional hemispherectomy"

          a) Central cortical resection, temporal lobectomy, corpus callosotomy

          b) Disconnects the hemisphere without leaving a cavity

    e. Corpus callosotomy

        1) Palliative, to decrease the generalization of seizures

        2) Reduces seizure intensity, frequency, and injuries

    f. Deep brain stimulation

        1) All forms are investigational

          a) Centromedian nucleus of thalamus

            i) The reticulothalamocortical pathway is thought to transmit discharges in generalized epilepsy

            ii) Stimulation may benefit generalized tonic-clonic and atypical absence seizures

          b) Subthalamic nucleus

            i) Stimulation used for Parkinson's disease

            ii) In animal models and small case series in humans, stimulation has decreased seizure activity

          c) Cortical stimulation: during cortical mapping, it was observed that afterdischarges provoked by cortical stimulation can be aborted by another brief pulse of stimulation

    g. Radiotherapy

        1) May be antiepileptic, under investigation

        2) Stereotactic radiosurgery is particularly useful for

certain focal lesions (arteriovenous malformations, tumors)

3) Stereotactic radiosurgery has been used successfully for mesial temporal sclerosis, but the disadvantage is that open surgery allows intracranial monitoring to localize more accurately the patient's seizures

3. Outcomes
   a. "Surgically privileged" seizure disorders
      1) About 80% probability of seizure-free outcome
      2) The lesion is characterized by the following
         a) Well-circumscribed on MRI: this is the most critical feature
         b) Well-localized interictal discharges
         c) Consistent focal onset by symptoms
         d) Focus is in noneloquent cortex: entire lesion can be removed without major morbidity
         e) No other possible seizure focus or foci
   b. Less ideal candidates who may still benefit
      1) Nonlesional epilepsy
         a) If work-up otherwise indicates the seizure is focal (e.g., video-EEG, SISCOM)
         b) In nonlesional epilepsy, the outcome is better for anterior temporal lobe (60%) than for extratemporal lobe (35%-40%)
      2) Bilateral mesial temporal sclerosis, if seizures originate primarily from one side
      3) Multiple lesions (e.g., cavernous angiomas, tuberous sclerosis) provided that seizures are primarily from one focus (Fig. 12-5)
      4) Focus near eloquent cortex: resection can be guided by cortical mapping or by operating on an awake patient
      5) Large or diffuse seizure focus or lesion
      6) Infantile spasms

Stereotactic radiosurgery has been used successfully for mesial temporal sclerosis, but the disadvantage is that intracranial monitoring cannot be performed

---

Patients whose seizures are associated with a single, well-circumscribed MRI lesion, have well-localized interictal discharges, produce consistent symptoms, and are located in noneloquent cortex have a high probability of freedom from seizures (~80%) after resection of the seizure focus

---

VI. THERAPY FOR STATUS EPILEPTICUS

A. Types of Status Epilepticus

1. Generalized convulsive status
   a. High mortality (20%)
   b. Mortality varies depending on the underlying cause
2. Nonconvulsive status
   a. Typically evolves from prolonged seizures
   b. Often requires EEG to differentiate it from other causes of unresponsiveness (postictal state, underlying neurologic disease)
3. Subtle nonconvulsive status
   a. Similar to nonconvulsive status
   b. There is subtle face, eyelid, or eye twitching
4. Focal status (simple or complex)
   a. Complex focal status has significant morbidity and mortality
   b. It merits aggressive treatment
5. Absence status
   a. Benign
   b. Brain damage is unlikely

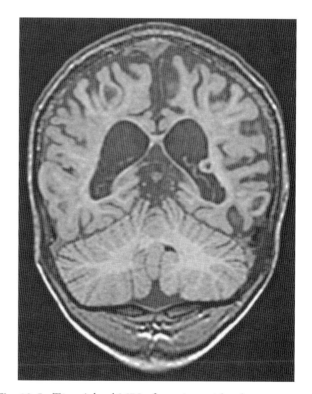

Fig. 12-5. T1-weighted MRI of a patient with tuberous sclerosis. Note the multiple tubers and subependymal nodule. Epilepsy surgery could be beneficial if surgical evaluation found that most seizures emanate from a single focus.

c. Responds to low-dose benzodiazepines

6. Myoclonic status
   a. Usually indicates severe neurologic injury (e.g., anoxic, degenerative)
   b. Thus, treatment response and prognosis are poor

B. Generalized Convulsive Status Epilepticus

1. Definition
   a. Classic definition: 30 minutes of continuous seizure activity or two or more seizures in 30 minutes without recovery of consciousness
   b. Controversial new definition: more than 5 minutes of seizure activity or two or more seizures without recovery of consciousness
   c. Advocates for old definition point out that neuronal damage begins after 30 minutes
   d. Advocates for new definition point out that seizures usually stop in less than 2 minutes
   e. All agree that early treatment is essential because longer seizures are more difficult to stop and can cause neuronal injury within 20 to 30 minutes, leading to mesial temporal sclerosis and epilepsy

2. Management (for algorithmic approach to treatment of status epilepticus, see Chapter 10)
   a. Initial management (adult)
      1) Airway, breathing, circulation
         a) Ventilation is usually adequate if an airway is maintained (e.g., with oral airway)
         b) Electrocardiographic and blood pressure monitoring: potential cardiac side effects of anticonvulsants (hypotension, arrhythmias)
      2) Oxygen, pulse oximetry
      3) If the intravenous route is not possible, consider the rectal or intramuscular route
      4) Intubation: usually required only after administration of large doses of anticonvulsants that have sedative properties
         a) If the patient is intubated, use short-acting nondepolarizing neuromuscular blockade (e.g., rocuronium)
         b) Avoid succinylcholine because it causes hyperkalemia and arrhythmias, especially if the patient has rhabdomyolysis from the convulsions
      5) Check blood glucose: if level is low, give 50 mL of

Myoclonic status epilepticus typically reflects severe neurologic injury (e.g., anoxic or degenerative)

Treatment response and prognosis are poor

Depolarizing neuromuscular blocking agents (e.g., succinylcholine) are contraindicated in patients with generalized convulsive status epilepticus because of the risk of hyperkalemia and arrhythmias

---

50% glucose with 100 mg thiamine
   b. Pharmacologic management: overview
      1) First-line agent: benzodiazepines
      2) Second-line agent: phenytoin
      3) Third-line agent: phenobarbital vs. anesthetic agent (midazolam, propofol)
      4) If refractory to midazolam or propofol, consider inhalent anesthetic (isoflurane is the first choice)

3. Medications for convulsive status epilepticus
   a. See above for further details about these drugs, this section reviews issues particularly relevant to their use in status epilepticus
   b. Lorazepam
      1) Probably the preferred benzodiazepine because it not only has an onset of action as fast as that of diazepam but also a longer duration of action (24 hours vs. 30 minutes)
      2) Dose (adults): 0.1 mg/kg intravenously at 1 mg/min
      3) Adverse effects: respiratory depression, hypotension, decreased level of consciousness
      4) Also rectal, sublingual, and intramuscular preparations
      5) Can also be given as a continuous intravenous infusion for refractory status epilepticus, like midazolam but with less tachyphylaxis, but long offset (especially with prolonged use)
   c. Diazepam
      1) Alternative to lorazepam but risk of recurrent seizure because of short duration of action
      2) Dose (adults): 0.2 mg/kg intravenously at 2 mg/min
      3) Rectal gel useful in children and infants or if there is no intravenous access
         a) 2 to 5 years old: 0.5 mg/kg
         b) 6 to 11 years old: 0.3 mg/kg
         c) 12 years and older: 0.2 mg/kg (adult intravenous dose)
      4) Adverse effects: respiratory depression, hypotension, decreased level of consciousness
   d. Phenytoin
      1) Standard second-line agent, but consider valproate if there are cardiac issues
      2) Water insoluble, so formulation is alkaline (pH 12) with propylene glycol and ethanol (responsible for

tissue toxicity and purple glove syndrome and, to some degree, cardiac effects)
  3) Dose (adults)
    a) 20 mg/kg intravenously at 50 mg/min
    b) May repeat an additional 10 mg/kg if seizures continue
  4) Note that administration is slow because of the risk of cardiovascular side effects (hypotension, arrhythmias, QT prolongation)
    a) For a 70-kg man receiving 1.4 g, administration would take 28 minutes
    b) Electrocardiographic and blood pressure monitoring are essential (intensive care unit or emergency department)
      i) Slow rate of administration if hypotension or cardiac effects occur
      ii) In part, cardiac effects are due to the propylene glycol diluent, so fewer cardiac effects occur with fosphenytoin
  5) Adverse effects: hypotension, QT prolongation, purple glove syndrome, others (see above)
e. Fosphenytoin
  1) More expensive than phenytoin, but better side-effect profile
  2) It is a phosphate ester prodrug of phenytoin
    a) It is water soluble, with no risk of purple glove syndrome and less risk of cardiac adverse effects
  3) Dose: 20 mg/kg phenytoin equivalents intravenously at 150 mg/min
    a) Despite faster infusion rate, time to onset of action is similar to that for phenytoin because of conversion time
    b) Cardiac monitoring is still needed, slow the rate of administration if hypotension or arrhythmia occurs
f. Valproate
  1) Alternative, second choice to phenytoin
  2) Loading dose: 15 to 20 mg/kg (over 5 minutes)
  3) Efficacy has been poorly studied, but side-effect

profile is favorable compared with phenytoin if patient has hemodynamic instability
g. Phenobarbital
  1) Dose: 20 mg/kg intravenously at 50 mg/min (same as for phenytoin)
  2) Marked side effects
    a) Use of phenobarbital after phenytoin fails to control seizures is controversial because of its adverse side-effect profile
      i) Depresses respiratory drive and consciousness
      ii) High risk of hypotension, decreased cardiac contractility
      iii) Because of the long half-life (48 hours), the effects are prolonged
h. Midazolam
  1) A benzodiazepine with a short half-life, used as an intravenous drip for its anesthetic properties in refractory status epilepticus
  2) Dose: 0.2 mg/kg load over 1 minute (*intubate*), then 0.05 to 2.0 mg/kg per hour
  3) Advantages: fast onset and offset, well tolerated, less hypotension than with phenobarbital or propofol
  4) Disadvantages: rapid onset of tachyphylaxis
i. Propofol
  1) Anesthetic: $GABA_A$ agonist (like benzodiazepines)
  2) Dose: 3 to 5 mg/kg load (intubate), then 1 to 15 mg/kg per hour
  3) Advantages: short onset and offset, effective
  4) Disadvantages: bradycardia, hypotension, high lipid content, slower offset after prolonged infusion, propofol infusion syndrome
  5) Propofol infusion syndrome
    a) Triad: severe hypotension, lipidemia, and metabolic acidosis
    b) Most common in children with metabolic enzyme deficiencies, but it can occur in adults

Lorazepam has an onset of action as fast as that of diazepam but has a longer duration of action

Although fosphenytoin can be administered more rapidly than phenytoin, the time to onset of action is similar because of fosphenytoin's conversion time

The use of phenobarbital as a third-line agent in status epilepticus (before anesthetics such as midazolam and propofol) is controversial because of the long half-life and the risks of hypotension and decreased cardiac contractility

Propofol infusion syndrome, most commonly seen in children with metabolic enzyme deficiencies, is the triad of hypotension, hyperlipidemia, and metabolic acidosis

VII. Epilepsy Issues for Women

A. Hormonal Abnormalities Related to Seizures and Anticonvulsants (infertility, menstrual irregularities, ovarian dysfunction, cosmetics)

1. Generalized or complex partial seizures can propagate to the hypothalamus, altering hormone release
2. Anticonvulsants can influence metabolism of sex hormones
   a. This is often mediated by cytochrome P-450 or by increased protein binding
   b. They can directly influence the cortical input to the hypothalamic-pituitary-ovarian axis
   c. Liver enzyme inducers (e.g., carbamazepine, phenytoin, phenobarbital, topiramate) reduce steroid hormone levels
3. Result of seizures or drug effects
   a. Anovulatory cycles, infertility, menstrual irregularities
   b. Polycystic ovary-like syndrome
4. Increased androgen levels can produce hirsutism, acne, excess facial hair, and weight gain
   a. Some debate about what hormonal dysfunction is attributable to drugs vs. epilepsy
   b. Polycystic ovary-like syndrome has been attributed to valproate, but some argue that the seizures are the culprit

B. Hormonal Exacerbation of Seizures

1. Estrogen has proconvulsant effects
   a. Estrogen downregulates $GABA_A$ and $GABA_A$ receptor synthesis, thus increasing neuronal excitability by decreasing GABA-mediated inhibition
   b. Estrogen also is an NMDA agonist in the hippocampus (excitatory)
2. Progesterone has anticonvulsant effects (opposite effects to estrogen)
   a. Upregulates $GABA_A$ and $GABA_A$ receptor synthesis
   b. Antagonist of hippocampus NMDA receptors
3. With increased estrogen, seizures may be triggered during menarche
4. Catamenial seizures: occur primarily during perimenstrual period when estrogen levels are high relative to progesterone levels
5. Progesterone therapy can be used in some circumstances of increased estrogen:progesterone ratio for antiepileptic properties
   a. Example: with anovulatory cycle, progesterone produc-

tion is inadequate because the corpus luteum (which produces progesterone) does not form from the follicle (which produces estrogen), so if a patient has seizures associated with anovulatory cycles, progesterone therapy can be helpful

C. Efficacy of Oral Contraceptives

1. Anticonvulsants that increase the metabolism of oral contraceptives reduce the efficacy of these medicines: carbamazepine, phenytoin, phenobarbital, oxcarbazepine, and topiramate (at high doses)
   a. Thus, the typical low-dose pills have a higher failure rate
   b. Higher dose pills or additional contraceptive methods are recommended
      1) Example: carbamazepine reduces estradiol by 40% to 50%
      2) Thus, an oral contraceptive pill containing 50 µg ethinyl estradiol is recommended instead of the typical "low-dose" 35 µg
2. The medicines that have no interaction with oral contraceptives are valproate, gabapentin, pregabalin, tiagabine, levetiracetam, zonisamide

D. Pregnancy: maternal issues

1. 25% of women have worsening of seizure frequency during pregnancy
   a. Increased risk if seizure frequency was high before pregnancy
   b. Pharmacokinetics change during pregnancy (e.g., increase in metabolism volume of distribution and protein binding), decreasing free drug levels
      1) Follow *free* drug levels during pregnancy
      2) Lamotrigine levels decrease markedly during pregnancy compared with those of other anticonvulsants
   c. The risk of eclampsia, preeclampsia, and other maternal complications of pregnancy is debated but may be increased

E. Pregnancy: fetal issues

1. Risks to the fetus
   a. Most (>90%) babies born to epileptic women are healthy
   b. Risks: miscarriage, prematurity, cerebral palsy, developmental delay, epilepsy, and major malformations (cardiac and neural tube defects)

Estrogen has proconvulsant effects and progesterone has anticonvulsant effects

---

Free anticonvulsant levels generally decrease during pregnancy because of increase in metabolism, volume of distribution, and protein binding

c. Previously referred to as "fetal hydantoin syndrome," now called "fetal anticonvulsant syndrome"

d. Risk of major fetal malformation is 4% to 8% (double the risk for the general population)

1) Various malformations are seen with most anticonvulsants

   a) Valproate and carbamazepine are associated particularly with spina bifida (1%-2% with valproate use, 0.5% with carbamazepine)

2) Greatest risk of cleft lip and palate, neural tube malformations, and congenital heart defects is during the first trimester

3) Note that the neural tube closes during weeks 3 to 4—a critical period

4) Folate supplementation decreases birth defects (especially neural tube defects) in the general population

   a) Whether folate also protects against defects related to anticonvulsants is not known

   b) The Centers for Disease Control and Prevention recommends 0.4 mg/day for all women planning pregnancy

   c) Higher doses are often recommended for women taking anticonvulsants (up to 5 mg/day, but the optimal dose is not known)

   d) Folate should be started while the woman is attempting pregnancy because the neural tube closes before many women know they are pregnant

e. Although anticonvulsants are associated with increased risks of congenital malformations, recurrent seizures are considered by most neurologists as unacceptable risks to the fetus and mother

f. Seizures can cause fetal and placental trauma and hypoxia

g. Risks of anticonvulsant-induced congenital malformations increase with the number of drugs used (5% for 1 drug, 23% for 4 drugs)

h. Goal: seizure control with the fewest anticonvulsants

> Folate use is recommended for epileptic women before conception and during the first trimester because the neural tube closes between weeks 3 and 4

> The goal in pregnancy is to control seizures with the fewest necessary antiepileptic drugs at the lowest doses needed
>
> Uncontrolled seizures are risky to the fetus

necessary and at the lowest dose

i. There may also be an increased risk of fetal hemorrhage from internal bleeding, thought possibly due to vitamin K-dependent clotting factor deficiency from anticonvulsants

1) Babies are routinely given vitamin K intramuscularly

2) Consider additional oral vitamin K during the last month of pregnancy

2. Breast-feeding

a. Highly protein-bound anticonvulsants are expressed to a greater degree in breast milk

1) These can cause sedation, especially barbiturates

2) Withdrawal symptoms can occur when nursing is discontinued

b. Anticonvulsants rarely cause hematologic and liver side effects

c. For newer anticonvulsants, the risks of nursing are uncertain

d. Benefits of nursing may outweigh potential neurologic consequences

F. Osteoporosis

1. Liver enzyme-inducing anticonvulsants decrease the level of active vitamin D, leading to premature osteoporosis and bone fractures

2. Epileptics are at risk for poor bone health independent of the effects of liver enzyme-inducing drugs

3. Bone densitometry is recommended for patients receiving long-term anticonvulsant therapy

4. Consider weight-bearing exercises, vitamin D and calcium supplementation, and bisphosphonate therapy

VIII. NEUROIMAGING IN PATIENTS WITH SEIZURES

A. Structural Imaging

1. MRI is more sensitive than CT (especially with 15-mm coronal cuts through temporal lobes)

a. MRI is useful for evaluating the cause of new-onset seizure disorder

b. Common lesional etiologies include stroke, traumatic injury, tumor, malformation of cortical development, cysticercosis, mesial temporal sclerosis (Fig. 12-6)

2. CT is useful in emergent settings to rule out acute blood

3. When structural imaging is indicated:

a. First-time seizure if focal lesion is suspected

1) Especially consider structural imaging if patient is older than 40 years (idiopathic epilepsy is unlikely in this age group)

2) Especially consider structural imaging if patient had a

focal seizure (suggests focal lesion)

b. Children with first nonfebrile seizure

   1) Urgent neuroimaging if there is focal deficit or prolonged confusion

   2) Nonurgent MRI if there is cognitive or motor impairment of unknown cause, abnormal neurologic findings, seizure of focal onset, EEG is not consistent with an idiopathic epilepsy syndrome, or patient is younger than 1 year

c. ILAE advocates imaging for all epilepsy patients at some point unless they clearly have an idiopathic epilepsy syndrome (consistent clinical story and EEG with normal examination findings)

B. Functional Imaging

1. Indicated in epilepsy surgical evaluation when primary means of seizure focus localization are inconclusive (history, examination, interictal EEG, MRI, video-EEG)
2. Is often used to provide a target for intracranial electrode placement
3. Positron emission tomography (PET) (Fig. 12-7)

   a. Images the degree of uptake of various radioactive ligands

   b. The usual glucose-uptake ligand is [18F]fluoro-2-deoxy-D-glucose

      1) Reflects metabolic activity

      2) Its short half-life limits use ictally

      3) Usually interictal, to search for hypometabolic regions that are potentially epileptogenic regions

      4) A seizure occurring during PET may show a hypermetabolic region

   c. Advantages

      1) If abnormal, high concordance with EEG

      2) Particularly useful in infants with infantile spasms because hypometabolic regions of these patients can be resected, with excellent surgical outcome despite normal structural imaging (80% in one study)

   d. Disadvantages

      1) Less likely to be abnormal if MRI is normal

      2) Interictal, so does not reflect seizure activity

      3) Expensive, need a cyclotron to generate radiotracer

      4) Abnormalities are often diffuse, e.g., abnormality often lateralizes to one hemisphere but not within the hemisphere

4. Single photon emission computed tomography (SPECT) and subtraction ictal SPECT coregistered to

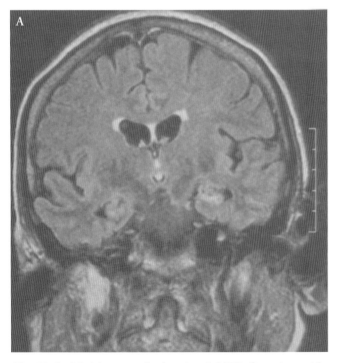

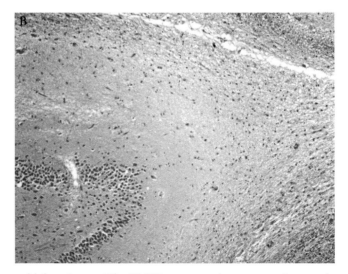

PET scans show interictal hypometabolism, whereas ictal SPECT scans show ictal increases in blood flow

Fig. 12-6. Mesial temporal sclerosis. *A*, MRI of a patient with temporal lobe seizures. The FLAIR sequence demonstrates increased signal in the left mesial temporal lobe and asymmetric hippocampal atrophy (L>R) best appreciated on quantitative MRI volumetry. *B*, Histopathologic section shows selective hippocampal neuronal loss and gliosis, with predominant loss of pyramidal cells in CA1. In this specimen, extensive gliosis has replaced the CA1 region.

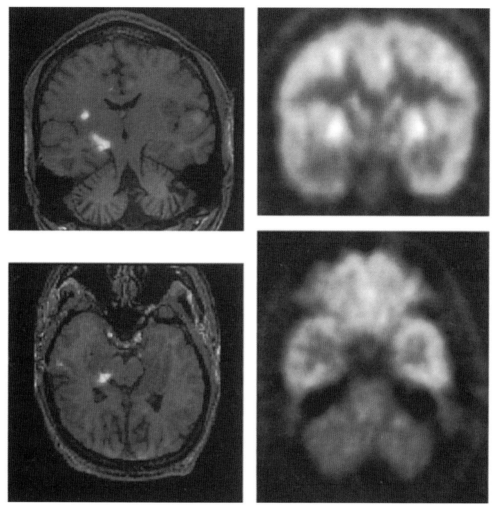

Fig. 12-7. SISCOM images (*left*) show a focal ictal area of hyperperfusion in the right mesial temporal lobe. PET images (*right*) obtained interictally in the same patient show hypoperfusion (decreased signal intensity) corresponding roughly to the same region in the SISCOM images. (From So EL. Role of neuroimaging in the management of seizure disorders. Mayo Clin Proc. 2002;77:1251-64. By permission of Mayo Foundation.)

MRI (SISCOM) (Fig. 12-7 and 12-8)
a. Ictal SPECT measures increased blood flow during a seizure
b. Unlike SISCOM, ictal SPECT is used at many institutions
c. Interictal SPECT measures decreased blood flow in an epileptogenic region
d. Interictal SPECT is less sensitive than ictal SPECT
e. Comparison of ictal and interictal SPECT facilitates identification of ictal abnormalities by contrast
f. SISCOM takes the ictal image and subtracts it digitally from the interictal image
   1) This "difference" image is coregistered to MRI to anatomically localize the seizure focus
   2) SISCOM localization is an independent predictor of epilepsy surgery outcome
   3) If EEG and MRI are nonlocalizing, the surgical outcome is better if the SISCOM abnormality is resected (60% vs. 20%)
g. Advantages
   1) Less expensive than PET, no cyclotron is needed
   2) Radiotracers have longer half-life, so ictal injections are feasible

SISCOM can often localize a seizure focus even when MRI and EEG are nonlocalizing

However, only a seizure focus active within 1 minute after injection is reflected

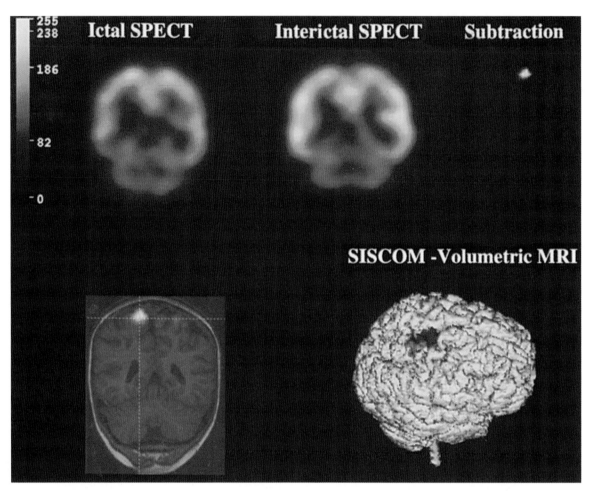

Fig. 12-8. To obtain a SISCOM image, ictal (*upper left*) and interictal (*upper middle*) SPECT images are "subtracted" to obtain a "difference" (*upper right*). The difference image is then coregistered with the MRI in two-dimensional planes (*lower left*) or on the surface of a three-dimensional MRI reconstruction (*lower right*). (From So EL. Role of neuroimaging in the management of seizure disorders. Mayo Clin Proc. 2002;77:1251-64. By permission of Mayo Foundation.)

h. Disadvantages
  1) Requires prompt injection during seizure, within 1 minute
  2) If the injection is delayed, then postictal hypoperfusion is imaged, which has a wider distribution
  3) Reflects only the seizure injected, not necessarily patient's every seizure type
5. Magnetic resonance spectroscopy (MRS)
  a. Noninvasive measurement of chemical composition of brain
  b. MRS measures hydrogen nucleus, thereby measuring metabolites such as *N*-acetylaspartate (NAA), creatine, and choline
    1) NAA reflects neuron abundance
    2) Creatine and choline are associated with glial cells

  3) NAA:creatine ratio
    a) If decreased in mesial temporal lobe, suggests mesial temporal sclerosis
    b) Especially helpful in temporal lobe resection candidates who do not have hippocampal atrophy
    c) Seizures usually arise from the side with relatively decreased NAA, reflecting mild mesial temporal sclerosis
    d) If MRS shows bilateral hippocampal abnormalities, seizure outcome of temporal lobectomy is less favorable and postoperative memory problems are more substantial
6. Functional cortex mapping
  a. Intracarotid injection of amobarbital (Wada's test)
    1) Depresses cortical function of hemisphere ipsilateral

to carotid artery injected
   2) Useful in identifying *hemisphere* of language
      localization, but poor identification of specific
      anatomical structures involved
 b. Functional MRI
   1) Can be used to measure task-activated cortex, thereby
      localizing function more accurately than with the
      amobarbital test
   2) It measures changes in deoxyhemoglobin on T2-
      weighted MRI
   3) A decrease of deoxyhemoglobin reflects an increase in
      blood flow in activated brain
   4) Functional MRI may be advantageous compared with
      electrocortical stimulation because it is noninvasive

IX. FEBRILE SEIZURES

A. Prevalence: 3% to 5% of all children, usually benign
   outcome

B. Age
1. Usually between 6 months and 5 years (range, 1 mo-10
   years)
2. 90% occur within the first 3 years of life

C. Typically Associated With Common Childhood
   Infections (including human herpesvirus-6)

D. Any Clinical Features Indicative of Central Nervous
   System Infection Preclude the Diagnosis

E. Recurrence
1. About 1/3 of patients with one febrile seizure have at
   least one additional seizure (higher risk if child is
   younger than 12 months at time of first febrile seizure)
2. Half of this group (15% of all patients) have a second
   seizure, and 9% of all patients have 3 or more recurrent
   seizures

F. Risk Factors for Developing Febrile Seizure
1. Family history
   a. Febrile seizures are 2 or 3 times more likely to occur in
      family members of affected children
   b. Increased risk with family history of febrile seizures (first-
      degree relatives), higher risk with family history in both
      parents
   c. Increased risk of afebrile epilepsy in first-degree relatives
      of patients with febrile seizures
2. Prolonged hospitalization in neonatal intensive care unit

3. Delayed development
4. Day-care attendance
5. Incidence does not increase in proportion to increase in
   temperature
6. No identifiable risk factor in approximately 50% of patients

G. Risk Factors For Developing Afebrile Epilepsy After
   Febrile Seizure
1. Developmental delay and abnormal neurologic
   examination
2. Family history of afebrile seizures
3. Complex febrile seizure

H. Risk of Recurrent Febrile Seizures Is Increased in
   Presence of
1. Family history of febrile or unprovoked seizures
2. Low temperature at time of initial febrile seizure
3. Initial febrile seizure when child is younger than 12
   months (50% of patients younger than 1 year presenting with a first febrile seizure will have recurrence, as
   compared with 20% of children older than 3 years at
   time of first febrile seizure)
4. Not increased with complex febrile seizure on presentation as compared with simple febrile seizure

I. Risk of Epilepsy
1. <5% of patients with febrile seizures develop epilepsy
2. About 15% of patients with epilepsy have a history of
   febrile seizures

J. Simple Febrile Seizure
1. Most febrile seizures
2. Brief (<15 minutes)
3. Generalized, lack focality
4. Occur in neurologically normal patients
5. Not associated with persistent deficits
6. Often have a familial predisposition: may be autosomal
   dominant with variable penetrance, polygenic, or autosomal recessive

K. Complex Febrile Seizure
1. 20% of febrile seizures
2. Prolonged (>15 minutes)
3. May have focal features
4. Seizure recurrence less than 24 hours
5. Abnormal neurologic examination
6. Postictal neurologic signs (e.g., Todd's paralysis)
7. Complex febrile seizures are more likely to be due to
   meningitis, encephalitis, or underlying seizure disorder
   than simple complex seizures

L. Prophylaxis After Febrile Seizure

1. Usually not indicated, but may be considered for recurrent or prolonged febrile seizures, later afebrile epilepsy, or after a complex partial seizure, especially in patients with abnormal neurologic examination and developmental delay
2. Chronic antiepileptic drug prophylaxis: phenobarbital and valproate
   a. Recurrence reduction; however, prophylaxis is usually avoided because drug side effects are a concern
   b. Phenobarbital can cause irritability, hyperactivity, somnolence, and possible interference with cognitive development
3. Short-term antiepileptic drug prophylaxis (prophylaxis during febrile illnesses only)
   a. Diazepam
      1) Studied in children (mean age, 2 years) with a history of febrile seizures
      2) Significant seizure reduction
      3) Significant side effects: irritability, lethargy, ataxia
      4) Useful if frequent or prolonged febrile seizures
   b. Ibuprofen: randomized placebo-controlled studies of ibuprofen use during febrile illnesses have failed to show statistically significant benefit

REFERENCES

Berkovic SF, Izzillo P, McMahon JM, Harkin LA, McIntosh AM, Phillips HA, et al. *LGI1* mutations in temporal lobe epilepsies. Neurology. 2004;62:1115-9.

Bradley WG, editor. Neurology in clinical practice. Vol 1 and 2. Philadelphia: Butterworth-Heinemann; 2004.

Browne TH, Holmes GL. Handbook of epilepsy. Philadelphia: Lippincott Williams & Wilkins; 2004.

Buchhalter JR, Jarrar RG. Therapeutics in pediatric epilepsy, part 2: epilepsy surgery and vagus nerve stimulation. Mayo Clin Proc. 2003;78:371-8.

Cascino GB, Britton JW, Buchhalter J, Shin C, So, EL. Advances in epilepsy surgery evaluation and treatment. Continuum: Lifelong Learning Neurol. 2000;6:45-65.

Cohen-Gadol AA, Britton JW, Wetjen NM, Marsh WR, Meyer FB, Raffel C. Neurostimulation therapy for epilepsy: current modalities and future directions. Mayo Clin Proc. 2003;78:238-48.

Cohen-Gadol AA, Stoffman MR, Spencer DD. Emerging surgical and radiotherapeutic techniques for treating epilepsy. Curr Opin Neurol. 2003;16:213-9.

Daube JR, editor. Clinical neurophysiology. 2nd ed. New York: Oxford University Press; 2002.

Depondt C, Van Paesschen W, Matthijs G, Legius E, Martens K, Demaerel P, et al. Familial temporal lobe epilepsy with febrile seizures. Neurology. 2002;58:1429-33.

Fenichel GM. Clinical pediatric neurology: a signs and symptoms approach. Philadelphia: Saunders; 2001.

Handforth A, DeGiorgio CM, Schachter SC, Uthman BM, Naritoku DK, Tecoma ES, et al. Vagus nerve stimulation therapy for partial-onset seizures: a randomized active-control trial. Neurology. 1998;51:48-55.

International League Against Epilepsy. Epilepsy syndromes and related conditions. 2004 [cited 2004 Dec]. Available from: http://www.ilae-epilepsy.org/Visitors/Centre/ctf/syndromes.cfm.

International League Against Epilepsy. Seizure types: epileptic seizure types and precipitating stimuli for reflex seizures. 2004 [cited 2004 Dec]. Available from: http://www.ilae-epilepsy.org/Visitors/Centre/ctf/seizure_types.cfm.

International League Against Epilepsy Task Force on Epilepsy Classification and Terminology. A proposed diagnostic scheme for people with epileptic seizures and with epilepsy. 2004 [cited 2005 Apr 19]. Available from: http://www.ilae-epilepsy.org/Visitors/Centre/ctf/overview.cfm.

Jarrar RG, Buchhalter JR. Therapeutics in pediatric epilepsy, part 1: the new antiepileptic drugs and the ketogenic diet. Mayo Clin Proc. 2003;78:359-70.

Manno EM. New management strategies in the treatment of status epilepticus. Mayo Clin Proc. 2003;78:508-18.

Noseworthy J, editor. Neurological therapeutics: principles and practice. Vol 1. London: Martin Dunitz; 2003.

Offringa M, Bossuyt PM, Lubsen J, Ellenberg JH, Nelson KB, Knudsen FU, et al. Risk factors for seizure recurrence in children with febrile seizures: a pooled analysis of individual patient data from five studies. J Pediatr. 1994;124:574-84.

Offringa M, Moyer VA. Evidence based paediatrics: evidence based management of seizures associated with fever. BMJ. 2001;323:1111-4.

Pennell PB. Antiepileptic drug pharmacokinetics during pregnancy and lactation. Neurology. 2003;61 Suppl 2:S35-42.

So EL. Classifications and epidemiologic considerations of epileptic seizures and epilepsy. Neuroimaging Clin N Am. 1995;5:513-26.

So EL. Role of neuroimaging in the management of seizure disorders. Mayo Clin Proc. 2002;77:1251-64.

So EL. Seizure type determination and localization by video-EEG (unpublished data).

So EL. Selection and adjustment of anti-epileptic drugs (unpublished data).

Tatum WO IV, Liporace J, Benbadis SR, Kaplan PW. Updates on the treatment of epilepsy in women. Arch Intern Med. 2004;164:137-45.

The Vagus Nerve Stimulation Study Group. A randomized controlled trial of chronic vagus nerve stimulation for treatment of medically intractable seizures. Neurology. 1995;45:224-30.

Wyllie E, editor. The treatment of epilepsy: principles and practice. 2nd ed. Baltimore: Williams & Wilkins; 1997.

Yerby MS. Management issues for women with epilepsy: neural tube defects and folic acid supplementation. Neurology. 2003;61 Suppl 2:S23-6.

QUESTIONS

1. In benign myoclonus of infancy, the EEG is characterized by:
   a. 3-Hz spike-and-wave pattern
   b. Atypical spike-and-wave pattern
   c. Normal pattern
   d. Polyspike-and-wave pattern
   e. Hypsarrhythmia

2. Mutations of *KCNQ2* on chromosome 20 are seen in:
   a. Early myoclonic encephalopathy
   b. Benign familial neonatal convulsions
   c. Aicardi's syndrome
   d. Benign childhood epilepsy with centrotemporal spikes
   e. Juvenile myoclonic epilepsy

3. Medications most likely to worsen absence seizures are:
   a. GABAergic agent
   b. Sodium channel inhibitor
   c. T-type calcium channel antagonist
   d. Glutamate antagonist
   e. Anesthetic agent

4. Automatisms can be seen in:
   a. Partial complex seizures
   b. Absence seizures
   c. Atypical absence seizures
   d. All the above
   e. a and b

5. A seizure beginning gradually with an early, nonforced left head turn, later followed by a forced right head turn, most likely localizes to the:
   a. Left frontal lobe
   b. Left temporal lobe
   c. Right frontal lobe
   d. Right temporal lobe
   e. a or b

6. Which of the following is suggestive of a nonepileptic behavioral event rather than a seizure?
   a. Thrashing of extremities
   b. Thrashing of head and neck
   c. Ictal laughter
   d. Ictal grunting or moaning
   e. Ictal spitting

7. If a patient's blood level of phenytoin is 2 mg/mL and the desired blood level is 12 µg/mL, what additional intravenous dose should be given?
   a. 20 mg/kg
   b. 14 mg/kg
   c. 8 mg/kg
   d. 6 mg/kg
   e. 4 mg/kg

8. Which of the following can reduce the effectiveness of low-dose oral contraceptives?
   a. Phenytoin
   b. Valproate
   c. Oxcarbazepine
   d. All the above
   e. None of the above

9. Drug concentrations of which of the following anticonvulsants are *not* affected by liver enzyme-inducing and inhibiting drugs?
   a. Lamotrigine and topiramate
   b. Oxcarbazepine and gabapentin
   c. Levetiracetam and gabapentin
   d. All the above
   e. None of the above

10. Felbamate is particularly associated with a high rate of complications due to:
    a. Liver autoinduction
    b. Stevens-Johnson syndrome
    c. Purple glove syndrome
    d. Worsening of absence seizures
    e. Aplastic anemia and severe hepatotoxicity

11. Hypotension, lipidemia, and metabolic acidosis can be seen with infusion of:
    a. Propofol
    b. Phenobarbital
    c. Lorazepam
    d. Fosphenytoin
    e. Midazolam

12. When advising an epileptic woman about pregnancy, which of the following would *not* be true?
    a. The benefits of nursing probably outweigh the risks for some anticonvulsants
    b. Most (>90%) babies born to epileptic women are healthy
    c. Free drug levels often decrease during pregnancy

d. The incidence of spina bifida is increased with valproate and carbamazepine therapy
e. Folate supplementation has been proved to prevent spina bifida caused by valproate

13. A SISCOM (subtraction ictal SPECT coregistered to MRI) focus reflects:
a. A hypermetabolic focus
b. A hyperperfused focus
c. A relative ictal focus of hyperperfusion, as compared with interictal SPECT
d. A relative ictal hypermetabolic focus, as compared with interictal SPECT
e. None of the above

14. All the following are positive predictors of freedom from seizures following epilepsy surgery except:
a. Circumscribed MRI lesion
b. Focus in eloquent cortex
c. Focal interictal discharges
d. Consistent semiology
e. Focal SISCOM abnormality

15. Antibodies to which of the following have been implicated in the pathogenesis of Rasmussen's encephalitis?
a. GABA receptors
b. Nicotinic acetylcholine receptors
c. Voltage-gated sodium channels
d. Glutamate receptors

ANSWERS

1. Answer: c.
Benign myoclonus of infancy is a nonepileptic disorder with a normal EEG. The symptoms can mimic infantile spasms. However, the characteristic interictal hypsarrhythmia pattern of infantile spasms is not present in benign myoclonus of infancy.

2. Answer: b.
Benign familial neonatal convulsions, or "fifth-day fits," are caused by a mutation in the voltage-gated potassium channel *KCNQ2* gene on chromosome 20. This mutation impairs potassium-dependent repolarization, leading to neuronal hyperexcitability.

3. Answer: a.
Absence seizures are driven by T-type calcium channels of the thalamus. Ethosuximide inhibits these channels, whereas GABAergic drugs, by promoting $GABA_B$ receptors, promote these channels. As a result, GABAergic drugs (vigabatrin, tiagabine) worsen absence seizures.

4. Answer: d.
Automatisms are seen most commonly in partial complex seizures but can also be seen in absence and atypical absence seizures.

5. Answer: b.
An early, nonforced head turn suggests seizure localization to the ipsilateral temporal lobe. Forced head turns suggest localization to the hemisphere contralateral to the direction of gaze. Forced head turns typically occur early, with explosive onset in frontal lobe seizures and later in temporal lobe seizures, as the focal seizure generalizes. An early nonforced left head turn, followed by a late forced right head turn, localizes best to the left temporal lobe.

6. Answer: b.
Frontal lobe seizures often involve violent thrashing of the extremities. Thrashing of the head and neck, in contrast, suggests a nonepileptic behavioral event (pseudoseizure). Ictal laughter is seen in gelastic seizures (hypothalamus or medial frontal lobe). Vocalizations, including grunting or moaning, are suggestive of frontal lobe seizures, whereas ictal spitting suggests right temporal lobe involvement.

7. Answer: c.
To estimate a loading dose in a patient with a subtherapeutic level, the additional dose (mg/kg) = volume of distribution

$(0.7) \times$ (phenytoin blood level desired – patient's current phenytoin blood level) μg/mL.
$$0.7 \times (12 - 2) = 7 \text{ mg/kg}$$

Note that this estimate does not hold true as the phenytoin level approaches zero-order kinetics. Therefore, above 10 μg/mL, small dosage increases can dramatically raise the blood level of phenytoin.

8. Answer: d.
The effectiveness of low-dose oral contraceptives is reduced by many anticonvulsants, including (but not limited to) liver enzyme-inducing anticonvulsants. Although oxcarbazepine exhibits less liver enzyme induction than carbamazepine, it can still reduce the effectiveness of low-dose oral contraceptives. Valproate, a liver enzyme inhibitor, is also associated with reduced effectiveness.

9. Answer: c.
Levetiracetam and gabapentin are excreted predominantly unchanged in the urine. Their concentrations are not affected by liver enzyme-inducing and inhibiting drugs.

10. Answer: e.
Felbamate is a broad-spectrum anticonvulsant. However, its use is limited by a relatively high rate of aplastic anemia and potentially fatal hepatotoxicity, requiring frequent blood monitoring.

11. Answer: a.
Propofol infusion syndrome is the triad of hypotension, lipidemia, and metabolic acidosis. This is seen most commonly in children who have metabolic enzyme deficiencies, but it can occur in adults.

12. Answer: e.
Most antiepileptic drugs are associated with an increased risk of neural tube defects. Specifically, valproate and carbamazepine have been associated with spina bifida. Folate supplementation has been proved to reduce the risk of neural tube defects in the general population. Although folate is recommended, it is not clear whether it has comparable protective benefits in women with epilepsy.

13. Answer: c.
SISCOM involves subtracting ictal SPECT from interictal SPECT. A seizure focus is typically reflected by a relative area of hyperperfusion in ictal SPECT compared with the interictal

study. PET scans using [^{18}F]fluoro-2-deoxy-D-glucose as the ligand reflect metabolic activity.

14. Answer: b.
A seizure focus in eloquent cortex is more challenging to remove in total without creating a neurologic deficit. Therefore, focal cortical resection of a focus in eloquent cortex has a lower success rate than resection in noneloquent cortex.

15. Answer: d.
Antibodies to glutamate receptor-3 (GLUR3) have been implicated in the pathogenesis of Rasmussen's encephalitis.

NEUROCUTANEOUS SYNDROMES

13

Lenora M. Lehwald, M.D.

Kelly D. Flemming, M.D.

I. DEFINITION

A. Neurocutaneous Disorders
1. Formerly called phakomatoses
2. Group of diseases with characteristic cutaneous and neurologic findings and most with familial tendencies
3. Often have dysplasia of other organ systems

B. Overview of Selected Neurocutaneous Disorders
(Table 13-1)

II. NEUROFIBROMATOSIS

A. Neurofibromatosis
1. Most common neurocutaneous disorder
2. Several distinctive types

B. Two Most Common Types: neurofibromatosis 1 (NF1) and 2 (NF2)

C. Less Common Variants
1. Familial café au lait spots
2. Familial schwannomatosis
3. Mosaic (segmental) NF1 and NF2: neurocutaneous involvement of limited region of body

D. Neurofibromatosis 1 (von Recklinghausen's disease, "peripheral neurofibromatosis")
1. Epidemiology
   a. NF1: 96% of all cases of neurofibromatosis
   b. Prevalence: 1:3,000
2. Genetics
   a. Autosomal dominant
      1) Variable expression
      2) Near complete penetrance
      3) Nearly 50% are new mutations
   b. *NF1* gene

1) Tumor suppressor gene (chromosome 17q11.2)
2) Codes for neurofibromin (protein involved in regulation of Ras signaling pathway)
   a) Loss of *NF1* gene expression: absence of neurofibromin
   b) Absence of neurofibromin leads to increased Ras activity and increased cell proliferation, resulting in neoplasms
   c) Neurofibromin may also regulate cyclic adenosine monophosphate levels
3. Presenting symptoms
   a. May be due to specific tumors, conditions associated with NF1, or overall disease
   b. Common symptoms
      1) Cognitive deficits and learning disabilities
      2) Pain in specific nerve distribution due to presence of a neurofibroma
      3) Visual complaints (may be related to optic glioma)
      4) Seizures (may be due to intracranial tumors)
      5) Headaches (may be migraine or intracranial pressure or mass)
      6) Pruritus
      7) Progressive neurologic deficits (due to neurofibroma or other tumors)
4. Neurofibromas
   a. Are peripheral nerve sheath tumors
   b. Are one of hallmark findings and *most* common tumor in NF1
   c. Often present in puberty and increase in number and size with age
   d. May be circumscribed (cutaneous or subcutaneous) or noncircumscribed (plexiform)
   e. Are typically benign, but plexiform neurofibromas may undergo malignant transformation
   f. May be asymptomatic or symptomatic (pain within a nerve distribution)
   g. Commonly located near a spinal nerve root
   h. Plexiform neurofibromas

Table 13-1. Review Table of Neurocutaneous Diseases and Syndromes

Syndrome	Inheritance	Genetics	Cutaneous findings	Neurologic findings	Other
Neurofibromatosis 1	Autosomal dominant	*NF1* gene (17q11)	Café au lait spots	Neurofibroma Lisch nodules Optic glioma May have learning disorder	MRI may show T2 signal change in subcortical regions in addition to tumors
Neurofibromatosis 2	Autosomal dominant	*NF2* gene (22q12)	May or may not have café au lait spots Cutaneous and subcutaneous schwannomas	Bilateral vestibular schwannoma Meningioma, ependymoma, and other nerve schwannomas common	Subcapsular cataracts common
Tuberous sclerosis complex	Autosomal dominant	*TSC1* gene (9q34.3) *TSC2* gene (16p13.3)	Ash-leaf spot Shagreen patches Adenoma sebaceum	Seizures (infantile spasm) Cortical tubers Subependymal giant cell astrocytoma	Vogt's triad: seizures, mental retardation, adenoma sebaceum Other affected organs: kidneys (angiomyoli-poma), heart (rhabdo-myoma), eyes (astrocytic hamartoma), lungs (LAM)
Sturge-Weber syndrome	Sporadic		Port wine stain (usually in ophthalmic division CN V region ipsilateral to angiomatosis)	Leptomeningeal angiomatosis Seizures Focal deficits	Skull X-ray or CT may show tram-track sign
Hereditary hemorrhagic telangiectasia	Autosomal dominant	*HHT1* gene (9q34) *HHT2* gene (12q13)	Mucocutaneous telangiectasias	Various types of cerebral vascular malformations Ischemic stroke	Epistaxis and gastro-intestinal tract bleeding are most common manifestations
Incontinentia pigmenti	X-linked dominant	NEMO/IKKγ gene (Xq28)	"Marble cake" hyperpigmentation Diffuse hypopig-mented retina	Mental retardation and seizures may occur	Abnormal dentition is common
von Hippel-Lindau disease	Autosomal dominant	*VHL* gene (3p26-p255)	Retinal heman-gioblastoma	Hemangioblastoma (most commonly cerebellum)	Renal cell carcinoma Pheochromocytoma
Cerebrotendinous xanthoma	Autosomal recessive	Chromosome 2q33	Tendon xanthoma	May develop mental retardation	Accelerated atherosclerosis Increased plasma and bile levels of cholestanol
Ehlers-Danlos syndrome type IV	Autosomal dominant	*COL3A1* gene (chromosome 2)	Skin hypermobility Easy bruising	Arterial dissection Carotid-cavernous fistula Intracranial aneurysm	Deficiency in type III collagen
Pseudoxanthoma elasticum	Autosomal recessive	*ABCC6* gene (16p13.1)	"Plucked chicken skin" appearance	Arterial disease from elastin degeneration Cerebral aneurysm	Angioid streaks of retina Retinal hemorrhage Cardiovascular and peripheral vascular disease

Table 13-1. **(continued)**

Syndrome	Inheritance	Genetics	Cutaneous findings	Neurologicv findings	Other
Menkes' syndrome (kinky hair disease)	X-linked recessive	*MNK* gene (Xq13)	Colorless, friable hair	Developmental delay and regression Tortuous arteries	Low serum levels of copper and ceruloplasmin
Epidermal nevus syndrome	Sporadic or autosomal dominant		Epidermal nevi	Mental retardation may occur Seizures may occur	Multiple subtypes
Xeroderma pigmentosa	Autosomal recessive	Heterogeneity of molecular defects	Photosensitivity Erythema and blistering of skin Excess freckling Prone to basal cell carcinoma	Some developmental retardation May develop ataxia Sensorineural hearing loss	Gene products involved in nucleotide excision repair mechanisms in DNA damaged by UV radiation Conjunctiva, eyelid, and retinal damage common
Hypomelanosis of Ito	Sporadic	Mosaicism at several loci	Macular hypo-pigmented areas May have abnor-malities of hair growth and color	Seizures Mental retardation	
Fabry's disease	X-linked recessive	*GAL* gene (Xq22)	Angiokeratoma	Ischemic stroke Small-fiber peripheral neuropathy Pain crises	α-Galactosidase A deficiency May have kidney, heart, and corneal manifesta-tions
Ataxia-telangiectasia	Autosomal recessive	*ATM* gene (11q22-23)	Oculocutaneous telangiectasia	Progressive ataxia	Immunodeficiency Malignancies

CN, cranial nerve; CT, computed tomography; LAM, lymphangioleiomyomatosis; MRI, magnetic resonance imaging.

1) Specific to NF1 and major cause of morbidity
   a) Irregular, thickened, noncircumscribed (Fig. 13-1)
   b) Can envelop vital structures, can involve orbit
   c) May be disfiguring
2) Malignant peripheral nerve sheath tumors may develop from plexiform neurofibromas
   a) 3% to 5% of NF1 patients develop malignant peripheral nerve sheath tumors
   b) Analysis of these tumors has shown epidermal growth factor receptor amplification and deletion of p16 tumor suppressor gene in addition to *NF1* deletion
   c) Difficult to treat because of invasive nature
5. Other tumors
  a. Optic nerve gliomas
   1) Second most common tumor in NF1
   2) A low-grade pilocytic astrocytoma arising from optic nerve or chiasm
   3) May be an incidental finding or present as progressive loss of vision and optic atrophy
  b. Intracranial tumors
   1) Hemispheric astrocytomas
   2) Solitary or multicentric meningiomas
   3) Pilocytic astrocytoma (hypothalamus, brainstem, cerebellum)
  c. Schwann-cell tumors on any nerve
  d. Pheochromocytoma (not in children)
  e. Malignant tumors may include
   1) Neuroblastoma
   2) Ganglioglioma
   3) Sarcoma
   4) Juvenile chronic myeloid leukemia
   5) Rhabdomyosarcoma
6. Other associated conditions and symptoms of NF1

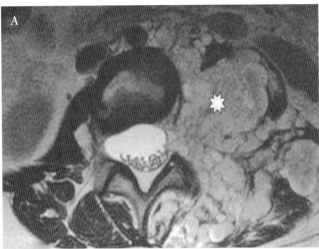

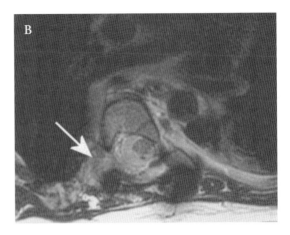

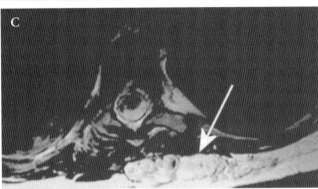

Fig. 13-1. MRI of thoracolumbar spine of a 5-year-old patient with neurofibromatosis type 1, showing plexiform neurofibromas at multiple levels. *A*, An extensive plexiform neurofibroma (*star*) extended from the lower thoracic-upper lumbar neural foramina on the left into the paraspinal muscles, left psoas muscle, and retroperitoneal space, displacing the left kidney laterally (not shown). *B*, The plexiform neurofibroma at mid-thoracic level extends from the right subpleural space into the neural foramen (*arrow*) and spinal canal around the thecal sac. Note that the patient had a decompressive laminectomy at this level. *C*, A subcutaneous plexiform neurofibroma (*arrow*) in same patient.

a. Macrocephaly
   1) Aqueductal stenosis
   2) Hydrocephalus
b. Kyphoscoliosis, often progressive (10% of cases)
c. Hypertension
d. Arterial occlusive disease
   1) Renal artery stenosis
   2) Moyamoya disease
e. Intracranial aneurysms (Table 13-2)
f. Migraine
g. Epilepsy (10% of cases)
h. Focal neurologic deficits
i. Learning disabilities (40%-60% of cases)
   1) Increased incidence of attention-deficit disorder
   2) Cognitive disabilities may include visuospatial problems, spatial-memory problems, and visuomotor integration skills
j. Proptosis
k. Glaucoma
l. Short stature
m. Constipation
7. Diagnosis

a. Diagnostic criteria require two or more of seven items
   1) At least six café au lait spots (hyperpigmented, oval, light brown skin macules)
      a) At least 5-mm diameter in prepubertal patients
      b) At least 1.5-cm diameter in postpubertal patients
      c) Typically located on trunk
   2) Axillary and/or inguinal freckling (usually present between ages 3 and 5 years)
   3) At least two Lisch nodules (iris hamartomas)
   4) Neurofibromas: more than one cutaneous neurofibroma or one plexiform neurofibroma
   5) Characteristic bone anomalies
   6) Optic nerve glioma
   7) Diagnosis of NF1 in first-degree relative
b. Mutation analysis available
8. Imaging
a. Magnetic resonance imaging (MRI) of head
   1) Shows nonenhancing, well-circumscribed hyperintense T2 signal lesions in several locations: basal ganglia (Fig. 13-2), cerebellum, brainstem
   2) No known prognostic significance
b. Other: cranial and spinal imaging may show incidental

Table 13-2. **Genetic Disorders Associated With Intracranial Aneurysms**

Disease	Inheritance pattern	Locus	Gene	Gene product
Achondroplasia	AD	4p16.3	FGFR3	Fibroblast growth factor receptor 3
Autosomal dominant polycystic kidney disease	AD	16p13.3	PKD1	Polycystin
Ehlers-Danlos syndrome type I	AD	9q	COL5A1	Collagen type V
Ehlers-Danlos syndrome type IV	AD	2q31	COL3A1	Collagen type III
Fabry's disease	XL-R	Xq22.1	GLA	α-Galactosidase A
Hereditary hemorrhagic telangiectasia	AD	9q34.1	HHT1, ENG	Endoglin
		12q13	HHT2, ALK-1	Activin receptor-like kinase
Marfan's syndrome	AD	15q21.1`	FBM1	Fibrillin-1
Neurofibromatosis type 1	AD	17q11.2	NF1	Neurofibromin
Noonan's syndrome	AD	12q22	NS1	Unknown
Osteogenesis imperfecta type 1	AD	17q22.1	COL1A1	Collagen type I
		7q22.1	COL1A2	Collagen type I
Pompe's disease	AR	17q23	GAA	α-Glucosidase
Pseudoxanthoma elasticum	AR	16p13.1	PXE	Transmembrane transport protein
Tuberous sclerosis complex	AD	9q34.3	TSC1	Hamartin
		16p13.3	TSC2	Tuberin
α1-Antitrypsin deficiency	ACoD	14q32.1	PI	α1-Antitrypsin

ACoD, autosomal codominant; AD, autosomal dominant; AR, autosomal recessive; XL-R, X-linked recessive.

NIH Diagnostic Criteria for Neurofibromatosis Type 1
Two or more of the following:
1. ≥6 café au lait spots
2. ≥2 neurofibromas of any type or ≥1 plexiform neurofibroma
3. Freckling (Crowe's sign) in axilla or groin
4. Optic glioma
5. ≥2 Lisch nodules (benign pigmented iris hamartomas)
6. Distinctive bony lesion
7. First-degree relative with neurofibromatosis type 1

or symptomatic neurofibromas or other tumors
9. Treatment
   a. Genetic counseling, anticipatory guidance, surveillance for treatable complications
   b. Annual physical examination (including blood pressure screening, growth, and pubertal status) and ophthalmologic examinations during school years
   c. Evaluate and treat for learning disabilities early
   d. Scoliosis and other skeletal abnormalities need observation, may require treatment

e. Surgical evaluation and treatment for symptomatic neurofibromas or other tumors

E. **Neurofibromatosis 2** (bilateral acoustic neurofibromatosis, "central neurofibromatosis")
1. Overview
   a. Autosomal dominant disorder
   b. Typical characteristics: bilateral vestibular schwannoma (acoustic neuroma), other nervous system tumors, ocular abnormalities
2. Epidemiology
   a. NF2: 3% of all cases of neurofibromatosis
   b. Prevalence: 1:40,000
3. Genetics
   a. Autosomal dominant: penetrance close to 100% by age 60 years
   b. NF2 gene
      1) Tumor suppressor gene (chromosome 22q12)
      2) Codes for merlin (also called schwannomin)
      3) Merlin
         a) Highly expressed in adult Schwann cells, meningeal cells, the lens, and nerve cells
         b) Structurally similar to family of proteins that link cytoskeleton to cell surface
      4) Patients with nonsense or frameshift NF2 mutations

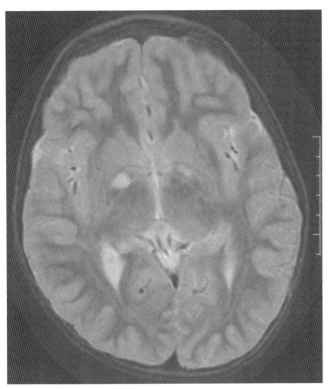

Fig. 13-2. MRI of brain of patient with neurofibromatosis 1. This T2-weighted image shows increased T2 signal in basal ganglia bilaterally.

have severe disease; those with missense mutations, in-frame deletions, or large deletions have mild disease

    5) Standard mutation detection

        a) Bilateral vestibular schwannomas

          i) Identify mutation in 66% of patients

          ii) Majority are truncated mutations

          iii) More severe clinical disease

        b) Without bilateral vestibular lesions

          i) Linkage analysis is test of choice

          ii) Provides more than 99% certainty

          iii) Patients tend to harbor missense mutations

          iv) Milder clinical disease

4. Clinical manifestations

  a. Symptoms often present in teenage years

  b. Symptoms depend on associated lesions (see below)

5. Vestibular schwannoma (also called acoustic neuroma)

  a. Nerve sheath tumor that typically occurs bilaterally in NF2

  b. Clinical presentation often includes progressive hearing loss, tinnitus, and imbalance

  c. MRI

    1) Technique: thin sections through internal auditory canals; performed with and without gadolinium contrast

    2) Appearance on MRI

      a) Extra-axial mass at cerebellopontine angle

      b) Typically hypointense or isointense on T1 images, with intense enhancement following contrast and mildly increased signal on T2

6. Other associated conditions or symptoms

  a. Spinal and cranial nerve (CN) schwannomas (CN V-XII)

  b. Intracranial meningiomas (often multiple)

  c. Spinal cord: ependymomas, gliomas

  d. Posterior subcapsular cataracts (85% of patients)

  e. Retinal hamartomas

  f. Occasional café au lait spots (45% of patients)

  g. Skin plaquelike lesion (70% of patients)

  h. Mononeuropathy (CN VII most common)

  i. Seizures

  j. Antigenic nerve growth factor is increased

7. Clinical criteria for diagnosis—NF2 is diagnosed in patients with one of the following:

  a. Bilateral vestibular schwannomas

  b. A first-degree relative with NF2 *and*

    1) Unilateral vestibular schwannoma *or*

    2) Any two of meningioma, schwannoma, glioma, neurofibroma, posterior subcapsular lenticular opacities

  c. Unilateral vestibular schwannoma *and* any two of meningioma, schwannoma, glioma, neurofibroma, posterior subcapsular lenticular opacities

  d. Multiple meningiomas *and*

    1) Unilateral vestibular schwannoma *or*

    2) Any two of schwannoma, glioma, neurofibroma, cataract

8. Clinical management

  a. Genetic counseling

  b. Anticipatory guidance and surveillance for treatable complications

  c. Baseline MRI of brain and spinal cord: reimage and monitor, especially if symptomatic

  d. Hearing and speech evaluation and augmentation

  e. Ophthalmologic evaluation

  f. Annually

    1) Neurologic evaluation

    2) Cranial MRI

    3) Audiography

9. Management of acoustic neuroma

  a. Observation

  b. Surgical management

  c. Stereotactic radiosurgery

  d. Fractionated radiotherapy

III. FAMILIAL SCHWANNOMATOSIS

A. Features
1. Rare form of neurofibromatosis characterized by multiple pathologically proven schwannomas on cranial, spinal, and peripheral nerves
2. Vestibular schwannomas or other kinds of tumors or manifestations of NF1 and NF2 do not develop

B. Genetics: autosomal dominant with incomplete penetrance and variable expression

C. Symptom: pain
1. In distribution of the schwannoma
2. Can occur in any part of the body
3. Only a single part of the body may be affected

D. Management
1. Surgical removal of symptomatic schwannoma if possible
2. If inoperable, multidisciplinary pain management

IV. TUBEROUS SCLEROSIS COMPLEX (BOURNEVILLE'S DISEASE)

A. Overview
1. Autosomal dominant
2. Often referred to as the tuberous sclerosis complex (TSC) because of involvement of multiple organ systems by development of distinctive tumors or hamartomas
3. Organs commonly involved: brain, kidney, skin, eye, heart
4. Classic triad (Vogt's triad): seizures, mental retardation, and adenoma sebaceum (less than 1/3 of patients display all three features)

B. Epidemiology
1. Prevalence: 1:6,000 to 1:9,000
2. Second most common neurocutaneous disorder

Hallmark Findings in Tuberous Sclerosis Complex
Mental retardation

Seizures

Adenoma sebaceum

C. Genetics
1. Autosomal dominant disorder with almost complete penetrance
2. Characterized by a wide phenotypic spectrum, even within same family
3. Mutations of two different genes can cause TSC
4. New mutations occur in 65% to 75% of cases
   a. Severely affected patients often have a new mutation
   b. No feature that distinguishes which of the two genes is defective
5. *TSC1* gene
   a. Tumor suppressor gene (chromosome 9q34.3)
   b. Codes for hamartin
   c. If this gene is affected, patient may have less risk of cognitive impairment than if *TSC2* gene is affected
6. *TSC2* gene
   a. Tumor suppressor gene (chromosome 16p13.3)
   b. Codes for tuberin
      1) Guanosine triphosphatase-activating leucine zipper protein
      2) Contiguous with adult polycystic kidney disease type 1 gene : may explain development of multiple renal cysts
7. Hamartin and tuberin bind to form a complex, explaining why a mutation in either gene may result in similar phenotype

D. Pathology
1. Hamartias, hamartomas, hamartoblastomas
   a. Hamartia
      1) Characterized by misaligned groups of dysplastic cells appropriate for the organ or tissue
      2) These undifferentiated cells do not multiply or grow more rapidly than normal cells of that particular organ
   b. Hamartoma
      1) Well-circumscribed group of dysplastic cells
      2) These cells have a propensity to multiply excessively, thus growing as benign tumors that may or may not become symptomatic
   c. Hamartoblastoma: rare malignant tumor derived from hamartoma
   d. Development and growth of hamartomas: age-dependent
   e. Brain hamartias and hamartomas include
      1) Most patients with TSC have at least one supratentorial brain lesion (infratentorial lesions less common)
      2) Cortical tubers (Fig. 13-3 and 13-4): common hamartia found in cortical gyri; may calcify over time
      3) White matter abnormalities: dysplastic changes of

white matter may occur; may have white matter linear migration lines

4) Subependymal nodules
   a) Hamartoma along ventricular surface
   b) Commonly located near caudate nucleus and just posterior to foramen of Monro
   c) May have the appearance of melting candle wax, so-called candle guttering, pathologically (Fig. 13-5) and on radiographs
   d) May be calcified

5) Subependymal giant cell astrocytoma (SEGA) (Fig. 13-6)
   a) Hamartoma located near foramen of Monro
   b) Often causes obstructive hydrocephalus
   c) May calcify and grow histologically benign

f. Other organs may be affected: kidneys, heart, eyes, lungs, skin (Table 13-3)

g. Not involved: muscles, peripheral nerves, craniospinal nerve roots

2. Rare malignancies can occur in TSC: renal malignancies (renal cell, malignant angiomyolipoma) and glioblastoma multiforme; may be more common in *TSC2* gene mutations

E. Symptoms
1. Epilepsy
   a. Most common neurologic manifestation
   b. Presenting complaint in majority of patients, more than 95% of infants
   c. Seizures
      1) Partial
      2) Generalized: if onset before age 5 years, Lennox-Gastaut syndrome may develop
      3) Often refractory
      4) Substantial risk of status epilepticus
   d. Infantile spasms
      1) Hypsarrhythmic electroencephalographic (EEG) pattern
      2) Poor prognosis
      3) Vigabatrin (not approved by U.S. Food and Drug Administration [FDA]) or ACTH may be efficacious

2. Obstructive hydrocephalus: caused by SEGA near foramen of Monro

3. Cognitive and behavior dysfunction (present in >50% of patients)
   a. Marked developmental delays
   b. Autism spectrum disorders

4. Other cerebral manifestations
   a. Pachygyria
   b. Subependymal nodules
   c. Intracranial aneurysms (Table 13-2)

5. Skin lesions
   a. Hypomelanotic skin macules (ash-leaf spot) (90% of patients) (Fig. 13-7)
   b. Facial angiofibromas (adenoma sebaceum) (75% of patients) (Fig. 13-8)

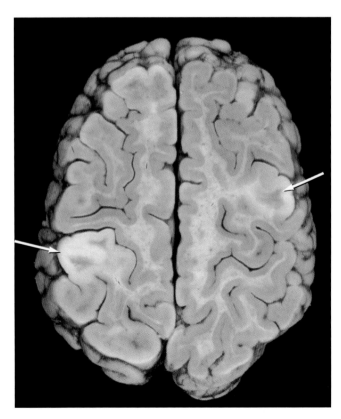

Fig. 13-3. Gross specimen of a cortical tuber (*arrows*) associated with tuberous sclerosis complex.

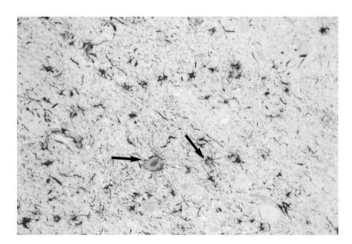

Fig. 13-4. Microscopic appearance of a cortical tuber. Note atypical astrocytes (*arrows*).

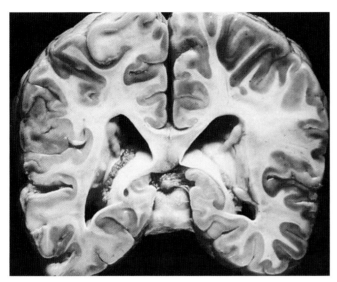

Fig. 13-5. "Candle guttering" of lateral ventricles in tuberous sclerosis complex. (From Scheithauer BW, Reagan TJ. Neuropathology. In: Gómez MR, Sampson JR, Whittemore VH, editors. Tuberous sclerosis complex. 3rd ed. New York: Oxford University Press; 1999. p. 101-44. Used with permission.)

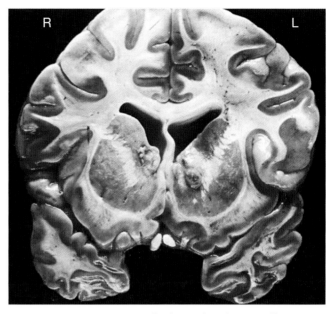

Fig. 13-6. Gross specimen of subependymal giant cell astrocytoma near foramen of Monro on right in patient with tuberous sclerosis complex. (From Scheithauer BW, Reagan TJ. Neuropathology. In: Gómez MR, Sampson JR, Whittemore VH, editors. Tuberous sclerosis complex. 3rd ed. New York: Oxford University Press; 1999. p. 101-44. Used with permission.)

    c. Ungual fibromas (21% of patients)
    d. Shagreen patches (19% of patients)
6. Cardiac manifestations
    a. Rhabdomyoma (50% of patients)
      1) May cause left ventricular outflow obstruction
      2) Majority are asymptomatic and spontaneously regress
    b. Dysrhythmias
      1) Wolff-Parkinson-White syndrome
      2) Ventricular arrhythmias
7. Ophthalmologic manifestations
    a. Most do not cause visual changes
    b. Retinal phakoma (mulberry lesions) (50% of patients)
    c. Astrocytomas of retina
8. Renal lesions (80% of patients)
    a. Pain: most frequent clinical symptom
    b. Second most common cause of morbidity in patients with TSC
    c. Simple cyst (25% of patients)
      1) Appear or disappear at any time
      2) May be multiple
    d. Angiomyolipomas (75% of patients)
      1) May be bilateral and multiple
      2) Increase in size with age
      3) Become symptomatic more commonly in females and with increasing age (by third decade)
      4) Clinical symptoms

        a) Lumbar pain
        b) Hematuria from slow bleeding
        c) Sudden hemorrhage (increased risk with increasing size >3.5 cm)
        d) Renal failure
        e) Arterial hypertension
      5) Treatment
        a) Options: observation, embolization, and total or partial nephrectomy
        b) Indication for treatment: if larger than 3.5 cm in diameter or symptomatic
9. Pulmonary manifestations (female predominance)
    a. Cystic lesions: may cause spontaneous pneumothorax
    b. Nodules
      1) Lymphangioleiomyomatosis (LAM)
        a) Rare disease can occur as isolated disorder (sporadic lymphangioleiomyomatosis)
        b) In TSC, exclusively affects females (34%)
        c) More common in women without mental retardation
        d) Present in third or fourth decade of life
        e) Severe symptoms (<1% of patients)
          i) Often fatal

Table 13-3.   Common Lesions in Patients With
Tuberous Sclerosis Complex

Organ	Hamartias	Hamartomas
Brain	Cortical tuber	Subependymal nodule
		Subependymal giant cell astrocytoma
Retina	Retinal depigmented spots	Astrocytic hamartoma
Skin	Hypomelanotic macules	Facial angiofibroma (adenoma sebaceum)
		Ungual fibroma
		Shagreen plaque
Heart		Rhabdomyoma
Kidney	Cysts	Angiomyolipoma
Lung		Lymphangioleiomyomatosis
Liver		Angiomyolipoma
Pancreas		Islet cell adenoma
Colorectal junction		Hamartomatous polyp
Adrenal gland		Angiomyolipoma
Thyroid gland		Papilliform adenoma
		Fetal thyroid adenoma
Gonads		Testicular angiomyolipoma
Bones	Cysts, osteomatous thickening	
Arteries	Wall defects (aneurysm)	

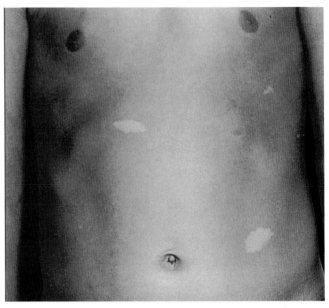

Fig. 13-7. Ash-leaf spot in a patient with tuberous sclerosis complex. These cutaneous findings may be seen best with a Wood's lamp examination.

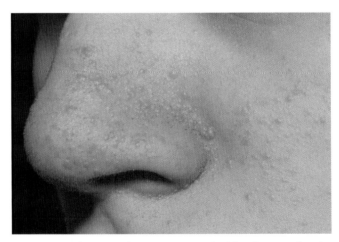

Fig. 13-8. Adenoma sebaceum associated with tuberous sclerosis complex.

    ii) Recurrent spontaneous pneumothorax
    iii) Hemoptysis
    iv) Chylothorax
    v) Respiratory failure
  c. Multifocal micronodular pneumocyte hyperplasia

F. **Diagnostic Criteria** (Table 13-4)
1. Definitive TSC: two major features or one major plus two minor features
2. Probable TSC: one major plus one minor feature
3. Possible TSC: one major or two minor features

G. **Imaging**
1. Plain skull radiographs: calcified subependymal nodules
2. Computed tomography (CT) of head: intracerebral calcifications
  a. Subependymal nodules along lateral ventricles

  b. Subependymal nodules may protrude into lateral ventricles producing candle-guttering appearance
3. MRI
  a. Supratentorial lesions (more common) may include
    1) Cortical tubers (Fig. 13-9)
    2) Subependymal nodules
    3) Subependymal giant cell astrocytoma
    4) Corpus callosum agenesis
    5) White matter linear migration lines
    6) Transmantle cortical dysplasia

Table 13-4. Diagnostic Criteria for Tuberous Sclerosis Complex

Major features	Minor features
Facial angiofibromas or forehead plaque	Multiple randomly distributed pits in dental enamel
Nontraumatic ungual or periungual fibroma	Hamartomatous rectal polyps
Hypomelanotic macules (>3)	Bone cysts
Shagreen patch (connective tissue nevus)	Cerebral white matter migration tracts
Cortical tuber	Gingival fibromas
Subependymal nodule	Nonrenal hamartoma
Subependymal giant cell astrocytoma	Retinal achromic patch
Multiple retinal nodular hamartomas	"Confetti" skin lesions
Cardiac rhabdomyoma, single or multiple	Multiple renal cysts
Lymphangioleiomyomatosis	
Renal angiomyolipoma	

  b. Infratentorial lesions may include
    1) Cerebellar calcifications
    2) Subependymal nodules or tubers within brainstem and fourth ventricle
    3) Agenesis or hypoplasia of cerebellum

H. Treatment
1. Genetic counseling
2. Anticipatory guidance and surveillance for treatable complications
  a. Seizures
    1) Antiepileptic drugs
    2) Infantile spasms: treated with ACTH or vigabatrin
    3) Partial seizures: epilepsy surgery should be considered
  b. Development should be followed closely
  c. Abdominal ultrasonography or CT every 1 to 3 years
  d. Chest radiographs at regular intervals
  e. Facial angiofibromas: treat with dermal abrasion
  f. Appropriate treatment of renal and pulmonary manifestations

V. STURGE-WEBER SYNDROME

A. Overview
1. Sporadic condition
2. Characterized by leptomeningeal angiomatosis and ipsilateral facial cutaneous vascular malformation called port-wine nevus, usually in distribution of ophthalmic division of CN V
3. Also known as encephalotrigeminal angiomatosis

B. Prevalence: 1:50,000

C. Pathology
1. Symptoms are generally related to leptomeningeal angiomatosis
2. Leptomeningeal angiomatosis
  a. A low-flow vascular malformation involving leptomeningeal vessels; often, poor superficial cortical venous drainage that can cause stasis and hypoxia
  b. Vascular malformation
    1) Usually unilateral (85% of patients), but can be bilateral
    2) Usually located in posterior parietal and occipital regions
  c. Leptomeningeal angiomatosis results in chronic ischemic damage to cerebral cortex because of repeated thrombosis; this may lead to progressive disease over time
  d. Although very rare, this type of vascular malformation does not typically cause subarachnoid hemorrhage
3. Port-wine nevus
  a. A cutaneous vascular malformation
  b. Distribution of ophthalmic division of CN V: forehead and upper eyelid or periorbital area
  c. Can be unilateral (more common) or bilateral; rarely, patients with Sturge-Weber syndrome may not have a port-wine nevus
  d. Note: most port-wine nevi are not due to Sturge-Weber syndrome
    1) Port-wine nevus involving the distribution of ophthalmic division of CN V increases probability of Sturge-Weber syndrome
    2) If child is born with nevus in ophthalmic division of CN V, head imaging should be considered

D. Clinical Manifestations
1. Seizures
  a. Occur in up to 75% to 90% of patients with Sturge-Weber syndrome by age 3 years
  b. Mean age at onset: 6 months
  c. Onset: during first year of life in 75% of patients, before age 2 years in 86%, and before age 5 years in 95%
  d. Typically focal motor, but secondary generalized tonic clonic seizures may develop; frequently, atonic, tonic, myoclonic, or infantile spasms

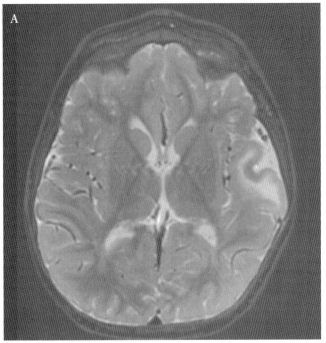 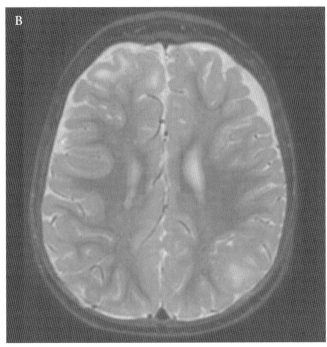

Fig. 13-9. T2-weighted MRI of brain with, *A*, mid and, *B*, upper axial sections from patient with tuberous sclerosis. Multiple cortical tubers involve both cerebral hemispheres. Note prominent involvement of the anterior left temporal lobe, with associated calvarial remodeling.

e. Associated with developmental delay and emotional and behavioral problems (higher incidence with earlier onset of seizures)

f. May be intractable (especially if seizure onset before age 2 years): these patients are more likely to have associated mental retardation

g. Seizures likely result from chronic hypoxia

2. Focal deficits

a. Hemiparesis

1) In 25% to 60% of patients with Sturge-Weber syndrome

2) Contralateral to leptomeningeal angiomatosis

3) Thought to be due to chronic hypoxia

b. Hemianopia can occur in up to 40% of patients with Sturge-Weber syndrome contralateral to leptomeningeal angiomatosis

c. Cerebral ischemia (transient or persistent)

1) Vascular steal phenomenon may develop around angioma, resulting in ischemia and parenchymal abnormalities

2) This may result in progressive calcification, gliosis, and atrophy

3) Dehydration or concurrent illness can increase chance of thrombosis

3. Vision and ocular abnormalities

a. Glaucoma can occur in eye ipsilateral to port-wine nevus

1) Glaucoma occurs only when the port-wine nevus involves eyelid; highest likelihood when both the upper and lower eyelids involved in the port-wine stain

2) May be present during infancy; highest incidence in first decade, although can occur at any age, even adults

b. Buphthalmos (enlargement of eye)

c. Choroidal hemangioma of eye

4. Headaches occur in about one-half of patients with Sturge-Weber syndrome

5. Developmental disorders

a. May occur in 50% to 75% of patients with Sturge-Weber syndrome

b. More common in patients with bilateral angiomatosis and onset of seizures before age 2 years

c. Developmental delay (although early development is usually normal)

d. Learning disorders, attention-deficit disorder, mental retardation

E. **Associated Conditions**

1. Extracranial angiomas

2. Macrocephaly

F. Subtypes

1. Type I: both facial and leptomeningeal angiomas; may have glaucoma
2. Type II: facial angioma alone; may have glaucoma
3. Type III: isolated leptomeningeal angiomatosis; usually no glaucoma

G. Diagnostic Testing

1. CT of head or skull radiography
   a. Calcification of the leptomeningeal angiomatosis produces so-called tram-track calcification, usually in the parieto-occipital area (Fig. 13-10)
   b. May not be seen in infancy, but 90% of patients with leptomeningeal angiomatosis have calcification noted by the end of second decade
2. MRI (Fig. 13-11)
   a. Atrophy ipsilateral to leptomeningeal angiomatosis
   b. Compensatory enlargement of ipsilateral lateral ventricle from cerebral atrophy
   c. Gadolinium-enhanced images show leptomeningeal angiomatosis
3. EEG: slowing over affected hemispheres and/or multifocal independent spikes

H. Treatment

1. Seizures
   a. Antiepileptic medications: carbamazepine and other medications used commonly for partial seizures
   b. If intractable to medications and unihemispheric, hemispherectomy may be considered in selected patients
2. Glaucoma: yearly ophthalmologic examination with treatment as necessary
3. Transient neurologic deficits: aspirin
4. Port-wine stain
   a. Laser therapy
   b. Cosmetic treatment has marked psychologic benefits

VI. HEREDITARY HEMORRHAGIC TELANGIECTASIA (HHT) (OSLER-WEBER-RENDU DISEASE)

A. Overview

1. Autosomal dominant
2. Characterized by mucocutaneous telangiectasias that occur in multiple organs
3. Epistaxis is most common presentation, followed by gastrointestinal bleeding
4. Neurologic manifestations: usually due to cerebral ischemia from paradoxical emboli through pulmonary fistulae

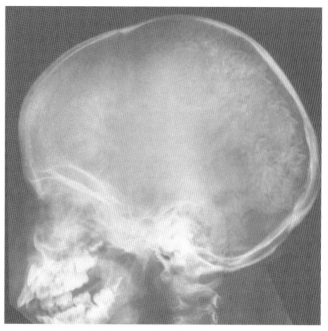

Fig. 13-10. Skull radiograph showing the tram-track sign. Calcification of leptomeningeal angiomatosis seen in Sturge-Weber syndrome.

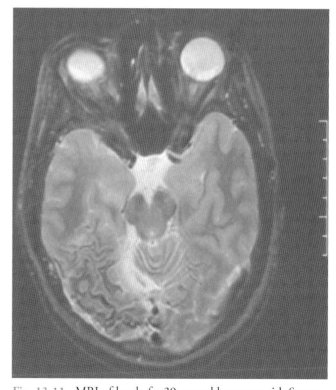

Fig. 13-11. MRI of head of a 39-year-old woman with Sturge-Weber syndrome. Note cortical calcification and atrophy involving the right posterior temporal and occipital lobes. Note also cerebellar atrophy, with prominent vessels superior to the right cerebellar hemisphere.

B. Epidemiology
1. Prevalence: 1:8,000
2. Clinical manifestations not generally present at birth; 71% of those with HHT have some manifestation of disease by age 16 years and 90% have or have had a manifestation by age 40 years

C. Genetics
1. Autosomal dominant
2. Variability of phenotype even among members of same family
3. Spontaneous mutation in 30% of patients
4. Subtypes
   a. HHT subtype 1
      1) *ENG* (endoglin) gene: chromosome 9q34
      2) 15 distinct mutations have been identified
      3) Higher incidence of pulmonary involvement
   b. HHT subtype 2
      1) *ALK-1* gene (activin receptor-like kinase): chromosome 12q13
      2) 12 distinct mutations have been identified
5. *ENG* and *ALK-1* encode proteins on vascular endothelial cells

D. Clinical Manifestations
1. Mucocutaneous telangiectasias: common locations are nasal cavity, oral cavity, lips, fingers
2. Most common presenting symptom (90% of patients): recurrent epistaxis
   a. Related to nasal cavity telangiectasia
   b. May require cauterization, embolization, or surgery
3. Gastrointestinal tract hemorrhage
   a. Related to gastrointestinal telangiectasia
   b. May present as iron deficiency anemia or overt gastrointestinal tract hemorrhage
   c. Occurs typically in mid-life
4. Pulmonary manifestations
   a. Typically develop and present after puberty
   b. Clinical symptoms as result of pulmonary arteriovenous malformations
      1) Dyspnea, cyanosis
      2) Hemoptysis
      3) Cerebral abscess, stroke, or transient ischemic attack (TIA) due to paradoxical shunting
5. Neurologic manifestations
   a. HHT should be considered in patients with multiple cerebral vascular malformations
   b. Cerebral and/or spinal arteriovenous malformations
   c. Cerebral aneurysms (Table 13-2)
   d. Cavernous angiomas
   e. Ischemic stroke (Table 13-5): most commonly from paradoxical embolus through pulmonary arteriovenous fistulae
   f. Brain abscess
   g. Migraine headache
6. Hepatic arteriovenous malformations may occur in up to 30% of HHT patients
7. Chronic anemia

E. Diagnosis (Table 13-6)
1. Definite: three criteria are present
2. Possible: two criteria are present
3. Unlikely: fewer than two criteria present

F. Management
1. Genetic counseling
2. Treatment of epistaxis and gastrointestinal tract bleeding
   a. Treat specific cause
   b. Transfusion as needed
   c. Iron supplementation
   d. Avoidance of anticoagulants, aspirin, and nonsteroidal anti-inflammatory drugs
   e. Hormone therapy (estrogen/progesterone) may have a role if patient is transfusion-dependent
3. Pulmonary arteriovenous malformations
   a. Can be detected on contrast echocardiography or thin-cut CT sections through chest
   b. Can be treated with embolization
   c. Subacute bacterial endocarditis antibiotic prophylaxis for dental or surgical procedure to prevent brain abscess formation
   d. Ischemic strokes are often due to paradoxical emboli, and evaluating for and treating pulmonary arteriovenous shunt should be considered
4. Cerebral arteriovenous malformations
   a. Debated whether asymptomatic patients with HHT should have screening tests for cerebral vascular malformations
   b. Treat individual malformation types (see Chapter 11, Cerebrovascular Disease)

VII. INCONTINENTIA PIGMENTI (BLOCH-SULZBERGER SYNDROME)

A. Overview
1. X-linked dominant disorder
2. Characterized by cutaneous lesions and abnormalities of teeth, eyes, central nervous system, and other organs

Table 13-5.   **Genetic Disorders Associated With Stroke**

Disease	Inheritance
Fabry's disease	X-linked recessive
	Xq22
	α-Galactosidase A deficiency
Hereditary hemorrhagic telangiectasia (HHT)	Autosomal dominant
	HHT type 1, endoglin gene, 9q
	HHT type 2, activin receptorlike kinase 1 (*ALK-1*), 12q
Mitochondrial encephalopathy, lactic acidosis, and stroke-like episodes (MELAS)	Maternally inherited
	Mitochondrial DNA mutation
	Respiratory chain enzymes, particularly complex I t-RNA$^{Leu(UUR)}$ (80% of patients)
Cereral autosomal dominant arteriopathy with subcortical infarcts and leukoencephalopathy (CADASIL)	Autosomal dominant
	Notch3 gene on chromosome 19
Sickle cell disease	Autosomal recessive
	β Globin gene
	Point mutation, glutamate to valine substitution
Homocystinuria	Autosomal recessive
	Cystathionine β-synthase (*CBS*) gene, 21q22.3
Factor V Leiden mutation	Autosomal dominant
	Factor V gene
Autosomal dominant polycystic kidney disease	Autosomal dominant
	Genetically heterogeneous
	PKD1, 16p
	PKD2, 4q
Carney's complex	Autosomal dominant
	Tumor suppressor gene
	Null mutation in type 1A subunit protein kinase A
Hereditary endotheliopathy with retinopathy, nephropathy, and stroke (HERNS)	Autosomal dominant
	Linked to locus on 3p21
Cerebral amyloid angiopathies	Autosomal dominant
Pseudoxanthoma elasticum	Autosomal recessive
	ABCC6 gene (chromosome 16p13.1)
Ehlers-Danlos disease type IV	Autosomal dominant
	COL3A1 gene on chromosome 2

B. Epidemiology

1. Prevalence unknown, but approximately 700 to 1,000 cases have been reported
2. Less than 30 reported cases in males

C. Genetics

1. X-linked dominant with high lethality in males; males surviving may have extra X chromosome or somatic mosaicism
2. Mutation of NEMO/IKKγ gene located on Xq28: NEMO/IKKγ is component in nuclear factor KB signaling pathway involved in expression of multiple genes protecting cells against apoptosis

D. Clinical Manifestations

1. Large range of findings that may vary even among family members
2. Dermatologic findings
   a. One of the first signs and highly prevalent
   b. Appears at or shortly after birth and evolves over time
   c. Four stages of cutaneous manifestation: 1) vesicular, 2) verrucous, 3) hyperpigmented, 4) atrophic, (Table 13-7)
   d. Alopecia
   e. Nail dystrophy
3. Neurologic features
   a. Majority of patients are intellectually normal
   b. Mental retardation

Table 13-6.   **Criteria for Diagnosis of Hereditary Hemorrhagic Telangiectasia**

1. Epistaxis: recurrent nose bleeds
2. Telangiectasias: multiple at characteristic sites
    a. Lips
    b. Oral cavity
    c. Fingers
    d. Nose
3. Visceral lesions
    a. Gastrointestinal telangiectasias
    b. Pulmonary arteriovenous malformations
    c. Hepatic arteriovenous malformations
    d. Cerebral vascular malformations
    e. Spinal vascular malformations
4. Family history of first-degree relative with hereditary hemorrhagic telangiectasia

      1) Males (25%)
      2) Females (1%)
   c. Seizures and infantile spasms (13% of patients)
   d. Microcephalus (5% of patients)
   e. Motor retardation (7.5% of patients)
4. Ophthalmologic findings
    a. Majority have normal vision, but up to 20% may have severe vision-threatening abnormalities
    b. Retinal or ocular lesions (35% of patients)
        1) Usually present within first year of life
        2) Generally result from vaso-occlusive ischemia, with compensatory vasoproliferation
        3) Findings can include mottled retinal pigment epithelium, neovascularization, vitreous hemorrhage, retinal detachment
    c. Nonretinal findings: strabismus, conjunctival pigmentation
5. Teeth
    a. Most common manifestation after skin findings
    b. Manifestations may include absent teeth or conical teeth and poor enamel quality
    c. Poor dentition may result in speech or nutritional difficulties
6. Other findings
    a. Leucocytosis, with up to 65% eosinophils
    b. Breast aplasia or hypoplasia, may have supernumerary nipple
    c. Skeletal changes uncommon but may include hemivertebrae, skull deformities, chondrodystrophy scoliosis, club foot, syndactyly

Table 13-7.   **Stages of Incontinentia Pigmenti**

Stage 1: Bullous stage (birth to first 8 weeks of life)
      Blisterlike eruptions
      Linear on extremities
      Circumferential on trunk
Stage 2: Verrucous stage (arises as stage 1 begins to resolve)
      Duration—2 months to years
      Hypertrophic, wartlike rash
      Linear on extremities
      Circumferential on trunk
      Dystrophic nails
      Tooth eruption abnormalities
Stage 3: Hyperpigmentation stage (6 months into adulthood)
      Macular, slate gray or brown hyperpigmentation
      Most characteristic stage
      "Marble cake" or swirled pattern
      Most frequent in groin and axilla
      Fades in second or third decade
      Linear on extremities
      Circumferential on trunk
Stage 4: Atrophic stage (does not occur in all patients)
      Linear hypopigmentation and alopecia

Characteristic Findings in Incontinentia Pigmenti
Dermatologic: "marble cake" hyperpigmentation often in groin and axilla

Dental: conical teeth and poor enamel

Neurologic: mental retardation and seizures (although majority of patients are intellectually normal)

E.   **Diagnosis**
1. Characteristic clinical findings of skin, teeth, hair, and nails
2. Proposed diagnostic criteria are listed in Table 13-8
3. MRI findings may include
    a. Diffuse atrophy
    b. Hypoplasia of corpus callosum
    c. Cysts
    d. Ventricular dilatation
4. Skin biopsy

F.   **Treatment**
1. Genetic counseling
2. Dental care
3. Ophthalmologic

a. Screening by retinal specialist after birth and frequent surveillance because early discovery and treatment may prevent blindness

b. Laser photocoagulation to treat proliferative retinopathy

4. Skin: skin lesions generally improve without treatment
5. Nail care
6. Brain
   a. Neurologic examination for patients with newly diagnosed incontinentia pigmenti
   b. Head imaging if examination or eye findings are abnormal

VIII. VON HIPPEL-LINDAU DISEASE

A. Overview

1. Autosomal dominant inheritance
2. A predisposition syndrome characterized by
   a. Hemangioblastomas of central nervous system and retina
   b. Renal cell carcinomas
   c. Pheochromocytomas
   d. Pancreatic islet cell tumors
   e. Endolymphatic sac tumors of middle ear
   f. Serous cystadenomas and neuroendocrine tumors of pancreas
   g. Papillary cystadenomas of epididymis and broad ligament
3. Hallmark lesions: retinal, cerebellar, and spinal cord hemangioblastomas

B. Epidemiology

1. Prevalence: approximately 1:40,000
2. Initial disease manifests in childhood, adolescence, or early adulthood
3. Shortened life span (median survival, 49 years); most deaths are due to renal cell carcinoma

C. Genetics

1. Autosomal dominant
   a. Reduced penetrance of clinical phenotype
   b. Marked phenotypic variability
   c. Classification of von Hippel-Lindau (VHL) phenotypes has been described on basis of likelihood of pheochromocytoma and renal cell carcinoma developing
   d. 80% of patients have affected parent
   e. 20% of patients have new gene mutation
2. von Hippel-Lindau (*VHL*) gene
   a. Tumor suppressor gene on chromosome 3p26-p255
   b. Numerous identified mutations
      1) Missense mutations are associated with pheochromocytoma

Table 13-8. Proposed Diagnostic Criteria for Incontinentia Pigmenti

Family history	Major criteria	Minor criteria
No evidence of incontinentia pigmenti in first-degree female relative*	1. Typical neonatal rash: erythema and vesicles with eosinophilia 2. Typical hyperpigmentation mainly on trunk, following lines of Blaschko, fading in adolescence 3. Linear, atrophic, hairless lesions	1. Dental anomalies 2. Alopecia 3. Abnormal nails 4. Retinal disease
Evidence of incontinentia pigmenti in first-degree female relative†	1. Suggestive history or evidence of typical rash, hyperpigmentation, atrophic hairless lesions 2. Vertex alopecia 3. Dental anomalies 4. Retinal disease 5. Multiple male miscarriages	

*At least one major criterion is necessary for diagnosis in cases with no apparent family history. Minor criteria support the diagnosis; complete lack thereof should induce degree of uncertainty.
†Presence of any one or more of the major criteria strongly suggests diagnosis of incontinentia pigmenti in cases with definitive family history.
From Berlin AL, Paller AS, Chan LS. Incontinentia pigmenti: a review and update on the molecular basis of pathophysiology. J Am Acad Dermatol. 2002;47:169-87. Used with permission.

      2) Nonsense, frame shift, splice site, and deletions not associated with pheochromocytoma
   c. VHL protein
      1) Appears to be related to tumor regulation
      2) Inactivation or loss of allele leads to tumor development
      3) Regulates expression of vascular endothelial growth factor

D. Symptoms: related to organ systems involved

E. Hemangioblastoma

1. Most common lesion associated with VHL disease
   a. 60% to 80% of patients with VHL disease develop hemangioblastoma
   b. Patients diagnosed with hemangioblastoma: 25% have VHL disease, 75% are sporadic

2. Mean age at onset: late 20s
3. Well-circumscribed, highly vascular benign neoplasms
4. Symptoms due to local mass effect of hemorrhage
   a. Central nervous system hemangioblastomas
      1) Common sites: cerebellum (usually hemisphere), followed by spinal cord (usually cervical or thoracic), and, least often, brainstem
      2) Symptoms at presentation depend on site
      3) Treatment: surgical removal of symptomatic and/or large lesions; surveillance of small, asymptomatic lesions
   b. Retinal hemangioblastomas: affect more than 50% of patients with VHL disease
      1) Retina or optic nerve hemangioblastomas can be bilateral and multiple lesions
      2) If untreated, can cause retinal detachment and hemorrhage, leading to blindness
      3) Age at onset varies from infancy to elderly (mean age at diagnosis, 25 years)
      4) Treatment of retinal lesions with laser coagulation and cryotherapy
      5) Initial ophthalmologic screening early (<6 years old)

F. **Associated Conditions**
1. Erythrocytosis (5%-20% of patients)
2. Pheochromocytoma
   a. In up to 15% of patients with VHL disease
   b. Can be multiple, may be extra-adrenal
3. Clear cell (renal cell) carcinoma
   a. Occurs in nearly 65% to 70% of patients with VHL disease
   b. Typically presents between ages 20 and 50 years
   c. May be bilateral or multifocal
4. Pancreatic lesions: may include cysts, serous cystadenoma, and neuroendocrine tumors
5. Endolymphatic sac tumors of middle ear
   a. Occur in up to 14% of patients with VHL disease
   b. Patient may present with hearing loss and tinnitus
6. Epididymal (men) and broad ligament (women) papillary cystadenomas

G. **Diagnostic Criteria**
1. Diagnosis usually based on clinical features
2. Family history and the finding of a single retinal or cerebellar hemangioblastoma, pheochromocytoma, or renal cell carcinoma are sufficient to justify the diagnosis
3. If no definite family history of VHL disease
   a. Two retinal or cerebellar hemangioblastomas *or*
   b. One hemangioblastoma plus one visceral tumor

H. **Treatment**
1. Genetic counseling for patient and family: molecular testing for suspected VHL disease
2. Annual monitoring for all patients
   a. Ophthalmologic examination for retinal hemangioblastomas
   b. Blood pressure
   c. Plasma catecholamines for pheochromocytoma (after age 10, begin abdominal CT screening)
3. After age 10 in patients with VHL disease: routine annual screening with MRI of brain and spinal cord for hemangioblastoma is recommended
4. Adults should also have screening for renal cell carcinoma and baseline hearing evaluation

I. **Chuvash Polycythemia**
1. Autosomal recessive disorder
2. Congenital disorder
3. Endemic to central Russia (Chuvashia)
4. *VHL* gene mutation
5. Symptoms
   a. Fatigue
   b. Headaches
   c. Pain
      1) Abdomen
      2) Lower extremities
      3) Chest
6. Signs
   a. Plethora (100% of patients)
   b. Mild hepatomegaly (33% of patients)
   c. Clubbing (30% of patients)
   d. Bleeding tendency or hemorrhage (24% of patients)

IX. **CEREBROTENDINOUS XANTHOMATOSIS**

A. **Overview**
1. Autosomal recessive disorder
2. Xanthomatous lesions form in brain, tendons, other tissues

B. **Genetics**
1. Autosomal recessive (chromosome 2q33)
2. Codes for mitochondrial sterol 27-hydroxylase

C. **Pathogenesis**
1. Impaired hepatic conversion of cholesterol to cholic and chenodeoxycholic acids
2. Accumulation of cholesterol and cholestanol in tissues

D. Pathology
1. Central nervous system
    a. Xanthomatous lesions and spindle-shaped lipid crystal clefts
        1) Cerebellum, adjacent to dentate nucleus
        2) Basal ganglia, brainstem, spinal cord
    b. Demyelination, gliosis, clusters of foam cells, neuronal loss
2. Peripheral nervous system: sensorimotor axonal polyneuropathy

E. Chronologic Order of Appearance of Clinical Hallmarks
1. Cataracts
    a. Bilateral
    b. Not congenital
    c. Mean age, 18 years (range, 4-40 years)
2. Chronic diarrhea
    a. Key symptom in all ages
    b. Typically apparent in first decade
    c. Pathogenesis not known
    d. Resolves within a few days after treatment is started
3. Tendon xanthomas
    a. Seldom before 20 years old
    b. Massive
    c. Achilles tendon
    d. Not obligatory for diagnosis of cerebrotendinous xanthomatosis
4. Progressive neurologic symptoms
    a. Mental retardation
    b. Pyramidal and cerebellar signs

F. Additional Conditions
1. Premature atherosclerosis
2. Osteoporosis
3. Repeated fractures
4. Pulmonary insufficiency

G. Diagnosis
1. Early diagnosis and treatment can prevent neurologic complications
2. Presence of two of four clinical hallmarks should prompt metabolic screening
    a. Increased plasma and bile cholestanol levels
    b. Increased urinary bile alcohol glucuronides associated with decreased biliary concentration of chenodeoxycholic acid
3. Normal lipoprotein profile despite increased cholesterol synthesis
4. Biochemical examination is recommended for all sib-

lings of patient with cerebrotendinous xanthomatosis
5. Imaging: MRI may show cerebral and cerebellar atrophy

H. Treatment
1. Chenodeoxycholic acid
    a. Bile acid replacement inhibits abnormal bile acid synthesis
    b. Reduces plasma cholestanol concentrations and bile alcohol
    c. Effective, affordable, safe
2. β-HMG-CoA reductase inhibitor
    a. Efficacy not clear
    b. On-going long-term treatment trials
3. Removal of Achilles tendon xanthomas for cosmetic reasons

X.   EHLERS-DANLOS SYNDROME

A. Overview
1. A heterogenous group of connective tissue disorders with at least 10 identified forms
2. Clinical features may include joint hypermobility, hyperelastic skin, easy bruising, abnormal scar formation
3. Neurologic dysfunction is unusual except for cerebrovascular lesions in individuals with type IV of the syndrome

B. Ehlers-Danlos Syndrome Type IV (vascular type)
1. Less common type, but most lethal because of arterial, intestinal, or uterine rupture
2. Genetics
    a. Autosomal dominant
    b. *COL3A1* gene on chromosome 2; encodes for type III procollagen synthesis
    c. Many different mutations
3. Pathogenesis
    a. Deficiency of collagen type III: major component of distensible tissues, including arteries and veins
    b. Pathology: arterial internal elastic membrane is fragmented and portions of wall fibrosed; microscopic ruptures between media and adventitia
4. Clinical presentation
    a. Easy bruising
    b. Arterial (dissection and aneurysm formation), intestinal, or uterine fragility
    c. Thin, translucent skin

d. Facial features: thin nose, hollow cheeks, and reduced adipose tissue

e. Other findings may include small joint hypermobility (rarely severe unlike other forms of the syndrome), skin hyperextensibility (also less severe than in other types of the syndrome), spontaneous pneumothorax, tendon rupture, and early varicose veins

f. Neurovascular complications
   1) Spontanenous rupture or dissection of arteries
   2) Carotid-cavernous fistula
   3) Intracranial aneurysm (Table 13-2)

5. Diagnosis
   a. Clinical manifestations
   b. Fibroblast culture to detect procollagen III molecules

6. Treatment
   a. Genetic counseling
   b. Avoid lifestyles with potential for trauma
   c. Noninvasive radiographic assessment of vessels, with close follow-up of asymptomatic patients
   d. Fragile vessels make angiography and surgery difficult
   e. Survival shortened with vascular complications

XI. PSEUDOXANTHOMA ELASTICUM (GRÖNBLAD-STRANDBERG SYNDROME)

A. Overview
1. Connective tissue disorder characterized by calcification of elastic fibers
2. Clinical manifestations involve skin, retina, and cardiovascular system
3. No direct involvement of nervous system

B. Epidemiology: rare

C. Genetics
1. Autosomal recessive
2. *ABCC6* gene (chromosome 16p13.1): encodes multidrug resistance-associated protein 6, which belongs to the ABC (ATP-binding cassette) transmembrane transporter family of proteins
3. Wide phenotypic variation

D. Pathology of Skin and Blood Vessels
1. Fragmented elastic tissues
2. Calcium deposits

E. Clinical Manifestations
1. Skin (average age at appearance, 10-15 years)
   a. Characteristic small, yellowish papules typically on the

---

> **Cerebrovascular Complications of Ehlers-Danlos Syndrome Type IV**
> Carotid-cavernous fistula
>
> Spontaneous arterial dissection
>
> Intracranial aneurysm formation

neck; may give appearance of "plucked chicken skin"
   b. May involve other flexural regions; skin may appear wrinkled

2. Eye
   a. Angioid streaks (brown lines radiating from optic disc)
      1) Represent degeneration and calcification of elastic fibers in retina due to choroidal neovascularization and subsequent leakage through defects in Bruch's membrane
      2) Develop months to years after skin lesions
      3) Occur in almost all patients, but present in conditions other than pseudoxanthoma elasticum
      4) Preceded by peau d'orange appearance of retina
   b. Retinal hemorrhages
      1) Feared complication of pseudoxanthoma elasticum
      2) Common at 40 years and older
      3) May result in loss of central vision

3. Cardiovascular manifestations due to generalized involvement of large- and medium-sized arteries or calcification of endocardium and valves
   a. Coronary artery disease: angina, myocardial infarction, sudden death
   b. Peripheral vascular disease: claudication
   c. Renovascular hypertension
   d. Mitral valve prolapse and stenosis

4. Cerebrovascular disease
   a. Arterial occlusion due to abnormal elastic lamina of arteries; may have appearance of severe atherosclerosis
   b. Aneurysms (Table 13-2)

5. Other
   a. Hemorrhage may occur from fragile, calcified vessels
   b. Gastrointestinal tract hemorrhage most common; can also occur in brain, uterus, joints

F. Diagnosis
1. Characteristic skin and ophthalmologic features
2. Skin biopsy, with special elastic fiber stains

G. Treatment: genetic counseling and anticipatory guidance and surveillance for treatable complications
1. Annual cardiac assessment

a. Assess clinical symptoms, blood pressure, peripheral pulses, cardiac examination
b. Treat risk factors for atherosclerosis (smoking cessation, lipid and blood pressure management, weight control)
2. Retinal specialist to follow eye examination every 6 to 12 months
3. Avoid excess calcium intake
4. Avoid contact sports
5. Avoid nonsteroidal anti-inflammatory drugs and warfarin; selective use of aspirin in patients at risk for thromboembolic events
6. First-degree relatives: screening tests

XII. MENKES' SYNDROME (KINKY HAIR DISEASE)

A. Overview
1. X-linked recessive
2. Lethal disorder, with progressive neurodegeneration and characteristic "kinky" hair neurocutaneous manifestation
3. Disease results from maldistribution of body copper
4. Rare: in 1:50,000 to 100,000 live-born males

B. Genetics
1. X-linked recessive
2. *MNK* gene on chromosome Xq13
   a. Encodes for energy-dependent copper-transporting membrane ATPase which is *expressed in all tissues except liver*
   b. Numerous mutations: may be splicing, duplication, nonsense, or missense mutations
   c. No correlation identified between mutation and clinical course

C. Copper Metabolism
1. Clinical manifestations due to defective incorporation of copper into essential enzymes because of maldistribution of copper
2. Copper-dependent enzymes are affected and contribute to clinical manifestations (Table 13-9)

D. Pathology
1. Skin: decreased number of elastic fibers
2. Brain
   a. Atrophy (diffuse)
   b. Focal degeneration of cortical gray matter, with neuronal loss and gliosis
   c. Loss of Purkinje cells in cerebellum
   d. Degeneration of thalamus
   e. Intramitochondrial "dense bodies" on electron microscopy
3. Arteries: tortuous vessels with fragmented internal elastic layer

E. Clinical Manifestations
1. Patients typically present in early infancy, but manifestations may be noted in neonatal period
   a. Most common initial symptoms: delayed development and seizures
   b. Hypothermia, hypotonia, and hypoglycemia may be noted in neonatal period
   c. Failure to thrive: poor feeding, poor weight gain
   d. Hair: characteristic, but not diagnostic; colorless, friable (pili torti = twisted hairs), trichorrhexis nodosa (fractures of hair shaft at regular intervals)
   e. Other organ involvement
      1) Long-bone abnormalities
      2) Osteoporosis
      3) Hydronephrosis, bladder rupture
2. Late manifestations
   a. Blindness
   b. Subdural hematoma
   c. Respiratory failure
3. Clinical course
   a. Progressive course: loss of acquired milestones
   b. Decreased life expectancy: majority die before age 2, although case reports of longer survival
   c. Cause of death may include
      1) Infection: respiratory, urinary, sepsis, meningitis
      2) Vascular complication such as cerebral hemorrhage
      3) Neurologic degeneration

F. Diagnosis
1. Clinical history and characteristic manifestations
2. Decreased serum levels of copper and ceruloplasmin
   a. Copper and ceruloplasmin levels are low in neonatal period in all infants
   b. Normal infants reach adult concentrations at 1 to 2 months of age, therefore test after this period
3. Neonatal diagnosis can be made by copper uptake studies in cultured fibroblasts
4. DNA mutation analysis if family gene defect previously known

G. Imaging
1. MRI of head
   a. Diffuse cortical atrophy
   b. Impaired myelination

Table 13-9. **Copper-Dependent Enzyme Dysfunction and Clinical Manifestations in Menkes' Syndrome (Kinky Hair Disease)**

Copper-containing enzyme	Function	Dysfunction (clinical result)
Cytochrome-*c* oxidase (complex IV)	Located in mitochondrial inner membrane	Impairment of myelination Mitochondrial abnormalities
Tyrosinase	Melanin biosynthesis	Decreased pigmentation of hair and skin
Superoxide dismutase	Catalyze conversion of superoxide to hydrogen peroxide and molecular oxygen	Cytotoxic effects
Lysyl oxidase	Deaminates lysine and hydroxylysine, a step in collagen crosslinkage	Defects in elastin and collagen crosslinkage
Peptidylglycine amidating mono-oxygenase	Removes carboxy-terminal glycine of several neuroendocrine peptide precursors	Reduction of neuroendocrine peptides (calcitonin, ADH, TRH, CRH, MSH)

ADH, antidiuretic hormone; CRH, corticotropin-releasing hormone; MSH, melanocyte-stimulating hormone; TRH, thyrotropin-releasing hormone.

c. Subdural effusions or hematoma may be seen
2. Angiography may show elongated, tortuous arteries

H. **Treatment**
1. Genetic counseling
2. Copper supplementation
   a. Patients absorb little or no oral copper
   b. Early intravenous copper therapy normalizes copper and ceruloplasmin levels (brain copper levels do not increase with treatment)
      1) May not change neurologic dysfunction
      2) Efficacy not clear
3. Copper-histidinate supplementation also advocated

I. **Menkes' Variants**
1. Occipital horn syndrome

a. Mildest recognized form of Menkes' syndrome (named from calcification in trapezius and sternocleidomastoid muscles at attachment to occipital bone)
b. Serum levels of copper and ceruloplasmin are decreased
c. Clinical manifestations
   1) Hyperelastic skin
   2) Hyperextensible joints
   3) Hernia: umbilical or inguinal
   4) Bladder diverticula
   5) Skeletal abnormalities
   6) Mental retardation may occur
2. Other phenotypes: symptoms may include ataxia and mild mental retardation

XIII. EPIDERMAL NEVUS SYNDROME

A. **Overview**
1. Heterogeneous group of congenital syndromes characterized by epidermal nevi associated with abnormalities of other organ systems
2. May be sporadic or autosomal dominant

B. **Epidemiology**
1. Rare: approximately 1:1,000 live births, males and females equally affected
2. Of patients with epidermal nevi, 10% to 18% have systemic developmental disorders

C. **Clinical Manifestations**
1. Epidermal nevi
   a. Majority of epidermal nevi appear during infancy
   b. Typically linear, do not cross midline
   c. Head and neck most common sites of occurrence
   d. Follow the lines of Blaschko
   e. Nevi may undergo malignant transformation
2. Other organ systems
   a. Nervous system
      1) Ocular defects
      2) Mental retardation
      3) Seizures (often associated with intracranial calcifications and vascular malformations)
   b. Cardiovascular
   c. Renal
   d. Skeletal: bone cysts, hypertrophies, bone deformities
   e. May be associated with malignancies

D. **Cutaneous Findings Depend on Predominant Cell Type Involved** (Table 13-10)

Table 13-10. **Cutaneous Findings and Subtypes of Epidermal Nevus Syndrome**

Disease	Appearance of skin lesion	Gene	Associated features
Sebaceous nevus syndrome (Schimmelpenning syndrome)	Salmon-tan plaques with smooth, waxy surface Face and neck Age-dependent appearance		Mental retardation Seizures Ocular and skeletal defects
Verrucous	Linear, whorled Skin-colored to hyperpigmented Change over time Uncommon on head and neck		
Inflammatory linear verrucous	Linear, erythematous, pruritic Hyperkeratotic papules Coalesce into plaques Unilateral and often lower half of body		Autoimmune thyroiditis Lichen amyloidosis Arthritis
Nevus comedonicus syndrome	Collections of dilated follicular pits Filled with keratin plugs Face, trunk, upper extremity	Fibroblast growth factor receptor 2 (FGFR2)	Ipsilateral cataracts Skeletal and cerebral anomalies
CHILD syndrome	Unilateral, erythematous patches Waxy scales Flexural areas	X-linked dominant Xq28 NSDHL	Ipsilateral bone and organ defects
Pigmented hairy epidermal nevus	Hyperpigmentation Hypertrichosis Shoulder most commonly affected More prominent after puberty		Androgen dependent Ipsilateral hypoplasia of breast Skeletal abnormalities
Proteus syndrome	Linear, flat, soft, velvety Papillomatous plaques	Tumor suppressor gene PTEN	Asymmetric hypertrophy and macrodactyly Skeletal abnormalities Vascular malformations Subcutaneous hamartomas
Phakomatosis pigmentokeratotica	Speckled lentiginous and epidermal nevus Checkerboard pattern		Hemiatrophy and muscular weakness Hypophosphatemic rickets

CHILD, congenital hemidysplasia with ichthyosiform nevus and limb defects.

E. Diagnosis

1. Presence of epidermal nevi in infant should prompt evaluation of other organ abnormalities
2. Evaluation may involve
   a. Skin biopsy
   b. Chest and skeletal radiography
   c. MRI of head
   d. Electrocardiography, echocardiography
   e. Abdominal ultrasonography
   f. Dilated eye examination
   g. Complete blood count, blood chemistry panel, urinalysis, serum and urine levels of calcium and phosphorus

XIV. XERODERMA PIGMENTOSUM

A. Overview

1. Autosomal recessive
2. Extreme photosensitivity of skin and eyes
3. Premature cutaneous aging
4. Photodamage and neoplasm formation (1,000-fold increased frequency of carcinomas and melanomas)
5. Neurologic abnormalities (mental retardation, deafness, spasticity, and ataxia) occur in 1/3 of patients

B. Epidemiology

1. Prevalence in USA: 1:1,000,000
2. Higher incidence in Israel, Japan, Egypt

C. Genetics
1. Autosomal recessive
2. Heterogeneity of molecular defects
3. Gene products involved in nucleotide excision repair mechanisms in DNA damaged by UV radiation
4. Xeroderma pigmentosum, Cockayne's syndrome, trichothiodystrophy: caused by mutations in genes involved in nucleotide excision repair and DNA transcription

D. Clinical Manifestations
1. Skin
    a. Median age at onset: 1 to 2 years
        1) By 18 months in 50% of patients
        2) By 4 years in 75% of patients
        3) By 15 years in 95% of patients
    b. Marked erythema and blistering of sun-exposed areas (sunburn)
    c. Excessive freckling
    d. Skin atrophy and telangiectasia of exposed areas (face, neck, ears, limbs)
    e. May later develop basal cell carcinoma and, less commonly, squamous cell carcinoma and melanoma
2. Eyes
    a. Median age at onset of damage: 4 years
    b. Conjunctiva: injection, pigmentation and telangiectasias form, basal cell or squamous cell carcinoma
    c. Lids: ectropion, entropion
    d. Cornea: keratitis, corneal scarring, basal cell or squamous cell carcinoma of cornea
    e. Epibulbar tumors and ocular melanomas
3. Neurologic manifestations
    a. De Sanctis-Cacchione syndrome (progressive neurologic degeneration)
    b. Develop in approximately 20% of patients, considerably higher percentage in Japan
    c. May occur in infancy or develop in second decade
    d. Manifestations may include
        1) Mental retardation (most common)
        2) Ataxia and/or spasticity
        3) Abnormal ocular motility
        4) Sensorineural deafness
        5) Seizures
        6) Axonal neuropathy
4. Malignancy
    a. By age 10 to 14 years: 50% incidence
    b. Squamous and basal cell carcinoma
    c. Malignant melanoma (5% of patients)
    d. Rare: keratoacanthoma, fibrosarcoma, angioma
    e. Increase risk of internal neoplasms

    f. Cause of death in 33% of patients
5. Clinical course
    a. Decreased life expectancy
    b. Carcinoma is most common cause of death, followed by infection

E. Treatment
1. Avoidance of sunlight or other sources of UV light
2. Monitoring and removal of skin neoplasms

XV. HYPOMELANOSIS OF ITO (INCONTINENTIA PIGMENTI ACHROMIANS)

A. Overview
1. The third most frequent neurocutaneous disease, exceeded by NF1 and TSC
2. Characterized by pigmentary anomalies, neurologic dysfunction (seizures and mental retardation), and structural malformations
3. Pigmentary disorder caused by genetic mosaicism

B. Prevalence: 1:8,000 to 10,000

C. Genetics
1. Heterogeneous, sporadic
2. Many different chromosomal abnormalities found in hypomelanosis of Ito; most common on chromosomes 18, 12, and X

D. Skin Manifestations
1. Macular hypopigmented areas
    a. Unilateral or bilateral
    b. Irregular borders
    c. Whorls and patches
    d. Linear white lines of Blaschko type
        1) Present within first 2 years of life in 90% of patients
        2) Lesion does not correlate with severity of disease
        3) Segmental nevi are typically benign
2. Other types of cutaneous lesions
    a. Café au lait spots
    b. Nevus marmorata
    c. Angiomatous nevi
    d. Mongolian blue spot
3. Hair: hypertrichosis and abnormalities of hair growth and color

E. Other Organ Manifestations
1. Neurologic
    a. Mental retardation: autistic behavior may be associated

with severe seizure disorder
  b. Seizures
  c. Abnormal head growth
  d. Motor retardation
2. Dental: dental hamartomatous tumors
3. Skeletal
  a. Scoliosis
  b. Thoracic deformities
  c. Finger and toe anomalies
  d. Limb asymmetry
4. Eye: strabismus, nystagmus, corneal opacification, cataracts

F. Treatment
1. Seizures treated with appropriate anticonvulsant
2. Cutaneous lesions do not need treatment

XVI. NEUROCUTANEOUS MELANOSIS

A. Overview
1. Congenital disorder of melanotic cell development and migration
2. Characterized by cutaneous melanocytic nevi and development of benign or malignant melanocytic tumors of central nervous system, especially leptomeninges
3. Greatest risk: high incidence of transformation of melanocytic cells into malignant melanoma

B. Pathogenesis
1. Sporadic condition
2. Failure of proper differentiation of neural crest cells into mature melanocytes
3. In patients with giant congenital melanocytic nevi, the risk of neurocutaneous melanosis developing is estimated at 2.5%, but true incidence not known

C. Pathology
1. Leptomeningeal melanosis
2. Accumulation of melanotic cells in arachnoid and pia mater
3. Common location of parenchymal melanocyte accumulation: amygdala, cerebellum, thalamus, frontal lobes, base of brain

D. Clinical Manifestations
1. Skin
  a. Two-thirds of patients with neurocutaneous melanosis have giant congenital melanocytic nevi and one-third have numerous nevi without a giant lesion

  b. Giant congenital melanocytic nevi
    1) Size defined in adult as more than 20 cm
    2) Congenital melanocytic nevi can occur without central nervous system involvement
    3) Giant nevus is absent in some patients
  c. Characteristic lesions
    1) Light brown to very dark hairy nevi
    2) Present at birth
    3) Location
    4) Head and scalp
    5) Upper arms and lower neck (cape nevus) (33% of patients)
    6) Back (80% of patients), dorsal spine (swimming trunk nevus)
  d. Likelihood of symptomatic neurologic involvement correlates with location of nevus
    1) Location on back: increased likelihood of neurologic symptoms
    2) Nevi restricted to the extremities: neurologic symptoms less likely
  e. Satellite nevi occur around giant nevus (80% of patients)
  f. Risk of melanoma or other neural crest malignancies: 5% to 15%
    1) Greatest risk in childhood; 50% to 60% before 5 years of age
    2) Axial more than extremities
2. Neurologic
  a. Symptoms most often present at age 2 years or younger
  b. Leptomeningeal melanosis
    1) Most common cause of neurologic symptoms (62% of patients)
    2) Most common at base of brain
  c. Intracranial melanoma
  d. Intracerebral or subarachnoid hemorrhage
  e. Present with signs and symptoms of increased intracranial pressure
    1) Hydrocephalus (64% of patients): result of accumulation of melanotic cells at basal subarachnoid cisterns
    2) Seizures (44% of patients)
    3) Cranial nerve palsies
    4) Papilledema (31% of patients)
    5) Headaches (31% of patients)
  f. Mental retardation (18% of patients)
  g. Malformation of vertebral column, spinal cord, cerebrum
  h. Dandy-Walker malformation
  i. Leptomeningeal proliferation affecting spinal cord function
    1) Myelopathy
    2) Cauda equina syndrome

E. Associated Conditions

1. Malignancies other than melanoma
   a. Pedunculated embryonal rhabdomyosarcoma
   b. Malignant schwannoma in retroperitoneum
   c. Neuroectodermal neoplasms
   d. Liposarcoma
   e. Peritoneal metastasis of leptomeningeal melanoma via ventriculoperitoneal shunt

F. Diagnostic Criteria

1. Large and/or multiple (≥3) congenital nevi in association with meningeal melanosis or melanoma
   a. Infant
      1) 9 cm or more on scalp
      2) 6 cm or more on the body
   b. Adult: 20 cm total
2. Absence of malignant melanoma in any organ (including skin) other than central nervous system

G. Imaging

1. Brain MRI may demonstrate T1 shortening in presence of melanin
2. Gadolinium enhancement of leptomeninges correlates with presence of melanin in leptomeninges
3. Occasionally may be difficult to distinguish melanoma from benign melanin deposits
4. If lesions are suspect, follow serial MRI

H. Treatment

1. Asymptomatic patient
   a. Baseline brain and spinal cord MRI
   b. Parent to evaluate skin for nevus changes monthly
   c. Physician to evaluate every 6 months
      1) Evaluate skin for nevus changes
      2) Follow with neurologic examination
2. Symptomatic patient
   a. Follow serial brain MRI
   b. Treat increased intracranial pressure
   c. Because poor prognosis in patients with symptomatic neurologic disease, treatment of skin lesions in this population is debated
3. Isolated skin lesions
   a. Many advocate early excision of nevi to reduce risk of malignant transformation
   b. Early surgery may decrease disfigurement

I. Prognosis

1. Poor with symptomatic neurologic involvement
2. Death generally within 3 years after presentation

XVII. Fabry's Disease (Anderson-Fabry Disease or Angiokeratoma Corporis Diffusum)

A. Overview

1. X-linked recessive lysosomal storage disease resulting from deficiency of α-galactosidase A
2. Often presents with painful paresthesias during childhood, and later progressive vasculopathy with occlusive cardiovascular, cerebrovascular, and renal disease
3. Skin manifestations include angiokeratoma

B. Epidemiology

1. Second most prevalent metabolic storage disease after Gaucher's disease
2. 1:40,000 to 60,000 males
3. Predominantly in Caucasians

C. Genetics

1. X-linked recessive
   a. Complete penetrance in males
   b. Heterozygous females may develop symptoms if uneven chromosome inactivation
   c. Variable penetrance
2. *GAL* gene localized to chromosome Xq22
3. Numerous (>300) causative mutations

D. Pathogenesis

1. α-Galactosidase A breaks down glycophospholipids
2. Defect of α-galactosidase A: progressive lysosomal accumulation of dihexoside ceramides, and trihexoside ceramides including globotriaosylceramide and globotetraosylceramide
3. Sphingolipid accumulation of product in vascular endothelial cells, smooth muscle cells, sweat gland cells, macrophages, central neurons, gastrointestinal ganglionic neurons, cardiac muscle, astrocytes, meningeal cells, autonomic ganglion cells

E. Clinical Manifestations

1. Pain crises
   a. Acute, episodic, neurogenic pain
   b. May begin as early as age 4 years; mean, 10 years
   c. Triggers: stress, heat, fatigue, exercise
   d. Hands and feet, may radiate proximally
   e. Acroparesthesia
      1) Often develops before cutaneous lesions
      2) Chronic burning or tingling pain in extremities
2. Skin: angiokeratoma
   a. Hyperkeratotic areas of dilated blood vessels

b. Typically purple-black color
c. Location
   1) Most commonly in "swim trunk" region
   2) May also be present in mucous membranes and conjunctiva
d. Increased number with age
e. Can be present in other lipid storage diseases

3. Eyes
   a. Corneal opacity by slit-lamp microscopy that does not affect vision (cornea verticillata)
   b. Tortuous retinal vessels

4. Neurologic manifestations
   a. Stroke or TIAs (Table 13-5)
      1) Small-vessel ischemic strokes
      2) Third or fourth decade of life
      3) Thrombosis due to globotriaosylceramide deposits
      4) Risk increases with age
   b. Small-fiber peripheral neuropathy (See also Chapter 21)
   c. Less commonly, headache, dementia, and aneurysm (Table 13-2)

5. Kidney
   a. Proteinuria
   b. Progressive renal failure
   c. Hypertension

6. Gastrointestinal tract
   a. Acute abdominal pain may be mistaken for appendicitis
   b. Abdominal discomfort
   c. Diarrhea, nausea, vomiting

7. Heart
   a. Myocardial infarction
   b. Valvulopathies
   c. Arrhythmias
   d. Cardiomyopathy

8. Other

Hallmark Characteristics of Fabry's Disease

Angiokeratoma

Episodic pain crises

Occlusive vasculopathy with resultant cardiovascular, peripheral vascular, and cerebrovascular manifestations

Small-fiber peripheral neuropathy

---

a. Depression, suicide
b. Retarded growth, delayed puberty

F. **Female Carriers**
1. Later onset, less severe disease, variable manifestations
2. Acroparethesia may occur in adolescence
3. May have angiokeratomas
4. Whorl keratopathy may be seen on slit-lamp examination

G. **Diagnosis**
1. Positive family history is helpful, but not always present
2. In affected males: low or absent α-galactosidase A enzyme level in plasma, serum, leukocytes, or cultured fibroblasts
3. Some females have normal enzyme level and require DNA analysis
4. Skin, kidney, or conjunctival biopsy may help

H. **Treatment**
1. Genetic counseling; prenatal testing for α-galactosidase deficiency can be performed on cultured amniotic cells or chorionic villus sample
2. Annual evaluation for renal and cardiac abnormalities
3. Pain crises
   a. Avoid triggers
   b. Consider medical treatment
      1) Phenytoin
      2) Carbamazepine
      3) Gabapentin
   c. Avoid narcotics
   d. Nonsteroidal anti-inflammatory drugs not effective
4. Enzyme replacement therapy
   a. Two enzymes: agalsidase alfa and agalsidase beta
   b. Has been shown to reduce pain and improve quality of life
   c. Goal: prevent development of neurologic, renal, and cardiac complications
5. Life span: about 50 years

XVIII. PROGRESSIVE FACIAL HEMIATROPHY (PARRY-ROMBERG SYNDROME)

A. **Craniofacial Condition:** manifests as progressive hemifacial atrophy of skin, soft tissue, and bone

B. **Epidemiology**
1. Typically presents in first or second decade
2. Sometimes begins after trauma to involved side
3. More common in females; F:M = 1.5:1

C. Etiology
1. Occurs sporadically
2. Cause unknown: theories include infection, trigeminal neuritis, scleroderma, cervical sympathetic loss

D. Clinical Manifestations
1. Progressive hemifacial atrophy, typically in distribution of CN V
2. Skin: linear scleroderma of forehead (en coup de sabre)
3. Central nervous system: rare

E. Treatment: surgical reconstruction

XIX. ATAXIA-TELANGIECTASIA

A. Neurodegenerative Disease
1. Characterized by: slowly progressive ataxia, telangiectasia, variable immunodeficiency, and ionizing radiation sensitivity
2. For details, see Chapter 9

B. Genetics
1. Autosomal recessive
2. Mutation of AT mutant (*ATM*) gene on chromosome 11q22-23

REFERENCES

Arun D, Gutmann DH. Recent advances in neurofibromatosis type 1. Curr Opin Neurol. 2004;17:101-5.

Baser ME, R Evans DG, Gutmann DH. Neurofibromatosis 2. Curr Opin Neurol. 2003;16:27-33.

Begbie ME, Wallace GM, Shovlin CL. Hereditary haemorrhagic telangiectasia (Osler-Weber-Rendu syndrome): a view from the 21st century. Postgrad Med J. 2003;79:18-24.

Berlin AL, Paller AS, Chan LS. Incontinentia pigmenti: a review and update on the molecular basis of pathophysiology. J Am Acad Dermatol. 2002;47:169-87.

Burstein F, Seier H, Hudgins PA, Zapiach L. Neurocutaneous melanosis. J Craniofac Surg. 2005;16:874-6.

DeBella K, Szudek J, Friedman JM. Use of the national institutes of health criteria for diagnosis of neurofibromatosis 1 in children. Pediatrics. 2000;105:608-14.

Desnick RJ, Brady RO. Fabry disease in childhood. J Pediatr. 2004;144 Suppl:S20-6.

Foster RD, Williams ML, Barkovich AJ, Hoffman WY, Mathes SJ, Frieden IJ. Giant congenital melanocytic nevi: the significance of neurocutaneous melanosis in neurologically asymptomatic children. Plast Reconstr Surg. 2001;107:933-41.

Friedman JM. Neurofibromatosis 1: clinical manifestations and diagnostic criteria. J Child Neurol. 2002;17:548-54.

Friedrich CA. Genotype-phenotype correlation in von Hippel-Lindau syndrome. Hum Mol Genet. 2001;10:763-7.

Goldberg MF. The skin is not the predominant problem in incontinentia pigmenti. Arch Dermatol. 2004;140:748-50.

Gómez MR, Sampson JR, Whittemore VH, editors. Tuberous sclerosis complex. 3rd ed. New York: Oxford University Press; 1999.

Gutmann DH, Gurney JG, Shannon KM. Juvenile xanthogranuloma, neurofibromatosis 1, and juvenile chronic myeloid leukemia. Arch Dermatol. 1996;132:1390-1.

Hunt JA, Hobar PC. Common craniofacial anomalites: conditions of craniofacial atrophy/hypoplasia and neoplasia. Plast Reconstr Surg. 2003;111:1497-508.

Hyman MH, Whittemore VH. National Institutes of Health consensus conference: tuberous sclerosis complex. Arch Neurol. 2000;57:662-5.

Inamadar AC, Palit A. Pseudoxanthoma elasticum. Postgrad Med J. 2004;80:297.

Jarrar RG, Buchhalter JR, Raffel C. Long-term outcome of epilepsy surgery in patients with tuberous sclerosis. Neurology. 2004;62:479-81.

Karnes PS. Neurofibromatosis: a common neurocutaneous disorder. Mayo Clin Proc. 1998;73:1071-6.

Kuster W, Konig A. Hypomelanosis of Ito: no entity, but a cutaneous sign of mosaicism. Am J Med Genet. 1999;85:346-50.

Landy SJ, Donnai D. Incontinentia pigmenti (Bloch-Sulzberger syndrome). J Med Genet. 1993;30:53-9.

Laube S, Moss C. Pseudoxanthoma elasticum. Arch Dis Child. 2005;90:754-6.

Lee A, Driscoll D, Gloviczki P, Clay R, Shaughnessy W, Stans A. Evaluation and management of pain in patients with Klippel-Trenaunay syndrome: a review. Pediatrics. 2005;115:744-9.

Maher CO, Piepgras DG, Brown RD Jr, Friedman JA, Pollock BE. Cerebrovascular manifestations in 321 cases of hereditary hemorrhagic telangiectasia. Stroke. 2001;32:877-82.

Makkar HS, Frieden IJ. Congenital melanocytic nevi: an update for the pediatrician. Curr Opin Pediatr. 2002;14:397-403.

Maria BL, Deidrick KM, Roach ES, Gutmann DH. Tuberous sclerosis complex: pathogenesis, diagnosis, strategies, therapies, and future research directions. J Child Neurol. 2004;19:632-42.

Masson C, Cisse I, Simon V, Insalaco P, Audran M. Fabry disease: a review. Joint Bone Spine. 2004;71:381-3.

Melean G, Sestini R, Ammannati F, Papi L. Genetic insights into familial tumors of the nervous system. Am J Med Genet C Semin Med Genet. 2004;129:74-84.

Menkes JH. Menkes disease and Wilson disease: two sides of the same copper coin. Part I: Menkes disease. Eur J Paediatr Neurol. 1999;3:147-58.

Meschia JF, Brott TG, Brown RD Jr. Genetics of cerebrovascular disorders. Mayo Clin Proc. 2005;80:122-32.

Moghadasian MH, Salen G, Frohlich JJ, Scudamore CH. Cerebrotendinous xanthomatosis: a rare disease with diverse manifestations. Arch Neurol. 2002;59:527-9.

Oderich GS, Panneton JM, Bower TC, Lindor NM, Cherry KJ, Noel AA, et al. The spectrum, management and clinical outcome of Ehlers-Danlos syndrome type IV: a 30-year experience. J Vasc Surg. 2005;42:98-106.

Plikaitis CM, David LR, Argenta LC. Neurocutaneous melanosis: clinical presentations. J Craniofac Surg. 2005;16:921-5.

Roach ES, Gomez MR, Northrup H. Tuberous sclerosis complex consensus conference: revised clinical diagnostic criteria. J Child Neurol. 1998;13:624-8.

Schievink WI. Genetics of intracranial aneurysms. Neurosurgery. 1997;40:651-62.

Sergeyeva A, Gordeuk VR, Tokarev YN, Sokol L, Prchal JF, Prchal JT. Congenital polycythemia in Chuvashia. Blood. 1997;89:2148-54.

Sims KB. von Hippel-Lindau disease: gene to bedside. Curr Opin Neurol. 2001;14:695-703.

Sparagana SP, Roach ES. Tuberous sclerosis complex. Curr Opin Neurol. 2000;13:115-9.

Stefansson K. Tuberous sclerosis. Mayo Clin Proc. 1991;66:868-72.

Thomas-Sohl KA, Vaslow DF, Maria BL. Sturge-Weber syndrome: a review. Pediatr Neurol. 2004;30:303-10.

Vujevich JJ, Mancini AJ. The epidermal nevus syndromes: multisystem disorders. J Am Acad Dermatol. 2004;50:957-61.

QUESTIONS

1. Routine follow-up care of a child with neurofibromatosis type 1 should include which of the following?
   a. Annual blood pressure monitoring
   b. Annual audiology
   c. Annual MRI of head
   d. Annual orthopedic evaluation

2. Neurofibromatosis is the most common neurocutaneous disease. Which of the following statements about neurofibromatosis is *incorrect*?
   a. Autosomal dominant inheritance
   b. Penetrance is nearly complete
   c. Family history is always positive for cutaneous findings and/or tumors
   d. Manifestations increase with age

3. Which neurocutaneous syndrome is distinguished from the others by its involvement of nearly all organ systems and tissues?
   a. Neurofibromatosis type 1
   b. Neurofibromatosis type 2
   c. Tuberous sclerosis complex
   d. von Hippel-Lindau syndrome
   e. Sturge-Weber syndrome

4. Which neurocutaneous disease does not affect peripheral nerves?
   a. Neurofibromatosis type 1
   b. Neurofibromatosis type 2
   c. Tuberous sclerosis complex
   d. Fabry's disease

5. Which is the only malignancy associated with tuberous sclerosis complex?
   a. Subependymal giant cell astrocytoma
   b. Renal cell carcinoma
   c. Rhabdomyoma
   d. Squamous cell carcinoma
   e. Small cell lung carcinoma

6. Seizure disorders associated with tuberous sclerosis complex are remarkable for the following *except*:
   a. Complex partial seizures only
   b. Risk of status epilepticus
   c. Seizures often refractory to antiepileptic drugs
   d. Infantile spasms with hypsarrhythmic EEG
   e. Most patients develop seizures, usually beginning before age 2 years

7. For which disease does the American Heart Association recommend antibiotic prophylaxis for dental and surgical procedures?
   a. Tuberous sclerosis complex
   b. Neurofibromatosis type 1
   c. Sturge-Weber syndrome
   d. Hereditary hemorrhagic telangiectasia
   e. Incontinentia pigmenti

8. Which of the following neurocutaneous diseases is *not* due to an identified genetic factor?
   a. Neurofibromatosis type 1
   b. Neurofibromatosis type 2
   c. Tuberous sclerosis complex
   d. Sturge-Weber syndrome
   e. Incontinentia pigmenti

9. von Hippel-Lindau disease is a neurocutaneous disease of autosomal dominant inheritance, which of the following is *not* associated with this disease?
   a. Hemangioblastomas of the retina and central nervous system
   b. "Marble cake" hyperpigmentation of the skin
   c. Pheochromocytoma
   d. Renal cell carcinoma
   e. Benign cysts

10. Each of the following syndromes or disorders may be associated with ischemic stroke *except*:
    a. Hereditary hemorrhagic telangiectasia (Osler-Weber-Rendu disease)
    b. Fabry's disease
    c. von Hippel-Lindau disease
    d. Mitochondrial encephalopathy, lactic acidosis, and stroke-like episodes (MELAS)
    e. Pseudoxanthoma elasticum

Answers

1. Answer: a.
These patients are at risk for developing hypertension. If a child develops hypertension, he or she should be evaluated to determine the cause. Adults most likely have essential hypertension. Because hearing loss due to tumor is not a feature of neurofibromatosis type 1, presymptomatic screening is not necessary. Annual MRI is not necessary if patient is asymptomatic unless an incidental tumor is discovered on screening MRI examination. Orthopedic evaluation is necessary at diagnosis if the patient has a bony lesion. Follow the orthopedic guidelines for follow-up care.

2. Answer: c.
Neurofibromatosis results from a new mutation in 30% to 50% of cases.

3. Answer: c.
Tuberous sclerosis complex is characterized by benign growths (hamartias and hamartomas) in multiple organ systems.

4. Answer: c.
Tuberous sclerosis complex is a systemic disorder involving multiple organs, including the brain, skin, heart, lungs, and kidneys. The muscle and peripheral nerve roots are not involved. The hallmark of neurofibromatosis type 1 (peripheral neurofibromatosis) is peripheral nerve neurofibromas. Neurofibromatosis type 2 (central neurofibromatosis) involves vestibular schwannomas of the peripheral nervous system. Fabry's disease can cause a small-fiber and autonomic neuropathy.

5. Answer: b.
Renal cell carcinoma, a tumor that originates in the same hyperplastic epithelium that forms renal cysts, occurs with increased frequency and at an earlier age in tuberous sclerosis complex. Subependymal giant cell astrocytoma and rhabdomyoma occur in tuberous sclerosis complex; however, they are not malignant.

6. Answer: a.
Seizures may be either partial, localization-related, or generalized.

7. Answer: d.
Patients with hereditary hemorrhagic telangiectasia can develop pulmonary arteriovenous malformations and are at risk for shunting of air, thrombus, and bacteria through a pulmonary arteriovenous malformation. This can cause a transient ischemic attack, embolic stroke, and cerebral abscess.

8. Answer: d.
Sturge-Weber syndrome occurs sporadically. Neurofibromatosis types 1 and 2 and tuberous sclerosis complex are autosomal dominant conditons. Incontinentia pigmenti is X-linked and often lethal to a male fetus.

9. Answer: b.
"Marble cake" hyperpigmentation of the skin is characteristic of incontinentia pigmenti.

10. Answer: c.
von Hippel-Lindau disease is characterized by hemangioblastomas of the central nervous system, retina, and skin; however, it is not associated with ischemic stroke. All the others listed are associated with ischemic stroke through various mechanisms.

INFLAMMATORY AND DEMYELINATING DISORDERS OF THE CENTRAL NERVOUS SYSTEM

14

Orhun H. Kantarci, M.D.

I. IDIOPATHIC INFLAMMATORY-DEMYELINATING DISORDERS OF CNS: SPECTRUM OF DISORDERS

A. Definitions

1. No identifiable cause, except for neuromyelitis optica (see below)
2. IIDDs need to be differentiated from other demyelinating disorders of known cause, such as leukodystrophies, progressive multifocal leukoencephalopathy, and central pontine myelinolysis
3. "Prototypical" IIDD is sometimes called "bout-onset" multiple sclerosis (BOMS) (this term is not preferred by some authorities, but implies a relapse at onset of the clinical disease)
4. Relapsing-remitting multiple sclerosis (RRMS) and secondary progressive multiple sclerosis (SPMS): the continuum of BOMS
5. In most texts and discussions, the name "multiple sclerosis" is "loosely" used to entail RRMS, SPMS, or primary progressive multiple sclerosis (PPMS)
6. Other definitions included in the category of multiple sclerosis: relapsing-progressive and progressive-relapsing multiple sclerosis (they have no known bearing on prognosis or treatment decisions and are not used in this chapter)
7. IIDDs vary in number, size, and distribution (focal, multifocal, or diffuse) of lesions in the CNS and in pathologic features
8. Acute syndromes may be classified according to severity of the initial clinical presentation and initial pathologic features (e.g., amount of inflammation, demyelination, and necrosis)
9. Chronic syndromes may be classified according to clinical evolution, with accumulating disability and chronic pathologic features (e.g., oligodendrocyte damage, demyelination, remyelination, axonal loss, gliosis) (Fig. 14-1)

10. Some focal isolated IIDDs, and even diffuse fulminant Marburg forms of multiple sclerosis have potential to show dissemination in time and space and convert to "prototypical" BOMS
11. RRMS often evolves into SPMS (Fig. 14-1)
12. Identification of individual disorders as they stand within the spectrum has prognostic and therapeutic implications

B. Isolated Syndromes

1. Focal isolated IIDDs
   a. Are restricted to one area of the CNS
   b. Are self-limited
   c. May be responsive to high-dose corticosteroid therapy during attacks (i.e., optic neuritis, acute transverse myelitis [ATM], and isolated brainstem or cerebellum inflammatory demyelination)
2. Isolated IIDDs may be postinfectious and postvaccinal like acute disseminated encephalomyelitis (ADEM) (see below)
3. May be recurrent (polyphasic) or nonrecurrent (monophasic) but not fulfilling the criteria for diagnosis of multiple sclerosis (Table 14-1)
   a. Neuroimaging (magnetic resonance imaging [MRI]) or paraclinical (evoked potential studies) evidence of dissemination in space and time suggests diagnosis of BOMS
      1) At 18 months from onset, 84% of patients with two or more enhancing lesions at presentation meet McDonald criteria for BOMS (Table 14-1)
      2) At 14 years from onset, only 19% who initially had normal MRI findings develop multiple sclerosis
   b. Recurrent optic neuritis, recurrent ATM, and neuromyelitis optica may be related (see below)
4. Optic neuritis: the most common and benign IIDD (see Chapter 3)
   a. Long intracanalicular lesions of the optic nerve seen on MRI are associated with poor recovery from attack of optic neuritis

NATURAL HISTORY OF MULTIPLE SCLEROSIS

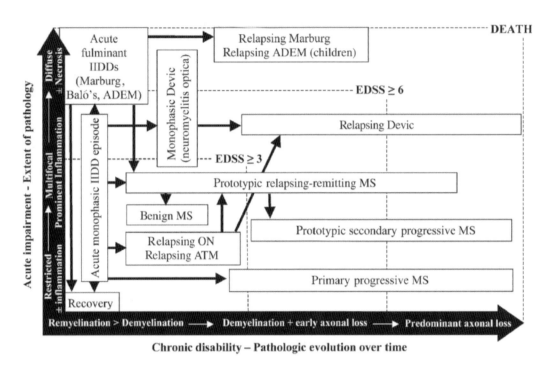

Fig. 14-1. Spectrum of idiopathic inflammatory demyelinating diseases (IIDDs). ADEM, acute disseminated encephalomyelitis; ATM, acute transverse myelitis; EDSS, Kurtzke Expanded Disability Status Scale; MS, multiple sclerosis; ON, optic neuritis. (From Kantarci OH, Weinshenker BG. Natural history of multiple sclerosis. Neurol Clin. 2005;23:17-38. Used with permission.)

b. For adults: overall risk of conversion to BOMS in 10 years, 38%
  1) If two or more MRI lesions suggestive of multiple sclerosis, 90% risk
  2) If one MRI lesion is suggestive of multiple sclerosis, 56% risk
  3) If normal MRI, 15% to 20% risk
  4) No conversion to BOMS in short term if normal MRI and no oligoclonal bands
  5) Factors associated with lower risk of conversion to BOMS: male sex, absence of pain, presence of optic disc swelling or peripapillary hemorrhages
5. ATM can be complete or partial
  a. Complete ATM
    1) Symmetric, combined sensory and motor syndrome with sausage-shaped, swollen, and elongated enhancing spinal cord lesions (Fig. 14-2)
    2) Presence of neuromyelitis optica antibodies (NMO IgG) predict evolution to neuromyelitis optica
  b. Partial ATM
    1) Asymmetric and generally milder multifocal myelitis

  2) 58% to 80% of cases evolve to multiple sclerosis (sensory symptoms, posterolateral location of lesion in spinal cord, abnormal brain MRI, and oligoclonal bands in cerebrospinal fluid [CSF] predict conversion)
6. Other noninflammatory isolated demyelinating syndromes
  a. Central pontine myelinolysis: associated with rapid correction of hyponatremia, alcoholism, malnutrition, and organ transplantation (see Chapter 17)
    1) Symptoms: decreased level of consciousness, tetraparesis, pseudobulbar palsy
    2) Symptoms may be mild in some patients (despite radiographic appearance)
    3) There may be extrapontine myelinolysis
    4) Fluid restriction is enough in some cases, but for saline infusion, the rate is 12 mEq/L per day or 0.5 mEq/L per hour
  b. Marchiafava-Bignami disease: focal demyelination of central area of corpus callosum seen in middle-aged chronic alcoholics (see Chapter 7)
    1) Symptoms: dementia, dysarthria, weakness, seizures, incontinence

Table 14-1. **Diagnostic Criteria for Multiple Sclerosis**

	Poser criteria				McDonald criteria (new)		
Category	Relapses	Clinical	Paraclinical*	CSF	Clinical (attacks)	Objective clinical lesion	Additional
Clinically definite					≥2	≥2	None
A1	2	2	NA	NA	≥2	1	Dissemination in space by MRI
A2	2	1	1	NA			*or*
							Positive CSF and ≥2 MRI lesions
							or
							Further attack involving a different site
Laboratory-supported definite					1	≥2	Dissemination in time by MRI
							or
							Second clinical attack
B1	2	1	1	+	1†	1	Dissemination in time by MRI
B2	1	2	NA	+			*or*
B3	1	1	1	+			Positive CSF and ≥2 MRI lesions
							and
							Dissemination in time by MRI
							or
							Second clinical attack
Clinically probable					0‡	1	Positive CSF
							and
C1	2	1	–	–			Dissemination in space by ≥9 T2 brain lesions *or*
C2	1	2	–	–			≥2 cord lesions *or*
C3	1	1	1	–			4-8 brain lesions and 1 cord lesion *or*
Laboratory-supported probable							4-8 brain lesions and positive VEPs *or*
							<4 brain lesions and 1 cord lesion and positive VEPs
D1	2	–	–	+			*and*
							Dissemination in time by MRI *or*
							Continued progression for 1 year

CSF, cerebrospinal fluid; MRI, magnetic resonance imaging; NA, not applicable; VEP, visual evoked potential.
*MRI or evoked potential studies.
†Monosymptomatic.
‡Progression from onset (primary progressive multiple sclerosis).

C. Neuromyelitis Optica (Devic disease, Asian type multiple sclerosis)

1. Distinct IIDD with multifocal lesions that follow a restricted pattern of optic nerve and spinal cord involvement
2. Antibodies specific to neuromyelitis optica have been described: antigenic stimulus is thought to be against aquaporin-4 molecule
3. May be misdiagnosed as RRMS by existing clinical criteria at presentation (optic neuritis and myelitis may occur in either condition) (Table 14-1)

4. Neuromyelitis optica is differentiated from RRMS by
   a. Predilection for Asians and African Americans as well as Caucasians in neuromyelitis optica
   b. Association with other systemic autoimmune disorders in neuromyelitis optica
   c. Restricted syndrome of optic neuritis and "complete" ATM (Fig. 14-2) generally lacking the typical brain lesions seen in RRMS
   d. CSF oligoclonal bands generally absent (a neutrophilic pleocytosis may occur during attacks in neuromyelitis optica)

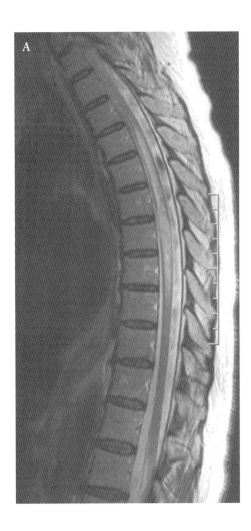

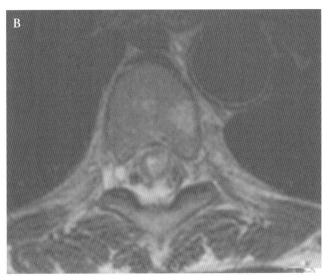

Fig. 14-2. MRI findings in complete acute transverse myelitis in sagittal (*A*) and axial (*B*) T2 images as seen in a patient with neuromyelitis optica. Note extensive T2 hyperintensity in the thoracic spinal cord, extending from T3-4 to T9.

D. Fulminant IIDDs

1. Acute, generally monophasic syndromes characterized by diffuse inflammatory demyelination of CNS that may be resistant to initial treatment with high-dose corticosteroids during attacks
2. Examples: ADEM, acute hemorrhagic leukoencephalitis (AHLE), Marburg variant of multiple sclerosis, Baló's concentric sclerosis, focal tumefactive demyelinating lesions that may simulate brain tumors, myelinoclastic diffuse sclerosis (Schilder's disease)
3. 44% of patients with acute fulminant attack unresponsive to corticosteroid therapy have moderate or marked improvement with plasma exchange
4. Specific diagnosis
   a. Based on clinical criteria
   b. There is no specific surrogate marker
5. ADEM
   a. Characterized by innumerable, diffusely enhancing, subcortical white matter lesions on MRI (Fig. 14-5)
   b. Often follows vaccination (rabies, diphtheria, pertussis, measles, rubella) or febrile illness (measles, *Enterovirus*, herpesvirus, influenza, Epstein-Barr virus, *Mycoplasma*, *Borrelia*)
   c. Occurs in adolescents or children
   d. CSF: absence of oligoclonal bands chronically (they may be present transiently), normal immunoglobulin content
   e. Clinical differentiation of ADEM from first attack of RRMS or other fulminant form of IIDD may be difficult

e. Specific neuromyelitis optica antibody absent in RRMS
f. Relatively homogeneous pathologic features of neuromyelitis optica, suggesting a B-cell–mediated disorder with characteristics distinct from multiple sclerosis (Fig. 14-3 and 14-4)
g. Attacks of neuromyelitis optica are more severe and less often responsive to corticosteroid therapy than RRMS (morbidity and mortality from respiratory failure due to cervical myelopathy)
   1) Monophasic course in 33% of patients (5-year survival, 90%); relapsing course in 67% (5-year survival, 68%)
   2) Simultaneous optic neuritis and myelitis (within 1 month) predict monophasic and relatively benign course
   3) Long interval between index events, female sex, older age at onset, and presence of other systemic autoimmune disease predict relapsing course and worse prognosis
5. Attacks of neuromyelitis optica may be resistant to initial high-dose corticosteroid therapy but may show improvement with plasma exchange

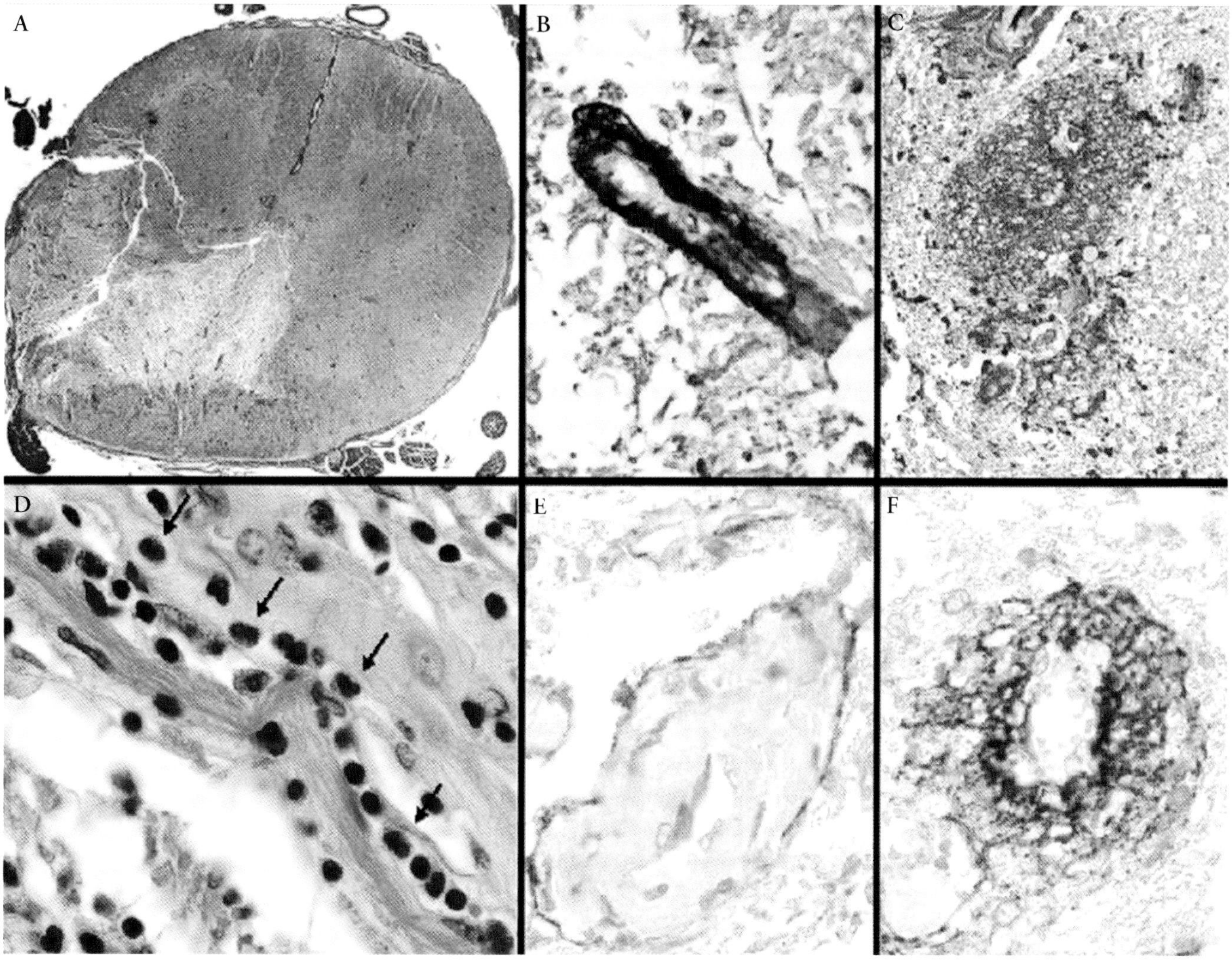

Fig. 14-3. Pathologic features of neuromyelitis optica. *A,* Spinal cord cross section demonstrating extensive demyelination in gray and white matter (Luxol fast blue and PAS myelin stain). *B,* Pronounced perivascular immunoglobulin reactivity (human Ig). *C,* IgM immunocytochemistry demonstrates a rosette perivascular staining pattern. *D,* Numerous perivascular eosinophils (*arrows*) are located within the lesion (Hematoxylin-eosin). Staining for complement activation with C9 neoantigen (*red*) demonstrates rim (*E*) and rosette (*F*) patterns of staining. (From Lucchinetti CF, Parisi J, Bruck W. The pathology of multiple sclerosis. Neurol Clin. 2005;23:77-105. Used with permission.)

    f. Pathology: predominant perivenular inflammation, with relative lack of confluent demyelination (Fig. 14-6)
    g. Most patients with ADEM recover
    h. Relapses and up to 20% mortality can occur in children
6. Acute hemorrhagic leukoencephalitis (Hurst disease)
    a. Characterized by abrupt fever, meningeal signs, seizures, and impaired level of consciousness following upper respiratory tract infection in 50% of patients from all age groups
    b. Possibly a form of ADEM
    c. Pathology: diffuse (sometimes asymmetric) edema and herniation associated with diffuse perivascular hemorrhages and demyelinating lesions with neutrophilic infiltration of perivascular cuffs surrounding necrotic venules with fibrinous exudates (Fig. 14-7)
    d. Usually fatal
7. Marburg variant of multiple sclerosis
    a. Characterized by confluent areas of enhancing hemispheric demyelination, typically asymmetric, on MRI, with mass effect and herniation, in the absence of oligoclonal bands
    b. Pathology: necrosis (Fig. 14-6), reflected in a more severe clinical course

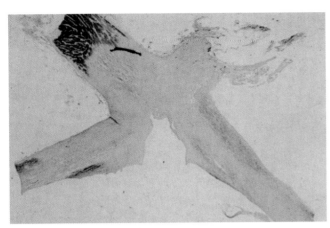

Fig. 14-4. Neuromyelitis optica. Gross specimen showing extensive demyelination through the optic chiasm. (From Okazaki H. Fundamentals of neuropathology. New York: Igaku-Shoin; 1983. p. 146. By permission of Mayo Foundation.)

    c. Patients may die, may recover with marked morbidity, or may remain free of relapse

    d. Disease may recur or evolve into RRMS after recovery from initial attack

8. Tumefactive multiple sclerosis
    a. Characterized by large tumor-like solitary demyelinating lesions with concentric whorled appearance in some cases (Baló's concentric sclerosis) (Fig. 14-6)
    b. Course may be monophasic, but may also evolve into RRMS
    c. Biopsy sometimes needed to differentiate from tumor (radiation is detrimental in demyelinating disease)
    d. Tumefactive multiple sclerosis without Baló's concentric sclerosis responds to corticosteroid therapy and has a more favorable course

9. Myelinoclastic diffuse sclerosis (Schilder's disease)
    a. Characterized by bilateral symmetric, hemispheric demyelinating lesions larger than 3×2 cm that can involve subcortical U fibers and adjacent cerebral cortex
    b. A rare syndrome of children, who present with visual problems, blindness, headache, vomiting, seizures
    c. Must be differentiated from leukodystrophy
    d. Pathology: mononuclear cellular infiltration maximal in the center rather than periphery, with axonal injury, tissue necrosis, and cavitation

E. Prototypical Bout-Onset Multiple Sclerosis
1. Epidemiology
    a. Prevalence decreases toward the equator and increases above 40 degrees north latitude and below 40 degrees south latitude

    b. High prevalence: defined as more than 30/100,000
    c. Based on population-based study in Olmsted County Minnesota, in 2000, age- and sex-adjusted prevalence rate is 191/100,000; crude annual incidence rates are 4.5/100,000 for men, 10.4/100,000 for women, 7.5/100,000 overall
    d. 250,000 to 350,000 cases of multiple sclerosis in U.S.
    e. Female-to-male ratio: 1.4 to 2.2/1
    f. Peak age at clinical onset of disease: 25 to 30

2. Etiology
    a. Epidemiologic evidence for complex interplay of genetics and environment but biologic relevance of individual genetic and environmental factors is not known
    b. Epidemiologic evidence for genetic basis
        1) Increased susceptibility in Caucasians
        2) Excess occurrence in Northern Europeans relative to indigenous populations of same region or virtual absence even in widely migrating populations such as gypsies
        3) 15% to 20% of patients have history of familial multiple sclerosis
        4) Excess concordance in monozygotic twins (31%) compared with dizygotic twins
        5) Increased recurrence in relatives (3% to 5%): 20 to 40 times more in first-degree relatives; rapid decrease by degree of relatedness
        6) No excess in adopted relatives of patients with multiple sclerosis
        7) Human leukocyte antigen (HLA)-DR2 (DRB1*1501,DQ1*0602—chromosome 6p21): associated with three- to fourfold increased risk of sporadic and familial cases of multiple sclerosis (in Sardinians, HLA-DR3 and HLA-DR4)
        8) Linkage to chromosome 12p12 in a large pedigree
    c. Epidemiologic evidence for environmental basis
        1) Geographic variation in prevalence and mutable risk with migration from low to high as well as high to low prevalence areas
        2) Pockets of increased prevalence and rare epidemics of multiple sclerosis (Faroe Islands, Iceland after World War II)
        3) Incomplete concordance (<30%) in monozygotic twins
        4) Emotional trauma: stress is associated with 1.9-fold increase in exacerbations of multiple sclerosis
        5) Physical trauma is not associated with onset or exacerbations of multiple sclerosis
        6) Associated with increased risk of multiple sclerosis
            a) Epstein-Barr virus: 2.1- to 5.5-fold
            b) Measles or mumps after age 15
            c) Insufficient vitamin D intake
            d) Smoking: 1.4- to 1.9-fold (dose effect of pack years)

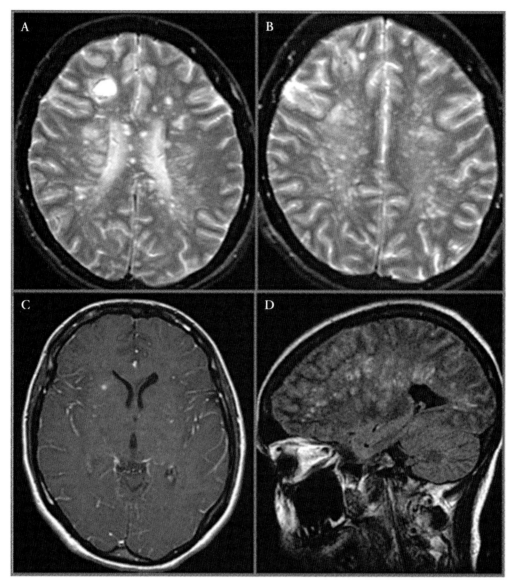

Fig. 14-5. MRI findings in biopsy-proven acute disseminated encephalomyelitis. (For contrast with typical multiple sclerosis lesions, see Figure 14-9.) *A* and *B,* Diffuse, punctate T2-weighted hyperintense lesions. *C,* Limited enhancement in T1-weighted image. *D,* Sagittal FLAIR-weighted image showing diffuse hyperintense lesions.

7) Decreased risk of multiple sclerosis: increased sun exposure between ages 6 and 15 and increased actinic sun damage

3. Pathology
   a. Early active lesion (Fig. 14-8)
      1) Perivascular inflammation
      2) Evidence of myelin breakdown, with lipid-laden macrophages
      3) Relatively preserved axons
      4) Presence or absence of oligodendrocytes
      5) Large hypertrophic-reactive astrocytes with eosinophilic cytoplasm and granular mitosis (Creutzfeldt-Peters cells) (these can be differentiated from glioma by even distribution rather than clumping together)
      6) Axonal ovoids indicative of newly transected axons may be seen in early active lesions
   b. Chronic inactive lesion (Fig. 14-9 and 14-10)
      1) Sharply circumscribed, hypocellular "plaque" with variable degree of perivascular inflammation, lack of active myelin breakdown, decreased or absent mature oligodendrocytes, incomplete remyelination restricted

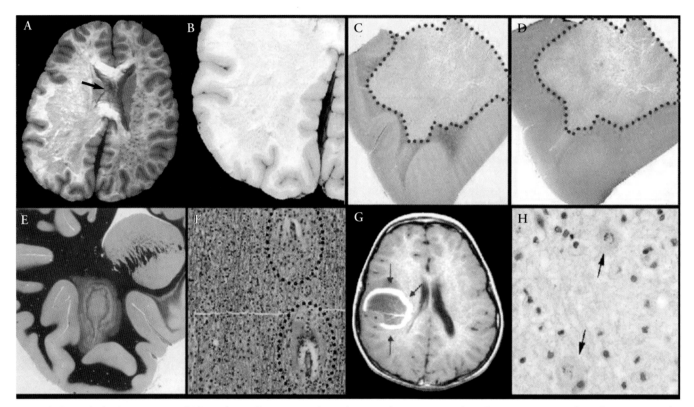

Fig. 14-6. Pathologic spectrum of idiopathic inflammatory demyelinating diseases. *A* and *B*, Gross specimens of Marburg type multiple sclerosis. Large confluent lesions lead to mass effect and herniation (*arrow* in *A*). *C* and *D*, Microscopic sections of lesion in *A* and *B* showing (*dotted area*) extensive demyelination (Luxol fast blue and PAS myelin stain) and axonal loss (Bielschowsky's silver impregnation). *E*, Baló's concentric sclerosis showing the characteristic alternating bands of demyelination and preserved myelin. *F*, Lesions of acute disseminated encephalomyelitis are characterized by perivascular inflammation and only minimal, mainly perivenular demyelination (*dotted circles*). *G*, Tumefactive lesion (*arrows*) with severe edema and mass effect. *H*, Hypertrophic astrocytes (*arrows*) (Creutzfeldt-Peters cell) in acute demyelinating lesion. (*A-D* and *F-H*, From Lucchinetti CF, Parisi J, Bruck W. The pathology of multiple sclerosis. Neurol Clin. 2005;23:77-105. Used with permission. *E*, From Okazaki H. Fundamentals of neuropathology. New York: Igaku-Shoin; 1983. p. 145. By permission of Mayo Foundation.)

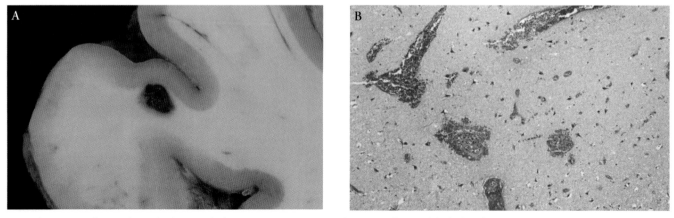

Fig. 14-7. Acute hemorrhagic leukoencephalitis. *A*, Gross specimen showing a focus of dark discoloration in juxtacortical white matter. *B*, Punctate perivascular hemorrhages in white matter.

to the edge of the "plaque," markedly reduced axonal density, and presence of fibrillary gliosis

    2) Oligodendrocyte precursor cells, extensive remyelination can be present in some lesions but with reduced staining for myelin "shadow plaques"

  c. Normal-appearing white matter is not disease-free

    1) Diffuse axonal injury and wallerian degeneration, diffuse lymphocytic infiltration (predominantly CD8+ T cells), and microglial activation

    2) Magnetic resonance spectroscopy evidence of reduced *N*-acetylaspartate-to-creatine ratios and brain atrophy that is independent of T2 lesion load in MRI (see below)

  d. Involvement of cerebral and cerebellar gray matter possible

4. Immunopathogenesis (Fig. 14-11)

  a. Current working hypothesis of pathogenesis in BOMS is based on evidence from human disease and animal models of experimental allergic encephalomyelitis (EAE), canine distemper virus–induced demyelination, and Theiler's virus–induced demyelination

    1) Human disease: four patterns of immunopathogenesis

      a) Pattern I: macrophage-associated demyelination

      b) Pattern II: antibody/complement-associated demyelination

      c) Pattern III: distal dying-back oligodendrogliopathy

      d) Pattern IV: primary oligodendrocyte degeneration

    2) The same pattern may persist in a patient

    3) Pattern I and pattern II lesions resemble the EAE

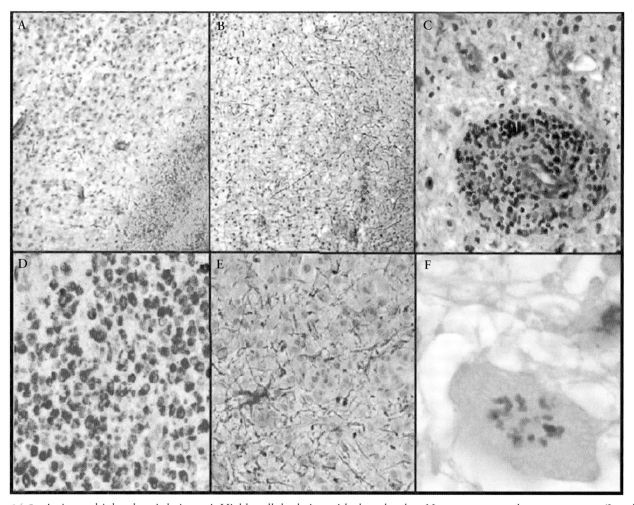

Fig. 14-8. Active multiple sclerosis lesion. *A*, Highly cellular lesion with sharp border. Numerous macrophages are present (Luxol fast blue and PAS myelin stain). *B*, Axons are reduced in number or lost and form so-called axonal balloons (Bielschowsky's silver impregnation). *C*, Dense perivascular infiltrate composed mainly of T cells (hematoxylin-eosin). *D*, Lesion is diffusely infiltrated by large number of macrophages removing the myelin debris (Ki-M1P). *E*, Astrocytes are hypertrophic, with increased multiple processes (glial fibrillary acidic protein). *F*, Hypertrophic astrocyte, so-called Creutzfeldt-Peters cell, with granular mitosis. (From Lucchinetti CF, Parisi J, Bruck W. The pathology of multiple sclerosis. Neurol Clin. 2005;23:77-105. Used with permission.)

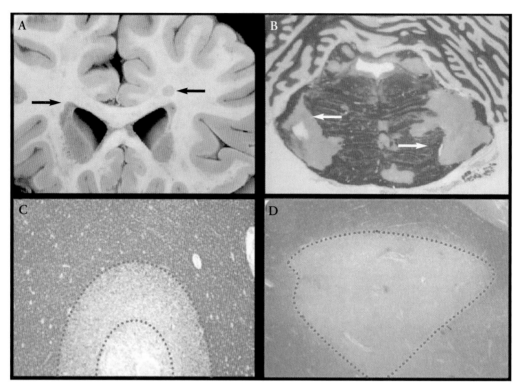

Fig. 14-9. Chronic multiple sclerosis lesions. *A*, Gross specimen showing periventricular plaques (*arrows*) typical of multiple sclerosis. *B*, Section through pons stained for myelin (Luxol fast blue and PAS myelin stain). Note numerous demyelinated lesions (*arrows*). *C* and *D*, Remyelinated so-called shadow plaques are characterized by reduced staining intensity of myelin. Remyelination is either restricted to the lesion edge (*dotted lines* in *C*, stained for MBP) or present throughout lesion (*dotted line*) (*D*, Luxol fast blue and PAS myelin stain). (From Lucchinetti CF, Parisi J, Bruck W. The pathology of multiple sclerosis. Neurol Clin. 2005;23:77-105. Used with permission.)

model of multiple sclerosis

b. Multiple sclerosis is a heterogeneous disease with multiple pathologic pathways leading to a similar clinical disease

c. One or more etiologic factors could be important in pathogenesis

　1) Evidence suggesting multiple sclerosis is a viral disease: evidence for endemics, susceptibility of CNS to acute and latent viral diseases that can also present as attacks, resemblance to canine distemper virus–induced or Theiler's virus–induced demyelination models

　2) Evidence suggesting multiple sclerosis is an autoimmune disease: presence of immune activation in the absence of a specific viral agent linked to causality, presence of abnormal T-cell clones, association with MHC class II molecules, resemblance to EAE

d. Common "autoimmune hypothesis" favoring the presence of Th1 over Th2 type T cells in the pathogenesis of autoimmune diseases and multiple sclerosis

　1) Protection from autoimmunity is achieved by self-tolerance mechanisms

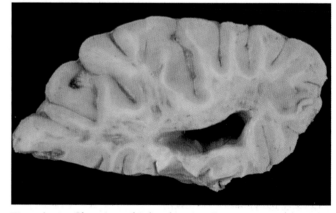

Fig. 14-10. Chronic multiple sclerosis. Gross specimen showing extensive confluent plaques in periventricular and juxtacortical white matter.

　　a) Central tolerance is achieved by thymic "negative-selection" of T cells sensitized to self (MHC class I molecules involved in recognition of self)

　　b) Peripheral tolerance is achieved by the type of the

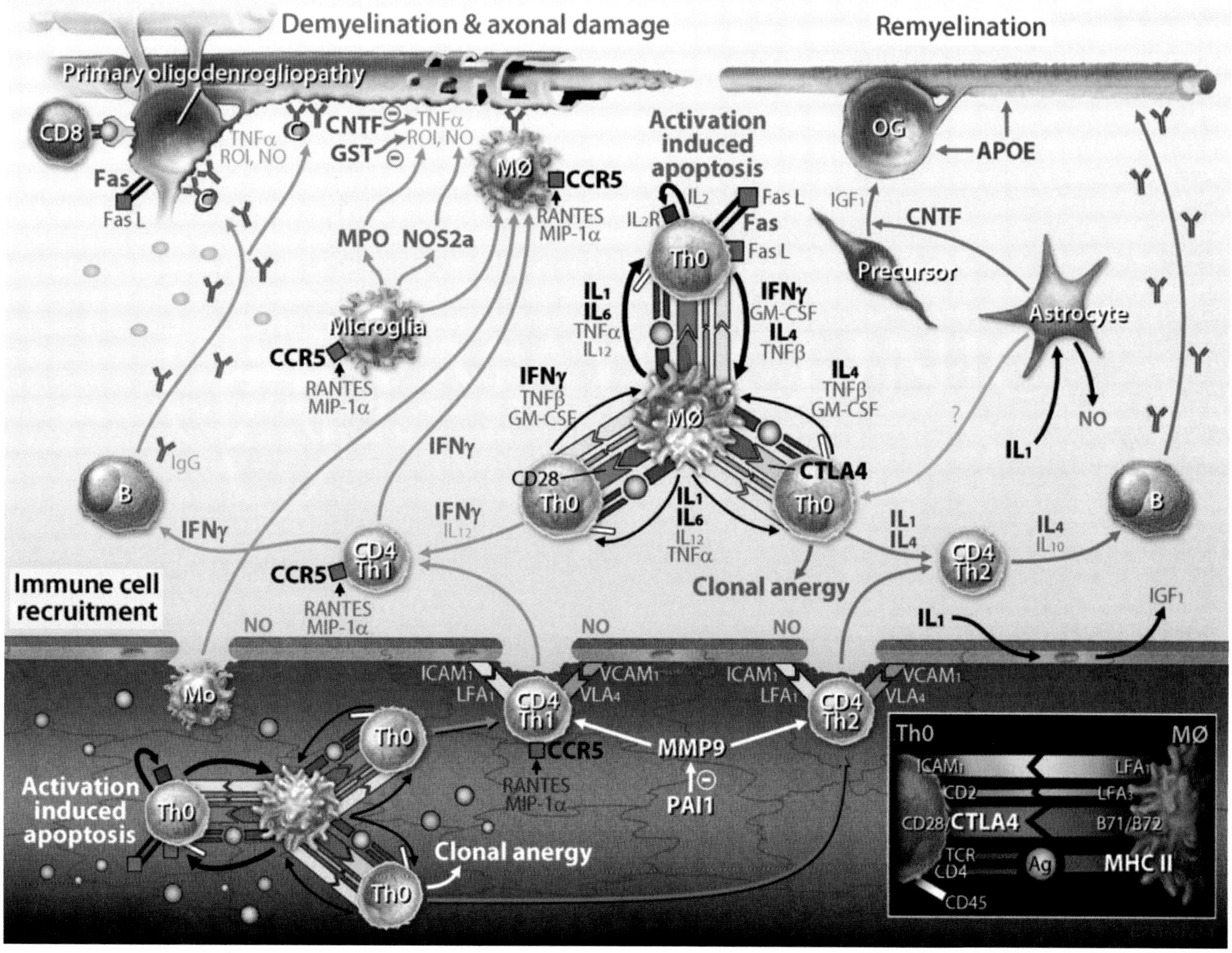

Fig. 14-11. Immunopathogenesis of multiple sclerosis and common autoimmune hypothesis, with immune cell recruitment and immune activation both peripherally and centrally leading to oligodendrocyte (*OG*) injury, demyelination, axonal damage. Favorable pathways and their end result of partial remyelination are in blue, and detrimental pathways and their end results are in red. *Inset*, T cell (*Th0*) and antigen-presenting cell (macrophage *MØ*) interaction and the involved molecules. Specific molecules involved in the T-cell macrophage interaction leading to activation-induced apoptosis, clonal anergy, or specific T-cell clonal expansion are shown both centrally and peripherally. Ag, antigen; APOE, apolipoprotein E; CNTF, ciliary neutrophilic factor; GM-CSF, granulocyte macrophage colony-stimulating factor; GST, glutathione-S-transferase; ICAM, intracellular adhesion molecule; IGF, insulin-like growth factor; IL, interleukin; INF, interferon; LFA, leukocyte function-associated antigen; MHC, major histocompatibility complex; MMP, matrix metalloproteinase; MPO myeloperoxidase; NO, nitric oxide; NOS, nitric oxide synthase; PAT, proton-coupled amino acid transporter; RANTES, regulated upon activated, normally T-cell expressed, and presumably secreted; ROI, reactive oxygen intermediate; TCR, T-cell receptor; TNF, tumor necrosis factor; VCAM, vascular cell adhesion molecule; VLA, very late activation protein.

costimulatory pathway used
  i) Th0 cell activation using CTLA4 can lead to clonal anergy or generate a Th2-cell response (thought to be protective)
  ii) Th0-cell activation using CD28 can lead to a Th1-cell response (thought to be detrimental)

c) Activation-induced apoptosis results from high intensity of the antigenic stimulus to Th0 cells, leading to increased production of interleukin (IL)-2 and activation of apoptotic Fas/FasL pathway
  i) Mutations in Fas lead to systemic autoimmunity in mice and men (autoimmune lymphoprolifer-

ative syndrome)
   d) Cells that escape central and peripheral tolerance become autoreactive T-cell clones, which are present in every person
2) A foreign antigen can lead to autoreactive T-cell activation due to molecular mimicry or a similar mechanism
   a) A uniform antigenic stimulus is not identified in multiple sclerosis—against the autoimmune hypothesis
   b) Initial event is presentation of an unknown antigen to naive Th0 cells by antigen-presenting cells (e.g., macrophages, microglia, B cells) via trimolecular complex (MHC class II, CD4, and T-cell receptor)
   c) Autoreactive T-cell activation can happen in CNS or in the periphery with recruitment through blood-brain barrier via integrin (endothelial surface) and adhesion molecule (lymphocyte surface) interactions (VCAM/VLA-4, ICAM/LFA-4) and matrix metalloproteinase-9 (MMP-9) stimulation
3) Proinflammatory cytokines secreted by Th1 cells initiate the detrimental cascade of events leading to myelin injury and/or primary oligodendrocyte degeneration
   a) Autoreactive antibodies produced by B cells, complement activation, microglia-induced myeloperoxidase (MPO) secretion and NOS2A activation, macrophage-induced demyelination, tumor necrosis factor α, nitric oxide (NO), reactive oxygen species (ROIs), and CD8 cell– or Fas-induced apoptosis
4) Anti-inflammatory cytokines (e.g., IL-1, IL-4, IL-10) secreted by Th2 cells initiate the protective cascade of events leading to myelin repair and/or oligodendrocyte precursor activation
   a) Remyelination depends on antibodies produced by B cells, ciliary neurotrophic factor produced by astrocytes, insulin-like growth factor-I produced by endothelial cells, apolipoprotein E, and glutathione synthetase family of molecules
5. Clinical syndromes and disease course
   a. An asymptomatic period of unknown duration precedes initial presentation with an isolated syndrome, as may be evidenced by neuroimaging
   b. Initial bout or attack: acute or subacute onset of isolated IIDD(s) evolving in several days, followed by stabilization and recovery (spontaneous or with treatment)
      1) No specific signs or symptoms of multiple sclerosis
      2) Typical onset: either monosymptomatic or polysymptomatic with sensory symptoms, unilateral optic neuritis (leading to relative afferent pupillary defect),

pyramidal symptoms, cerebellar symptoms, brainstem signs such as internuclear ophthalmoplegia (involvement of medial longitudinal fasciculus, most common reason in young adults), and bladder-bowel incontinence or retention
      3) Less common presentations: Lhermitte's sign (flexion of neck induces back or extremity paresthesias), cortical symptoms (aphasia, apraxia, recurrent seizures, visual field defects), or extrapyramidal syndromes (chorea and rigidity) presenting as individual attacks
   c. Relapses, with complete remission or stepwise accumulation of deficit
      1) Occurrence (on average): once every 2 years
      2) Frequency decreases with time
   d. Fatigue: worse in the afternoon with physiologic increase in body temperature
   e. Uhthoff's phenomenon: all symptoms may be exacerbated by overheating
   f. Pseudoexacerbations: appear like a new "attack" and may occur with fever, exhaustion, or metabolic upset
   g. Pain syndromes associated with multiple sclerosis: neuralgias (e.g., trigeminal neuralgia), dysesthesia, radicular pain, flexor and extensor spasms, optic neuritis, low back pain, osteoporosis-associated fractures
   h. Recurrent, brief stereotypic paroxysmal symptoms (e.g., paroxysmal limb pain and paresthesias, myokymia, hemifacial spasm, trigeminal neuralgia, episodic clumsiness and dysarthria, tonic limb posturing) are likely due to ephaptic transmission and may respond to antiepileptic agents
   i. Spasticity is a major problem in multiple sclerosis
   j. Overt dementia: present in about 5% of patients; neuropsychometric test abnormalities suggestive of subcortical dementia in 50% of patients
6. Diagnosis
   a. Based on clinical and paraclinical criteria of "dissemination in time and space" (Table 14-1)
   b. Differential diagnosis of BOMS: nongranulomatous vasculitides, granulomatous disorders (Wegener's granulomatosis, sarcoidosis), connective tissue disorders (rheumatoid arthritis, systemic lupus erythematosus, Sjögren's syndrome) Behçet's syndrome, infections (Lyme disease, human T-cell lymphoma virus, human immunodeficiency virus, progressive multifocal leukoencephalopathy, neurosyphilis, Epstein-Barr virus, cytomegalovirus), CNS lymphoma
   c. Paraclinical (laboratory) studies used in diagnosis: MRI, evoked potentials, CSF studies
   d. Paraclinical studies may indicate disease activity even in absence of clinical activity

1) MRI
   a) 90% to 97% sensitive
   b) Typical lesions: localized to juxtacortical and periventricular white matter, corpus callosum, brainstem, cerebellar peduncles (Fig. 14-12)
   c) Lesions are usually ovoid
   d) "Dawson's fingers": lesions follow deep white matter medullary veins from ventricle into centrum semiovale, best seen in sagittal images as flame-like lesions perpendicular to lateral ventricles
   e) Acute multiple sclerosis lesions: typically isointense in T1-weighted images, hyperintense in FLAIR images (helpful in visualizing periventricular and juxtacortical lesions due to fluid suppression), and hyperintense in T2-weighted images (more sensitive than FLAIR for posterior fossa lesions)
   f) Active lesions: enhancement
      i) Characteristic enhancement pattern with open ring toward cerebral cortex, but can be solid
      ii) Enhancement represents blood-brain barrier breakdown and may persist for up to 2 to 6 weeks without acute treatment
   g) Chronic lesions: typically hypointense in T1-weighted images (black holes); not usually seen in posterior fossa and should be differentiated from strokes (which are isointense with CSF in all sequences)
      i) Chronic corpus callosal atrophy, whole-brain atrophy and ex-vacuo dilatation of ventricles correlate with disability and cognitive decline
      ii) "Multiple sclerosis-like" lesions may be seen with hypertension or migraine headaches: typically, lesions are distributed randomly throughout white matter
2) Evoked potentials
   a) Sensitivity of evoked potentials in diagnosis of multiple sclerosis
      i) Visual evoked potentials, 80% to 85%
      ii) Sensory evoked potentials, 75%
      iii) Brainstem auditory evoked potentials, 65%
   b) Visual evoked potentials are abnormal in more than 90% of patients with previous optic neuritis despite normal visual acuity
3) CSF
   a) Usually normal cell count or mild lymphocytosis (<50 cells) with normal or slightly increased protein and presence of oligoclonal bands (90%-95% sensitive) and increased IgG index (sign of intrathecal antibody secretion independent of blood-brain barrier breakdown)
   b) Oligoclonal bands may not be present initially but can appear later in the disease course
   c) Oligoclonal bands can also be present in other conditions (7%) (e.g., subacute sclerosing panencephalitis, CNS measles and rubella, chronic meningitis, neurosyphilis, neurosarcoidosis, paraneoplastic disorders, acute idiopathic demyelinating polyneuropathy [Guillain-Barré syndrome] and sometimes stroke)
   e. Diagnostic criteria for multiple sclerosis
      1) Former diagnostic criteria (Poser criteria) did not allow for diagnosis of RRMS in the setting of only one clinical attack or diagnosis of PPMS
      2) Recently modified diagnostic criteria (McDonald criteria) included neuroimaging to expand clinical definition of dissemination in space or time that is required to diagnose prototypic RRMS
      3) This modification helps with earlier diagnosis of RRMS and yields a fourfold increase in the diagnosis of definite RRMS in first 12 months after a clinically isolated event
7. Natural history and prognosis
   a. Benign multiple sclerosis: in about 15% of patients, all neurologic systems remain fully functional 15 years after disease onset
   b. Accumulation of disability over time
      1) Disability is caused by progressive cognitive impairment, depression, emotional lability, dysarthria, dysphagia, vertigo, progressive quadriparesis, sensory loss, ataxic tremors, pain, sexual dysfunction, spasticity, severe sphincter problems
      2) Disability can accumulate in absence of clinical activity because of subclinical disease activity
      3) Most commonly accepted clinical scales for defining disability in multiple sclerosis are Kurtzke Expanded Disability Status Scale (EDSS) and Multiple Sclerosis Functional Composite (MSFC)
      4) MSFC includes cognitive dysfunction and correlates better with MRI changes
   c. Clinical predictors of relatively favorable course
      1) Female sex
      2) Young age at onset (<40)
      3) Optic neuritis or sensory symptoms at onset
      4) Monosymptomatic onset
   d. Clinical predictors of unfavorable course
      1) Male sex
      2) Older age at onset (>40)
      3) Motor, cerebellar, or sphincter symptoms at initial presentation
      4) Multifocal (polysymptomatic) disease at onset

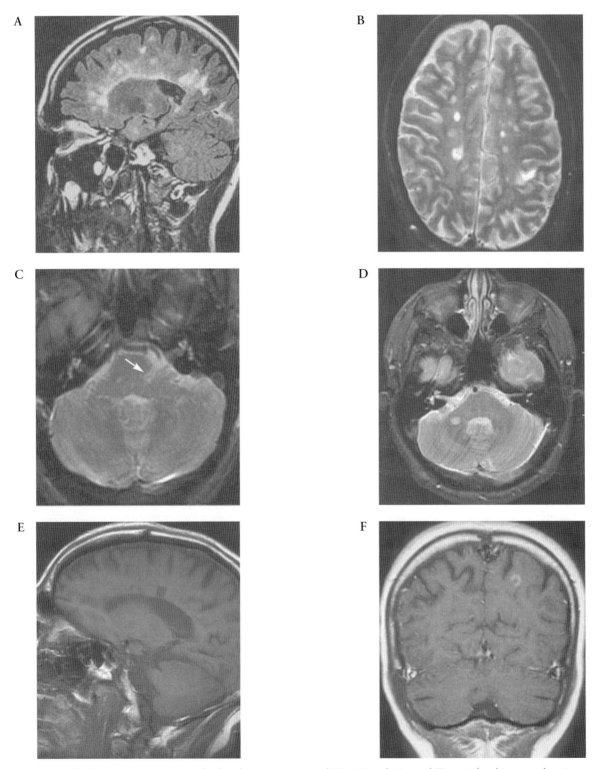

Fig. 14-12. MRI findings in bout-onset multiple sclerosis. *A*, Sagittal FLAIR and, *B*, axial T2-weighted images showing multiple rounded areas of increased T2 signal in deep and periventricular white matter, some perpendicular to lateral ventricles (*A*). *C*, T2-weighted image from multiple sclerosis patient presenting with facial sensory symptoms; image shows increased signal along left trigeminal nerve (*arrow*). *D*, T2-weighted image of a plaque in middle cerebellar peduncle, typical for multiple sclerosis. *E*, T1-weighted sagittal image with old periventricular "Dawson's finger" lesion appearing hypointense ("black hole") and perpendicular to lateral ventricle. *F*, Gadolinium-enhanced T1-weighted image showing typical enhancement pattern (open-ring enhancement) of a juxtacortical lesion.

5) Relatively frequent attacks within first 5 years
6) Short interval between first two attacks
7) Relatively short time to reach EDSS level 4 (out of 10)
8) Progressive course
9) High lesion load, apparent on early neuroimaging
10) Incomplete remission after first relapses
  e. Course in first 5 years usually predicts outcome
  f. During pregnancy: relapse rate decreases but postpartum relapse rate initially increases and later decreases to pre-conception disease frequency
  g. Cross-sectional MRI does not reliably predict long-term outcome (brain atrophy correlates with long-term cognitive dysfunction)
  h. *APOE* genotype may correlate with long-term outcome (ε4 allele unfavorable, ε2 allele favorable)
  i. Homozygosity for HLA-DR1501 alleles may be associated with more severe disease
  j. Development of SPMS
    1) May represent crossing of a clinical threshold of axonal damage resulting from previous or ongoing inflammatory demyelinating episodes
    2) SPMS evolves from RRMS after a highly variable period
    3) 75% of RRMS patients develop SPMS disease course by 25 years
    4) Predictors of conversion to SPMS: male sex, older age at onset, polysymptomatic onset, sphincter symptoms at onset, recurrent motor or sphincter symptoms, early attainment of disability
  k. 50% of multiple sclerosis patients die of causes other than multiple sclerosis
  l. Mean survival: more than 25 years after disease onset

F. Primary Progressive Multiple Sclerosis
1. Characterized by insidious, progressive course and lack of definite exacerbations, paucity of radiographic findings (e.g., gadolinium-enhancing lesions), laboratory, or pathologic evidence of inflammation
2. Differential diagnosis when presenting as progressive myelopathy: progressive myelopathic disorders, disorders with deficiency states (such as vitamin B_{12} deficiency), Arnold-Chiari malformation with syrinx, dural arteriovenous fistulas, spinocerebellar ataxias, hereditary spastic paraparesis, presenilin-1 mutation associated with spastic paraparesis, adrenomyeloneuropathy, and primary lateral sclerosis
3. Second most common form of IIDD after BOMS (7% in hospital-based cases and 20% in population-based cases of multiple sclerosis)
  a. Features distinguishing PPMS from prototypical BOMS:

older age at onset, lack of female preponderance, predilection for chronic progressive myelopathy, paucity of intracranial lesions (only in 60%-70% and few lesions) found on MRI
  b. PPMS has worse prognosis than BOMS (one-half of patients with PPMS require at least unilateral gait assistance by 8 years)
    1) Involvement of three or more functional systems (motor, cerebellar, sensory, or other) predicts a significantly worse outcome than involvement of two or fewer systems

G. Treatment of Idiopathic Inflammatory Demyelinating Diseases
1. Treatment of relapses
  a. High-dose corticosteroid therapy
    1) Alleviates symptoms faster than natural history of the attack
    2) Transiently restores blood-brain barrier
    3) Does *not* affect long-term outcome
      a) Two or three annual courses of methylprednisolone intravenously may slow accumulating clinical disability or cerebral atrophy seen on MRI
    4) Intravenous "pulse" of methylprednisolone 500 to 1,000 mg daily for 3 to 7 days with gastrointestinal prophylaxis is the accepted practice
    5) Tapered oral dose may be continued but is not necessary
    6) Lower dose oral prednisone alone may increase the risk of recurrent episodes of disease activity in optic neuritis
    7) Other intravenous corticosteroids such as dexamethasone or adrenocorticotropic hormone may be administered instead
    8) Minimally symptomatic attacks limited to nondisabling systems (e.g., sensory symptoms) do not need to be treated
    9) Chronic or frequent use of corticosteroids may increase the risk of osteoporosis, but osteoporosis may develop independently of corticosteroid use in prototypical RRMS
  b. Natalizumab (Tysabri) is a humanized anti-α4-integrin antibody that inhibits the trafficking of leukocytes across endothelium: approved but marketing was suspended in March 2005 because of cases of progressive multifocal leukoencephalopathy
  c. Plasma exchange may benefit patients with severe attacks with marked acute disability in whom acute corticosteroid therapy fails
    1) 7.1-fold increased chance of moderate or better recovery over sham treatment

2) Seven exchanges administered every other day is accepted regimen

2. Chronic immunomodulatory and immunosuppressant treatments

   a. Several immunomodulatory treatments are available (Table 14-2): none are curative

   b. All the listed medications are approved by U.S. Food and Drug Administration (FDA)

   c. Interferons and glatiramer acetate: approved for RRMS but not any of the progressive forms

   d. Mitoxantrone hydrochloride (immunosuppressant)

     1) Approved for SPMS and worsening RRMS, specifically during rapid progression from RRMS to SPMS

     2) Important dose-dependent cardiotoxicity, which is less than its analogue, doxorubicin

     3) The risk for chronic cardiomyopathy limits the approved cumulative dose of mitoxantrone for treatment of multiple sclerosis to 140 mg/m^2

   e. Effects of immunomodulatory treatments

     1) Decreased number of attacks (variable rate, approaching 30% for interferons)

     2) Decreased number of enhancing lesions on MRI

     3) Reduced enlargement rate of lesions on MRI

     4) Likely help to decrease long-term atrophy

     5) None have been studied long enough to address long-term clinical benefit

   f. Interferons produce neutralizing antibodies that may hamper their effectiveness; the frequency of this differs by agent

   g. Mechanism of action of these agents is incompletely understood

     1) Interferons

       a) Reduce overall T-cell proliferation and production of tumor necrosis factor α

       b) Decrease antigen presentation

       c) Shift T-cell response to a Th2 type response

       d) Increase IL-10 and IL-4 secretion

       e) Reduce immune cell trafficking through the blood-brain barrier by inhibiting adhesion molecules, chemokines, and proteases involved in the trafficking

     2) Glatiramer acetate

       a) Synthetic polypeptide mix containing alanine, lysine, tyrosine

       b) May promote proliferation of Th2 cytokines

       c) Competes with myelin basic protein for presentation on MHC class II molecules

       d) Alters macrophage function

       e) Induces antigen-specific suppressor T cells

     3) Mitoxantrone hydrochloride

       a) Potent immunosuppressant with important dose-dependent cardiotoxicity, which is less than its analogue, doxorubicin

       b) Suppresses proliferation of T cells, B cells, and macrophages

       c) Impairs antigen presentation

       d) Decreases secretion of proinflammatory cytokines

       e) Enhances T-cell suppressor function

       f) Inhibits B-cell function and antibody production

       g) Inhibits macrophage-mediated myelin degradation

   h. Controlled High-Risk Subjects Avonex Multiple Sclerosis Study (CHAMPS) and Early Treatment of Multiple Sclerosis (ETOMS) trial

     1) Onset of treatment with interferon beta-1a after the first attack of isolated demyelinating syndrome delays conversion to clinically definite multiple sclerosis by Poser criteria (Table 14-1) and lowers the risk of subsequent attack from 50% (placebo treated) to ~35% (low-dose interferon–treated) over 2 to 3 years

Table 14-2. **Chronic Treatment Options for Multiple Sclerosis**

Multiple sclerosis type	Therapeutic agent	Dose
Isolated IIDDs RRMS	Interferon beta-1a (Avonex)	30 μg, IM, weekly
	Interferon beta-1a (Rebif)	22 μg, SC, weekly
	Interferon beta-1b (Betaseron)	8 million IU, SC, every other day
	Interferon beta-1a (Avonex)	30 μg, IM, weekly
	Interferon beta-1a (Rebif)	22 or 44 μg, SC, every other day
	Glatiramer acetate (Copaxone)	20 μg, SC, every day
	Immunoglobulin	0.15-0.20 g/kg body weight, IV, monthly × 2 years
SPMS	Interferon beta-1b (Betaseron) (controversial)	8 million IU, SC, every other day
	Mitoxantrone hydrochloride	5 or 12 mg/m^2 body surface area, IV, every 3 months × 2 years
PPMS	None	

IIDD, idiopathic inflammatory demyelinating disease; IM, intramuscularly; PPMS, primary progressive multiple sclerosis; RRMS, relapsing-remitting multiple sclerosis; SC, subcutaneously; SPMS, secondary progressive multiple sclerosis.

2) Beneficial effect in CHAMPS is different for different clinically isolated syndromes and should not be generalized

  a) Prevention of conversion to clinically definite multiple sclerosis is evident in an isolated spinal cord syndrome more than a brainstem-cerebellar syndrome

  b) In case of isolated optic neuritis, the effect is marginal

  c) For patients defined as "high risk" for converting to multiple sclerosis by having at least nine T2-weighted hyperintense lesions and at least one enhancing lesion in initial MRI study, predicts a two-thirds reduction in conversion to definite multiple sclerosis in 2 years, but 44% in this group do not convert to definite multiple sclerosis in 2 years without any treatment

3) Follow-up time is short for both studies and there is no evidence that delayed conversion to BOMS prevents long-term disability

3. Symptomatic treatment

  a. Fatigue

    1) Mainstay treatment: organization of daily chores with intermittent rest periods

    2) First-choice medical treatment: amantadine 100 mg twice daily

    3) Alternatives: modafinil 200 mg once or twice daily, pemoline 18.75 mg daily (short-term use associated with liver toxicity, often not recommended), or selective serotonin reuptake inhibitors (SSRIs) (little evidence for the latter)

    4) Aspirin has been suggested recently

  b. Spasticity

    1) Mainstay treatment: physical and occupational therapy

    2) Overtreatment of spasticity may lead to loss of beneficial posture to overcome weakness

    3) First choice: oral baclofen 10 mg daily before sleep and titrated to 60 mg daily or higher; if refractory, intrathecal baclofen pump

    4) Alternatives: tizanidine up to 8 mg four times daily, dantrolene 25 mg daily and titrated to symptoms, or benzodiazepines

  c. Paroxysmal symptoms and pain

    1) First choice: carbamazepine

    2) Alternatives: phenytoin, gabapentin, or other antiepileptics

    3) Tricyclic antidepressants

    4) Rhizotomy for refractory trigeminal neuralgia

    5) Hydroxyzine for itching

    6) Botox injections for spasms

  d. Depression: SSRIs or tricyclic antidepressants

  e. Cerebellar tremor

    1) Clonazepam, valproic acid, or isoniazid

    2) Thalamic stimulator for contralateral tremor for refractory cases

    3) Overall, difficult to manage effectively

  f. Bladder dysfunction

    1) Characterized by urodynamic studies (and urology consultation if necessary)

    2) Most common urologic issue: frequency and urgency due to hyperreflexic bladder with small capacity and early detrusor contraction

      a) Chronic medical management with anticholinergics: oxybutynin (Ditropan), tolterodine (Detrol), or hyoscyamine (Levsinex)

    3) Less common urologic issue: flaccid bladder

      a) Mainstay treatment: self-catheterization

      b) Medical treatments: cholinergic agents (bethanechol and baclofen can be used)

    4) Sphincter-detrusor dyssynergia: α-adrenergic blockers such as prazosin (Minipress) used to relax the sphincter

    5) Acute worsening could be due to urinary tract infections and should be managed appropriately

II. AUTOIMMUNE CONNECTIVE TISSUE DISORDERS (TABLE 14-3)

A. Systemic Lupus Erythematous (SLE)

1. Systemic manifestations of SLE: malar rash, photosensitivity, arthritis, serositis (pleuritis or pericarditis), nephritis, mucosal ulcers, hematologic depression (anemia, leukopenia, thrombocytopenia), hypocomplementemia, false-positive VDRL (differentiate from neurosyphilis)

2. Neuropsychiatric presentation (50% of SLE patients) can be acute (e.g., antiphospholipid antibody syndrome and stroke), subacute, or chronic progressive with relapses

  a. 30% reduced 5-year survival for patients with neurologic involvement

  b. Psychiatric and behavioral CNS manifestations (most common): acute confusional states, psychosis, dementia (must rule out opportunistic infections)

  c. Stroke (arterial and venous)

    1) Most important neurologic manifestation

    2) Due to cardiac emboli, coagulopathy, degenerative vasculopathy, venous sinus thrombosis

Table 14-3. Common Systemic Autoimmune Vasculitis and Nonvasculitic Inflammatory Disorders With Neurologic Complications*

Type	Systemic	Symptoms CNS	PNS	Diagnosis	Treatment
			Connective tissue diseases		
SLE	Rash (malar or discoid), photosensitivity, oral ulcers, arthritis, serositis, nephropathy, Libman-Sacks endocarditis	Seizures, stroke,[†] chorea, parkinsonism, ataxia, vasculitis (rare), APL syndrome, behavioral,[‡] transverse myelitis	Axonal sensori-motor neuropathy, mononeuritis multiplex, trigeminal sensory neuropathy	Lab: ANA, anti–double-stranded DNA, anti-RNP, anti-SM, APL, ↓ RBCs, ↓ platelets, ↓ WBCs CSF: pleocytosis, ↑ protein, OCBs MRI Cerebral angiography and/or biopsy if necessary	NSAIDs, steroids if end-organ damage, anticoagulants if stroke, steroids & immunosuppressants
Rheumatoid arthritis	Symmetric polyarthritis, subcutaneous nodules, pulmonary nodules, interstitial fibrosis, pleuritis, pneumonitis, pericardial effusions, skin lesions, Felty's syndrome	CNS vasculitis (rare), rheumatoid extradural spinal or leptomeningeal nodules (rare), brainstem syndromes (rare), myelopathy (atlantoaxial dislocation)	Compression neuropathy, distal sensori-motor or sensory polyneuropathy, mononeuritis multiplex		NSAIDs, COX-2 inhibitors, gold, penicillamine, sulfasalazine, hydrochloroquine, immunosuppressive agents
Sjögren's syndrome	Exocrine gland (lacrimal/salivary), arthritis (80%), interstitial nephritis (40%), lymphoproliferative, lymphadenopathy, purpura	Aseptic meningitis, seizures, vasculitis, transverse myelitis (myelopathy) Rare: optic neuropathy, ataxia, INO, movement disorder	Polyganglionopathy (neuronopathy), trigeminal neuropathy, sensory or sensorimotor neuropathy, entrapment neuropathy, mononeuritis multiplex	Xeropthalmia: Schirmer's test (rose Bengal)/slit-lamp test Xerostomia: nuclear scan of salivary gland, radiologic sialography, salivary gland biopsy Lab: ↑ ESR, anemia, leukopenia, (+)RF, hypergammaglobulinemia, (+)SSB, (+)SSA CSF: lymphocytic pleocytosis, ↑ protein & protein synthesis, IgG, OCBs	
Systemic sclerosis	Raynaud's phenomenon, glomerulonephritis, GI mucosal lesions, keratoconjunctivitis, fibrosis (heart, lung, pleura, pericardium)		Trigeminal neuropathy, multiple mononeuropathies		Penicillamine, colchicine, prednisone, immunosuppressants tried with success Prognosis: 10-year survival, 50%

Table 14-3. (**continued**)

Type	Symptoms			Diagnosis	Treatment
	Systemic	CNS	PNS		
Mixed connective tissue disease	Arthralgia/arthritis, sclerodactyly, rash, lymphadenopathy, pericarditis, Raynaud's phenomenon, esophageal dysmotility, pulmonary hypertension	Aseptic meningitis, psychosis, seizures Rare: stroke, optic neuritis, chorea, ataxia, transverse myelitis (occur with active disease and are steroid-responsive)	Trigeminal sensory neuropathy, vasculitic neuropathy, myositis (occur at any time & are steroid resistant)	Clinical: >1 type of connective tissue disease & characteristic serologic markers CSF: lymphocytic pleocytosis or ↑ protein Creatine kinase/electromyography Biopsy: inflammatory myositis	Steroids, IVIG, pheresis or immunosuppressants for CNS disorders Myositis: steroid-responsive Trigeminal neuropathy and peripheral neuropathy: not steroid responsive

Systemic vasculitis

Type	Systemic	CNS	PNS	Diagnosis	Treatment
Behçet's disease	Uveitis/retinitis, oral or genital ulcers, skin ulcers or erythema nodosum, claudication (vasculitis), pulmonary infarct or myocardial (vasculitis), pulmonary aneurysms, gastrointestinal ulcers	Diencephalic-mesencephalic meningo-encephalitis/venulitis and associated MRI lesions, aseptic meningitis, focal brain lesion (white matter), venous thrombosis	Peripheral neuropathy, myopathy	No diagnostic test History of ulcers, skin lesions Lab: ESR (can be ↑ if large-vessel vasculitis), platelets (may be ↑), APL (↑ 15%-35% of patients) Skin biopsy Pathergy: nodular reaction at needle puncture site Eye exam MRI: white matter, brainstem, & deep gray lesions; *do not* have predilection for periventricular area CSF: ↑ cells (mean, 82) with predominantly lymphocytes, ↑ protein, may or may not be ↑ IgG & OCBs	Steroids: not effective in preventing neurologic morbidity Alkylating agents Chlorambucil: for uveitis or meningoencephalitis, risk of sterility with use Cyclosporine if chlorambucil doesn't work (side effect, renal disease) Azathioprine, methotrexate, colchicine For venous thrombosis: prednisone & alkylating agent (warfarin if no pulmonary vasculitis or low-dose aspirin)
Temporal arteritis	Fever, anorexia, weight loss, malaise, anemia, jaw claudication	Headache (72%), ± transient monocular blindness (anterior ischemic optic neuropathy, 10%-12%), stroke (rare)	Proximal muscle pain, & stiffness	↑ ESR, C-reactive protein, biopsy	Prednisone

Table 14-3. (continued)

| Type | Symptoms | | | Diagnosis | Treatment |
	Systemic	CNS	PNS		
Takayasu's arteritis		Stroke/transient ischemic attack, monocular blindness, dizziness Aorta (65%) > carotid (58%) > renal (38%) > vertebral (35%) artery		Physical exam: check pulse & blood pressure in both arms, check for bruits Lab: CBC, chemistry, ESR (>20 = active disease; used to monitor; ↑ in 72% with active and 44% with inactive disease), ultrasonography, MRI, angiography (cannot use to assess disease activity; long stenotic lesions)	Prednisone, other immunosuppressants (methotrexate, azathioprine) Surgery/PTCA (renal, carotid, aorta) *Note*: antiplatelet *not* necessary because native vessel thrombosis is uncommon Monitoring: inactive (no symptoms, normal ESR, no change on angiography), ESR can be ↑ without active disease but is useful in individual patient
Wegener's granulomatosis	Upper & lower airway problems (90%), nasal sinus, ear (70%), glomerulonephritis (77%)	Headache (vasculitis, sinusitis, pachymeningitis), cranial neuropathies (due to mononeuritis multiplex or pachymeningitis), ophthalmoplegia & proptosis (due to granulomas, can be presenting sign), poor visual acuity (optic nerve granuloma), intracranial vasculitis is uncommon, (small vessels)	Mononeuritis multiplex (may be presenting sign), distal polyneuropathy, arthralgia/myalgia, myopathy (rare)	Lab: CBC (leukocytosis, anemia), ESR (usually >70 mm/1 h, correlates with disease activity), (+)cANCA (sensitivity depends on disease activity) Lung biopsy: granulomatous vasculitis with necrosis, giant cells, microabscesses	Prednisone, cyclophosphamide Mortality rate, 20%
Churg-Strauss syndrome		Upper respiratory (sinusitis, rhinitis), skin, heart	Mononeuritis multiplex, distal symmetric polyneuropathy, radiculopathy	Lab: CBC (eosinophilia), (+)pANCA (70%) Skin biopsy	Steroids (neurologic symptoms may improve), cytotoxic agents if needed

Table 14-3. (**continued**)

Type	Symptoms			Diagnosis	Treatment
	Systemic	CNS	PNS		
Poly-arteritis nodosa	Fever, arthralgia, weakness, abdominal pain, pericarditis, nodular skin rash/livedo reticularis	Stroke (rare), delirium, seizures, myelopathy	Mononeuritis multiplex, asymmetric polyneuropathy, myopathy	Skin biopsy Lab: ESR (↑ at 60 mm/1 h), CBC (anemia, leukocytosis), urinalysis (abnormal sediment), pANCA (20%), (+)hepatitis B antibody Electromyography Sural nerve biopsy MRI/angiography (may have aneurysms)	Steroids, other immunosuppressants (cyclophosphamide, vidarabine [if hepatitis B]), aspirin
Primary CNS angiitis		Headache, nausea, vomiting, diffuse encephalopathy, focal deficits		Lab: CBC, chemistry, ESR (>44 mm/1 h in 66%) CSF: abnormal in 81%, mixed or lymphocytic pleocytosis in 68%, elevated protein in 70% EEG: diffuse slowing in 81% Imaging: multifocal infarcts (normal imaging is rare) Angiography: normal (13%), use cut films if possible Leptomeningeal/cortical biopsy (diagnostic sensitivity of biopsy compared with path studies, 74.4%)	Steroids and cyclophosphamide Monitoring: clinical symptoms are best, pick out marker to follow Postpartum disease: treat with prednisone & calcium channel blocker
Buerger's disease (male smokers)	Intermittent claudication, ischemic pain, Raynaud's phenomenon		Sensory polyneuropathy	Lab: ESR (↑ in 15%) Angiography: segmental occlusions of medium-sized vessels	Smoking cessation, anticoagulant/antiplatelet, steroids do not help, iloprost (prostacyclin analogue) improves leg pain

ANA, antinuclear antibody; ANCA, antineutrophil cytoplasmic antibody (c, cytoplasmic; p, perinuclear); APL, antiphospholipid antibodies; CBC, complete blood count; CNS, central nervous system; CSF, cerebrospinal fluid; ESR, erythrocyte sedimentation rate; INO, internuclear ophthalmoplegia; MRI, magnetic resonance imaging; NSAID, nonsteroidal antiinflammatory drug; OCB, oligoclonal band; PTCA, percutaneous transluminal coronary angioplasty; PNS, peripheral nervous system; RBC, red blood cell; RF, rheumatoid factor; SLE, systemic lupus erythematosus; SSA, Sjögren's syndrome A; SSB, Sjögren's syndrome B; WBC, white blood cell.
*Neurosarcoidosis is not considered here.
†Can be due to emboli, atherosclerosis (steroids), dissection, coagulopathy, Libman-Sacks endocarditis.
‡Opportunistic infection: cytomegalovirus, Listeria, Aspergillus, Strongyloides.

3) One cause of cardiac emboli in this setting: Libman-Sacks endocarditis
d. Aseptic meningitis: rare (has been described in association with use of nonsteroidal antiinflammatory drugs or azathioprine)
e. "Cerebral lupus": direct antibody-mediated angiitis of CNS with fibrinoid necrosis of small vasculature, is rare

f. Noncompressive myelopathy and transverse myelitis (must rule out opportunistic infections)
g. Cranial neuropathies (e.g., optic neuritis, trigeminal sensory neuropathy)
h. Movement disorders: parkinsonism, ataxia, chorea (see Chapter 8)
i. Seizures

1) May occur from foci of infarction, opportunistic infection, drug intoxication, others
2) 30% to 54% of SLE patients have seizures at some point

3. Neuromuscular manifestations of SLE
   a. Vasculitis-induced mononeuropathies (mononeuritis multiplex)
   b. Symmetric, axonal, distal sensorimotor (or primarily sensory) neuropathy
   c. Polyradiculopathy
   d. Polyradiculoneuropathy (a chronic inflammatory demyelinating polyradiculoneuropathy)
   e. Myositis or vasculitic myopathy

4. Serologic features
   a. Antinuclear antibody (ANA): nonspecific
   b. Extractable nuclear antigen (ENA)
      1) Constitutes antibodies to native double-stranded DNA, Sm antigen, and ribonucleoprotein antigen
      2) Good evidence for SLE in appropriate clinical context
   c. Antiphospholipid antibodies with procoagulant properties: lupus anticoagulant and anticardiolipin antibodies
   d. Antiphospholipid antibodies are present in all patients with antiphospholipid syndrome and in 30% of patients with SLE, but may also be present in up to 29% of patients with BOMS
   e. Presence of antiphospholipid antibodies predicts 50% chance of recurrence of SLE and greater likelihood of valvular and cardiac disease
   f. Presence of antiphospholipid antibodies and active SLE during second trimester predict increased risk of abortion and stroke
   g. Low complement levels: may be used to determine disease activity

5. Treatment
   a. High-dose intravenous corticosteroids, followed by oral prednisone
   b. Immunosuppressant, steroid-sparing agents: cyclophosphamide, azathioprine, methotrexate
   c. Antimalarial agents (e.g. hydroxychloroquine) not well-studied in the peripheral nervous system or CNS disease

B. Rheumatoid Arthritis

1. The most common connective tissue disorder, rare CNS involvement
2. Most common mechanism of disease: widespread arthropathy with secondary compression neuropathies
3. Course: chronic, progressive
4. Systemic manifestations
   a. Symmetric polyarthritis
   b. Subcutaneous nodules
   c. Pulmonary nodules
   d. Interstitial fibrosis
   e. Pleuritis
   f. Pneumonitis
   g. Pericardial effusions
   h. Skin lesions

5. Cervical compression myelopathy due to atlantoaxial subluxation (anterior, posterior, ventral, lateral)—careful with hyperextension of neck during endotracheal intubation

6. Rheumatoid nodules: extradural spinal canal, leptomeningeal

7. Neuromuscular involvement
   a. Chronic progressive compression neuropathies (most common)
   b. Most common compression neuropathy: median neuropathy at the wrist
   c. Distal symmetric sensory polyneuropathy
   d. Distal symmetric sensorimotor polyneuropathy
   e. Asymmetric axonal polyneuropathy, mononeuritis multiplex
   f. Vasculitic peripheral nerve manifestations are secondary to systemic fulminant vasculitis or obliterative vasculitis (microvascular occlusive disease) and secondary ischemia: acute or subacute presentation
   g. Muscle disease: vasculitic myositis, idiopathic overlap polymyositis syndrome, steroid-induced myopathy

8. Neurologic complications of specific rheumatoid arthritis treatments: gold (neuropathy), penicillamine (drug-induced myasthenia gravis, myopathy), chloroquine (retinopathy, neuropathy, myopathy)

9. Treatment: no standard treatment, corticosteroids and immunosuppressant agents such as cyclophosphamide, azathioprine, methotrexate, or mycophenolate may be tried (controlled trials lacking)

C. Sjögren's Syndrome

1. Systemic manifestations: xerostomia and keratoconjunctivitis sicca (due to destructive lymphocytic inflammation of exocrine glands), arthritis, interstitial nephritis, skin involvement

2. Neurologic manifestations: predominantly involvement of peripheral nervous system
   a. High frequency of positive anti-Ro (SSA) antibodies (sensitive and specific to general autoimmunity), present in SLE, Sjögren's syndrome, SLE-Sjögren overlap syndrome, and primary biliary cirrhosis
   b. Low frequency of anti-La (SSB) antibodies are more specific to Sjögren's syndrome
   c. Therefore, presence of only anti-Ro antibodies marks general systemic autoimmunity but not Sjögren's syndrome as the cause of neurologic complications

d. Peripheral nervous system manifestations: sensory ataxic neuronopathy (ganglionopathy), sensory or sensorimotor symmetric polyneuropathy, cranial neuropathies (most commonly trigeminal neuropathy); high female prevalence

e. CNS manifestations (less common): aseptic meningoencephalitis, diffuse and focal CNS syndromes (including myelopathy) should be considered in the differential diagnosis of recurrent isolated transverse myelitis

f. Trimethoprim-sulfamethoxazole (Bactrim)–associated aseptic meningitis is more common in patients with Sjögren's syndrome

3. Associated with other autoimmune neurologic disorders (e.g., myasthenia gravis, polymyositis)

D. Progressive Systemic Sclerosis

1. Systemic manifestations
   a. Raynaud's phenomenon
   b. Renal involvement, including glomerulonephritis: leading cause of death
   c. Diffuse or limited cutaneous scleroderma: symmetric skin thickening
   d. Systemic fibrosis: cardiac, pulmonary (interstitial pulmonary fibrosis, pericarditis, congestive heart failure)
   e. Gastrointestinal mucosal lesions
   f. Keratoconjunctivitis
   g. Associated with CREST (calcinosis, Raynaud's phenomenon, esophageal dysmotility, sclerodactyly, telangiectasias) syndrome

2. CNS involvement: rare

3. Peripheral nervous system involvement: most common neurologic involvement
   a. Fibrosis can cause cranial neuropathies: most common, isolated trigeminal neuropathy
   b. Peripheral neuropathy: rare, often due to other organ involvement
   c. Compression mononeuropathies (e.g., median neuropathy at the wrist) from fibrotic thickening of surrounding tendon sheaths
   d. Mononeuropathy multiplex most frequently with CREST (vasculitic neuropathy with perivascular inflammation) syndrome

4. May present as part of mixed connective tissue disorder

5. Mechanism of damage due more often to fibrosis than vasculitis

6. Treatment: penicillamine, azathioprine, colchicine, corticosteroids (short-term only)

E. Mixed Connective Tissue Disease: heterogeneous, variable features of other connective tissue disorders (Table 14-3)

III. Systemic Vasculitides Affecting CNS

A. Polyarteritis Nodosa, Churg-Strauss Syndrome, and Wegener's Granulomatosis

1. All are necrotizing vasculitides

2. Polyarteritis nodosa and Churg-Strauss syndrome involve small- and medium-sized vessels; Wegener's granulomatosis involves smaller vessels

3. Polyarteritis nodosa
   a. CNS manifestations
      1) Common (40%-45% of patients) but have delayed onset after initial symptoms of the disease (2-3 years)
      2) Diffuse encephalopathy with seizures (40%), hypertensive encephalopathy, focal vasculitic lesions (50%), isolated cranial neuropathies (most common, cranial nerves II, III, VIII) (10%-15%)
   b. Peripheral nervous system manifestations
      1) Common and early (50%-60% of patients)
      2) Predominantly mononeuritis multiplex, mixed sensorimotor distal symmetric polyneuropathy, plexopathy, radiculopathy, inflammatory myopathy
   c. Systemic vasculitic manifestations: most commonly kidneys, skin, mesenteric vessels
   d. Gastrointestinal tract angiography: sometimes needed to make diagnosis
   e. 30% of patients may have hepatitis B surface antigen
   f. Polyarteritis nodosa is *not* associated with antineutrophil cytoplasmic antibodies (ANCA)

4. Churg-Strauss syndrome
   a. Asthma, allergic rhinitis, and nasal polyposis
   b. Peripheral eosinophilia, increased IgE levels
   c. Extravascular granulomas
   d. Granulomatous or nongranulomatous eosinophilic necrotizing vasculitis (involving arteries and veins)
   e. Higher predilection for hemorrhages than polyarteritis nodosa (more venous involvement)
   f. Associated with perinuclear ANCA

5. Wegener's granulomatosis
   a. Classic triad: segmental glomerulonephritis, granulomas of respiratory tract, necrotizing vasculitis
   b. Nervous system involvement
      1) Granulomatous spread from paranasal sinuses leading to exophthalmos (ocular pseudotumor), optic nerve involvement, oculomotor and other cranial neuropathies, cavernous sinus syndrome, pituitary syndromes
      2) Granulomatous vasculitis: peripheral neuropathy, vasculitic stroke, encephalopathy, intracerebral or subarachnoid hemorrhage, optic neuritis
   c. Approximately 5% of patients have intracranial hemorrhage
   d. Associated with cytoplasmic ANCA against proteinase-3

in most patients

6. Renal failure: most common cause of death in necrotizing vasculitides

7. Treatment: corticosteroids, cyclophosphamide

B. Giant Cell Arteritis: temporal arteritis and Takayasu's arteritis

1. Temporal arteritis
   a. Systemic panarteritis affecting older adults (almost all older than 50)
   b. Affects medium- or large-sized arteries, primarily the intracranial and extracranial vessels
   c. Visual disturbance
   d. Temporal throbbing headache with radiation to the ear, jaw, tongue, and ipsilateral or contralateral bifrontal or occipital head regions
   e. Scalp tenderness
   f. Jaw claudication
   g. Constitutional symptoms (low-grade fever, fatigue, night sweats, anorexia)
   h. Other symptoms: blindness due to optic neuropathy, ocular muscle dysfunction, strokes, seizures
   i. Other intracranial vessels (vertebral and carotid arteries) can be involved
   j. Half of the patients have polymyalgia rheumatica
   k. Diagnosis: erythrocyte sedimentation rate more than 50 mm/h and temporal artery biopsy (in 70% of cases diagnosis is made after biopsy) even if the disease involves other parts of CNS vasculature
   l. Treatment
      1) Oral prednisone should be started without awaiting biopsy results because of risk of blindness
      2) Treatment usually continued for 2 years

2. Takayasu's arteritis
   a. Large-vessel arteritis involving aorta and its branches
   b. Predominantly affects young Asian women
   c. May present with unexplained systemic illness and fever of unknown origin
   d. Often, nonspecific symptoms at presentation: headaches, dizziness, arthralgias
   e. Features related to the large-vessel arteritis: stroke, syncope, subclavian steal syndrome, amaurosis fugax and other transient ischemic events, claudication, chest and abdominal angina
   f. Bruits often heard from involved vessels
   g. Treatment: oral prednisone, cyclophosphamide, methotrexate, or cyclosporine

C. Behçet's Disease

1. Endemic in countries along the ancient "Silk Road"

(Japan, Korea, Middle East, Mediterranean basin), with highest incidence in Turkey

2. Associated with HLA-DR5

3. Affects men more than women

4. A systemic vasculitis characterized by arterial and venular involvement of different size vessels

5. Systemic manifestations: predominantly venulitis leading to hallmark oral and genital aphthous ulcers
   a. Ocular manifestations: uveitis, retinal vasculitis
   b. Cutaneous manifestations: oral and genital ulcers, erythema nodosum, papulopustular lesions
   c. Venous involvement: superficial thrombophlebitis, deep venous thrombosis, cerebral venous sinus thrombosis, superior vena cava syndrome
   d. Pulmonary vascular complications can be fatal
   e. Gastrointestinal tract ulcers (need to be differentiated from inflammatory bowel disease)
   f. Arthritis
   g. Diagnostic hallmark: a skin reaction called "pathergy phenomenon," which is also responsible for delayed wound healing
   h. Diagnostic criteria: recurrent oral ulcers plus two of the following:
      1) Recurrent genital ulcers
      2) Uveitis, retinitis
      3) Skin lesions, including erythema nodosum

6. CNS complications affect 10% to 30% of patients and are common causes of morbidity and mortality
   a. Most common presentation: headache followed by long tract signs
   b. Aseptic meningitis (rare, but before MRI era, it was thought to be common)
   c. Venous sinus thrombosis and resultant intracranial hypertension
   d. CNS parenchymal disease likely due to venulitis involving diencephalic regions with characteristic MRI findings of inflammation and edema responsive to corticosteroids
   e. Spinal cord involvement (predilection for thoracic cord)
   f. Brainstem involvement: cranial neuropathies (e.g., recurrent facial palsies), long tract signs
   g. Peripheral neuropathy
   h. Necrotizing myopathy (sometimes due to chemotherapeutic agents)
   i. CNS arterial involvement: rare; may cause stenosis, aneurysm formation, dissection of intracranial vessels

7. Disease course: single attack, relapsing-remitting, or secondary progressive

8. MRI: T2 hyperintense lesions in brainstem, basal ganglia, internal capsule, subcortical white matter (no

predilection for periventricular regions, as in multiple sclerosis)

9. CSF: elevated opening pressure (may be only abnormality with isolated venous sinus thrombosis), pleocytosis, increased protein level, normal glucose, and, infrequently, oligoclonal bands
10. Treatment (Table 14-3)

D. Isolated CNS Vasculitis (see Chapter 11)

IV. NEUROSARCOIDOSIS

A. Features
1. Multisystem, idiopathic, noncaseating granulomatous disease
2. Most prevalent in African Americans and women
3. 50% of patients with neurologic involvement present with neurologic disease

B. Systemic Manifestations
1. Pulmonary involvement: bilateral hilar adenopathy and pulmonary infiltrates
2. Cutaneous manifestations: erythema nodosum
3. Uveitis
4. Arthritis

C. Nervous System Involvement (3%-5% of patients): diverse, may affect CNS, peripheral nervous system, and muscle
1. Cranial neuropathies (from basal meningitis)
   a. Facial neuropathy: most common
   b. Optic neuropathy: may be acute and resemble idiopathic, demyelinating optic neuritis (to be differentiated from uveitis, which may also be present)
   c. Rarely due to cerebellopontine angle mass lesion
2. Pituitary-hypothalamic dysfunction (e.g., diabetes insipidus, somnolence, obesity, hypopituitarism)
3. Meningoencephalitis: usually aseptic meningitis with increased opening CSF pressure, mononuclear CSF pleocytosis, increased CSF protein level, possibly oligoclonal bands
4. Increased intracranial pressure (often with aseptic meningitis), and, occasionally, hydrocephalus
5. Intracranial parenchymal disease: may be due to inflammatory infiltration of parenchyma from leptomeningeal and/or ependymal surfaces
6. Spinal cord parenchymal disease
   a. Transverse myelitis due to sarcoidosis should be differentiated from isolated transverse myelitis, neuromyelitis

optica, multiple sclerosis, human T-cell lymphotropic virus-1 (HTLV1), and Sjögren's syndrome
   b. Resistance to steroids and plasma exchange, with persistent inflammation, should further suggest sarcoidosis especially in African American patients
7. Peripheral nerve involvement
   a. Symmetric distal polyneuropathy or, less commonly, polyradiculoneuropathy (especially with cauda equina leptomeningeal involvement)
   b. Asymmetric polyneuropathy: mononeuritis multiplex
8. Myopathy
   a. More than 50% of patients have muscle involvement, most are asymptomatic
   b. Acute or chronic myositis (with proximal more than distal muscle weakness), pain, tenderness
   c. Nodular, patchy myositis

D. Histopathology (Fig. 14-13)
1. Noncaseating granulomas consisting of epithelioid macrophages, monocytes, lymphocytes, fibroblasts; sometimes have fibrotic (rarely necrotic) centers
2. Perivascular inflammation may cause thickening of intima and media of affected vessels and tissue ischemia; may spread to involve parenchyma
3. Fibrosis may eventually develop: treatment goal is to diminish irreversible fibrosis and resultant ischemia

E. Ancillary Testing
1. MRI: parenchymal lesions with increased T2 signal and leptomeningeal, parenchymal, and nerve root enhancement
2. CSF examination may show any combination of the following: increased opening pressure, increased protein level, decreased glucose level, mononuclear pleocytosis, elevated IgG index and oligoclonal bands, and increased CSF angiotensin-converting enzyme (nonspecific marker, with questionable sensitivity because negative CSF angiotensin-converting enzyme does not exclude the diagnosis)
3. Evoked potentials, electromyography, nerve conduction studies in selected cases
4. 30% to 70% of patients have increased serum levels of angiotensin-converting enzyme (nonspecific)
5. Endocrine testing
6. Serum and urine calcium: concentration may be increased
7. Kveim testing: not available
8. Biopsy of relevant tissues (skin, conjunctiva, lymph node, lung) necessary for diagnosis in clinically suspected cases

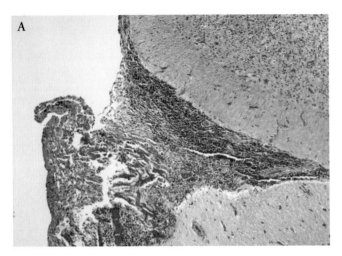
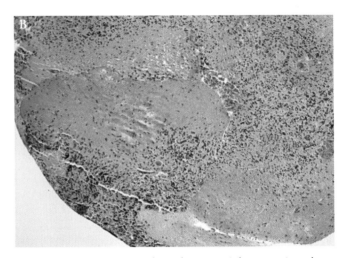

Fig. 14-13. Histopathologic sections of cerebellum of patient with central nervous system sarcoidosis showing, *A*, leptomeningeal mononuclear infiltrates and *B*, adjacent noncaseating sarcoid granulomas.

9. Nerve root or nerve biopsy may be necessary for diagnosis in selected cases

F. **Disease Course**
1. Monophasic in two-thirds of patients, progressive or relapsing-remitting course in one-third
2. Poor prognostic factors: hydrocephalus; spinal cord, brainstem, or cerebral mass lesions; epilepsy; encephalopathy; optic nerve involvement

G. **Treatment**
1. Prednisone
2. Methotrexate, azathioprine, cyclosporine, cyclophosphamide

V. **AUTOIMMUNE PARANEOPLASTIC DISORDERS OF CNS** (SEE CHAPTER 16)

REFERENCES

Beck RW, Chandler DL, Cole SR, Simon JH, Jacobs LD, Kinkel RP, et al. Interferon β-1a for early multiple sclerosis: CHAMPS trial subgroup analyses: CHAMPS Study Group. Ann Neurol. 2002;51:481-90.

Freedman MS, Blumhardt LD, Brochet B, Comi G, Noseworthy JH, Sandberg-Wollheim M, et al. International consensus statement on the use of disease-modifying agents in multiple sclerosis: Paris Workshop Group. Mult Scler. 2002;8:19-23.

Kantarci OH, Weinshenker BG. Natural history of multiple sclerosis. Neurol Clin. 2005;23:17-38.

Lucchinetti CF, Parisi J, Bruck W. The pathology of multiple sclerosis. Neurol Clin. 2005;23:77-105.

Noseworthy JH. Treatment of multiple sclerosis and related disorders: what's new in the past 2 years? Clin Neuropharmacol. 2003;26:28-37.

Noseworthy JH, editor. Neurological therapeutics: principles and practice.

London: Martin Dunitz; 2003.

Noseworthy JH, Lucchinetti C, Rodriguez M, Weinshenker BG. Multiple sclerosis. N Engl J Med. 2000;343:938-52.

O'Connor PW, Goodman A, Willmer-Hulme AJ, Libonati MA, Metz L, Murray RS, et al. Randomized multicenter trial of natalizumab in acute MS relapses: clinical and MRI effects: Natalizumab Multiple Sclerosis Trial. Neurology. 2004;62:2038-43.

O'Riordan JI, Thompson AJ, Kingsley DP, MacManus DG, Kendall BE, Rudge P, et al. The prognostic value of brain MRI in clinically isolated syndromes of the CNS: a 10-year follow-up. Brain. 1998;121:495-503.

Rolak LA, editor. Neurology secrets. 3rd ed. Philadelphia: Hanley & Belfus; 2001.

Stern BJ. Neurological complications of sarcoidosis. Curr Opin Neurol. 2004;17:311-6.

QUESTIONS

1-5. Match the disease (1-5) with the corresponding feature (a-e)

1. Systemic lupus erythematosus

2. Wegener's granulomatosis

3. Takayasu's arteritis

4. Giant cell arteritis

5. Polyarteritis nodosa

a. Predominantly affects aortic arch in young Asian women

b. Associated with seropositivity for hepatitis B

c. Associated with cytoplasmic (c)-ANCA reactivity

d. Occurs in patients older than 50 years, often with an increased erythrocyte sedimentation rate

e. Aseptic meningitis may be induced by use of non-steroidal anti-inflammatory drugs

6. All the following are typical brain MRI lesions of multiple sclerosis *except*:
   a. Well circumscribed
   b. Appear hyperintense (bright) on T1- and T2-weighted MRI
   c. Round or ovoid appearance
   d. Typically are a few millimeters to 1 cm in diameter

7. Patients with a clinically isolated symptom of demyelination:
   a. Have clinically definite multiple sclerosis regardless of what MRI demonstrates
   b. Have approximately an 85% chance of developing clinically definite multiple sclerosis in the next 10 years if two or more cerebral lesions are seen on MRI at onset
   c. Have approximately a 45% chance of developing clinically definite multiple sclerosis in the next 10 years if two or more cerebral lesions are seen on MRI at onset
   d. Have approximately a 50% chance of developing clinically definite multiple sclerosis in the next 10 years if two or less cerebral lesions are seen on MRI at onset

e. MRI is not indicated because it has no prognostic value for these patients

8. Which of the following is associated with a favorable long-term prognosis for patients with multiple sclerosis?
   1) Male sex
   2) Onset before age 30
   3) T1 hypointense lesions on initial MRI of head
   4) Optic neuritis as presenting symptom
   Choices are a=1,3; b=2,4; c=1,2,3; d=4 only

9. Interferon beta therapy for multiple sclerosis is *not* associated with:
   a. Injection site reactions
   b. Pancreatitis
   c. Increased liver enzyme levels
   d. Risk of worsening depression
   e. Flulike symptoms

10. Glatiramer acetate is:
    a. Composed of amino acids making up myelin basic protein
    b. Approved for treating secondary progressive multiple sclerosis
    c. Associated with worsening of attacks of multiple sclerosis
    d. Associated with flulike symptoms after injection
    e. Used to alter the predominant immune response from Th2 to Th1 type

For questions 11-13, mark *all* responses that are correct.

11. Which of the following is/are true about the use of mitoxantrone (Novantrone)?
    a. May cause a dose-dependent, irreversible reduction in cardiac output
    b. May stain the skin if allowed to enter the interstitial space during infusion
    c. Is usually well tolerated, with only mild nausea and hair loss
    d. Shown to reduce clinical progression in primary and secondary progressive multiple sclerosis

12. Which of the following is/are true about the management of tremor in multiple sclerosis?
    a. Upper limb tremor and ataxia present for 4 months or more commonly subsides without treatment

b. Weighted bracelets are often helpful in improving quality of life

c. Valproic acid may benefit up to one-third of patients with upper limb ataxia

d. Thalamotomy and thalamic stimulation may reduce tremor but have less effect on limb ataxia

13. Which of the following is/are true about fatigue in multiple sclerosis?

a. Fatigue is the most common disabling symptom of multiple sclerosis

b. Worsens in a circadian fashion in most patients

c. Responds often to either amantadine or modafinil

d. Commonly resolves when underlying depression is recognized and treated effectively

14. Which of the following has been approved for treating secondary progressive multiple sclerosis?

a. Betaseron

b. Cyclophosphamide

c. Avonex

d. Mitoxantrone

Answers

1. Answer: e.

2. Answer: c.

3. Answer: a.

4. Answer: d.

5. Answer: b.

6. Answer: b.
Multiple sclerosis lesions appear hypointense or isointense on T1-weighted imaging.

7. Answer: b.

8. Answer: b.

9. Answer: b.

10. Answer: a.

11. Answer: a,b,c.

12. Answer: d.

13. Answer: a,b,c.

14. Answer: d.
Mitoxantrone is the only agent approved for treatment of secondary progressive multiple sclerosis.

Neurology of Infectious Diseases

15

Jennifer A. Tracy, M.D.

Nima Mowzoon, M.D.

I. Bacterial Infections of the Nervous System

A. Bacterial Meningitis

1. Epidemiology
   a. Incidence: 3 to 5/100,000 persons annually
   b. Most likely pathogen: depends on patient age and other risk factors
   c. Common pathogens by age
      1) Neonates: group B streptococcus (*Streptococcus agalactiae*), *Escherichia coli*, *Listeria monocytogenes*
      2) Children 1 month or older: *Streptococcus pneumoniae* and *Neisseria meningitidis*
      3) Adults (in order of frequency): *S. pneumoniae* and *N. meningitidis*, followed by *L. monocytogenes*, staphylococci, gram-negative bacilli (including *E. coli*, *Klebsiella*, *Enterobacter*, *Pseudomonas aeruginosa*), and *Haemophilus influenzae* (the incidence of the latter is <3% since advent of *H. influenzae* vaccine)
      4) *L. montocytogenes* infections: more common with extremes of age
   d. Common pathogens by other risk factors
      1) Trauma/neurosurgery procedure: staphylococci, gram-negative bacilli, *S. pneumoniae*
      2) Immunocompromised: *S. pneumoniae*, *L. monocytogenes*, gram-negative bacilli
2. Pathophysiology
   a. Infection and secondary inflammation of leptomeninges and cerebrospinal fluid (CSF) by bacterial pathogen
   b. Initially, increase in polymorphonuclear infiltrates, followed within a few days by lymphocytes and histiocytes
   c. Infection may arise from
      1) Hematogenous spread, bacteremia, and seeding of the meninges
      2) Parameningeal infection: sinusitis, otitis media, brain abscess, mastoiditis, others
      3) Abscess rupture into CSF space
      4) Trauma/surgery with disruption of blood-brain barrier

   d. CSF is "immunodeficient" media: poor availability of immunoglobulins and components of complement cascade
   e. Endothelial dysfunction and loss of autoregulation of cerebral vasculature result in vasogenic edema and increased intracranial pressure (ICP), may induce herniation
3. Clinical presentation
   a. Subacute onset, rapid progression of symptoms within hours to days
   b. Symptoms
      1) Fever
      2) Meningismus (may be absent in extreme ages)
         a) Neck pain
         b) Kernig's sign (discomfort induced by extending the leg with the thigh flexed)
         c) Brudzinski's sign (when the neck is flexed, patient develops hip and knee flexion)
      3) Headache
      4) Nausea and/or vomiting
      5) Photophobia
      6) Other cerebral symptoms: seizures, confusion, cranial nerve palsies, possible focal deficits
      7) Systemic symptoms
      8) Rash may be present with *N. meningitidis*
   c. Neonatal presentation
      1) Classic symptoms may be absent
      2) May have irritability, inconsolable crying, decreased or absent feeding, fever
4. Complications
   a. Cerebritis and abscess formation
   b. Subdural effusions and/or empyema
   c. Vasogenic edema
   d. Hydrocephalus with or without transependymal flow of intraventricular CSF
   e. Ventriculitis
   f. Arteritis, vasospasms, possible infarcts
   g. Venous sinus thrombosis

h. Increased ICP due to any or all the above

i. Systemic complications: acute respiratory distress syndrome (ARDS), septic shock (the combination of hypotension due to septic shock and increased ICP can potentiate further decrease in perfusion pressure)

5. Diagnosis
   a. Neuroimaging
      1) Head computed tomography (CT) without contrast is usually normal, but may show hydrocephalus: performed before CSF examination, especially if focal neurologic deficit or signs or symptoms suggestive of increased ICP
      2) Head magnetic resonance imaging (MRI) with gadolinium: may show enhancement of leptomeninges
   b. CSF examination (Table 15-1)
      1) Opening pressure often increased
      2) Increased CSF protein (>120 mg/dL), decreased glucose (<30 mg/dL and <30% of plasma glucose), neutrophilic pleocytosis (100-10,000 white blood cells [WBCs]/mm³)
      3) Cell count: usually more than 1,000 cells/μL, but may be less than 1,000 cells/μL early in disease, in partially treated bacterial meningitis, or in immunosuppressed patients
      4) Isolation of microorganism by Gram stain, culture, and sensitivities (CSF and blood) and antigen detection with latex particle agglutination
      5) Bacterial antigen testing (latex particle agglutination) available for *S. pneumoniae*, *N. meningitidis*, *H. influenzae* type b, *E. coli* K1, and group B streptococci
   c. Increased number of peripheral blood WBCs

d. Blood cultures: positive in 50% of cases

e. Differential diagnosis (Table 15-1)

6. Pathology (Fig. 15-1)
   a. Macroscopic appearance: diffuse edema, purulent exudates accumulating in subarachnoid space, over cerebral convexities and sulci, and at base of the brain
   b. Microscopic appearance
      1) Polymorphonuclear exudates within the leptomeninges, invading perivascular spaces and infiltrating the walls of leptomeningeal and cortical arteries and veins
      2) Fibrinoid necrosis of leptomeningeal and cortical arteries and veins
      3) Thrombosis of leptomeningeal and cortical blood vessels: may cause focal infarcts

7. Treatment
   a. Early treatment is important and should be initiated as soon as blood is drawn for culture
   b. Initial, empirical treatment
      1) Neonates: third-generation cephalosporin and ampicillin
      2) Infants, children, adults: third-generation cephalosporin (such as ceftriaxone) or fourth-generation cephalosporin (cefepime) and vancomycin
      3) Ampicillin should be added for treatment in elderly patients, infants, immunocompromised patients, and in the setting of alcoholism or pregnancy, because *L. monocytogenes* is potential pathogen
      4) Bacterial meningitis as a complication of head trauma or neurosurgical procedure (shunt infections): cephalosporin plus vancomycin; metronidazole to be added if anaerobic contamination is suspected

Table 15-1. **Cerebrospinal Fluid Characteristics of Different Types of Meningitis**

Meningitis type	Pressure	Glucose	Protein	Cells	Cell type
Bacterial	Elevated	Decreased	Increased	Increased, usually >1,000/mm³	Polymorphonuclear
Viral	Normal or elevated	Normal	Normal or increased	Increased, usually <1,000/mm³	Mononuclear, may be polymorphonuclear predominance in first 48 hours
Fungal	Normal or elevated	Normal or decreased	Increased	Increased, usually <1,000/mm³	Mononuclear in most cases
Tuberculous	Elevated	Decreased	Increased	Increased	Mononuclear
Lyme	Normal or elevated	Normal or decreased	Increased	Increased	Mononuclear
Syphilis	Normal or elevated	Normal or decreased	Increased	Increased	Mononuclear

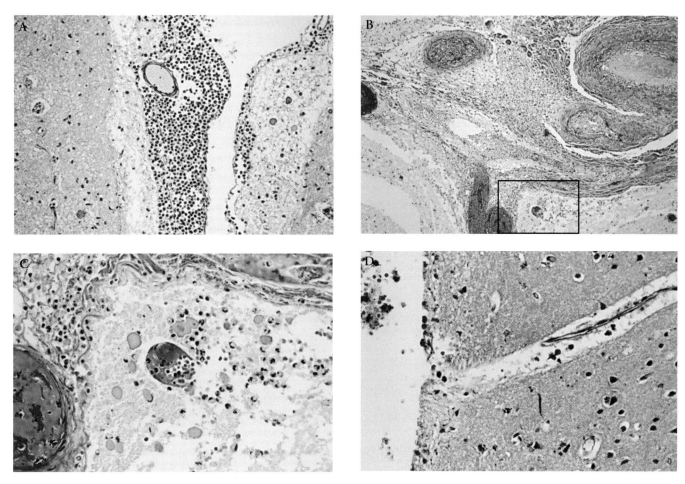

Fig. 15-1. Histopathology of acute bacterial meningitis is characterized by leptomeningeal exudates, consisting predominantly of polymorphonuclear cells with strands of fibrin (*A* and *B*) and infiltration of the walls of leptomeningeal and cortical arteries and veins, sometimes superimposed with thrombosis of these blood vessels, as in *B*. *C*, Higher magnification of the box in *B* showing polymorphonuclear cells penetrating disrupted walls of a small cortical vein that has undergone fibrinoid necrosis. *D*, Polymorphonuclear cellular infiltrates also invade Virchow-Robin spaces and infiltrate cortical blood vessels.

5) Intraventricular vancomycin recommended for intra-ventricular catheter-associated meningitis
c. Specific treatment
   1) Penicillin G, ampicillin, or ceftriaxone for penicillin-susceptible *S. pneumoniae*
   2) Third-generation cephalosporin for *N. meningitidis*
   3) Cefepime (or alternatively, ceftriaxone) plus vancomycin for penicillin-resistant *S. pneumoniae*
   4) Ceftriaxone, cefepime, or cefotaxime for *H. influenzae* or Enterobacteriaceae
   5) Meropenem, cefepime, ceftazidime for *P. aeruginosa*
   6) Nafcillin or oxacillin for treatment of methicillin-susceptible staphylococci
   7) Vancomycin for treatment of methicillin-resistant

staphylococci or *Staphylococcus epidermidis*
   8) Ampicillin for *L. monocytogenes* or group B strepto-cocci (*Streptococcus agalactiae*)
   9) Bacterial meningitis due to *N. meningitidis*: 5- to 7-day course of antibiotics
   10) Bacterial meningitis due to *S. pneumoniae*, *H. influen-zae*, and group B streptococci: 10- to 14-day course of antibiotics
   11) Bacterial meningitis due to Enterobacteriaceae or *L. monocytogenes*: 3- to 4-week course of antibiotics
d. Adjunctive therapy
   1) Corticosteroid therapy
      a) Reduces vasogenic edema, meningeal inflamma-tion, and inflammatory response of meningitis

Bacterial Meningitis

S. pneumoniae and *N. meningitidis*: most common pathogens in adults

L. monocytogenes: possible pathogen in neonates, the elderly, alcoholics, and immunosuppressed patients; these patients need empiric treatment with ampicillin

An appropriate empiric treatment for adults with acute bacterial meningitis is vancomycin and a third-generation cephalosporin, such as ceftriaxone, with or without ampicillin

(provoked by bacterial lysis and release of bacterial cell wall contents into CSF)

   b) Potential to reduce CSF penetration by some antibiotics by "stabilizing" blood-brain barrier
   c) Improves outcome and reduces mortality in infants, children, and adults with bacterial meningitis
   d) Reduces incidence of neurologic sequelae, includ ing sensorineural hearing loss in infants and children
   e) Best if reserved for severely ill patients or those with complications of meningitis such as hydrocephalus or increased ICP
   2) Management of increased ICP: elevate head of the bed, hyperosmolar agents, hyperventilation
   3) Anticoagulation of septic venous sinus thrombosis: controversial, has been associated with increased risk of bleeding
 e. Prevention
   1) Pneumococcal vaccine recommended for patients older than 65 years, asplenic patients, or those with human immunodeficiency virus (HIV) infection or other chronic debilitating illness
   2) *H. influenzae* type b vaccination beginning at age 2 to 6 months
   3) Chemoprophylaxis with rifampin recommended for persons in contact with patients with meningococcal meningitis

B. **Bacterial Brain Abscess**
1. Pathophysiology
 a. Mechanism of abscess formation

   1) Hematogenous spread (typically from pulmonary infection): gray-white matter junction is the most likely site for abscess
   2) Direct contiguous spread from nearby structures: sinusitis, mastoiditis, otitis media
   3) Seeding due to cranial trauma, e.g., bullet fragments, neurosurgical procedures
 b. Focal infectious site or sites within brain: usually spread from local infection such as dental, sinus, ear, bone; can also be hematogenous spread
 c. Site of origin can often be inferred by location of abscess, e.g., temporal lobe abscess from ear infection
 d. Frontal and temporal lobes are most common sites for abscess
 e. Most likely pathogens: microaerophilic streptococci and anaerobes
 f. Four major stages in formation of brain abscess
   1) Early cerebritis (days 1-3): perivascular polymorpho-nuclear inflammatory infiltration around core of coagulation necrosis
   2) Late cerebritis (days 4-9): newly formed, thin rim of fibroblasts, neovascularization, and inflammatory infiltrates (consisting predominantly of macrophages), bordering a more defined necrotic center and sur-rounded by vasogenic edema
   3) Early capsule formation (days 10-13): increased number of fibroblasts and macrophages, thickening collagenous capsule
   4) Late capsule formation (day 14 and later): dense col-lagenous capsule surrounding a necrotic center, and regression of surrounding vasogenic edema
2. Clinical presentation: fever, headache, focal neurologic deficits, and focal seizures
3. Diagnosis
 a. Leukocytosis may be present
 b. Blood cultures often unremarkable
 c. Lumbar puncture generally contraindicated
 d. MRI of brain (Fig. 15-2 and 15-3)
   1) Early cerebritis stages: T1-hypointense and T2-hyperintense mass lesion with poor margins and sur-rounding vasogenic edema, which also appears as high signal on T2 sequences
   2) Capsular stages: development of T2-hypointense capsular ring around lesions with characteristic ring enhancement with administration of contrast
4. Treatment
 a. Antibiotics: considered for early cerebritis stage, patients who are poor surgical candidates, or deep location of abscess
 b. External drainage, CT-guided stereotactic aspiration

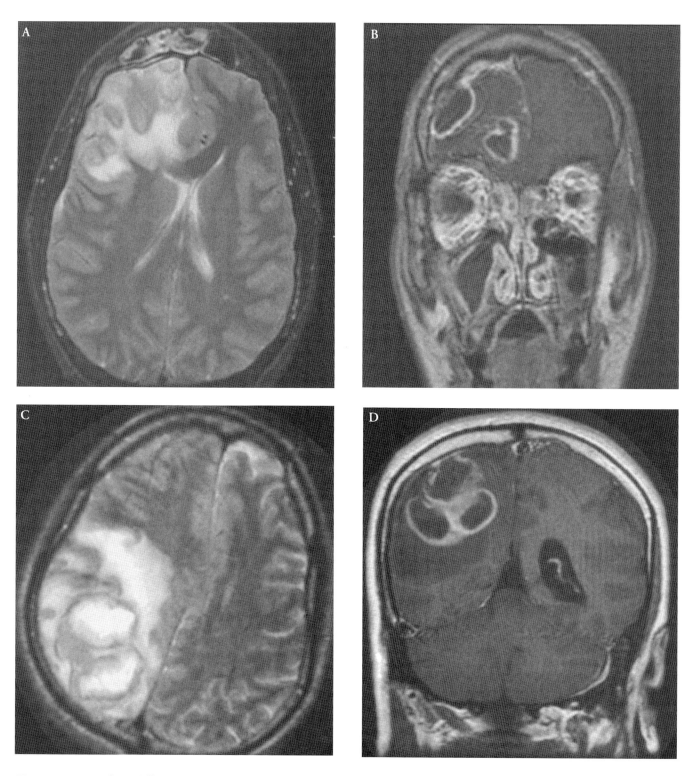

Fig. 15-2. MRI of two different patients with brain abscess. *A* and *B*, A 16-year-old patient who has severe sinusitis with intracranial extension producing subdural empyema and abscesses. There is opacification of the right frontal air cells with membrane thickening (*A*) and intracranial extension with diffuse dural enhancement on the right and collection of empyema in the right epidural space and along the falx cerebri (*B*). There is also formation of an intraparenchymal abscess, with surrounding ring enhancement and mass effect (*A* and *B*). *C* and *D*, Patient with a partially cystic, loculated, and necrotic mass with surrounding vasogenic edema and mass effect with mild midline shift. (*A* and *C*, axial T2-weighted images; *B* and *D*, postcontrast coronal T1-weighted images.)

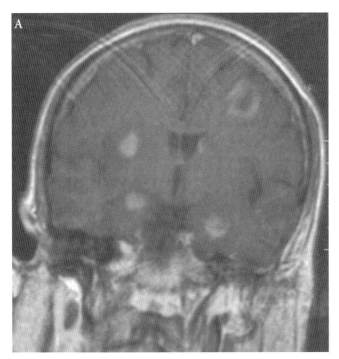
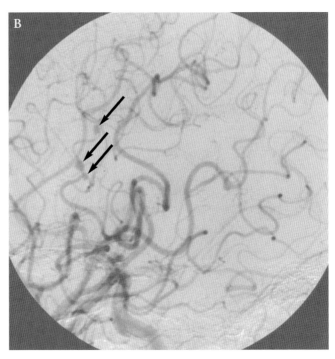

Fig. 15-3. *A*, MRI of a patient with infective endocarditis (postcontrast) T1-weighted image showing multiple brain abscesses due to hematogenous spread of septic emboli. The abscesses appear as small enhancing lesions, some with ring enhancement. *B*, Cerebral angiogram from same patient showing small dilatations, termed mycotic aneurysms (*arrows*).

(through a burr hole) or excision, followed by prolonged course of antibiotics
  c. Corticosteroids for marked surrounding vasogenic edema, mass effect, or increased ICP
  d. Antiepileptic medicines for treatment of seizures

C. Cranial Epidural Abscess
1. Develops between inner aspect of the skull and dura mater
2. Typically, local spread from cranial infection (orbit, ear, sinus, mastoid process, surrounding bone), but can also develop postoperatively (craniotomy) or after trauma
3. Usual pathogens: *Staphylococcus aureus*, aerobes, anaerobes, and gram-negative organisms
4. Clinical presentation: fever, severe unilateral headache, focal neurologic signs
5. Diagnosis: characteristic MRI features—epidural collection, increased signal on both T1 and T2 sequences, often with marked dural enhancement
6. Treatment
  a. Neurosurgical drainage: culture and Gram staining of collection should be performed
  b. Empirical treatment with antibiotics: third- or fourth-generation cephalosporin and vancomycin

D. Subdural Empyema
1. Collection of pus between dura mater and arachnoid
2. Typically due to local spread from cranial infection, e.g., paranasal sinusitis, mastoiditis, or otitis media
3. Usual pathogens: aerobic, microaerophilic, and anaerobic streptococci
4. Clinical presentation: fever, headache, increased ICP and change in level of consciousness, focal brain ischemia, focal neurologic deficits, seizures
5. Diagnosis
  a. Lumbar puncture contraindicated
  b. MRI characteristics: crescent-shaped fluid collections in subdural space, with increased signal intensity on T1 and T2 sequences
6. Treatment: neurosurgical evacuation and empirical treatment with antibiotics to include penicillin G or third- or fourth-generation cephalosporin, metronidazole, and vancomycin

E. Spinal Epidural Abscess
1. Bacterial infection in spinal epidural space
2. Pathogenesis often involves spread from local infection (e.g., osteomyelitis, soft tissue infection), trauma, intravenous drug use, postoperative, or after epidural

catheter placement
3. Most epidural abscesses: posterior to spinal cord
4. Most common pathogens: *Staphylococcus aureus*, then gram-negative bacilli, and *Streptococcus*
5. Clinical presentation: subacute (hours-days) or more chronic (several weeks) localized back pain, radicular symptoms, myelopathy, paralysis, fever
6. Most common location: thoracic spine (>50% of cases)
7. Diagnosis with emergent MRI showing an enhancing epidural collection, often posterior to spinal cord, with varying degrees of mass effect
8. Treatment: surgical drainage of abscess and empirical treatment with antibiotics

F. **Most Common Pathogens of Meningitis and Abscess**
1. *Streptococcus pneumoniae*
   a. Gram-positive coccus
   b. Acquired via inhalation
   c. Causes disease in immunocompetent patients, but higher risk if immunocompromised
   d. Most common cause of bacterial meningitis
   e. Treatment: vancomycin and cefepime (or ceftriaxone) for penicillin-resistant organisms, and penicillin G for the penicillin-sensitive organisms
   f. Vaccination available
2. *Neisseria meningitidis*
   a. Gram-negative diplococcus
   b. Second most frequent cause of bacterial meningitis in adults
   c. Also very frequent in young adults
   d. Petechial rash (usually in lower trunk, lower extremities) is common
   e. Treatment: third-generation cephalosporin or penicillin G or ampicillin
   f. Close contacts should be treated with ciprofloxacin or rifampin
   g. Vaccine is available
   h. Increased risk in patients with complement deficiency
3. *Haemophilus influenzae*
   a. Gram-negative coccobacillus
   b. Acquired via inhalation
   c. Much less common cause of meningitis since advent of vaccine
   d. Optimal treatment: ceftriaxone, cefotaxime, or cefepime
   e. Rifampin prophylaxis for household contacts if other young children
4. *Listeria monocytogenes*
   a. Gram-positive bacillus, found widely in nature
   b. May cause acute or chronic meningitis
   c. Most common in children younger than 1 year, adults older than 60 years, immunosuppressed patients, and in the setting of alcoholism and pregnancy
   d. Best covered by ampicillin
5. Group B streptococcus (*Streptococcus agalactiae*)
   a. Gram-positive coccus
   b. Most common in infants, usually within first month of life (may occur in immunosuppressed elderly)
   c. Pathogenesis typically involves passage through colonized birth canal (note: *many* asymptomatic women have vaginal colonization)
   d. Treatment: ampicillin or penicillin G
6. Enterobacteriaceae (such as *Klebsiella* or *E. coli*)
   a. Gram-negative bacillus
   b. Most common in infants within first month of life
   c. Treatment: ceftriaxone, cefotaxime, or cefepime

G. **Lyme Disease:** neuroborreliosis
1. Pathogenic agent: *Borrelia burgdorferi* (a spirochete)
2. Transmitted via bite of *Ixodes* tick in nymph stage, usually acquired in the summer
3. Regional predilection for the Northeast, Midwest, and Northwest United States
4. Early infection (3-32 days): erythema migrans
   a. "Bull's-eye rash": center of the lesion is site of tick bite, surrounded by a migrating erythematous ring that expands outward
   b. Present in most, but not all patients
   c. Often nonspecific symptoms such as fever, malaise, muscle aches, headache
5. Second stage (several weeks after onset of the rash)
   a. Systemic signs: additional skin lesions, arthralgias, and cardiac abnormalities (arrhythmias, myopericarditis, ventricular dysfunction)

Lyme Disease
Caused by *B. burgdorferi*

Three major stages:
1st (primary) stage: erythema migrans (bulls-eye rash)

2nd stage: systemic manifestations, including arthralgias, cardiac involvement, and multiple types of neuropathies and/or meningitis

3rd stage: neuropathy, encephalopathy, encephalomyelopathy

b. Headache, stiff neck, aseptic meningitis

c. Radiculitis: dermatomal distribution of pain and sensory loss, and corresponding myotomal weakness and reflex changes

d. Cranial neuropathies: especially cranial nerve (CN) VII (facial nerve)

e. Polyneuropathy (peripheral neuropathy, polyradiculo-neuropathy, or mononeuritis multiplex)

f. Brachial plexopathy or lumbosacral plexopathy may be first manifestation

6. Third stage (many months after second stage)

a. Systemic features, including large-joint arthritis, carditis

b. Any of the aforementioned peripheral nerve manifestations, especially long-standing and indolent length-dependent, symmetric peripheral neuropathy

c. Neurologic features may also include chronic encephalomyelopathy: many cases termed "mild encephalopathy" may encompass "memory dysfunction" that may be attributed to other causes, including psychiatric disease rather than organic brain disease

7. Diagnosis

a. Serologic testing is negative early in disease course: patients with classic skin lesions and negative for antibodies should be treated

b. Enzyme-linked immunosorbent assay (ELISA): high false-positive rate because of cross-reactivity

c. Western blot: higher specificity than ELISA (less sensitivity), used as a confirmatory test for positive ELISA

d. CSF: lymphocytic pleocytosis (mean cell count, 166 WBCs/mm^3), normal or increased protein (8-400 mg/dL), and oligoclonal bands (may remain positive for decades while the other markers normalize)

e. CSF polymerase chain reaction (PCR): high specificity, limited sensitivity

f. MRI: normal or may show leptomeningeal enhancement in patients with meningitis

8. Treatment

a. Doxycycline for patients with nonneurologic manifestations only

b. Ceftriaxone (intravenous) for neuroborreliosis (better central nervous system [CNS] penetration)

H. Neurosyphilis

1. Pathogen: *Treponema pallidum* (a spirochete)

2. Transmission through exposure to infected skin or mucous membrane lesion (usually during sexual contact); may also occur from passage through birth canal

3. Clinical features

a. Primary syphilis

1) Usually occurs within few weeks after exposure

2) Manifests as painless chancre at initial site of infection (usually genitalia)

b. Chancre

1) Painless

2) Appears at site of inoculation, with raised border and ulcerated center (resolves without intervention)

c. Most patients with primary syphilis develop secondary syphilis

d. Secondary syphilis (weeks to months after primary syphilis): nonspecific symptoms—fever, headache, rash (including palms and soles), condyloma latum, generalized lymphadenopathy (resolves without intervention)

e. Syphilitic meningitis may occur in secondary syphilis stage (within first 2 years after primary infection) and responds well to treatment

f. Syphilitic meningitis is often characterized by headache, nausea, vomiting, meningismus, altered mentation, seizures, cranial neuropathies

g. Latent syphilis: absence of clinical signs and symptoms, but persistent serologic evidence (may last several years, and may eventually progress to tertiary syphilis)

h. Tertiary syphilis: gummatous syphilis, cardiovascular (including aortitis) and CNS complications, iritis

i. Major neurologic complications occur in tertiary syphilis, which can occur up to decades after primary infection

j. CNS involvement

1) Tabes dorsalis (involvement of posterior columns of spinal cord)

a) Usually manifests as proprioceptive loss, sensory ataxia, lancinating and lightning-like pains, and areflexia

b) Patients may develop trophic changes because of sensory loss, including Charcot joints

2) Meningovascular syphilis (peaks about 7 years after primary infection): characterized by inflammation of intracerebral blood vessels, which can lead to strokes in different arterial distributions (may also affect arterial vasculature of spinal cord)

3) Parenchymatous neurosyphilis (paretic neurosyphilis, general paresis of the insane): chronic meningoencephalitis characterized by slowly progressive syndrome of dementia and neuropsychiatric symptoms with prominent personality change, emotional lability, easy fatigability, sleep disturbance, and poor judgment (with progression)

4) Gummatous neurosyphilis

a) Rare

b) CNS gummas often arise from meninges

c) Symptoms often due to local mass effect or parenchymatous extension

5) Argyll Robertson pupils
   a) Result from brainstem damage
   b) Poor direct and consensual pupillary reflexes, but preserved constriction to accommodation
4. Diagnosis
   a. Dark field microscopy: used for direct examination of infective organisms in chancre of primary syphilis (insensitive for demonstrating organism in CSF)
   b. CSF in acute syphilitic meningitis: mild mononuclear pleocytosis, mildly increased protein, normal or slightly decreased glucose, positive VDRL
   c. CSF in meningovascular syphilis: mild lymphocytic pleocytosis with increased protein
   d. Magnetic resonance angiography or conventional cerebral angiography in meningovascular syphilis: may show focal narrowing of affected vasculature
   e. CSF VDRL
      1) High specificity with low sensitivity for CNS syphilis (in the absence of blood contamination by traumatic lumbar puncture)
      2) Not reliable for following treatment response
   f. Rapid plasma reagin (RPR) test: variation of VDRL (used only in serum, not suitable for CSF)
   g. Fluorescent treponemal antibody (FTA) test
      1) Is called "FTA-ABS" when antigen preparation is absorbed
      2) High false-positive rate when used on CSF: very little blood contamination can cause positive reaction
      3) More sensitive than VDRL
      4) Negative CSF FTA test essentially excludes neurosyphilis, but a positive test is not diagnostic
      5) May remain positive for many years: a positive FTA-ABS and negative VDRL may be seen in successfully treated syphilis
   h. *T. pallidum* hemagglutination assay: another treponemal serologic test
5. Pathology
   a. Parenchymatous neurosyphilis (paretic neurosyphilis, general paresis of the insane): thickened leptomeninges, atrophied gyri, granular appearance of ependymal lining, scanty meningeal and perivascular lymphocytic infiltrates
   b. Meningovascular neurosyphilis: leptomeningeal and perivascular parenchymal lymphocytic infiltrates
6. Treatment
   a. Aqueous crystalline penicillin G 18 to 24 million units daily, administered as 3 to 4 million units intravenously every 4 hours for 2 weeks or a continuous infusion, *or*
   b. Procaine penicillin 2.4 million units intramuscularly once daily *and* probenecid 500 mg orally 4 times daily for 10 to 14 days

I. CNS Tuberculosis
1. Pathogen: *Mycobacterium tuberculosis*, a gram-positive aerobic bacterium with very slow growth and associated with subacute to chronic meningitis
2. Usual route of transmission: inhalation of aerosolized droplet nuclei; may spread hematogenously to extrapulmonary sites, including CNS
3. Incidence of tuberculosis in United States has increased since advent of HIV
4. Subacute to chronic meningitis
   a. Clinical features
      1) Most common CNS presentation
      2) Prodrome of 2 to 4 weeks: nonspecific symptoms of fatigue, malaise, and possibly fever
      3) Mental status
         a) Fully alert and oriented (first stage)
         b) Confused, disoriented, and inattentive (second stage)
         c) Comatose or stuporous (third stage)
      4) Fever, meningismus, headache, nausea, vomiting, and often basilar signs, such as cranial nerve palsies (CN VI most commonly affected)
      5) Ophthalmoscopic examination may show papilledema or choroidal tubercles (latter observed only in small fraction of patients)
      6) Other possible features: seizures, hydrocephalus (more frequently in children than adults)
      7) Similar presentation for CNS tuberculosis in setting of HIV infection
      8) Complications may include hydrocephalus and cerebral infarctions (the latter due to vascular involvement of the leptomeningeal and pachymeningeal inflammation)
   b. Diagnosis
      1) Acid-fast bacilli (AFB) smear: positive in 10% to 30% of cases
      2) Purified protein derivative (PPD): false positive in patients who have received the BCG vaccine, and false negative in patients with severe immunosuppression
      3) Chest radiograph: possible presence of lymphadenopathy and Ghon's complex or miliary lesions
      4) Neuroimaging: meningeal enhancement of basal cisterns, especially interpeduncular fossa and ambiens cisterns
      5) CSF profile: lymphocytic pleocytosis, decreased glucose, increased protein
      6) CSF PCR: specificity, 94% to 100%; sensitivity, 54% to 100%
      7) CSF amplified *Mycobacterium tuberculosis* direct test:

rapid (available within 24 hours) and probably highly specific and sensitive nucleic acid amplification assay

c. Treatment

1) First-line antimicrobial agents: isoniazid (INH), rifampin, ethambutol, pyrazinamide, streptomycin

2) Second-line antimicrobial agents: ethionamide, cycloserine

5. Parenchymal tuberculosis: tuberculoma and tuberculoid abscess

a. Clinical features

1) May be found in cerebral or cerebellar parenchyma and deep gray matter; may involve epidural, subdural, or subarachnoid space

2) Clinical presentation

a) Depends on location of lesion

b) May include headaches, seizures, increased ICP, and papilledema

3) Clinical course of an underlying tuberculoid abscess is usually more precipitous and marked with rapid progression compared with indolent chronic progression of tuberculoma

b. Diagnosis

1) Neuroimaging

a) Tuberculomas: appear as isointense to parenchyma on T1-weighted images; may have central hyperintense region on T2-weighted images, with surrounding ring enhancement characteristics; there may be central calcification in mature tuberculomas (Fig. 15-4)

b) Multiple small lesions: characteristic of miliary spread

2) CSF may be normal

3) Response to antituberculosis antibiotics

c. Pathology: central caseation necrosis surrounded by collagenous capsule with multinucleated giant cells, epithelioid cells, fibroblasts, and mononuclear inflammatory infiltrates (to be differentiated from acute tuberuous abscess, which is liquefactive necrosis with neutrophilic inflammatory infiltrates); vasogenic edema and gliosis may occur outside the tuberculoma

d. Treatment

1) Antimicrobial agents and dexamethasone

2) Surgical resection when medical treatment fails or if diagnosis is uncetain

6. Spinal tuberculosis

a. Spinal tuberculous meningitis

1) Rare, may be caused by dissemination of disease in context of intracranial meningitis

2) Subacute or chronic onset of radiculomyelitis, due to involvement of the spinal cord and roots

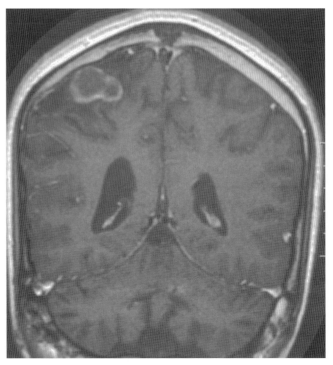

Fig. 15-4. MRI of a 17-year-old boy with tuberculoma (post-contrast T1-weighted image) showing a loculated mass with surrounding ring enhancement and no mass effect.

3) Imaging characteristics: leptomeningeal enchancement; clumping and enhancement of the roots

4) May rarely present as tuberculomas in the intradural or intramedullary space

b. Pott's disease: vertebral tuberculosis infection

1) Most often involves low thoracic and thoracolumbar region

2) Usually starts in anterior aspect of vertebral bodies (often more than one segment) and spreads to adjacent intervertebral disks, causing softening and collapse of the vertebrae, producing kyphosis

3) May involve paravertebral tissues; may give rise to paravertebral abscesses

4) May result in pronounced spondylosis and spinal cord compromise: myelopathic or radicular symptoms and signs

5) Clinical features

a) Gradual onset

b) Back pain: may be present for several weeks before presentation

c) Paraspinal muscle spasms

d) Kyphotic deformity of spine

e) Constitutional symptoms may be present: fever, weight loss

f) Retropharyngeal abscess when upper cervical spine is involved

6) Treatment: antimicrobial agents; surgical treatment for patients with progressive neurologic deficits, spinal instability, and poor response to antimicrobial agents

J. Leprosy (Hansen's disease)
1. Pathophysiology
   a. Etiologic agent: *Mycobacterium leprae*, AFB, responsible for infection of peripheral nerves and overlying skin
   b. Most likely route of transmission: respiratory or cutaneous
   c. Directly infects Schwann cells, producing demyelination of peripheral nerves
   d. There may be granulomatous damage of the perineurium
   e. Rare in United States, usually occurs in immigrants from endemic areas (e.g., Southeast Asia)
2. Clinical features
   a. Chronic infection, marked by very slow growth of the bacillus
   b. Peripheral nerve trophism with preference for cooler body regions, 7-10°C cooler than core temperatures
   c. Skin lesions: multiple, multifocal hypopigmented, anesthetic patches
   d. Peripheral nerve involvement: loss of pain and temperature and soft sensation in the hypopigmented, anhidrotic skin lesions involving the distal cutaneous sensory branches, with relative preservation of vibratory and proprioceptive sensation
   e. Clinical syndrome of mononeuritis multiplex occurs when there is proximal involvement of the individual peripheral nerves
   f. Peripheral nerves are more predisposed to entrapment at the common sites of compression
   g. Tuberculoid leprosy
      1) Occurs in setting of good host immunity

Mycobacteria
M. tuberculosis can present neurologically with chronic basilar meningitis

M. leprae presents with hypopigmented, anesthetic patches of skin and multiple mononeuropathies

Both types of mycobacteria require long-term multidrug therapy

---

2) Well-demarcated lesions with raised erythematous borders and central clearing
3) Limited form of leprosy, but antibiotic treatment is often required
4) Most frequently affected peripheral nerve is ulnar nerve
   h. Lepromatous leprosy
      1) Occurs in setting of inadequate host immunity
      2) Ongoing bacteremia, organisms deposit throughout the body and establish infection in cooler body regions
      3) Skin lesions are poorly demarcated and may appear as diffuse, infiltrative, nodular, and erythematous lesions
      4) Initially, often a painful, purely sensory neuropathy, with preferential involvement of extensor surfaces of upper and lower limbs, pinnae of the ears, and zygomatic arch bilaterally
      5) With progression: nerve trunk involvement, with enlargement and damage of peripheral nerves; motor and sensory loss in the distribution of individual nerves
   i. Intermediate form: features of both tuberculoid and lepromatous types
3. Diagnosis
   a. Tissue diagnosis with skin smears or nerve biopsies: weakly AFB positive
   b. Lepromin skin test: similar to PPD, Fernandez reaction read at 48 hours (indicative of infection), and Mitsuda reaction read at 4 to 5 weeks (indicative of resistance)
4. Treatment: dapsone, clofazimine, rifampin

K. Rickettsial Infections
1. Pathogens: *Rickettsia rickettsii, R. conorii, R. prowazekii,* and *Orientia tsutsugamushi*
2. Clinical features of neurologic disease
   a. Headaches, altered mentation, coma, seizures, focal neurologic deficits
   b. Aseptic meningitis is a common presentation; CSF polymorphonuclear cells may be prominent in some patients
   c. Rocky Mountain spotted fever
      1) Pathogen: *R. rickettsii*
      2) Headache, high fever, nausea, myalgias, arthralgias, malaise, conjunctival injection
      3) Maculopapular, petechial, and ecchymotic rash (often first appearing as macular, "small red dots," then becoming petechial): appears first on wrists and ankles, then spreads to involve the soles and palms, and then the trunk
      4) Meningitis or meningoencephalitis may follow severe cases

5) Organisms are angioinvasive and may cause microangiopathy
   a) May produce CNS microinfarcts, retinal vasculitis
   b) Conjunctival injection and skin rash may be explained on basis of this microangiopathy

  d. Scrub typhus
   1) Pathogen: *O. tsutsugamushi*
   2) Transmitted by bites of larvae of mites (larvae live in soil and mites live in rodents)
   3) Two-week incubation period
   4) Fever, headache, painful adenopathy, scab at original bite site
   5) Neurologic complications uncommon, but may cause aseptic meningitis

  e. Endemic, or murine, typhus
   1) Pathogen: *R. typhi*
   2) Presentation: fever, nausea, maculopapular truncal rash, myalgias, and malaise
   3) Neurologic complications uncommon

  f. Epidemic typhus
   1) Pathogen: *R. prowazekii*
   2) Clinical features: 12- to 14-day incubation period followed by
    a) Headache, fever, macular rash first appearing in upper trunk and axillae and sparing the face, palms, and soles
    b) Meningitis, meningoencephalitis: unrelenting fever, delirium, confusion, coma, focal deficits
    c) Organisms invade endothelial cells
    d) May be complicated by brainstem microinfarctions

3. Treatment: chloramphenicol, tetracycline, doxycycline

L. Whipple's Disease

1. Pathogen: *Tropheryma whippelii*
2. Multisystem involvement, but almost always involves gastrointestinal tract: arthralgias, weight loss, diarrhea, abdominal pain, low-grade fever, lymphadenopathy
3. Neurologic manifestations
  a. Altered mentation, encephalopathy, coma, seizures
  b. Dementia from chronic and recurrent meningitis
  c. Involvement of hypothalamic-pituitary axis: polydipsia, polyuria, hypogonadism, hyperinsomnia
  d. Supranuclear ophthalmoplegia
  e. Cerebellar ataxia
  f. Myelopathy
  g. Oculomasticatory myorhythmia: characterized by slow and smooth convergent-divergent pendular nystagmus associated with synchronous rhythmic myoclonic movements of tongue and mandible
  h. Oculofacial-skeletal myorhythmia: similar rhythmic

movements involving different muscle groups in face and limbs

4. Diagnosis
  a. CSF PCR for *T. whippelii*
  b. Small-bowel biopsy
  c. Neuroimaging: often normal, may show parenchymal T2 hyperintensities in middle cerebellar peduncle and other parenchyma

5. Treatment
  a. Trimethoprim-sulfamethoxazole: for initial therapy, also for recurrent disease
  b. Alternative treatments: combination of penicillin and streptomycin or parenteral ceftriaxone

II. VIRAL INFECTIONS OF THE NERVOUS SYSTEM

A. Viral Meningitis (aseptic meningitis)

1. Clinical features: fever, chills, headaches, photophobia, nuchal rigidity, nausea, anorexia, myalgias, with or without rash
2. Most common pathogens and specific features
  a. Enteroviruses
   1) Most common cause of aseptic meningitis
   2) Coxsackieviruses, echoviruses, polioviruses, and human enteroviruses 68 to 71
   3) Infection transmitted by fecal-oral contamination, respiratory droplets
   4) Seasonal peak in late summer
   5) May be a respiratory or gastrointestinal prodrome
   6) Benign form of viral meningitis, except in immunosuppressed patients (in which case may be protracted or recurrent)

  b. La Crosse (California) encephalitis
   1) Most common cause of arbovirus meningoencephalitis in United States
   2) Clinical presentation is aseptic meningitis, often occurring concurrently with encephalitis
   3) Mild disease, predominantly affecting children (>85% of cases in children <12 years old)
   4) Seizures are common (distinguishing feature): generalized and partial seizures develop with approximately equal frequency; status epilepticus occurs in 25%
   5) Focal signs or symptoms in 20%
   6) Serologic tests may not be positive until 2 to 4 weeks after acute illness
   7) Seasonal peak in late summer
   8) Usually self-limited and uncomplicated: mortality less than 1%, persistent sequelae in ~10% to 15%

(memory and behavioral disturbance, aphasia, seizures, cranial nerve palsies)

9) Rarely may have fulminant presentation, with fever, headache, obtundation progressing to coma, and sometimes status epilepticus

c. Mumps (see below, under "C. Specific Viral Entities")

d. Herpes simplex type 2

1) Herpesvirus, a DNA virus

2) May cause viral meningitis concurrent with, or after, primary genital infection by reactivation from sacral dorsal root ganglia

3) The most common agent believed to cause benign recurrent lymphocytic meningitis (Mollaret's meningitis)

4) Genital lesions may not be observed in recurrent meningitis

5) Diagnosis

a) CSF: positive PCR for herpes simplex virus (HSV) type 2, protein normal or mildly increased, glucose normal or mildly decreased, lymphocytic pleocytosis (may be mainly polymorphonuclear neutrophils if CSF obtained within first 48 hours), usually WBC <1,000 cells/mm^3

b) Neuroimaging: may be normal or show lepto-meningeal enhancement

e. Varicella-zoster virus (VZV)

1) Syndrome of meningoencephalitis, usually in context of zoster, with dermatomal distribution of vesicular rash, accompanying pain, and possibly dermatomal neurologic deficits (most often as a complication of ophthalmic zoster)

2) May also cause self-limited cerebellar ataxia, brainstem encephalitis, transverse myelitis, granulomatous arteritis, and small-vessel angiopathy, sometimes producing cerebral infarction

3) Mild lymphocytic pleocytosis may be present in context of uncomplicated dermatomal zoster, without clinical features of aseptic meningitis

4) Good prognosis

5) Recommended treatment with acyclovir, especially in immunosuppressed patients

f. HIV-1: may spread to CSF and meninges during time of acute infection and cause aseptic meningitis

g. Lymphocytic choreomeningitis

1) Rodent-borne virus transmitted to humans through exposure to rodent urine, feces, saliva, or blood

2) Often asymptomatic or mild but can cause aseptic meningitis, encephalitis, life-threatening infections in immunosuppressed persons

3) May cause severe congenital defects

h. Arboviruses (other than La Crosse encephalitis): much more common cause of encephalitis or meningoencephalitis (discussed below)

B. Viral Encephalitis

1. Viral infection of brain parenchyma

2. Most common nonepidemic viral cause: HSV-1

3. Pathogenesis

a. Viruses may penetrate mucosal surfaces, skin, or gastro-intestinal or genitourinary barriers

b. Pathogens seed CNS via hematogenous (most common route) or neuronal spread by reactivation from neural ganglia, followed by retrograde axonal transmission

c. Hematogenous dissemination is most common method of viral entry to CNS; involves transient viremia shortly after inoculation and viral replication at site of inoculation

d. Pathogenic virus tends to spread to reticuloendothelial organs (lymph nodes, liver, spleen, bone marrow), where viral replication continues and second wave of increased viremia occurs

4. Clinical features

a. Encephalitis usually occurs concurrent with meningitis as meningoencephalitis

b. Acute onset of febrile illness, headache, nuchal rigidity, altered mental status with disorientation, and behavioral disturbance

c. HSV encephalitis: aphasia, complex partial seizures, characteristic electroencephalographic (EEG) findings (periodic lateralized epileptiform discharges [PLEDs])

5. Pathology

a. Lymphocytic infiltration of brain parenchyma and meninges, with edema and necrosis

b. Microglial nodules

c. There may be virus-specific inclusions

d. Immunohistochemistry for organism identification

6. Most common pathogens and specific features

a. HSV-1

1) Most common nonepidemic cause of viral encephalitis

2) Predilection for inferior frontal and temporal lobes: causes behavioral dysfunction, personality change, aphasia, complex partial seizures, and PLEDs localized to involved parenchyma

3) Fever with or without nuchal rigidity

4) CSF may show red blood cells (because of underlying hemorrhagic necrosis of involved parenchyma)

5) CSF PCR

a) Highly sensitive and specific; useful for early detection

b) Influenced by antiviral therapy: 98% remain positive within first week of treatment (47% with 1-2 weeks of treatment, 21% with >2 weeks of treatment)

6) Serologic testing
   a) May be used after at least 2 weeks of illness; largely replaced by CSF PCR
   b) Increased serum titers: nonspecific
   c) Serum:CSF ratio less than 20:1 (after at least 2 weeks of infection) strongly favors primary CNS antibody production and indicates CNS infection

7) Pathology (Fig. 15-5)
   a) Perivascular mononuclear infiltrates
   b) Necrotizing inflammation
   c) Foci of hemorrhage
   d) Intranuclear viral inclusions

8) Neuroimaging (Fig. 15-6): T2 hyperintense lesions predominantly involving frontotemporal regions, variable enhancement, with or without hemorrhagic component

9) Treatment: intravenous acyclovir should be started as soon as possible because of high mortality rate

10) Mortality: 70% of untreated patients

b. Arboviruses
   1) Arthropod-borne
   2) Common epidemic encephalitis of summer months
   3) Usually cause meningoencephalitis: seizures, focal neurologic deficits
   4) Benign illness without sequelae, good prognosis
   5) La Crosse (California) encephalitis (discussed above)
   6) Japanese encephalitis virus (*Flavivirus*)
      a) Most common cause of arbovirus encephalitis worldwide
      b) Route of transmission: from *Culex* mosquito bite (mosquitoes acquire it from infected birds or pigs), hematogenous spread to CNS
      c) Predominantly affects children in endemic regions
      d) Most infected patients do not develop CNS symptoms
      e) Typical clinical presentation in symptomatic cases: febrile headache, aseptic meningitis, or encephalitis
      f) Prodrome of viral illness: headache, nausea, vomiting, low-grade fever, other constitutional symptoms, behavioral change, and often seizures
      g) Virus can spread to and establish infection in various regions of brain via hematogenous dissemination: cerebral cortex, deep gray matter (thalamus, basal ganglia, substantia nigra), brainstem, and cerebellum
      h) Clinical features depend on part of CNS involved

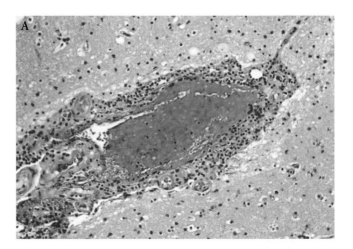

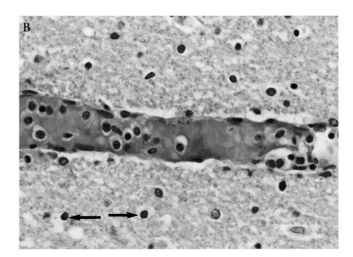

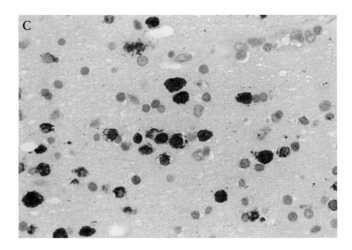

Fig. 15-5. Perivascular mononuclear infiltrates (*A*) and homogenous-appearing viral inclusions (*B, arrows*) are characteristic histopathologic features of herpes encephalitis. *C*, Viral inclusions are demonstrated better with immunohistochemical staining of herpes simplex virus antigens.

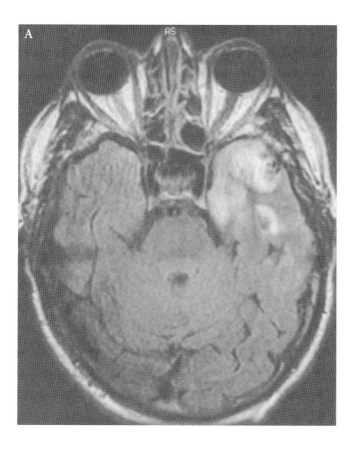

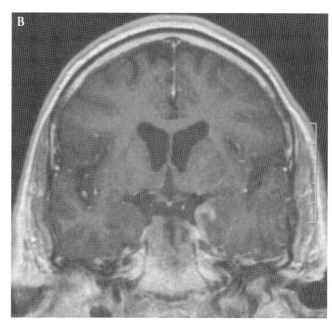

Fig. 15-6. *A* and *B*, MRI of a 69-year-old man with HSV encephalitis showing multifocal signal abnormality involving anterior left temporal lobe and consisting of foci of blood surrounded by edema with patchy gadolinium enhancement. (*A*, Axial FLAIR sequence; *B*, coronal postcontrast T1 sequence.)

i) Extrapyramidal features: tremors, axial rigidity, cogwheel appendicular rigidity, choreoathetosis from involvement of basal ganglia

j) Spinal cord involvement: asymmetric flaccid paralysis from involvement of anterior horn cells, affecting lower more than upper extremities

k) Brainstem involvement (rhombencephalitis): cranial nerve palsies, diffuse weakness, long tract signs

l) Cerebellar involvement: ataxia

m) Mortality is 30%; approximately half of survivors continue to have severe neurologic sequelae

7) St. Louis encephalitis virus (SLEV)

a) Most common in southern, western, and midwestern United States; mainly occurs in late summer and autumn months

b) Route of transmission: from *Culex* mosquito bite

c) Patients are usually older than those with other arboviral illnesses

d) Frank encephalitis with psychotic features occurs in older patients

e) Aseptic meningitis in 25% of patients, usually in younger patients

f) Labial, lingual, and hand tremors in 50% of patients

g) Slow progression of encephalitis, generalized fatigue, malaise, and tremors characterize syndrome

h) Mortality rate: 20%

8) West Nile virus

a) Usually asymptomatic in areas of endemic disease

b) Elderly and immunosuppressed persons are at risk for encephalitis

c) Severe neurologic manifestations are more common in young children and elderly

d) Febrile viral illness occurs after incubation period of 3 to 15 days: pharyngitis, headache, conjunctivitis, malaise and fatigue, back pain

e) May be gastrointestinal symptoms: nausea, abdominal pain, diarrhea

f) Prominent and distinguishing feature of West Nile virus infection: tremor (up to 94% of patients)

g) May be other extrapyramidal symptoms: myoclonus (40%) and parkinsonism (75%)

h) Direct infection of anterior horn cells causes poliomyelitis-like acute flaccid paralysis characterized by acute onset of asymmetric muscle weakness and hyporeflexia with minimal sensory abnormalities

---

West Nile Encephalitis

Two most common presentations

Meningoencephalitis: typical encephalitic features

Flaccid paralysis: poliolike clinical features with anterior horn cell damage

Rare cases of parkinsonism, myoclonus, and other clinical presentations

---

    i) CSF profile: mild lymphocytic pleocytosis (27-51 cells), normal or increased protein (38-899 mg/dL), usually normal glucose

    j) CSF anti–West Nile virus IgM antibodies by ELISA: IgM antibodies do not cross blood-brain barrier; their presence indicates intrathecal antibody production and CNS infection

    k) CSF PCR: low sensitivity, high specificity

    l) Neuroimaging: may show meningeal, thalamus, or basal ganglia abnormalities

  9) Eastern equine encephalitis virus

    a) Responsible for most severe arboviral encephalitis

    b) Clinical presentation marked by abrupt onset of fever, convulsions, altered mentation, with rapid progression to coma

    c) Encephalitis may be preceded by viral prodrome of constitutional symptoms

    d) There may be focal lesions in basal ganglia and thalamus (less often, brainstem)

  10) Western equine encephalitis virus

    a) Asymptomatic infections are common

    b) Viral prodrome, presenting with pharyngitis, myalgias, fever, and other constitutional symptoms

    c) Convulsions and progression to coma develops in some patients

  11) Epstein-Barr virus (EBV) (see below)

  12) Cytomegalovirus (CMV) (see below)

C. Specific Viral Entities

1. Herpesviruses

  a. HSV-1 and HSV-2 (discussed above)

  b. VZV

    1) Chickenpox: primary infection, usually without neurologic sequelae; the virus becomes latent in dorsal root ganglia

    2) Pathogenesis of herpes zoster virus infection

      a) Due to reactivation of latent virus in dorsal root ganglia

      b) Reactivation after trauma or with reduced cell-mediated immunity with age or concurrent immunosuppression

      c) Radicular pain and paresthesias in cranial or spinal dermatomes, followed by vesicular rash involving same distribution

      d) Usually involves mid to low thoracic (less commonly, cranial and lumbosacral) segments

      e) Possible sequelae: postherpetic neuralgia

      f) Ophthalmic zoster: involvement of first division of trigeminal ganglion, may be complicated by aseptic meningitis or granulomatous arteritis

      g) Ramsey Hunt syndrome: painful facial weakness accompanied by vesicular eruption involving external auditory canal

      h) Cranial nerve involvement in older patients: high risk for developing meningoencephalitis, all should be treated with antiviral agents

    3) Aseptic meningitis and meningoencephalitis (discussed above)

    4) Zoster myelitis (spinal cord involvement): poor prognosis for recovery of encephalomyelitis, especially if underlying immunosuppression

    5) Self-limited cerebellar ataxia

    6) Granulomatous arteritis and small-vessel microangiopathy

      a) May complicate ophthalmic zoster

      b) Multifocal ischemic and occasional hemorrhagic infarcts

      c) Hyperplasia of blood vessel intima and media and superimposed thrombus formation

      d) Small-vessel arteritis, microangiopathy: may cause multifocal deep white matter lesions

    7) Reye's syndrome: may rarely occur in children, particularly with use of aspirin; characterized by encephalopathy, renal failure, and liver dysfunction

    8) Postinfectious multifocal, demyelinating leukoencephalomyelitis: rare, demyelination due to infection of oligodendrocytes, with Cowdry type A intranuclear inclusions

    9) Treatment: supportive measures, intravenous acyclovir or famciclovir

  c. CMV

    1) Largest human herpesvirus

    2) A DNA virus

    3) Ubiquitous presence in asymptomatic persons, with widespread exposure among population: 80% of individuals are seropositive for CMV by adulthood

4) Predominantly a disease of immunocompromised host and infected newborns

5) Can infect several organs, including nervous system; infection may remain latent or be persistent

6) Immunocompetent persons: acute infection may be asymptomatic or, uncommonly, person may present with aseptic meningitis or mononucleosis syndrome

7) Acute meningitis of CMV

8) CMV encephalitis
   a) Occurs in immunocompromised adults (rare in immunocompetent patients)
   b) Fever, headache, mental status changes, cranial nerve palsies, cognitive dysfunction
   c) Multifocal CNS disease with involvement of spinal cord, nerve roots, ventricular and subependymal regions, and both gray and white matter (with predilection for deep gray matter structures)
   d) Variable presentation: acute encephalitis or slowly progressive ventriculoencephalitis with necrotizing ependymitis or ventriculitis
   e) Myeloradiculitis: patients may have predominance of polymorphonuclear cells and low glucose level (a profile more typical of bacterial infections)
   f) Common presentation in context of HIV: ventriculitis or ependymitis with subacute progression, polymorphonuclear CSF pleocytosis with low CSF glucose level

9) Diffuse ependymitis and ventriculitis
   a) Presentation: subacute to chronic meningitis
   b) Cauda equina may be involved
   c) CSF: prominent mononuclear pleocytosis and increased protein
   d) Subependymal enhancement outlining ventricular system

10) CMV polyradiculopathy (discussed below)

11) Congenital CMV
   a) Most common congenital infection
   b) Transmission to infant from infected mother: vertical transmission through birth canal at time of delivery or breast milk in perinatal period
   c) Most primary maternal infections transmitted to infants are acquired in first trimester
   d) 90% of CMV-infected infants born to mothers with primary CMV infection have no clinical features of infection at birth; these infants carry lifetime risk up to 15% for sensorineural hearing loss
   e) 10% of CMV-infected infants have clinical features of infection at birth: jaundice, hepatosplenomegaly, petechial rash, growth retardation, sensorineural hearing loss, microcephaly, micro-

gyria, seizures, cerebral calcifications, choreoretinitis, and death in perinatal period (5% of patients)
   f) Children with very mild disease may only have sensorineural hearing loss

12) Pathology (Fig. 15-7)
   a) Involvement predominantly of ependymal cells and microglia
   b) Cowdry type A intranuclear inclusions
   c) Microglial nodules (dense focal aggregates of microglial cells and macrophages)
   d) Severity of inflammatory infiltrates depends on degree of immunocompetence
   e) CMV ventriculitis: necrosis of ventricular surface
   f) CMV polyradiculopathy: necrosis of nerve roots, inflammatory infiltrate

13) Diagnosis
   a) Serologic testing: unreliable because of fluctuating titers
   b) CSF PCR: sensitivity reported up to 95%, specificity of 99%
   c) Infants symptomatic with congenital CMV: thrombocytopenia, direct hyperbilirubinemia, abnormal liver function enzymes, periventricular calcifications on CT (50% of symptomatic infants), and sometimes parenchymal neural migration abnormalities (when infection occurs during period of neural migration, e.g., polymicrogyria, lissencephaly, schizencephaly)
   d) Other radiographic characterics: ventriculomegaly because of parenchymal loss; focal areas of contrast enhancement (especially periventricular) apparent in the active infection, replaced later by nonenhancing calcification

14) Treatment: ganciclovir with or without foscarnet

d. EBV
   1) Infection spread through saliva; establishes latent infection in B cells
   2) Acute infection

Congenital cytomegalovirus infection
   Phenotype varies from very mild (only sensorineural hearing loss) to severe cerebral injury, including developmental delay, microcephaly, microgyria, seizures, cerebral calcifications, choreoretinitis, and death in the perinatal period in 5% of patients

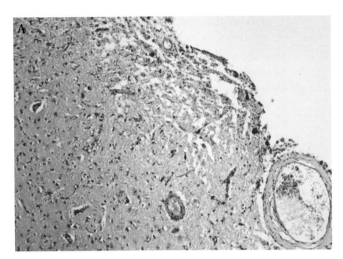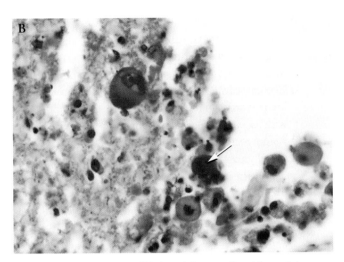

Fig. 15-7. Cytomegalovirus ventriculitis. Necrosis and rarefraction of ventricular surface (*A*), filled with large cells with nuclei containing the typical inclusion bodies (Cowdry type A intranuclear inclusions [*arrow*]) with the surrounding pale halo (*B*), characteristic of cytomegalovirus infection.

a) Asymptomatic

b) Nonspecific febrile viral illness

c) Infectious mononucleosis: cervical lymphadenopathy, pharyngitis, and splenomegaly

3) Neurologic complications in less than 1% of acute EBV infections

a) Aseptic meningitis: may occur at time of primary infection, along with acute mononucleosis

b) Encephalitis

c) Cerebellitis

d) Transverse myelitis

e) Guillain-Barré syndrome

f) Optic neuritis

g) Cranial neuropathies, including facial palsy

4) May have a pathogenic role in development of primary CNS lymphoma in immunocompromised patients: EBV genome has been found in up to 100% of lymphomas in immunocompromised patients, including those with HIV infection (only 16% of lymphomas in immunocompetent patients)

5) Diagnosis by serologic studies

a) Acute, acquired infection: presence of IgM antibodies against EBV viral capsid antigen (VCA) or combination of IgG antibodies against both VCA and early antigen (EA-diffuse)

b) CSF IgM antibodies persist for several months and are sensitive and specific markers for acute CNS infection

c) Past exposure: presence of IgG antibodies against VCA and EBV nuclear antigen (EBNA), observed in serum specimens collected as early as approximately 1 month after onset of illness

d) EBNA antibodies may remain positive for person's lifetime; when present alone, they indicate remote infection

e) Heterophil antibody and Monospot tests: are unreliable and frequently negative in patients with EBV infections of CNS

6) Diagnosis by CSF PCR

a) Not positive in patients with latent EBV infection

b) Sensitivity and specificity for diagnosis of acute EBV infections of the CNS: unknown

c) EBV CSF PCR: often positive in patients with acquired immunodeficiency syndrome (AIDS)-associated primary CNS lymphoma (PCNSL); test appears to be sensitive indicator of the presence of tumor

7) Treatment: data are largely anecdotal, successful use of ganciclovir has been reported

e. Human herpesvirus 6 (HHV-6)

1) Ubiquitous virus: 2/3 of children are seropositive by 1 year and up to 95% by adulthood

2) Responsible for roseola infantum in infants and young children (also called sixth disease or exanthema subitum): high fever, malaise, irritability, and pharyngitis, followed by macular or maculopapular rash that starts on trunk

3) ~1/3 of babies with primary HHV-6 infection have seizures; common presentation is febrile seizures some time before the characteristic rash appears

4) After acute primary infection, HHV-6 becomes latent; it can reactivate in infants and young children, causing recurrent febrile seizures; can reactivate during immunosuppression

5) Recurrent HHV-6 should be considered as pathogenic agent in setting of recurrent febrile seizures (even without the characteristic rash)

6) Meningoencephalitis may occur in immunocompromised patients; can be severe in this setting

7) Most primary HHV-6 infections are self-limited and do not require treatment

8) HHV-6 infection has been associated with multiple sclerosis, but its pathogenic role has not been established

f. HHV-7

1) Clinical features of the acute infection are similar to those of HHV-6 infection

2) Treatment: most isolates resistant to acyclovir but sensitive to cidofovir, foscarnet, and ganciclovir (foscarnet may be more efficacious than ganciclovir)

2. Rabies virus

a. Caused by rabies virus (an RNA virus) in genus *Lyssavirus*, in rhabdovirus family

b. Pathophysiology

1) Often due to bite of infected animal (e.g., skunk, bat, or raccoon); risk of CNS disease is 50 times higher with bite than scratch

2) Many cases do not have known exposure; this may be secondary to prolonged incubation of virus

3) Virus multiplies in muscle at inoculation site and is taken up by nerve endings in muscle spindles or at neuromuscular junction; is retrogradely transported to CNS

4) Centripetal spread to CNS: fast retrograde axonal transport results in widespread CNS infection; symptoms can occur years after infection

5) Some evidence that virus undergoes replication in dorsal root ganglia and anterior horn cells

6) Centrifugal spread from CNS: after infection is established in CNS, the virus can spread to different regions of head and neck

7) Bites at sites with high concentrations of nicotinic acetylcholine receptors (e.g., head or face) have greater chance of causing CNS infection and have shorter incubation periods

c. Clinical features

1) Incubation period: usually 1 to 2 months after exposure (may be as early as 5 days if peripheral nerves directly inoculated)

2) Prodrome: nonspecific illness with fever, headache,

myalgias; possibly with local symptoms of paresthesias, numbness, dysesthesias, pruritis at site of exposure

3) Local symptoms start at site of the bite and spread to involve entire limb or ipsilateral face

a) Onset of local symptoms marks end of incubation period

b) Condition progresses into acute neurologic infectious phase, and most patients die within next 2 weeks

4) Acute neurologic phase: takes the form of two different syndromes, either classic or nonclassic rabies

5) Classic rabies is categorized as furious rabies and paralytic rabies

a) Furious classic rabies

i) Fluctuations in mentation, behavior, and consciousness

ii) Persistent fever

iii) Psychiatric disturbance, including depression and agitation

iv) Hydrophobia or aerophobia due to spasms of pharyngeal muscles (which may be triggered by swallowing or environmental stimuli)

v) Hypersalivation: combination of autonomic hyperactivity and dysphagia

vi) Other autonomic features: hyperhidrosis, priapism, spontaneous ejaculation, anisocoria, fixed pupils

b) Paralytic classic rabies

i) Ascending weakness, axonal polyradiculoneuropathy

ii) Weakness in both lower extremities in ascending fashion develops in all patients, with early loss of tendon reflexes

iii) Myoedema

6) Nonclassic rabies: various symptoms localizing to CNS, including signs of brainstem deficits, hemiparesis, hemisensory loss, ataxia, and vertigo

7) Coma: associated with inspiratory spasms and tachycardia

8) MRI: normal or nonspecific T2 hyperintense lesions, with or without enhancement

9) Skin biopsy from neck: frozen sections of skin with fluorescent antibody technique show rabies virus antigen in subcutaneous nervous tissue

10) CSF: normal or minimal pleocytosis

11) Pathology

a) Leptomeningeal and perivascular lymphocytic infiltrates, relative paucity of inflammatory response

b) Inclusion bodies: Negri bodies usually found in

Purkinje cells and in hippocampus

   12) Postexposure prophylaxis

     a) Immediate cleansing site of the wound

     b) Rabies immune globulin: inject locally around wound and at intramuscular site close to wound

     c) Vaccination: intramuscular and intradermal

3. Measles

  a. Pathogen: measles virus, a paramyxovirus (an RNA virus)

  b. Virus generally spreads through infected respiratory secretions; may cause neurologic manifestations through spread to CNS during initial infection, but also may have CNS effects years after initial infection

  c. Acute infection

    1) Constitutional symptoms, including fever

    2) Maculopapular rash: appears first on head and shoulders and spreads downward (and disappears in same sequence)

    3) Koplik's spots: small erythematous lesions with pale centers in mucosal surface of oropharynx; develop shortly after onset of the rash

    4) Cough, coryza

    5) Incidence has decreased significantly with advent of vaccination, but new cases possibly due to immunization have been reported

    6) May be associated with acute encephalitis, aseptic meningitis, transverse myelitis

  d. Measles inclusion body encephalitis: rapidly progressive dementing illness developing 1 to 6 months after inoculation; associated with myoclonus, seizures, coma

  e. Subacute sclerosing panencephalitis

    1) Rare, delayed complication: 5 to 10 of every 1 million cases of measles

    2) Delayed onset after acute infection: 2 to 12 years (median, 8 years)

    3) Gradual onset of behavioral disturbance, followed by seizures, dementia, spasticity, and various movement disorders (myoclonus, choreoathetosis, ataxia) and progressing to akinetic mutism and eventually coma and death

    4) EEG: generalized, stereotyped, repetitive, polyphasic sharp and slow wave-high voltage complexes, 0.5 to 2 seconds in duration and usually recurring every 4 to 15 seconds (usually bisynchronous, but may be asymmetric), often occurring in conjunction with myoclonic jerks

    5) Pathology: parenchymal and leptomeningeal perivascular lymphocytic infiltrates in cerebral cortex, white matter, thalamus, and basal ganglia, with loss of neurons and myelinated fibers, gliosis, and intranuclear inclusions (Fig. 15-8)

4. Mumps

  a. Pathogen: mumps virus, a paramyxovirus

  b. Replicates in respiratory tract and regional lymph nodes; hematogenous spread to distant sites

  c. May infect parotid gland (parotitis) and testes (orchitis)

  d. Aseptic meningitis or encephalitis may occur in nonimmunized persons

  e. Prevention with live, attenuated vaccine

5. Papovaviruses and progressive multifocal leukoencephalopathy (discussed below)

6. Human T-lymphotropic virus (discussed in Chapter 20)

7. HIV infection (discussed below)

8. Poliovirus (discussed in Chapter 20)

III. NEUROLOGIC MANIFESTATIONS OF HUMAN IMMUNODEFICIENCY VIRUS INFECTION

A. Pathogen

1. Retrovirus in the lentivirus family

  a. Two forms are pathogenic in humans: HIV-1 and HIV-2

  b. HIV-1 is more common in United States; HIV-2 has been identified mainly in West Africa and Indian subcontinent

2. Major components include the p24 antigen (most HIV tests detect antibodies to p24), reverse transcriptase, integrase, protease, and RNA; its lipid layer comes from host cells

3. Preferential infection of CD4$^+$ cells; typically affects T cells (CD4$^+$), dendritic cells, and macrophages

4. An HIV envelope protein, gp120, binds to CD4; next step is binding of gp120 to either CCR5 or CXCR4 receptors on host cell, giving virus ability to enter host cell

5. Virus then spreads to other host cells; death of host cells leads to development of severe immunodeficiency

6. Virus migrates into CNS early in course of infection; major viral reservoirs in CNS are macrophages and microglia

B. Routes of Transmission

1. Main routes of transmission are via blood and genital secretions, typically by sexual contact, intravenous drug use, or maternal-fetal transfer

2. Currently, sexual contact is most common mode of transmission

3. Many hemophiliacs developed disease before blood products were screened for HIV

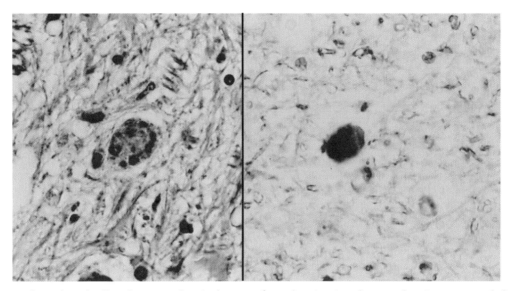

Fig. 15-8. *Left*, A multinucleated cell with intranuclear inclusions of measles virus in subacute sclerosing panencephalitis. *Right*, Immunohistochemistry staining for the viral antigens is better for demonstrating the viral inclusions.

4. May also spread through breast milk and, in rare cases, via occupational exposure

C. Epidemiology
1. Over 60 million people have been infected with HIV worldwide; currently over 40 million people worldwide are HIV infected
2. Almost 1 million of these cases are in United States

D. Natural History
1. At time of primary infection, there may be seroconversion-related illness, which can include fever, maculopapular rash, malaise, myalgias, primary meningitis
2. Usually a subsequent clinical, but not virologic, latent period of 10 years (average); many patients develop lymphadenopathy during this period
3. Eventually, fevers, mild signs, and symptoms suggestive of reduced cell-mediated immunity develop
4. With progressive decrease of CD4 count, opportunistic infections and AIDS develop
5. Most neurologic complications of HIV are symptomatic during latter stages of infection; about 50% of people with HIV develop related neurologic symptoms in the course of disease

E. Aseptic Meningitis
1. Monophasic illness that occurs within first 6 weeks after seroconversion or later in course of HIV infection
2. Acute viral syndrome of constitutional symptoms of fever, headache, lethargy, nausea, anorexia; also diffuse

arthralgias, maculopapular rash, pharyngitis, lymphadenopathy
3. Neurologic syndromes other than aseptic meningitis: encephalitis, meningoencephalitis, seizures, myelopathy, peripheral neuropathy
4. CSF in aseptic meningitis of acute HIV infection is marked by mild lymphocytic pleocytosis (<25 cells/μL), increased protein, and normal glucose
5. May have HIV antibodies in blood, but may only be positive for p24 antigen if early in the course of infection
6. MRI of head: normal or shows meningeal enhancement
7. Typically self-limited disease, recovery expected within a few months

F. HIV-Associated Dementia
1. Thought to be related to HIV infection rather than opportunistic infection
2. Usually occurs late in HIV infection, when CD4 count is <200 cells/mm^3
3. Incidence among HIV-infected patients: about 1% since HIV treatment has been available
4. Minor cognitive motor disorder: a mild form occurs in approximately 20% of patients with HIV infection (not necessarily progressive)
5. Based on one review, 35% of asymptomatic HIV-infected patients have been shown to have neuropsychologic deficits (compared with 12% of seronegative controls) (Grant and White et al, HNRC group)

6. Before era of HIV treatment: up to 60% of patients developed some cognitive impairment

7. Prevalence may be increasing because more HIV-infected patients live longer

8. Risk factors for HIV-associated dementia: anemia, low peripheral blood CD4 T-cell count, high viral load (i.e., high plasma HIV RNA), history of injection drug use, history of hepatitis C infection, female gender, and older age

9. Clinical features
   a. Cognitive impairment, behavioral changes, and motor dysfunction
   b. Cognitive impairment: slowness in thinking (bradyphrenia), poor attention and concentration, impairment in short-term and working memory, and reduced psychomotor speed and cognitive flexibility on formal testing
   c. Personality changes: apathy, inertia, social withdrawal, irritability; occasionally, agitation, psychosis, mania, obsessive-compulsive behavior
   d. Motor impairment: nonspecific gait disturbance characterized by "clumsiness," incoordination, and slowed movements; usually develops after onset of cognitive deficits
   e. Progressive syndrome: at end stage, patient can become bedbound, severely demented, with minimal responsiveness and profoundly slow psychomotor function
   f. Minor cognitive motor disorder: mild or equivocal neurocognitive symptoms, patients need to be monitored closely and periodically for development of HIV-associated dementia
   g. Children infected with HIV: onset as early as age 2 months, with microcephaly, developmental delay and regression, progressive encephalopathy, weakness, ataxia, hyperreflexia, and spasticity; basal ganglia calcification

10. Pathology (Fig. 15-9)
    a. Diffuse, patchy, and confluent rarefaction and pallor of white matter, due to neuronal loss
    b. Microglial nodules
    c. Activated macrophages and astrocytes and multinucleated giant cells with immunophenotype of microglia or macrophages; predilection for perivascular aggregation
    d. Perivascular and periventricular parenchymal lymphocytic infiltrates

11. Diagnosis
    a. Clinical examination and formal neuropsychologic testing: opportunistic infections or drug effects must be excluded
    b. CSF analysis: may be mild lymphocytic pleocytosis, nonspecific
    c. MRI of head: diffuse, confluent periventricular white matter T2 hyperintense lesions, with normal T1 images (Fig. 15-10)

G. **HIV-Associated Vacuolar Myelopathy**

1. Observed in 50% of autopsies of all patients with AIDS
2. Most common cause of myelopathy in HIV-infected persons
3. Uncommon in HIV-infected children
4. Subacute onset and progression of spastic paraparesis
   a. Painless upper motor neuron pattern of weakness (especially legs), spasticity, urinary incontinence, erectile dysfunction, Babinski's sign
   b. Progressive sensory deficits in lower extremities, although a sensory level often cannot be determined
5. Often occurs concomitantly with HIV-associated dementia
6. HIV-associated vacuolar myelopathy needs to be differentiated from the rare acute or subacute HIV (transverse) myelitis
7. Pathology
   a. Spongiform change with vacuolization of myelin sheaths
   b. Lipid-laden macrophages
   c. Aggregation of activated and foamy macrophages and microglia
   d. Multinucleated giant cells
   e. Changes predominantly involve posterior and lateral columns (anterolateral tracts with progression), most commonly in thoracic segments
8. Treatment: predominantly symptomatic; highly active antiretroviral therapy (HAART) usually indicated because of profound immunosuppression at this stage of infection

H. **HIV-Associated Neuromuscular Disease**

1. Distal sensory polyneuropathy
   a. Painful, symmetric, predominantly sensory axonal polyneuropathy
   b. Gradual onset of pain, dysesthesias, paresthesias, deep pain, hyperalgesia in feet (distal > proximal); predominantly decreased pain, temperature, and vibratory sensation and relatively preserved proprioception until later in disease course
   c. Progression marked by gradual proximal spread of symptoms
2. Acute inflammatory demyelinating polyradiculoneuropathy (AIDP)
   a. Distinguishing feature from idiopathic Guillain-Barré syndrome: lymphocytic pleocytosis
   b. Usually occurs in early stages of HIV infection as result of immune dysregulation

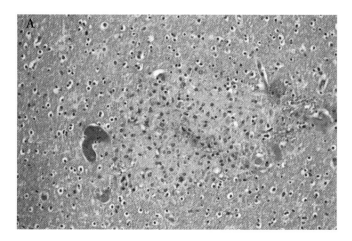

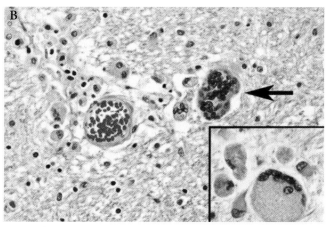

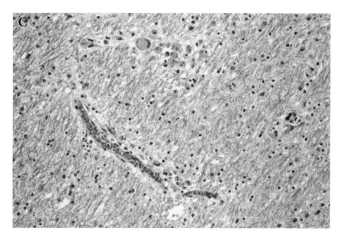

Fig. 15-9. Histopathologic features of human immunodeficiency virus encephalitis. Microglial nodules (*A*) are nonspecific and may be seen in encephalitis caused by other viral pathogens, including cytomegalovirus. Multinucleated giant cells may have abundant eosinophilic cytoplasm that displaces the multiple nuclei to the periphery (*B, inset*) or have a morular appearance, with nuclei clustered in the center (*B, arrow*). The enlarged, activated macrophages and multinucleated giant cells tend to cluster around blood vessels (*B* and *C*).

c. Clinical presentation in HIV patients similar to that of noninfected patients: may have lower extremity sensory paresthesias, followed by progressive ascending weakness and areflexia

d. Predominantly sensory symptoms, infrequently causes sphincter disturbance

e. CSF: increased protein, but often also mild mononuclear pleocytosis

f. Nerve conduction studies (NCS) and electromyography (EMG): demyelinating features, with prolonged distal latencies and F-wave latencies and slowed conduction velocities

g. Treatment
   1) Intravenous immunoglobulin or plasma exchange may be given to patients with AIDP: recovery is the norm but may be slow
   2) Chronic inflammatory demyelinating polyradiculopathy may require longer term treatment, but benefits of iatrogenic immunosuppression must be weighed against the risks in these patients

3. Antiretroviral-associated neuropathy

a. Pathophysiology
   1) Often associated with use of nucleoside analog HIV treatment, such as ddI (didanosine), ddC (zalcitabine), or d4T (stavudine); may occur in up to 1/3 of patients taking these agents
   2) Believed to be related to mitochondrial dysfunction induced by these agents

b. Clinical presentation: length-dependent peripheral neuropathy, with primarily sensory symptoms; weakness is less common

c. Electrophysiologic characteristics: axonal length-dependent neuropathy, decreased sural amplitude, may show mild EMG changes of denervation in distal leg muscles

d. Often can be distinguished from primary HIV neuropathy only by withdrawal of drug: there may be significant lag time between drug withdrawal and symptom improvement

e. Treatment: symptomatic treatment and withdrawal of offending agent if possible

4. Cranial mononeuropathies or mononeuritis multiplex occur early in course of HIV infection

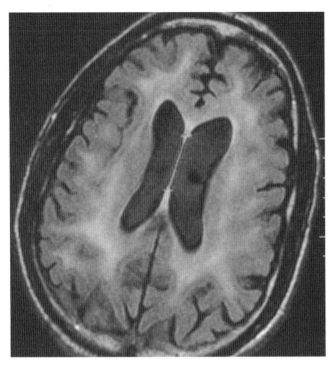

Fig. 15-10. MRI of a patient with human immunodeficiency virus–associated dementia. The characteristic feature is diffuse, confluent, ill-defined periventricular white matter hyperintense lesions on axial FLAIR sequences.

5. HIV-associated lumbosacral plexopathy
6. Motor neuron disease-like illness may occur late in course of HIV infection
7. CMV polyradiculopathy
   a. Caused by CMV, usually reactivation of latent virus in patient
   b. Usually occurs in severe immunosuppression, with CD4 count <50 cells/mm^3
   c. Clinical features: slow onset of progressive flaccid paraparesis (often rapidly evolving and asymmetric), sphincter dysfunction, lower extremity sensory loss (in absence of definite sensory level), and pain in back and radicular distributions
   d. NCS/EMG: active denervation and axonal loss in polyradicular distribution, usually only in lumbosacral roots
   e. CSF: increased protein, polymorphonuclear pleocytosis; positive CMV PCR and/or viral cultures
   f. Neuroimaging: normal or thickened lumbosacral nerve roots seen with gadolinium enhancement
   g. Pathology: necrotizing inflammation of nerve roots, with positive CMV immunohistochemistry staining of Schwann cells

8. HIV-associated myopathy
   a. Pathophysiology: cause of this rare disorder is unclear, but may be muscle fiber damage from immune dysregulation or inflammatory cytokines
   b. Characterized by proximal weakness and myalgias
   c. Variable increase in creatine kinase
   d. NCS/EMG: consistent with myopathy, short-duration motor unit potentials in proximal musculature
   e. Pathology: degeneration of muscle fibers, with variable amounts of mononuclear inflammation
9. AZT-associated myopathy
   a. Caused by exposure to antiretroviral drug zidovudine
   b. Believed to be caused by mitochondrial damage from zidovudine

I. Progressive Multifocal Leukoencephalopathy (PML)
1. Caused by JC virus, a human polyomavirus, that exists asymptomatically in up to 70% of immunocompetent persons
2. PML: thought to result from reactivation of virus in most cases, not new infection
3. PML is either result of reactivation of virus in the brain or of virus transported from other organs to brain
4. Often occurs in immunosuppressive illness (e.g., AIDS or other immunocompromised states)
5. Affects approximately 4% of AIDS patients, usually occurs when CD4 count is <200 cells/mm^3
6. Pathology and pathogenesis (Fig. 15-11)
   a. Caused by direct lytic infection of brain oligodendrocytes and astrocytes; produces multifocal and confluent demyelinating lesions
   b. Predominantly involves frontal, parietal, and occipital lobes (predilection for parieto-occipital region); also described in cerebellum and brainstem (80%-90% are supratentorial lesions, 10%-20% are infratentorial)
   c. Viral products may be seen as "inclusions" within oligodendrocytes
7. Clinical features
   a. Variable, depends on localization and extent of lesions
   b. Unusual to present with fever or headache; absence of mass effect or meningitis
   c. Most common features: altered mentation and cognitive deficits, focal paralysis or generalized weakness, homonymous hemianopia (most common manifestation in AIDS patients: hemiparesis)
   d. Visual disturbance (e.g., visual field deficits); posterior subcortical white matter frequently affected
   e. Other neurologic deficits: gait abnormalities, sensory deficits

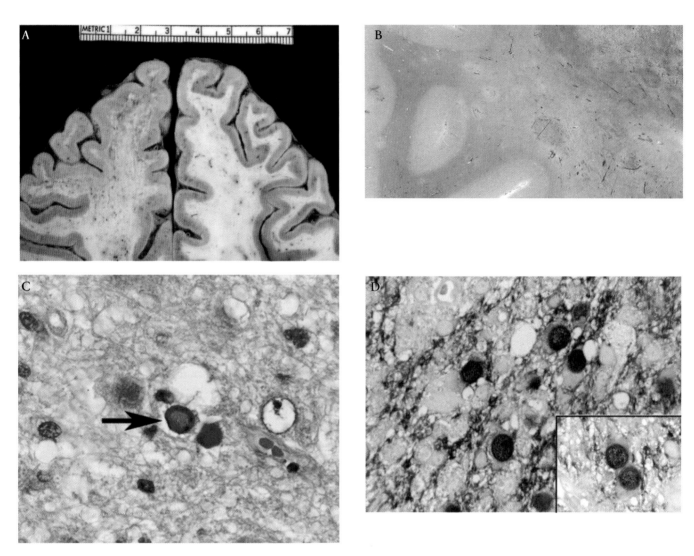

Fig. 15-11. Progressive multifocal leukoencephalopathy. *A*, Macroscopic examination of a postmortem specimen from a 35-year-old patient with acquired immunodeficiency syndrome shows extensive granular cavitation of the juxtacortical white matter in right frontal lobe. *B*, The granular appearance of the white matter is due to confluence of multiple foci of demyelination. *C*, Oligodendrocytes with intranuclear inclusions (*arrow*) filled with virions is a pathologic hallmark of this condition. *D*, Immunohistochemistry staining for JC virus antigens is better for demonstrating the inclusions.

8. Diagnostic evaluation
   a. CT: multiple foci of hypoattenuation, insensitive
   b. MRI
      1) Hyperintense T2 superficial, subcortical white matter multifocal lesions beginning at gray-white matter junction and coalescing to form confluent lesions
      2) Lesions appear hypointense in T1 images; may appear bright on diffusion-weighted imaging
      3) Typically, there is little or no enhancement
   c. EEG: diffuse or focal slowing, nonspecific
   d. CSF: normal or nonspecific mild mononuclear pleocytosis and increased protein
   e. CSF JC virus PCR: sensitivity of more than 80%, specificity of more than 90%; a negative test does not exclude diagnosis
9. Pathology
   a. Macroscopic appearance: confluent demyelination predominantly at juxtacortical white matter or near the deep gray matter (in contrast to multiple sclerosis lesions, which have predilection for periventricular white matter)
   b. Enlarged oligodendrocytes (filled with virions)
   c. Relative sparing of axons in areas of demyelination
   d. Reactive astrocytosis, with bizarre appearance of giant astrocytes

10. Treatment
    a. HAART: mainstay of treatment; concomitant use of other therapies is debated
    b. Some success reported with other agents: cytosine arabinoside, amantadine, vidarabine, acyclovir, and interferon alpha

J. **Cytomegalovirus** (discussed above)

K. **Toxoplasmosis**
1. Pathogenic agent: *Toxoplasma gondii*, an obligate intracellular protozoa
2. Usually occurs in patients with CD4 count <100 cells/mm^3, resulting from reactivation of latent infection
3. Approximately 1/3 of adult population is seropositive for *T. gondii*: seroprevalence varies from country to country
4. May be acquired in utero: congenital toxoplasmosis
5. Pathogenesis
    a. Primary mode of inoculation is oral-fecal: ingestion of oocytes or cysts in feline feces-contaminated food or uncooked meet (usually pork or lamb)
    b. Parasites are released from cysts after ingestion and are disseminated via hematogenous and lymphatic spread to different organs
    c. Organism may remain latent and cause infection when person is immunocompromised
6. Clinical presentation varies, depending on the location of lesion or lesions
    a. Acute mass lesion with focal (or multifocal) signs and symptoms due to focal parenchymal abscess or abscesses: headache, seizures, hemiparesis, hemianopia, aphasia, ataxia
    b. Subacute encephalitis (with or without acute mass lesions): fever, headaches, subacute onset of confusion, inattention, disorientation, and behavioral disturbance
7. Diagnosis
    a. IgG antibodies to *T. gondii* at time of presentation (IgM antibodies are uncommon); may be difficult to interpret because of seroprevalence in general population
    b. CSF: increased protein, lymphocytic pleocytosis, PCR for *T. gondii* very specific (>95%), but not very sensitive (only about 50%-60%)
    c. Lumbar puncture may be contraindicated in the setting of focal mass lesion with mass effect
    d. Neuroimaging: one or more ring-enhancing lesions (about 2/3 of patients have multiple lesions at presentation), often with central necrosis and mass effect, with ring enhancement and surrounding vasogenic edema

e. Main differential diagnosis: PCNSL
    1) Thallium-201 single photon emission CT (SPECT) and positron emission tomography (PET) may distinguish the two conditions
    2) Most clinicians decide to treat for toxoplasmosis and consider alternate diagnosis in nonresponders
8. Pathology (Fig. 15-12)
    a. Toxoplasmic abscess is referred to as "gold coin lesion" because of discoloration from central coagulative or hemorrhagic necrosis
    b. Microscopic appearance: encysted *T. gondii* bradyzoites or free organisms (tachyzoites) typically found at borders of the lesions
    c. Organized abscesses have typical histologic appearance of coagulative necrosis
9. Treatment
    a. Primary induction therapy with oral pyrimethamine and oral sulfadiazine for minimum of 6 weeks, followed by maintenance therapy of reduced doses of same regimen
    b. Folinic acid is often added to counteract bone marrow toxicity of pyrimethamine
    c. Relapses are very common if maintenance therapy is discontinued (persistence of parenchymal cysts despite treatment may be responsible for reactivation and may be cause of relapses)
    d. Maintenance therapy may be continued for life in absence of retroviral therapy (may be discontinued when the CD4 counts are sustained above 200 cells/μL)
    e. Primary prophylaxis with trimethoprim-sulfamethoxazole indicated for severely immunocompromised patients with CD4 cell counts less than 100 cells/μL
    f. Primary prophylaxis should also include avoidance of ingestion of uncooked meat, contact with material potentially contaminated with cat feces

L. **Cryptococcal Meningitis**
1. Most frequent primary cause of meningitis in AIDS patients (affects approximately 10% of these patients)
2. Caused by *Cryptococcus neoformans*, an encapsulated yeast widely present in nature (often found in soil and pigeon droppings)
3. Clinical features
    a. Chronic basilar meningitis with cranial neuropathies and slow onset of altered mentation, behavioral disturbance, change in personality, psychiatric manifestations, obtundation, and coma
    b. Other manifestations: focal signs and symptoms (e.g., hemiparesis, seizures)
    c. Relative absence of nuchal rigidity because of mild inflammatory reaction

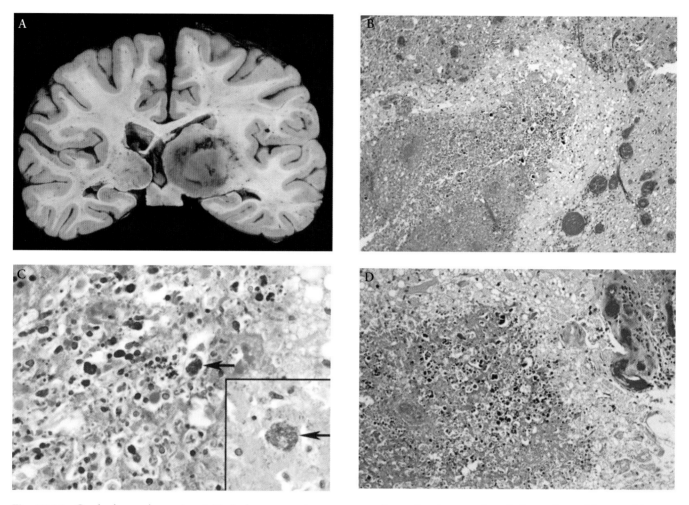

Fig. 15-12. Cerebral toxoplasmosis. *A*, Typical macroscopic appearance of toxoplasmic parenchymal abscess (resembling a gold coin), with foci of hemorrhagic necrosis. *B*, Toxoplasmic abscess with nonspecific features of central necrosis surrounded by rim of neovascularization, vasogenic edema, and inflammatory infiltrates. *Toxoplasma* organisms are usually found at advancing edges of the lesion. Higher magnification shows typical histologic features of aggregates of *Toxoplasma* organisms at outer edge of the abscess, including microcysts containing *Toxoplasma gondii* bradyzoites (*C, arrows*) or free organisms as tachyzoites (*C* and *D*).

4. Diagnostic evaluation
   a. CSF profile: normal or mild mononuclear pleocytosis with slightly increased protein and decreased glucose
   b. CSF fungal cultures: high sensitivity (>90%) and specificity (almost 100%), but may take several weeks; sensitivity of serum fungal cultures is much less
   c. Increased serum and CSF cryptococcal capsular polysaccharide antigen titer (often determined by latex agglutination)
   d. India ink stain: detects pathogen and demonstrates typical morphology in 70% to 90% of cases; positive test is helpful, but negative test does not exclude diagnosis
   e. Neuroimaging characteristics: normal or nonspecific abnormalities, including nonspecific small T2 hyperin-

tense lesions (typically nonenhancing); there may or may not be sulcal or basilar leptomeningeal enhancement, with occasional parenchymal involvement (Fig. 15-13)

5. Pathology
   a. Macroscopic appearance: thick, fibrotic, and opacified meninges of chronic meningitis covering the brain; there may be multiple small cysts and cryptococcomas (Fig. 15-14)
   b. Leptomeningeal inflammatory infiltrates in cryptococcal meningitis (mononuclear inflammatory cells and multinucleated giant cells)
   c. Cryptococcal cysts: enlarged cystic spaces (often perivascular) filled with the organism; may be encapsulated or in form of budding yeast

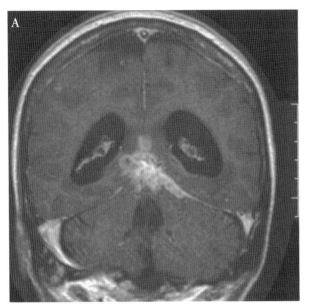

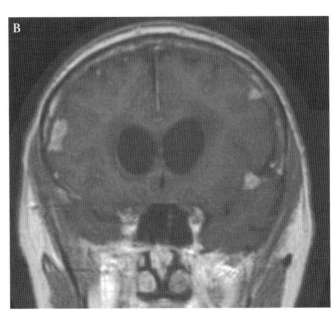

Fig. 15-13. *A*, MRI of a patient with cryptococcosis showing diffuse nodular enhancement within the quadrigeminal plate cistern and extending along dorsolateral aspect of cerebral peduncles bilaterally and tentorium cerebelli. *B*, Nodular foci of enhancement may represent cryptococcomas. (*A* and *B*, gadolinium-enhanced coronal T1-weighted images.)

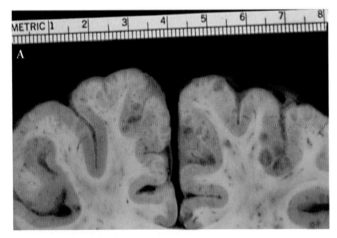

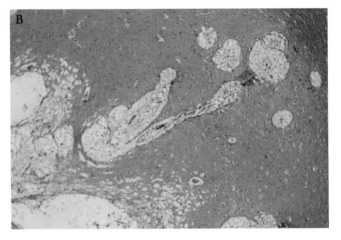

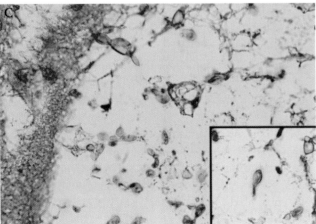

Fig. 15-14. Cryptococcosis. *A*, Typical macroscopic appearance of multiple small intraparenchymal gelatinous cysts involving cerebral cortex. *B*, Parenchymal lesions are cystic spaces filled with colonies of cryptococci, often appearing as enlarged perivascular spaces. *C*, Higher magnification showing encapsulated organisms, which appear as round basophilic structures.

6. Treatment
   a. Induction therapy with intravenous amphotericin B for 2 weeks (with or without flucytosine), followed by 8 to 10 weeks of maintenance therapy with oral fluconazole

M. **Primary CNS Lymphoma** (discussed in Chapter 16)

IV. Fungal Infections

A. Pathogenesis
1. Fungal meningitis is characterized by infection of pia mater and arachnoid membrane by a fungus, without associated involvement of brain parenchyma
2. Primary inoculation usually by inhalation, often followed by hematogenous spread to CNS; an exception is *Candida*, which penetrates mucosal surface it normally colonizes and gains access to deep tissue
3. Much more common in immunocompromised patients, either by primary disease (e.g., HIV/AIDS, diabetes mellitus) or by iatrogenic immunosupression (corticosteroid use, chemotherapy, transplant recipients who receive immunosuppressant therapy)
4. Recent surgery or foreign body (e.g., ventriculoperitoneal shunt) can provide direct means of fungal entry

B. Clinical Features
1. Subacute to chronic meningitis: malaise, fever, headaches, nausea, meningismus, failure to thrive, cranial nerve findings, seizures
2. Usually not as ill as patient with bacterial meningitis
3. Lethargy and confusion with progression
4. Immunocompromised patients have more rapid course than immunocompetent patients and may have rapid progression to severe, permanent neurolgic deficits, coma, or death

C. Diagnosis
1. Typical CSF profile
   a. Lymphocytic pleocytosis (usually <1,000 cells/mm^3), increased protein, decreased glucose
   b. Eosinophilic pleocytosis: suggests coccidioidal meningitis
2. India ink stain to observe encapsulated yeasts of *Cryptococcus* (discussed above)
3. Cryptococcal antigen test: sensitive and specific, rapid test
4. Fungal cultures
   a. Most useful in cryptococcal meningitis
   b. Time-consuming, often do not yield the organism

(growth occurs in 50% of cases of blastomycosis, histoplasmosis, or coccidioidomycosis)
   c. Cultures of large volume of CSF may have better yield
   d. Limited by contamination by normal flora
5. Serologic testing
   a. Nonspecific, there is cross-reactivity
   b. Difficult to interpret
6. Neuroimaging (MRI more sensitive than CT)
   a. Leptomeningeal enhancement, often involving basal cisterns
   b. Space-occupying lesions with mass effect (abscess or granulomas)
   c. Hemorrhagic infarcts may indicate underlying vasculitis

D. Pathology
1. Varies greatly depending on organism
2. Abscesses, with necrotic centers and hemorrhage, in cases of angioinvasive fungi
3. Thick exudates, inflammatory meningeal infiltrates consisting of neutrophils, plasma cells, lymphocytes, and macrophages
4. Caseating or noncaseating granulomas with multinucleated giant cells, epithelioid cells, and activated macrophages
5. Yeasts, hyphae, molds are often visible with PAS or silver stain
6. Endospores of *Coccidioides immitis* within spherules: rupture of the spherules may induce acute inflammatory response

---

Fungal meningitis
Usually subacute or chronic

Cerebrospinal fluid usually has mononuclear pleocytosis, increased protein, and normal or decreased glucose

Most infections acquired via inhalation

More common in immunosuppressed patients

Common pathogens to be considered are *Cryptococcus*, *Histoplasma*, *Aspergillus*, *Coccidioides*, *Blastomyces*, *Candida*

Usual treatment is amphotericin B (watch for renal toxicity)

7. Aspergillosis: infiltraton of blood vessels by fungal hyphae (Fig. 15-15)

E. **Treatment**
1. Amphotericin B
   a. Usually first-line agent for fungal infections of CNS
   b. Administration: systemic or intrathecal (latter reserved for refractory cases)
   c. Broad antifungal spectrum
   d. Associated with nephrotoxicity (minimized by use of lipid preparations)
   e. Lipid preparations have reduced CSF penetrance compared with standard formulations
2. Flucytosine
   a. Good antimicrobial activity against *Candida* and *Cryptococcus neoformans*
   b. Drug resistance may develop
   c. Often given in conjunction with amphotericin B
   d. Eliminated unchanged in urine: renal insufficiency can cause drug accumulation
   e. Adverse effects: rash, diarrhea, eosinophilia, liver dysfunction, bone marrow toxicity when given in combination with amphotericin B
3. Fluconazole and itraconazole
   a. Not recommended as first-line agents, inferior to amphotericin for primary therapy
   b. Main role as maintenance therapy and lifelong secondary preventive therapy for immunocompromised patients
   c. Advantages: good CNS penetration, few adverse effects

F. **Individual Pathogens**
1. Aspergillosis (Fig. 15-15)
   a. Causative agents: *Aspergillus fumigatus* or *A. flavus*
   b. Filamentous fungus (mold)
   c. Acquired through inhalation, then subsequent fungemia, which may spread to CNS; may also spread directly from *Aspergillus* sinusitis
   d. Angioinvasive, infiltration of blood vessels by hyphae; associated with blood vessel thrombosis, infarcts, parenchymal and subarachnoid hemorrhages
   e. Neurologic disease most common in immunosuppressed patients
   f. Almost all patients have associated pulmonary manifestations
   g. Neurologic manifestations
      1) Result from direct, contiguous parenchymal invasion (e.g., from focus of sinusitis) or intravascular invasion (vasculitis)
      2) Usually consist of multiple focal deficits with fever (multiple infarcts, abscesses)

3) Potential for rapid progression in immunocompromised host
2. Yeasts
   a. *Cryptococcal neoformans* (discussed above)
   b. *Candida*
      1) Yeast, in form of coherent budding, oval chains, or pseudohyphae; may also produce true hyphae
      2) Normal flora of mucosal and skin surfaces in the immunocompetent host
      3) Systemic infection may follow penetration of fungus into deeper tissues
      4) Predisposing factors: underlying immunosuppression and neutropenia (neutrophils are primary effector cells), indwelling ventriculostomy tubes or shunts
      5) Angioinvasive: associated with blood vessel thrombosis, infarcts, parenchymal and subarachnoid hemorrhages
3. Systemic fungal infections
   a. Pathogens: *Coccidioides immitis, Blastomyces dermatitidis, Histoplasma capsulatum*
   b. Dimorphic fungi: found as mycelia (at room temperature) and yeasts (at core body temperature)
   c. Primary inoculation by inhalation, local pulmonary infection, followed by hematogenous dissemination
   d. Majority of infected patients are asymptomatic
   e. May present with pulmonary infection (calcified granulomas may follow primary infection)
   f. Disseminated disease: commonly occurs in immunocompromised host; may cause fungal infection of CNS and subacute to chronic meningitis; may occur after primary infection or reactivation of old infection
   g. May be mass lesions and granulomas along neuroaxis
   h. *C. immitis*
      1) Most prevalent in southwestern U.S. and Mexico
      2) Common symptom at presentation: headache, often accompanying other symptoms of chronic meningitis
   i. *H. capsulatum*
      1) Nonencapuled organism
      2) Endemic areas: Mississippi and Ohio River valleys, Central and South America
      3) Present in bird and bat droppings; primary infection by inhalation of aerosolized contaminated soil
      4) Most cases are self-limiting
      5) Systemic manifestations: hepatosplenomegaly, lymphadenopathy, diffuse pulmonary infiltrates, mucosal ulcerations
      6) CNS disease usually in form of subacute meningitis and/or cerebral abscess
   j. *B. dermatitidis*
      1) Neurologic involvement seen in up to 1/3 of cases of

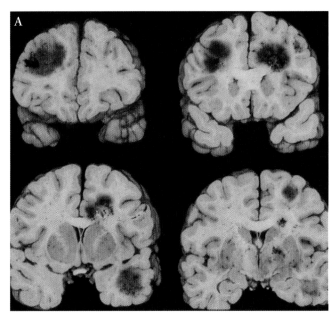

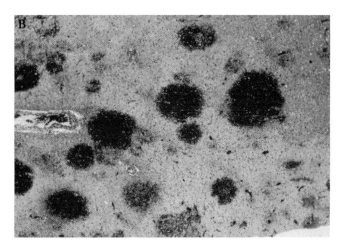

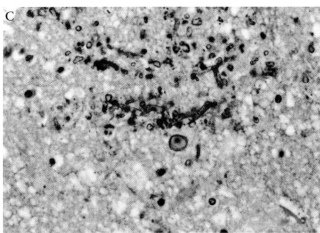

Fig. 15-15. Aspergillosis. *A*, Multiple hemorrhagic and necrotic mass lesions characteristic of cerebral aspergillosis. *B*, Numerous microscopic hemorrhages occur from invasion of blood vessels. *C*, Numerous hyphae are seen at high magnification. (PAS stain.)

tously; high index of suspicion and urgent surgical removal of infected tissue are required
   f. Presentation may be that of cerebral infarction: angio-invasive hyphae causing arterial thrombosis and hemorrhagic infarctions and direct parenchymal invasion causing brain abscess
   g. Presentation may also be that of cavernous sinus syndrome due to thrombosis of cavernous sinus
   h. Only effective therapy: surgical removal of the infected tissue; amphotericin B may be used as adjunctive therapy

V. PARASITIC INFECTIONS

A. Cerebral Malaria
1. Protozoal infection caused by *Plasmodium*, species; in most cases, CNS involvement is due to *P. falciparum* (rare cases of cerebral malaria due to *P. vivax* have been reported)
2. Life cycle
   a. Sporozoites: carried by mosquito, injected into host, enter bloodstream, and invade and inhabit hepatocytes
   b. Each sporozoite then undergoes multiple nuclear divisions, forming a multinuclear body (schizont)
   c. Each nucleus inside the schizont acquires cytoplasm and becomes a small body (merozoites)
   d. Merozoites rupture and enter other hepatocytes and bloodstream

disseminated disease; meningitis may be marked by rapid deterioration; some patients may develop blastomycomas (mass lesions, abscess)
      2) Osteolytic lesions of vertebral bodies may occur
      3) Infection not significantly more frequent in immunocompromised hosts
4. Mucormycosis
   a. Opportunistic, aggressive infection of brain vessels
   b. Caused by zygomycete fungi, including *Rhizopus arrhizus* and *Mucor* species
   c. Predisposing conditions: diabetes mellitus, organ transplant recipient, hematologic malignancies, intravenous drug use, AIDS
   d. CNS infection often due to contiguous spread from adjacent paranasal sinuses or orbital or retro-orbital space
   e. Rhinocerebral infection may progress slowly or precipi-

> **Mucor**
>
> Most commonly causes disease in immunosuppressed persons; common in diabetes mellitus
>
> Usually has rhinocerebral presentation, with sinusitis and local extension into bone, brain, and involvement of cranial nerves
>
> Usually requires debridement and amphotericin B

    e. After entering bloodstream, merozoites invade erythrocytes and form a trophozoite

    f. Trophozoite undergoes nuclear division and is transformed into a multinuclear schizont, containing multiple merozoites

    g. Erythrocyte ruptures and merozoites enter bloodstream, eliciting immune reaction responsible for recurrence of fever and constitutional symptoms

    h. Phagocytic cells of reticuloendothelial system, including liver and spleen, engulf debris from the destroyed erythrocytes; this produces hepatosplenomegaly

3. Incubation period: depends on immune status and *Plasmodium* species, usually 1 to 2 weeks (may vary from 9 days to >3 months)

4. Prodrome of headache, malaise, chills

5. Periodic high-grade fever (one every third day) associated with chills and diaphoresis

6. Systemic manifestations: nausea, abdominal pain, hepatosplenomegaly, jaundice, azotemia, anemia, tachycardia, arthralgias

7. Neurologic manifestations: focal deficits, retinal hemorrhages, abnormal extraocular movement, focal or generalized seizures, status epilepticus, delirium, proceeding to coma

8. Mortality: up to 50% reported

9. Diagnosis
    a. Examine peripheral blood smear for trophozoites; if initial smear is negative, repeat smear
    b. CSF: usually normal, may show mild lymphocytic pleocytosis
    c. Increased serum and CSF levels of lactate
    d. MRI: usually normal

10. Treatment: quinine, quinidine, and artemisinin derivatives

B. Amebic Infections of CNS
1. Often fatal protozoa infection

2. Primary amebic meningoencephalitis
    a. The protozoa is found in warm freshwater
    b. Trophozoite and flagellate forms enter nasal cavity, penetrate epithelium and cribriform plate, and enter parenchyma causing necrotizing inflammation
    c. Meningoencephalitis: acute onset of fever, headache, photophobia, stiff neck, impaired consciousness, seizures
    d. May be focal signs and symptoms
    e. Possible complications: hydrocephalus, diffuse brain edema, increased ICP
    f. Death may occur within 1 week after onset of symptoms
    g. Treatment
        1) Poor therapeutic response
        2) Best with combination of antimicrobial agents amphotericin B, rifampin, miconazole

3. Granulomatous amebic encephalitis
    a. Predisposing factors: immunocompromised state, HIV infection, splenectomy, long-term corticosteroid therapy, diabetes mellitus, chronic alcoholism
    b. Primary infectious focus may be skin or respiratory or olfactory epithelium
    c. Trophozoites invade CNS by hematogenous spread and set up multiple necrotic abscesses, with some predilection for posterior fossa
    d. Clinical features: often nonspecific but may include focal signs and symptoms (focal seizures) or deficits related to focal lesions
    e. Progression is gradual, but disease often progresses to coma and death in 2 to 3 weeks

4. Amebic brain abscess
    a. Rare, late complication of intestinal, pulmonary, or hepatic amebiasis
    b. Metastatic CNS abscess produced by hematogenous spread of organism, usually at gray-white matter junction
    c. Fever, altered mentation, focal signs and symptoms, seizures
    d. Treatment: both medical (metronidazole) and surgical resection

C. Toxoplasmosis (discussed above)

D. American Trypanosomiasis: Chagas' disease
1. Protozoal pathogen is *Trypanosoma cruzi*: disease of the Americas, including southern U.S. and Central and South America

2. Vector: reduviid bug (kissing bug)

3. Organism multiplies in intestinal tract of vector and transforms in rectum into infective trypomastigotes, which are abundant in feces

4. When the vector takes a blood meal, it also defecates

and releases trypomastigotes, which enter bloodstream of human host (Fig. 15-16)

5. Shortly after entering the bloodstream, the organism transforms into the amastigote form after losing the undulating membrane and flagellum and rapidly multiplies, forming pseudocyst

6. Pseudocysts are present in multiple host tissues, including skeletal muscle, reticuloendothelial cells, and CNS

7. Acute illness: marked by erythema and swelling at site of inoculation (chagoma), cardiac involvement (including arrhythmias), and, uncommonly, meningoencephalitis (more common in infected children or HIV-infected persons)

8. Chronic phase: dilated cardiomyopathy (most common neurologic manifestation of chronic phase is cardioembolic stroke); megacolon and megaesophagus (from involvement of enteric nervous system); organisms leave the bloodstream but serologic tests remain positive

E. **African Trypanosomiasis:** sleeping sickness

1. Protozoal pathogen, *T. brucei* subspecies, transmitted by tsetse fly

2. Following the bite, flagellated motile trypomastigote form of the organism travels in bloodstream to lymph nodes and reticuloendothelial system and CNS

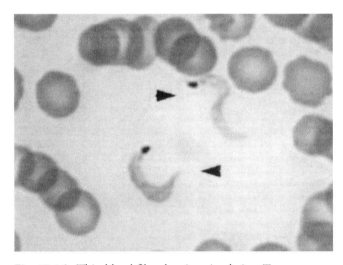

Fig. 15-16. Thin blood film showing circulating *Trypanosoma cruzi* trypomastigotes (*arrowheads*) in bloodstream. (From Barreira AA, Nascimento OJM. Peripheral neuropathies in Chagas disease. In: Noseworthy JH, editor-in-chief. Neurological therapeutics: principles and practice. Vol 2. New York: Martin Dunitz; 2003. p. 1992-8. By permission of Mayo Foundation.)

3. Initial manifestations

   a. Erythematous, painful skin ulcer (chancre) at bite site

   b. Appearance of chancre is followed by systemic illness occurring after incubation period of less than 3 weeks: cyclic fever, headache, lymphadenopathy, malaise (fever occurs in cycles of hours to days)

   c. Initial stage may last for several months

4. Second stage of meningoencephalitis

   a. Organism crosses blood-brain barrier and causes CNS infection marked by headaches, ataxia, extrapyramidal symptoms, slurred speech, behavioral changes, dementia, lethargy and hypersomnolence (hence, "sleeping sickness")

   b. May be rapid deterioration to coma and death

   c. Duration of this stage may be as long as 1 year

F. **Cysticercosis**

1. Helminthic infection

2. Pathogen is pork tapeworm, *Taenia solium*

3. Acquired via fecal-oral route from other infected individuals or by ingestion of food contaminated with the eggs

4. Eggs are ingested by human host; in small intestine, hatch into larvae, which migrate in bloodstream to effector organs, including CNS

5. Cysticerci may remain in vesicular state for years and either induce an inflammatory reaction or undergo destruction and calcification by host's immune response

6. Degeneration of the cysts induces inflammatory response (more severe with large parasitic load); inflammatory response is accompanied by vasogenic edema and reactive gliosis

7. Intense inflammatory reaction may cause fulminant meningoencephalitis

8. Neurologic manifestations

   a. Most common: seizures (partial or generalized)

   b. Increased ICP: headaches, vomiting, neurocognitive deficits

   c. Infarcts: may be due to vasculitis

   d. Obstructive hydrocephalus may be due to intraventricular cysts or proliferation of ependymal cells or thickened leptomeninges due to local inflammatory response at foramina

9. Neuroimaging may show characteristic cystic lesions, with or without enhancement or surrounding edema (active disease), characteristic parenchymal calcifications (of the cysts), hydrocephalus, possibly leptomeningeal enhancement; cyst location may be meningobasal, parenchymal, or intraventricular

10. Treatment

a. Antiparasitic agents for active parenchymal disease: albendazole or praziquantel
b. Surgical resection may be required

c. Supportive therapy, including ventriculoperitoneal shunt for hydrocephalus
d. Long-term anticonvulsant

References

Berger JR, Kaszovitz B, Post MJ, Dickinson G. Progressive multifocal leukoencephalopathy associated with human immunodeficiency virus infection: a review of the literature with a report of sixteen cases. Ann Intern Med. 1987;107:78-87.

Bleck TP. Central nervous system involvement in Rickettsial diseases. Neurol Clin. 1999;17:801-12.

Cinque P, Casari S, Bertelli D. Progressive multifocal leukoencephalopathy, HIV, and highly active antiretroviral therapy. N Engl J Med. 1998;339:848-9.

Citizens Development Corps. Available from: http://www.cdc.gov.

Coyle PK. Overview of acute and chronic meningitis. Neurol Clin. 1999;17:691-710.

Davis LE. Fungal infections of the central nervous system. Neurol Clin. 1999;17:761-81.

de Gans J, van de Beek D, European Dexamethasone in Adulthood Bacterial Meningitis Study Investigators. Dexamethasone in adults with bacterial meningitis. N Engl J Med. 2002;347:1549-56.

deShazo RD, Chapin K, Swain RE. Fungal sinusitis. N Engl J Med. 1997;337:254-9.

Di Rocco A, Tagliati M, Danisi F, Dorfman D, Moise J, Simpson DM. A pilot study of L-methionine for the treatment of AIDS-associated myelopathy. Neurology. 1998;51:266-8.

Di Rocco A, Werner P, Bottiglieri T, Godbold J, Liu M, Tagliati M, et al. Treatment of AIDS-associated myelopathy with L-methionine: a placebo-controlled study. Neurology. 2004;63:1270-5.

Durand ML, Calderwood SB, Weber DJ, Miller SI, Southwick FS, Caviness VS Jr, et al. Acute bacterial meningitis in adults. A review of 493 episodes. N Engl J Med. 1993;328:21-8.

Ellison D, Love S, Chimelli L, Harding B, Lowe JS, Vinters H. Neuropathology: a reference text of CNS pathology. 2nd ed. Edinburgh: Mosby; 2004.

Fishbein DB, Robinson LE. Rabies. N Engl J Med. 1993;329:1632-8.

Garcia-Monco JC. Central nervous system tuberculosis. Neurol Clin. 1999;17:737-59.

Grant I, Heaton RK, Atkinson JH, HNRC Group, HIV Neurobehavioral Research Center. Neurocognitive disorders in HIV-1 infection. Curr Top Microbiol Immunol. 1995;202:11-32.

Greenlee JE. Progressive multifocal leukoencephalopathy—progress made and lessons relearned. N Engl J Med. 1998;338:1378-80.

Hall CD, Dafni U, Simpson D, Clifford D, Wetherill PE, Cohen B, et al, AIDS Clinical Trials Group 243 Team. Failure of cytarabine in progressive multifocal leukoencephalopathy associated with human immunodeficiency virus infection. N Engl J Med. 1998;338:1345-51.

Harrison MJG, McArthur JC. AIDS and neurology. Edinburgh: Churchill Livingstone; 1995.

Johnson RT, Gibbs CJ Jr. Creutzfeldt-Jakob disease and related transmissible spongiform encephalopathies. N Engl J Med. 1998;339:1994-2004.

Leis AA, Stokic DS, Polk JL, Dostrow V, Winkelmann M. A poliomyelitis-like syndrome from West Nile virus infection. N Engl J Med. 2002 Oct 17;347:1279-80. Epub 2002 Sep 23.

Mandell GL, Bennett JE, Dolin R, editors. Mandell, Douglas, and Bennett's principles and practice of infectious diseases. 6th ed. Philadelphia: Elsevier Churchill Livingstone; 2005.

McArthur JC. Neurologic manifestations of AIDS. Medicine (Baltimore). 1987;66:407-37.

McArthur JC, Hoover DR, Bacellar H, Miller EN, Cohen BA, Becker JT, et al. Dementia in AIDS patients: incidence and risk factors: multicenter AIDS cohort study. Neurology. 1993;43:2245-52.

McArthur JC, Nance-Sproson TE, Griffin DE, Hoover D, Selnes OA, Miller EN, et al. The diagnostic utility of elevation in cerebrospinal fluid beta 2-microglobulin in HIV-1 dementia: multicenter AIDS cohort study. Neurology. 1992;42:1707-12.

McJunkin JE, de los Reyes EC, Irazuzta JE, Caceres MJ, Khan RR, Minnich LL, et al. La Crosse encephalitis in children. N Engl J Med. 2001;344:801-7.

Noah DL, Drenzek CL, Smith JS, Krebs JW, Orciari L, Shaddock J, et al. Epidemiology of human rabies in the United States, 1980 to 1996. Ann Intern Med. 1998;128:922-30.

Noseworthy JH, editor. Neurological therapeutics: principles and practice. London: Martin Dunitz; 2003.

Petersen LR, Roehrig JT, Hughes JM. West Nile virus encephalitis. N Engl J Med. 2002 Oct 17;347:1225-6. Epub 2002 Sep 23.

Prusiner SB. Shattuck lecture: neurodegenerative diseases and prions. N Engl J Med. 2001;344:1516-26.

Quagliarello VJ, Scheld WM. Treatment of bacterial meningitis. N Engl J Med. 1997;336:708-16.

Redington JJ, Tyler KL. Viral infections of the nervous system, 2002: update on diagnosis and treatment. Arch Neurol. 2002;59:712-8.

Richardson-Burns SM, Kleinschmidt-DeMasters BK, DeBiasi RL, Tyler KL. Progressive multifocal leukoencephalopathy and apoptosis of infected oligo-dendrocytes in the central nervous system of patients with and without AIDS. Arch Neurol. 2002;59:1930-6.

Roos KL. Encephalitis. Neurol Clin. 1999;17:813-33.

Sampathkumar P. West Nile virus: epidemiology, clinical presentation, diagnosis, and prevention. Mayo Clin Proc. 2003;78:1137-43.

Selwyn PA, Hartel D, Lewis VA, Schoenbaum EE, Vermund SH, Klein RS, et al. A prospective study of the risk of tuberculosis among intravenous drug users with human immunodeficiency virus infection. N Engl J Med. 1989;320:545-50.

Solomon T. Flavivirus encephalitis. N Engl J Med. 2004;351:370-8.

Spach DH, Jackson LA. Bacterial meningitis. Neurol Clin. 1999;17:711-35.

Steere AC. Lyme disease. N Engl J Med. 2001;345:115-25.

Stevens DA. Coccidioidomycosis. N Engl J Med. 1995;332:1077-82.

Tan SV, Guiloff RJ. Hypothesis on the pathogenesis of vacuolar myelopathy, dementia, and peripheral neuropathy in AIDS. J Neurol Neurosurg Psychiatry. 1998;65:23-8.

Tyler KL. Creutzfeldt-Jakob disease. N Engl J Med. 2003;348:681-2.

Weihl CC, Roos RP. Creutzfeldt-Jakob disease, new variant Creutzfeldt-Jakob disease, and bovine spongiform encephalopathy. Neurol Clin. 1999;17:835-59.

White DA, Heaton RK, Monsch AU, The HNRC Group, HIV Neurobehavioral Research Center. Neuropsychological studies of asymptomatic human immunodeficiency virus-type-1 infected individuals. J Int Neuropsychol Soc. 1995;1:304-15.

Whiteman ML, Post MJ, Berger JR, Tate LG, Bell MD, Limonte LP. Progressive multifocal leukoencephalopathy in 47 HIV-seropositive patients: neuroimaging with clinical and pathologic correlation. Radiology. 1993;187:233-40.

Wilson WR, Sande MA, editors. Current diagnosis and treatment in infectious diseases. New York: Lange Medical Books; 2001.

Woo HH, Rezai AR, Knopp EA, Weiner HL, Miller DC, Kelly PJ. Contrast-enhancing progressive multifocal leukoencephalopathy: radiological and pathological correlations: case report. Neurosurgery. 1996;39:1031-4.

World Health Organization. Available from: www.who.int.

QUESTIONS

1. A 32-year-old man, human immunodeficiency virus (HIV)-positive, presents with a 3-week history of upper quadrantanopia, right arm weakness, and fatigue. His recent laboratory evaluation shows a CD4 count of 50 cells/mm³. Brain MRI shows multiple areas of white matter lesions, mostly posterior, without mass effect, and nonenhancing. What is the most likely cause of this man's symptoms?
   a. Cytomegalovirus (CMV) ventriculitis
   b. Progressive multifocal leukoencephalopathy (PML)
   c. Primary central nervous system lymphoma
   d. Toxoplasmosis

2. A 28-year-old woman, human immunodeficiency virus (HIV)-positive, presents with a several-week history of mild bifrontal headache, neck stiffness, and low-grade fevers. Also a facial palsy developed sometime before she presented. Brain MRI shows mild enhancement of the basilar cisterns. The CD4 count is 150 cells/mm³. What organism is of particular concern in this patient and why?
   a. *Toxoplasma gondii*
   b. *Staphylococcus aureus*
   c. *Neisseria meningitidis*
   d. *Cryptococcus neoformans*

3. A 13-year-old boy has a 4-day history of headache, mild neck stiffness, vomiting, and diarrhea. Cerebrospinal fluid (CSF) examination at presentation showed a mild lymphocytic pleocytosis and mild increase in protein. Neuroimaging findings are unremarkable. A viral meningitis is diagnosed. What are the most common etiologic agents?
   a. Herpes simplex virus type 2
   b. Cytomegalovirus
   c. Non-polio enterovirus
   d. Varicella-zoster virus

4. A 62-year-old woman from New York experienced fevers, skin rash, and myalgias for 1 week. West Nile virus infection was diagnosed. What is the chance that this will progress to neurologic disease?
   a. 1%
   b. 10%
   c. 50%
   d. 75%

ANSWERS

1. Answer: b.

PML is an opportunistic infection caused by JC virus. Multifocal, confluent signal abnormality related to demyelination is the most typical neuroimaging characteristic. It usually occurs in late stages of HIV infection, and the prognosis is poor, with no known effective long-term treatment. CMV also tends to be pathogenic in patients with low CD4 counts, notoriously causing ventriculitis. Primary central nervous system lymphoma and cerebral toxoplasmosis can appear as mass lesions, often with enhancement.

2. Answer: d.

The subacute presentation, pattern of enhancement of the basilar cisterns, cranial nerve palsy, and underlying immuno-compromised state are all indicative of infection with *Cryptococcus neoformans*. This is treated with amphotericin B and flucytosine; the risk of relapse can be significantly reduced by prophylaxis with fluconazole.

3. Answer: c.

Non-polio enteroviruses are the most common cause of viral meningitis. Supportive care is required because the condition usually resolves without complication. Herpes simplex virus type 2 and varicella-zoster virus infection can also cause aseptic meningitis, but these are encountered less frequently than the enteroviruses. Cytomegalovirus infection is usually encountered as ventriculitis or encephalitis in immunocompromised patients.

4. Answer: a.

There is only a 1% chance of neurologic disease developing as part of a West Nile virus infection. The most common syndrome reported is meningoencephalitis, which can be particuarly severe in children and the elderly. Another syndrome is a poliolike syndrome with flaccid paralysis. Parkinsonian syndromes and myoclonus have also been reported to be associated with West Nile virus infection.

Neoplasms of the Nervous System and Related Topics

16

Nima Mowzoon, M.D.

Steven Vernino, M.D., Ph.D.

I. GENERAL CONCEPTS

A. Epidemiology and Statistics
1. Common tumors *in childhood*
   a. Most common brain tumor: cerebellar astrocytoma
   b. Second most common brain tumor: medulloblastoma
   c. Third most common brain tumor: ependymoma
   d. Most common intramedullary spinal cord tumor: astrocytoma
2. Common tumors *in adulthood*
   a. Most common intracranial tumor: metastatic tumor
   b. Most common primary central nervous system (CNS) tumor: glioblastoma multiforme (50% of all gliomas)
   c. Most common low-grade gliomas (in decreasing order): astrocytoma, oligodendroglioma, mixed oligoastrocytoma
   d. Most common intramedullary spinal cord tumor: ependymoma
   e. Most common spinal cord tumor *in elderly*: epidural metastases
3. Pilocytic astrocytomas have the best prognosis of all primary brain tumors
4. Most common brain tumor in patients with acquired immunodeficiency syndrome (AIDS): primary CNS lymphoma
5. Most common neoplasm in pineal region: germinoma
6. Most common tumor of filum terminale and cauda equina: myxopapillary ependymoma
7. Most common primary tumors for brain metastasis (in decreasing order): non–small cell lung carcinoma, breast, small cell lung carcinoma, malignant melanoma, renal cell carcinoma, gastrointestinal
8. Most common nerve sheath tumor: schwannoma

B. Clinical Manifestations of CNS Tumors
1. Signs and symptoms of raised intracranial pressure
   a. Headache: nocturnal or worse when waking up, may improve over the course of the day, worsen with coughing, Valsalva maneuver, or postural change
   b. Nausea, vomiting
   c. Papilledema
   d. Altered mental status
   e. False localizing signs (such as cranial nerve [CN] VI palsy)
   f. Increased intracranial pressure may be due to mass effect attributable to tumor, surrounding edema and hemorrhage, and hydrocephalus
2. Focal neurologic dysfunction
   a. Seizures: most often partial, some with secondary generalization, common with temporal lobe tumors
   b. Focal signs and symptoms are highly dependent on localization of the tumor
3. Pain also may result from local invasion of pain-sensitive structures, e.g., dura mater, intracranial vasculature, and periosteum

II. NEOPLASMS BY LOCATION PREDILECTION

A. Temporal Lobe
1. Dysembryonic neuroepithelial tumor (DNET), ganglioglioma, pleomorphic xanthoastrocytoma, astrocytoma, oligodendroglioma

B. Pituitary Fossa and Sellar and Suprasellar Regions
1. Pituitary gland tumors: pituitary adenoma, Rathke's cyst, granular cell tumors
2. Suprasellar region: germ cell tumors, craniopharyngioma, olfactory neuroblastoma, optic nerve gliomas, colloid cyst, epidermoid cyst, dermoid, lymphoma, hamartoma (hypothalamus), metastasis
3. Clivus: chordoma, osteosarcoma, chondrosarcoma
4. Differential diagnosis should also include nonneoplastic causes: carotid or cavernous aneurysm or fistula, sarcoidosis, cavernous sinus thrombosis

C. Pineal Region
1. Germ cell tumors (germinoma, teratoma), pineal cell

tumors (pineocytoma, pineoblastoma), meningioma, astrocytoma, pineal cysts, metastasis, lipoma, epidermoid and dermoid cysts (also arachnoid cyst)

2. Germ cell tumors occur in childhood

D. Intraventricular

1. Lateral ventricles: astrocytoma, central neurocytoma, oligodendroglioma, subependymoma, meningioma, choroid plexus papilloma, subependymal giant cell astrocytoma (most commonly at foramen of Monro)
2. Third ventricle: the above plus colloid cyst
3. Fourth ventricle (special considerations): ependymoma, subependymoma, medulloblastoma, exophytic brainstem gliomas, pilocytic cerebellar astrocytoma, hemangioblastoma

E. Corpus Callosum

1. Lymphoma, glioblastoma multiforme

F. Cerebellopontine Angle

1. Schwannoma (acoustic neuroma), meningioma, epidermoid, metastasis
2. Rare: paraganglioma, choroid plexus papilloma

G. Foramen Magnum

1. Astrocytoma, meningioma, ependymoma, medulloblastoma, metastasis
2. Mostly involving the clivus: chordoma, osteosarcoma, chondrosarcoma

H. Spinal Cord (discussed below)

III. GLIAL TUMORS

A. General Characteristics

1. Derived from neuroglia and progenitor cells (stem cells)
2. Include astrocytomas, oligodendrogliomas, mixed oligoastrocytomas, pleomorphic xanthoastrocytomas, ependymomas
3. Prognostic factors for gliomas
   a. Age at diagnosis
   b. Karnofsky performance status (KPS)
   c. Histologic grade provides helpful prognostic information (see classification below)
      1) Astrocytomas (from worse to better prognosis): glioblastoma multiforme, anaplastic astrocytoma, low-grade (World Health Organization [WHO] grade II) astrocytoma
      2) Anaplastic astrocytomas: worse prognosis than

anaplastic oligodendrogliomas

4. Other possible prognostic factors
   a. Extent of surgical resection
   b. Mental status changes at onset
   c. Short duration of symptoms before diagnosis
   d. Tumor size

B. Associated Inherited Syndromes

1. Li-Fraumeni syndrome
   a. Rare autosomal syndrome associated with familial clustering of soft tissue and bone sarcomas, breast carcinomas, and CNS neoplasms
   b. Often diagnosed before age 45 years
   c. Associated with germline mutation of $p53$
   d. Reported brain tumors include astrocytoma (anaplastic and glioblastoma multiforme) and diffuse B-cell lymphoma
   e. Possible association with Sturge-Weber syndrome (no adequate data)
2. Familial polyposis syndromes
   a. Turcot's syndrome: adenomatosis polyposis coli associated with gliomas and primitive neuroepithelial tumors
   b. Gardner's syndrome: osteomas and soft tissue tumors
3. Neurofibromatosis type 1 (NF1)
   a. Neurocutaneous syndrome associated with low-grade gliomas (including optic gliomas), neurofibromas
   b. Linked to a mutation of tumor suppressor gene (*NF1*) on chromosome 17q11.2 (see Chapter 13)
4. Neurofibromatosis type 2 (NF2)
   a. Neurocutaneous syndrome associated with meningiomas, astrocytomas, and bilateral schwannomas
   b. Linked to a mutation of tumor suppressor gene (*NF2*) on chromosome 22q11.2 (see Chapter 13)
5. Cowden's disease (multiple hamartoma syndrome)
   a. Autosomal dominant inheritance with variable penetrance
   b. Associated with Lhermitte-Duclos disease and characterized by various mucocutaneous papules, noncutaneous benign hamartomatous tumors, and carcinomas
   c. Most common malignant tumors are breast and thyroid carcinomas

C. Astrocytoma Classifications (Table 16-1)

1. WHO classification
2. St. Anne/Mayo grading

D. Diffuse (fibrillary) Astrocytomas

1. Low-grade (WHO grade II) diffuse astrocytomas
   a. Associated with mutations of the tumor suppressor gene $p53$ on chromosome 17p13.1 in two-thirds of cases and

Table 16-1. WHO Classification and St. Anne/Mayo Grading of Astrocytic Tumors

WHO		St. Anne/Mayo	
Designation	Classification	Grade (based on criteria)*	Criteria*
Pilocytic astrocytoma	I	1 (no criteria)	No criteria
Astrocytoma	I, II	1 (no criteria, WHO I)	No criteria
		2 (1 criterion)	Nuclear atypia
Anaplastic astrocytoma	III	3 (2 criteria)	Nuclear atypia
			Mitosis
Glioblastoma	IV	4 (3 criteria)	Nuclear atypia
			Mitosis
			Endothelial proliferation and/or necrosis

WHO, World Health Organization.
*St. Anne/Mayo criteria: nuclear atypia, mitosis, and capillary endothelial proliferation and/or necrosis. Grade = number of criteria + 1; maximum grade, 4.

overexpression of proto-oncogene encoding platelet-derived growth factor (PDGF)
  b. Occur typically in either first decade or between third and fourth decades
  c. Usually hemispheric location, with predilection for temporal and posterior frontal lobes more than anterior parietal lobe
  d. Tends to be infiltrative, with no well-defined borders
  e. Seizure is common presentation
  f. Pathology
    1) Pattern (from most common to least common): often fibrillary, protoplasmic, gemistocytic astrocytomas
    2) Fibrillary astrocytomas (Fig. 16-1)
       a) Well-differentiated astrocytes with scant cytoplasm; atypical and hyperchromatic nuclei; fine, fibrillary processes
       b) Microcysts containing mucinous material
       c) Scant to absent mitotic figures and vascular proliferation
       d) Calcification is rare but may occur in up to 10% to 20% of cases
    3) Protoplasmic astrocytomas
       a) Hypocellular
       b) Cells with small round nuclei, sparse cytoplasm
       c) Prominent characteristic microcystic spaces
    4) Gemistocytic astrocytomas (Fig. 16-2)
       a) Large cells with abundant eosinophilic cytoplasm and eccentrically placed nuclei
       b) Usually worse prognosis
       c) Malignant transformation: more often than other pathologic subtypes

  g. Neuroimaging characteristics: T2 hyperintense lesions with little to no enhancement, edema, or hemorrhage
  h. Prognosis
    1) Survival is variable (at least 3-5 years is expected)
    2) Most low-grade astrocytomas undergo malignant transformation with time
    3) Risk factors for malignant transformation: tumor size, gemistocytic pathology, presentation in first decade or after age 50 years, increased enhancement
2. Anaplastic (WHO grade III) astrocytoma
  a. Associated with mutations of the tumor suppressor gene *p53* on chromosome 17p13.1 (as with the low-grade astrocytomas), mutation of the retinoblastoma (*RB*) tumor suppressor gene on chromosome 13q14 in 1/3 of cases, and loss of heterozygosity (LOH) of chromosome 19q (the latter two are involved in transformation from a low-grade to an anaplastic astrocytoma)
  b. Presentation is often between 40 and 60 years of age (younger patients have longer survival)
  c. Mascroscopic features
    1) Diffusely infiltrating heterogeneous neoplasm
    2) Tumor may appear cystic and/or contain hemorrhagic foci
  d. Microscopic features
    1) Cellular proliferation is more prominent than in low-grade astrocytomas
    2) Often, frequent mitotic figures and endovascular proliferation
    3) No necrosis
  e. Seeding of the neuroaxis by cerebrospinal fluid (CSF) dissemination and ependymal spread may occur but are rare

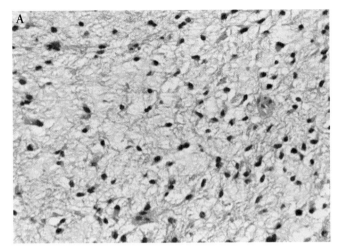

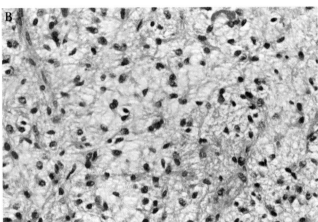

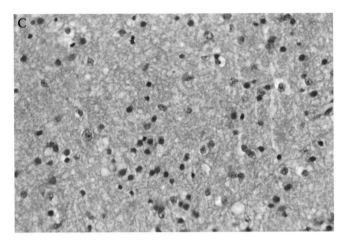

Fig. 16-1. Fibrillary astrocytoma. *A* and *B*, Fibrillary astrocytomas are characterized by well-differentiated astrocytes with hyperchromatic nuclei and scant cytoplasm; fine fibrillary processes make up the background. *C*, The fibrillary background is often interrupted by microcysts.

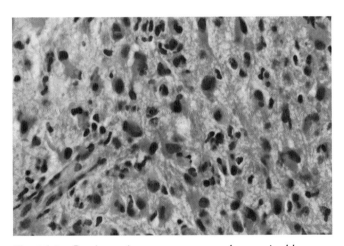

Fig. 16-2. Gemistocytic astrocytomas are characterized by large, plump eosinophilic cell bodies with abundant eosinophilic cytoplasm displacing nuclei eccentrically.

    f. Median survival: usual estimate, about 2 to 3 years after presentation
3. Glioblastoma multiforme
    a. Most common primary brain tumor, 50% of all gliomas
    b. Presentation: typically after age 50
    c. With the aggressive nature and rapid progression, presenting symptoms include increased intracranial pressure, seizures, and focal neurologic symptoms
    d. Genetics
      1) Secondary glioblastomas (malignant transformation of lower grade glioma to glioblastoma) can be associated with mutation of gene encoding PDGF-α, loss of tumor suppressor gene *PTEN* (LOH at chromosome 10q)
      2) Primary (de novo) glioblastomas
        a) Have no apparent antecedent low- or intermediate-grade tumor history
        b) Are often associated with amplification of the proto-oncogenes epidermal growth factor receptor (*EGFR*) and *MDM2*, loss of tumor suppressor

gene *PTEN*, LOH at chromosome 10, and mutation involving the *RB* gene
    e. Most common locations: deep white matter and deep gray matter, including thalamus and basal ganglia
    f. Macroscopic and neuroimaging features
      1) Heterogeneous-appearing mass with foci of necrosis, hemorrhage, and peritumoral edema (Fig. 16-3)
      2) Neuroimaging often confirms the heterogeneous appearance, with central area of necrosis and a ring-enhancing rim
      3) Despite the circumscribed gross appearance, the

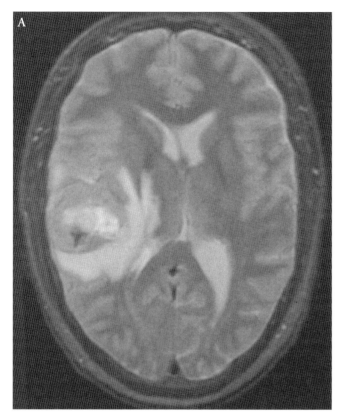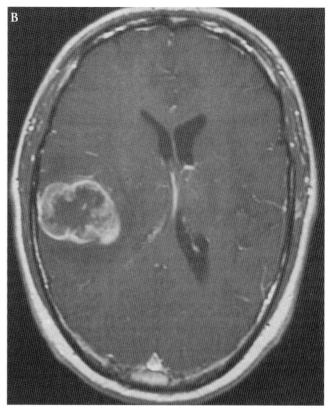

Fig. 16-3. MRI of 33-year-old patient with glioblastoma multiforme. *A*, T2-weighted and, *B*, contrast-enhanced T1-weighted images show peripherally enhancing mass with a heterogeneous signal within the lesion, situated in the junction of right posterior frontotemporal operculum and insula. Note vasogenic edema in the white matter surrounding lesion, associated with mass effect and right-to-left midline shift.

tumor is highly infiltrative and may also spread to opposite hemisphere through the corpus callosum ("butterfly gliomas")

4) Glioblastoma multiforme tumors may arise from malignant transformation of separate regions of the tumor and appear multifocal

5) Contrast enhancement and vasogenic edema occur from disrupted blood-brain barrier (BBB)

6) Treatment with corticosteroids assists in reestablishment of BBB and can yield almost immediate improvement of symptoms

g. Microscopic features

1) All the features of anaplastic astrocytomas in addition to prominent endothelial proliferation and/or necrosis, surrounded by pseudopalisading of cells (Fig. 16-4)

2) Neovascularization and endothelial hyperplasia may be due to production of angiogenic factors such as vascular endothelial growth factor (VEGF)

h. Natural history and spread

1) Typical: spread of tumor along white matter tracts and around the ependyma

2) Atypical: CSF dissemination through neuroaxis (occurs in 10%-20% of cases), may include pachymeningeal spread

3) Almost never occur: invasion of dura mater and metastasis outside of CNS

4) Meningeal invasion is sometimes called "meningeal gliomatosis," occurs more frequently with malignant gliomas

i. Treatment

1) Usually includes surgical debulking aimed at relieving mass effect and increasing effectiveness of adjunctive therapy (also sometimes to obtain pathology specimen)

2) Complete resection is not possible because tumor is diffusely infiltrative and multifocal

3) Stereotactic biopsy: reserved for deep and inaccessible

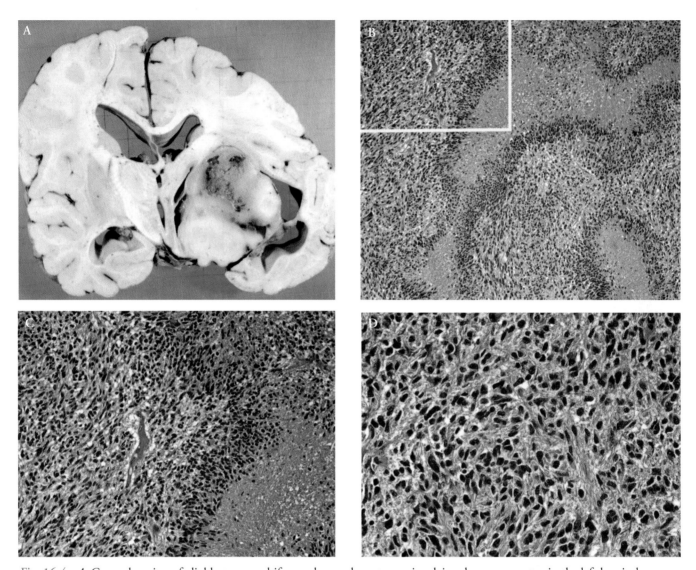

Fig. 16-4. *A*, Coronal section of glioblastoma multiforme shows a large tumor involving deep gray matter in the left hemisphere, with a large heterogeneous central area of cystic necrosis. Histopathologic characteristics of glioblastoma multiforme include pseudopalisading cells around necrotic regions (*B*), neovascularization, cellular pleomorphism (*C* and *D*), and mitotic figures. (*C* is higher magnification of inset in *B*.)

tumors and comorbidities precluding general anesthesia
  4) Most effective adjunctive therapy: external beam radiotherapy administered to limited field, up to 60 Gy given in conjunction with temozolomide chemotherapy—median survival, about 14 months; 2-year survival, about 27%
4. Gliomatosis cerebri (Fig. 16-5)
  a. Diffuse, infiltrative glial tumor (usually astrocytoma) causing diffuse expansion of a portion of or entire cerebral hemisphere; may spread to one or both cerebral hemispheres

  b. Microscopic features (Fig. 16-6)
    1) Resembles low-grade glioma
    2) Mild increase in cellularity and pleomorphism
    3) Rare mitotic figures
    4) No hemorrhage or necrosis
    5) Neoplastic glial cells cluster around neurons
  c. Treatment
    1) Some benefit from chemotherapy (as with PCV or temozolamide)
    2) No role for surgery because of infiltrative nature of tumor

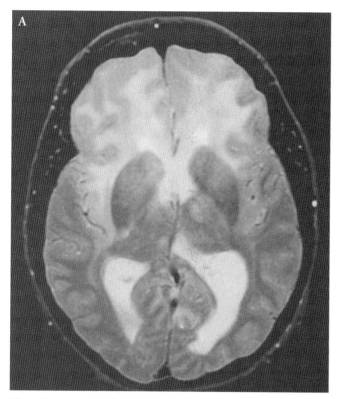
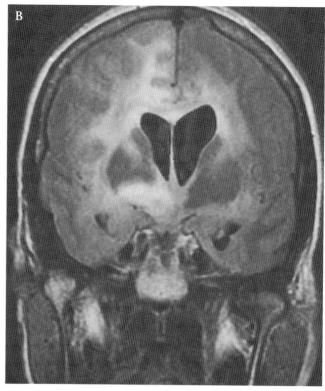

Fig. 16-5. MRI of gliomatosis cerebri. *A*, Axial T2-weighted and *B*, coronal FLAIR images show extensive confluent abnormal nonenhancing increased T2 signal involving white matter of both frontal lobes, notably the corpus callosum anteriorly. Additional abnormal signal is seen in hypothalamus (*B*), notably in region of anterior commissure on the right. There is obstructive hydrocephalus of the lateral ventricles and severe mass effect.

3) Marginal benefit from radiotherapy
d. 2-Year survival after treatment, 5% to 10%

E. Circumscribed Astrocytomas

1. Pilocytic astrocytomas (WHO grade I)
   a. Usually occur in first or second decade of life
   b. Better prognosis than diffuse astrocytomas
   c. Common locations: cerebellum (hemispheres > vermis), optic chiasm, hypothalamus, and periventricular area of third and fourth ventricles (Fig. 16-7 *A*)
   d. Less common locations: spinal cord (Fig. 16-7 *B* and *C*), brainstem, cerebral hemispheres (temporal lobe is most common hemisphere site); tend to occur in older age group (young adults)
   e. Cerebellar hemisphere tumors: often large cystic, fluid-filled masses appearing hyperintense on T2-weighted images, with strongly (but somewhat heterogeneously) contrast-enhancing mural nodule
   f. Optic and hypothalamic gliomas: tend to be solid, pilocytic tumors
   g. Brainstem gliomas: likely to be solid, diffuse fibrillary astrocytomas (rarely pilocytic tumor arising from fourth ventricle with "dorsally exophytic" growth, which may portend better prognosis)
   h. Macroscopic features: unencapsulated, but well-circumscribed (there may be limited degrees of infiltration) heterogeneous mass; may have a mural nodule associated with a cyst
   i. Microscopic features
      1) Compact pilocytic arrangements of elongated (sometimes stellate) cells admixed with microcystic areas
      2) Classic feature: abundant Rosenthal fibers, may be slight nuclear pleomorphism and rare mitoses
   j. 5-Year postoperative survival: 85% to 100% (95%-100% for cerebellar pilocytic astrocytomas)
   k. Cerebellar pilocytic astrocytomas have the best prognosis of all primary brain tumors
   l. Treatment
      1) Maximal surgical excision of tumor
      2) Surgical excision of the mural nodule may be

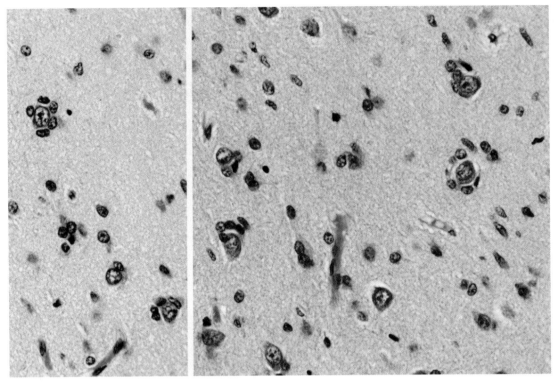

Fig. 16-6. Gliomatosis cerebri is characterized histopathologically by mildly pleomorphic cells tending to cluster around neurons (perineural satellitosis) and relative absence of mitosis, necrosis, and neovascularization.

adequate and cystic wall need not be removed
  3) With increasing thickness or enhancement of nodule wall, the cystic wall also needs to be removed
  4) Nonresectable tumors or recurrence with malignant transformation may require adjuvant radiotherapy
2. Pleomorphic xanthoastrocytomas (WHO grade II or III)
  a. Occur in second or third decade of life (average age at diagnosis, 26 years)
  b. Often a history of seizures
  c. May originate from subpial astrocytes
  d. Macroscopic features
    1) Well-encapsulated tumor frequently containing a mural nodule within a cyst
    2) Often located superficially in temporal lobe
  e. Microsocopic features
    1) Large cells with eosinophilic cytoplasm, some containing lipid droplets
    2) Nuclear pleomorphism
    3) Rare mitoses
  f. Neuroimaging: well-circumscribed cystic lesions appearing isointense or hypointense to brain parenchyma on T1-weighted and hyperintense on T2-weighted images,

> Large cells with cytoplasmic eosinophilic granular bodies are a characteristic feature of pleomorphic xanthoastrocytoma, which is a low-grade glioma

often with intense contrast enhancement of nodule
  g. Treatment
    1) Often includes complete resection
    2) Radiation and chemotherapy often reserved for recurrent or malignant tumors
  h. Postresection survival rates: 81% at 5 years, 70% at 10 years; relatively benign prognosis
3. Subependymal giant cell astrocytomas (WHO grade I)
  a. Very slow-growing tumors, always associated with tuberous sclerosis (found in up to 14% of patients with tuberous sclerosis)
  b. Presentation: usually in first or second decade of life
  c. Usually originate near foramen of Monro, blocking CSF outflow and causing hydrocephalus
  d. Macroscopic features: well-circumscribed, lobulated red mass (vascular tumor), often calcified and cystic

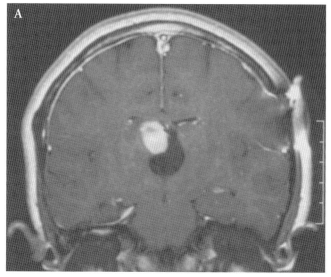

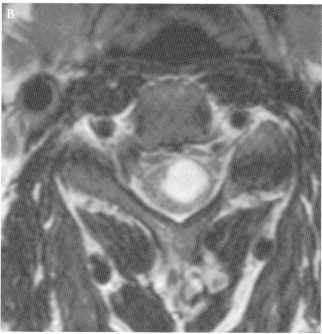

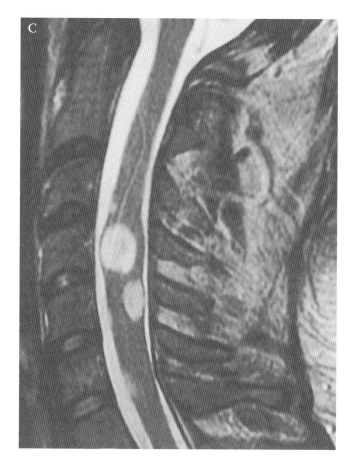

Fig. 16-7. MRI of pilocytic astrocytoma. *A*, MRI (T1-weighted image) with contrast shows enhancing tumor nodule near left foramen of Monro. Incidentally, there are bilateral shunt tubes at the lateral ventricles and diffuse dural enhancement. *B*, Axial and, *C*, coronal T2-weighted sequences of cervical spine of a different patient with pilocytic astrocytoma of cervical spinal cord. Note multiple intradural, intramedullay T2 hyperintense lesions. The largest lesions were identified at C4 and C5. In both cases, biopsy showed pilocytic astrocytoma.

e. Microscopic features
   1) Large, oval cells with abundant eosinophilic cytoplasm and large, eccentric nucleus; often surround blood vessels in this vascular tumor
   2) Pleomorphism is often present
   3) Mitoses and necrosis are unusual
f. Neuroimaging: isointense or hyperintense on T2-weighted images; intense, heterogeneous enhancement on T1-weighted imaging with contrast
g. Definitive treatment for symptomatic patients (i.e., hydrocephalus) or extensive tumors: surgical resection

h. Unless symptomatic, patients are only followed with periodic neuroimaging

F. **Special Considerations**
1. Optic gliomas (Fig. 16-8)
   a. 3% to 5% of all childhood brain tumors
   b. 2% of gliomas in adults
   c. Female predominance (female:male = 2:1)
   d. More common in children: 50% of patients present before age 5, 90% before age 20
   e. Tumors involving optic nerve alone have a better

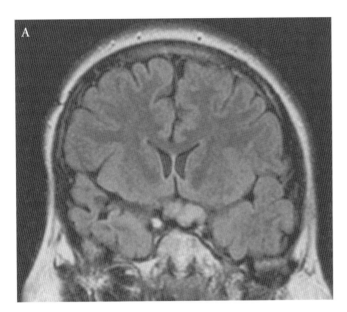

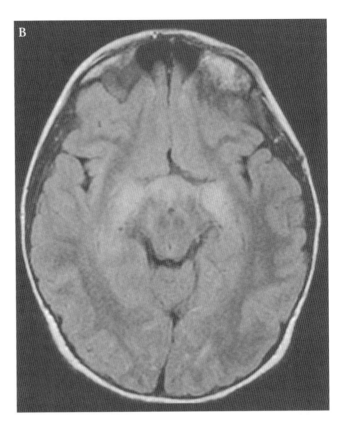

Fig. 16-8. MRI of optic glioma. *A*, Coronal FLAIR MRI of an 18-year-old girl shows a multilobular mass centered on the optic chiasm. *B*, Axial FLAIR MRI of a 5-year-old boy with neurofibromatosis type 1 and bilateral optic nerve gliomas extending along the optic tracts to the lateral geniculate bodies and further posteriorly along the optic radiations.

prognosis than those involving optic chiasm (which have better prognosis than hypothalamic gliomas, although aggressive tumors involving optic chiasm may spread to involve hypothalamus)

   f. Associated with NF1

      1) Occur in 1% to 7% of children with NF1

      2) As many as 50% of patients with optic gliomas have NF1

      3) Almost all patients with bilateral optic nerve tumors sparing optic chiasm have NF1

   g. Slow-growing tumors; malignant histologic features or aggressive behavior are rare (reported in cases of optic chiasm and hypothalamic gliomas)

   h. Usually pilocytic astrocytomas causing either diffuse expansion without subarachnoid involvement or primary subarachnoid spread with minimal involvement of optic nerve

   i. Symptoms unique to optic nerve gliomas

      1) Visual loss, visual field defects, painless proptosis, and symptoms related to increased intracranial pressure

      2) Symptoms of hypothalamic involvement

         a) Endocrinopathies: precocious puberty, diabetes insipidus, other related endocrinopathies

         b) Gelastic seizures: characterized by involuntary

laughter, more common with hypothalamic hamartomas

         c) "Diencephalic syndrome": emaciation, cachexia and loss of subcutaneous fat, emesis, pallor, hyper-activity, inappropriate behavior, euphoria

   j. Treatment

      1) Considered for tumors with aggressive behavior, espe-cially for patients presenting with visual deterioration

      2) Radiotherapy considered for patients older than 5 years presenting with tumors in locations other than intraorbital (intracranial locations such as chiasmal or retrochiasmal) and when total resection is not possible

      3) Chemotherapy considered for patients younger than 5 years

      4) Surgical excision may be limited to biopsy, especially for tumors involving optic chiasm

2. Brainstem gliomas

   a. Account for 10% to 15% of brain tumors in children (<5% of gliomas in adults)

   b. Age at diagnosis: often between 5 and 10 years

   c. Heterogeneous group of neoplasms: all grades of pathol-ogy observed, but most are malignant, with poor prognosis

   d. Symptoms: usually related to ataxia and other cerebellar

features, long tract signs, or cranial nerve deficits
  e. Neuroimaging (can predict prognosis better than pathologic features)
     1) Lesions appear as a high T2 signal with variable degrees of enhancement
     2) May contain a cystic component (Fig. 16-9)
     3) Diffuse pontine gliomas: all are malignant
     4) Most gliomas involving cervicomedullary junction are low-grade gliomas
     5) Tumors of midbrain usually have a better prognosis than those involving medulla or pons
     6) Dorsal exophytic tumors tend to have better prognosis
  f. Prognosis
     1) Best for focal lesions, dorsal exophytic tumors, low histologic grade, longer period from onset of symptoms to diagnosis, adult age group, and in context of neurofibromatosis

     2) 5-Year survival: 5% to 30%
  g. Treatment
     1) Best: radiotherapy
     2) Surgical resection usually involves stereotactic biopsy; is best performed on focal, cystic, or exophytic tumors

G. **Rare Astrocytic Variants**
1. Gliosarcomas: high-grade gliomas admixed with sarcoma (variant of glioblastoma multiforme, with same prognosis)
2. Gliofibroma
   a. Glioma admixed with population of cells resembling fibroblasts
   b. Usually present in the first decade

H. **Oligodendroglioma**
1. From cells of oligodendroglial origin (O2A progenitor cells)

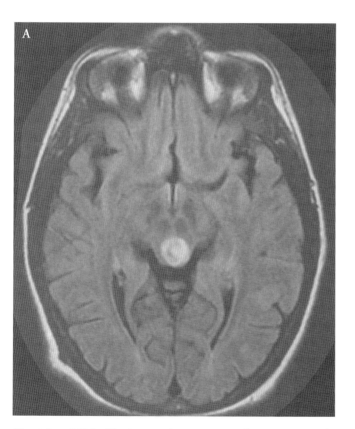 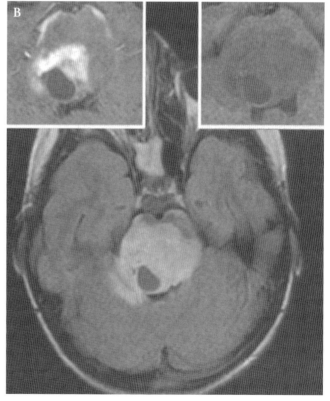

Fig. 16-9. MRI of brainstem glioma. *A,* Axial FLAIR image shows a tectal plate mass that is likely low-grade glioma. *B,* Axial FLAIR image of a 7-year-old girl with brainstem gliomas shows a cystic, enhancing expansive mass (*upper left* inset, contrast-enhanced T1-weighted image) in the posterior fossa extending from pons to midbrain, abutting the anterior surface of the fourth ventricle and cerebral aqueduct, causing moderate noncommunicating hydrocephalus (not shown). The large tumor appears to be of high T2 and low T1 signal (*upper right* inset, T1-weighted image). Although the radiographic appearance of this lesion is suggestive of pilocytic astrocytoma, biopsy showed high-grade brainstem glioma.

2. Genetics
   a. Development of low-grade oligodendrogliomas: associated with loss of heterozygosity of chromosomes 1p, 19q, and 4q
   b. Development of high-grade oligodendrogliomas from the low-grade tumors: associated with loss of heterozygosity of chromosomes 9p and 10q
   c. Both are associated with overexpression of EGFR
3. Account for 5% of all primary brain tumors and 30% of all intracranial gliomas
4. May be a male predominance (male:female = 3:2)
5. More often presents in adults: usually present between third and fifth decades
6. Small earlier peak in childhood between 6 and 12 years; thalamic location at presentation is common in children
7. Seizures are often the initial presentation in up to 75% of patients because tumor commonly involves cerebral cortex
8. Most common location: frontal lobe, followed by temporal and parietal lobes; rarely brainstem or spinal cord
9. Slow-growing, infiltrative gliomas: may start in subcortical white matter, tend to spread along white matter tracts and corpus callosum
10. Better prognosis than astrocytomas
11. 5-Year survival rate, 75%
12. Mean postoperative survival, 4 to 11 years

13. Macroscopic features: well-circumscribed, unencapsulated mass with cystic degeneration and calcification (necrosis and hemorrhage are rare)
14. Microscopic features (Fig. 16-10)
    a. Variable
    b. Homogeneously appearing cells with sparse cytoplasm and round, uniform nuclei
    c. Cells may appear elongated, with a displaced nucleus; because of fixation artifact, there may be artifactual clearing of the cytoplasm, resembling fried eggs
    d. There may be mucin-rich microcystic spaces
    e. Capillaries interposed between uniform-appearing cells may form a delicate vascular "chicken-wire" pattern
    f. Pleomorphism and endothelial hyperplasia (less commonly, necrosis) indicate high-grade oligodendroglioma
15. Neuroimaging: heterogeneous appearing T2 hyperintense mass often involving cerebral cortex with variable, heterogeneous enhancement pattern, cystic component, and calcification (in up to 90% of cases)
16. Classified into high-grade and low-grade tumors
17. Features associated with high-grade tumors and less favorable prognosis
    a. Contrast enhancement
    b. Endothelial proliferation
    c. Mitotic figures
    d. More than 5% of MIB-1 staining
    e. Astrocytic component (with oligoastrocytomas, as

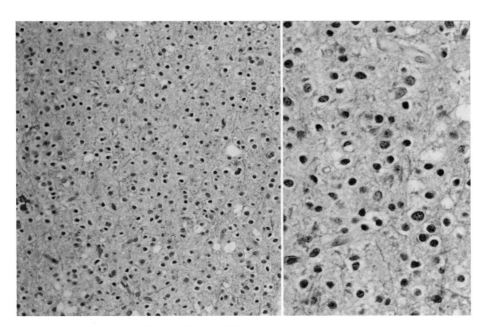

Fig. 16-10. Oligodendroglioma. Sheets of uniform cells with "fried egg" appearance due to artifactual clearing of the cytoplasm (best seen in higher magnification on the right).

discussed below)
18. Treatment
    a. Gross total resection when possible (because tumor is infiltrative, microscopic infiltrates always remain)
    b. Primary adjuvant therapy: chemotherapy with alkylating agent such as temozolomide (before development of temozolomide, procarbazine/lomustine/vincristine [PVC] were used)
    c. Loss of heterozygosity of chromosome 1p or combined loss of heterozygosity of chromosomes 1p and 19q (50%-80% of cases) portend better prognosis, prolonged survival, and better response to chemotherapy
    d. Although intermediate-grade oligodendrogliomas are often chemotherapy-responsive (e.g., 1p/19q deleted tumors), radiation (often in combination with chemotherapy) is still the mainstay of treatment to achieve maximal survival advantage

I.   Oligoastrocytoma
1. Composed of different populations of cells, some resembling astrocytes, some oligodendrocytes, and some indeterminate
2. A common progenitor cell that differentiates into two different cell lines is likely
3. Glial tumors with predominant oligodendrocytic population of cells are often interpreted as oligodendrocytes
4. Increasing proportion of oligodendroglial component generally portends better prognosis (chromosome 1p and 19q deletions signify greater sensitivity of tumor to chemotherapy)

J.   Ependymoma
1. Epidemiology
    a. 5% to 8% of all primary intracranial tumors
    b. Age at presentation often in the first decade, with a second peak in the fourth decade (prognosis worse for patients younger than 3 years)
    c. Third most common brain tumor in children
    d. Location (pediatric population): intracranial (90%) or spinal cord (10%)
    e. 2/3 of intracranial ependymomas occuring in children are infratentorial and about 1/3 supratentorial
    f. 2/3 of intracranial ependymomas occur in children (mostly infratentorial), and more than 90% of spinal cord ependymomas occur in adults (mostly myxopapillary ependymomas)
2. Symptoms at presentation (depend largely on tumor location)
    a. Intracranial tumors often occur on floor (more frequent than roof or lateral recesses) of fourth ventricle (medul-

loblastomas tend to arise most frequently from roof of fourth ventricle)
    b. May present with obstructive hydrocephalus and associated symptoms of headache, nausea, vomiting, ataxia, vertigo, nystagmus
3. Potential for CSF dissemination: because of close contact with CSF, there may be "drop metastasis" in 5% of cases
4. Myxopapillary ependymomas
    a. Well-encapsulated, indolent, slow-growing vascular tumors arising from filum terminale
    b. Occur most often in adults
    c. Associated with good prognosis
5. Posterior fossa ependymomas
    a. Well-demarcated tumors that tend to fill fourth ventricle and extend through foramen magnum
    b. Appear as T2 hyperintense masses with heterogeneous signal that may represent tumor vascularity (or necrosis)
    c. Often a heterogeneous pattern of enhancement
6. Microscopic features (Fig. 16-11)
    a. Sheets of uniform cells with round nuclei and variable cytoplasm among perivascular anuclear fibrillary processes: "pseudorosettes" (fine cellular fibrillary processes that radiate toward blood vessel)
    b. Myxopapillary ependymomas are characterized by sheets of uniform columnar or cuboidal cells admixed with pools of mucin often bordered by tumor cells and containing a central blood vessel
    c. Cytologic pleomorphism, necrosis, mitotic figures, and giant cells often signify anaplastic ependymomas
7. Treatment: surgical resection and/or adjuvant radiotherapy (optimal outcome with doses between 5,000 cGy and 5,500 cGy)
    a. Higher survival with gross total resection: goal is to obtain maximal possible resection
    b. For low-grade ependymomas of spine parenchyma or filum terminale (myxopapillary ependymoma): surgical resection is mainstay of treatment, radiation is considered if residual tumor is present postoperatively
    c. Extensive craniospinal radiation to entire neuroaxis required for patients presenting with CSF dissemination
    d. Response to chemotherapy is suboptimal; this treatment modality is considered for patients with contraindications to radiation (e.g., children younger than 3 years or patients with recurrent disease)
8. Prognosis: generally favorable, especially adults with myxopapillary ependymomas (except for 10%-20% of cases that have CSF dissemination)
9. Reduced survival has been associated with young age at onset and anaplastic histopathologic features, and higher risk of recurrence with partial resections

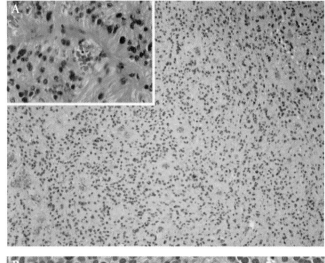

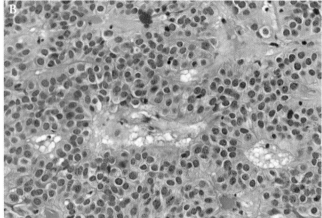

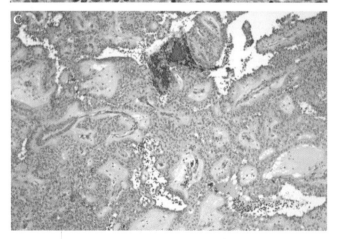

Fig. 16-11. Ependymoma. *A*, Sheets of cells with regular, round, uniform nuclei interrupted by characteristic perivascular acellular areas called pseudorosettes. These consist of fibrillary processes projecting toward the central vessel (*inset*). *B* and *C*, Myxopapillary ependymoma is characterized by clusters of uniform columnar or cuboidal cells with round uniform nuclei (*B*), interrupted by pools of mucin, which comprise the myxopapillary appearance, better seen at lower magnification (*C*).

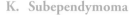

K. Subependymoma

1. Slow-growing large firm masses most often occurring in fourth ventricle, arising from medulla or lateral ventricles attached to septum pellucidum
2. Age at presentation: usually between 40 and 60 years
3. Microscopic features (Fig. 16-12): cells with round nuclei and sparse cytoplasm; admixed with microcystic clusters and foci of calcification on a fibrillary background
4. Neuroimaging characteristics: mildly hyperintense lesions on T2-weighted images often with heterogeneous appearance and little to no enhancement

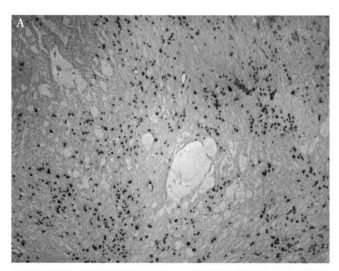

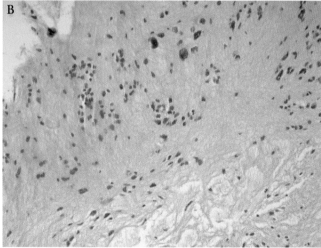

Fig. 16-12. Subependymoma. *A*, Low and *B*, high magnification showing scattered groups of cells interspersed with microcystic clusters on a dense fibrillary background.

IV. NEUROEPITHELIAL TUMORS WITH NEURONAL FEATURES

A. Ganglion Cell Neoplasms

1. Rare, slow-growing, benign well-circumscribed firm tumors often occurring in temporal lobes, sometimes with cystic or calcified foci
2. Age at presentation: first 3 decades
3. Most common presentation: seizures (often intractable)
4. Predilection for temporal lobes (followed by frontal and parietal lobes); much less common, cerebellum and spinal cord
5. Neuroimaging characteristics: classically appear as well-circumscribed cystic mass (hyperintense on T2-weighted images) with a mural nodule with variable enhancement
6. Microscopic features
   a. Presence of both neuronal (ganglion) and glial neoplastic cells
   b. Gangliocytoma: tumors with predominance of neoplastic ganglion cells without an obvious astrocytic component
   c. Ganglioglioma: tumors containing neoplastic glial cells that often outnumber ganglion cells
   d. Some neoplastic ganglion cells are binucleated or multi-nucleated (unfortunately not always present, but quite helpful when present) (Fig. 16-13)
7. Treatment
   a. Resection
   b. Radiotherapy: reserved for recurrent tumor or those with anaplastic histopathologic features
8. Prognosis
   a. Most carry benign prognosis with total or subtotal resection
   b. Anaplastic histopathologic features: less favorable prognosis

B. Central Neurocytomas

1. Neoplasms of neuronal differentiation
2. Rare (about 0.5% of all primary CNS tumors), occur primarily in young adults between second and fourth decades
3. Commonly present with symptoms of increased intracranial pressure (most commonly, headaches)
4. Most commonly an intraventricular location, often at foramen of Monro: 50% of all intraventricular tumors in adults
5. Microscopic features: sheets of uniform cells with round nuclei; immunoreactive for synaptophysin

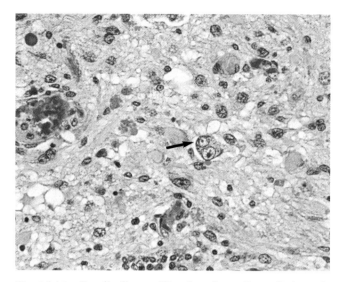

Fig. 16-13. Ganglioglioma. Binucleated ganglion cells (*arrow*) are a characteristic feature and pathognomonic of gangliogliomas, but not always present. (From Okazaki H, Scheithauer BW. Atlas of neuropathology. New York: Gower Medical Publishing; 1988. p. 103. By permission of Mayo Foundation.)

6. Neuroimaging: heterogeneous signal (isointense or hyperintense on T2-weighted images) with hetero-geneous enhancement (Fig. 6-14)
7. Treatment often involves resection (total, if possible)
8. Benign prognosis with total or subtotal resection, with long survival rates

C. Dysembryoplastic Neuroepithelial Tumor (DNET)

1. Rare, slow-growing (sometimes cystic) tumors with predilection for temporal lobes
2. Most common presentation: complex partial seizures (often intractable)
3. Microscopic features
   a. Mucin-rich cellular glial nodules containing masses of oligodendrocyte-like cells
   b. Specific glioneuronal elements
   c. Adjacent foci of cortical dysplasia
   d. Dystrophic calcification
4. Neuroimaging characteristics: hyperintense on T2-weighted images (hypointense on T1-weighted images)
5. Benign prognosis
6. Surgical resection usually reserved for symptomatic cases (e.g., intractable seizures)

D. Lhermitte-Duclos Disease (dysplastic gangliocytoma of cerebellum)

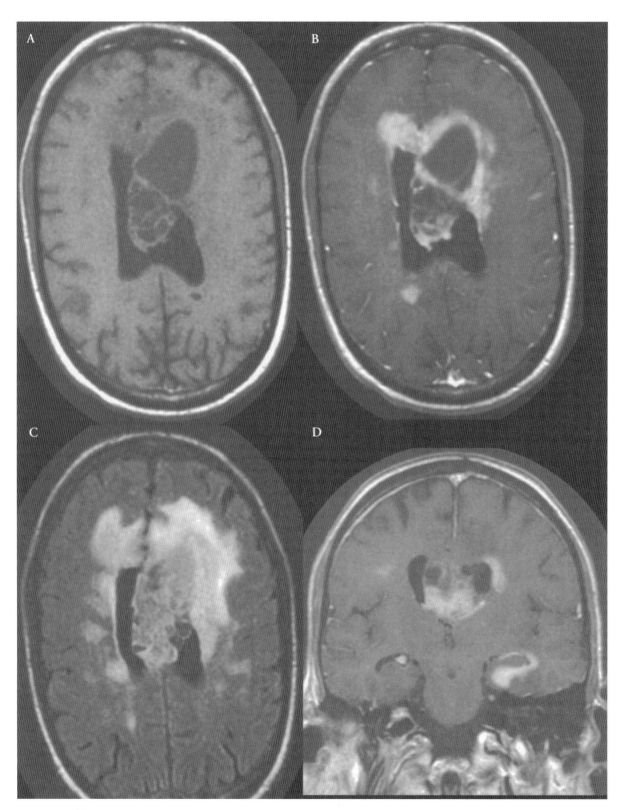

Fig. 16-14. MRI of biopsy-proven central neurocytoma shows a heterogeneous, complex mass involving lateral and third ventricles, with peritumoral edema best appreciated in FLAIR sequences, and circumferential heterogeneous enhancement. *A,* Axial T1-weighted image; *B,* axial gadolinium-enhanced T1-weighted image; *C,* axial FLAIR image; and *D,* coronal gadolinium-enhanced T1-weighted image.

1. Commonly presents as slow-growing cerebellar mass with increased intracranial pressure
2. Commonly presents in the fourth decade
3. Associated with Cowden's disease (about 50% of patients with dysplastic gangliocytoma have clinical stigmata of Cowden's disease)
4. Macroscopic features: hypertrophied, thickened cerebellar folia (Fig. 16-15)
5. Microscopic features
   a. Enlarged ganglion cells (neurons) replace granule cells, atrophy of granular layer
   b. Loss of Purkinje cells
   c. Reduction and cavitation of cerebellar white matter
6. Neuroimaging: laminated increased T2 signal without enhancement

E. Desmoplastic Infantile Astrocytoma (DIA) and Ganglioma (DIG)

1. Rare, often occurring in the first 2 years of life
2. Large, cystic tumors with dural attachments, and predilection for frontal and parietal areas
3. DIG has male predominance, DIA female predominance
4. DIG associated with LOH for chromosomes 17p and 10q
5. Good prognosis with surgical resection (adjuvant therapy often not needed)

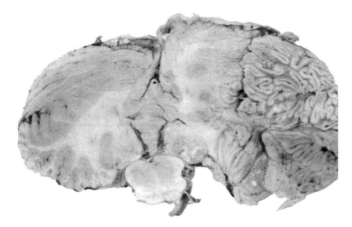

Fig. 16-15. Lhermitte-Duclos disease (dysplastic gangliocytoma of cerebellum). Note focal thickening and hypetrophy of cerebellar folia. (From Okazaki H, Scheithauer BW. Atlas of neuropathology. New York: Gower Medical Publishing; 1988. p. 106. By permission of Mayo Foundation.)

V. Primitive (Embryonal) Neuroectodermal Tumors (PNETs): Small Blue Cell Tumors

A. Medulloblastoma

1. Most common PNET
2. Arises from cerebellar external granular layer precursor cells
3. Age at presentation: often between 5 and 9 years old, with second smaller peak between 20 and 24 years
4. 20% of all intracranial tumors in children
5. 75% of tumors arise from midline cerebellum or vermis
6. 25% of tumors arise from cerebellar hemispheres (more commonly in adults with medulloblastoma)
7. Most common presentation: signs of increased intracranial pressure such as nausea, vomiting, nocturnal headache, CN VI palsy ("nonlocalizing" sign due to hydrocephalus); common cerebellar findings of ataxia, titubation, and others
8. Early dissemination through CSF and metastasis
   a. Leptomeningeal metastasis may occur with CSF dissemination
   b. Parenchymal metastasis occurs from spread to Virchow-Robin spaces
   c. Thus, magnetic resonance imaging (MRI) of entire neuroaxis should be part of the work-up
9. Macroscopic features: firm tumors that may contain foci of hemorrhage, necrosis, calcification (rare), or cysts
10. Microscopic features (Fig. 16-16)
    a. Densely packed, undifferentiated cells with dark, small oval nuclei and sparse cytoplasm, abundant mitotic figures and apoptosis among small foci of necrosis
    b. Homer Wright rosettes in 40% of cases, represent attempts at neuroblastic differentiation
    c. There may be immunoreactivity to synaptophysin
11. Histologic variants
    a. Desmoplastic (nodular) variant
       1) Characterized by clusters of neoplastic cells contained within reticulin-rich firbrous septa
       2) Often more neuronal differentiation within center of

Medulloblastoma is associated with relatively high incidence of widespread leptomeningeal dissemination. This occasionally occurs with glioblastoma and ependymoma

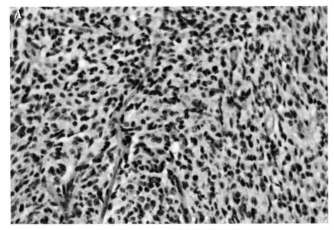

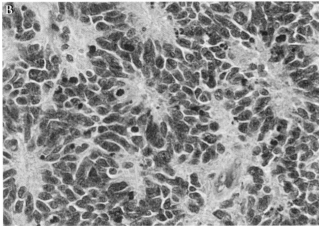

Fig. 16-16. Medulloblastoma. *A*, Densely packed, undifferentiated cells with hyperchromatic pleomorphic nuclei and sparse cytoplasm. *B*, Neuronal differentiation into neuroblastic (Homer Wright) rosettes (lacking a central vascular component) is common. (*B* from Okazaki H, Scheithauer BW. Atlas of neuropathology. New York: Gower Medical Publishing; 1988. p. 111. By permission of Mayo Foundation.)

the "nodules," which implies better prognosis
   3) This variety may be seen more frequently in adults and those with nevoid basal cell carcinoma syndrome (Gorlin's syndrome)
  b. Melanotic medulloblastoma: contains focal, limited melanin production
  c. Medullomyoblastoma: contains striated muscle differentiation, immunoreactive for myoglobin; less favorable prognosis
12. Neuroimaging: hyperintense on T2-weighted images with a heterogeneous signal and enhancement pattern, often filling fourth ventricle and extending to cisterns
13. Treatment
  a. Often surgical resection for relief of symptoms of hydro-

cephalus and to establish diagnosis: gross total resection when possible
  b. Surgical resection is often followed by craniospinal radiotherapy because of early risk of CSF dissemination
14. Prognosis
  a. 5-Year survival rate, often more than 50%
  b. Children older than 3 years often have 5-year survival better than 75%
  c. Infants and those with disseminated tumor have 5-year survival rates between 30% and 40%
15. Collin's law for medulloblastoma
  a. Period of risk for recurrence for tumor is patient's age at diagnosis plus 9 months
  b. If no recurrence within period of risk, tumor is cured

B. Ependymoblastoma
1. Large masses
2. Undifferentiated small cells with hyperchromatic nuclei ("small blue cells," as with the rest of PNETs)

C. Esthesioblastoma
1. Originates from neuroepithelial cells of upper nasal cavity
2. Locally invasive tumor
  a. Tends to invade skull through the cribriform plate
  b. May invade subarachnoid space and brain parenchyma
3. Treatment usually involves gross total resection, often followed by adjuvant radiation (external beam radiotherapy) and chemotherapy
4. Good prognosis with complete resection

D. Pinealoblastoma (see below)

E. Retinoblastoma

F. Cerebral Neuroblastoma (referred to as supratentorial PNET)
1. Peak incidence: in first decade of life, usually before age 5
2. Much less common than neuroblastomas arising from sympathetic chain
3. Presentation: often increased intracranial pressure
4. Associated with opsoclonus, myoclonus, and encephalopathy
5. Predilection for frontal and parietal lobes
6. Macroscopic features
  a. Large, heterogeneous-appearing enhancing mass with predilection for deep white matter and periventricular areas of frontal and parietal lobes
  b. Also possible: cystic, hemorrhagic, or necrotic regions

c. CSF dissemination may occur
7. Microscopic features
   a. Small cells with hyperchromatic nuclei and sparse cytoplasm
   b. High mitotic activity, with scattered Homer Wright rosettes representing some neuronal differentiation
8. Poor prognosis

VI. MENINGEAL AND MESENCHYMAL TUMORS

A. Meningioma
1. Most common nonglial primary CNS tumor
2. Most common *benign* brain tumor
3. Second most common primary brain tumor after gliomas: 15% to 20% of all primary brain tumors
4. Female:male = 2:1
5. Peak incidence: in fifth to seventh decades, rare in children
6. 40% to 80% of meningiomas: associated with mutation involving gene responsible for NF2 on chromosome 22 and a tumor suppressor gene on chromosome 22q
7. Tumors contain hormone receptors (such as progesterone) and tend to grow during pregnancy
8. Well-circumscribed, slow-growing, dural-based benign tumors arising from arachnoid cap cells
   a. Tend to compress or envelop (not invade) surrounding nervous tissue
   b. May infrequently invade the surrounding bone and soft tissue
9. Almost 90% are asymptomatic
10. Clinical presentation depends on tumor location
11. Predilection (in order of occurrence): parasagittal > convexity > sphenoid ridge > tuberculum sellae and olfactory groove > falx cerebri > lateral ventricle (other locations such as the optic nerve sheath, spinal, and extradural/extracranial are much less frequent)
12. 1% to 10% of cases may have mulitple meningiomas: consider NF2
13. Parasagittal and falx cerebri meningiomas may present with weakness and seizures, and olfactory groove meningiomas may present with Foster Kennedy syndrome (ipsilateral optic atrophy, contralateral papilledema, anosmia)
14. Macroscopic features: well-circumscribed firm (sometimes soft) tumors with smooth surface (Fig. 16-17 *A*)
15. Microscopic features (Fig. 16-17)
   a. WHO classification: typical, atypical, and anaplastic meningiomas

b. Meningothelial: sheets or lobules of arachnoid epithelioid oval cells appearing to have inclusions (are essentially nuclear membrane invaginations of the cytoplasm)
   c. Fibrous (fibroblastic)
      1) Elongated spindle cells with background of collagen fiber deposition
      2) Whorl formation and psammoma bodies are not characteristic features
   d. Transitional
      1) Features of both the meningothelial and fibrous types
      2) Contains abundant whorls and occasional psammoma bodies
   e. Psammomatous: transitional meningioma with many psammoma bodies
   f. Secretory: meningothelial or transitional meningioma, characterized by cytoplasmic PAS-positive eosinophilic globules
   g. Clear cell meningioma: clusters of elongated cells with increased cytoplasmic glycogen embedded in a matrix of fibrous septa
   h. Microcystic meningioma: foamy cells on a microcystic background
   i. Anaplastic meningioma: highly cellular, rapidly progressive tumor with excessive mitotic activity, nuclear atypia, and necrosis
16. Neuroimaging characteristics
   a. Skull plain films: hyperostosis and bony erosion of surrounding bony structures
   b. MRI of head
      1) Lesion is isointense with gray matter on T1-weighted and T2-weighted images (the latter is more variable), enhances strongly, and most have a "dural tail" (Fig. 16-18)
      2) Variable degree of peritumoral vasogenic edema noted as increased T2 signal around tumor
17. Metastasis: rare (benign meningiomas may also rarely metastasize)
18. Treatment
   a. Primary mode is surgical resection
   b. Asymptomatic tumors or patients with well-controlled seizures may be observed with serial scans
   c. Complete resection is not always possible; risk of recurrence depends on amount of residual tumor and histologic grade
   d. Stereotactic radiosurgery is considered for partially resected tumors, "difficult-to-reach" places such as falx cerebri, and recurrent tumors
   e. For tumors not amenable to stereotactic radiation (e.g., too large, odd shape, proximity to optic apparatus), fractionated radiation can be used

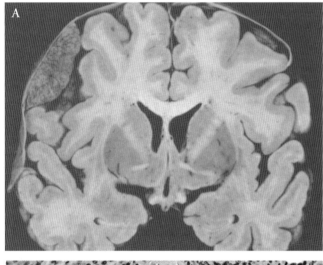

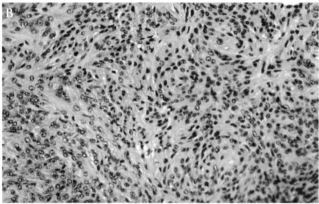

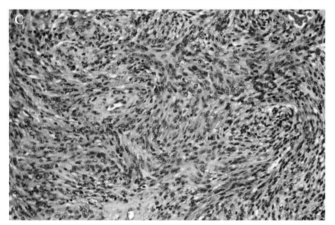

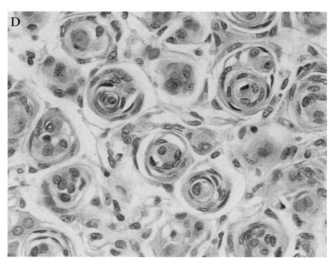

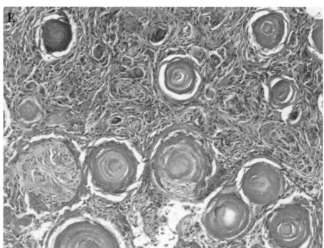

Fig. 16-17. *A*, Well-circumscribed meningioma attached to dura mater overlying left cerebral convexity. *B* and *C*, Meningothelial meningioma consists of sheets of cells, some with pseudoinclusions that are nuclear membrane invaginations of the cytoplasm. *D*, An abundance of whorls is seen with transitional meningioma. *E*, Psammomatous meningioma is characterized by abundant psammoma bodies on a background filled with whorls. (*A* from Okazaki H. Fundamentals of neuropathology: morphologic basis of neurologic disorders. 2nd ed. New York: Igaku-Shoin; 1989. p. 203-74. By permission of Mayo Foundation. *D* and *E* from Okazaki H, Scheithauer BW. Atlas of neuropathology. New York: Gower Medical Publishing; 1988. p. 131. By permission of Mayo Foundation.)

   f. Chemotherapy (including treatment with sex steroid receptor antagonists) has been disappointing

B. **Hemangioblastoma**
1. Rare vascular neoplasm (1% of all primary CNS tumors)
2. Often presents as cystic lesion of cerebellum with an enhancing nodule
3. Peak incidence: fifth to seventh decades
4. 10% of cases occur in context of von Hippel-Lindau disease (90% are sporadic)
5. Predilection for cerebellum (may also occur in spinal cord, in which it tends to cause syringomyelia)

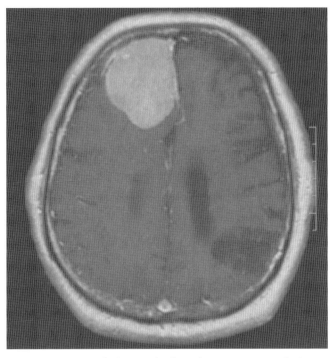

Fig. 16-18. MRI of a large right frontal meningioma with characteristic dural tail and near homogeneous enhancement (gadolinium-enhanced axial T1-weighted sequence).

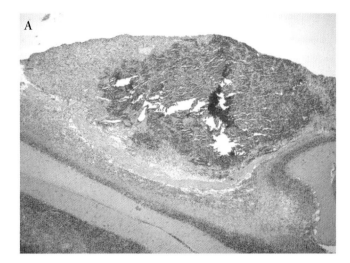

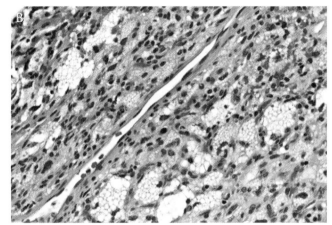

Fig. 16-19. Hemangioblastoma. *A*, Low-power view showing profoundly vascular tumor overlying the cerebellum. *B*, Fine vascular network of small capillaries and arterioles make this a vascular tumor. In the space between vascular channels are stromal cells with hyperchromatic nuclei and abundant cytoplasm containing lipids and glycogen.

6. Macroscopic features
   a. 2/3 are cystic with enhancing mural nodule
   b. 1/3 are solid
   c. Cystic wall is often lined by nonneoplastic tissue
   d. Because of the tumor's vascular nature, it may grossly appear as a red cystic mass
7. Microscopic features (Fig. 16-19)
   a. Numerous fine vascular channels
   b. In space between vascular structures are interstitial, stromal cells with hyperchromatic nuclei and abundant cytoplasm filled with lipid and glycogen
8. Neuroimaging (Fig. 16-20)
   a. Cystic lesions often appear hyperintense on T2-weighted images (hypointense to brain parenchyma on T1-weighted images), with intensely enhancing mural nodule
   b. When tumor involves spinal cord, it almost always is intramedullary, expansile lesion often associated with syrinx
9. Treatment
   a. Surgical resection may be curative; this is to include resection of mural nodule (if one is present)
   b. CSF dissemination may occur postoperatively

C. Hemangiopericytoma
1. Aggressive vascular tumor of undetermined origin, but believed to be a dural-based sarcoma
2. Is *not* a variant of meniongiomas, as once believed
3. Macroscopic features: well-circumscribed, encapsulated mass that may resemble a meningioma but is often vascular
4. Microscopic features (Fig. 16-21 *A* and *B*)
   a. Sheets of uniform cells interspersed within matrix of small capillaries and larger blood vessels with a branching, "staghorn" appearance and a dense reticulin pattern
   b. Increased mitosis, necrosis, or hemorrhage seen in

anaplastic variety

5. Neuroimaging (Fig. 16-21 *C*): strongly enhancing masses with hyperintense signal on T2-weighted images, appearing isointense to surrounding cerebral cortex on T1-weighted images, often with flow voids representing large vascular structures

6. Treatment
   a. Surgical resection
   b. Limited experience with radiation
   c. No defined role for chemotherapy
7. Recurrence rate: may be as high as 60% to 80%; may be higher with high-grade histology (rare)

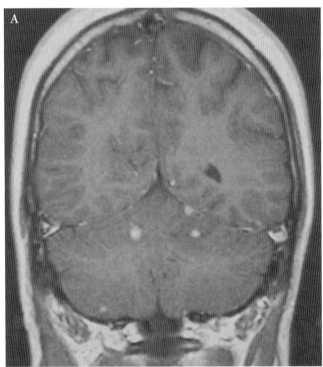

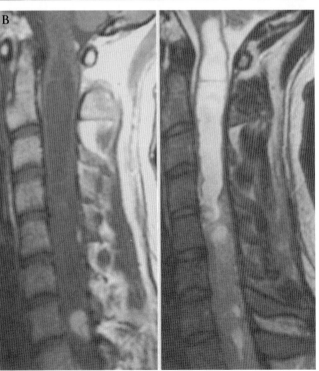

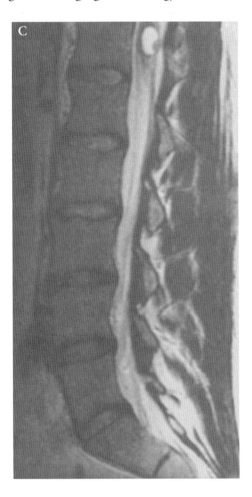

Fig. 16-20. MRI of hemangioblastoma. *A*, Gadolinium-enhanced T1-weighted image showing multiple hemangioblastomas within cerebellar hemispheres bilaterally. *B*, Sagittal MRI images (T2-weighted image on *right* and enhanced T1-weighted image on *left*) of cervical spine of patient with multiple hemangioblastomas showing strongly enhancing tumor nodule at level of vertebra C7 (*left*) and the associated large syrinx extending rostrally into the medulla (best seen on the *right*). *C*, More typical appearance is that of a cystic lesion with a tumor nodule (strongly enhancing) (T2-weighted image).

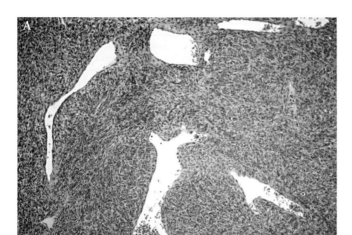

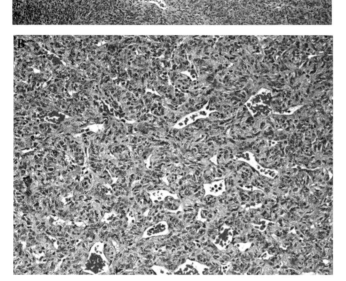

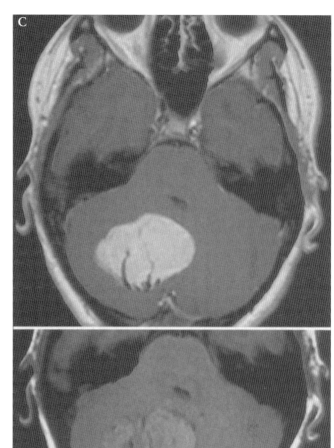

Fig. 16-21. Hemangiopericytoma. *A*, Sheets of densely packed cells with little cytoplasm are interrupted by small vascular (capillary) channels and larger vascular channels that have a branching "stag-horn" appearance, characteristic of this tumor. *B*, Higher magnification showing small vascular structures interrupting sheets of neoplastic cells. *C*, Well-circumscribed cerebellar tumor appearing isointense with the cerebellar cortex on nonenhanced T1-weighted image (*bottom*) and displaying intense enhancement on enhanced T1-weighted image (*top*), with prominent flow voids representing vascular channels.

VII. LYMPHOMA

A. Systemic Lymphoma

1. Nervous system is eventually involved in up to 10% of cases (rarely at onset of presentation) (leukemics have a very high incidence of leptomeningeal involvement [up to 70% of patients], although incidence of symptomatic cases has decreased with prophylactic CNS treatment)

2. Primary lymphoma that most commonly spreads to nervous system: usually non-Hodgkin's lymphoma

3. Nervous system involvement most commonly includes leptomeningeal spread, presenting with

   a. Cranial nerve palsies
   b. Increased intracranial pressure and associated symptoms
   c. Spinal root involvement (e.g., polyradiculopathy)

4. Systemic lymphomas that spread to the spine usually have contiguous spread into epidural space

5. CSF examination: often abnormal; first lumbar puncture is diagnostic in up to 80% of cases

B. Primary Central Nervous System Lymphoma (PCNSL)

1. Epidemiology
   a. Predilection for immunocompromised patients (most commonly AIDS)

b. Most common brain tumor in setting of AIDS; second most common intracranial lesion in this population

c. Peak incidence: sixth to seventh decades (younger peak with immunocompromised patients)

d. Male predominance (male:female = 3:2)

2. Location

a. Predilection for frontal lobes and deep periventricular regions (may access CSF and subarachnoid space)

b. Infratentorially, more often in the cerebellum than brainstem

c. Leptomeningeal involvement is eventually demonstrated in up to 40% of CSF examinations, but primary leptomeningeal lymphoma is less common

3. Association with Epstein-Barr virus (EBV)

a. Almost 100% of PCNSLs occurring in setting of AIDS are EBV-driven

b. EBV genome has been found in only 16% of PCNSLs in immunocompetent patients

c. Although EBV may induce B-cell neoplastic transformation in AIDS, it probably has little role in pathogenesis in immunocompetent patients

4. Clinical presentation

a. Symptoms at presentation depend mainly on the area involved

b. With predilection for frontal lobes, psychiatric symptoms, change in personality and behavior, and altered mentation are common

c. Other less common presentations: signs and symptoms of increased intracranial pressure, cranial nerve palsies, seizures, ataxia

5. Ocular involvement is common

a. Most patients with ocular involvement also eventually have cerebral involvement

b. Presents as chronic uveitis

c. Diagnosis can be confirmed by vitreous biopsy

6. Primary intramedullary spinal cord parenchymal involvement is rare

7. CSF should be tested for cytology, and EBV polymerase chain reaction (PCR), among other tests, to rule out conditions in differential diagnosis

8. Macroscopic features: tumor is usually well-demarcated despite microscopic infiltrative nature

9. Microscopic features (Fig. 16-22)

a. Sheets of neoplastic cells often occupy the perivascular space and tend to penetrate and destroy walls of surrounding small vessels

b. Most tumors are diffuse large B-cell lymphomas, as noted on immunohistochemistry

c. Foci of necrosis tend to be more common with diffuse large B-cell lymphomas; hemorrhagic infarcts may be

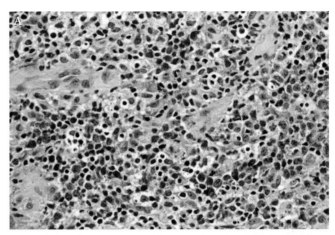

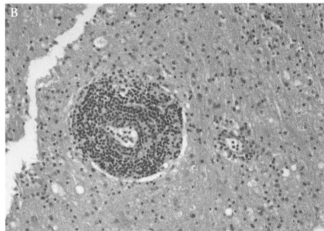

Fig. 16-22. Primary central nervous system lymphoma. *A*, Sheets of polymorphous large cells resembling immunoblasts are admixed with smaller cells resembling lymphocytes and are interrupted by areas of necrosis. *B*, Typical angiocentric pattern due to propensity of angioinvasive cells to accumulate in perivascular spaces and invade vascular walls.

seen with rare angiotropic lymphoma

10. Neuroimaging characteristics (Fig. 16-23)

a. Lesions tend to be isointense or hyperintense on T2-weighted images

b. Somewhat specific for lymphoma: mirror-image lesions in deep gray matter, including thalamus and basal ganglia

c. Immunocompromised patients: heterogeneously enhancing mass with sometimes hemorrhagic or necrotic foci

d. Immunocompetent patients: enhancement is often intense and homogeneous; ring enhancement is rare

11. Prognosis

a. Age and Karnofsky performance score are important prognostic indicators

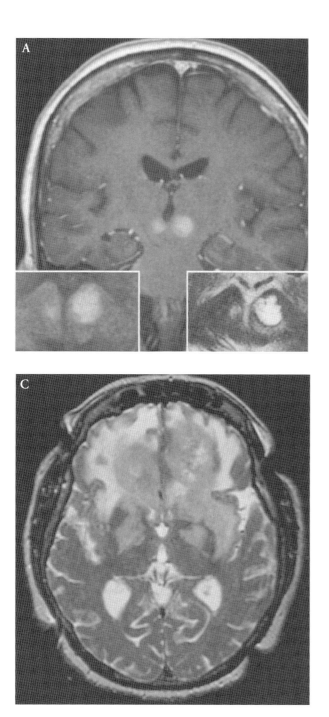

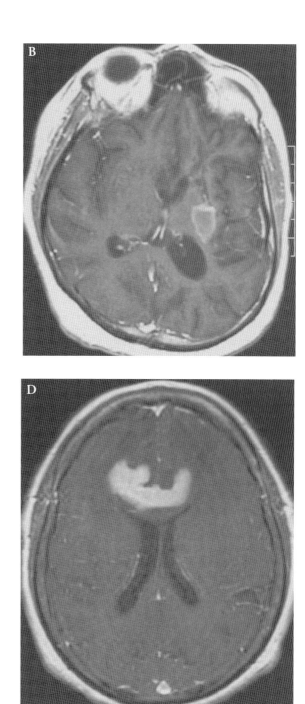

Fig. 16-23. MRI of primary central nervous system lymphoma. *A*, A 64-year-old woman with diffuse large B-cell lymphoma presented with worsening mental status. Gadolinium-enhanced T1-weighted image shows lesions in deep gray matter appearing as mirror images. Both pregadolinium T1- (*left inset*) and T2- (*right inset*) weighted images showed increased signal, suggestive of subacute hemorrhage into the mass. *B*, Gadolinium-enhanced T1-weighted image of an 18-year-old girl with diffuse large B-cell lymphoma shows ring-enhancement outlining the lesion in deep gray matter (common location for lymphoma). *C*, T2-weighted image and, *D*, gadolinium-enhanced T1-weighted image of a different patient with diffuse large B-cell lymphoma shows large intraparenchymal mass in frontal lobes bilaterally, extending through genu of corpus callosum and involving deep gray matter. There appears to be extensive perilesional vasogenic edema and mass effect on the frontal horns of the lateral ventricles.

b. Median survival is usually only 3 months without treatment

12. Treatment
   a. Characteristic ring enhancement in setting of AIDS is more common with toxoplasmosis, and patients traditionally have initially received treatment for toxoplasmosis
   b. Nonresponders usually undergo diagnostic work-up, including biopsy
   c. With recent advent of functional imaging, hypermetabolic positron emission tomography (PET) or single photon emission computed tomography (SPECT) plus positive EBV PCR are highly suggestive of lymphoma and occasionally preclude need for brain biopsy
   d. Corticosteroids
      1) Dramatic response
      2) Corticosteroids have both cytotoxic effect on lymphoma neoplastic cells and act to decrease peritumoral vasogenic edema
      3) Withhold corticosteroid therapy until diagnosis is confirmed because of unacceptable rate of false-negative results on biopsy obtained after corticosteroid therapy is initiated
   e. Chemotherapy
      1) Mainstay of treatment for PCNSL is generally systemic high-dose methotrexate
      2) Most effective agents are those with better penetrance of BBB, such as procarbazine and high-dose methotrexate and cytarabine
      3) Elderly patients are prone to neurotoxic effects of radiation, but long-term chemotherapy is also complicated by neurotoxicity, including encephalopathy
      4) Cytotoxic effects of chemotherapy makes this treatment less desirable for AIDS-associated lymphoma
      5) Despite this, combination of chemotherapy and radiotherapy has been reported to prolong survival in a proportion of AIDS patients to at least 2 years
   f. Radiation is usually saved for palliative situations

VIII. PINEAL REGION TUMORS

A. Clinical Presentations
1. Increased intracranial pressure from noncommunicating hydrocephalus such as headaches, false-localizing signs (CN VI palsy)
2. Local mass effect: compression on midbrain causing upper brainstem signs, including dorsal midbrain syndrome (Parinaud's syndrome)—loss of upward gaze and convergence, pupillary abnormalities such as nonreactive pupils
3. Extension into thalamus (may cause motor or sensory deficits) and hypothalamus (may cause diabetes insipidus, precocious puberty)

B. Germ Cell Tumors
1. Common presentations
   a. Symptoms of increased intracranial pressure
   b. Symptoms of direct brainstem and cerebellar compression
   c. Endocrine dysfunction
      1) Usually secondary to hydrocephalus or hypothalamic involvement
      2) Precocious puberty in boys may occur with tumors of syncytiotrophoblastic cells that secrete β-human chorionic gonadotropin (βhCG) (choriocarcinomas and some germinomas)
      3) Secondary sexual characteristics are due to excessive androgens secreted by Leydig cells, stimulated by βhCG
2. Germinomas
   a. Arise from developmental rests of primordial germ cells, which may occur in gonads, midline structures of CNS, or elsewhere in the body, such as mediastinum
   b. Epidemiology
      1) Commonly occur in first to third decades (almost always occur in boys)
      2) 2/3 of pineal region germ cell tumors
      3) Most common tumor in pineal region
      4) Tumors from different sites of origin are identical histologically
   c. Occur in midline: most common site is pineal gland, followed by suprasellar or hypothalamic region
   d. Diabetes insipidus: common presenting syndrome of suprasellar and hypothalamic tumors
   e. Propensity for CSF dissemination
   f. Survival rate: better than for other germ cell tumors
   g. CSF: increased placental alkaline phosphatase, and increased βhCG in 10% of cases (the latter occurs in germinomas with syncytiotrophoblastic cells and portends a slightly worse prognosis)
   h. Macroscopic features: soft, well-circumscribed midline masses that may be cystic
   i. Microscopic features: sheets of large cells with glycogen-rich clear cytoplasm and prominent nucleoli, surrounded by fibrovascular stroma containing abundant reactive T lymphocytes
   j. MRI characteristics: isointense to cerebral cortex with strong enhancement (also on contrast-enhanced computed tomography [CT])

k. Sensitive to radiotherapy and chemotherapy: almost 100% curable
3. Teratomas
   a. Male predominance
   b. Commonly occur in childhood, as with germinomas
   c. Well-circumscribed masses (lobulated, cystic) containing elements from all three embryonic cell lines (endoderm, ectoderm, mesoderm), often nonfunctional, and arranged in a haphazard way
   d. Commonly contain neural tissue
   e. Mature teratomas (predominantly adult tissue)
   f. Immature teratomas (predominantly embryonic tissue)
4. Other germ cell tumors
   a. Embryonal carcinoma
      1) Poorly differentiated carcinoma composed of sheets of large, pleomorphic, totipotential cells
      2) Elevated CSF placental alkaline phosphatase (as well as βhCG and alpha-fetoprotein)
   b. Endodermal sinus tumor (yolk sac tumor)
      1) Lacy structure, Schiller-Duval bodies, PAS-positive eosinophilic bodies
      2) CSF elevation of alpha-fetoprotein (and placental alkaline phosphatase)
   c. Choriocarcinoma
      1) Characterized by multinucleate syncytiotrophoblasts (immunoreactive for βhCG), interspersed with mononucleated syncytiotrophoblastic elements and foci of necrosis and hemorrhage: highly vascular
      2) CSF elevation of βhCG (predominantly)

C. Pineal Cell Tumors
1. Present with increased intracranial pressure or signs of brainstem compression such as Parinaud's syndrome
2. Age at presentation usually between third and fourth decades (younger age at onset of symptoms for pinealoblastomas)
3. 1/3 of cases are pineocytomas, 1/3 are pinealoblastoma, 1/3 are mixed pathology
4. Pineocytoma
   a. Benign, slow-growing firm tumor composed of mature pineal cells (small monomorphic cells) arranged in pineocytomatous rosettes, often identical to normal pineal gland histology
   b. Resembles pineal cysts on MRI
   c. CSF dissemination is rare
5. Pinealoblastoma
   a. A PNET composed of large undifferentiated pineal cells
   b. More gelatinous than pineocytoma
   c. Rarely associated with retinoblastoma in children
   d. CSF dissemination is common

D. Pineal Cysts
1. Benign, nonneoplastic
2. Often found incidentally
3. Usually observed with serial MRI studies

E. Treatment
1. Treatment of hydrocephalus with CSF shunting
2. Diagnostic stereotactic needle biopsy: predisposed to sampling error but ideal if CSF dissemination
3. Open biopsy or resection using microsurgery
4. Radiotherapy
   a. Most effective for germinomas
   b. Irradiation of entire neuroaxis indicated if CSF dissemination

IX. PITUITARY ADENOMAS (FIG. 16-24)

A. Clinical Presentation of Pituitary Region Tumors
1. Mass effect and pituitary hormone excess or deficits
2. Extension of tumor to involve cranial nerves occurs with pituitary apoplexy or aggressive tumors (not slow-growing pituitary adenomas)

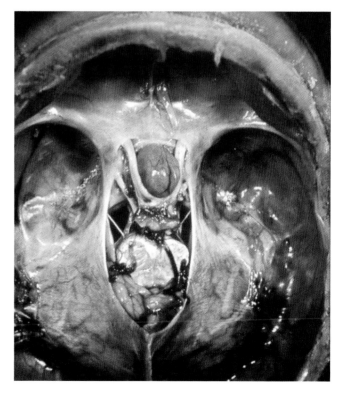

Fig. 16-24. Pituitary macroadenoma in situ (postmortem examination).

B. Pituitary Apoplexy (Fig. 16-25)
1. May occur from combination of high metabolic demand of pituitary tumor and marginal blood supply
2. Often presents as sudden onset of headaches, signs of compression of cranial nerves (ophthalmoplegia, facial pain), cavernous sinus hypertension (proptosis, chemosis), and altered mentation (especially with hydrocephalus)
3. Pituitary apoplexy may occur in normal pituitary gland or Rathke's cleft cyst
4. Sheehan's syndrome: development of apoplexy at time of delivery, possibly induced by transient hypotension and hypoperfusion of physiologically hypertrophied (and otherwise normal) pituitary gland (no underlying neoplasm)

C. Functional Classification of Pituitary Adenomas
1. With the pituitary tumors as a whole, pituitary hormonal deficits are generally more common than hormonal excess

2. Nonfunctional tumors
   a. More likely to present from mass effect
   b. May be signs of hypopituitarism: hypothyroidism, hypogonadism, diabetes insipidus, hyperprolactinemia (with pituitary stalk syndrome discussed below)
3. Functional tumors
   a. Most common: prolactinomas presenting with gynecomastia, galactorrhea, hypogonadism
   b. Nonfunctional pituitary tumors or neoplasms of other origins in this region may cause hyperprolactinemia as result of compression of pituitary stalk and reduction of hypothalamic dopaminergic inhibition of prolactin-producing cells
   c. In the latter situation, plasma prolactin level is often less than 150 ng/mL, which is less than level diagnostic of prolactinomas (>200 ng/mL)
   d. Other functional tumors present with gigantism and acromegaly (growth hormone excess before or after closure, respectively, of long-bone epiphyses), Cushing's disease (elevated corticotropin [ACTH]), etc.

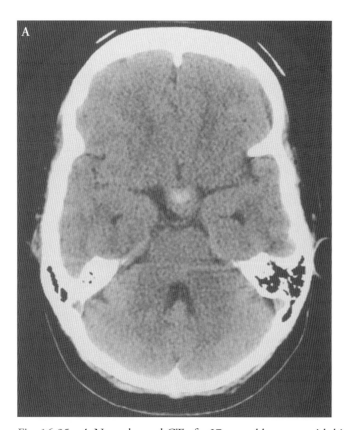
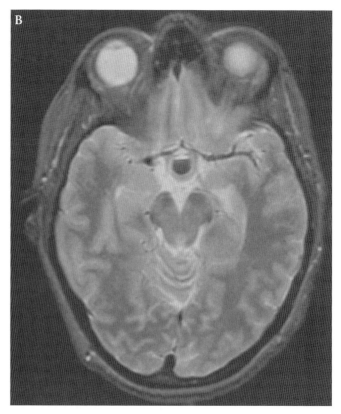

Fig. 16-25. *A*, Nonenhanced CT of a 37-year-old woman with history of sudden-onset headache, nausea, and vomiting shows area of high attenuation in sella turcica. The presentation is that of pituitary apoplexy, and the area of hyperintensity is actual hemorrhage into pituitary macroadenoma. *B*, T2-weighted MRI shows a "level" of decreased T2 signal within pituitary gland consistent with the hemorrhage.

D. Treatment
1. Specific medical treatment of hormonal disorder for functional tumors, such as dopamine agonists (e.g., bromocriptine) for prolactinomas
2. Surgery: most often initial treatment of choice, especially in treating pituitary apoplexy and macroadenomas (prolactinomas nonresponsive to medical treatment, tumors secreting excess growth hormone or ACTH)

X. Miscellaneous Brain Tumors

A. Craniopharyngiomas
1. Suprasellar mass arising from superior aspect of pituitary and believed to be an embryonal rest or remnant of Rathke's pouch, although there may be factors that promote its growth during adulthood
2. Most commonly presents in childhood (peak around 10 years of age): the most common supratentorial brain tumor in children
3. A second peak occurs in adults between fifth and sixth decades
4. Clinical presentations
   a. Signs of extension of tumor to involve optic chiasm, resulting in visual field defects (bitemporal hemianopsia)
   b. Craniopharyngiomas tend to compress optic chiasm from superior and posterior directions, compressing first the crossing nasal fibers that travel in the superior portion of optic nerve and chiasm; this may first manifest as bitemporal lower quadrantanopia, with eventual involvement of superior temporal quadrants
   c. In contrast, pituitary tumors tend to compress optic chiasm from inferior and anterior directions, compressing first the crossing nasal fibers that travel in the inferior portion of optic nerve and chiasm; this may manifest first as bitemporal upper quadrantanopia, with eventual involvement of inferior temporal quadrants
   d. Signs of increased intracranial pressure
      1) Result of extension into third ventricle
      2) Often occur in older patients
      3) Headache is most common presenting sign of hydrocephalus
   e. Endocrinopathies as a result of tumor compression of pituitary gland or pituitary stalk
   f. Chemical meningitis from seeding of craniopharyngioma cyst material into subarachnoid space: rare
5. Macroscopic features
   a. Well-delineated tumors with both cystic and solid components
   b. Solid component may contain calcifications; may be a solid mural nodule within cystic component
   c. Calcification is often confined to edge of tumor ("rim calcification")
   d. Cystic component contains dark, viscous, cholesterol-rich fluid
6. Microscopic features
   a. Adamantinomatous ("classic craniopharyngioma"): aggregates of squamous cells interspersed with cystic areas lined by stratified epithelium as well as foci of keratinized anuclear ghost-like keratinocytes (wet keratin), and calcification and "cholesterol clefts"
   b. Papillary
      1) Much less common variant, often occurs in third ventricle of adults
      2) Characterized by groups of squamous cells within connective tissue stroma, with other features of adamantinomatous craniopharyngiomas (calcification, cholesterol deposits, and keratinized foci) being much less common
7. Neuroimaging characteristics: hyperintense on T2-weighted images, with nodular or rim strong enhancement—may be due to peritumoral inflammatory response to cholesterol-rich cystic fluid (Fig. 16-26)
8. Treatment: optimally treated with surgical resection with or without radiotherapy
   a. Surgical resection
      1) Required for establishing diagnosis for decompression and treatment of mass effect, and for definitive treatment
      2) Urgent surgery is indicated for progressive compromise of vision
      3) Is often challenging because tumor adheres strongly to surrounding structures
      4) Also, cystic fluid may spill into subarachnoid space, causing chemical meningitis
   b. Radiotherapy including stereotactic radiotherapy
      1) Considered when complete surgical resection is not possible
      2) Reported complications: radiation-induced vasculopathy and endocrinopathies (may also occur with surgical resection), and long-term side effects (e.g., cognitive decline and learning disability)
9. Excellent prognosis, with survival rates more than 90% 10 years after diagnosis

B. Choroid Plexus Tumors
1. Epidemiology
   a. Less than 1% of all brain tumors
   b. May occur at any age

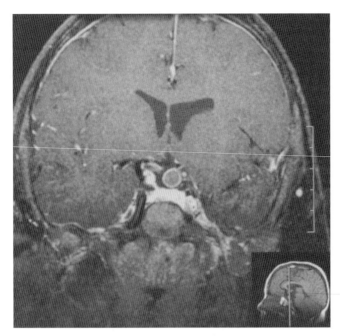

Fig. 16-26. Craniopharyngioma. Gadolinium-enhanced T1-weighted MRI shows ring-enhancing, partially cystic soft tissue nodule in left lateral aspect of suprasellar cistern. Pathologic features were consistent with craniopharyngioma. The ring enhancement may be due to peritumoral inflammatory response to cholesterol-rich cystic fluid.

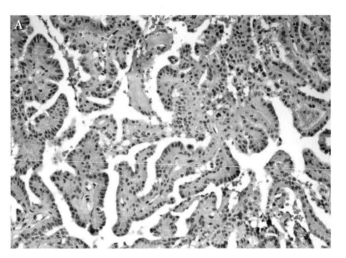

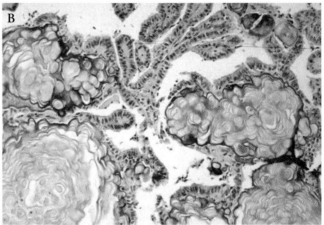

Fig. 16-27. Choroid plexus papilloma. *A*, Fibrovascular papillary structures characteristic of choroid plexus papilloma are lined with columnar epithelium. *B*, Stroma often contains foci of calcification, which is also observed on CT. (*B* from Okazaki H, Scheithauer BW. Atlas of neuropathology. New York: Gower Medical Publishing; 1988. p. 99. By permission of Mayo Foundation.)

    c. Majority of cases present in first 2 years of life
2. Location
    a. In children: predilection for lateral ventricles
    b. In adults: predilection for fourth ventricle
3. Possible association with Li-Fraumeni syndrome and von Hippel-Lindau disease
4. Pathology
    a. Choroid plexus papilloma (Fig. 16-27)
       1) Vascular well-circumscribed tumors
       2) Columnar epithelium lining fibrovascular papillary structures, characterized by increased nuclear cytoplasmic ratio and nuclear pleomorphism
       3) May be stromal calcification (may be observed on CT, see Neuroimaging below)
       4) Mitotic figures are sparse
       5) Foci of hemorrhage not uncommon
    b. Choroid plexus carcinoma
       1) Vascular, invasive tumor
       2) Highly pleomorphic cells with large number of mitotic figures and foci of necrosis
5. Most common presenting symptom: headache
6. Neuroimaging
    a. Calcification (noted on CT)

    b. Enhancing intraventricular masses
    c. Possibly flow voids reflecting tumor vascularity
7. Leptomeningeal seeding may occur
8. Often cured surgically with resection; no role for chemotherapy or radiotherapy

XI. NONNEOPLASTIC TUMORS

A. Epidermoid Tumors
1. Rare: less than 1% of primary intracranial tumors
2. May present anytime between the third and seventh decades

3. Usually developmental (inclusion of nonneoplastic ectodermal tissue formed at time of neural tube closure)

4. May be acquired (traumatic): much less common than developmental inclusion cysts, do not occur intracranially, and may be a complication of lumbar puncture when seen in the lumbosacral spine

5. Usually located off midline: predilection for cerebellopontine angle, parasellar region, and cranial diploë

6. Third most common cerebellopontine angle tumor

7. Rarely rupture, but aseptic chemical meningitis is the presentation when rupture occurs

8. Macroscopic features: pearly white lobulated surface

9. Microscopic features (Fig. 16-28): lining of keratinizing squamous epithelium containing degenerate keratinocytes and cellular debris, keratin, and crystalline cholesterol

10. Neuroimaging
   a. Usually are isointense to brain parenchyma on both T1- and T2-weighted images, but some tumors with high lipid content are hyperintense on T1-weighted images
   b. Possibly occasional peripheral enhancement

B. Dermoid Tumors

1. Usually developmental: ectodermal inclusion cyst, same as epidermoid cyst

2. Less common than epidermoid tumors

3. Age at presentation peaks between fourth and sixth decades (younger than with epidermoid tumors)

4. Usually midline location: predilection for lumbosacral spine and conus medullaris (most common), parasellar area, and midline cerebellar vermis and fourth ventricle

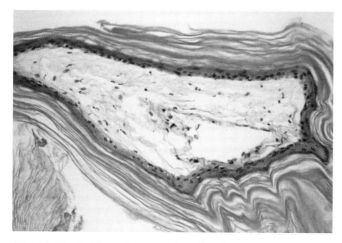

Fig. 16-28. Epidermoid cyst. Note the characteristic keratinizing squamous epithelium lining the cyst.

5. Rupture is common
   a. Tumors disseminate widely through subarachnoid space and present with aseptic meningitis
   b. Supratentorial tumors often present with headaches and seizures

6. Macroscopic features: well-circumscribed inclusion cysts with same contents as epidermoid cysts, plus occasionally hair and sebaceous and sweat glands

7. Microscopic features (Fig. 16-29): dense fibrous tissue lining outer wall and squamous epithelium with adnexal appendages (hair follicles, sebaceous and sweat glands) lining inner wall of the cyst, unlike epidermoid tumors

8. MRI characteristics: hyperintense on T1-weighted imaging, variable signal on T2-weighted imaging (signal may be heterogeneous and dependent on tumor contents)

9. Treatment: often surgical

C. Colloid Cysts

1. Round cystic mass composed of fibrous capsule and inner cuboidal or columnar epithelial surface, contains gelatinous material

2. Age at presentation in adulthood: peaks between third and fifth decades

3. Rare: less than 1% of all primary intracranial tumors

4. Location: always anterior third ventricle at foramen of Monro, between columns of fornix (Fig. 16-30)

5. Clinical presentation: often acute or recurrent hydrocephalus (blockage of foramen of Monro) often presenting with sudden-onset headaches (intermittent and onset or exacerbation with Valsalva manuever and bending down), papilledema, sometimes mental status change, drop attacks, and rarely sudden death

6. Neuroimaging characteristics: quite variable, usually nonenhancing

7. Treatment
   a. Serial neuroimaging and observation for small, asymptomatic cysts
   b. Surgical resection and ventriculoperitoneal shunt if indicated

D. Lipomas

1. Rare, benign, well-demarcated midline lesions often associated with other developmental anomalies (e.g., corpus callosum agenesis)

2. Often occur in midline and on surface of corpus callosum; may also occur as intradural or epidural spinal tumor, midline brainstem tumor, cerebellar vermis tumor

3. Microscopic appearance resembles normal adipose tissue

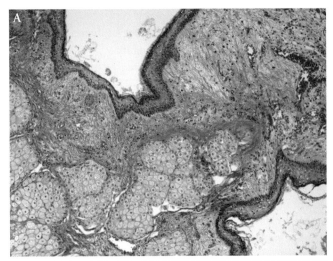

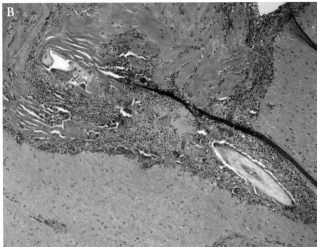

Fig. 16-29. Dermoid cysts are lined with stratified squamous cell epithelium (*A*), as are epidermoid cysts (Fig. 16-28). However, the distinguishing histologic features of dermoid cysts are the presence of sebaceous glands (*A*) and hair follicles (*B*, oblique section of hair follicle).

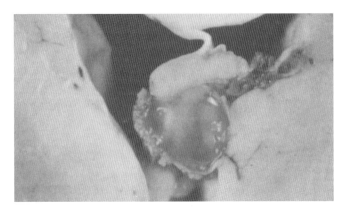

Fig. 16-30. Colloid cyst of third ventricle. (From Okazaki H. Fundamentals of neuropathology: morphologic basis of neurologic disorders. 2nd ed. New York: Igaku-Shoin; 1989. p. 203-74. By permission of Mayo Foundation.)

4. Neuroimaging: same characteristics as fat (hyperintense on T1-weighted images and hypointense on T2-weighted images) (Fig. 16-31)
5. Almost always an incidental finding: patients are asymptomatic and do not require surgical treatment

XII. SKULL-BASED TUMORS

A. Chordoma
1. Rare tumor of remnants of primitive notochord
2. Tends to occur most often at either end of notochord:

clivus and sacral-coccygeal regions (much less common elsewhere in vertebral column, often involving multiple vertebral bodies)
3. Male predominance (2:1) for the sacral-coccygeal tumors (males=females for cranial tumors)
4. Peak incidence: 50 to 60 years
5. Presentation: depends on location and extent of tumor
6. Usual presenting symptoms of clivus tumors: headaches and neck pain
7. Tumor tends to grow very slowly and extend to involve and destroy contiguous bone
   a. May involve sphenoid sinus, cavernous sinus, pituitary fossa, and diencephalon
   b. May present with cranial nerve symptoms, visual field defects, and endocrinopathies if diencephalon is involved
8. Metastasis and malignant transformation are rare and usually late when they occur; systemic metastasis to liver, lungs, and lymph nodes may occur
9. High recurrence rate
10. Microscopic features (Fig. 16-32)
    a. Vacuolated physaliphorous cells on mucinous background
    b. Chondroid chordomas often have cartilaginous foci
11. Neuroimaging
    a. Heterogeneous-appearing mass in typical locations, higher signal intensity to CSF on T2-weighted images
    b. Heterogeneous pattern of enhancement
    c. Tumors are often calcified, bony destruction is often apparent on CT
12. Treatment
    a. Combination of en bloc surgical resection and radiation
    b. Complete surgical resection is often difficult; postopera-

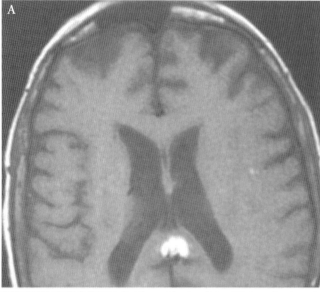

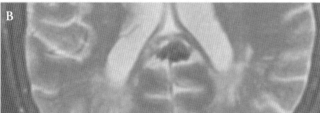

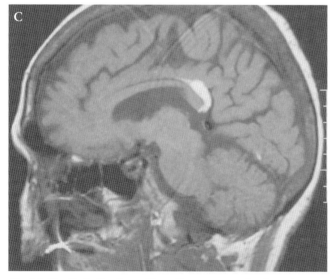

Fig. 16-31. Pericallosal curvilinear lipoma appearing hyperintense on T1-weighted image (*A* and *C*) and hypointense on T2-weighted image (*B*). *C*, Sagittal T1-weighted image better illustrates the position of the tumor, which encases the corpus callosum.

tive radiation is often needed to treat residual disease

    c. Proton beam therapy or stereotactic radiotherapy may be more effective

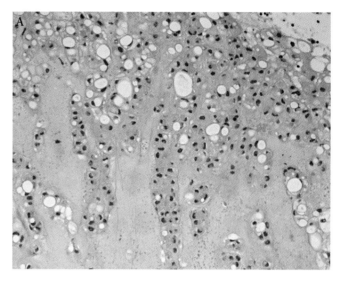

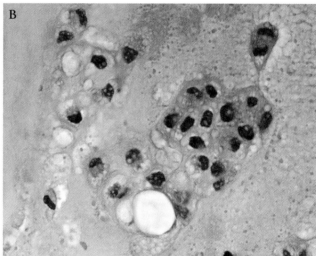

Fig. 16-32. *A*, Chordoma consists of strands of physaliphorous cells within a basophilic mucinous background. *B*, The cell cytoplasm contains vacuoles of various sizes.

B. Osteoma
1. Most common primary calvarial tumor
2. Multiple cranial osteomas may be seen in Gardner's syndrome
3. Asymptomatic tumors may simply be monitored

C. Chondrosarcoma
1. Rare
2. Predilection for temporal bone of middle cranial fossa
3. Slow-growing locally destructive cartilaginous tumor
4. Neurologic dysfunction common from involvement of bony structures around the parenchyma and cranial nerves

5. Neuroimaging
   a. MRI: hyperintense on T2-weighted images, with heterogeneous pattern of enhancement
   b. CT: calfication common
6. Treatment: total gross resection (difficult because of invasive character of tumor), followed by postoperative radiotherapy

D. Glomus Tumors

1. Paraganglioma: polyhedral cells with granular cytoplasm demarcated by fibrovascular network in richly vascular matrix
2. Slow-growing, highly vascular tumors arising from paraganglion cells
3. Presentation depends on location
   a. Glomus jugulare tumors
      1) Arise at jugular bulb
      2) Involve glossopharyngeal nerve (CN IX), vagal nerve (CN X), and spinal accessory nerve (CN XI): may present with pulsatile tinnitus
      3) May also involve adjacent facial nerve (CN VII)
      4) "Glomus jugulare" often refers to tumor arising from superior vagal ganglion; "glomus intravagale," to tumor arising from inferior vagal ganglion
   b. Glomus tympanicum tumors
      1) Associated with conductive (obstruction of external ear canal) or sensorineural hearing loss
      2) Pulsatile mass may be seen on otoscopic examination; biopsy should not be performed because of vascular nature of tumor
   c. Carotid body tumors at the carotid bifurcation: compression of internal carotid artery may cause carotid stenosis and, thus, transient ischemic attacks or infarcts
   d. Tumors of sympathetic chain and adrenal medulla: pheochromocytoma
   e. Paraganglioma of filum terminale is not categorized as a glomus tumor (discussed below, Fig. 16-33 elsewhere)
4. Occasionally, a tumor secretes catecholamines, especially norepinephrine
5. Neuroimaging
   a. Conventional angiography: vascular lesion with primary vascular supply usually from external carotid artery
   b. MRI or CT can localize the tumor and demarcate its extent
6. Treatment
   a. Surgical resection, usually immediately following ligation of feeding and draining vessels (usually external carotid artery)
   b. Preoperative embolization of main feeding arteries may be favored for richly vascular tumors

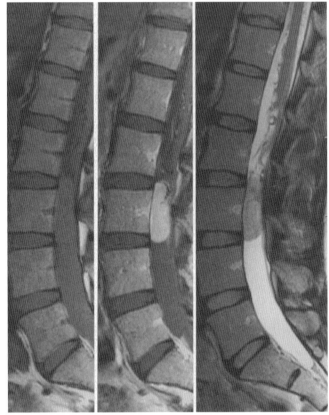

Fig. 16-33. MRI of spinal paraganglioma. Sagittal views (*left*, T1-weighted, *middle*, gadolinium enhanced T1-weighted, *right*, T2-weighted) show a uniformly enhancing intrathecal and extramedullary mass extending from level L2-3 to L3-4 within spinal canal. Note prominent tortuous flow voids above the mass.

   c. Radiotherapy is reserved as alternative for large tumors or poor surgical candidates

XIII. Neoplasms of the Spinal Cord

A. Extradural Tumors

1. Hemangioma: often involves vertebral bodies, especially lumbar and thoracic
   a. Common, slow-growing, benign tumors (most commonly, cavernous hemangioma) appearing as high signal on T1- and T2-weighted images
   b. Vascular and fatty stroma
   c. Most tumors are asymptomatic, may cause pathologic compression fracture of vertebral bodies, compression of spinal cord
2. Osteoid osteomas

a. Benign lesions of young patients, male predominance

b. Predilection for neural arch of vertebrae (most commonly, lumbar)

3. Osteochondromas: common tumors with predilection for the spinous and transverse processes

4. Aneurysmal bone cysts

   a. Rare

   b. Often occur in first two decades

   c. Benign, multiloculated, expansile, vascular osteolytic nonneoplastic lesions

   d. Frequently involve long bones and posterior elements of cervical and thoracic spine

   e. Neurologic manifestations such as spinal cord compression from expansile mass are rare

5. Epidural lipomatosis: excessive deposition of epidural fat, often occur with chronic corticosteroid use, frequently resolve after discontinuation of corticosteroid use

6. Lymphomas: extradural lymphoma, often non-Hodgkin lymphoma with contiguous spread (see above)

7. Sarcomas

8. Chordomas

9. Nerve sheath tumors: may be extradural (paraspinous "dumbbell-shaped"), but most often intradural extramedullary tumors (see below)

10. Epidural metastases are the most common spinal tumors in the elderly

B. Intradural Extramedullary Tumors

1. Extramedullary tumors can cause radicular pain or vertebral pain (focal pain localized to area of spinal cord compression by the tumor); extramedullary lesions may also cause Brown-Séquard syndrome

2. Nerve sheath tumors: most common intradural extramedullary tumors

   a. Neurofibroma, schwannoma, ganglioneuroma, neurofibrosarcoma

   b. Symptoms depend on location; are often radiculopathic, myelopathic

3. Neuroimaging: hyperintense on T2-weighted images, strong enhancement apparent on T1-weighted images with contrast (periphery of tumor may be more intensely enhancing than the center)

   a. Because of the chronicity and slow growth of the tumors, osseous changes such as erosion and enlargement of neural foramina may be seen

   b. Schwannomas may have a cystic component and, less frequently, a hemorrhagic or necrotic component

4. Meningiomas

a. Predilection for thoracic spine

b. Neurologic manifestations depend on location of tumor and rate of growth and degree of displacement of spinal cord and roots

5. Paragangliomas

   a. Arise from filum terminale or one of lumbosacral roots of cauda equina

   b. Well-encapsulated, highly vascular tumors appearing hyperintense on T2-weighted images and strongly enhance on T1-weighted images with contrast, with flow voids (which enhance with contrast) above and below tumor (Fig. 16-33)

   c. Pathology: well-encapsulated vascular neoplasm; sheets of uniform cells with granular cytoplasm surrounded by delicate fibrovascular network (Fig. 16-34)

6. Dermoid tumors (see above)

   a. Congenital midline cystic lesion often occurring in lumbosacral spine and conus medullaris

   b. May be intramedullary or intradural extramedullary tumor

   c. Same appearance as fat on neuroimaging

7. Epidermoid (see above)

   a. Congenital or acquired (trauma or late complication of lumbar puncture)

   b. Symptomatic cases present with radiculopathies and gait abnormalities

C. Intradural Intramedullary Tumors

1. Ependymomas

   a. Most common intramedullary spine tumor in adults

   b. Myxopapillary ependymoma: most common tumor of filum terminale and cauda equina

   c. Well-demarcated slow-growing tumors, may erode bone

   d. May have cystic or hemorrhagic components

   e. Myxopapillary ependymomas arise from ependymal cells in fibrous band of filum terminale

   f. Cellular ependymomas arise most often from cervical cord

   g. Clinical presentation

      1) Back pain (most common), neck pain, sphincter dysfunction, dysesthesias, leg weakness

      2) Funicular (central) pain characteristic of intramedullary expansile masses: deep and poorly localized dysesthetic discomfort that may be related to involvement of spinothalamic tracts or dorsal columns

   h. Ependymomas arise around the central canal and often cause a centrifugal intramedullary expansion of spinal cord

      1) This expansile mass can involve the crossing fibers of spinothalamic tracts (pain and temperature sensations) and cause dysesthesias in upper extremities

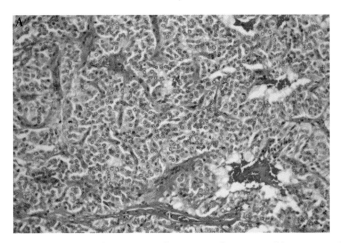
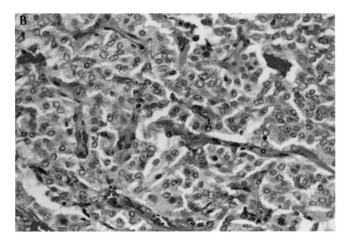

Fig. 16-34. *A* and *B*, Paragangliomas are characterized by groups of homogeneous-appearing cells encased within a sinusoidal vascular network of capillaries (better seen at highter magnification in *B*).

2) Involvement of corticospinal tracts and upper motor neuron signs occur late in the course
3) Capelike loss of pain and temperature senstation in upper extremities may be seen in cervical cord lesions
4) Sacral-sparing sensory loss occurs with more extensive lesions sparing far laterally located sacral spinothalamic fibers
5) With involvement of dorsal column, vibratory sensation is involved often more than joint position sensation
i. Myxopapillary ependymomas may cause urinary incontinence and saddle anesthesia; tumors of cauda equina can also impair neurologic function in distribution of a single root
j. MRI characteristics
1) Isointense with spinal cord on T1-weighted images and hyperintense on T2-weighted images; enhancement is heterogeneous and intense
2) Commonly a rim of hypointense signal surrounding the intramedullary tumor on T2-weighted images
k. Tend not to invade adjacent normal tissue and may be easily resected or debulked, in contrast to more infiltrative astrocytomas
l. Postresection radiotherapy may be given for residual tumors but usually is not recommended
2. Astrocytomas
a. Most common intramedullary spine tumors in children (twice as common as ependymomas in children)
b. Intratumoral cystic component or syringomyelia in up to 40% of tumors
c. Most are low grade and slow growing (in contrast to intracranial astrocytomas)

d. Cervical cord (then thoracic) is most common site
e. Most common presentation: focal axial pain, followed by weakness and paresthesias
f. MRI characteristics: hyperintense T2 lesions, heterogeneous pattern of enhancement (almost all enhance, even low-grade astrocytomas, in contrast to intracranial astrocytomas)
3. Intramedullary metastasis
a. Most often affects conus medullaris
b. Small cell lung carcinoma, breast cancer, lymphoma, colorectal carcinoma, renal cell carcinoma
c. Prognosis: usually poor

D. Treatment
1. Surgical resection: generally the mainstay treatment, even for intramedullary tumors, because of avascular character of tumors and well-defined surgical resection planes
2. Radiotherapy: often not recommended; prognosis is generally good

XIV. PERIPHERAL NERVE TUMORS

A. Schwannomas
1. Epidemiology
a. Most common nerve sheath tumors
b. Benign (often single) tumors
c. Peak incidence in fourth to fifth decades of life
d. Higher incidence in women
2. Usually present as asymptomatic, often superficial and palpable mass with Tinel's sign (pain less common)

3. May arise from
   a. Cranial nerve
      1) Most common: CN VIII, "acoustic neuroma," an enhancing lesion that may or may not have cystic component
      2) Bilateral acoustic neuromas are suggestive of NF2
   b. Spinal nerve root
      1) Extramedullary intradural (sometimes extradural), appear as dumbbell-shaped tumor as it encases spinal cord and expands through foramina bilaterally
      2) Spinal schwannomas may occur at multiple levels in patients with NF2
      3) Signs and symptoms of radiculopathy, myelopathy, etc.
   c. More distal peripheral nerve location
   d. Plexiform schwannomas are usually cutaneous in location and rare
4. High-resolution MRI may aid in defining presence of the tumor and anatomic location
5. Pathology (Fig. 16-35)
   a. Macroscopic features
      1) Well-encapsulated, nodular growths appearing to encase one or two nerve fascicles, displacing the remaining fascicles
      2) May be lobulated or cystic
      3) Plexiform schwannomas may involve multiple fascicles
   b. Microscopic features
      1) Antoni A pattern (spindle-shaped cells arranged in compact fascicles with dense reticulin) and Antoni B pattern (stellate- or spindle-shaped cells arranged in loose, myxomatous, microcystic stroma with sparse reticulin), and Verocay bodies (appearing as columns of nuclei present in the palisading arrangement of Antoni A pattern)
      2) May be hyalinized, thickened blood vessels
6. Treatment
   a. Asymptomatic tumors may be followed with serial imaging; resection is considered if there is growth or increasing neurologic symptoms; recurrence is rare
   b. Malignant transformation of the tumor is rare (much less common than that of neurofibroma)

B. Neurofibromas
1. Higher incidence in women
2. Often present with pain, dysesthesias, or paresthesias in the distribution involved nerve, often with Tinel's sign
3. May be cutaneous or plexiform (intraneural)
4. Associated with NF1
5. Macroscopic features (Fig. 16-36 A)

   a. Likely arise from perineural fibroblasts
   b. Well-circumscribed (but not encapsulated)
   c. A tumor intimately infiltrates the nerves from which it arises
   d. Tumors often appear as symmetric, fusiform nerve expansions (rather than well-encapsulated nodular schwannomas that displace nerve fascicles)
6. Microscopic features (Fig. 16-36 B)
   a. Haphazard arrangement of spindle-shaped cells in myxomatous-mucoid stroma or in between collagen fibers, infiltrating nerve fascicles (not displacing them as do schwannomas)
   b. Blood vessels tend to be less hyalinized and thickened than schwannomas
7. High-resolution MRI may help define presence and anatomic localization of tumor
8. Asymptomatic lesions that remain stable need to be followed because they can undergo malignant transformation (5%-10% of tumors)
9. Low threshold for surgical resection is often practiced for symptomatic tumors (pain, neurologic deficits) or for growing tumors

C. Neurothekomas
1. Benign, slow-growing soft, mobile nerve sheath tumors often located in the dermis, may originate from Schwann cells or perineural cells
2. Peak incidence: first three decades of life
3. Recurrence is rare

D. Intraneural Perineuromas (Fig. 16-37)
1. Rare, benign masses arising in extremities
2. Peak incidence: first two decades of life
3. Patients may present with motor mononeuropathy
4. Affected nerve becomes enlarged
5. Microscopic features: intrafascicular proliferation of perineurial cells appearing to surround single nerve fibers, forming pseudo-onion bulbs
6. Curative treatment: complete resection

E. Malignant Nerve Sheath Tumors
1. May arise de novo or from malignant transformation (usually of plexiform neurofibroma, much less commonly schwannoma)
2. Associated with NF1
3. Usual presentation: pain, often with progressive neurologic deterioration and rapidly growing mass
4. Treatment
   a. Wide local resection (limb amputation may be needed)
   b. External radiotherapy (with or without chemotherapy)

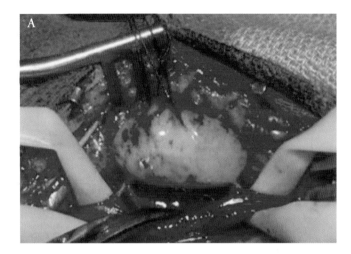

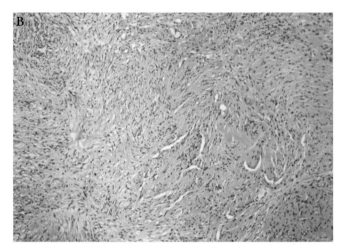

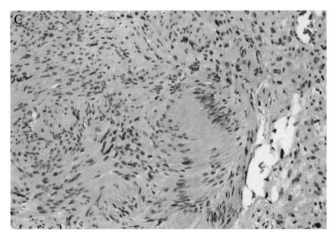

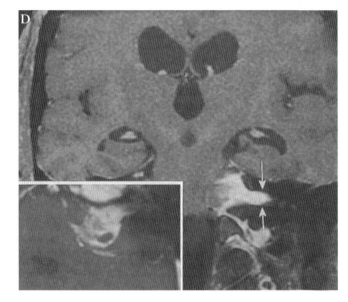

Fig. 16-35. Schwannoma. *A*, Schwannoma in situ appearing as well-encapsulated mass encasing nerve fascicle adjacent to preserved main nerve trunk. *B*, Histopathologic features include random Antoni A pattern (*right*) and Antoni B pattern (*left*) of cell arrangement. Antoni A pattern refers to palisading arrangement of spindle-shaped cells with elongated nuclei within tightly packed fascicles. Antoni B pattern is more loose, random arrangment of spindle-shaped cells within microcystic and myxoid background. *C*, Verocay bodies are columns of spindle-shaped cells with nuclear palisading, characteristically in Antoni A areas. *D*, Typical MRI features of acoustic neuroma (vestibular schwannoma). This tumor is in left cerebellopontine angle and enlarges left internal auditory canal (*vertical arrows*). (There is intense, heterogeneous enhancement of the tumor on contrast-enhanced T1-weighted image [*A* courtesy of Robert J. Spinner, MD.])

5. Prognosis
    a. High recurrence rate despite therapy
    b. 5-year survival rate: 10% to 50%
    c. Distal metastasis is rare
    d. Patients with NF1 usually have worse prognosis

XV. METASTASIS

A. Most Common Intracranial Tumor of Adults

B. Skull Metastases

1. Most common tumors to metastasize to skull (in descending order of frequency): breast, lung, prostate, renal, thyroid, melanoma
2. Half of cases are asymptomatic (especially calvarial-based metastases)
3. Calvarial metastases may produce focal neurologic symptoms related to focal area of involvement
4. Invasion of cerebral venous sinuses predisposes to veno-occlusive disease and related complications such as venous infarction and increased intracranial pressure
5. Tumor extent and involvement of underlying parenchyma

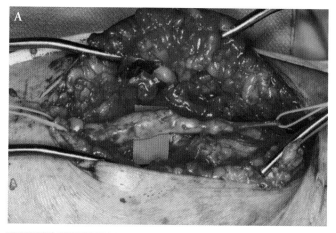

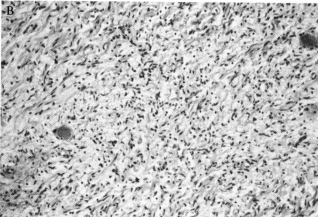

Fig. 16-36. Neurofibroma. *A*, Neurofibroma in situ. Note fusiform enlargement of affected nerve from infiltrative nature of tumor (sural nerve; *left*, proximal; *right*, distal). *B*, Histopathologic features include haphazard arrangement of spindle-shaped wavy cells in myxomatous and mucoid stroma or in between collagen fibers. (*A* courtesy of Robert J. Spinner, MD.)

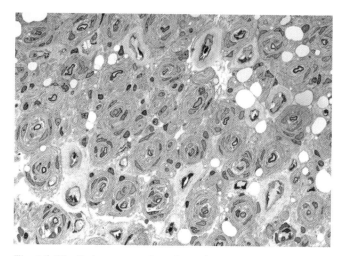

Fig. 16-37. Perineuroma. Intrafascicular proliferation of perineurial cells appear to surround single nerve fibers, forming pseudo-onion bulbs.

are better delineated with gadolinium-enhanced MRI
6. Radiotherapy often used for symptomatic patients

C. **Dural Metastases**
1. Often extension of adjacent calvarial metastasis
2. Most common cancers to cause dural metastasis: non–small cell carcinoma, prostate cancer, breast cancer
3. Often become symptomatic by compressing adjacent parenchyma or venous sinuses or by producing subdural hygromas or fluid collections
4. Treatment
   a. Often focal radiotherapy
   b. Whole-brain radiation reserved for leptomeningeal metastasis

c. Surgical resection is often indicated for large symptomatic tumors

D. **Leptomeningeal Metastases**
1. Often associated with solid tumors (especially adenocarcinomas such as breast, lung, and gastrointestinal), non-Hodgkin's lymphoma, and leukemia
2. May arise from hematogenous (or alternatively, epidural) spread
3. Once leptomeninges are involved, metastatic cells can spread via CSF; have a propensity for cauda equina and basal cisterns because of gravity and slow CSF flow
4. Tumor cells may invade Virchow-Robin spaces; with extensive perivascular infiltration, tumor nodules may take on a "miliary" pattern
5. When subarachnoid space is involved, presentation is often that of carcinomatous meningitis, symptoms related to cranial nerve (most commonly CNs III, IV, and VI) or spinal root (most commonly lumbosacral) involvement, and hydrocephalus, which may result from occlusion of CSF outflow by tumor cells
6. Positive CSF cytologic findings are diagnostic and helpful; may also occur with parenchymal metastases without leptomeningeal involvement
   a. CSF examination yield can be increased from 50% with first lumbar puncture to about 90% with repeated punctures
   b. In other 10% of cases, malignant cells are often strongly adherent to leptomeninges and do not shed into CSF

E. Parenchymal Metastases

1. 80% of metastases occur supratentorially and 20% infratentorially (distribution of cerebral blood supply)
2. Up to 75% of patients have neuroimaging evidence of multiple metastases at presentation
   a. This value was almost 50% before widespread use of MRI
   b. Lung cancer and melanoma are most likely to produce multiple metastases
   c. Renal cell carcinoma, breast cancer, and colon cancer are most likely to produce single brain metastasis
3. Retroperitoneal, pelvic, gastrointestinal primary tumors have predilection for posterior fossa
4. For patients presenting with brain metastasis with no known primary tumor
   a. Most common type of primary neoplasm: non–small cell carcinoma
   b. Next most common: breast cancer, small cell carcinoma, malignant melanoma (second, third, and fourth most common, respectively)
   c. These are followed by renal cell carcinoma and gastrointestinal tract cancers
5. Most common tumor with metastasis to brain in children: neuroblastoma, Wilms' tumor, sarcomas
6. Neoplasm with highest tendency for CNS metastasis: malignant melanoma
7. Metastasis occurs with hematogenous spread and typically land at gray matter–white matter junction because of abrupt change in blood vessel caliber
8. Except for certain neoplasms such as malignant melanomas that can penetrate arterial (arteriolar) walls and are often hemorrhagic, most tumors usually penetrate capillary beds to arrive at their destination
9. Malignant melanoma, choriocarcinoma, non–small cell lung carcinoma, and renal cell carcinoma are most common metastatic malignancies that have a tendency to present as hemorrhagic lesions
10. Clinical presentation
    a. Incidental finding in about 1/3 of patients
    b. Is variable and dependent mainly on tumor location
    c. Includes unilateral weakness, focal seizures, etc.

Primary cancers that commonly metastasize to the spinal cord (in order of occurrence): lung (49%), breast (15%), lymphoma (9%), colorectal (7%), renal (6%), and head and neck tumors (6%)

d. Headache is most common complaint; is sometimes due to increased intracranial pressure from hydrocephalus
e. Altered sensorium and hemiparesis are most common clinical sings on presenting examination
f. Other symptoms: gait ataxia and dysarthria
g. Onset of symptoms: subacute or chronic, progressive; sometimes, acute onset due to hemorrhage, seizure, transient ischemic attack, or cerebral infarction (marantic [nonbacterial] endocarditis, hypercoagulability with arterial or venous thrombotic disease)
h. Dural-based metastatic tumors may invade venous sinuses, predisposing to veno-occlusive disease
11. Neuroimaging characteristics (Fig 16-38)
    a. Single or multiple lesions at the gray matter–white matter junction with various degrees of surrounding vasogenic edema, hemorrhage, or necrosis
    b. Most often appear hyperintense on T2-weighted images and hypointense on T1-weighted images (except for hemorrhage)
    c. Most metastases strongly enhance (often ring enhancement, sometimes enhancement of entire lesion, which is frequently heterogeneous)

F. Management of Metastatic Neoplasm

1. All patients with single (or multiple) brain tumor should have metastatic work-up to search for primary tumor
2. Morbidity and mortality may be less if tissue biopsy specimens are obtained from primary extracranial tumor instead of brain
3. Goal of treatment: improve quality of life and improve or stabilize neurologic condition
4. Corticosteroid therapy (lymphoma must be reasonably excluded)
   a. Reduces peritumoral vasogenic edema and induces rapid improvement in symptoms
   b. Corticosteroids improve median survival by 1 or 2 months and should always be used
   c. Many authorities prefer dexamethasone to other corticosteroids
5. Except for metastatic melanoma, tumors involving motor cortex, and parenchymal tumors with leptomeningeal involvement, anticonvulsant therapy is often not indicated as prophylactic treatment
6. Treatment often involves resection of surgically accessible single lesion, followed by radiation
7. Radiotherapy
   a. Marginal improvement in overall survival rates
   b. Important role in tumor shrinkage and palliation
   c. Whole-brain radiation often given to patients with

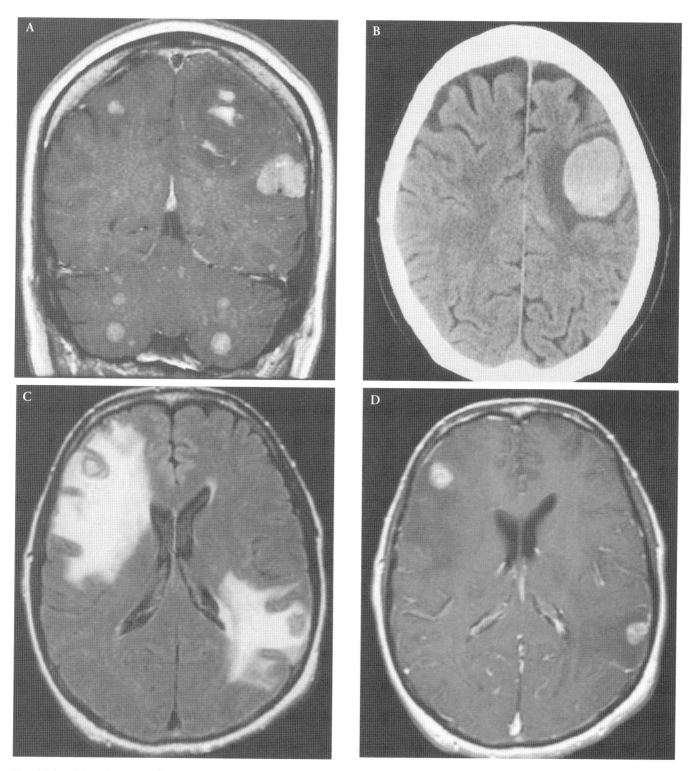

Fig. 16-38. Neuroimaging of metastatic cancer shows single or multiple enhancing lesions at junction of gray and white matter with various degrees of surrounding vasogenic edema, hemorrhage, or necrosis. *A*, Gadolinium-enhanced coronal T1-weighted image of metastatic melanoma shows numerous enhancing masses throughout brain. *B*, Unenhanced CT of a different patient with metastatic melanoma shows subacute hemorrhage into the metastatic focus at parasagittal posterior left frontal cortex. *C*, Axial FLAIR and, *D*, enhanced axial T1-weighted images show two enhancing foci of metastasis at junction of gray and white matter, with surrounding vasogenic edema The primary tumor was metastatic lung adenocarcinoma.

radiosensitive tumors with multiple metastases such as non–small cell carcinoma of lung

d. Prophylactic cranial radiation reduces risk of metastasis and increases survival rates; should be considered for radiosensitive tumors that commonly metastasize, such as small cell lung carcinoma

e. Stereotactic radiosurgery
  1) Prolongs survival similar to surgical resection and radiotherapy
  2) May be used for surgically inaccessible lesions
  3) Not ideal for large or radioresistant tumors

f. Recent clinical studies by RTOG group have suggested that whole-brain radiation combined with stereotactic radiation to tumor bed is superior (survival) to whole-brain radiation alone; however, survival advantage, although statistically significant, is marginal at best in practical terms

8. Chemotherapy
  a. Questionable role
  b. Sometimes not effective because patient may have already received chemotherapy for treatment of primary tumor
  c. Temozolomide, with high CNS penetration, is sometimes used for brain metastases

9. Small cell lung carcinoma: surgical resection, radiotherapy, prophylactic cranial radiation, and possibly chemotherapy

10. Non–small cell lung carcinoma and breast cancer
  a. Surgical resection for single, surgically accessible metastasis, followed by radiation (continuing controversy about whole-brain radiation vs. stereotactic radiation vs. both)
  b. Radiation without surgical resection for multiple metastases

11. Melanoma
  a. Surgical resection for single, accessible tumors
  b. This may be followed by postoperative radiotherapy, which may be palliative and slow neurologic progression, despite radioresistance of the tumors
  c. Melanoma tends to be chemotherapy-resistant

12. Multiple metastases
  a. Whole-brain radiation is typically recommended; however, can consider stereotactic radiation of individual lesions, depending on number of lesions or targets
  b. Surgical resection (as palliative treatment) of symptomatic lesions may improve quality of life and survival

XVI. COMPLICATIONS OF CHEMOTHERAPY

A. Cisplatin
1. Platinum-based alkylating agent, renally excreted, may cause renal toxicity
2. Neurotoxicity
  a. Peripheral neuropathy and ganglionopathy (predominantly sensory neuropathy with evidence of axonal loss with demyelinating features, affecting both peripheral nerves and dorsal root ganglia)
  b. Ototoxicity and vestibulopathy
  c. Lhermitte's sign in absence of other myelopathic features
  d. Rarely, reversible leukoencephalopathy

B. Methotrexate
1. Antifolate agent that acts to inhibit dihydrofolate reductase; may cause kidney or liver toxicity
2. Used in treatment of PCNSL, primary sarcomas of CNS, leptomeningeal metastasis
3. Neurotoxicity: aseptic meningitis (with intrathecal administration), acute encephalopathy (may be marked by transient symptoms, normal MRI, slow electroencephalogram [EEG]), chronic leukoencephalopathy (most common delayed complication with variable degrees of dementia, diffuse white matter disease and atrophy), and myelopathy

C. Cytarabine (cytosine arabinoside, ARA-C)
1. Pyrimidine analogue; active metabolite inhibits DNA polymerase A and chain elongation
2. Used to treat lymphoma, leptomeningeal carcinomatosis, leptomeningeal lymphoma; intrathecal administration ideal for leptomeningeal neoplastic disease
3. Neurotoxicity
  a. Acute cerebellar syndrome with variable degrees of ataxia occurs in 10% to 25% of cases
  b. Aseptic (chemical) meningitis and reversible myelopathy with intrathecal route are rare

D. Vinca Alkaloids (e.g., vincristine)
1. Mechanism of action: inhibition of microtubule assembly and arrest of cell cycle
2. Effective for lymphomas, leukemia, sarcomas; vincristine used in oligodendrogliomas (vincristine is part of PCV regimen for oligodendroglial tumors)
3. Neurotoxicity
  a. Primarily axonal sensorimotor peripheral neuropathy, often painful neuropathies
  b. Vincristine may also produce autonomic neuropathy, cranial neuropathies, and, less commonly, syndrome of inappropriate antidiuretic hormone secretion (SIADH) and related hyponatremia
  c. Vinblastine, vindesine, and vinorelbine are less toxic

E.   Fluorouracil (5 FU)
1. Inhibits thymidylate synthase and disrupts DNA synthesis
2. Used to treat breast cancer and colon cancer
3. Neurotoxicity
   a. 5% of patients may have acute cerebellar syndrome characterized by acute onset of appendicular and axial/midline (gait) ataxia (including cerebellar dysarthria, which may occur several weeks to months after initiation of treatment)
   b. These symptoms usually are completely reversible with discontinuation of the agent

F.   Procarbazine
1. Part of PCV regimen for oligodendroglial tumors
2. Inhibitor of monoamine oxidase; may not be used concomitantly with tyramine-rich diet or tricyclic antidepressants
3. Oral dose may produce mild reversible encephalopathy and intravenous route may yield severe encephalopathy
4. Other side effects include peripheral neuropathy and autonomic neuropathy
5. These adverse effects are usually transient and/or reversible

G.   Nitrosoureas
1. Lipid-soluble alkylating agents that easily cross BBB
2. Carmustine (BCNU), lomustine (CCNU)
3. May be used in treatment of high-grade gliomas or glioblastoma and lymphoma
4. High-dose intravenous carmustine may cause encephalomyelopathy and seizures
5. Intra-arterial carmustine may cause retinopathy and blindness, headaches, and progressive encephalopathy

XVII. Complications of Radiotherapy

A.   Usually Dose-Dependent
1. Total dose, daily fractions, and treatment duration are proportional to radiation-induced injury in sigmoid-shaped curve (small increments above critical level greatly increase rate of cerebral necrosis)

B.   Encephalopathy
1. Acute
   a. Sudden onset of altered mental status, headache, fever, and possibly worsening of neurologic deficits attributable to tumor
   b. Presumably result of diffuse edema, and tends to occur in patients with large tumors receiving high doses of whole-brain radiotherapy
   c. Acute encephalopathy should be treated with high doses of dexamethasone
   d. Prophylaxis includes administration of dexamethasone to patients with large tumors before large doses of whole-brain radiation
2. Early delayed
   a. Characterized by worsening of neurologic function, headaches, fever, somnolence, several months after completion of radiotherapy
   b. This is characterized by worsening edema and mass effect, sometimes with increased enhancement
   c. This complication usually occurs about 3 to 8 weeks after completion of radiotherapy
3. Late delayed
   a. Chronic progressive dementia with deficits primarily of attention and problem-solving, also gait disturbance, occasionally diffuse atrophy, ventriculomegaly, white matter changes
   b. Changes in neuroimaging characteristics accumulate over time
   c. This complication usually occurs approximately 16 to 18 months after the completion of radiotherapy
   d. Less common delayed complication is focal cerebral necrosis, which usually occurs at the site of tumor

C.   Myelopathy
1. Acute myelopathy due to spinal cord infarction
2. Transient myelopathy
   a. Usually occurs about 3 to 6 months after completion of radiotherapy (range, 1-30 months)
   b. Symptoms often limited to Lhermitte's sign and paresthesias in the extremities
   c. Transient syndrome with good prognosis
   d. Patients receiving 4,000 cGy to spinal cord are at higher risk
3. Delayed myelopathy
   a. Gradual onset of symptoms often about 14 months (4 months-19 years) after completion of radiotherapy: sensory symptoms in the legs (paresthesias and dysesthesias), followed by urinary incontinence and weakness
   b. Most patients experience *progressive* weakness and some become paraplegic or quadriplegic
   c. MRI shows spinal cord enlargement and edema, with abnormal intramedullary T2 hyperintensity and sometimes enhancement
   d. With chronic myelopathy and progression, spinal cord may atrophy
   e. Higher risk associated with higher dosage per fraction and total dose

D. Optic Neuropathy

1. Usually delayed onset (about 1 year) of rapidly progressive painless severe vision loss (reduced visual acuity or visual fields, monocular or binocular) in patients receiving radiation to orbits, paraorbital regions, or pituitary region or stereotactic radiosurgery

E. Motor Lumbosacral Polyradiculopathy and Lower Motor Neuron Syndrome

1. Subacute onset and gradual progression of unilateral or bilateral leg weakness with atrophy and fasciculations
2. Occurs about 4 months to 1 year after completion of spinal radiotherapy
3. Often, progression eventually reaches plateau

XVIII. PARANEOPLASTIC SYNDROMES

A. General Principles and Definitions

1. Broadest definition: any indirect effects of systemic malignancy, including vascular disorders, side effects of chemotherapy, metabolic disorder, or nutritional deficiency
2. More exclusively, a clinical syndrome produced by remote effect of a systemic malignancy that cannot be attributed to direct invasion by tumor or its metastasis, infection, ischemia, surgery, related metabolic or nutritional disorder, or toxic effects of therapy
3. Two broad categories of paraneoplastic syndrome in its most exclusive definition
   a. Paraneoplastic syndromes related to ectopic hormone production (e.g., SIADH, ACTH)
   b. Paraneoplastic neurologic syndromes (focus of the rest of this section)
4. Rare
   a. Much less common than metastatic disease
   b. About 0.01% of cancer patients, but as many as 3% of patients with small cell lung carcinoma
5. Median age at onset: about 65 years
6. Strong female predominance (female:male = 2:1), even if sex-specific tumors are excluded
7. Subacute presentation of typical syndrome is a clue: worsening over weeks to months, but more rapid progression (over a few days) or more insidious course may occur
8. Clinical syndromes are often multifocal in localization; clinical manifestations are heterogeneous
9. Clinical syndromes may be
   a. Indistinguishable from common neurologic syndromes (e.g., peripheral neuropathy, myasthenia gravis) *or*
   b. Very characteristic of a particular paraneoplastic syndrome to prompt aggressive search for occult malignancy (e.g., limbic encephalitis or paraneoplastic cerebellar degeneration)
10. Identical syndromes may occur in absence of cancer (e.g., sensory neuronopathy due to Sjögren's syndrome)
11. Neurologic syndrome is often the presenting symptoms of an underlying occult malignancy (predates the diagnosis of cancer), and an initial comprehensive search for malignancy may be unrevealing
12. Neurologic syndrome generally occurs when malignancy is in a limited stage: an effective anti-tumor immune response or earlier diagnosis; patients with paraneoplastic syndromes appear to have more favorable oncological outcome than those with similar stage tumors
13. Paraneoplastic syndrome may also herald recurrence of a known malignancy or develop after treatment of malignancy (not attributed to the treatment by the strict definition)
14. Often cause severe and permanent neurologic morbidity
15. Must be considered in differential diagnosis of a neurologic syndrome in a patient with known underlying cancer
16. Response of neurologic syndrome to treatment is often unsatisfactory
17. Early diagnosis is essential for more successful treatment of underlying malignancy and better neurologic outcome (high index of suspicion is required)

B. Proposed Pathogenesis

1. Neuroendocrine tumors may express neuronal nuclear, cytoplasmic, or membrane proteins that serve as antigens triggering autoimmune phenomenon
2. Immune system identifies cancer and mounts an immune response against malignant cells: response is both cell-mediated and humoral, although cytotoxic T cells appear to be primary mediators
3. Once activated, immune system may target normal cells (in nervous system) as well as malignant cells
4. Often a personal or family history of autoimmunity and higher incidence of other autoantibodies
5. Autoimmune attack is specific, and a more widespread systemic inflammatory response is often lacking; CSF may be normal or only show mildly increased protein level
6. Antibodies are highly sensitive and specific markers of underlying paraneoplastic syndrome (although may not be highly specific to particular syndromes)

7. Antibodies may not be pathogenic but a marker of autoimmunity (nuclear and cytoplasmic antibodies)
8. Passive transfer of some disorders by serum or IgG (ion channel antibodies)
9. Immunosuppression or removal of tumor in early stage of neurologic syndrome may improve neurologic symptoms
10. Nonspecific inflammatory changes in CNS: perivascular lymphocytic infiltration (predominantly T cells) and microglial nodules

C. **Malignancies Relatively More Likely To Be Associated With Paraneoplastic Neurologic Syndromes**
1. Small cell carcinoma (most commonly, lung)
2. Gynecologic malignancies (breast, ovary, fallopian tube, peritoneum)
3. Hodgkin's and non-Hodgkin's lymphoma
4. Testicular cancer
5. Neuroblastoma

D. **Specific Syndromes of CNS**
1. Paraneoplastic cerebellar degeneration
   a. Subacute onset of gait unsteadiness progressing over weeks to disabling ataxia and severe pancerebellar syndrome
   b. Severe ataxic dysarthria progressing to inability to communicate
   c. Nystagamus, vertigo, diplopia, titubation
   d. Symptoms are restricted to cerebellum and related pathways
   e. Imaging: normal early on, cerebellar atrophy in advanced disease
   f. Pathology: loss of Purkinje cells
   g. Purkinje cell antibody type-1(PCA-1 or anti-Yo, serum or CSF) predicts ovarian cancer (80% of cases) or breast cancer (10% of cases) in women
   h. Positive PCA-1 antibodies warrant exploratory laparotomy if imaging findings are negative
   i. Other antibodies are associated with small cell lung carcinoma (ANNA-1 or anti-Hu, P/Q-type calcium channel, CRMP-5) or lymphoma (anti-Tr)
   j. No effective treatment, but immunosuppression and cancer treatment may arrest progression
2. Paraneoplastic encephalomyelitis
   a. Constellation of CNS syndromes, two or more of which may occur concurrently or each may occur in isolation
   b. These include limbic encephalitis, brainstem encephalitis, stiff-person syndrome, optic neuritis, transverse myelopathy, motor neuron disease (each of these is discussed separately except for latter two)

3. Paraneoplastic limbic encephalitis
   a. From short-term memory loss to frank dementia
   b. Psychiatric symptoms: personality changes, depression, anxiety psychosis with delusions and hallucination
   c. Seizures (complex partial temporal lobe seizures)
   d. Lesions localized to limbic structures bilaterally (often asymmetric) and also to anteromedial temporal lobes, hippocampus, insula, hypothalamus, amygdala
   e. MRI: enhancing or nonenhancing high T2 signal in mesial temporal lobes (seen best on coronal FLAIR sequences) and in any other areas that may be affected such as brainstem (with concurrent brainstem encephalitis, see below) or hypothalamus (Fig. 16-39)
   f. CSF may have transient lymphocytic pleocytosis, increased protein, and increased oligoclonal bands
   g. EEG shows generalized or focal slowing
   h. Most common associated tumor: small cell lung carcinoma
   i. Most common associated antibody markers: ANNA-1/anti-Hu (small cell lung carcinoma), anti-Ma (lung, breast, testicular tumors), and anti-Ta (reactive with Ma2 protein, associated with testicular germ cell tumors)
   j. Patients with anti-Hu antibodies and lung cancer (small cell lung carcinoma) often have other nervous system involvement in addition to limbic system
   k. Patients may respond to tumor treatment or corticosteroid therapy
   l. Eventually, mesial temporal atrophy and permanent cognitive impairment ensue
   m. Nonparaneoplastic limbic encephalitis may be associated with antibodies against voltage-gated potassium channel
4. Paraneoplastic brainstem encephalitis
   a. With or without cerebellar degeneration
   b. Prominent abnormalities of eye movements: diplopia and supranuclear and infranuclear gaze palsy, especially vertical gaze palsy
   c. Bulbar involvement: flaccid dysarthria, dysphagia, jaw dystonia
   d. Ptosis and facial weakness
   e. Spastic quadriparesis, ataxia
   f. Dysregulation of sleep, hypersomnolence
   g. Other paraneoplastic neurologic syndromes may be present concurrently (e.g., limbic encephalitis, cerebellar degeneration)
   h. MRI may be normal or show increased signal in affected brainstem
5. Opsoclonus and myoclonus
   a. Random high-amplitude, arrhythmic, multidirectional involuntary conjugate eye movements and focal or diffuse myoclonus (often involving trunk, limbs,

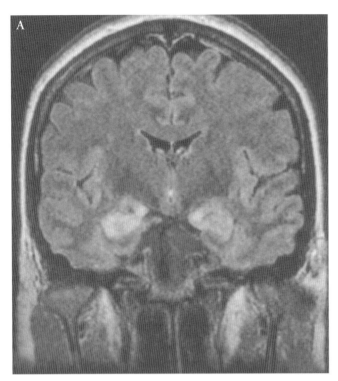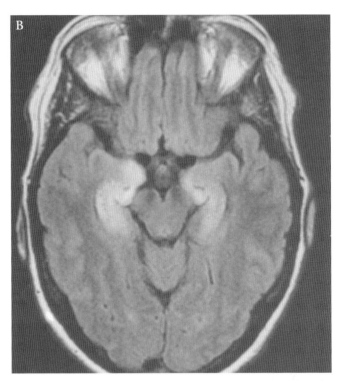

Fig. 16-39. MRI characteristics of paraneoplastic limbic encephalopathy in a patient with small cell lung carcinoma. Coronal (*A*) and axial (*B*) FLAIR sequences show increased signal within mesial temporal lobes bilaterally. The lesions were nonenhancing (not shown).

diaphragm, larynx, pharynx)
b. In children
1) May be self-limiting disease not associated with tumor and epiphenomenon of underlying viral encephalitis or drug intoxication: good prognosis and response to treatment
2) When occurs in the setting of neuroblastoma: good prognosis and cancer survival
3) Associated with anti-Hu (ANNA-1) antibodies (neuroblastoma)
c. In adults (many cases are nonparaneoplastic)
1) Associated with anti-Hu (ANNA-1 antibodies often associated with small cell lung carcinoma) and anti-Ri (ANNA-2 antibodies, which may be associated with small cell lung carcinoma or breast carcinoma)
2) With or without other concurrent syndromes (including cerebellar degeneration)
d. Treatment
1) When associated with neuroblastoma in children: improves with removal of tumor and with ACTH, corticosteroids
2) Good recovery in patients without cancer
3) Worse prognosis for adult-onset paraneoplastic syndrome

6. Paraneoplastic chorea
a. Subacute onset of generalized or focal chorea or choreoathetosis
b. High index of suspicion required, especially if disease is associated with other neurologic symptoms
c. MRI may show increased signal in striatum (caudate and anterior putamen)
d. Confirmed by CRMP-5 IgG
e. Highly associated with small cell lung carcinoma (less commonly, lymphoma or renal cell carcinoma)
f. May improve with treatment of underlying cancer and/or corticosteroid therapy
7. Cancer-associated retinopathy
a. Subacute progressive painless unilateral or bilateral loss of vision, abnormalities of color vision, or photosensitivity
b. Night blindness
c. Positive visual symptoms
d. Abnormal electroretinogram
e. Associated with small cell lung carcinoma (much less commonly, breast cancer)
8. Paraneoplastic optic neuritis
a. Ophthalmoscopic examination: possible papillitis or papilledema (or normal)
b. Afferent pupillary defect

c. Clinical presentation may be indistinguishable from that of idiopathic or demyelinating optic neuritis

d. Normal electroretinogram

e. Associated with small cell lung carcinoma and CRMP-5 antibodies

9. Stiff-person syndrome (see also Chapter 8)

a. Painful rigidity and spasms (predominantly axial and hip girdle areas), may then slowly affect proximal limb muscles

b. Exaggerated lumbar lordosis

c. Paraneoplastic syndrome is only a subset of stiff-person syndrome

d. Idiopathic stiff-person syndrome is associated with antibodies against glutamic acid decarboxylase

e. Continuous involuntary motor activity on needle electromyography (EMG) examination, especially in paraspinal muscles

f. Encephalomyelitis with rigidity

   1) Rapidly progressive course, ending in death within few months after onset

   2) Usually paraneoplastic

   3) Often associated with disease of brainstem or spinal cord

   4) Painful spasms lasting seconds to days

   5) May be associated with myoclonus

g. Paraneoplastic stiff-person syndrome that occurs in context of more widespread progressive encephalomyelopathy: often associated with small cell lung carcinoma and ANNA-1 antibodies

h. May occur as an isolated syndrome in association with anti-amphiphysin antibodies and breast cancer, and, less commonly, Hodgkin's lymphoma or other lymphomas, also reported with small cell lung carcinoma

E. **Paraneoplastic Syndromes of Peripheral Nervous System**

1. Isaacs' syndrome

a. Syndrome of peripheral nerve hyperexcitability

b. Associated with autoantibodies directed against voltage-gated potassium channels on peripheral nerve terminals

c. Associated tumor in 15% of cases: most commonly, small cell lung carcinoma or thymoma; less commonly, Hodgkin's lymphoma, breast carcinoma

d. Needle EMG: cramp discharges, fasciculation potentials, myokymic discharges, complex repetitive discharges, neuromyotonia

e. May respond to anticonvulsants (carbamazepine or phenytoin) or to plasma exchange

2. Peripheral neuropathy

a. Most common pattern is length-dependent, predomi-

nantly axonal, mixed sensory and motor neuropathy

b. Often rapid progression of clinical symptoms and electrophysiologic findings

c. Incidence is unknown because of many potential explanations for peripheral neuropathy in patients with cancer

d. May present as syndrome of acute or chronic inflammatory polyradiculoneuropathy (commonly associated with Hodgkin's and non-Hodgkin's lymphoma) or an asymmetric neuropathy resembling mononeuritis multiplex

e. May present in the context of neoplasms associated with paraproteinemias, such as myeloma, POEMS syndrome, monoclonal gammopathy of undetermined significance, and Waldenström's macroglobulinemia

f. Associated with many cancers: small cell lung carcinoma, non–small cell lung carcinoma, breast cancer, thymoma

g. Associated with several antibodies: ANNA-1, ANNA-2, CRMP-5, amphiphysin, and N-type calcium channel antibodies

3. Paraneoplastic sensory neuronopathy (sensory ganglionopathy)

a. 20% of sensory neuronopathies are paraneoplastic

b. Usual symptoms at onset: subacute onset and progression of symmetric or asymmetric pain, dysesthesias, hyperesthesias, paresthesias, numbness involving distal upper and/or lower limbs

c. Sensory ataxia and "pseudoathetosis" may develop from loss of joint position sense

d. Normal motor function, absent reflexes

e. Mean time from diagnosis to death: 14 months

f. Removal of tumor may halt progression, but no recovery is the rule

g. May be associated with encephalomyelitis

h. Most common associated tumor: small cell lung carcinoma (often with positive ANNA-1 and/or CRMP-5)

i. Also associated with breast cancer and lymphoma

j. Pathology

   1) Loss of cells from dorsal root ganglia with inflammation (large myelinated fibers damaged more than small fibers)

   2) Nondiagnostic sural nerve biopsies (not primary site of lesion)

k. CSF: mild pleocytosis early on, elevated protein level

l. Electrophysiology: absent sensory nerve action potentials, preserved motor responses

m. Immunotherapy shows no clear benefit, although some reports of response to intravenous immunoglobulin

4. Paraneoplastic autonomic neuropathy

a. Targeted cells are those of autonomic nervous system; motor and sensory nerves are relatively spared

b. Variable degree of autonomic failure causing orthostatic

hypotension, anhidrosis (and heat intolerance), dry mouth, gastroparesis, impotence in men

c. Gastrointestinal symptoms are very prominent; severe gastroparesis and constipation

d. Most common associated tumor: small cell lung carcinoma

e. Most common associated antibodies: ANNA-1 (anti-Hu), neuronal ganglionic acetylcholine receptor (AChR) antibodies

f. Autonomic symptoms are common in patients with Lambert-Eaton syndrome

g. Patients with ganglionic AChR antibodies may improve with cancer treatment, intravenous immunoglobulin, or plasma exchange

F. **Paraneoplastic Disorders of Neuromuscular Transmission** (see also Chapter 23)

1. Myasthenia gravis
   a. Paraneoplastic in 15% of patients
   b. Most commonly associated tumor: thymoma (less commonly, small cell lung carcinoma)
   c. Thymoma has been associated with
      1) High titers of anti-striational antibodies in young patients (<45 years old)
      2) High titers of modulating AChR antibodies (>90% loss of AChRs)
   d. Usually respond to immunosuppressive treatment (e.g., corticosteroids, intravenous immunoglobulin, plasma exchange, azathioprine), but the syndrome may be difficult to treat unless underlying thymoma is removed
   e. Symptomatic therapy with pyridostigmine

2. Lambert-Eaton myasthenic syndrome
   a. Associated with antibodies against P/Q-type voltage-gated calcium channels on motor nerve terminal
   b. Most commonly associated tumor: small cell lung carcinoma (60% of adults with the syndrome)
   c. Immunosuppression usually effective, in addition to pyridostigmine and 3,4-diaminopyridine
   d. Symptoms generally improve after underlying cancer is removed

G. **Paraneoplastic Disorders of Muscle**

1. Malignancy-associated necrotizing polymyositis
   a. Rare
   b. Rapid progressive presentation of proximal-predominant symmetric weakness (developing in less than 2-3 months), with increased creatine kinase levels (often marked)
   c. Associated with small cell lung carcinoma, breast cancer, gastrointestinal adenocarcinoma

2. Dermatomyositis

a. Debate about whether it is true paraneoplastic syndrome

b. Associated with anti–Jo-1 antibodies

c. Proposed mechanism of injury: antibody-mediated muscle angiopathy

d. Associated with adenocarcinoma (ovarian, lung, pancreatic, stomach, colorectal), and non-Hodgkin's lymphoma

H. **Paraneoplastic Autoantibodies**

1. Nuclear and cytoplasmic antibodies (Table 16-2)
   a. Screening method: detection of serum antibody binding to section of nervous system tissue (immunohistochemistry) or by Western blot
   b. Results confirmed by detecting serum antibody binding to recombinant proteins in Western blot
   c. Antibodies are very specific (but not highly sensitive) markers of paraneoplastic disease (e.g., more than 80% of patients with ANNA-1/anti-Hu antibody have lung cancer, but among patients with small cell lung carcinoma–related limbic encephalitis, <50% have ANNA-1)
   d. Antibody type usually correlates with the malignancy type and, to lesser extent, type of neurologic syndrome (highly specific for presence of cancer and predictive of type of cancer, but usually less specific for the type of neurologic syndrome)
   e. Exceptions to this rule are as follows:
      1) PCA-1 (anti-Yo) antibodies in ovarian or breast cancer almost always associated with paraneoplastic cerebellar degeneration
      2) Anti-Ma antibodies in lung, breast, and testicular cancers usually associated with limbic and brainstem encephalitis
      3) Anti-retinal antibodies in small cell lung carcinoma and melanoma usually associated with cancer–associated retinopathy
      4) PCA-Tr (anti-Tr) antibodies in Hodgkin's lymphoma associated with paraneoplastic cerebellar degeneration

2. Ion channel (membrane) antibodies (Table 16-3)
   a. Method: immunoprecipitation of radiolabeled ion channel proteins
   b. Antibodies often correlate with specific neurologic syndromes but are not always markers of cancer (e.g., 99% of patients with Lambert-Eaton syndrome have P/Q-type calcium channel antibodies but about 40% do not have cancer)
   c. Exception: N-type calcium channel antibody is a sensitive marker of paraneoplastic autoimmunity but is not associated with a single syndrome or cancer
   d. Unlike nuclear and cytoplasmic antibodies: antibody may be cause of the disorder, and antibody titers correlate better with clinical course

Table 16-2. Neuronal Nuclear and Cytoplasmic Antibodies

Antibody	Antigen characteristics	Neoplasm	Paraneoplastic neurologic syndrome
ANNA-1 (anti-Hu)	Nucleus, all neurons	SCLC	EM, CD, SN, AN, MMPLX, SMN
ANNA-2 (anti-Ri)	Nucleus, neuronal	Lung or breast cancer	CD, OM, SMN
ANNA-3	Antigen not defined, observed in nuclei of Purkinje cells & renal glomerular podocytes	SCLC	EM, SMN, CD, myelopathy
Anti-amphiphysin	Vesicle-associated protein amphiphysin	Breast, SCLC	EM, SPS
CRMP-5 (anti-CV2)	Neuronal cytoplasmic	SCLC or thymoma	EM, ON, retinitis, chorea, SMN
Anti-Ma	Nuclear & cytoplasmic proteins in germ line tumors (Ma1 & Ma2)	SCLC, breast, testicular germ cell tumors (may also occur in ectopic sites)	EM
PCA-1 (anti-Yo)	Purkinje cell cytoplasm	Ovarian or breast cancer	CD
PCA-2	Not defined	SCLC	EM
PCA-Tr (anti-Tr)	Purkinje cell cytoplasm, antigen not defined	HL	CD (30% of patients with CD associated with HL have anti-Tr)
Anti-retinal (anti-recoverin)	Multiple antigens including *Recoverin* on photoreceptors and ganglion cells	SCLC, melanoma (less common)	CAR

AN, autonomic neuropathy; ANNA, antineuronal nuclear antibody; BE, brainstem encephalitis; CAR, cancer-associated retinopathy; CD, cerebellar degeneration; CRMP, collapsing response-mediator protein antibody; EM, encephalomyelitis; HL, Hodgkin's lymphoma; MMPLX, mononeuritis multiplex; OM, opsoclonus-myoclonus; ON, optic neuritis; PCA, Purkinje cell antibody; PR, polyradiculoneuropathy; SCLC, small cell lung carcinoma; SMN, sensorimotor neuropathy; SN, sensory neuronopathy; SPS, stiff-person syndrome.

Table 16-3. Ion Channel Antibodies

Antibody	Antigen characteristics	Paraneoplastic neurologic syndrome	Neoplasm
P/Q-type VGCC	Neuronal calcium channels	LEMS (60% are paraneoplastic), EM (less common)	SCLC (60%)
N-type VGCC	Neuronal calcium channels	EM (nonspecific)	Lung or breast cancer (may not be associated with cancer)
VGKC	Shaker-type potassium channels in nerve terminals	IS, CFS, EM (limbic encephalitis), Morvan's syndrome (insomnia, neuromyotonia, EM [Chapter 19])	SCLC, thymoma
Muscle AChR	Nicotinic acetylcholine receptors at postsynaptic muscle membrane	MG	Thymoma (15% of MG patients, also associated with anti-striational antibodies)
Ganglionic AChR	Nicotinic acetylcholine receptors at autonomic ganglia	AN, IS or CFS (less common)	SCLC (15%)
mGluR1	Metabotropic glutamate receptor	CD	HL

AChR, acetylcholine receptor antibody; AN, autonomic neuropathy; CD, cerebellar degeneration; CFS, cramp-fasciculation syndrome; EM, encephalomyelitis; HL, Hodgkin's lymphoma; IS, Isaacs' syndrome; LEMS, Lambert-Eaton myasthenic syndrome; MG, myasthenia gravis; SCLC, small cell lung carcinoma; VGCC, voltage-gated calcium channel antibody; VGKC, voltage-gated potassium channel antibody.

Questions

1-4. Match the antibodies in the right column with the appropriate clinical syndrome in the left column

1. Sensory neuronopathy
2. Lambert-Eaton myasthenic syndrome
3. Paraneoplastic cerebellar degeneration
4. Stiff-person syndrome

a. Calcium channel antibodies
b. Anti-Hu antibodies
c. Anti-amphiphysin antibodies
d. Anti-Yo (PCA-1) antibodies

5-9. Match the description presented in the left column with the tumor in the right column. Note that an answer may be used once, more than once, or not at all.

5. Common tumor of the cerebellopontine angle
6. Positive immunohistochemistry for epithelial membrane antigen (EMA)
7. Positive immunohistochemistry for S-100 protein
8. Cells are joined by many desmosomes in the elongated intertwined cell processes
9. "Antoni A" and "Antoni B" areas and Verocay bodies

a. Meningioma
b. Schwannoma
c. Both

10-13. Match the brain neoplasm or condition associated with brain neoplasms in the left column with the genetic mutation in the right column.

10. Neurofibromatosis type 1
11. Neurofibromatosis type 2
12. Astrocytic tumors (40% of all subtypes)
13. Retinoblastoma

a. p53 gene (chromosome 17p)
b. pRB gene (chromosome 13q)
c. Gene encoding for neurofibromin
d. Gene encoding for merlin (chromosome 22q)

14. Which of the following tumors is more likely to be multiple?
    a. Meningioma
    b. Lipoma
    c. Primary central nervous system lymphoma
    d. Glioblastoma multiforme

15. Which of the following tumors commonly occurs in children younger than 2 years and has dural attachments?
    a. Meningioma
    b. Desmoplastic ganglioglioma
    c. Dysembryoplastic neuroepithelial tumors (DNETs)
    d. Central neurocytoma

16. Which of the following statements is *true*?
    a. Prostate neoplasms commonly metastasize to the brain
    b. Malignant melanomas commonly occur in African Americans
    c. Meningiomas are dural-based and always enhance with contrast
    d. Cerebellum is a less frequent site of central nervous system metastases than the leptomeninges, thalamus, or brainstem
    e. Glioblastoma occurs in older age groups and is the most common glial tumor, accounting for more than 50% of all primary brain tumors

17. All the following pathologic diagnoses would be considered in the differential diagnosis of a solitary tumor of the lumbar cistern *except*:
    a. Schwannoma
    b. Meningioma
    c. Paraganglioma
    d. Myxopapillary ependymoma
    e. Central neurocytoma

18. Which of the following is *true* about Cowden's disease?
    a. Autosomal dominant inheritance
    b. Associated with hamartomas in multiple organ systems, including hamartomatous colon polyps
    c. Associated with dysplastic gangliocytoma of the cerebellum as the primary central nervous system manifestation
    d. 50% of patients with dysplastic gangliocytoma of the cerebellum have clinical stigmata of Cowden's disease
    e. *All* of above.

19. Which of the following tumor types usually produce diffuse infiltration of the central nervous system?
    a. Gliomas
    b. Metastatic carcinomas
    c. Central astrocytomas
    d. Meningiomas
    e. Pleomorphic xanthoastrocytomas

ANSWERS

1. Answer: b.

2. Answer: a.

3. Answer: d.

4. Answer: c.

5. Answer: c.

6. Answer: a.

7. Answer: b.

8. Answer: a.

9. Answer: b.

10. Answer: c.

11. Answer: d.

12. Answer: a.

13. Answer: b.

14. Answer: c.
Primary central nervous system lymphoma tends to be multiple in 50% of cases. Meningiomas are multiple in less than 10% of cases. Glioblastoma multiforme appears multicentric in less than 5% of cases. Lipomas are usually incidental findings and almost never multiple.

15. Answer: b.
Meningiomas are rare in children younger than 2 years. Desmoplastic infantile ganglioglioma and desmoplastic infantile astrocytoma are large cystic tumors with dural attachments. They occur in infants, and the prognosis is generally good after resection. DNET do not have dural attachments and tend to occur in older children and young adults, often with seizures. Central neurocytomas occur in adults (mean age, 29 years).

16. Answer: e.
Brain metastases are rare from prostatic neoplasms. Malignant melanoma is uncommon in African Americans. Meningiomas are often dural-based but may not enhance with contrast. The cerebellum is a more frequent site of central nervous system metastasis than the leptomeninges, thalamus, brainstem, or spinal cord. Glioblastoma multiforme occurs in older age groups, is the most common glial tumor, and accounts for more than 50% of all primary brain tumors.

17. Answer: e.
The differential diagnosis of a solitary tumor of the lumbar cistern includes schwannoma, meningioma, myxopapillary ependymoma, and paraganglioma of the filum terminale. The latter two arise from the film terminale. Central neurocytomas are often located in the third and lateral ventricles.

18. Answer: e.

19. Answer: a.
Gliomas and lymphoma are capable of diffuse infiltration of the central nervous sytem. Metastatic carcinomas usually have a sharp border with the surrounding brain parenchyma. Meningiomas and pleomorphic xanthoastrocytomas are usually well circumscribed.

17

TOXIC AND METABOLIC DISORDERS OF THE NERVOUS SYSTEM

Nima Mowzoon, M.D.

I. NUTRITIONAL DEFICIENCIES AND TOXICITIES

A. Folate and Vitamin B₁₂ Deficiencies (see Chapter 20)

B. Vitamin E Deficiency (see Chapter 9)
1. Associated with
   a. Cystic fibrosis in children
   b. Severe malabsorption because of disease of the alimentary tract
   c. Inherited conditions, including ataxia with isolated vitamin E deficiency (due to mutation of α-tocopherol transfer protein gene on chromosome 8q) or abetalipoproteinemia (see Chapter 9)
2. Vitamin E: radical scavenger and antioxidant
3. Clinical features: spinocerebellar syndrome (cerebellar ataxia and large-fiber sensory loss), areflexia, ataxic dysarthria, cerebellar and sensory gait ataxia, extensor plantar responses, acanthocytosis, hemolytic anemia, retinitis pigmentosa
4. Pathology: acanthocytosis (peripheral blood smear); swollen axons in affected central nervous system (CNS) structures, including posterior columns

C. Niacin (nicotinic acid) Deficiency (pellagra)
1. Niacin
   a. Nicotinic acid and nicotinamide (latter is readily deaminated in the body to form nicotinic acid)
   b. Nicotinic acid and nicotinamide form nicotinamide adenosine dinucleotide (NAD^+) and NAD phosphate ($NADP^+$), important coenzymes in carbohydrate metabolism
   c. Niacin is derived from enriched grains and cereals, milk, meat and, in small quantities, as end product of tryptophan metabolism
2. Prevalence of pellagra has decreased with fortification of bread and cereals with niacin
3. Nonendemic pellagra may occur in context of alcoholism or nutritional deficiency due to gastrointestinal tract disease

4. Clinical triad of "3Ds": dermatitis, diarrhea, dementia
5. Gastrointestinal features: stomatitis, diarrhea, abdominal pain, vomiting
6. Neurologic: myelopathy and spastic paraparesis, irritability, depression, apathy, memory loss
7. Dermatitis: hyperkeratotic, hyperpigmented, diffuse, extensive rash
8. Treatment: oral or parenteral nicotinic acid or nicotinamide

D. Vitamin B₆
1. Vitamin B_6: pyridoxine, pyridoxal, pyridoxamine—all are precursors of coenzyme pyridoxal phosphate
2. Ubiquitous in corn, wheat, egg yolk, and lean meat
3. Clinical syndrome of deficiency
   a. Infantile onset
      1) Occurs in setting of syndrome of pyridoxine deficiency-related seizures (due to malnutrition of mothers) or congenital dependency on pyridoxine (not true deficiency) (see Chapter 12)
      2) Normal prenatal and peripartum course, followed by poor feeding, irritability, exaggerated startle, and abrupt onset of seizures (may be intractable and lead to status epilepticus)
   b. Adult onset
      1) Rare: adults are much more resistant to vitamin B_6 deficiency
      2) Often due to intake of isoniazid, hydralazine, or penicillamine
      3) Distal sensorimotor peripheral neuropathy (predominant features of sensory symptoms and axonal degeneration)
      4) Treatment: slow improvement with withdrawal of offending drug or initiation of low-dose vitamin B_6 supplementation
      5) Primary prevention: coadministration of vitamin B_6 prevents this neuropathy
4. Pyridoxine excess

a. Sensory polyneuropathy: length-dependent axonal neuropathy with predominant features of sensory loss or sensory ataxia due to polyganglionopathy (see Chapter 21)

b. Partial or complete resolution with withdrawal of offending agent

E. Vitamin A

1. Hypervitaminosis A (vitamin A toxicity) may cause
   a. Pseudotumor cerebri
   b. Birth defects and pervasive developmental disorders in children born to mothers with this condition
2. Vitamin A deficiency: rare, may present with night blindness

F. Thiamine Deficiency

1. Most frequently occurs in setting of alcoholism
2. Thiamine is a precursor for the biologically active thiamine pyrophosphate
3. Thiamine pyrophosphate acts as a coenzyme for
   a. Transketolase reaction in hexose monophosphate shunt
   b. Oxidative decarboxylation of pyruvate to form acetyl coenzyme A (CoA) by pyruvate dehydrogenase
   c. Conversion of α-ketoglutarate to succinyl CoA by α-ketoglutarate dehydrogenase
4. Thiamine requirements are greatest during periods of high metabolic demand and/or high glucose intake: this may partly explain occurrence of Wernicke's encephalopathy with administration of intravenous glucose to a thiamine-deficient patient
5. Beriberi
   a. Length-dependent, axonal, sensorimotor peripheral neuropathy with distal sensory loss, paresthesias, weakness (termed "dry beriberi" in absence of cardiac involvement)
   b. Associated with cardiac involvement: cardiomyopathy, arrhythmias, congestive heart failure (termed "wet beriberi")
   c. Laboratory diagnosis
      1) Decreased serum and urine levels of thiamine
      2) Decreased erythrocyte transketolase activity (functional assay)
      3) Increased serum pyruvate levels
      4) Electromyographic evidence of axonal, distal peripheral neuropathy
6. Wernicke-Korsakoff syndrome (see Chapter 7)

G. Other Nervous System Conditions Associated With Alcoholism

1. Alcoholic neuropathy
   a. Associated with severe, prolonged alcohol use
   b. Predominantly sensory neuropathy: painful neuropathy, painful dysesthesias, paresthesias, allodynia

c. Weakness is mild, usually involves distal lower extremity
d. Autonomic involvement
e. Predisposition to compression mononeuropathies
f. Associated with other alcohol-related complications: Wernicke-Korsakoff syndrome and cerebellar degeneration
g. Patients should receive parenteral thiamine supplementation

2. Ethanol-induced myopathy
   a. Usually develops in setting of chronic, heavy ethanol intake and binge drinking
   b. Occurs as acute necrotizing myopathy or chronic myopathy with muscle wasting
   c. Acute necrotizing myopathy
      1) Acute onset of myonecrosis, often in the midst of heavy bout of drinking (in context of chronic alcoholism)
      2) Acute onset of muscle pain and myoedema, often associated with myoglobinuria
      3) Weakness: often proximal and symmetric or there may be focal weakness of the quadriceps or calves
      4) Pathology: patchy, segmental necrotizing process, with degeneration and regeneration of the muscle fibers
   d. Chronic alcoholic myopathy
      1) Gradual onset and progression of proximal weakness, muscle wasting, cramps, and myalgias
      2) Increased serum levels of creatine kinase and myoglobinuria
3. Marchiafava-Bignami disease (see Chapter 7)
4. Alcoholic dementia (see Chapter 7)
5. Acute withdrawal syndrome, including delirium tremens and alcohol withdrawal seizures
6. Alcohol-related cerebellar degeneration
   a. Usually in context of long-standing alcohol abuse
   b. Insidious and gradual onset and progression of cerebellar ataxia
   c. Often associated with alcoholic neuropathy and withdrawal seizures
   d. Abstinence may yield improvement: gradual, often incomplete
   e. Pathology
      1) Cerebellar atrophy: predilection for anterior and superior vermis
      2) Diffuse loss of Purkinje cells, patchy loss of granule cells
      3) Often concomitant diffuse cerebral atrophy
7. Fetal alcohol syndrome
   a. Occurs in infants whose mothers drink alcohol during pregnancy: most afflicted infants are born to mothers with alcohol-related complications during pregnancy,

but there is no minimum safe amount of alcohol intake during the gestational period; expectant mothers must abstain completely

b. Intrauterine growth retardation: low birth weight, small head circumference

c. Craniofacial and joint deformities

d. Congenital developmental malformations of brain, including microcephaly, agenesis of corpus callosum, cerebellar dysplasia, heterotopic gray matter

e. Afflicted infants: irritability, poor feeding

f. High infant mortality rate: 1 in 6 afflicted infants die

g. Many infants who survive infancy have psychomotor developmental delay, mental retardation, and pervasive developmental disorders marked by poor learning, memory, attention, and problem solving; social and behavioral problems

H. Copper Deficiency

1. Acquired (see Chapter 20)
2. Congenital: Menke syndrome

I. Postgastroplasty Polyneuropathy

1. Associated with jejunoileal bypass, gastrojejunectomy, gastric stapling, gastroplasty, gastrectomy with Roux-en-Y anastomosis
2. Neurologic syndrome always follows intractable vomiting and precipitous weight loss
3. Acute or subacute onset of symmetric sensory loss and paresthesias, distal and/or proximal weakness, which may progress to quadriparesis
4. Few patients develop encephalopathy

II. ACQUIRED METABOLIC DISORDERS RELATED TO TOXINS

A. Metal Intoxication

1. Arsenic
   a. Usually associated with deliberate poisoning, may also occur in the context of accidental exposure
   b. Shortly after ingestion, arsenic is stored in reticuloendothelial system, kidney, and intestines; is slowly released
   c. Slow excretion via kidney and feces
   d. Deposited in hair within 2 weeks; remains in the hair for years
   e. Clinical features vary, depending on the dose
      1) Acute or subacute exposure: abdominal pain, nausea, vomiting, hyperthermia, headaches, anxiety, vertigo, possibly seizures, encephalopathy, and coma (if severe)

2) Fatal acute poisoning: precipitous development of lethargy and coma, followed by death in few days, may be due to diffuse edema and/or hemorrhagic encephalopathy

3) Low-dose chronic exposure: similar clinical features but much less severe; abdominal pain, vertigo, long-standing cognitive disturbance, persistent headaches, and development of peripheral neuropathy

4) Sphincter dysfunction

5) Optic neuropathy: possible delayed manifestation

6) Mees' lines: white lines in nails, usually appear 2 to 3 weeks after acute exposure

7) Peripheral neuropathy
   a) Painful, distal peripheral neuropathy (axonopathy)
   b) Distal pansensory loss in a glove-stocking distribution involving both small-fiber and large-fiber modalities and causing dense proprioceptive loss and pseudoathetosis, reduced temperature sensation, hyperesthesia, dysesthesia, and allodynia
   c) Weakness involving the distal extremity, hand, and foot muscles: effort may be poor because of dense proprioceptive loss
   d) Hyporeflexia or areflexia distally
   e) Associated with exfoliative dermatitis

f. Diagnosis
   1) 24-Hour urine heavy metal arsenic levels: may be falsely elevated by ingestion of shellfish
   2) Increased arsenic levels in nail clippings or pubic hair (preferable to scalp hair because of less chance of environmental contamination)

g. Treatment
   1) Acute treatment: supportive measures, including hydration and morphine for abdominal pain, gastric lavage
   2) Chelation therapy with dimercaprol or its water-soluble derivative, dimercaptosuccinic acid (DMSA); or penicillamine (best if started early)

2. Inorganic lead
   a. Toxicity due to occupational or nonoccupational exposure or, in children, old lead-based paint
   b. Lead inhibits erythrocyte γ-aminolevulinic acid dehydratase in biochemical pathways of porphyrin metabolism
   c. Children
      1) Acute intoxication: acute gastrointestinal illness, confusion, lethargy, seizures, coma, and respiratory arrest with high levels of exposure
      2) Chronic, low-level exposure: gradual onset of listlessness, behavioral changes, psychomotor slowing, sleep disturbance, seizures, gait disorder characterized by clumsiness or frank ataxia

d. Adults
   1) Polyneuropathy: predominantly motor neuropathy, with distal weakness, atrophy, and fasciculations (pain uncommon)
   2) Motor manifestation may be more prominent in upper extremities: may present with bilateral wrist-drop, with or without distal lower limb weakness
   3) Motor neuropathy commonly involves radial nerve (wristdrop is most common)
   4) There may or may not be sensory symptoms, predominantly paresthesias (allodynia and dysesthesias are uncommon)
e. Laboratory diagnosis
   1) Microcytic, hypochromic anemia
   2) Basophilic stippling of red blood cells on peripheral blood smear
   3) Renal insufficiency, azotemia
   4) Elevated blood and urine levels of lead
f. Treatment: chelation with DMSA, intravenous calcium disodium-EDTA, or penicillamine

3. Manganese
   a. Exposure
      1) Primary source of exposure (occupational): inhalation, primarily mine workers
      2) Patients receiving total parenteral nutrition containing manganese
   b. Pathology: neuronal loss and gliosis affecting the globus pallidus and subthalamic nucleus; uncommon involvement of substantia nigra
   c. Main source of disposal is biliary excretion: patients with biliary atresia or chronic liver disease are prone to develop manganese toxicity (may explain high T1 signal in pallidum observed in chronic liver disease)
   d. Clinical features
      1) Onset of symptoms may occur early (1-2 months after exposure) or may be delayed (about 20 years after exposure)
      2) Headaches, neuropsychiatric manifestations (memory disturbance, hallucinations, aggressive behavior, apathy, irritability, social withdrawal, personality changes, and psychosis, referred to as "manganese madness")
      3) Extrapyramidal symptoms: parkinsonism with hypomimia (decreased facial expression), bradykinesia, micrographia
      4) Hypophonic and monotonous speech
      5) Absence of typical parkinsonian rest tremor, but there may be a fine, low-amplitude, high-frequency tremor
      6) Gait: retropulsion, propulsion, often tendency to walk on toes with elbows flexed and erect posture
   e. Diagnosis

1) Brain MRI: high T1 signal in the globus pallidus (also striatum and midbrain) bilaterally because of manganese accumulation
   f. Treatment
      1) Levodopa: partial to no benefit
      2) Chelation with EDTA: improvement in some patients

4. Inorganic mercury
   a. Acute intoxication: acute colitis, vomiting, renal failure, stomatitis, little cognitive impairment except for irritability and delirium with acute poisoning
   b. Chronic, low-grade toxicity: tremor, peripheral neuropathy
   c. Personality changes, anxiety, but little cognitive impairment
   d. Peripheral neuropathy: sensorimotor axonopathy, associated with sensory loss, sensory ataxia, pain, paresthesias, distal weakness, atrophy

5. Organic mercury
   a. Methylmercury: better penetrance of blood-brain barrier
   b. Predilection for dorsal root ganglia, calcarine cortex, and cerebellar granular layer (may also affect parietal cortex)
   c. Clinical features
      1) Cerebellar and sensory ataxia
      2) Peripheral neuropathy
      3) Cortical blindness from involvement of the calcarine cortex
      4) Sensory disturbance due to involvement of dosal root ganglia and sensory cortex
      5) Deafness, dysarthria
      6) Choreoathetosis
      7) Motor neuron syndrome resembling amyotrophic lateral sclerosis, with both lower motor neuron features (atrophy and fasciculations) and upper motor neuron features (hyperreflexia)
      8) Cognitive impairment ("mad as a hatter"): short-term memory loss, depression, hallucinations, other features of psychosis
   d. Diagnosis
      1) Elevated mercury levels in serum, urine, saliva, hair samples
      2) Urine mercury levels: poor correlation with clinical severity
      3) Serum mercury levels: variable, unpredictable
   e. Treatment: chelation with penicillamine or DMSA

6. Thallium
   a. Competes with potassium ions in transport by the Na/K adenosine triphosphatase (ATPase) system
   b. Used in pesticides
   c. Acute intoxication from exposure to large quantities: acute gastrointestinal illness with nausea, vomiting, and diarrhea; irritability, confusion, and coma (severe cases)
   d. Ingestion of large quantities: a painful, predominantly

sensory neuropathy may occur, possibly with autonomic features

   e. Initial stage may be followed by progressive weakness, ataxia, chorea

   f. Respiratory weakness and cranial neuropathies may occur in severe cases

   g. Chronic, low-grade exposure: distal, predominantly sensory, large-fiber more than small-fiber peripheral neuropathy with or without mild distal weakness (axonopathy)

   h. Alopecia: occurs about 2 to 4 weeks after acute intoxication

   i. Diagnosis: measurement of urine thallium levels

B. Organic Chemicals

1. Acrylamide
   a. Monomeric acrylamide (not polyacrylamide) is neurotoxic
   b. Acute intoxication with severely high exposure: seizures, encephalopathy
   c. Chronic, moderately high exposure: gradual onset of encephalopathy and peripheral neuropathy
   d. Chronic, low-grade exposure: peripheral neuropathy
   e. Features of peripheral neuropathy
      1) Predominantly axonal, distal neuropathy
      2) Preceded by skin irritation and peeling
      3) Neurotoxicity may occur in abnormalities of axonal (retrograde) transport; accumulation of neurofilaments and axonal loss are evident in sural nerve biopsy specimens
      4) Predominantly sensory neuropathy, involving both small-fiber and large-fiber modalities
      5) Reduced proprioceptive and vibratory sensation, sensory ataxia, hyporeflexia, numbness, paresthesias, incoordination
      6) Motor involvement (distal weakness) may be present with repetitive, high-grade exposure

2. Hexacarbon solvents (*n*-hexane and methyl *n*-butyl ketone)
   a. *n*-Hexane and methyl *n*-butyl ketone are both converted to 2,5-hexanediol, which is toxic to peripheral nerve axons and affects axonal transport (hence, giant multifocal axonal enlargements from accumulation of neurofilaments)
   b. Used as paint, varnish, and glue (exposure may occur in person sniffing glue)
   c. Acute exposure: euphoria, hallucinations, headaches (encephalopathy does not occur)
   d. Progressive sensorimotor peripheral neuropathy with slowed conduction velocities on electrodiagnostic testing

3. Carbon disulfide
   a. Used in manufacturing rayon and cellophane
   b. Primary route of intoxication: inhalation (or ingestion)
   c. Acute inhalation of large amounts of the compound can produce encephalopathy (varying severity)
   d. Sensorimotor peripheral neuropathy with chronic exposure: predominantly sensory involvement, with paresthesias and numbness and some motor involvement
   e. Peripheral nerve histologic characteristics of long-term exposure to carbon disulfide: focal paranodal axonal swellings, accumulation of neurofilaments, and secondary demyelination
   f. Long-term exposure could also possibly cause: minor affective or cognitive disorder, pyramidal or extrapyramidal symptoms (parkinsonism), optic neuropathy
   g. Diagnosis: urine metabolite 2-thiothiazolidine-4-carboxylic acid

4. Carbon monoxide
   a. Pure form: odorless, colorless gas
   b. Produced by combustion of carbon-based fuels
   c. Mechanism of action
      1) Binds to hemoglobin with greater affinity than oxygen (forming carboxyhemoglobin), competes with binding of oxygen to hemoglobin
      2) Impairs release of oxygen from oxyhemoglobin
      3) In essence, prevents oxygenation of tissues
   d. Severity of clinical presentation depends on concentration of the gas in the exposed environment and duration of exposure
   e. Clinical features of acute intoxication may range from headaches, nausea, dizziness to confusion, encephalopathy, pyramidal and extrapyramidal symptoms (including tremors), seizures, coma, death
   f. Survivors of acute intoxication who have partial or complete recovery may suffer from delayed deterioration and recurrence of the aforementioned symptoms; some may progress to persistent vegetative state
   g. Pathology of acute or subacute stage (Fig. 17-1): diffuse cerebral edema, scattered petechial hemorrhages in white matter and more prominent hemorrhagic foci in the globus pallidus bilaterally
   h. Pathology of chronic stage: necrosis and cavitation of the globus pallidus, confluent foci of necrosis in subcortical white matter

5. Toluene
   a. Used as solvent in paint, varnishes, thinners, glues, dyes; used to synthesize benzene
   b. Acute intoxication: euphoria, incoordination and ataxia, confusion, headache
   c. Chronic use: euphoria, disihibition, memory and attentional deficits, tremor, cerebellar symptoms (intention tremor, titubation, truncal ataxia), optic neuropathy and other cranial neuropathies
   d. Diagnosis: hippuric acid (urine metabolite)

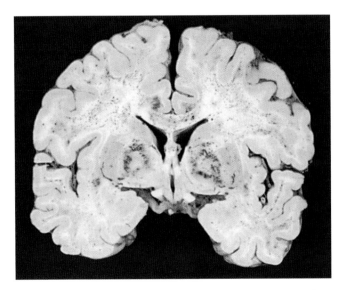

Fig. 17-1. Macroscopic appearance of early carbon monoxide toxicity. Note diffuse, scattered, and confluent foci of petechial hemorrhages throughout white matter, with more prominent hemorrhagic foci in the globus pallidus bilaterally. (From Okazaki H, Scheithauer BW. Atlas of neuropathology. New York: Gower Medical Publishing; 1988. p. 262. By permission of Mayo Foundation.)

6. Trichloroethylene
   a. Typical presentation with high-level exposure: cranial neuropathies, especially trigeminal neuropathy
   b. Trigeminal neuropathy: typically facial numbness, followed by weakness of muscles of mastication
   c. There may also be ptosis, weakness of muscles of facial expression, abnormalities of extraocular movements
   d. Other nonspecific symptoms: headaches, dizziness, fatigue, insomnia
7. Methanol toxicity
   a. Causes necrosis of optic nerves and putamina bilaterally
   b. Acute intoxication
      1) Presentation often delayed for several hours until methanol is metabolized to formaldehyde and formic acid
      2) Headache, dizziness, nausea, blurred vision
      3) Permanent visual loss may occur
      4) Severe effects: encephalopathy, seizures, cardiopulmonary failure, coma, death
   c. Pathology: likely caused by formate metabolites, hypoxemia, and metabolic acidosis
   d. 4-Methyl-1H-pyrazole (fomepizole) may be used to treat patients older than 12 years: acts as effective inhibitor of alcohol dehydrogenase
8. Organophosphates

a. Mainly used in insecticides
b. Absorbed through gastrointestinal or respiratory tract or skin
c. Act as acetylcholinesterase inhibitors
d. Acute cholinergic toxicity (type I syndrome): nausea, hypersalivation, increased bronchial secretions, bronchospasms, increased lacrimation, diarrhea, miosis, fasciculations, pulmonary edema, bradycardia, seizures, coma
e. Intermediate (type II) syndrome
   1) Occurs within 12 to 96 hours after exposure and resolves in 2 to 3 weeks
   2) Cholinergic stimulation of nicotinic receptors
   3) Characterized by respiratory, bulbar, and proximal limb weakness, fasciculations, tachycardia, hypertension, and cardiac failure in severe cases
f. Delayed polyneuropathy may occur after 2 to 3 weeks
   1) Subacute onset
   2) Early cramps in calves and paresthesias in feet, followed by weakness (predominantly in feet and ascending proximally)
   3) Predominantly motor and few sensory symptoms
   4) Depressed Achilles reflexes, relatively preserved reflexes proximally
   5) May be concurrent involvement of spinal cord, with long tract signs

C. **Plant and Animal Neurotoxins**
1. Snake
   a. Toxins
      1) α-Bungarotoxin and cobrotoxin: postsynaptic blockade of acetylcholine receptors (AChRs)
      2) β-Bungarotoxin and crotoxin: presynaptic inhibition of acetylcholine (ACh) release
   b. Local pain, swelling, and erythema at site of the bite
   c. Focal weakness or compartment syndrome
   d. Diffuse proximal weakness resembling myasthenia gravis
   e. Ptosis, cranial neuropathies, dysphagia, areflexia, fasciculations, respiratory distress
   f. Systemic manifestations, including hypotension and shock
2. Female black widow spider (*Latrodectus mactans*)
   a. Most important spider to cause potentially significant morbidity
   b. Toxin: α-latrotoxin, causing presynaptic facilitation of ACh release and depletion of ACh
   c. Erythema at site of the bite, intense pain, and involuntary muscle spasms involving the limbs, truncal muscles, and diaphragm (latter causing respiratory arrest)
   d. Autonomic symptoms: hypertension, piloerection, diaphoresis, brochospasm
3. Scorpion

a. Tityustoxin, produced by *Tityus serrulatus*, causes presynaptic facilitation of ACh release and postsynaptic activation of voltage-gated sodium channels

b. Local pain and erythema at site of the bite, local paresthesias, followed by diffuse paresthesias, fasciculations, tremors, hyperreflexia

c. Pandysautonomia: hypertension, hyperthermia, hypersalivation, diaphoresis, urinary frequency, fecal urgency

4. *Amanita* mushrooms

a. Potent anticholinergic effects; block both cholinergic and γ-aminobutyric acid (GABA) synapses

b. Acute intoxication (6-8 hours after ingestion): intractable emesis and bloody diarrhea, altered mentation, agitation, convulsions, muscle spasms

c. Hepatotoxicity and renal failure develop in the next 3 to 5 days, followed by secondary metabolic encephalopathy

D. Marine Neurotoxins

1. Ciguatera fish poisoning

a. Most common nonbacterial form of food poisoning related to seafood ingestion in the United States, Canada, and Europe

b. Caused by ciguatera toxins produced by dinoflagellates in different species of reef fish

1) Ciguatoxins: increase sodium permeability via tetrodotoxin-sensitive voltage-gated sodium channels in nerves and muscles, causing membrane depolarization

2) Maitotoxin: increases calcium permeability of voltage-gated calcium channels

c. Clinical symptoms at onset: abdominal pain and cramps, hypersalivation, nausea, vomiting, diarrhea

d. Neurologic manifestations typically follow: dysesthesias of extremities, spreading paresthesias (including circumoral), pruritis (either generalized or on palms and soles)

e. Other: inverted sensory phenomenon (e.g., cold objects feel warm), sensation of having loose teeth, headache, vertigo, dizziness, dry mouth, metallic taste

f. Cardiovascular manifestations: hypotension, bradycardia, hypertension, tachycardia, arrhythmias, heart block, pulmonary edema, congestive heart failure

g. Most symptoms remit in 1 week after exposure, but certain symptoms may persist for years after original exposure

2. Paralytic shellfish poisoning

a. Caused by saxitoxins and related compounds from dinoflagellates found in certain shellfish

b. Toxin blocks voltage-dependent sodium channels in nerve and muscle

c. Abrupt onset (within 30-60 minutes after ingestion) of

symptoms: paresthesias of face, tongue, perioral areas, and lips; numbness; vertigo; dysarthria; ophthalmoplegia; pupillary abnormalities; ataxia

d. Weakness does not occur in every patient (despite name): when present, may involve the limbs, cranial musculature, swallowing, and respiratory muscles

e. Lack of gastrointestinal illness at onset: toxin has some anticholinergic activity and may act to slow gastric emptying; this, together with absence of emesis, may enhance absorption of the toxin

3. Neurotoxic shellfish poisoning

a. Caused by brevetoxins, polyether neurotoxin produced by the marine dinoflagellate *Karenia brevis* and found in shellfish

b. Brevetoxins

1) Potent lipid-soluble neurotoxins that bind to sodium channels on nerve and muscle cell membranes

2) Produce excessive influx of sodium ions across membranes, causing cellular dysfunction or death

c. Similar to, but less severe than, ciguatera

d. Onset of symptoms: minutes to several hours after ingestion of contaminated food

e. Illness begins with gastrointestinal symptoms: nausea, vomiting, diarrhea, abdominal pain and cramping, rectal burning

f. Neurologic manifestations occur concurrently with gastrointestinal illness: circumoral paresthesias progressing to involve pharynx, torso, and extremities; muscle weakness; myalgias; tremor; dysphagia; mydriasis; inverted temperature sensory phenomenon (as with ciguatera fish poisoning)

g. ELISA assay available for diagnosis

4. Amnestic shellfish poisoning

a. Caused by domoic acid: glutamate receptor agonist, excitatory neurotoxin acting on various CNS glutamate receptors, especially those of hippocampus

b. Source of domoic acid: diatoms

c. Domoic acid: found in shellfish, including certain species of mussel

d. Initial gastrointestinal symptoms, usually within first 24 hours after ingestion: nausea, vomiting, abdominal cramps, diarrhea

e. Neurologic symptoms within 48 hours after ingestion: seizures, hemiparesis, ophthalmoplegia, neuropathy, altered mentation, coma

f. Memory impairment: anterograde and, less common but more severe, retrograde

g. Gradual improvement over 3 months

5. Pufferfish poisoning

a. Most cases associated with consumption of pufferfish

from waters of Indo-Pacific ocean regions

b. Due to tetrodotoxins in various fish, including puffer fish; block voltage-gated sodium channels

c. First symptom of intoxication: perioral paresthesias, appearing 20 minutes to 3 hours after consuming contaminated food

d. Paresthesias spread to face and limbs

e. Other symptoms: headaches, sensation of floating, epigastric pain, nausea, vomiting, diarrhea

f. Following these symptoms: paralysis

g. May be respiratory distress, dysarthria, dyspnea, convulsions, altered mentation, and death within 4 to 6 hours

h. Coma and seizures may occur

i. High mortality rate

j. Death may be due to cardiac arrhythmias or respiratory paralysis; patients may remain completely alert and lucid until death

III. SYSTEMIC METABOLIC DISEASE

A. Nonketotic Hyperosmolar State

1. Hyperglycemia without ketosis, dehydration
2. Reduced level of consciousness, progressing to coma
3. Focal signs or symptoms, including hemiparesis or focal seizures: unique to nonketotic hyperosmolar state, absent in other metabolic derangements; occurrence of focal deficits may be due to previous silent cerebrovascular events
4. Transient T2 signal changes may be present in deep gray matter

B. Diabetic Ketoacidotic Coma

1. Hyperglycemia with ketosis, acidosis, and hyperosmolarity
2. Focal signs uncommon; should raise the possibility of alternative etiology
3. Most patients have benign prognosis, with no residual neurologic deficits
4. May be complicated by diffuse cerebral edema, which presents as recurrence of coma after initial improvement; patients may rapidly lose all brainstem reflexes, including pupillary responses, and meet criteria for brain death within 1 to 2 hours
5. May be associated with abrupt onset of predominantly motor polyneuropathy, with improvement expected some time after treatment of ketoacidosis

C. Hepatic Encephalopathy

1. Pathophysiology

a. Hyperammonemia

  1) Increased ammonia production due to excess dietary protein, constipation, gastrointestinal hemorrhage

  2) Liver: important role in detoxification of ammonia

  3) Degree of encephalopathy: related to blood ammonia levels

b. Endogenous benzodiazepines

  1) Excess endozepine-4 in serum and cerebrospinal fluid; also occurs in relapsing coma due to idiopathic recurring stupor, i.e., spontaneous stupor or coma not associated with known metabolic, toxic, or structural abnormalities but reversed with flumazenil, a pure benzodiazepine antagonist

  2) Cause CNS inhibition by stimulating GABA-benzodiazepine complex

c. Decreased liver metabolism of toxins due to portal-systemic shunting or reduced liver parenchymal reserves because of liver damage

d. Deposition of manganese in brain, especially in deep gray matter

2. Fulminant hepatic failure

a. Often no previous history of liver disease, may be precipitated by viral illness or hepatotoxin

b. Common presenting symptoms: abdominal pain, nausea, vomiting

c. Precipitous onset of mania, hyperexcitability, and delirium, which may rapidly progress to coma if untreated

d. Low incidence of seizures, possibly because of presence of endogenous benzodiazepines

e. Characterized by diffuse brain edema, increased intracranial pressure, possibly brain herniation

3. Chronic hepatic encephalopathy

a. Grade I

  1) Insomnia and abnormal sleep pattern, apathy, irritability, anxiety, inattention, agitation, depression

  2) Fine postural tremor, poor coordination

b. Grade II

  1) Lethargy, disorientation, inappropriate behavior

  2) Asterixis, dysarthria, paratonia, ataxia, hypoactive reflexes, disorientation, personality change, poor recall

c. Grade III

  1) Somnolent, arousable, disorientation

  2) Signs of hyperexcitability: asterixis, myoclonus, exaggerated startle response, hyperactive reflexes, extensor plantar responses, rigidity and paratonia, hyperventilation

d. Grade IV: coma, posturing

e. Asterixis: nonspecific; may be seen in other metabolic conditions, including uremia and dialysis-related encephalopathy, pulmonary disease, nonketotic hyperglycemia, hypokalemia, hypomagnesemia, drugs (lithium, carbamazepine, phenytoin, barbiturates), recovery phase following general anesthesia, structural lesions (typically unilateral asterixis)

    f. Unilateral asterixis
       1) Always raises possibility of structural lesion involving genu and anterior portion of internal capsule or ventrolateral thalamus and, less commonly, midbrain, parietal cortex, medial frontal cortex
       2) Most common cause: thalamic hemorrhage

4. Brain magnetic resonance imaging (MRI): increased T1 signal in globus pallidus, likely from increased concentrations of manganese

5. Electroencephalography (EEG): slowing of background activity (delta slowing when advanced grade encephalopathy) or triphasic waves

6. Blood ammonia levels: arterial blood must be drawn and hand-carried to laboratory for immediate analysis; ammonia levels from venous blood may be artificially increased because applying a tourniquet causes local ischemia of the underlying muscle tissue, from which excess ammonia is released

7. Pathology
    a. Alzheimer type II cells: in neocortex, deep gray matter, brainstem, dentate nucleus
    b. May be microcavitation with gliosis and neuronal loss in these regions

8. Treatment
    a. Symptomatic treatment, including management of intracranial hypertension in cases of fulminant hepatic failure
    b. Specific treatment of precipitating factor or cause
    c. Lactulose, dietary protein restriction, antibiotics (against urea-producing organisms, e.g., neomycin)
    d. Flumazenil (benzodiazepine receptor antagonist)
    e. Embolization or surgical ligation of portal-systemic shunts
    f. Liver transplantation: generally needed for fulminant hepatic failure

D. Neurologic Manifestations of Renal Failure and Dialysis

1. Uremic encephalopathy
    a. Encephalopathy in setting of renal failure, often with multiple concomitant metabolic derangements, including hyponatremia, hypocalcemia, hyperkalemia, hypermagnesemia, metabolic acidosis
    b. Headache, fatigue, malaise, apathy, poor concentration, sleep disturbance, decreased libido, irritability, paranoid ideation, slurred speech, and abnormal movements, including postural tremor, myoclonus (multifocal

myoclonus or minipolymyoclonus), asterixis
    c. Frank delirium may occur
    d. Persistent focal deficits suggest alternate diagnosis
    e. To be differentiated from dialysis dementia (discussed below)
    f. EEG: diffuse slowing, triphasic waves when advanced
    g. Improved with dialysis (as opposed to dialysis encephalopathy, which is worsened by dialysis)

2. Dialysis encephalopathy
    a. Characterized by progressive cognitive decline, nonfluent aphasia and dysarthria (aphasia uncommon in uremic encephalopathy), myoclonus, tremor, asterixis, seizures, and improvement with diazepam (uremic encephalopathy does not respond to diazepam)
    b. Associated with proximal myopathy
    c. Rare entity since establishment of limitations on use of aluminum in dialysis

3. Dialysis disequilibrium syndrome
    a. Occurs with institution of dialysis in setting of chronic renal failure
    b. Pathophysiology
       1) Cytotoxic edema due to osmotic shifts of water, which may be caused by reverse osmotic shift induced by urea and decrease in cerebral intracellular pH
       2) Hemodialysis rapidly removes small solutes such as urea from plasma; permeation of urea molecules across plasma membranes may take several hours to occur
       3) Reduction in plasma urea decreases plasma osmolality and produces transient osmotic gradient that promotes movement of water molecules into cells
    c. Symptoms often occur during or shortly after hemodialysis
    d. Clinical features
       1) Mild disease: headaches, nausea, vomiting, malaise, myalgias, anorexia, restlessness, blurred vision
       2) More severe disease: movement disorders (myoclonus, tremors), seizures, coma, possibly death
    e. Treatment: gentle initial dialysis with goals of slow urea removal and gradual reduction in blood urea nitrogen (BUN)

4. Uremic polyneuropathy
    a. Distal sensorimotor peripheral neuropathy, with predominant electrophysiologic features of axonal loss (predominantly sensory neuropathy until advanced)
    b. Occurs in 60% of patients with end-stage chronic renal failure requiring dialysis
    c. Most common initial clinical features: paresthesias, dysesthesias, burning feet, restless legs syndrome, cramps (latter two may be present without neuropathy)

d. Mild autonomic symptoms

e. Weakness develops with progression (often first involving lower extremities and ascending)

f. Incidence of severe disease reduced with advent of dialysis

g. Uremic mononeuropathies: higher incidence of entrapment neuropathies and occurrence of ischemic monomelic neuropathy in patients with arteriovenous fistula for dialysis (see Chapter 21, Part B)

h. A fulminant, severe, and rapidly progressive, predominantly motor polyneuropathy may occur, often in setting of concomitant sepsis; critical illness polyneuropathy (see Chapter 21)

E. Central Pontine and Extrapontine Myelinolysis

1. Usually occurs in alcoholics

2. Risk factors: chronic liver disease, chronic illness, malnutrition, anorexia, diuretic use, cancer, liver transplantation

3. Pathophysiology likely associated with rapid correction of hyponatremia, but undefined

4. Monophasic demyelinating illness, predominantly involving basis pontis, with or without extrapontine lesions in subcortical white matter, cerebellum, lateral geniculate body, basal ganglia, thalamus, internal capsule (Fig. 17-2)

5. Clinical features: spastic paraparesis, pseudobulbar palsy and dysarthria (from involvement of corticobulbar tracts), lethargy, confusion, locked-in-syndrome, and coma (in most severe form)

6. Clinical course may be complicated by superimposed Wernicke's encephalopathy, ethanol withdrawal, hepatic encephalopathy

F. Hypertensive Encephalopathy

1. Occurs in setting of hypertensive emergency (defined as severely increased blood pressure in presence of end-organ damage)

2. May occur in eclampsia (hypertensive emergency of pregnancy), associated with peripheral edema and proteinuria

3. Usually occurs in context of abrupt increase in blood pressure in normotensive patients

4. May be precipitated by use of stimulant drugs such as cocaine or amphetamines

5. Pathophysiology

a. Vasogenic edema (cytotoxic edema may also occur when there is concomitant cerebral ischemia)

b. There may be a component of vasoconstriction and resultant hypoperfusion

c. Seems to be predilection for involvement of parenchyma supplied by posterior circulation; may be related to relatively deficient sympathetic innervation of posterior circulation compared with that of anterior circulation

d. Predilection for posterior circulation explains the common occurrence of reversible posterior leukoencephalopathy (RPLE) in this setting

e. RPLE may also occur from immunosuppressive drugs such as cyclosporine, likely due to direct toxic effect on vascular endothelium, vasoconstriction caused by endothelin, and formation of microthrombi

f. Predisposing (or causative) factors: eclampsia, pheochromocytoma, acute glomerulonephritis, sympathomimetic agents (e.g., cocaine, amphetamines), vasculitis and collagen vascular disease, withdrawal from antihypertensive agents

6. Neuroimaging characteristics

a. T2-hyperintense (T1-hypointense) lesions, with predilection for occipital and posterior parietal lobes (RPLE)

b. Increased values on acute diffusion coefficient (ADC) mapping (in contrast to decreased values seen in cytotoxic edema of subacute infarcts): indicative of vasogenic edema

c. Changes may also be present in cerebral white matter and basal ganglia

7. Clinical features

a. Headaches, nausea, seizures, altered mentation

b. Visual obscurations or loss of vision (due to papilledema secondary to increased intracranial pressure or RPLE)

c. Upward transtentorial herniation and hydrocephalus due to cerebellar edema has rarely been reported

8. Treatment

a. Discontinuation of offending agent, if there is one (e.g., immunosuppresants)

b. Emergent initiation of antihypertensives: goal should be baseline blood pressure before presentation

c. If untreated, cerebral ischemia and hemorrhage may occur, producing irreversible brain injury

d. "Set point" for autoregulation of cerebral vasculature changes within several hours: aggressive and rapid control of hypertension could potentially precipitate cerebral ischemia

e. β-Blockers or calcium channel blockers (particularly those with rapid onset and short duration of action) are preferred agents (e.g., labetalol or esmolol, nicardipine)

f. Vasodilators such as nitroglycerine should be avoided because they can increase intracranial pressure

g. Hydralazine (arterial vasodilator) also has potential to increase intracranial pressure

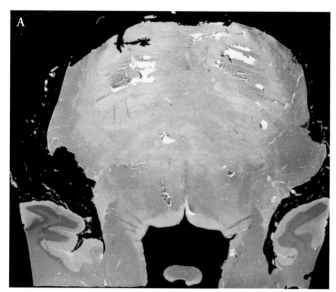

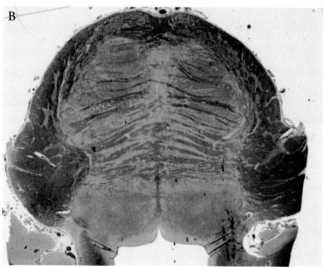

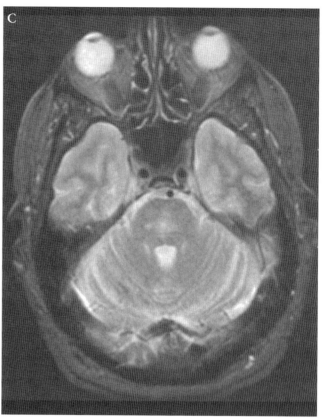

Fig. 17-2. Central pontine myelinolysis (CPM). *A*, Symmetric and extensive loss of myelin in basis pontis, with relative sparing of subpial tissue and small patches within substance of the pons. (Klüver stain.) *B*, Remarkable preservation of axons in region of extensive demyelination. (Silver stain.) *C*, MRI of a different patient with CPM shows symmetric increased T2 signal in pons, corresponding to region of demyelination. (Axial T2 MRI sequence.)

REFERENCES

Engleberg NC, Morris JG Jr, Lewis J, McMillan JP, Pollard RA, Blake PA. Ciguatera fish poisoning: a major common-source outbreak in the U.S. Virgin Islands. Ann Intern Med. 1983;98:336-7.

Gijtenbeek JM, van den Bent MJ, Vecht CJ. Cyclosporine neurotoxicity: a review. J Neurol. 1999;246:339-46.

Morris JG Jr, Lewin P, Hargrett NT, Smith CW, Blake PA, Schneider R. Clinical features of ciguatera fish poisoning: a study of the disease in the US Virgin Islands. Arch Intern Med. 1982;142:1090-2.

Pearn J. Neurology of ciguatera. J Neurol Neurosurg Psychiatry. 2001;70:4-8.

Perl TM, Bedard L, Kosatsky T, Hockin JC, Todd EC, McNutt LA, et al. Amnesic shellfish poisoning: a new clinical syndrome due to domoic acid. Can Dis Wkly Rep. 1990;16 Suppl 1E:7-8.

Teitelbaum JS, Zatorre RJ, Carpenter S, Gendron D, Evans AC, Gjedde A, et al. Neurologic sequelae of domoic acid intoxication due to the ingestion of contaminated mussels. N Engl J Med. 1990;322:1781-7.

Vaughan CJ, Delanty N. Hypertensive emergencies. Lancet. 2000;356:411-7.

QUESTIONS

1. A 62-year-old woman with hypertension presents with unilateral asterixis. The most likely cause is:
   a. Uremia
   b. Nonketotic hyperglycemic state
   c. Reversible posterior leukoencephalopathy
   d. Thalamic hemorrhage
   e. Pontine infarct

2. *All* the following clinical features may be used to distinguish between uremic encephalopathy and dialysis encephalopathy (dementia) *except*:
   a. Clinical response to dialysis
   b. Aphasia
   c. EEG characteristics
   d. Response to diazepam

MATCHING. Match the toxins in the left column with the syndrome in the right column. A choice from the right column may be usued once, more than once, or not at all.

3. Organic mercury
4. Trichloroethylene
5. Thallium
6. Methanol
7. Carbon monoxide
8. Inorganic lead

a. Alopecia
b. Predilection for dorsal root ganglia, calcarine cortex, and cerebellar granular layer
c. Necrosis of optic nerves and putamina bilaterally
d. Trigeminal neuropathy
e. Basophilic stippling of red blood cells on peripheral blood smear
f. Pallidal hemorrhages

MATCHING. Match the toxin in the left column with the pathogenic mechanism of action in the right column. A choice from the right column may be used once, more than once, or not at all.

9. Saxitoxin
10. *Amanita* toxins
11. α-Latrotoxin
12. Tityustoxin
13. Tetrodotoxin
14. Domoic acid

a. Postsynaptic activation of voltage-gated sodium channels
b. Block voltage-gated sodium channels
c. Block cholinergic synapses
d. Glutamate receptor agonist
e. Acute release of acetylcholine from synaptic terminals

ANSWERS

1. Answer: d.
Thalamic hemorrhage is the most common cause of unilateral asterixis. Uremia, nonketotic hyperglycemic state, and use of drugs (e.g., phenytoin, lithium, carbamazepine, and barbiturates) are more commonly associated with bilateral asterixis. Reversible posterior leukoencephalopathy has not been associated with unilateral asterixis.

2. Answer: c.
EEG characteristics do not distinguish between the two entities. There may be diffuse slowing with or without triphasic waves in both circumstances. Patients with uremic encephalopathy tend to respond to dialysis, whereas patients with dialysis encephalopathy experience clinical worsening when treated with dialysis. Aphasia occurs commonly in patients with dialysis encephalopathy and only rarely in those with uremic encephalopathy. Treatment with diazepam produces clinical improvement in patients with dialysis dementia but rarely in those with uremic encephalopathy.

3. Answer: b.

4. Answer: d.

5. Answer: a.

6. Answer: c.

7. Answer: f.

8. Answer: e.

9 and 13. Answer: b.
Saxitoxin and tetrodotoxin both block voltage-gated sodium channels.

10. Answer: c.
Mushroom toxins, such as those from *Amanita muscaria*, block both cholinergic and GABA synapses.

11. Answer: e.
Latrotoxin, the venom of the black widow spider, produces acute release of acetylcholine from synaptic terminals.

12. Answer: a.
Tityustoxin, produced by *Tityus serrulatus* scorpion, causes presynaptic facilitation of acetylcholine release and postsynaptic activation of voltage-gated sodium channels.

14. Answer: d.
Domoic acid, an excitatory neurotoxin produced by diatoms, is a glutamate receptor agonist, which acts on hippocampal glutamate receptors to produce amnestic shellfish poisoning.

HEADACHE 18

Kelly D. Flemming, M.D.

I. CLASSIFICATION AND APPROACH

A. International Headache Society (IHS) Criteria

1. IHS has developed criteria to divide headaches into primary and secondary types
2. Primary type: headaches without specific cause (migraine, tension, cluster, miscellaneous)
3. Secondary type: headaches with underlying structural or metabolic cause

B. Headache History and Physical Examination

1. Headache history
   a. Aimed at distinguishing between primary and secondary types of headache
   b. Typical questions to consider
      1) Prodrome or aura
      2) Onset and course
      3) Duration and frequency
      4) Pain quality and severity
      5) Associated features
      6) Precipitating factors
      7) Ameliorating factors
      8) Family and social history
   c. Worrisome features in history for secondary type
      1) Thunderclap (acute) onset
      2) Late-onset headache with no previous headache history
      3) Systemic disease (infectious, metabolic, toxic)
      4) Patient with history of cancer
      5) Patient with history of immunosuppressed state
      6) Headache worsens with cough or strain, especially worrisome if associated with transient visual obscurations
2. Physical examination
   a. Aimed at distinguishing between primary and secondary types of headache
   b. Worrisome features in physical examination suggesting a secondary type

1) Focal neurologic deficits
2) Papilledema

II. ACUTE HEADACHE

A. Clinical Presentation

1. Determine onset and course
   a. Did the headache reach maximum severity in seconds, minutes, hours, or days—thunderclap presentation (maximum severity within seconds) is particularly worrisome
   b. Is the headache improving, stable, worsening
2. Determine associated symptoms
   a. Nausea or vomiting
   b. Photophobia
   c. Visual phenomena
   d. Focal limb deficits (sensory or motor): can be suggestive of intracranial lesion
   e. Visual obscurations: may be suggestive of increased intracranial pressure
3. Determine if there were or are any provoking factors
   a. Postural: upright vs. laying down (if headache worse in upright position, may suggest low-pressure headache syndrome)
   b. Coughing, sneezing, or straining: may suggest increased intracranial pressure
   c. Exertion

B. Differential Diagnosis of Acute Thunderclap Headache (Table 18-1)

C. Diagnostic Approach

1. Subarachnoid hemorrhage must be ruled out in all patients presenting with a thunderclap headache
2. Sensitivity of computed tomography (CT) of the head for subarachnoid hemorrhage
   a. CT without contrast is 92% sensitive in detecting

Table 18-1.   Differential Diagnosis of Acute Thunderclap Headache

Subarachnoid hemorrhage

Intracerebral hemorrhage

Pituitary apoplexy

Venous sinus thrombosis

Arterial dissection

Acute meningitis

Hypertensive crisis

Low-pressure headache

Call-Fleming syndrome (reversible segmental cerebral vasoconstriction)

Glaucoma

Migraine

Benign thunderclap headache

Cluster headache

Exertional headache (exertional, cough, or coital headache)

subarachnoid hemorrhage if performed within 24 hours

   b. Sensitivity falls to approximately 50% by end of day 5 after symptom onset

   c. If CT is negative and clinical suspicion high, lumbar puncture is necessary

3. Cerebrospinal fluid (CSF) examination

   a. Best to perform at least 6 hours after symptom onset, but no more than 2 to 3 weeks after symptom onset

   b. Variables evaluated: opening pressure, cell counts in tube 1 and tube 4, protein, glucose, Gram stain, xanthochromia

   c. Interpretation of CSF findings (see Chapter 10)

4. Magnetic resonance imaging (MRI) and magnetic resonance (MR) venography: may be performed to exclude venous sinus thrombosis when CSF is normal or shows increased opening pressures and is otherwise normal, thus excluding subarachnoid hemorrhage and meningitis

5. Consideration of additional tests

   a. MR or conventional angiography

     1) If suspicion for subarachnoid hemorrhage or sentinel leak of aneurysm is high

     2) Conventional angiography has greater sensitivity for small aneurysms than MR angiography

   b. MRI head: if increased intracranial pressure, hypertensive crisis, or intracranial hemorrhage suspected

D. Treatment: specific to the cause

III. MIGRAINE HEADACHE

A. Epidemiology

1. Lifetime prevalence: estimated to be approximately 20% to 25% for women, 8% to 10% for men

2. Begins in males earlier than females

3. Positive family history for migraine is common

B. Pathophysiology

1. Etiology: may have genetic component, for example, P type calcium channels may be implicated in cause of migraine headaches (involved with 5-hydroxytryptamine [5HT] release)

2. Migraine aura

   a. Hypoperfusion of blood flow is seen often before headache begins and in association with aura

   b. This wave of reduced cerebral blood flow travels across cerebral cortex 2 to 3 mm/min

3. Headache

   a. Intracranial blood vessels innervated by pain-sensitive fibers of trigeminal nerve (supratentorial area) and cervical nerves (posterior fossa)

   b. One theory: antidromic stimulation of trigeminal nerve releases substance P, calcitonin gene-related peptide (CGRP), and neurokinin A, producing neurogenic inflammation

   c. Neurogenic inflammation results in vessel dilatation and plasma protein extravasation

   d. Central processing of pain

     1) Afferent projections to trigeminal spinal nucleus

     2) Synaptic relay from trigeminal spinal nucleus is in thalamus: ventral posteromedial (VPM), intralaminar, and posterior nuclei

     3) Thalamic projections to cerebral cortex

     4) Influence from the dorsal raphe nucleus and locus ceruleus

   e. $5HT_{1b}$ receptor: responsible for cranial vasoconstriction

     1) Three receptor types: G protein–coupled receptors, ligand-gated ion channels, and transporters

     2) Seven classes of receptors (1-7)

     3) $5HT_1$: five receptor subtypes (Table 18-2)

   f. Triptan medications are $5HT_{1b/1d}$ agonists

     1) Inhibit release of vasoactive peptides

     2) Promote vasoconstriction

     3) Affect modulating pain pathways in brainstem

C. Clinical Presentation

1. Prodrome

   a. Hours to days before headache

   b. Occurs in more than 50% of patients with migraine

Table 18-2.　5-Hydroxytryptamine (5HT) Subclass 1 Receptors

Subtype of 5HT$_1$ receptor	Agonist	Location	Function
A	Dihydro-ergotamine		Behavioral (satiety)
B	Dihydro-ergotamine	Extracerebral cranial vessels	Cerebrovascular receptor
	Eletriptan	Trigeminal ganglion	
	Naratriptan		
	Rizatriptan	Coronary vessels	
	Sumatriptan		
	Zolmitriptan		
D	Dihydro-ergotamine	Trigeminal ganglion	Trigeminal neuronal receptor
	Eletriptan	Cerebral microvessels	
	Naratriptan		
	Rizatriptan		
	Sumatriptan		
	Zolmitriptan		
E	Rizatriptan		Not clear
F	Dihydro-ergotamine		Not clear
	Naratriptan		
	Rizatriptan		
	Sumatriptan		
	Zolmitriptan		

Modified from Silberstein SD, Lipton RB, Goadsby PJ. Headache in clinical practice. Oxford: Isis Medical Media; 1998. p. 41-58. Used with permission.

   c. Can consist of mental state changes, poor concentration, food cravings, gastrointestinal and urinary symptoms

2. Aura
   a. Focal neurologic symptoms preceding headache typically lasting less than 1 hour
   b. Most commonly consist of visual disturbances but also can include sensory (second-most common), motor, language dysfunction
   c. May occur alone or associated with headache

3. Location
   a. Unilateral more often than bilateral
   b. Often frontal

4. Quality: throbbing, pounding (not always)

5. Associated symptoms
   a. Nausea and/or vomiting
   b. Photophobia and/or phonophobia
   c. Anorexia
   d. Worse with exertion, better in dark room

6. Duration: hours to days

7. Precipitating factors
   a. Variable
   b. May include
     1) Food and/or drink (red wine, monosodium glutamate)
     2) Stress
     3) Certain odors
     4) Minor trauma
     5) Menses

D. Differential Diagnosis
1. Structural lesions (secondary headaches)
2. Metabolic disorders (secondary headache syndromes), including **m**itochondrial myopathy, **e**ncephalopathy, **l**actic **a**cidosis, **s**troke (MELAS) syndrome
3. **C**erebral **a**utosomal **d**ominant **a**rteriopathy with **s**ub-cortical **i**nfarcts and **l**eukoencephalopathy (CADASIL)
4. Tension headaches

E. Diagnostic Approach
1. IHS criteria for migraine are listed in Table 18-3
2. Diagnosis is based on clinical symptomatology
3. Neurologic examination and head neuroimaging are usually negative

F. Treatment
1. Acute treatment
   a. Early treatment: should be given soon after symptom onset
   b. Options for acute treatment
     1) General analgesics
     2) Migraine-specific remedies (serotonergic ["triptan"] medications and dihydroergotamine)
   c. Management of associated symptoms (e.g., nausea and vomiting)
   d. Treatments available for acute migraine headache are reviewed in Table 18-4
   e. Current triptan medications are reviewed in Table 18-5

2. Prophylaxis
   a. Should be considered for patients whose headache frequency is functionally disabling
   b. Prophylactic options are listed in Table 18-6

3. Nonmedication therapy
   a. Biofeedback
   b. Physical therapy
   c. Acupuncture

Table 18-3. **International Headache Society Criteria for Migraine Headaches**

Migraine without aura
  A. At least 5 attacks fulfilling criteria B-D
  B. Headache lasting 4-72 hours (untreated or unsuccessfully treated)
  C. Headache has at least 2 of the following characteristics:
       1. Unilateral location
       2. Pulsating quality
       3. Moderate or severe intensity (inhibits or prohibits daily activities)
       4. Aggravation by walking stairs or similar routine physical activity
  D. During headache at least 1 of the following:
       1. Nausea and/or vomiting
       2. Photophobia and phonophobia
  E. Not attributed to another disorder
Migraine with aura
  A. At least 2 attacks fulfilling criteria B-D
  B. Aura consisting of at least 1 of the following, but no motor weakness:
       1. Fully reversible visual symptoms, including positive features (e.g., flickering lights, spots, or lines) and/or negative features (i.e., loss of vision)
       2. Fully reversible sensory symptoms, including positive features (e.g., pins and needles) and/or negative features (e.g., numbness)
       3. Fully reversible dysphasic speech disturbance
  C. At least 2 of the following:
       1. Homonymous visual symptoms and/or unilateral sensory symptoms
       2. At least 1 aura symptom develops gradually over 5 or more minutes and/or different aura symptoms occur in succession over 5 or more minutes
       3. Each symptom lasts at least 5 minutes and no more than 60 minutes
  D. Headache fulfilling criteria B-D for migraine without aura begins during the aura or follows aura within 60 minutes
  E. Not attributed to another disorder
Basilar migraine
  A. At least 2 attacks fulfilling criteria B-D
  B. Aura consisting of at least 2 of the following fully reversible symptoms, but no motor weakness:
       1. Dysarthria
       2. Vertigo
       3. Tinnitus
       4. Decreased hearing
       5. Double vision
       6. Visual symptoms simultaneously in both temporal and nasal fields of both eyes
       7. Ataxia
       8. Bilateral paresthesias
       9. Decreased level of consciousness
  C. At least 1 of the following:
       1. At least 1 aura symptom develops gradually over 5 or more minutes and/or different aura symptoms occur in succession over 5 or more minutes
       2. Each aura symptom lasts at least 5 minutes and no more than 60 minutes
  D. Headache fulfilling criteria B-D for migraine without aura begins during the aura or follows aura within 60 minutes
  E. Not attributed to another disorder
Familial hemiplegic migraine
  A. At least 2 attacks fulfilling criteria B and C
  B. Aura consisting of fully reversible motor weakness and at least 1 of the following:
       1. Fully reversible visual symptoms, including positive features (e.g., flickering lights, spots, or lines) and/or negative features (e.g., loss of vision)
       2. Fully reversible sensory symptoms, including positive features (e.g., pins and needles) and/or negative features (e.g., numbness)
       3. Fully reversible dysphasic speech disturbance

Table 18-3. **continued**

Familial/hemiplegic migraine (continued)
   C. At least 2 of the following:
      1. At least 1 aura symptom develops gradually over 5 or more minutes and/or different aura symptoms occur in succession over 5 or more minutes and less than 24 hours
      2. Headache fulfilling criteria B-D for migraine without aura begins during the aura or follows onset of the aura within 60 minutes
   D. At least 1 first-degree or second-degree relative has had attacks fulfilling criteria A-E
   E. Not attributed to another disorder
Chronic migraine
   A. Headache fulfilling criteria C and D for migraine without aura on at least 15 days per month for more than 3 months
   B. Not attributed to another disorder

Table 18-4. **Treatments for Acute Migraine Headache**

Medication	Side effects	Contraindications (relative and absolute)
General analgesics		
Acetaminophen	Well tolerated Hepatotoxicity with excess use	Liver disease
Nonsteroidal anti-inflammatory drugs	Gastrointestinal symptoms: abdominal pain, constipation, diarrhea, dyspepsia, heartburn, nausea, stomatitis, vomiting Neurologic symptoms: dizziness, drowsiness, headache Other: rash	Severe liver or kidney disease Peptic ulcer disease Pregnancy
Aspirin	Gastritis/peptic ulcer disease Renal insufficiency Toxicity	Renal insufficiency Peptic ulcer disease
Narcotics	Constipation Respiratory suppression	Abuse history Severe respiratory disease
Isometheptene	Dizziness	Severe hypertension Renal or hepatic disease Concurrent MAOI therapy Glaucoma
Migraine-targeting medications		
Dihydroergotamine	Altered taste (nasal spray) Dizziness Nausea/vomiting Vascular ischemia (rare, but serious) Ergotism (rare)	Severe hypertension Use with other pressor/vasoconstrictive medications Hemiplegic/basilar migraine Hypersensitivity to ergot alkaloid products Previous vascular disease Pregnancy and lactation Prolonged hypotension, shock Impaired liver and kidney function
Ergotamine	Similar to dihydroergotamine Retroperitoneal fibrosis (rare, but serious)	Same as for dihydroergotamine
Triptan	Flushing Chest pain Dizziness, fatigue, asthenia Dyspnea Nausea/vomiting, diarrhea Precipitate vascular disease (rare, but serious)	Vascular disease or patients at risk for vascular disease Coadministration with other triptan or ergotamine derivative Recent MAOI therapy Hemiplegic or basilar migraine Hypersensitivity to triptan Uncontrolled hypertension Severe liver disease

MAOI, monoamine oxidase inhibitor.

Table 18-5.   **Comparison of Triptan Agents (Selective Serotonin Agents)**

Triptan	Dosage forms	Onset of action	Duration (half-life)
Sumatriptan	Subcutaneous	10-60 min	2 h
	Oral	1-2 h	
	Intranasal	60 min	
Zolmitriptan	Oral	Within 1 h	2.5-3 h
	Oral disintegrating	...	
	Intranasal	...	
Almotriptan	Oral	1-2 h	3-4 h
	Subcutaneous	1-2 h	
Naratriptan	Oral	1 h	5-6 h
Eletriptan	Oral	Within 1 h	4-5 h
Rizatriptan	Oral	30 min	2-3 h
Frovatriptan	Oral	2 h	25 h

G. Status Migraine

1. Definition: severe persistent migraine headache often with intractable nausea and vomiting
2. Management
   a. Rule out secondary causes of headache
   b. Hydrate patient with intravenous fluids
   c. Specific treatment (administered individually)
      1) Dihydroergotamine
      2) Valproate intravenous
      3) Chlorpromazine or prochlorperazine intravenous
      4) Ketorolac intravenous
      5) Metoclopramide
      6) Corticosteroids
      7) Narcotic medication

H. Transformed Migraine (see section VI)

I. Familial Hemiplegic Migraine (FHM)

1. Definition: diagnostic criteria listed in Table 18-3
2. Clinical description
   a. Typically begins in childhood
   b. Hemiplegia may precede or occur concomitantly with headache or headache may be absent
   c. Hemiplegia may last hours to days
3. Genetics and pathophysiology
   a. Hemiplegic migraine may be sporadic or familial
   b. Autosomal dominant with variable penetrance
   c. Three types have been identified
      1) FHM1, linked to chromosome 19p13 in majority of

families (*CACNA1A* gene): results in defect in P/Q calcium channel subunit
      2) FHM2, linked to chromosome 1q23 (*ATP1A2* gene): results in defect in A1A2 sodium-potassium ATPase channel
      3) FHM3, linked to chromosome 2q24 (*SCN1A* gene): results in cortically expressed presynaptic and post-synaptic voltage-gated sodium channel

J. Migrainous Cerebral Infarction (see section IX)

IV. Tension Headache

A. Epidemiology

1. Up to 80% of people experience one tension headache in their lifetime
2. More common in women than men
3. Peak prevalence: between age 20 and 50 years

B. Clinical Presentation

1. Location: majority are bilateral occipital, frontal, or fronto-occipital, but may occur in any location
2. Quality: dull ache or pressure
3. Severity: often mild to moderate
4. Associated symptoms
   a. Tenderness to palpation
   b. Absence of nausea, vomiting, photophobia
   c. Not aggravated by physical activity
5. Precipitating factors include sleep deprivation

C. Diagnostic Approach

1. Diagnosis is based on clinical criteria and evaluating for secondary causes
2. IHS criteria are noted in Table 18-7

D. Chronic Tension Headache (see section VI)

E. Treatment

1. Pharmacologic
   a. Abortive
      1) Nonsteroidal anti-inflammatory drugs
      2) Aspirin
      3) Acetaminophen
   b. Prophylactic
      1) Tricyclic antidepressants
      2) Antiepileptic medications (most commonly, topiramate, valproic acid, gabapentin)
      3) Selective serotonin reuptake inhibitors
      4) β-Blockers
      5) Calcium channel blockers

Table 18-6. **Migraine Prophylactic Regimens***

Medication	Contraindications	Recommended for patient	Examples
β-Blockers	Obstructive pulmonary disease Hypotension Bradycardia Heart block	With concurrent hypertension	Propranolol, nadolol
Calcium channel blockers	Hypotension Bradycardia Heart block	With concurrent hypertension	Verapamil
Antidepressants			
Tricyclic and tetracyclic	Concomitant MAOI therapy Severe urinary retention Cardiac dysthymia	With concurrent depression or insomnia	Amitriptyline, nortriptyline, mirtazapine
MAOIs	Many drug and food interactions Congestive heart failure Certain anesthetics Liver disease Uncontrolled hypertension Pregnancy	With concurrent depression	Phenelzine
Selective serotonin reuptake inhibitors	Concurrent MAOI use Liver disease Seizure disorder (precaution) Mania	With concurrent depression	Sertraline, fluoxetine
Anticonvulsants			
Divalproate	Liver disease Urea cycle disorders Pancreatitis	With concurrent mood disorder With concurrent seizure disorder	
Topiramate	Kidney or liver disease	With concurrent seizure disorder	
Gabapentin	Hypersensitivity Renal insufficiency	With concurrent seizure disorder	
Herbal/nutritional remedies			
Riboflavin (vitamin B_2)	Hypersensitivity to vitamin	Intolerant to systemic side effects of medication Who is not willing to take prescription medications	
Butterbur root extract (Petadolex)	Hypersensitivity to butterbur Pregnancy	Intolerant to systemic side effects of medication Who is not willing to take prescription medications	
Injections			
Botulinum toxin type A (Botox)	Infection in area where injections to be given Hypersensitivity to drug	With severe systemic side effects with medication trials With severe comorbidities with contraindications to medications	

MAOI, monoamine oxidase inhibitor.
The list is not exhaustive and one should consult a medication reference before prescribing any of these drugs.

Table 18-7. International Headache Society Criteria for Tension-Type Headaches

Episodic tension headache
  A. At least 10 previous headaches fulfilling criteria B-D; must have fewer than 180 headache episodes per year (<15/month)
  B. Headache lasting from 30 minutes to 7 days
  C. At least 2 of the following characteristics:
      1. Pressing/tightening (nonpulsating) quality
      2. Mild or moderate intensity (may inhibit, but does not prohibit, activities)
      3. Bilateral location
      4. Not aggravated by climbing stairs or similar routine physical activity
  D. Both of the following:
      1. No nausea or vomiting (anorexia may occur)
      2. Photophobia and phonophobia are absent or one but not the other is present
Chronic tension-type headache
  A. Average headache frequency more than 15 days/month (180 days/year) for more than 6 months fulfilling criteria B-D above

2. Nonpharmacologic: behavioral treatment, biofeedback, treatment of concurrent depression

V. CLUSTER HEADACHE

A. Epidemiology
1. Incidence: 15.6/100,000 person-years for men; 4.0/100,000 person-years for women
2. Mean age at onset: 20s to 30s

B. Pathophysiology
1. Unknown
2. Because of episodic clustering of headaches and cyclical bouts on yearly basis, hypothalamus (suprachiasmatic nucleus) may be involved
3. Retro-orbital pain suggests involvement of the trigeminal nerve (ophthalmic division)
4. Sympathetic dysfunction and parasympathetic overactivity suggest role of autonomic system

C. Clinical Presentation
1. Timing
   a. Cluster periods may last weeks to months
   b. Cluster periods often separated by remission (if not, may represent chronic cluster)
   c. Attacks within a cluster period may be daily to several times daily, each lasting 15 to 180 minutes
2. Location: unilateral, orbital, or temporal pain
3. Quality: often severe
4. Precipitating factors: alcohol and other solvents, nitrates
5. Patients tend to pace, rather than lay down (as with patients with migraine headaches)
6. Associated symptoms
   a. Conjunctival injection
   b. Lacrimation
   c. Nasal congestion
   d. Rhinorrhea
   e. Forehead and facial sweating
   f. Miosis
   g. Ptosis
   h. Eyelid edema

D. Diagnostic Approach and Differential Diagnosis
1. Diagnosis is generally a clinical one
2. Important distinction is eliminating potential secondary causes
3. Differential diagnosis: trigeminal autonomic cephalgias, cavernous sinus disease, sinusitis, vertebral arterial dissection, Raeder's paratrigeminal syndrome, temporal arteritis, Tolosa-Hunt syndrome

E. Treatment
1. Abortive (of individual attacks)
   a. Oxygen
      1) Use oxygen by face mask at flow rate of 7 to 10 L/minute for 15 minutes
      2) May help in up to 60% to 70% of patients
   b. Sumatriptan
      1) 6 mg subcutaneously has rapid onset and is effective in most patients within 15 minutes
      2) Contraindications (Table 18-4)
   c. Lidocaine: intranasal lidocaine drops may be used
   d. Dihydroergotamine (DHE): 1 mg intramuscularly or intravenously is effective rapidly
2. Prophylaxis (prevention of cluster periods and reduce length of present attacks)
   a. Consider if
      1) Frequent attacks would require overusing certain abortive agents
      2) Attacks are too short lived for abortive treatment
      3) Frequent cluster periods
   b. Treat throughout cluster period and 2 weeks after last headache
   c. Options are noted in Table 18-8

Table 18-8.   **Prophylaxis for Cluster Headaches***

Medication	Starting dose	Typical maintenance dose	Side effects
Verapamil	80 mg PO 3 times daily	120-480 mg daily in 3-4 divided doses	Constipation Edema Hypotension
Ergotamine	1 mg PO 3 times daily	4 mg daily in divided doses	Nausea Paresthesias Itching

Lithium carbonate	300 mg PO twice daily	300-900 mg daily in 2-3 divided doses
		Serum concentration should be
		   <1.2 mEq/L
			Nausea
			Diarrhea
			Muscle weakness
			Visual scotoma
			Rare, but serious: cardiac
			   dysrhythmia, ataxia,
			   increased intracranial
			   pressure, polyuria

Corticosteroids
  (dexamethasone
  or prednisone)
		Dexamethasone: 4 mg twice daily
		  for 2 weeks, then taper
		Prednisone: 60 mg for 3-5 days and
		  taper by 10 mg every 3 days
			Euphoria
			Osteoporosis (long term)
			Immunosuppression
			Hypertension
			Hyperglycemia

Methysergide	2 mg PO daily	4-8 mg daily in divided doses	Facial flushing
			Weight gain
			Diarrhea
			Nausea/vomiting
			Rare, but serious: vaso-
			  spasm, retroperitoneal
			  fibrosis, pulmonary
			  fibrosis, ergotism

Valproic acid	250 mg PO twice daily	500-2,000 mg daily	Alopecia
			Weight gain
			Nausea, diarrhea
			Rare, but serious: pancrea-
			  titis, thrombocytopenia,
			  liver failure

PO, orally.
*The list is not exhaustive and one should consult a medication reference before prescribing any of these drugs.

    d. Choice of medication may depend on comorbid
       conditions
    e. Avoidance of known triggers

VI. Chronic Daily Headache

A. Overview

1. A group of headache disorders that occur most days per
   month lasting 4 hours or more
2. May include both primary and secondary headache types

    a. Primary: transformed migraine, chronic tension, new
       daily persistent headache (NDPH), and hemicrania
       continua
    b. Secondary: cerebral venous thrombosis, increased or
       decreased intracranial hypertension, lesion in cervical or
       trigeminal distribution, space-occupying mass, central
       nervous system (CNS) or sinus infection, cervical spine
       disorders, post-traumatic, Arnold-Chiari malformation,
       sleep apnea
3. Primary types may be seen with or without medication
   overuse (rebound)

B. Transformed Migraine

1. Definition
   a. Patients have previous episodes of migraine headache that increase in frequency to daily or near daily
2. Common features
   a. Patients have history of episodic migraine that increases in frequency over time
   b. Associated symptoms such as nausea, photophobia, and phonophobia decrease but headache becomes constant, occurring more than 15 days per month
   c. Headache may take on a chronic tension-type quality
   d. Increased frequency commonly occurs in setting of overuse of analgesics
   e. Depression is common
3. Differential diagnosis: includes other chronic daily headaches (primary and secondary)
4. Treatment
   a. If medication overuse, withdrawal of (taper) or limiting offending agent is important
   b. Preventive medications include those commonly used for migraine prophylaxis

C. Chronic Tension Headache

1. Clinical features
   a. Patients may have had a previous history of episodic tension headaches that increased in frequency to occur 15 or more days per month
   b. Headache characteristics similar to episodic tension headache but may include nausea
   c. Headache duration: generally more than 4 hours
   d. Criteria require these characteristics to be present for at least 6 months
   e. Transformation to chronic daily headache may or may not be associated with increased analgesic use
2. Differential diagnosis
   a. Includes other chronic daily headaches (primary and secondary)
   b. IHS criteria are listed in Table 18-7
3. Treatment: prophylactic agents and nonpharmacologic treatment similar to that of tension headaches

D. New Daily Persistent Headache (NDPH)

1. Clinical features
   a. Headache typically develops within 1 to 3 days and persists
   b. Headache characteristics similar to those of tension headache
   c. May or may not be associated with medication overuse
2. Differential diagnosis
   a. Includes other chronic daily headaches (primary and secondary)

   b. Criteria for NDPH are listed in Table 18-9
3. Treatment: strategies similar to those for transformed migraine and chronic tension headache

E. Hemicrania Continua (see section VII)

F. Medication Overuse Headache (rebound headache)

1. Epidemiology
   a. Offending agents: many types, including narcotics, barbiturates or barbiturate-containing combination medications, general analgesics, triptans, ergotamine, caffeine
   b. Common presentation in headache clinics
2. Pathophysiology
   a. Can occur in patients taking offending agents as few as 2 times weekly to several times daily
   b. Some believe this represents a withdrawal syndrome of offending agent
3. Clinical features
   a. Headache is generally described as a constant, diffuse, dull headache
   b. Anxiety and depression are common
4. Treatment
   a. Prevention is important in patients being prescribed any analgesic, including triptans
   b. Refractory to prophylactic medications until offending analgesic is tapered and limited or withdrawn
   c. Offending agent should be tapered by 10% to 25% per week
   d. Prophylactic agents used for other chronic daily headaches can be considered

---

Table 18-9. **International Headache Society Criteria for New Daily Persistent Headache**

A. Headache for more than 3 months fulfilling criteria B-D
B. Headache is daily and unremitting from onset or for less than 3 days from onset
C. At least 2 of the following pain characteristics:
   1. Bilateral location
   2. Pressing and/or tightening quality
   3. Mild or moderate intensity
   4. Not aggravated by routine physical activity such as walking or climbing stairs
D. Both of the following:
   1. No more than 1 of photophobia, phonophobia, or mild nausea
   2. Neither moderate/severe nausea nor vomiting
E. Not attributed to another disorder

VII. Trigeminal Autonomic Cephalgias and Indomethacin-Responsive Headaches

A. **Trigeminal Autonomic Cephalgia:** definitions
1. Unifying features include pain in distribution of trigeminal nerve and autonomic signs reflecting activation of cranial parasympathetic systems (superior salivatory nucleus innervation of lacrimal glands and nasal mucosa via sphenopalatine and otic ganglia)
2. Includes cluster, paroxysmal hemicrania, short-lasting unilateral neuralgiform headache with conjunctival injection and tearing (SUNCT) syndrome
3. Hemicrania continua was thought a trigeminal autonomic cephalgia, but recently was designated as "other primary headache"
4. Because many of these syndromes are unilateral and associated with autonomic symptoms, neuroimaging is often necessary to rule out structural causes
5. Differential diagnosis is listed in Table 18-10

B. **Paroxysmal Hemicrania**
1. Epidemiology
   a. Female:male is 2:1
   b. Onset: generally in 30s, but range can be wide
   c. Two types: episodic and chronic
2. Clinical presentation
   a. Headache
      1) Unilateral, temporal, or orbital
      2) Severe, boring, throbbing, stabbing pain
      3) Short lasting (average, 30 minutes)

Table 18-10. Differential Diagnosis of Trigeminal Autonomic Cephalgias (Secondary Causes)

Chronic paroxysmal hemicrania	SUNCT syndrome
Cavernous sinus lesion (tumor, aneurysm, inflammation and/or granulomas)	Cerebellopontine lesions (arteriovenous malformations)
Sella turcica/pituitary lesions (tumors)	Brainstem lesions (infarction, pontine cavernoma, basilar impression)
Pancoast's tumor	Craniosynostosis
Vasculitis	
Occipital infarction	
Head trauma	

SUNCT, short-lasting unilateral neuralgiform headache with conjunctival injection and tearing.

4) Multiple attacks daily common (often 10-20 daily)
5) Episodes can last weeks to months, with remissions in between
6) Can occur at night
   b. Associated features
      1) Lacrimation
      2) Nasal congestion
      3) Conjunctival injection
      4) Rhinorrhea
   c. Episodic and chronic types have similar clinical features, but episodic paroxysmal hemicrania has clear pain-free periods between attacks, typically lasting months to years
3. Diagnosis
   a. Diagnostic criteria are listed in Table 18-11
   b. Neuroimaging, complete blood count, erythrocyte sedimentation rate are important to rule out secondary causes
4. Treatment
   a. Indomethacin
   b. Other potential treatments: alternative nonsteroidal anti-inflammatory drugs, verapamil or other calcium channel blockers

C. **Hemicrania Continua**
1. Epidemiology
   a. More common in females than males
   b. Presentation age variable, but mean age in the 30s
2. Clinical presentation
   a. Headache
      1) Unilateral
      2) Moderate to severe throbbing pain
      3) Often continuous pain, but may occur in episodes lasting weeks to months with pain-free periods
   b. Associated symptoms
      1) Autonomic features similar to paroxysmal hemicranias and SUNCT
      2) Nausea, vomiting
      3) Photophobia, phonophobia, osmophobia
3. Diagnosis: depends on ruling out secondary causes (Table 18-12)
4. Treatment
   a. Response to indomethacin is diagnostic
   b. May also respond to alternative nonsteroidal anti-inflammatory drugs, corticosteroids, dihydroergotamine, gabapentin, lithium, methysergide, and lamotrigine

D. **SUNCT Syndrome**
1. Characterized by brief, unilateral attacks of stabbing pain with ipsilateral autonomic manifestations
2. Epidemiology

Table 18-11. International Headache Society Criteria for Paroxysmal Hemicrania

Paroxysmal hemicrania
- A. At least 20 attacks fulfilling criteria B-D
- B. Attacks of severe unilateral orbital or temporal pain or both, lasting 2-30 minutes
- C. Pain is associated with at least 1 of the following signs or symptoms on the side ipsilateral to pain:
    1. Conjunctival injection and/or lacrimation
    2. Nasal congestion and/or rhinorrhea
    3. Ptosis or miosis
    4. Eyelid edema
    5. Forehead and facial sweating
- D. Attacks have a frequency of more than 5/day for more than half the time, although periods with lower frequency may occur
- E. Attacks are prevented completely by therapeutic doses of indomethacin
- F. Not attributed to another disorder

Episodic paroxysmal hemicrania
- A. Attacks fulfilling criteria A-F for paroxysmal hemicrania
- B. At least 2 attack periods lasting 7-365 days and separated by pain-free remission periods of at least 1 month

Chronic paroxysmal hemicrania
- A. Attacks fulfilling criteria A-F for paroxysmal hemicrania
- B. Attacks recur over more than 1 year without remission periods or with remission periods lasting less than 1 month

Table 18-12. International Headache Society Criteria for Hemicrania Continua

- A. Headache for more than 3 months fulfilling criteria B-D
- B. All the following characteristics:
    1. Unilateral pain without side shift
    2. Daily and continuous, without pain-free periods
    3. Moderate intensity, but with exacerbations of severe pain
- C. At least 1 of the following autonomic features occurs on the side of the pain:
    1. Conjunctival injection and/or lacrimation
    2. Nasal congestion and/or rhinorrhea
    3. Ptosis and/or miosis
- D. Complete response to therapeutic doses of indomethacin
- E. Not attributed to another disorder

Table 18-13. International Headache Society Criteria for SUNCT Syndrome

- A. At least 20 attacks fulfilling criteria B-D
- B. Attacks of unilateral moderately severe orbital, supraorbital, or temporal stabbing or throbbing pain lasting 5-240 seconds
- C. Pain is associated with ipsilateral conjunctival injection and lacrimation
- D. Attacks occur with a frequency from 3 to 200 per day
- E. Not attributed to another disorder

SUNCT, short-lasting unilateral neuralgiform headache with conjunctival injection and tearing.

- a. More common in males than females
- b. Clinical presentation: mean age, 45 years
3. Clinical presentation
    - a. Headache
        1) Strictly unilateral
        2) Localized to orbit or frontal region
        3) Characterized by stabbing or burning pain
        4) Paroxysms of pain can occur 5 times per hour with each paroxysm lasting 15 to 120 seconds
    - b. Associated symptoms
        1) Autonomic symptoms similar to paroxysmal hemicranias, with conjunctival injection and tearing being common
4. Diagnosis (Table 18-13): Neuroimaging may be needed to exclude structural causes found in secondary cases
5. Treatment
    - a. Difficult to treat; indomethacin is not useful
    - b. Medications tried with variable efficacy: sumatriptan, dihydroergotamine, prednisone, verapamil, valproate, carbamazepine, lithium

VIII. OTHER PRIMARY HEADACHE DISORDERS

A. **Trigeminal Neuralgia** (tic douloureux)
1. Epidemiology
    - a. Male:female is 2:3
    - b. Idiopathic trigeminal neuralgia typically presents in older patients
    - c. Trigeminal neuralgia presenting in young patients should raise concern for potential structural lesion
2. Pathophysiology
    - a. Irritation of trigeminal nerve
    - b. Usually idiopathic but may be related to structural causes: multiple sclerosis, aneurysm, arterial compression, tumor, dental problem
    - c. Vascular compression may cause demyelination of trigeminal nerve, producing pain

3. Clinical presentation
   a. Lancinating (electric shocklike) pain within trigeminal nerve distribution
   b. Most commonly unilateral, rarely bilateral
   c. May be provoked by wind, touch, talking, brushing teeth
   d. Episodes typically occur several times daily and last seconds to less than 2 minutes
   e. Idiopathic trigeminal neuralgia: physical examination is generally normal; concern for structural cause if trigeminal sensory loss or motor dysfunction
4. Diagnostic approach
   a. Diagnosis can be made by clinical history (IHS criteria are listed in Table 18-14)
   b. MRI of brain: rule out structural, compressive cause (Fig. 18-1)
5. Treatment
   a. Factors affecting treatment decisions
      1) Age of patient: younger age, may favor surgical intervention if intolerant or not controlled with pharmacologic treatment; older age, may favor pharmacologic management or ablative procedures over surgery
      2) Etiology (e.g., if multiple sclerosis is the cause, the headache does not respond well to microvascular decompression)
      3) Atypical face pain does not respond well to ablative procedures or surgery
   b. Pharmacologic treatment
      1) Carbamazepine (first-line treatment)
      2) Phenytoin
      3) Gabapentin
      4) Baclofen
      5) More recently, lamotrigine, oxcarbazepine, and topiramate
      6) Narcotics, nonsteroidal anti-inflammatory drugs not generally useful
   c. Ablative procedures
      1) Procedure choices include
         a) Alcohol block
         b) Glycerol block
         c) Balloon compression
         d) Radiofrequency ablation
         e) Gamma knife radiosurgery
      2) These procedures are compared in Table 18-15
   d. Surgery-microvascular decompression
      1) Efficacious, with immediate pain relief reported in as many as 90% of patients
      2) Recurrence rate of pain: 3.5% annually
      3) Less efficacious for trigeminal pain that is atypical or due to multiple sclerosis
      4) Advantages: preservation of facial sensation, highly efficacious
      5) Disadvantages
         a) Complications can include cranial nerve deficits, CSF leak, hemorrhage
         b) Anesthesia dolorosa (continuous burning pain) can develop in approximately 5% of patients

B. Geniculate Neuralgia
1. Pathophysiology
   a. Irritation of facial nerve
   b. May be idiopathic or related to structural irritation (tumor, aneurysm, trauma)

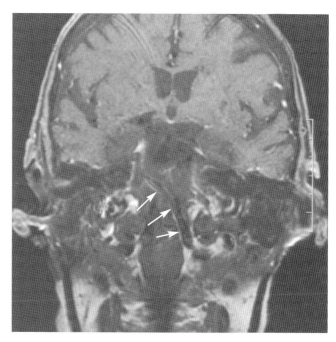

Fig. 18-1. Coronal T1-weighted MRI showing dolichoestatic basilar artery (*arrows*) compressing left trigeminal nerve in a patient with left-sided trigeminal neuralgia.

Table 18-14. **International Headache Society Criteria for Idiopathic Trigeminal Neuralgia**

A. Paroxysmal attacks of pain lasting 1 second to less than 2 minutes and affecting 1 or more divisions of the trigeminal nerve and fulfilling criteria B and C
B. Pain has at least 1 of the following characteristics:
   1. Intense, sharp, superficial, or stabbing
   2. Precipitated from trigger areas or by trigger factors
C. Attacks are stereotyped in the individual patient
D. No neurologic deficit found on examination
E. Not attributed to another disorder

Table 18-15. **Comparison of Ablative Therapies for Trigeminal Neuralgia**

Procedure	Description	Efficacy	Side effects
Alcohol block	Injection of alcohol into painful peripheral nerve branch	Temporary effect Duration of pain relief: 2-30 months Recurrence rate: 50%	Numbness in trigeminal distribution Skin necrosis (rare)
Glycerol block	Percutaneous stereotactic delivery of glycerol to trigeminal ganglion via foramen ovale	Initial pain relief: 80%-96% of patients Recurrence rate: 10%-72%	Numbness in trigeminal distribution Meningitis (rare)
Balloon compression	Percutaneous stereotactic balloon compression of trigeminal ganglion via foramen ovale	Initial pain relief: 90%-100% of patients Recurrence rate: 10%-56%	Numbness in trigeminal distribution (less risk of facial or corneal anesthesia than with glycerol or radiofrequency ablation) Weakness of trigeminal motor root Bradycardia (trigeminal vagal reflex)
Radiofrequency ablation	Percutaneous stereotactic radiofrequency thermo-coagulation of trigeminal ganglion via foramen ovale	Initial pain relief: 91%-99% of patients Recurrence rate: 10%-25%	Numbness in trigeminal distribution Motor weakness possible (rare) Diplopia (proximity of abducens nerve; rare) Ophthalmic division lesions carry risk of corneal anesthesia, which can lead to keratitis
Gamma knife radiosurgery	Stereotactic radiosurgery with partial ablation of trigeminal nerve root	Onset of pain relief: within 3 months after treatment Initial pain relief: 75% of patients Recurrence rate: 50% in 3 years	Numbness in trigeminal distribution (9%-16% of patients) May be useful if trigeminal neuralgia is associated with multiple sclerosis

2. Clinical presentation
   a. May present as unilateral lancinating pain within the ear, episodes last seconds to minutes and may occur several times daily
   b. Can also develop into chronic, dull pain within the ear
3. Diagnostic approach
   a. Clinical diagnosis
   b. Rule out glossopharyngeal neuralgia
   c. Rule out herpes zoster oticus (Ramsay Hunt syndrome)
      1) Reactivation and migration of varicella-zoster virus latent in geniculate, auditory, and vestibular ganglia
      2) Usual manifestations: pain and small vesicles in external ear, with or without facial paralysis, and inner ear symptoms

   d. Appropriate neuroimaging (head MRI) to rule out structural cause
4. Treatment
   a. Pharmacologic: similar to that for trigeminal neuralgia
   b. Surgical: reserved for intractable pain despite pharmacologic treatment (several options)
      1) Surgical excision of nervus intermedius
      2) Microvascular decompression
      3) Geniculate ganglionectomy

C. **Glossopharyngeal Neuralgia**
1. Pathophysiology
   a. Irritation of glossopharyngeal nerve, thought to be due to blood vessel compression in idiopathic cases

b. Structural causes: tumors, aneurysms, trauma
2. Clinical presentation
   a. Unilateral lancinating pain in throat, which may radiate to ear
   b. Episodes last seconds to minutes, can occur multiple times daily
   c. Triggers: chewing, swallowing, coughing, yawning
   d. Rarely, syncope may result from hypersensitivity of baroreceptor reflex
3. Diagnostic approach
   a. Clinical diagnosis
   b. Rule out structural lesion with neuroimaging (may need to image head and neck)
   c. Application of local anesthetic to throat can be diagnostic
4. Treatment
   a. Pharmacologic: similar to that for trigeminal neuralgia
   b. Surgical: section glossopharyngeal nerve and portion of vagus nerve at the level of jugular foramen

D. Occipital Neuralgia
1. Unilateral or bilateral occipital pain that may or may not radiate to vertex
2. Continuous dull and/or throbbing pain often superimposed by sharp, sometimes lancinating, pain
3. Pain may be reproduced or exacerbated by applying pressure (or percussion) over occipital nerves
4. Pathophysiology may be related to
   a. Chronic, excessive contraction of neck and scalp muscles
   b. Trauma or compression
   c. Entrapment of the greater and/or lesser occipital nerves
5. Treatment
   a. Local massage and rest
   b. Anticonvulsants
   c. Tricyclic antidepressants
   d. Local nerve blocks and injection of corticosteroids: both diagnostic and therapeutic measures

E. Hypnic Headache
1. Mean age at onset: about 63 years
2. Clinical presentation (IHS criteria are listed in Table 18-16)
   a. Also called "alarm clock" headache because of nocturnal nature of headache
   b. Moderate to severe pain variably described as dull, throbbing, or sharp that typically occurs after falling asleep (most commonly during REM sleep)
   c. May be unilateral or bilateral
   d. Associated with nausea (20% of patients)
   e. Can occur several times per night, typically lasting 1 hour per episode (some longer)

Table 18-16. International Headache Society Criteria for Hypnic Headache

A. Dull headache fulfilling criteria B-D
B. Develops only during sleep and awakens patient
C. At least 2 of the following characteristics:
   1. Occurs more than 15 times per month
   2. Lasts for at least 15 minutes after waking
   3. First occurs after age 50 years
D. No autonomic symptoms and no more than 1 of nausea, photophobia, or phonophobia
E. Not attributed to another disorder

3. Pharmacologic treatment
   a. Sumatriptan and oxygen have been tried with little benefit
   b. Aspirin may provide some benefit
   c. Lithium may be helpful prophylaxis

F. Exertion-Induced Headaches
1. Epidemiology
   a. More common in men than women
   b. Typically occurs in middle age
   c. Overall prevalence: about 1%
2. Clinical presentation (Table 18-17)
   a. Classified by type of exertion that precipitates headache
   b. Benign cough headache
      1) Precipitated by cough (also any Valsalva maneuver-related activity)
      2) Sudden, severe bilateral headache within seconds after Valsalva maneuver
      3) Rare to have nausea or vomiting in benign types
      4) Differential diagnosis of cough headache: mass in posterior fossa (cyst or tumor), increased intracranial pressure, Chiari malformation
   c. Benign exertional headache
      1) Precipitated by physical exercise
      2) Pain onset with exertion lasting minutes to hours
      3) Differential diagnosis of exertional headache
         a) Mass lesion, sinus disease
         b) If sudden, severe onset, consider differential diagnosis of a sudden, acute headache noted in Table 18-1
         c) Other possibilities: pheochromocytoma, migraine, increased intracranial pressure
   d. Headache associated with sexual activity (Table 18-17)
      1) Headache is often bioccipital or holocephalic; may last minutes to 24 hours (mean duration of severe

Table 18-17. **International Headache Society Criteria for Benign Exertional Headaches**

Primary cough headache
  A. Headache fulfilling criteria B and C
  B. Sudden onset, lasting from 1 second to 30 minutes
  C. Brought on by and occurring only in association with coughing, straining, or Valsalva maneuver
  D. Not attributed to another disorder
Primary exertional headache
  A. Pulsating headache fulfilling criteria B and C
  B. Lasting from 5 minutes to 48 hours
  C. Brought on by and occurring only during or after physical exertion
  D. Not attributed to another disorder
Headaches associated with sexual activity (type 2, explosive type)
  A. Sudden severe (explosive) headache fulfilling criterion B
  B. Occurs at orgasm
  C. Not attributed to another disorder

pain, 4 hours), often followed by a longer-lasting (up to 72 hours) pain of milder severity
  2) Precipitated by sexual activity
  3) Three types
     a) Type 1 (dull type): starts early as mild headache and slowly intensifies as sexual excitement increases, onset before orgasm (may be tension type headache with pathophysiology related to excessive muscle contractions during early phase of coitus)
     b) Type 2 (explosive type): sudden onset of severe throbbing pain with orgasm (pathophysiology may be related to Valsalva maneuver during coitus)
     c) Type 3: postural headache occurring after orgasm (debatable entity)
  4) Associated with migraine headache disorders
  5) Differential diagnosis of the explosive type includes entities listed in Table 18-1
3. Diagnostic approach: exclusion of structural causes with neuroimaging and/or lumbar puncture if sub-arachnoid hemorrhage is a consideration
4. Treatment
  a. Trial of prophylactic indomethacin if headaches are frequent; may require concurrent gastritis prophylaxis
  b. Alternative: naproxen, other nonsteroidal anti-inflammatory drugs

G. **Idiopathic Stabbing Headache** (ice-pick headache)
1. Associated with migraine, cluster, and other trigeminal autonomic cephalgia headaches

2. Clinical presentation
  a. Characterized by stabs of sudden, severe pain located commonly in orbit, temple, or parietal region
  b. Pain episodes generally less than 1 second
  c. Pain episodes can occur 1 to 50 times daily, episodes can occur in clusters throughout the year
3. Treatment
  a. Treatment requires prophylaxis because of brevity of pain episode
  b. May respond to indomethacin

H. **Cold-Stimulus Headache** (ice cream headache)
1. Induced by cold stimulus (e.g., ice cream) touching trigeminal-innervated pharynx and mouth
2. Most often mid-frontal localization
3. Occurs more often in migraineurs than general population

IX. Secondary Headache Disorders

A. **Neoplasm**
1. Epidemiology
  a. Headache is present in up to 50% of patients with brain tumors
  b. Depends on location and type of tumor and associated mass effect and/or hydrocephalus
     1) Posterior fossa tumors commonly associated with headache
     2) Pituitary tumor, craniopharyngioma, and cerebello-pontine angle infrequently produce headache
  c. More common in children with brain tumor than adults (likely because of prevalence of posterior fossa tumors in children)
2. Pathophysiology: may be related to increased intracranial pressure, impingement of dural structures, hydrocephalus
3. Clinical presentation
  a. Headache may be unilateral, bilateral, or generalized
  b. Often of moderate severity and constant
  c. May be present upon awakening
  d. May have nausea and vomiting
  e. Some worsen with bending or straining
  f. Examination may show papilledema and/or focal neurologic symptoms based on tumor location
4. Treatment: diagnosis and treatment of tumor based on type and location (see Chapter 16)

B. **Infection**
1. Overview

a. Wide variety of intracranial and extracranial infections and systemic infection can lead to headache
b. Intracranial: meningitis, encephalitis, abscesses with mass effect, empyema
c. Extracranial: sinusitis, tooth abscess, orbital cellulitis

2. Pathophysiology
   a. Febrile illnesses may produce interferons that have a role in generating headache
   b. Infections may irritate meninges, producing headache
   c. Some infections such as abscesses may be associated with mass effect and increased intracranial pressure

3. Clinical presentation
   a. Acute meningitis
      1) Rapidly progressive severe generalized headache with radiation to neck
      2) Pain may worsen with eye movement
      3) Nausea and vomiting are common
      4) Photophobia may occur
      5) Fever
      6) Alteration of consciousness may occur
      7) Cranial nerve palsies may occur
      8) Examination
         a) May confirm above
         b) Kernig's sign and Brudzinski's sign may be present
   b. Chronic meningitis
      1) Subacute, progressive generalized headache may be only sign
      2) Intermittent fever and neurologic focal signs may also be present

4. Diagnostic approach and treatment (see Chapter 15 on management of infectious conditions)

C. Chiari Malformation

1. Definition
   a. Chiari I malformation: tonsillar herniation below the level of foramen magnum
   b. May be associated with syringomyelia (50%-70% of patients) and hydrocephalus

2. Pathophysiology of headaches associated with Chiari I malformation: compression of neural tissues and alteration of CSF dynamics

3. Clinical presentation
   a. May present in adulthood or childhood
   b. Headaches located typically in occipital region, often precipitated by cough
   c. Many patients may have posterior fossa symptoms from brainstem compression: vertigo, ataxia, hoarseness, dysphagia, nystagmus, hearing loss, spasticity
   d. Patients with syrinx may have weakness, sensory loss, and atrophy at segmental level

4. Diagnostic approach: MRI of brain (sagittal) can help detect Chiari malformations
   a. Definition of Chiari I is age-dependent because cerebellar tonsils ascend with age
   b. Degree of herniation of cerebellar tonsils below foramen magnum considered to be abnormal, by age
      1) First decade: 6 mm
      2) Second and third decades: 5 mm
      3) Fourth–eighth decades: 4 mm
      4) Ninth decade: 3 mm

5. Treatment
   a. Observation if asymptomatic
   b. Surgical: suboccipital craniectomy considered for definitely symptomatic patients, especially those with brainstem signs or symptoms

D. Stroke and Migraine

1. Introduction
   a. Case control studies have suggested patients younger than 45 years with history of migraine have increased risk of ischemic stroke compared with controls (especially for women)
   b. Ischemic stroke may be related to migraine because of
      1) Regional blood flow changes related to migraine pathophysiology
      2) Alteration in platelet function
      3) Possible association with diseases that have concomitant migraine and stroke, such as CADASIL, MELAS, antiphospholipid antibody syndrome

2. Classification
   a. Coexisting stroke and migraine: patient has stroke and history of migraine, but migraines are remote from time of stroke
   b. Stroke with clinical features of migraine
      1) "Symptomatic migraine": patients with structural vascular lesion that presents with features of migraine
      2) "Migraine mimic": acute stroke accompanied by headache that acts similar to migraine with aura
   c. Migraine-induced stroke (migrainous cerebral infarction)
      1) Patient must have previous history of migraine with aura
      2) Cerebral infarction occurs during course of typical migraine with aura but aura not reversible, resulting in infarction
      3) Other causes of ischemic infarction are ruled out with appropriate clinical studies
   d. Uncertain: patient has migraine and stroke, but causal relationship cannot be established

3. Evaluation includes clinical testing for causes of ischemic stroke (see Chapter 11)

E. Sinus Disease

1. Clinical presentation
   a. Facial tenderness and pain
      1) Maxillary: localized to upper jaw teeth and cheek
      2) Frontal: localized to forehead
      3) Sphenoid: generalized or posteriorly localized pain
      4) Ethmoid: localized between orbits
   b. Nasal congestion (with ethmoid and maxillary involvement)
   c. Purulent nasal discharge
   d. Anosmia
   e. Fever (50%-60% of patients)
2. Diagnostic approach: pain associated with purulent discharge and abnormal sinus imaging findings suggests the diagnosis
3. Treatment
   a. Treat bacterial infection
   b. Decongestants

F. Obstructive Sleep Apnea (Table 18-18)

1. Epidemiology: headache may present in up to 50% of patients with obstructive sleep apnea
2. Pathophysiology: hypotheses on relation of headache to obstructive sleep apnea
   a. Fluctuation of oxygen saturation during night, with hypercapnia, vasodilatation, and increased in intracranial pressure
   b. Degree of oxygen desaturation may be risk factor (debated)
   c. Obstructive sleep apnea may precipitate idiopathic migraine headaches
3. Clinical presentation
   a. Headaches commonly occur in morning (upon awakening) and last several hours

---

Table 18-18. International Headache Society Criteria for Headache Associated With Sleep Apnea

---

A. Recurrent headache with at least 1 of the following characteristics and fulfilling criteria C and D
   1. Occurs on >15 days per month
   2. Bilateral, pressing quality and not accompanied by nausea, photophobia, or phonophobia
   3. Each headache resolves within 30 minutes
B. Sleep apnea (respiratory disturbance index of 5 or more) demonstrated by overnight polysomnography
C. Headache is present on awakening
D. Headache ceases within 72 hours, and does not recur, after effective treatment of sleep apnea

---

b. May be unilateral or bilateral, variable location
c. Typical quality of pain is described as tight or squeezing pain of mild to moderate severity
4. Treatment: primarily treatment of underlying disorder

G. Post-traumatic

1. Clinical presentation
   a. Headache present within 14 days after injury
   b. Trauma may be minor (*without* loss of consciousness) or major (*with* loss of consciousness)
   c. Headaches often have features of either migraine or tension headache
   d. Associated symptoms: dizziness, blurred vision, memory and other cognitive complaints, alteration of taste and smell, depression, sleep disturbances
   e. Specific syndromes associated with trauma
      1) Low-pressure headaches (see below)
      2) Temporomandibular joint pain
      3) Carotidynia due to arterial dissection
      4) Increased intracranial pressure due to cerebral edema
2. Diagnostic approach
   a. Appropriate neuroimaging and spine films in acute setting are important
   b. IHS criteria (Table 18-19)
3. Treatment
   a. Appropriate management of fractures, intracranial pressure, arterial dissection
   b. Tailored to headache characteristics
   c. If cervical component, some patients may benefit from physical therapy

H. Intracranial Hypertension

1. Definition
   a. May be idiopathic or secondary cause
   b. Secondary (structural or nonstructural): intracranial mass, infection, hypertensive encephalopathy, trauma, hydrocephalus
   c. Causes of increased intracranial pressure without structural abnormalities seen on neuroimaging are listed in Table 18-20
   d. Idiopathic intracranial hypertension (pseudotumor cerebri): may or may not be associated with papilledema (rest of discussion below is on pseudotumor cerebri)
2. Epidemiology of pseudotumor cerebri
   a. More common in women than men
   b. Often occurs in young women in 20s
   c. Obesity is risk factor
3. Pathophysiology of pseudotumor cerebri (several hypotheses)
   a. Increased CSF formation

Table 18-19. International Headache Society Criteria for Post-traumatic Headache

Acute post-traumatic headache *with significant* head trauma and/or confirmatory signs
  A. Headache, no typical characteristics known, fulfilling criteria C and D
  B. Head trauma with at least 1 of the following:
    1. Loss of consciousness for more than 30 minutes
    2. Glasgow Coma Scale less than 13
    3. Post-traumatic amnesia for more than 48 hours
    4. Imaging demonstration of traumatic brain lesion (cerebral hematoma, intracerebral and/or subarachnoid hemorrhage, brain contusion and/or skull fracture)
  C. Headache develops within 7 days after head trauma or after regaining consciousness following head trauma
  D. One of the following:
    1. Headache resolves within 3 months after head trauma
    2. Headache persists but 3 months have not yet passed since head trauma
Acute post-traumatic headache *with minor* head trauma and no confirmatory signs
  A. Headache, no typical characteristics known, fulfilling criteria C and D
  B. Head trauma with all the following:
    1. Either no loss of consciousness or loss of consciousness for less than 30 minutes
    2. Glasgow Coma Scale 13 or more
    3. Symptoms and/or signs diagnostic of concussion
  C. Headache develops within 7 days after head trauma
  D. One of the following:
    1. Headache resolves within 3 months after head trauma
    2. Headache persists but 3 months have not yet passed since head trauma
Chronic post-traumatic headache *with significant* head trauma and/or confirmatory signs
  Similar criteria to those for acute post-traumatic headache with significant head trauma, but the headache continues for more than 3 months after head trauma
Chronic post-traumatic headache *with minor* head trauma and no confirmatory signs
  Similar criteria to those for acute post-traumatic headache with minor head trauma, but headache continues for more than 3 months after head trauma

    b. Decreased CSF absorption
    c. Increased venous pressure (congenital stenoses of venous sinuses)
  4. Clinical presentation of pseudotumor cerebri
    a. Clinical symptoms
     1) Majority, but not all, patients have headache
      a) Unilateral or bilateral
      b) Frontal or occipital
      c) Quality similar to tension headache
      d) May be worse in morning
     2) Associated symptoms may include
      a) Transient (seconds) visual obscurations: temporary graying of vision, especially with straining
      b) Bilateral pulsatile tinnitus
      c) Diplopia (abducens palsy)
      d) Visual loss
      e) Nausea and vomiting
    b. Physical examination
     1) Papilledema
     2) Abducens palsy
     3) Visual loss (enlarging blind spot)

    c. Subgroup of idiopathic intracranial hypertension without papilledema
     1) Similar symptomatology except no visual loss or papilledema
     2) Elevated opening pressure diagnosed with lumbar puncture
  5. Diagnostic approach
    a. Clinical symptomatology
    b. Visual field examination
    c. Neuroimaging to rule out secondary causes of increased intracranial pressure (including veno-occlusive disease)
    d. Laboratory studies to rule out secondary causes of increased intracranial pressure
    e. CSF examination to measure opening pressure and rule out secondary causes (meningitis)
     1) Normal CSF pressure: 40 to 200 mm H_2O
     2) Abnormal CSF pressure in nonobese patients: >200 mm H_2O
     3) Abnormal CSF pressure in obese patients: >250 mm H_2O
  6. Treatment of pseudotumor cerebri

Table 18-20. **Differential Diagnosis of Increased Intracranial Pressure in Absence of a Structural Lesion**

Venous sinus thrombosis
Systemic lupus erythematosus
Hematologic
    Polycythemia vera
    Acute iron deficiency
Toxic-metabolic
    Vitamin A toxicity
    Vitamin D deficiency
    Medications (nalidixic acid, danazol, minocycline, tetracycline, corticosteroids, cyclosporine, isotretinoin)
Endocrine
    Corticosteroid withdrawal
    Hypothyroidism
    Addison's disease
    Hypoparathyroidism
Kidney disease

    a. Nonpharmacologic: weight loss
    b. Pharmacologic
        1) If no evidence of visual loss, consider treatment of headache alone; if evidence of visual loss, consider carbonic anhydrase inhibitor
        2) Carbonic anhydrase inhibitor (e.g., acetazolamide)
           a) Common side effects: weight loss, diarrhea, nausea and/or vomiting, altered taste sensation, paresthesias, confusion, polyuria
           b) Serious side effects: metabolic acidosis, tinnitus, sulfonamide adverse reaction
           c) Contraindications: adrenal gland failure, angle-closure glaucoma, cirrhosis, hyponatremia and/or hypokalemia, hyperchloremic acidosis, severe hepatic or renal disease, sensitivity to sulfonamides
        3) Topiramate
           a) Common side effects: nausea, confusion, dizziness, memory impairment, nystagmus, paresthesias, somnolence, motor retardation, tremor, poor concentration, anxiety, angle-closure glaucoma, fatigue
           b) Serious side effects: metabolic acidosis, pancreatitis, nephrolithiasis, renal tubular acidosis, hyperchloremia, hyperammonemia, hepatitis, liver failure, anemia, leukopenia
           c) Contraindications: sensitivity to topiramate
           d) Use with precaution in behavioral disorders or cognitive deficits, medical conditions or therapies that

predispose to acidosis, patients with inborn errors of metabolism, renal or hepatic impairment
        4) Short course of high-dose prednisone (controversial)
    c. Procedures (serial high-volume lumbar punctures)
    d. Surgery
        1) Reserved for failure of conservative treatment and progressive clinical symptoms or signs
        2) Lumboperitoneal shunt or ventriculoperitoneal shunt (used to reduce severe headaches not amenable to conservative treatment or progressive visual loss despite conservative treatment)
        3) Optic nerve fenestration: incision of dural covering of intraorbital optic nerve, used to prevent progressive visual loss
7. Outcome of pseudotumor cerebri
    a. Early treatment prevents visual loss
    b. Blindness may occur in up to 10% of patients
    c. Can spontaneously remit

I.   **Low CSF Pressure Headaches**
1. Pathophysiology
    a. Etiology: hypovolemic state, CSF shunt overdrainage, CSF leak (may be iatrogenic or spontaneous)
    b. Iatrogenic CSF leaks occur with trauma, lumbar puncture, epidural catheterization, spinal or cranial neurosurgical procedures
    c. Spontaneous CSF leaks may occur in setting of dural tear due to spondylosis or dural weakness due to meningeal diverticuli
    d. Spontaneous CSF leaks most often occur at level of thoracic spine
    e. Low CSF pressure results in traction on supporting structures (including pain-sensitive meninges and venous sinuses) resulting in pain, occasionally subdural hematoma (stretching of bridging veins), and rarely cerebral venous thrombosis
2. Clinical presentation
    a. Headache occurs with upright posture and is relieved with supine posture
        1) Typically bilateral (not always)
        2) May be bifrontal, bioccipital, fronto-occipital, or holocephalic
        3) Over time, chronic daily headache may also evolve and not worsen with positional changes or to a lesser extent
    b. Associated symptoms may include
        1) Stiff neck (sometimes orthostatic)
        2) Nausea and vomiting (often orthostatic)
        3) Horizontal diplopia (unilateral or bilateral abducens palsy)
        4) Distortion of hearing

5) Visual blurring

6) Photophobia

7) Visual field defect (superior binasal)

8) Dizziness

9) Back pain, radicular pain

10) Rare complications: subdural hematoma, coma, encephalopathy, dementia, parkinsonism

3. Diagnosis

a. Clinical symptomatology

b. Diagnostic criteria (Table 18-21)

c. MRI of head with gadolinium may show findings suggestive of low-pressure syndrome (Fig. 18-2)

1) Dural (pachymeningeal) enhancement

2) Downward displacement of brain: downward displacement of cerebellar tonsils, caudal displacement of pons, effacement of pontine cistern, caudal displacement of optic chiasm and hypothalamus

3) Pituitary enlargement

4) Ventricular size may be decreased

5) Engorgement of venous sinuses

6) Subdural fluid collections

d. CSF

1) Opening pressure is typically very low and rarely normal

2) CSF protein may be normal or high (up to 100 mg/dL)

3) CSF leukocyte count may be normal or mildly elevated

e. Radioisotope cisternography

1) Indium-111 is placed into the spinal subarachnoid space and movement followed with sequential scans for up to 24 to 48 hours

2) In normal patients, indium-111 can be detected over the cerebral convexities by 24 hours

3) In presence of CSF leak, indium-111 does not reach the convexities by 24 to 48 hours and appears early in kidneys and bladder

f. CT myelography

1) May detect region of spinal leak showing extradural egress of contrast or meningeal diverticulum

2) Most common site of leak is thoracic spine

4. Treatment

a. First-line symptomatic measures

1) Bed rest with hydration

2) Caffeine: effectiveness is questionable and short-lasting

Table 18-21. **International Headache Society Criteria for Headache Attributed to Spontaneous Low CSF Pressure**

A. Diffuse and/or dull headache that worsens within 15 minutes after sitting or standing, with at least 1 of the following and fulfilling criterion D:

   1. Neck stiffness

   2. Tinnitus

   3. Hypacusia

   4. Photophobia

   5. Nausea

B. At least 1 of the following:

   1. Evidence of low CSF pressure on magnetic resonance imaging (e.g., pachymeningeal enhancement)

   2. Evidence of CSF leakage on conventional myelography, computed tomographic myelography, or cisternography

   3. CSF opening pressure less than 60 mm H_2O in sitting position

C. No history of dural puncture or other cause of CSF fistula

D. Headache resolves within 72 hours after epidural blood patching

CSF, cerebrospinal fluid.

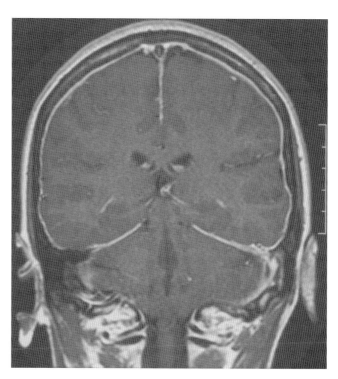

Fig. 18-2. Patient with low cerebrospinal fluid pressure headache syndrome. Gadolinium-enhanced coronal T1-weighted MRI shows diffuse enhancement of both supratentorial and infratentorial pachymeninges.

3) Corticosteroids: anecdotal evidence only; partial, temporary improvement only
4) Intrathecal or epidural fluid infusions of crystalloids may be considered (potential for infectious complications)

b. Epidural blood patch (second-line therapy): may need more than one attempt

c. Surgery
1) Reserved for patients in whom conservative treatment failed and area of spinal leak has been identified
2) Repair of dural defect or packing the defect with fibrin glue or an absorbable gelatin sponge (Gelfoam) has been performed

REFERENCES

Alberti A, Mazzotta G, Gallinella E, Sarchielli P. Headache characteristics in obstructive sleep apnea syndrome and insomnia. Acta Neurol Scand. 2005;111:309-16.

Cheshire WP. Trigeminal neuralgia: diagnosis and treatment. Curr Neurol Neurosci Rep. 2005;5:79-85.

Dodick DW. Indomethacin-responsive headache syndromes. Curr Pain Headache Rep. 2004;8:19-26.

Evers S, Goadsby PJ. Hypnic headache: clinical features, pathophysiology, and treatment. Neurology. 2003;60:905-9.

Headache Classification Subcommittee of the International Society. The International Classification of Headache Disorders: 2nd edition. Cephalalgia. 2004;24 Suppl 1:9-160.

Mokri B. Spontaneous low cerebrospinal pressure/volume headaches. Curr Neurol Neurosci Rep. 2004;4:117-24.

Saper JR, Dodick D, Gladstone JP. Management of chronic daily headache: challenges in clinical practice. Headache. 2005;45 Suppl 1:S74-85.

Silberstein SD, Lipton RB, Goadsby PJ. Headache in clinical practice. Oxford: Isis Medical Media; 1998.

Taylor FR, Larkins MV. Headache and Chiari I malformation: clinical presentation, diagnosis, and controversies in management. Curr Pain Headache Rep. 2002;6;331-7.

Trucco M, Mainardi F, Maggioni F, Badino R, Zanchin G. Chronic paroxysmal hemicrania, hemicrania continua and SUNCT syndrome in association with other pathologies: a review. Cephalalgia. 2004;24:173-84.

Young RF. Geniculate neuralgia (letter to the editor). J Neurosurg. 1992;76:888.

QUESTIONS

1. A 38-year-old woman who takes oral contraceptives presented with a 2-week history of progressive dull headache, then sudden severe worsening. This is the worst headache she has experienced. The neurologic examination is unremarkable. Computed tomography (CT) of the head is unremarkable. Cerebrospinal fluid examination shows the following: leukocyte and no erythrocytes per high-power field; glucose, 50 mg/dL; protein, 40 mg/dL; and no evidence of xanthochromia. Opening pressure was 30 cm H_2O. What is the next best management strategy?
   a. Obtain magnetic resonance (MR) venogram
   b. Treat patient with sumatriptan and discharge
   c. Admit patient for observation
   d. Obtain conventional angiogram to rule out cerebral aneurysm

2. A female patient presents with headache that immediately worsens in the upright position and improves in the supine position. Also, she has neck pain, nausea, and vomiting when upright. Which of the following radiographic findings might you see on magnetic resonance imaging (MRI) of the brain?
   a. Pachymeningeal enhancement
   b. Engorgement of venous sinuses
   c. Cerebellar tonsillar ectopia
   d. All the above

3. Which of the following headache types is commonly associated with autonomic features?
   a. Exertional headache
   b. Hypnic headache
   c. SUNCT (short-lasting unilateral neuralgia form headache with conjunctival injection and tearing) headache
   d. Trigeminal neuralgia

4. A 60-year-old man with a history of coronary artery disease and hypetension has developed severe unilateral right retro-orbital pain that lasts 30 minutes at a time and occurs several times a day, but mainly at night. He has tearing of his right eye and nasal congestion. Secondary causes were ruled out. The best abortive treatment to try first in this patient is:
   a. Sumatriptan subcutaneous at onset of headache
   b. Oxygen 2 L/min by nasal cannula at onset of headache
   c. Dihydroergotamine injection at onset of headache
   d. Lithium carbonate 300 mg orally

5. A 25-year-old man presents with jabbing pain in the throat often triggered by chewing or yawning. In addition, he has had one episode of unexplained loss of consciousness. The headache syndrome described here is:
   a. Trigeminal neuralgia
   b. Geniculate neuralgia
   c. Glossopharyngeal neuralgia
   d. Occipital neuralgia

6. A serious, preventable complication of untreated pseudotumor cerebri is:
   a. Chronic daily headache
   b. Cerebral hemorrhage
   c. Venous thrombosis
   d. Visual loss

7. For a patient with rapidly escalating migraine headaches, the quickest acting oral medication may be:
   a. Rizatriptan
   b. Frovatriptan
   c. Propoxyphene
   d. Almotriptan

8. What is a common complication of nonoperative procedures for trigeminal neualgia (such as balloon compression and radiofrequency ablation)?
   a. Infection
   b. Facial weakness
   c. Anesthesia dolorosa
   d. Numbness in distribution of treated trigeminal subdivision

9. What primary headache type is characterized by moderate bilateral head pain that occurs at night, resulting in awakening, and has no associated autonomic symptoms?
   a. Idiopathic stabbing headache
   b. Hypnic headache
   c. Cluster headache
   d. Exertional headache

10. The designation "post-traumatic headache" requires that the person suffered major head trauma with loss of consciousness.
    a. True
    b. False

ANSWERS

1. **Answer: a.**
Venous sinus thrombosis can present with acute headache, but it often has a subacute, progressive course. CT and neurologic examination findings can be normal. The high opening pressure in this situation should make you consider venous sinus thrombosis. MR venography is an appropriate next step.

2. **Answer: d.**

3. **Answer: c.**

4. **Answer: b.**
Sumatriptan and dihydroergotamine are contraindicated in patients with coronary artery disease. Lithium is a medication for prevention of cluster headaches, not for acute therapy.

5. **Answer: c.**

6. **Answer: d.**

7. **Answer: a.**

8. **Answer: d.**

9. **Answer b.**

10. **Answer: b.**

NEUROLOGY OF SLEEP DISORDERS 19

Timothy J. Young, M.D.

Maja Tippmann-Peikert, M.D.

I. INTRODUCTION

A. **Sleep:** characterized by the complex interplay of physiologic and behavioral factors

B. **Behavioral Definition of Sleep:** a reversible physiologic state of decreased perception of and responsiveness to external stimuli

II. FUNCTION OF SLEEP

A. **No Single Accepted Model**

B. **Several Proposed Theories**
1. Body repair
2. Brain restoration
3. Thermoregulation and energy conservation
4. Maintenance of immunocompetence
5. Memory consolidation and learning
6. Unlearning

III. SLEEP DEPRIVATION

A. **Animal Experiments**
1. Total sleep deprivation in rats resulted in death of unclear cause after a mean of 21 days
   a. Proposed mechanism: bacteremia, sepsis
   b. High metabolic rate, weight loss, decreased body temperature, and ulcerative skin lesions on tail and extremities preceded death
2. Partial sleep deprivation: similar changes but slower rate of progression (death occurred after a mean of 37 days)
3. Recovery sleep resulted in survival

B. **Human Experiments**
1. Most normal adults need 7.5 to 8 hours of nocturnal sleep

2. Total sleep deprivation of 5 to 10 days: development of tremor, ptosis, diminished corneal reflex, hyperreflexia, nystagmus
   a. Electroencephalography (EEG): increased theta and delta frequencies while awake with eyes closed and diminished alpha activity
   b. During recovery sleep: large amounts of slow wave sleep (SWS), i.e., SWS rebound, occur during first night; large amounts of rapid eye movement (REM) sleep occur during second night
3. Partial sleep deprivation of 2 hours or more per night: impaired psychomotor function, mood changes, increased risk of falling asleep while driving, motor vehicle accidents
   a. Chronic partial sleep deprivation (4-6 hours nocturnal sleep) for 2 weeks: cumulative deficits on objective cognitive testing
   b. Recent studies on sleep-deprived medical and surgical residents showed increased medical errors: impairment of electrocardiogram interpretation, longer time to complete procedures, surgical errors, increased complication rate
   c. Sleep-deprived residents also showed deterioration of performance on psychomotor testing, increased risk of falling asleep while driving, increased number of traffic citations and accidents
   d. Selective REM sleep deprivation leads to REM rebound during recovery sleep
4. Subjective sleepiness increases with acute sleep loss but does not worsen significantly further with persistent sleep deprivation

IV. SLEEP PHYSIOLOGY

A. **Sleep-Wakefulness Control Mechanisms:** exerted by specific neuronal groups of brainstem ascending reticular activating system (ARAS) (Table 19-1)

1. Pedunculopontine nucleus (cholinergic)
2. Laterodorsal tegmental nuclei (cholinergic)
3. Locus ceruleus (noradrenergic)
4. Raphe nuclei (serotonergic)

B. **ARAS:** projects to intralaminar thalamic nuclei, posterior hypothalamus, basal forebrain

C. **Additional Neurotransmitters Involved in Sleep-Wake Regulation**
1. Histamine (tuberomamillary nucleus): promotes arousal and wakefulness
2. Dopamine (ventral tegmental area): promotes wakefulness
3. Hypocretin (dorsolateral hypothalamus): promotes arousal
4. Other sleep-promoting neurochemicals: γ-amino-butyric acid (GABA) (ventrolateral preoptic area), galanin, adenosine, cytokines (interleukins, C-reactive protein, tumor necrosis factor α), prostaglandin D_2, delta sleep-inducing peptide, muramyl peptides, growth hormone-releasing factor, cortistatin, opioid peptides

D. **Sleep Stages:** non–rapid eye movement (NREM) sleep and REM sleep
1. Normal sleep
   a. 4-6 cycles per night of NREM sleep, followed by REM sleep
   b. Cycle duration: about 90 minutes
   c. NREM sleep consists of stages I, II, III, and IV
   d. NREM sleep gets progressively deeper and arousal threshold increases from stage I to IV
   e. Stage I is typically followed sequentially by stages II, III, and IV (stages III and IV = SWS) and again stage II before REM sleep
   f. Throughout the night

   1) SWS periods shorten
   2) REM sleep periods lengthen
   3) Thus, most NREM sleep occurs during first half of the night, followed by predominantly REM sleep in the second half
2. Typical sleep architecture in a young adult (Fig. 19-1)
   a. Stage I: <5%
   b. Stage II: 40% to 60%
   c. Stage III/IV (SWS): 10% to 20%
   d. REM sleep: 20% to 25%

E. **NREM Sleep:** general characteristics
1. Synchronized, rhythmic EEG activity
2. Decreased cerebral blood flow
3. Decreased skeletal muscle tone
4. Decreased heart rate, blood pressure, respiratory tidal volume

F. **Stage I**
1. Dropout of occipital alpha rhythm
2. Low-amplitude theta activity
3. Positive occipital sharp transients of sleep (POSTS)
4. Vertex waves (V waves) over frontocentral leads
5. Slow rolling eye movements (horizontal)
6. Partial relaxation of voluntary muscles

G. **Stage II** (Fig. 19-2)
1. K complexes: central high-amplitude, diphasic waves, >0.5 second in duration
2. Sleep spindles: central 12 to 14-Hz activity of 0.5 to 2 seconds' duration
3. POSTS, V waves, slow rolling eye movements may occasionally persist

H. **Stage III:** synchronized, high-amplitude delta activity (≤2 Hz, ≥75 µV, 20%-50% of a 30-second epoch)

Table 19-1. **Neurotransmitter Activity of ARAS in Sleep and Wakefulness**

| State | Neurotransmitter | | |
	Acetylcholine	Noradrenaline	Serotonin
NREM sleep	–	+ (slow)	+
REM sleep	+ (intermittent)	–	–
Wakefulness	+ + (tonic)	+ + (rapid)	+ +

–, quiescence; +, activation; ARAS, ascending reticular activating system; NREM, non-REM; REM, rapid eye movement.

Sleep is a physiologic state, and deprivation leads to derangements of cognitive and psychomotor function.

Control mechanisms of sleep and wakefulness include the brainstem and ascending reticular activating system and its projections.

Cholinergic, noradrenergic, serotonergic, and other neuronal groups control sleep and wakefulness, with projections from brainstem to thalamus, hypothalamus, and basal forebrain.

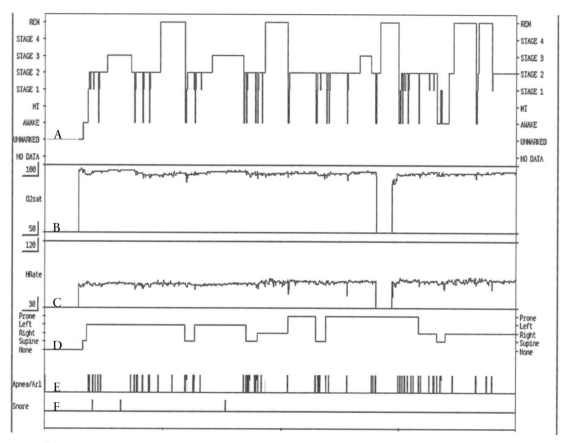

Fig. 19-1. Normal hypnogram. *A*, Distribution of individual sleep stages throughout the night. *B*, Oxygen saturation. *C*, Heart rate. *D*, Body position. *E*, Number of sleep-disordered breathing events and arousals. *F*, Snoring. Note the transient signal dropout of oxygen saturation and heart rate due to displacement of the recording probe in the second half of the tracing (third REM sleep period).

I. **Stage IV:** synchronized, high-amplitude delta activity (≤2 Hz, ≥75 µV, >50% of a 30-second epoch) (Fig. 19-3)

J. **REM Sleep:** general characteristics (Fig. 19-4)
1. Generalized skeletal muscle atonia
   a. Exceptions: diaphragm and extraocular muscles
   b. Atonia may conserve energy and/or protect person from acting out dreams
2. First REM period: usually occurs about 90 minutes after sleep onset
3. Increased cerebral blood flow (compared with NREM)
4. Dreaming occurs
5. Tonic REM phenomena
   a. Desynchronized, low-amplitude, mixed frequency cortical EEG
   b. Atonia of voluntary skeletal muscles
   c. Impaired thermoregulation
   d. Penile erections, clitoral engorgement
6. Phasic REM phenomena

Sleep is divided into non–rapid eye movement (NREM) and rapid eye movement (REM) stages.

NREM sleep is divided further into four stages (I-IV), and these alternate with REM sleep in four to six cycles per night.

NREM sleep is characterized by decreased heart rate and cerebral blood flow, with generalized slowing of the EEG.

REM sleep is characterized by skeletal muscle atonia (excluding the diaphragm and extraocular muscles) and a desynchronized EEG pattern.

During REM sleep, dreaming typically occurs and there is greater autonomic instability.

Circadian rhythms are mediated through the suprachiasmatic nucleus and are primarily controlled by exposure to light.

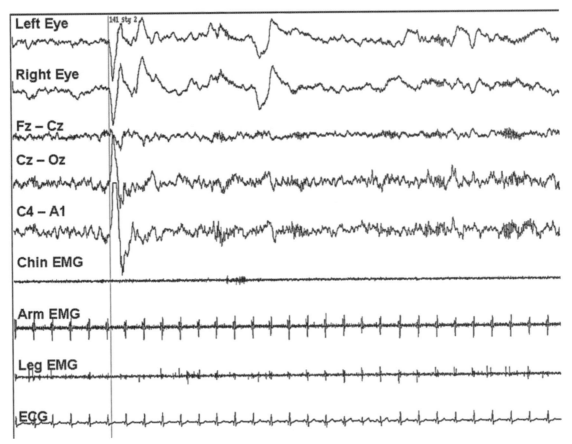

Fig. 19-2. Stage II sleep. Note the K complex on the left of the tracing and several sleep spindles on the right (30 second epoch). Left eye/right eye: eye leads applied to left and right outer canthus and referenced to Fpz (frontopolar midline electrode). Fz – Cz, frontal midline to central midline electrode; C4 – A1, right parasagittal to left ear electrode; Cz – Oz, central midline to occipital midline electrode; chin EMG, EMG lead on chin muscles; arm EMG, upper extremity EMG; leg EMG, anterior tibialis EMG.

a. Rapid eye movements
b. Phasic muscle twitches
c. Irregular acceleration of heart rate and respiratory rate
d. Sawtooth waves in central EEG leads
e. Rhythmic hippocampal theta activity

V.　CIRCADIAN RHYTHMS

A. Biological Rhythms That Repeat Approximately Every 24 Hours

1. Suprachiasmatic nucleus in the anterior hypothalamus: circadian pacemaker that regulates the sleep-wake cycle
2. Suprachiasmatic nucleus projects to areas of brain involved in sleep-wake regulation: basal forebrain, thalamus, hypothalamus, pineal gland
3. Human circadian rhythms have a cycle length of 24.2 hours and are synchronized with environmental stimuli (24-hour day period) via optic nerve and other pathways ("entrainment")
4. Regulating factors
   a. Circadian clock genes determine internal circadian rhythmicity
   b. Light: the most effective stimulus for the internal clock, via the retinohypothalamic tract
   c. Other stimuli: food, exercise, activity, hormones, social cues

VI. SLEEP TESTING

A. Polysomnography (PSG): usually performed in a sleep laboratory with multiple channel recording of

1. EEG
2. Electro-oculogram
3. Surface electromyogram (EMG) on chin and legs

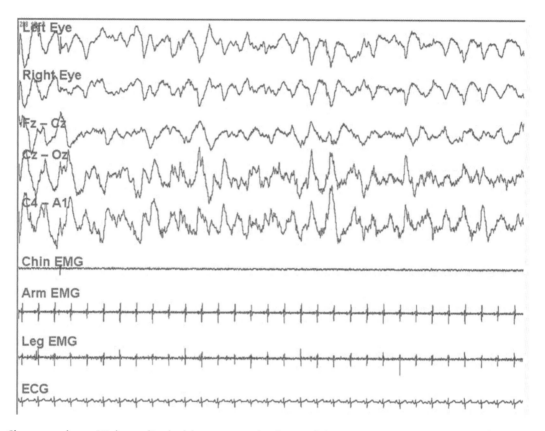

Fig. 19-3. Slow wave sleep. High-amplitude delta waves predominate. (Montage as in Fig. 19-2; 30-second epoch.) Note ECG artifact in arm and leg EMG channels.

4. Electrocardiogram (ECG)
5. Nasal and oral airflow
6. Oxygen saturation
7. Video and audio recording of behavior and snoring
8. May involve trial of continuous positive airway pressure (CPAP) or other interventions during testing

B. **Multiple Sleep Latency Test** (MSLT)
1. Patients are provided four or five sequential napping opportunities 2 hours apart starting 2 hours after awakening from their nocturnal sleep period
2. Measures degree of sleepiness
3. Performed in sleep laboratory the day after PSG
4. Only valid following documented adequate sleep time by PSG and preferably after 7 to 14 days of wrist actigraphy and/or sleep logs
5. Sleep latency
   a. Less than 5 minutes: pathologic
   b. 5 to 10 minutes: diagnostic "gray zone"
   c. More than 10 minutes: normal
6. Two or more sleep-onset REM periods are considered

abnormal but are nonspecific. Can be seen in
a. Narcolepsy
b. Other states of prior REM sleep deprivation
   1) Insufficient sleep syndrome
   2) Sleep apnea syndromes
   3) Withdrawal from REM sleep–suppressing medications (selective serotonin reuptake inhibitors [SSRIs], tricyclic antidepressants)
   4) Major depression
7. REM-suppressing agents (SSRIs, tricyclic antidepressants, monoamine oxidase inhibitors) need to be discontinued at least 2 weeks before MSLT; and if long-acting agent (fluoxetine), 4 weeks

C. **Maintenance of Wakefulness Test** (MWT)
1. Four opportunities to assess patient's ability to stay awake in a quiet dark room for 20 to 40 minutes (40 minutes preferred)
2. Used to assess treatment effect in patients with hypersomnia of various causes
3. No consensus about normal sleep latencies on MWT

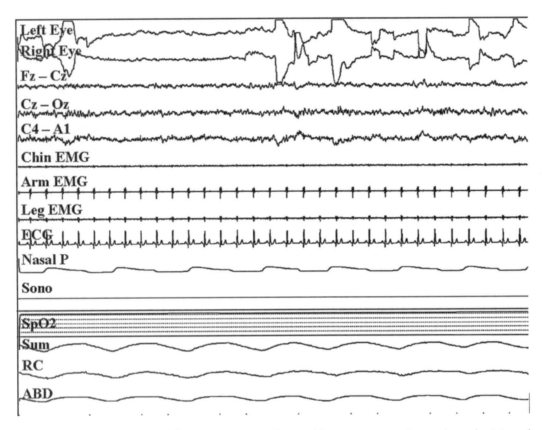

Fig. 19-4. REM sleep. Low-voltage mixed frequency pattern. Note rapid eye movements in eye channels. Normal muscle atonia in chin, arm, and leg (anterior tibialis) EMG channels (30-second epoch). Montage as in Fig. 19-2, additional leads include ABD, abdominal respiratory band; Nasal P, nasal airflow; RC, rib cage respiratory band; Sono, snore microphone; SpO2, oxygen saturation; Sum, sum of the rib cage and abdominal respiratory bands.

4. American Academy of Sleep Medicine practice parameters recommend the 40-minute test to obtain objective data on ability to stay awake
   a. Mean sleep latency of less than 8 minutes: abnormal
   b. Mean sleep latencies of 8 to 40 minutes: of unknown significance
   c. Mean sleep latency for normal subjects: 30.4±11.2 minutes
5. No proven correlation between MWT data and performance and vigilance; being able to stay awake during the MWT provides no guarantee that the subject will not experience sleepiness in the work environment

D. Actigraphy (Fig. 19-5)
1. Records activity level resulting from movements
2. Paucity of movements results in absence of signal and is assumed to represent sleep periods
3. Patients wear the actigraph on the wrist for up to 1 month to evaluate circadian activity and duration of sleep and wake periods

VII. Sleep Disorders

A. **Sleep-Related Breathing Disorders**
1. Obstructive sleep apnea (OSA)
   a. Features
      1) Recurrent partial or complete upper airway obstruction resulting in decreased (hypopnea) or absent

---

Polysomnography (PSG) evaluates sleep characteristics and disorders.

PSG incorporates EEG, surface EMG, and respiratory parameters.

Multiple sleep latency test (MSLT) is performed after PSG to detect mean sleep latency and sleep-onset REM periods.

Actigraphy estimates a person's circadian rhythm.

Time of day

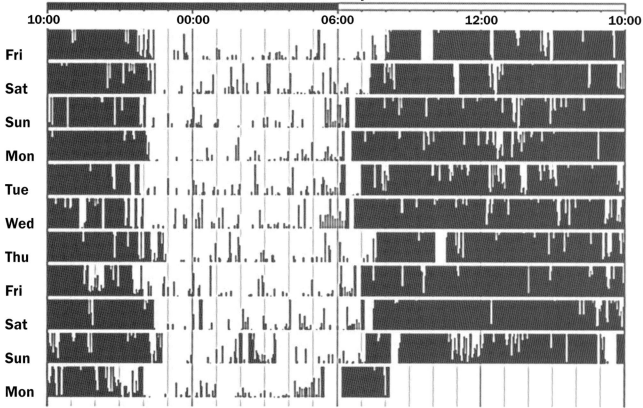

Fig. 19-5. Actigraphy recording. Dark areas, movements or increased activity; white areas, presumed sleep or quiescence. Normal circadian rhythm with quite regular bed and somewhat variable wake times. Occasional decrease in activity levels may represent nap periods.

(apnea) airflow in setting of persistent respiratory effort
2) Associated with oxygen desaturation, arousals, sleep fragmentation
3) Obesity: the major predisposing factor
4) A narrow upper airway is often present
5) Other anatomical risk factors: retrognathia, macroglossia, enlarged tonsils (children), craniofacial malformations
6) Other risk factors leading to decreased upper airway muscle activity: alcohol, benzodiazepines, narcotics, other sedatives
b. Pathophysiology
1) Reduced cross-sectional upper airway diameter
2) Inadequate respiratory reflex response mechanisms of the upper airway musculature (hypotonia of pharyngeal dilator muscles) to exaggerated upper airway negative pressures during inspiration
c. Clinical features
1) Nonrestorative sleep, dry and sore mouth and throat

at night or in morning, morning headache and excessive daytime sleepiness
2) Nocturnal choking or gasping events, insomnia, nocturia, impotence, fatigue, cognitive dysfunction, and irritability
3) Bed partners report snoring, apneas, gasping, restless sleep
4) Patients are often unaware of the high frequency of arousals but occasionally experience considerable insomnia
d. Epidemiology
1) Prevalence of OSA in U.S. population: at least 2% in women, 4% in men
2) Recent estimates suggest an even higher prevalence of sleep-disordered breathing without daytime hypersomnolence: 24% of men and 9% of women have an apnea-hypopnea index (AHI) of 5/h or more, 9% of men and 4% of women have AHI greater than 15/h
e. Diagnosis
1) History

2) PSG
   a) Duration of apneas and hypopneas are characterized by reduction or complete cessation of airflow signal for at least 10 seconds with persisting respiratory effort
   b) Respiratory events are often accompanied by bradyarrhythmias and tachyarrhythmias
   c) Apneas and hypopneas recorded per hour during PSG provide an index (AHI) as a measure for severity of OSA: 5 to 15/h, mild OSA; 15 to 30/h, moderate; more than 30/h, severe
   d) If no daytime symptoms are reported by the patient, AHI must be more than 15/h to diagnose OSA
   e) Degrees of recurrent nocturnal desaturation, hypoxia, sleep disruption, and daytime sleepiness: additional important determinants of severity of obstructive sleep apnea-hypopnea syndrome (OSAHS)

f. Associated features: hypertension, pulmonary hypertension, arrhythmias, cardiovascular disease, congestive heart failure, and possibly stroke via secondary mechanisms, type 2 diabetes mellitus

g. Treatment
   1) Weight loss
   2) Positional therapy
   3) Avoidance of sedatives and alcohol
   4) Oral appliance
   5) Positive airway pressure therapy: CPAP (preferred treatment for most patients) and bilevel positive airway pressure (BiPAP)
   6) In selected cases, surgical options include tonsillectomy (especially in children), uvulopalatopharyngoplasty, tongue-base reduction surgery, genioglossus advancement, maxillary and mandibular advancement, tracheostomy

2. Upper airway resistance syndrome
   a. Features and clinical symptoms
      1) Similar to OSA
      2) Increased respiratory effort during sleep is due to increased upper airway resistance resulting in arousals (>10-15/h), but without apneas or hypopneas
   b. Diagnosis: requires documentation of increasingly negative esophageal pressures before the arousal
   c. Treatment: similar to OSA

3. Central sleep apnea syndromes
   a. Primary central sleep apnea (CSA)
      1) Features
         a) Recurrent episodes of diminished or absent airflow without upper airway obstruction; unlike OSA, absence of respiratory effort during apneas and hypopneas

         b) Associated with oxygen desaturation, arousals, sleep fragmentation
      2) Clinical symptoms
         a) Sleep disruption, insomnia, excessive daytime sleepiness
         b) Nocturnal dyspnea, witnessed apneas
      3) Epidemiology
         a) Less common form of sleep-disordered breathing
         b) Etiology unknown (idiopathic)
      4) Pathophysiology
         a) Heightened ventilatory response to CO_2 leads to instability of respiratory control during wake-sleep transition and may persist into NREM sleep, this typically ceases in REM sleep
         b) $PaCO_2$ levels tend to be lower (close to apnea threshold), thus a small increase in ventilation leads to apnea
      5) PSG
         a) Recurrent cessation of respiration during sleep without ventilatory effort
         b) Sleep fragmentation
      6) Associated features: can be seen in neurologic disorders with associated autonomic nervous system dysfunction (multiple system atrophy, Parkinson's disease)
      7) Diagnosis
         a) History
         b) PSG
            i) Central sleep apneas of at least 10 seconds' duration occur more than 5/h (simultaneous cessation of ventilation and respiratory effort)
            ii) Usually associated with mild oxygen desaturation
      8) Treatment
         a) Oxygen
         b) Positive airway pressure therapy
   b. Cheyne-Stokes respiration
      1) Features
         a) Cyclical crescendo-decrescendo breathing pattern, with central apneic pauses followed by hyperpnea
         b) Arousals occur at the peak of the hyperpneic phase
         c) Associated with recurrent oxygen desaturations
         d) Mostly during wake-sleep transition and lighter NREM sleep
      2) Clinical symptoms
         a) Nocturnal dyspnea, insomnia, excessive daytime sleepiness
         b) May be asymptomatic
      3) Associated features
         a) Most common in congestive heart failure, occasionally in central nervous system disease

b) Often coexists with CSA

c) Waking PaCO$_2$: usually less than 45 mm Hg

4) Epidemiology

   a) Typically seen in patients older than 60 years

   b) More common in men

   c) 25% to 40% of patients with congestive heart failure have Cheyne-Stokes breathing

   d) 10% of stroke patients have Cheyne-Stokes breathing

5) Pathophysiology

   a) Due to instability in ventilatory control during wake-sleep transition in association with increased circulation time in patients with congestive heart failure and increased responsiveness of respiratory drive to rising CO$_2$ levels

   b) PaCO$_2$ is close to the apneic threshold

   c) Small increases in ventilation lead to central apnea by lowering PaCO$_2$ and are followed by arousals leading to hyperventilation

   d) Mechanism in patients with stroke: unknown

6) PSG

   a) Recurrent central apneas and hypopneas alternate with a crescendo-decrescendo ventilatory pattern

   b) Associated with mild oxygen desaturations

   c) May show associated arousals

7) Diagnosis

   a) History

   b) PSG

      i) Periodic breathing pattern with more than 10/h central apneas/hypopneas

      ii) Cycle length longer than 45 seconds

8) Treatment

   a) Optimization of cardiac function

   b) Oxygen (especially Cheyne-Stokes respiration with congestive heart failure) with close monitoring of pCO$_2$

   c) CPAP, BiPAP

   d) Less commonly, respiratory stimulants: acetazolamide, progesterone; theophylline is rarely used because of narrow therapeutic window

c. High-altitude periodic breathing

   1) Features and clinical symptoms: periodic cycling of recurrent central apneas and hyperpneas

      a) Cycle length is shorter than in Cheyne-Stokes breathing (<35 seconds)

      b) Normal adaptation to altitude after a recent ascent to at least 4,000 m

      c) Insomnia, nonrestorative sleep, dyspnea

   2) Pathophysiology

      a) Hyperventilation in response to hypoxia at high altitudes leads to a decrease in PaCO$_2$ inducing central apneas

      b) Often in association with heightened ventilatory responses to hypoxia

   3) PSG: recurrent apneas and hypopneas alternate with hyperventilatory pattern during NREM sleep

   4) Treatment

      a) Oxygen

      b) Acetazolamide

d. CSA due to drug or substance

   1) Features and clinical symptoms

      a) Central apneas occurring while person is taking long-acting opioids

      b) May also see periodic breathing, hypoventilation

      c) May lead to increased mortality

   2) Pathophysiology

      a) Respiratory depression

      b) Depression of hypercapnic ventilatory response

   3) Treatment: discontinuation of causative agent

4. Sleep-related hypoventilation/hypoxemic syndromes

   a. Idiopathic sleep-related nonobstructive alveolar hypoventilation

      1) Other names: central alveolar hypoventilation, primary alveolar hypoventilation, idiopathic central alveolar hypoventilation

      2) Features

         a) Decreased alveolar ventilation resulting in oxygen desaturation despite normal mechanical lung function

         b) Decreased tidal volume leading to abnormal increase in PaCO$_2$ during sleep, hypoxemia, and oxygen desaturation not associated with apneas or hypopneas

      3) Clinical symptoms

         a) Sleep fragmentation leads to insomnia and excessive daytime sleepiness

         b) Morning headaches

      4) Epidemiology

         a) Rare

         b) Variable onset, often in adolescence or early adulthood

         c) Slowly progressive

      5) Pathophysiology: reduced response to hypoxia and hypercapnia thought to be due to dysfunction of medullary chemoreceptors involved in ventilatory control

      6) Associated features

         a) Often coexists with OSA and/or CSA

         b) Can lead to severe hypoxemia and hypercapnia resulting in cardiac arrhythmias, pulmonary hypertension, cor pulmonale, biventricular heart failure, respiratory failure, impaired quality of life, death

7) PSG
  a) Recurrent episodes of decreased tidal volume with associated oxygen desaturation and increase in CO_2, worse during REM sleep
  b) Duration: longer than 10 seconds
  c) Sleep fragmentation
8) Diagnosis
  a) History
  b) PSG
  c) Evaluate for primary underlying disorders: pulmonary, neuromuscular, skeletal
  d) Arterial blood gases to evaluate for daytime hypercapnia, blood count to evaluate for erythrocytosis
  e) Consider magnetic resonance imaging (MRI) of brain to rule out medullary lesions
  f) Cardiac work-up to evaluate for associated problems
9) Treatment
  a) CPAP, BiPAP, noninvasive positive pressure ventilation
  b) Oxygen
  c) Respiratory stimulants (progesterone)
b. Congenital central alveolar hypoventilation syndrome
  1) Other names: central alveolar hypoventilation syndrome, primary alveolar hypoventilation syndrome
  2) Features
    a) Failure of automatic central control of respiration resulting in hypoventilation in absence of underlying neurologic, pulmonary, or metabolic disorder
    b) Absence of ventilatory response to hypoxia and hypercapnia
    c) Hypoventilation is worse during sleep because of lack of voluntary respiratory control
  3) Clinical symptoms
    a) Shallow breathing and/or apneas during sleep and, occasionally, wakefulness
    b) May be present from birth
    c) Cyanosis
    d) Consequences of chronic hypoxemia: pulmonary hypertension, cor pulmonale, developmental delay, seizures, growth retardation, and others
    e) Intercurrent infections may lead to respiratory failure
  4) Epidemiology
    a) Rare, prevalence is unknown
    b) Congenital, mostly sporadic mutations
    c) Onset: usually at birth or in infancy, occasionally later (including adulthood)
    d) Unremitting, leads to death if not treated
  5) Pathophysiology
    a) Unknown

b) Thought to be due to disorganization or dysfunction of brainstem chemoreceptors controlling respiration
6) Associated features: autonomic dysfunction, Hirschsprung's disease, tumors (neuroblastoma, neuroganglioma)
7) PSG
  a) Hypoxemia and hypercapnia without arousals, worse during SWS
  b) May show associated central apneas
8) Diagnosis
  a) History
  b) PSG
  c) Arterial blood gases: hypoxemia, hypercapnia
9) Treatment: mechanically assisted noninvasive positive pressure ventilation during sleep and, occasionally, during wakefulness
c. Secondary forms of sleep-related hypoventilation/ hypoxemia
  1) Features: sleep-related hypoxemia occurs in association with morbid obesity (body mass index >34), neuromuscular disorders, chest wall restriction, high spinal cord or brainstem lesions, lower airway obstruction, and pulmonary parenchymal or vascular idiopathic disorders
  2) Treatment: depends on underlying cause
    a) Treat the underlying condition
    b) Weight loss
    c) CPAP, BiPAP
    d) Noninvasive positive pressure ventilation
    e) Oxygen
    f) Respiratory stimulants (progesterone)

B. Hypersomnias of Central Origin
1. Narcolepsy
  a. Features and clinical symptoms
    1) Classic tetrad: excessive daytime sleepiness, cataplexy, hypnagogic or hypnopompic hallucinations, sleep paralysis
    2) Excessive daytime sleepiness
      a) Occurs in about 90% of patients with narcolepsy
      b) Usually the first symptom, onset in adolescence or early adulthood
      c) When severe, the patient frequently falls asleep under inappropriate circumstances
      d) Exacerbated by sedentary activities
      e) Sleep attacks: sudden sleep episodes without preceding drowsiness
      f) Short naps are often refreshing
    3) Cataplexy
      a) Occurs in 75% to 80% of patients

The most common sleep disturbance is obstructive sleep apnea (OSA), which is recurrent upper airway obstruction resulting in apneas, hypopneas, and arousals.

Risk factors for OSA include obesity and narrowed upper airway.

Features of OSA are excessive daytime sleepiness and headache.

Management of OSA involves weight loss, avoiding sedatives, positive airway pressure, and, occasionally, surgery.

Central sleep apnea is more rare and can be primary or secondary.

b) Most specific symptom of narcolepsy
c) Sudden, transient loss of muscle tone with associated hyporeflexia or areflexia, provoked by an emotional stimulus such as laughter, surprise, anger
d) Partial or complete muscle atonia (sparing of respiratory and extraocular muscles)
e) Duration: seconds to minutes
f) Occasionally accompanied by hypnagogic hallucinations
g) In contrast to seizures, consciousness is preserved during cataplexy and there is no postictal state
h) Represents an intrusion of REM sleep atonia into state of wakefulness
4) Sleep paralysis
a) Occurs in 40% to 80% of patients
b) Brief transient skeletal muscle atonia (sparing only diaphragm and extraocular muscles)
c) Occurs mostly upon awakening but also at sleep onset
d) Resolves spontaneously or with sensory stimuli (touching patient, calling person's name)
5) Hypnagogic and hypnopompic hallucinations
a) Occur in about 40% to 80% of patients
b) Mostly visual hallucinations at transition between sleep and wakefulness; auditory, tactile, vestibular hallucinations also possible
c) Difficult to distinguish from dreams
6) Many patients do not have all four symptoms: up to 20% of patients have all the cardinal symptoms except cataplexy (= "narcolepsy without cataplexy")
7) Proposed fifth symptom: disturbed nocturnal sleep occurs in 50% of patients

8) Despite excessive daytime sleepiness, total amount of sleep over 24 hours is not increased and patients often experience poor nocturnal sleep with insomnia, poor sleep consolidation, and sleep fragmentation
b. Associated features
1) Sleep disorders
a) REM sleep behavior disorder (RBD)
b) Periodic limb movements of sleep
c) Obstructive sleep apnea
2) Obesity or increased body mass index
3) Depression
c. Epidemiology
1) Prevalence: from 0.02% in Israel to 0.18% in Japan
2) Onset peaks in second and third decades of life
3) Genetic predisposition
a) 85% to 95% of patients with narcolepsy with cataplexy are positive for HLA-DQB1*0602 gene on chromosome 6
b) Patients who have narcolepsy without cataplexy are only 40% HLA-DQB1*0602-positive (normal population: 24% HLA-DQB1*0602-positive)
c) Only 1% to 2% of cases are familial: patients with familial narcolepsy are less likely to be HLA-DQB1*0602-positive
4) Lifelong disorder with serious personal and social consequences: motor vehicle accidents (34% of patients), poor school and work performance (92%), depressive disorders (30%)
d. Pathophysiology
1) Disorder of sleep-wake regulation
2) Proposed disease mechanism: autoimmune destruction of hypocretin-secreting cells in posterolateral hypothalamus
a) Hypocretin-secreting neurons promote wakefulness via extensive projections throughout the central nervous system: cerebral cortex, basal forebrain, amygdala, brainstem reticular formation, raphe nuclei, locus ceruleus, spinal cord
b) Loss of 85% to 95% of hypocretin-producing neurons in dorsolateral hypothalamus reported in autopsy studies
c) Low or absence of cerebrospinal fluid (CSF) hypocretin levels have been found in more than 90% of patients with narcolepsy with cataplexy
d) Weaker association of low CSF hypocretin levels for narcolepsy without cataplexy
3) Canine models of narcolepsy show hypocretin receptor-2 gene deletions as the disease mechanism; autosomal recessive inheritance; no similar mechanism has been reported for humans

e. Symptomatic (secondary) narcolepsy
  1) Infrequent
  2) Occurs in setting of hypothalamic-pituitary abnormalities: tumors, vascular malformations, sarcoidosis, head injury, after cranial irradiation
f. Diagnosis
  1) Clinical history: most specific feature is cataplexy in the setting of daytime sleepiness and abnormal MSLT
  2) PSG
    a) Short sleep latency: less than 10 minutes
    b) May show short REM sleep latency or sleep-onset REM sleep
    c) May show increased muscle tone in REM sleep, RBD, periodic limb movements during sleep, sleep fragmentation
  3) MSLT
    a) Ideally performed after overnight PSG to ensure adequate sleep time and rule out other sleep disorders
    b) Mean sleep latency: <5 minutes and 2 or more sleep-onset REM periods
g. Treatment
  1) Nonpharmacologic
    a) Regular sleep-wake schedule
    b) Scheduled naps
    c) Avoidance of sleep deprivation
    d) Avoidance of sedentary work environment and shift work
  2) Pharmacologic: excessive daytime sleepiness
    a) Stimulants such as methylphenidate, dextroamphetamine, methamphetamine, or modafinil to improve alertness
    b) Modafinil is often first choice because of longer half-life and duration of action and favorable side effect profile, but has less alerting effect than traditional stimulants
    c) Mechanism of action
      i) Stimulants: dopamine release and reuptake inhibition
      ii) Modafinil: unknown, dopamine reuptake inhibition (?)
    d) Side effects of stimulants
      i) Irritability, agitation, headache, insomnia, peripheral sympathetic stimulation
      ii) Tolerance develops in one-third of patients
      iii) Potential for abuse
  3) Pharmacologic: cataplexy
    a) Sodium oxybate (γ-hydroxybutyrate [GHB]), tricyclic antidepressants, or SSRIs to reduce frequency and severity of cataplexy

    b) GHB is first FDA-approved drug for treatment of cataplexy, effective for 70% to 80% of patients
      i) Mechanism of action: not known
      ii) Side effects: central nervous system depression, respiratory depression, dizziness, headaches, nausea, vomiting, sleepwalking, nocturnal confusion
      iii) Complicated dosing schedule: one-half of dose given at bedtime, second half 2.5 to 4 hours later
    c) Tricyclic antidepressants: probably effective by suppressing REM sleep
    d) SSRIs are less potent than tricyclics but have fewer side effects
  4) Pharmacologic: sleep paralysis and hypnagogic hallucinations
    a) Drug therapy not usually required
    b) Try REM sleep suppressants (tricyclic antidepressants, SSRIs); if severe insomnia, try short-acting hypnotics, GHB
2. Idiopathic hypersomnia
  a. Features and clinical symptoms
    1) Severe persistent excessive daytime sleepiness with (>10 hours) or without (<10 hours) long nocturnal sleep episodes without evidence of cataplexy
    2) Symptoms lasting more than 6 months
    3) No evidence of other causes of sleepiness by history or on PSG
    4) Naps typically are not refreshing
  b. Epidemiology
    1) Less common than narcolepsy
    2) Onset: adolescence, early adulthood
    3) Chronic course
  c. Pathophysiology: unknown
  d. Diagnosis
    1) History
    2) Actigraphy, sleep logs for at least 1 week to document duration of nocturnal sleep period and daytime naps
    3) PSG to ensure adequate sleep time before MSLT and rule out other sleep disorders as a cause of excessive daytime sleepiness
    4) MSLT with mean sleep latency less than 8 minutes and fewer than two sleep-onset REM periods
  e. Differential diagnosis: insufficient sleep syndrome, delayed sleep phase syndrome, narcolepsy, untreated sleep-disordered breathing, medication effect, status post head injury, psychiatric disorders
  f. Treatment: similar to narcolepsy (good sleep hygiene and stimulants) with various degrees of success
3. Recurrent hypersomnia (Kleine-Levin syndrome)
  a. Features and clinical symptoms

Narcolepsy is characterized by the clinical tetrad of excessive daytime sleepiness, cataplexy, hypnagogic hallucinations, and sleep paralysis.

There is a genetic predisposition to narcolepsy in persons with the HLA-DQB1*0602 allele.

Not all narcoleptics have cataplexy.

Most narcoleptics with cataplexy have low CSF levels of hypocretin (orexin).

Hypocretins are produced in posterolateral hypothalamus and coordinate transitions between sleep and wakefulness.

Narcolepsy is diagnosed by history and by MSLT demonstrating two or more sleep-onset REM periods.

Treatment consists of stimulants such as methylphenidate or modafinil for hypersomnolence and γ-hydroxybutyrate, tricyclics, or selective serotonin reuptake inhibitors for cataplexy.

   1) Recurrent periods of hypersomnolence with transient cognitive, mood, or behavioral disturbance; hyperphagia; hypersexuality
   2) Each episode lasts 1 to 2 weeks, followed by return to normal cognitive and psychosocial function for several weeks or months
   b. Epidemiology
      1) Uncommon disorder usually affecting teenage boys
      2) Benign course, with decreasing frequency and severity of episodes over time
   c. Pathophysiology
      1) Unclear
      2) Possible hypothalamic dysfunction
      3) Possibly autoimmune mediated because of frequent association with HLA-DQB1*0201
   d. Diagnosis
      1) History
      2) PSG during attacks: prolonged sleep time with decreased sleep efficiency, increased wake time after sleep onset, decreased SWS, increased light sleep
      3) MSLT during attacks: decreased mean sleep latency, may show sleep-onset REM periods
   e. Treatment
      1) Self-limited condition
      2) No proven therapy
      3) Stimulants tend to be ineffective
      4) Lithium may prevent recurrences

C. Insomnia
1. Features
   a. Perception of insufficient total sleep or unsatisfactory sleep
   b. Divided into several categories
      1) Delay in falling asleep (sleep-onset insomnia)
      2) Frequent awakenings throughout the night (sleep-maintenance insomnia)
      3) Early morning awakening without return to sleep
   c. Insomnia severity
      1) Mild: symptoms almost nightly but normal daytime function
      2) Moderate: nightly symptoms with mild-moderate impairment of daytime function
      3) Severe: nightly symptoms with severe impairment of daytime function
   d. Insomnia duration: variable definitions
      1) Adjustment (acute): days to weeks
      2) Chronic: more than 1 to 3 months
2. Clinical symptoms
   a. Insomniacs tend to underestimate the time they actually spend asleep
   b. In addition to difficulties falling asleep and maintaining sleep, patients may report the following:
      1) Nonrestorative sleep, light sleep, short sleep
      2) Impaired cognition, attention, mood, daytime functioning
      3) Fatigue and reduced motivation
      4) Excessive daytime sleepiness
      5) Social dysfunction
      6) Headaches, gastrointestinal tract distress, anxiety over sleep loss
3. Associated features
   a. Often influenced by environmental factors and/or psychologic disturbance, especially stress, anxiety, depression, drug dependence, or other mental illness
   b. A specific trigger may be identified
4. Primary insomnias
   a. Characterized by state of hyperarousal
   b. Types
      1) Idiopathic insomnia
         a) Onset: early childhood
         b) Proposed mechanisms: abnormal sleep-wake regulation, organic hyperarousal state
         c) Lifelong condition
      2) Psychophysiologic insomnia
         a) Patient does not associate bedroom and bedtime with sleep, usually as a learned behavior that prevents sleep from occurring
         b) Frustration and anxiety develop from inability to

sleep, leading to state of increased arousal and tension that prevents sleep, thereby, perpetuating the insomnia

c) Can develop from transient or chronic insomnia of any cause

d) Patient usually sleeps better in a different environment than own bedroom

3) Paradoxical insomnia (sleep-state misperception)

a) Subjective complaint of insomnia in which the patient misperceives the amount of time spent asleep

b) No PSG evidence of sleep disturbance; objectively normal sleep duration

5. Behavioral insomnias

a. Are due to learned behaviors or voluntary actions inconsistent with sleep

1) Sleep-onset association disorder: child learns to fall asleep only under certain conditions, for example, when being rocked or in parents' bed

2) Limit-setting sleep disorder: child refuses to go to bed when asked to

3) Inadequate sleep hygiene: consumption of caffeine, nicotine, other stimulants, or vigorous exercise shortly before bedtime, watching TV in bed, frequent daytime naps

6. Secondary insomnia

a. Underlying factors or conditions

1) Environmental factors: bedroom environment, noise, temperature, sleep surface, high altitude

2) Psychologic factors: stress, life events

3) Abnormal sleep schedule: shift work, jet lag

4) Circadian rhythm disorders: delayed sleep phase preference, irregular sleep-wake disorder, non–24-hour sleep disorder

5) Medication effect: stimulants, β-agonists, methylxanthines, dopaminergic agents (and others); rebound insomnia following abrupt discontinuation of benzodiazepines

6) Medical conditions: especially pain syndromes, respiratory disorders, gastroesophageal reflux

7) Psychiatric disorders: depression, anxiety, posttraumatic stress disorder (PTSD), nocturnal panic attacks, drug or alcohol abuse, psychotic disorders

8) Primary neurologic diseases: fatal familial insomnia, Morvan's fibrillary chorea (discussed below), others

9) Fatal familial insomnia (see Chapter 7)

a) Features and clinical symptoms

i) Begins with difficulty initiating sleep and leads to severe complete insomnia within several months

ii) Rapid progression to coma and death within about 2 years

iii) Other symptoms: ataxia, tremor, myoclonus, dystonic posturing, pyramidal signs, cognitive changes, sympathetic nervous system hyperactivity, episodic stupor

b) Epidemiology

i) Prion disease

ii) Autosomal dominant

iii) Onset: fifth or sixth decade

c) PSG: no SWS, decreased stage II NREM sleep, dissociated REM sleep without muscle atonia

d) Imaging studies

i) Computed tomography (CT) and MRI: normal brain

ii) Positron emission tomography (PET): decreased glucose metabolism in thalamus and putamen

e) Autopsy: anterior and dorsomedial thalamic nuclei atrophy with neuronal loss and reactive gliosis

f) Treatment: barbiturates and benzodiazepines may induce EEG sleep patterns

10) Morvan's fibrillary chorea

a) Features and clinical symptoms: severe insomnia, fluctuating encephalopathy, peripheral nerve hyperexcitability, weakness, cramping, neuromyotonia, dysautonomia (hypertension, tachycardia, profuse perspiration, increased body temperature)

b) Pathophysiology

i) Unknown

ii) Possible autoimmune mechanism or paraneoplastic phenomenon (associated with myasthenia gravis, malignancy; positive antibodies to voltage-gated potassium channels)

c) Laboratory data

i) PSG: no NREM sleep features (absence of K complexes, spindles, delta waves), "subwakefulness" state characterized by EEG theta activity associated with behavioral sleep, brief REM sleep periods without atonia

ii) EMG: spontaneous repetitive discharges (doublets, triplets, multiplets, and myokymia)

iii) Lab test: increased plasma norepinephrine level

d) Treatment

i) Improvement with plasma exchange, immune-modulating agents, or thymectomy in the presence of thymoma, including normalization of EEG, PSG, and EMG

ii) Opioids

7. Diagnosis of insomnia

a. Based on clinical history: identify predisposing and perpetuating factors

b. PSG and actigraphy are rarely used to rule out primary

sleep disorders leading to insomnia (sleep apnea, restless legs syndrome, periodic limb movement disorder) or sleep-state misperception
8. Treatment of insomnia
   a. Depends on underlying cause: treat underlying conditions
   b. Cognitive behavioral therapy, biofeedback, relaxation techniques, stimulus control, sleep restriction
   c. Good sleep hygiene (e.g., dark, quiet environment, no television in bedroom)
   d. Short-term pharmacologic therapy with hypnotics
   e. Physician reassurance after serious underlying disorders have been ruled out

D. Sleep-Related Movement Disorders
1. Restless legs syndrome
   a. Features and clinical symptoms
      1) Irresistible urge to move the legs associated with leg discomfort that is often described as a creepy, crawling sensation but also aching, cramping, or unable to describe
      2) Exacerbated by rest (lying down or sitting quietly); temporarily relieved by movement
      3) Usually bilateral and symmetric; asymmetric or unilateral involvement is possible
      4) Arms can be affected
      5) Symptoms: most prominent in evening and nighttime
      6) Often results in sleep-onset or sleep-maintenance insomnia
      7) Some patients also complain of excessive daytime sleepiness or fatigue
   b. Epidemiology
      1) Prevalence: 5% to 15%, more common in women
      2) All age groups
      3) 80% of patients have associated periodic limb movements of sleep

---

> Insomnia is a perceived state of insufficient or unsatisfying sleep.
>
> Insomnia may be triggered by a stressful life event, with subsequent reinforcement of disturbed sleep.
>
> Neurologic, psychiatric, and medical causes must be ruled out and addressed if present.
>
> Treatment includes management of underlying conditions, behavior modification, and short-term medication.

---

4) Primary restless legs syndrome
   a) Positive family history of similar symptoms, including adolescent "growing pains"
   b) Autosomal dominant inheritance
   c) Onset: early, before age 45 years, often childhood, adolescence
5) Secondary restless legs syndrome
   a) Associated with pregnancy, peripheral neuropathy, chronic renal failure, iron deficiency anemia, latent iron deficiency (correlates with low ferritin levels [<50 µg/L]), folate deficiency
   b) Linked to several medications: antidepressants, neuroleptics, dopamine antagonists, sedating antihistamines
   c. Pathophysiology: cerebral iron and dopamine pathways have been implicated (iron deficiency state theory)
      1) Low serum levels of ferritin
      2) Decreased CSF levels of ferritin
      3) MRI: shows decreased iron content in substantia nigra and putamen
      4) Iron is a cofactor of tyrosine hydroxylase and synthesis of dopamine
      5) Excellent treatment response to dopamine agonists and levodopa
   d. Diagnosis
      1) History: restless legs syndrome is a clinical diagnosis and PSG is generally unnecessary
      2) Laboratory evaluation for predisposing conditions: ferritin, folate, vitamin B_{12}
   e. Differential diagnosis: insomnia, nocturnal leg cramps, akathisia, painful legs moving toes, peripheral neuropathy, radiculopathy, restlessness associated with anxiety disorders
   f. Treatment
      1) First-line agents: dopaminergic agonists
      2) Pramipexole, ropinirole, or pergolide
         a) If given 2 hours before bedtime, low risk of augmentation
         b) Treatment of choice for moderate to severe restless legs syndrome
      3) Levodopa
         a) Low dose (25 mg) at bedtime
         b) Over time, patients taking levodopa frequently develop augmentation, with increasing severity of symptoms, occurrence of symptoms earlier in the day, and spread to involve other body parts
      4) Gabapentin, benzodiazepines, or low-potency opioids if dopaminergic agents are ineffective or cause side effects
      5) Iron replacement therapy if serum ferritin level is less than 50 µg/L

6) If symptoms are mild and infrequent, intermittent use of low-potency opioids can be tried

7) Nonpharmacologic measures: regularly scheduled exercise, hot or cold baths

2. Periodic limb movement disorder

  a. Features

    1) Repetitive, stereotyped movement of extremities with extension of big toe, ankle dorsiflexion, flexion of knee and hip of one or both legs during sleep (= periodic limb movements of sleep)

    2) Upper extremities can be involved less frequently

    3) Occurs mostly during NREM sleep

  b. Clinical symptoms

    1) Patients may complain of insomnia and sleep disruption from resulting arousals, nonrestorative sleep, excessive daytime sleepiness

    2) Clinical significance of periodic limb movements of sleep is debated because

      a) High prevalence of asymptomatic periodic limb movements of sleep in the elderly

      b) Symptomatic periodic limb movements of sleep is rare

  c. Epidemiology

    1) Typical age at onset: unknown

    2) Prevalence: increases with age

    3) Often seen with restless legs syndrome, RBD, narcolepsy

  d. Diagnosis

    1) Requires a suggestive history and PSG (Fig. 19-6)

    2) A periodic limb movement index (= periodic limb movements per sleep hour) of more than 5 to 15 is considered abnormal in the presence of clinical symptoms (in the elderly population, a higher PLM index should be considered abnormal)

    3) Duration of a single movement: 0.5 to 5 seconds, occurring 4 to 90 seconds apart

  e. Pathophysiology

    1) Decreased brain iron and dopaminergic pathways have been implicated

---

Restless legs syndrome is discomfort in the legs, with an irresistible need to move the limbs, typically at night.

Treatment consists of dopamine agonists and iron supplements.

Over time, treatment with levodopa-carbidopa can result in augmentation of the symptoms.

---

2) Serum ferritin level can be low

  f. Differential diagnosis: sleep starts, propriospinal myoclonus, spinal myoclonus, myoclonic epilepsy

  g. Treatment

    1) Only indicated if marked sleep fragmentation results from periodic limb movements of sleep–associated arousals

    2) Similar to restless legs syndrome; dopaminergic agents are first-line treatment

3. Rhythmic movement disorder

  a. Features and clinical symptoms

    1) Stereotyped, repetitive, rhythmic movements of body parts, most commonly head, neck, trunk that occur either before sleep onset and persist into light sleep or occur only during sleep (all sleep stages)

    2) Movements include head banging, head rolling, and body rocking

    3) Is considered a disorder only if the behaviors

      a) Interfere with sleep

      b) Result in daytime sleepiness

      c) Lead to head trauma or other injuries

  b. Epidemiology

    1) Mostly in infants and young children (used as a sleep aid), also mentally handicapped patients

    2) Mean age at onset: 6 months

    3) Typically resolves spontaneously by age 2 or 3 years

    4) May persist into adulthood

  c. Pathophysiology: unknown

  d. Diagnosis

    1) History

    2) PSG

  e. Treatment

    1) Reassurance of caregivers

    2) Padding of crib or bed

    3) Protective head gear

    4) If necessary, try benzodiazepines, tricyclic antidepressants

4. Bruxism

  a. Features and clinical symptoms

    1) Stereotyped, intermittent, rhythmical teeth grinding and clenching during any sleep stage

    2) Patient may present with soreness of jaw muscles and joints in the morning, headache, facial pain, abnormal dental wear

    3) Can lead to sleep disturbance of patient and bed partner

  b. Epidemiology

    1) Most common in childhood (about 15% of children)

    2) About 5% of adults

    3) Familial occurrence

  c. Pathophysiology

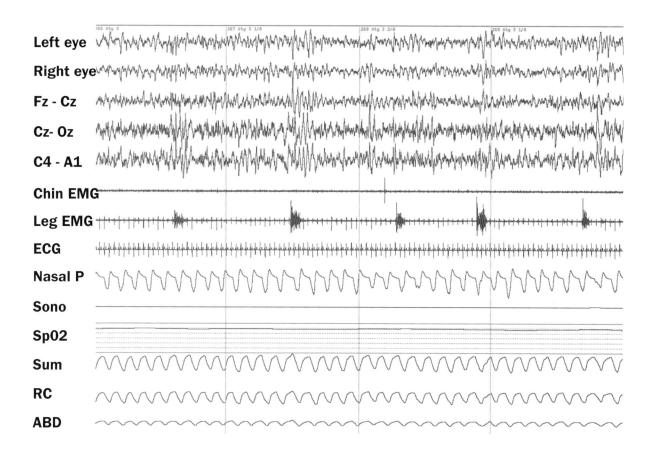

Fig. 19-6. Periodic limb movements of sleep. Note the periodicity; no associated arousals are seen (120-second epoch). Montage as in Fig. 19-2, additional leads include ABD, abdominal respiratory band; Nasal P, nasal airflow; RC, rib cage respiratory band; Sono, snore microphone; SpO_2, oxygen saturation; Sum, sum of the rib cage and abdominal respiratory bands.

1) Unknown
2) May be worsened by stress
  d. Treatment
    1) Dental appliance
    2) Relaxation techniques
    3) Stress management

E. Circadian Rhythm Disorders (Fig. 19-7)
1. Features
  a. Persistent inability to sleep at desired or expected time and/or excessive sleepiness during the wake period as defined by environmental and societal factors
  b. Due to alteration of the person's circadian system
  c. Results in occupational and/or social dysfunction
2. Delayed sleep phase disorder
  a. Features
    1) Delayed sleep onset and wake times in relation to societal norms
    2) When allowed to sleep at own schedule, total sleep duration and alertness during the wake period are normal
  b. Clinical symptoms: complaints of sleep-onset "insomnia," difficulties waking at the desired time in the morning, daytime sleepiness
  c. Epidemiology
    1) Most common in adolescents and young adults in whom a delayed sleep phase tendency is physiologic
    2) Genetic predisposition, familial occurrence
    3) Chronic course into late adulthood in some patients
  d. Pathophysiology
    1) Delayed circadian rhythms, including body temperature and melatonin secretion
    2) Environmental and behavioral factors
      a) Bright light exposure in evening delays internal circadian rhythms
      b) Caffeine and other stimulant use late in the day
  e. Diagnosis: sleep logs, actigraphy for at least 1 week
  f. Treatment

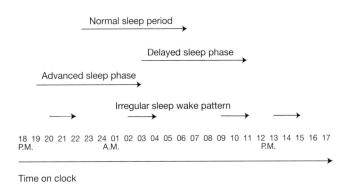

Fig. 19-7. Circadian rhythm disorders. Sleep periods for normal subjects and several circadian rhythm disorders.

1) Chronotherapy
   a) Progressive gradual phase delay with later bedtimes until acceptable bedtime is reached
   b) Alternatively, gradual daily advancement of bedtime may be attempted
2) Light therapy: early morning bright light (10,000 lux) exposure for 30 to 60 minutes after awakening
3) Melatonin 1 to 3 hours before desired bedtime
4) Strict adherence to sleep-wake schedules

3. Advanced sleep phase disorder
   a. Features
      1) Sleep onset and wake times are several hours earlier than societal norms
      2) Sleep duration is normal per 24-hour period and sleep schedule is stable but advanced
   b. Clinical symptoms
      1) Excessive sleepiness in late afternoon and early evening hours
      2) "Insomnia" complaints because of early morning awakenings with inability to reinitiate sleep
   c. Epidemiology
      1) More common in the elderly
      2) Genetic predisposition, familial occurrence
      3) Chronic course
   d. Diagnosis: sleep logs, actigraphy for at least 1 week
   e. Differential diagnosis
      1) Major depression may lead to early morning awakenings
      2) Insomnia of various causes
   f. Treatment
      1) Light therapy in early evening
      2) Can try melatonin in morning
4. Circadian rhythm sleep disorder, nonentrained type (non–24-hour sleep-wake disorder)
   a. Features: internal circadian rhythm either lacks synchronization with 24-hour environmental rhythms or is free running at a non–24-hour rhythm (typically longer than 24 hours)
   b. Clinical symptoms: complaints of variable sleep patterns with intermittent insomnia and excessive daytime sleepiness
   c. Epidemiology
      1) Rare
      2) Observed most often in visually impaired patients, also seen in mental retardation
      3) Occasionally due to behavioral patterns, environmental factors in sighted people
      4) Chronic course
   d. Pathophysiology: lack of light stimulus to the suprachiasmatic nucleus in blind persons leads to absence of entrainment of internal circadian rhythm to environmental rhythms
   e. Diagnosis: sleep logs, actigraphy for at least 1 week
   f. Treatment
      1) Melatonin before bedtime
      2) Light therapy can be tried but may be ineffective
5. Irregular sleep-wake rhythm
   a. Features
      1) Severely disturbed sleep-wake rhythm
      2) Sleep is fragmented into several naps throughout the 24-hour period
      3) Total 24-hour sleep duration is normal
   b. Clinical symptoms: may complain of insomnia and excessive daytime sleepiness
   c. Epidemiology
      1) Rare
      2) Occurs mostly in patients with cerebral dysfunction or those who choose an inconsistent sleep-wake schedule but are capable of entrainment
   d. Pathophysiology: abnormal circadian clock function
   e. Diagnosis
      1) Sleep logs, actigraphy for at least 1 week
      2) Prolonged PSG recording (>24 hours) shows loss of the normal sleep-wake rhythm with multiple short sleep periods
   f. Treatment
      1) Light therapy
      2) Melatonin
      3) Strict adherence to schedules
6. Other circadian rhythm disorders
   a. Jet lag syndrome
      1) Features and clinical symptoms
         a) Insomnia, excessive daytime sleepiness, fatigue, somatic complaints in relation to travel across time zones

b) Severity depends on the number of time zones crossed during travel

c) Eastward travel requires a phase advance

d) Westward travel requires a phase delay of circadian rhythms

e) On average, one day per time zone is required to adjust to local time

2) Epidemiology

a) Temporary condition

b) More severe and longer duration in the elderly

3) Diagnosis: no sleep tests required

b. Shift-work sleep disorder

1) Features and clinical symptoms

a) Insomnia, excessive daytime sleepiness in the setting of a work schedule that entails late, night, early morning, or rotating shifts

b) Reduced 24-hour sleep time

c) Sleep may be fragmented

d) Duration of symptoms: at least 1 month

e) Can have significant social consequences because patients have to balance between the need for daytime sleep and family and social activities that often lead to further voluntary sleep curtailment

2) Epidemiology

a) Course: variable depending on work schedule

b) Sleep parameters and daytime alertness tend to normalize when conventional bed times are kept

3) Diagnosis: sleep log, actigraphy for at least 1 week

c. Circadian rhythm sleep disorder due to medical condition

1) Features and clinical symptoms

a) In setting of primary medical or neurologic disorders, for example, blindness, encephalopathies, dementia, movement disorders

b) Insomnia, excessive daytime sleepiness

c) Wide range of sleep-wake patterns

d) Possibly due to altered circadian rhythm related to the underlying disorder

2) Diagnosis: sleep log, actigraphy for at least 1 week

F. **Parasomnias**

1. Types

  a. NREM sleep parasomnias

  b. REM sleep parasomnias

  c. Other parasomnias

2. NREM sleep parasomnias (disorders of arousal)

  a. Types

   1) Sleepwalking

   2) Sleep terrors

   3) Confusional arousals

b. Features common to all NREM parasomnias

1) Abnormal behaviors occur with sudden partial arousals from NREM sleep

2) Typically arise from SWS

3) Most frequent during the first one-third of the night when most NREM sleep occurs

c. Clinical symptoms common to all NREM parasomnias

1) Patients usually are not responsive to external stimuli and appear confused when awakened during an episode

2) Often no recall in the morning

d. Triggers

1) Sleep deprivation and stress

2) Environmental (e.g., sudden loud noises), medical, psychiatric conditions leading to increased number of arousals

3) Central nervous system depressant medications and substances (e.g., sedatives, hypnotics, alcohol) that prevent complete arousal from sleep by increasing SWS and/or arousal threshold

e. Pathophysiology: abnormal arousal mechanism from SWS

f. Epidemiology

1) Most common in childhood (maturational factors)

2) Genetic predisposition (familial occurrence)

3) Psychologic factors (adults without a childhood history of arousal disorder may occasionally have psychiatric disease)

g. Diagnosis

1) Generally a clinical diagnosis

2) PSG may show sudden arousals from SWS

h. Differential diagnosis: REM sleep parasomnias, untreated sleep apnea, nocturnal panic attacks, seizures

i. Sleep walking (somnambulism)

1) Complex motor behavior, including ambulation during altered state of consciousness

a) Behaviors are often inappropriate (e.g., urinating in a closet, moving objects randomly) and can be as complex as driving a car

b) May result in injury

c) Patients may exhibit violent behavior, especially adults, when attempts are made to wake them; homicide has been reported on very rare occasions

d) Usually arises from SWS

2) Epidemiology

a) Most common in children (6%-17%)

b) 2% to 4% of adults sleepwalk

c) 20% of children who sleepwalk continue to do so in adulthood

3) Diagnosis

a) History (per patient, spouse, family)

b) Time-synchronized video PSG recording, additional limb EMG leads, especially if behaviors have been or are potentially injurious

   i) Recurrent arousals from SWS with or without typical complex motor behaviors

   ii) Partial or complete persistence of SWS patterns or mixed frequencies on EEG during motor activities

4) Treatment

a) Reassurance

b) Secure sleeping environment (e.g., alarms on doors)

c) Eliminate precipitants

d) If behaviors are potentially injurious or problematic, benzodiazepines or tricyclic antidepressants can be prescribed

e) Can also try hypnosis, psychotherapy, relaxation therapy, stress management strategies, particularly in adults with comorbid psychiatric disorders

j. Sleep terrors (pavor nocturnus)

1) Features

a) Abrupt arousal from SWS in first hours of sleep, with signs of intense fear and inconsolable crying, screaming, hyperventilation, tachycardia

b) Patient is difficult to awaken, confused once awake

c) No recollection of preceding nightmare or the event itself

d) Benign condition

2) Epidemiology: more common in children (estimated prevalence, 1%-6%) than adults

3) Diagnosis

a) History (per spouse, family)

b) Time-synchronized video PSG recording can support the diagnosis: arousals from SWS with or without the typical behaviors

4) Treatment

a) Reassurance

b) Avoidance of precipitants

c) Behavioral therapy such as scheduled awakenings

d) If severe, benzodiazepines, tricyclic antidepressants

5) Confusional arousals

a) Features

   i) Least dramatic form of arousal disorders

   ii) Patient awakens partially and shows confusion and disorientation

   iii) Poor response to external stimuli

   iv) No associated prominent vocalization, motor activity, or fear

   v) No memory of the event

b) Epidemiology: more common in children (17%)

than adults (3%-4%)

c) Diagnosis

   i) History

   ii) Time-synchronized video PSG can support the diagnosis

   iii) Arousals from SWS with or without the typical confusional behavior

   iv) During the episode, EEG shows delta, theta, or poorly reactive alpha pattern and microsleeps

d) Treatment: usually not required

3. REM sleep parasomnias

a. RBD

1) Features: abnormal skeletal muscle tone (absence of atonia and increased phasic activity) during REM sleep, resulting in complex motor activity and dream enactment behavior that may lead to injury

2) Epidemiology

a) Prevalence: estimated at 0.38% to 0.5%

b) 90% of patients are men in the sixth to seventh decade

3) Clinical symptoms

a) Distinctly altered, unpleasant, vivid dreams of intruders or attackers (people or animals) occur in 87% of patients and are recalled immediately after the event

b) Dream enactment behavior that is often violent occurs in about 90% of patients

c) Frequent behaviors: vocalization, laughing, reaching, punching, kicking, jumping/falling out of bed, running, striking furniture

d) Frequent injuries to self (79%-96%) or bed partner: bruises, lacerations, fractures, subdural hematomas

e) No dream recall the following morning

f) May occasionally complain of disruptive sleep and excessive daytime sleepiness

4) PSG (Fig. 19-8)

a) Overall normal sleep architecture

b) Loss of normal skeletal muscle atonia or excessive phasic muscle twitching in REM sleep

c) Increased occurrence of classic periodic leg movements (up to 75% of patients) during NREM sleep, prominent aperiodic movements (37% of patients)

d) May show excessive simple or complex motor behaviors during REM sleep

5) Associated features

a) A less frequent acute form may be caused by structural brainstem lesions (e.g., infarction, demyelinating disease, tumor) or may be induced by

certain medications, drug intoxication, withdrawal from certain substances (alcohol, sedative hypnotics)
b) The more common chronic form is frequently associated with neurologic disorders (>50% of patients at initial presentation)
c) Most commonly, neurodegenerative diseases pathologically characterized by α-synuclein–positive intracellular inclusions (synucleinopathies: Parkinson's disease, dementia with Lewy bodies, multiple system atrophy)
d) 92% to 94% of patients with dementia and RBD meet clinical criteria for possible or probable dementia with Lewy bodies
e) 69% to 90% of patients with multiple system atrophy have RBD, as do 15% to 33% of patients with Parkinson's disease
f) Most patients (65%) originally thought to have idiopathic RBD subsequently develop a parkinsonian or dementing disorder
g) All autopsies of patients with a history of RBD have shown changes characteristic of synucleinopathies
h) RBD can precede onset of parkinsonian or dementia symptoms by years or decades
i) RBD is associated more frequently with narcolepsy than in general population
6) Imaging studies
a) MRI: usually normal in idiopathic RBD or may show findings specific for the associated neurodegenerative disorder; occasional cases have visible brainstem lesions (pons) due to infarcts, demyelination, or tumors
b) PET and single photon emission (SPE)CT: decreased striatal dopamine activity
7) Pathophysiology
a) Unclear, possibly due to lesions in pontomedullary pathways promoting REM sleep muscle atonia in combination with increased activity in locomotor generators
b) Brainstem lesion studies have shown abnormal motor behaviors in REM sleep in cats
c) Close association between synucleinopathies and RBD
d) Association with narcolepsy and periodic limb movements of sleep suggests motor control dysfunction
8) Diagnosis
a) History
b) Time-synchronized video PSG is essential to document abnormal muscle tone in REM sleep and absence of epileptiform discharges on EEG

9) Differential diagnosis
a) Nocturnal seizures (especially of frontal lobe origin)
b) Untreated OSA
c) NREM sleep parasomnias
d) Periodic limb movement disorder
e) Psychiatric disorders: nocturnal panic attacks, PTSD, dissociative states, malingering
10) Treatment
a) Bedroom safety (e.g., removal of nightstands, sharp objects, addition of padding)
b) Clonazepam
i) Effective in up to 90% of patients
ii) Watch for side effects (nocturnal confusion!) in elderly patients with cognitive impairment (dementia with Lewy bodies)
c) Melatonin
i) Has been effective in few small uncontrolled series
ii) Can be tried in patients with side effects from or inadequate control with clonazepam
b. Nightmares
1) Features and clinical symptoms
a) Frightening dreams resulting in awakenings
b) No prominent associated motor activity or vocalization
c) Usually full alertness and dream recall immediately after awakening
d) Difficulty reinitiating sleep
2) Epidemiology
a) More frequent in children and patients with psychiatric disorders (substance abuse, PTSD)

Parasomnias occur in NREM and REM sleep and include abnormal movements or behaviors such as sleepwalking and night terrors.

REM sleep behavior disorder is a parasomnia that occurs primarily in older men, often with an underlying synucleinopathy such as Parkinson's disease, MSA, or dementia with Lewy bodies.

Skeletal muscle tone in REM sleep is increased in REM sleep behavior disorder, and patients act out dreams, often violently.

Bedroom safety of REM sleep behavior disorder patients and bed partners must be considered; treatment with clonazepam can be effective.

A

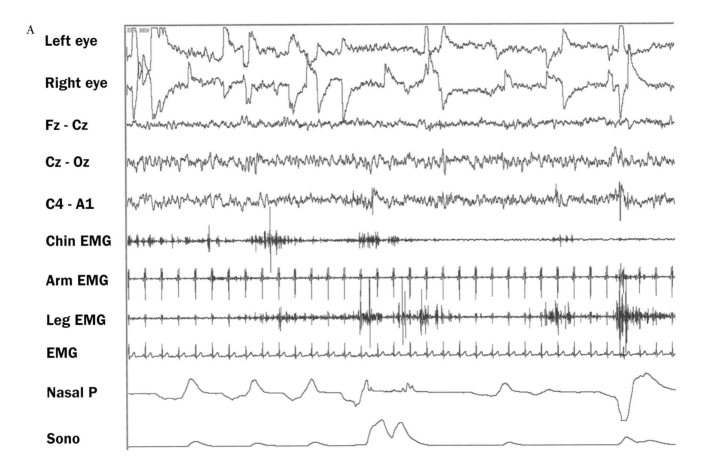

| Left eye |
| Right eye |
| Fz - Cz |
| Cz - Oz |
| C4 - A1 |
| Chin EMG |
| Arm EMG |
| Leg EMG |
| EMG |
| Nasal P |
| Sono |

b) Probable lifetime prevalence: almost 100% in the general population

c) Recurrent nightmares are estimated to affect 2% to 8% of the population

3) Treatment
   a) Treat the underlying disorder
   b) If necessary, psychotherapy, behavioral therapy, hypnosis

c. Sleep paralysis
  1) Features
    a) Transient partial or complete skeletal muscle paralysis at sleep onset or upon awakening with preserved consciousness
    b) Spared muscles: diaphragm, extraocular muscles
  2) Clinical symptoms
    a) Usually frightening experience of paralysis lasting seconds to several minutes
    b) Can be accompanied by hallucinations
    c) Attacks can be aborted by sensory stimuli (e.g., calling or touching the patient)
  3) Triggers: sleep deprivation, irregular sleep-wake schedule
  4) Epidemiology

a) Isolated episodes may have a lifetime prevalence of up to 40% in normal subjects

b) Recurrent attacks are more frequent in narcoleptics

c) Familial occurrences have been described

d) Onset: often in adolescence

5) Pathophysiology: thought to represent intrusion of REM sleep muscle atonia into wakefulness

6) Diagnosis: history

7) Treatment
   a) Often unnecessary
   b) REM sleep suppressants: SSRIs, tricyclic antidepressants

4. Other parasomnias
  a. Catathrenia
    1) Features
     a) Unusual expiratory sound, "nocturnal groaning," during a prolonged expiration following deep inspiration
     b) Bradypnea during those episodes without evidence of respiratory distress
     c) Typically arises from REM sleep but may persist into NREM stage II
     d) Clusters of individual sounds, each lasting for 5 to

B

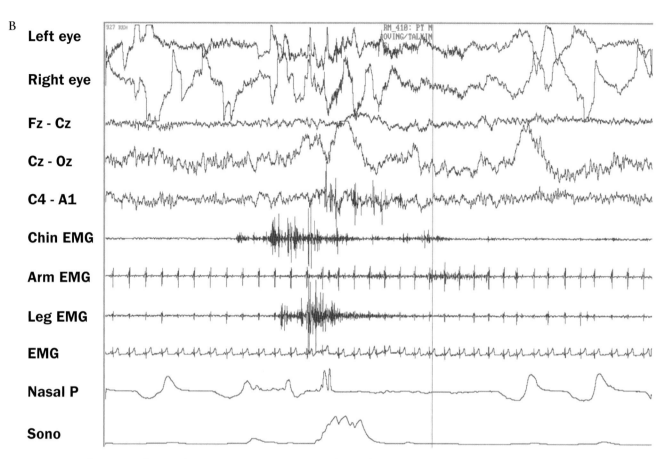

Left eye

Right eye

Fz - Cz

Cz - Oz

C4 - A1

Chin EMG

Arm EMG

Leg EMG

EMG

Nasal P

Sono

Fig. 19-8. *A* and *B*, REM sleep without atonia. *A*, Note increased muscle tone in chin, arm, and anterior tibialis EMG leads. Some of the periods of loss of muscle atonia were associated with video evidence of excessive movements (punching in the air, kicking) and talking, laughing, and screaming (*B*), which made the diagnosis of REM sleep behavior disorder possible. Muscle artifact is also present in the eye and EEG channels (30-second epochs).

      50 seconds, may recur for minutes up to 1 hour
2) Clinical symptoms
  a) Loud groaning noises without associated motor activity
  b) Patient is usually unaware of sounds
  c) May cause considerable sleep disturbance of bed partner
3) Epidemiology
  a) Most often affects young men
  b) Prevalence: unknown
  c) Can persist for years
4) Pathophysiology
  a) Unknown
  b) Normal laryngoscopic findings in awake patients
5) Diagnosis
  a) History
  b) PSG with respiratory sound monitoring: bradypnea, decreased respiratory signal amplitude in expira-

tion associated with groaning sound
6) Differential diagnosis
  a) CSA
  b) Stridor
  c) Asthma
  d) Sleep talking
7) Treatment
  a) None proven effective; CPAP does not eliminate the sound
  b) Can try REM sleep suppressants if bed partner complains of sleep disruption
b. Sleep-related hallucinations
  1) Features and clinical symptoms
    a) Mostly visual hallucinations that occur upon falling asleep (hypnagogic) or waking (hypnopompic)
      i) Hallucinations may also be auditory, tactile, kinetic
      ii) May be associated with sleep paralysis

b) Complex nocturnal visual hallucinations occur after sudden awakenings from sleep
   i) May be a separate entity
   ii) Immobile images of animals or people
   iii) Can last for minutes
   iv) Images disappear when lights are turned on
   v) Often frightening experience
2) Epidemiology
   a) Hypnagogic and hypnopompic hallucinations are more common in young people (30% and 10%, respectively) and occur with higher frequency in patients with narcolepsy
   b) Complex nocturnal visual hallucinations are rare, usually found with visual and neurologic disorders (narcolepsy, dementia with Lewy bodies) but can be idiopathic
3) Pathophysiology: hypnagogic and hypnopompic hallucinations are thought to represent intrusion of REM sleep phenomena into wakefulness
4) PSG
   a) Hypnagogic and hypnopompic hallucinations arise mostly from sleep-onset REM sleep periods
   b) Complex nocturnal visual hallucinations appear to occur out of NREM sleep
5) Diagnosis: history
6) Treatment: not usually necessary
c. Sleep-related eating disorder
   1) Features and clinical symptoms
      a) Recurrent involuntary episodic eating during nocturnal sleep period
      b) Level of consciousness is impaired at least partially
      c) Food is usually high in calories, odd concoctions may be prepared, inedible substances
      d) Morning anorexia
      e) Dangerous behaviors and injuries may occur during food preparation (e.g., fires, burns)
      f) No or only partial recall in morning
      g) Associated weight gain can be a problem
      h) Complaints of insomnia, nonrestorative sleep, excessive daytime sleepiness
   2) Epidemiology
      a) More common in women
      b) Onset: most often in third decade
      c) Idiopathic or in setting of other sleep disorders (most often sleepwalking, also periodic limb movement disorder, restless legs syndrome, OSA), can be medication-induced (zolpidem, triazolam)
      d) Unremitting course
   3) Pathophysiology: unknown
   4) PSG

a) Often shows frequent confusional arousals with or without the eating behavior
b) Episodes arise most often from SWS, can be triggered by other sleep disorders
c) Alpha rhythm during the eating behavior
5) Treatment
   a) Treat associated sleep disorder if present
   b) Try clonazepam, combinations of levodopa with clonazepam or codeine, or topiramate
d. Hypnic jerks ("sleep starts")
   1) Features and clinical symptoms
      a) Sudden brief jerks occurring upon falling asleep
      b) Usually involve the extremities
      c) May be associated with a sensation of falling
      d) May lead to sleep-onset insomnia if repetitive
      e) May worsen with caffeine consumption or after exercise
   2) Epidemiology
      a) Prevalence: 60% to 70%
      b) Benign course
   3) Pathophysiology: unknown
   4) PSG: brief jerk (<250 ms) during drowsiness/stage I sleep, often followed by arousal
   5) Diagnosis: history
   6) Treatment: usually not required
e. Exploding head syndrome ("sensory starts")
   1) Features and clinical symptoms
      a) Sudden loud noise or painless sensation of the head exploding upon falling asleep or waking
      b) Often frightening
      c) May be accompanied by visual phenomena (light flashes)
   2) Epidemiology
      a) Prevalence: unknown
      b) More common in women than men
      c) Mean age at onset: sixth decade
      d) Benign course
   3) Pathophysiology: unknown, may represent a variant of hypnic jerks
   4) Diagnosis: history
   5) Treatment
      a) Reassurance
      b) Otherwise, not usually necessary
f. Sleep enuresis
   1) Features and clinical symptoms: recurrent involuntary nocturnal micturition at least twice per week persisting beyond age 5 years
   2) Epidemiology
      a) Prevalence: depends on age (3%-30% for children 4-12 years old, 2% for adults)

b) Typically occurs in younger children

c) More common in boys

d) Mostly due to primary enuresis (dryness in sleep was never accomplished), only 10% secondary (recurrence of enuresis after being dry for a 3-month period)

e) Course depends on underlying cause

3) Pathophysiology

a) Primary enuresis: failure of arousal from sleep in response to a full bladder sensation and/or failure of inhibition of bladder contraction during sleep

b) Secondary enuresis: due to various medical disorders leading to inability to concentrate urine, increased urine production, urinary tract disorders, neurologic disorders, sleep disorders (OSA), psychologic stressors, caffeine and diuretic use

4) Diagnosis

a) History

b) Must rule out organic causes

c) PSG is indicated only if sleep-related epilepsy or OSA is suspected

5) Treatment

a) Behavioral techniques: scheduled awakenings, retention control training, urine alarm devices

b) Desmopressin intranasally at bedtime if necessary

g. Parasomnia overlap disorder

1) Features

a) Combination of RBD and NREM parasomnias

b) Most often sleep walking or sleep terrors

c) Possibly represents a disorder of generalized motor dyscontrol in sleep

2) Epidemiology

a) Usually presents in childhood or adolescence

b) Mean age at onset: 15 years

3) Treatment

a) Same as for REM sleep or NREM sleep parasomnias

b) Benzodiazepines are most effective

G. **Sleep Disorders Associated With Neurologic Conditions**

1. Neurologic conditions with prominent features during sleep: behavioral and neurodegenerative disorders, epilepsy, headache

2. Behavioral and neurodegenerative conditions

a. Specific neurodegenerative disorders known as α-synucleinopathies have the highest incidence of REM sleep behavior disorder, including Parkinson's disease, dementia with Lewy bodies, and multiple system atrophy

b. RBD is estimated to be present in 69% to 90% of patients with multiple system atrophy and 15% to 33% of patients with Parkinson's disease

c. Neurologic exam may show evidence of these disorders, but RBD can precede the diagnosis by years or decades

d. Of 29 patients thought to have idiopathic RBD, 65% developed parkinsonism or dementia up to 13 years after the onset of symptoms of RBD

e. Treatment

1) Safe bedroom environment

2) Low-dose benzodiazepines (clonazepam): use with caution in elderly and demented patients because agents may cause confusion and worsening cognitive function

3) Melatonin

3. Parkinson's disease

a. Sleep problems are frequent in Parkinson's disease (60%-86% of patients)

b. Sleep problems result from positive and negative symptoms of the disorder

1) Rigidity, bradykinesia, tremor

2) Difficulties turning over in bed

3) Early morning dystonia

4) Treat with extended release levodopa or dopamine agonists at bedtime

c. Medication effects (L-dopa, dopamine agonists)

1) Insomnia: treatment is to reduce dopaminergic dose, add hypnotic

2) Hallucinations, nightmares, confusion: treatment is to reduce dopaminergic dose

3) Excessive daytime sleepiness

4) Sleep attacks (dopamine agonists), unknown mechanism

d. Dyskinesia: treatment is to reduce dopaminergic dose

e. Comorbid depression

f. Sleep-maintenance insomnia: treat with antidepressants

g. Primary sleep disorders: higher incidence of restless legs syndrome, periodic limb movement disorder, RBD (up to 33% of patients)

h. Hypersomnia

1) Can occur independently of medication effects

2) In one study, 25% of patients had excessive daytime sleepiness independent of dopamine agonist use but correlating with severity of Parkinson's disease

3) Rule out coexisting primary sleep disorders

4. Multiple system atrophy: sleep problems result from

a. Nocturnal stridor

1) Occurs in up to 30% of patients

2) Possible cause: vocal cord dystonia, vocal cord paralysis, paradoxical vocal cord adduction with inspiration

3) May cause sudden death in sleep

4) If patient has suggestive history, PSG
5) Treatment
   a) Tracheostomy
   b) More recently, nasal CPAP titrated to eliminate stridor has shown some promise
  b. Other respiratory disturbances
   1) Sleep apnea: obstructive and central
   2) Respiratory rhythm disturbances: Cheyne-Stokes breathing, apneustic breathing, cluster breathing, irregular breathing
   3) Respiratory failure
   4) Treatment: consider positive airway pressure device, tracheostomy, nocturnal ventilation depending on type of abnormality
  c. RBD
   1) REM sleep without atonia occurs in 95% of patients with multiple system atrophy
   2) Frank RBD occurs in 69% to 90% of patients
5. Dementia
  a. Disturbed circadian rhythms
  b. Inability to sleep at night and frequent daytime dozing and napping result in sleep fragmentation
  c. Nocturnal wandering, confusion, agitation are frequent
6. Epilepsy
  a. Sleep is associated with increased frequency of epileptiform discharges and seizures in NREM sleep, particularly during stages III and IV, and become more widespread
  b. Epileptiform discharges are suppressed in REM sleep and become more focal
  c. 15% to 30% of patients with epilepsy have seizures exclusively or predominantly during sleep
  d. Certain seizure types are more closely related to sleep
   1) Frontal lobe epilepsy
   2) Temporal lobe epilepsy
   3) Juvenile myoclonic epilepsy
   4) Benign childhood epilepsy with centrotemporal spikes
   5) Epilepsy with generalized tonic-clonic seizures on awakening
  e. Effects of nocturnal seizures on sleep
   1) Increased nocturnal awakenings and sleep fragmentation
   2) Increased percentage of lighter sleep stages
   3) Decreased REM sleep
   4) May cause excessive daytime sleepiness
  f. Effects of sleep on seizures: sleep deprivation
   1) Lowers seizure threshold
   2) Increases frequency of interictal discharges
   3) Is used to enhance detection of epileptiform activity during EEG
  g. Anticonvulsants

1) Tend to consolidate sleep
2) May cause excessive daytime sleepiness (benzodiazepines, carbamazepine, phenobarbital, topiramate, gabapentin)
3) May cause insomnia (felbamate)
  h. OSA and seizures
   1) OSA is frequent in patients with epilepsy
   2) OSA occurs in up to 30% of patients with medically refractory epilepsy
   3) Patients with OSA are more likely to have seizures
   4) Seizure control tends to improve with treatment of OSA
7. Headache
  a. Migraine
   1) Can be provoked by sleep disturbance (deprivation or excess)
   2) Headache typically develops in REM sleep in patients with nocturnal migraine
   3) Sleep has long been recognized as therapeutic in migraine
   4) The relation is thought to be due to serotonin effects
  b. Cluster headache and chronic paroxysmal headache
   1) Can occur predominantly or exclusively at night
   2) Often arise from REM sleep
  c. Hypnic headache
   1) Rare
   2) Recurrent headache syndrome affecting the elderly
   3) Diffuse, moderately severe headache occurs exclusively during sleep
    a) No associated autonomic findings
    b) Occurs usually at the same time each night
    c) Duration: 30 minutes to 2 hours

Neurologic diseases that commonly disrupt sleep include Parkinson's disease, dementia, epilepsy, and headache.

Sleep lowers seizure threshold, and some seizure syndromes such as juvenile myoclonic epilepsy and benign childhood epilepsy with centrotemporal spikes arise primarily out of sleep.

Certain headache types arise from sleep, particularly during REM sleep periods, whereas sleep can be therapeutic for migraine and other headache patterns.

Morning headache occurs frequently with obstructive sleep apnea but also with other sleep disorders.

4) May respond to lithium and indomethacin

d. Morning headache

    1) Occurs frequently in patients (36%-58%) with OSA

       a) Mostly upon awakening, may also occur during the night

       b) Mechanism: unknown

       c) Typically dull in character, diffuse

       d) Duration: short, resolves upon getting up

    2) Possibly correlated with severity of oxygen desaturation and hypercapnia, possibly also frequency of apneas and hypopneas, and number of nocturnal arousals

    3) Usually improves with CPAP therapy

    4) Morning headache can also result from various other causes of sleep disruption: restless legs syndrome, insomnia, chronic pain syndromes, depression, anxiety

REFERENCES

Abrahamson EE, Leak RK, Moore RY. The suprachiasmatic nucleus projects to posterior hypothalamic arousal systems. Neuroreport. 2001;12:435-40.

Albin RL, Koeppe RA, Chervin RD, Consens FB, Wernette K, Frey KA, et al. Decreased striatal dopaminergic innervation in REM sleep behavior disorder. Neurology. 2000;55:1410-2.

Allen RP, Barker PB, Wehrl F, Song HK, Earley CJ. MRI measurement of brain iron in patients with restless legs syndrome. Neurology. 2001;56:263-5.

Allen RP, Picchietti D, Hening WA, Trenkwalder C, Walters AS, Montplaisi J. Restless legs syndrome: diagnostic criteria, special considerations, and epidemiology: a report from the Restless Legs Syndrome Diagnosis and Epidemiology Workshop at the National Institutes of Health. Sleep Med. 2003;4:101-19.

American Academy of Sleep Medicine. The international classification of sleep disorders: diagnostic and coding manual. 2nd ed. Westchester (IL): American Academy of Sleep Medicine; 2005.

American Academy of Sleep Medicine Task Force. Sleep-related breathing disorders in adults: recommendations for syndrome definition and measurement techniques in clinical research. Sleep. 1999;22:667-89.

Berger RJ, Oswald I. Effects of sleep deprivation on behaviour, subsequent sleep, and dreaming. J Ment Sci. 1962;108:457-65.

Boeve BF, Silber MH, Ferman TJ, Kokmen E, Smith GE, Ivnik RJ, et al. REM sleep behavior disorder and degenerative dementia: an association likely reflecting Lewy body disease. Neurology. 1998;51:363-70.

Boeve BF, Silber MH, Parisi JE, Dickson DW, Ferman TJ, Benarroch EE, et al. Synucleinopathy pathology and REM sleep behavior disorder plus dementia or parkinsonism. Neurology. 2003;61:40-5.

Bonnet MH, Arand DL. Sleep loss in aging. Clin Geriatr Med. 1989;5:405-20.

Bonnet MH, Arand DL. 24-Hour metabolic rate in insomniacs and matched normal sleepers. Sleep. 1995;18:581-8.

Bradley TD, Floras JS. Sleep apnea and heart failure: part II. Central sleep apnea. Circulation. 2003;107:1822-6.

Bucher SF, Seelos KC, Oertel WH, Reiser M, Trenkwalder C. Cerebral generators involved in the pathogenesis of the restless legs syndrome. Ann Neurol. 1997;41:639-45.

Carskadon MA, Dement WC. Effects of total sleep loss on sleep tendency. Percept Mot Skills. 1979;48:495-506.

Carskadon MA, Dement WC, Mitler MM, Roth T, Westbrook PR, Keenan

S. Guidelines for the multiple sleep latency test (MSLT): a standard measure of sleepiness. Sleep. 1986;9:519-24.

Cortelli P, Parchi P, Contin M, Pierangeli G, Avoni P, Tinuper P, et al. Cardiovascular dysautonomia in fatal familial insomnia. Clin Auton Res. 1991;1:15-21.

Dauvilliers Y, Mayer G, Lecendreux M, Neidhart E, Peraita-Adrados R, Sonka K, et al. Kleine-Levin syndrome: an autoimmune hypothesis based on clinical and genetic analyses. Neurology. 2002;59:1739-45.

Dexter JD. The relationship between stage III + IV + REM sleep and arousals with migraine. Headache. 1979;19:364-9.

Dexter JD. Headache as a presenting complaint of the sleep apnea syndrome [abstract]. Headache. 1984;24:171.

Dexter JD, Weitzman ED. The relationship of nocturnal headaches to sleep stage patterns. Neurology. 1970;20:513-8.

Dodick DW. Polysomnography in hypnic headache syndrome. Headache. 2000;40:748-52.

Dodick DW, Eross EJ, Parish JM, Silber M. Clinical, anatomical, and physiologic relationship between sleep and headache. Headache. 2003;43:282-92. Erratum in: Headache. 2004;44:384.

Doghramji K, Mitler MM, Sangal RB, Shapiro C, Taylor S, Walsleben J, et al. A normative study of the maintenance of wakefulness test (MWT). Electroencephalogr Clin Neurophysiol. 1997;103:554-62.

Earley CJ, Connor JR, Beard JL, Malecki EA, Epstein DK, Allen RP. Abnormalities in CSF concentrations of ferritin and transferrin in restless legs syndrome. Neurology. 2000;54:1698-700.

Edgar D. Functional role of the suprachiasmatic nuclei in the regulation of sleep and wakefulness. In: Guilleminault C, Montagna P, Gambetti P, editors. Fatal familial insomnia: inherited prion disease, sleep and the thalamus. New York: Raven Press; 1994. p. 203-14.

Eisensehr I, Linke R, Noachtar S, Schwarz J, Gildehaus FJ, Tatsch K. Reduced striatal dopamine transporters in idiopathic rapid eye movement sleep behaviour disorder: comparison with Parkinson's disease and controls. Brain. 2000;123:1155-60.

Ferman TJ, Boeve BF, Smith GE, Silber MH, Kokmen E, Petersen RC, et al. REM sleep behavior disorder and dementia: cognitive differences when compared with AD. Neurology. 1999;52:951-7.

Franklin KA, Eriksson P, Sahlin C, Lundgren R. Reversal of central sleep apnea with oxygen. Chest. 1997;111:163-9.

Garcia-Rill E. Disorders of the reticular activating system. Med Hypotheses. 1997;49:379-87.

Guilleminault C, van den Hoed J, Mitler MM. Clinical overview of the sleep apnea syndromes. Vol 11. In: Guilleminault C, Dement WC, editors. Sleep apnea syndromes. New York: Alan R. Liss; 1978. p.1-12.

Hagan JJ, Leslie RA, Patel S, Evans ML, Wattam TA, Holmes S, et al. Orexin A activates locus coeruleus cell firing and increases arousal in the rat. Proc Natl Acad Sci U S A. 1999;96:10911-6.

Hauri P, Fisher J. Persistent psychophysiologic (learned) insomnia. Sleep. 1986;9:38-53.

Hillman DR. Sleep apnea and myocardial infarction. Sleep. 1993;16 Suppl:S23-4.

Hoffstein V, Mateika S. Cardiac arrhythmias, snoring, and sleep apnea. Chest. 1994;106:466-71.

Horner RL. Motor control of the pharyngeal musculature and implications for the pathogenesis of obstructive sleep apnea. Sleep. 1996;19:827-53.

Hung J, Whitford EG, Parsons RW, Hillman DR. Association of sleep apnoea with myocardial infarction in men. Lancet. 1990;336:261-4.

Iranzo A, Santamaria J, Tolosa E, Vilaseca I, Valldeoriola F, Marti MJ, et al. Long-term effect of CPAP in the treatment of nocturnal stridor in multiple system atrophy. Neurology. 2003;63:930-2.

Javaheri S. A mechanism of central sleep apnea in patients with heart failure. N Engl J Med. 1999;341:949-54.

Javaheri S, Parker TJ, Liming JD, Corbett WS, Nishiyama H, Wexler L, et al. Sleep apnea in 81 ambulatory male patients with stable heart failure: types and their prevalences, consequences, and presentations. Circulation. 1998;97:2154-9.

Javaheri S, Parker TJ, Wexler L, Liming JD, Lindower P, Roselle GA. Effect of theophylline on sleep-disordered breathing in heart failure. N Engl J Med. 1996;335:562-7.

Kales A, Tan TL, Kollar EJ, Naitoh P, Preston TA, Malmstrom EJ. Sleep patterns following 205 hours of sleep deprivation. Psychosom Med. 1970;32:189-200.

Kilduff TS, Peyron C. The hypocretin/orexin ligand-receptor system: implications for sleep and sleep disorders. Trends Neurosci. 2000;23:359-65.

Koehler U, Schafer H. Is obstructive sleep apnea (OSA) a risk factor for myocardial infarction and cardiac arrhythmias in patients with coronary heart disease (CHD)? Sleep. 1996;19:283-6.

Kollar EJ, Namerow N, Pasnau RO, Naitoh P. Neurological findings during prolonged sleep deprivation. Neurology. 1968;18:836-40.

Krahn LE, Black JL, Silber MH. Narcolepsy: new understanding of irresistible sleep. Mayo Clin Proc. 2001;76:185-94.

Kryger MH, Roth T, Dement WC, editors. Principles and practice of sleep medicine. 3rd ed. Philadelphia: WB Saunders; 2000.

Lammers GJ, Arends J, Declerck AC, Ferrari MD, Schouwink G, Troost J. Gammahydroxybutyrate and narcolepsy: a double-blind placebo-controlled study. Sleep. 1993;16:216-20.

Lee EK, Maselli RA, Ellis WG, Agius MA. Morvan's fibrillary chorea: a paraneoplastic manifestation of thymoma. J Neurol Neurosurg Psychiatry. 1998;65:857-62.

Liguori R, Vincent A, Clover L, Avoni P, Plazzi G, Cortelli P, et al. Morvan's syndrome: peripheral and central nervous system and cardiac involvement with antibodies to voltage-gated potassium channels. Brain. 2001;124:2417-26.

Lugaresi A, Baruzzi A, Cacciari E, Cortelli P, Medori R, Montagna P, et al. Lack of vegetative and endocrine circadian rhythms in fatal familial thalamic degeneration. Clin Endocrinol (Oxf). 1987;26:573-80.

Lugaresi E. The thalamus and insomnia. Neurology. 1992;42 Suppl 6:28-33.

Lugaresi E, Coccagna G, Mantovani M, Lebrun R. Some periodic phenomena arising during drowsiness and sleep in man. Electroencephalogr Clin Neurophysiol. 1972;32:701-5.

Mahowald MW, Schenck CH. NREM sleep parasomnias. Neurol Clin. 1996;14:675-96.

Malow BA, Levy K, Maturen K, Bowes R. Obstructive sleep apnea is common in medically refractory epilepsy patients. Neurology. 2000;55:1002-7.

Meijer JH, Rietveld WJ. Neurophysiology of the suprachiasmatic circadian pacemaker in rodents. Physiol Rev. 1989;69:671-707.

Mendelson WB. Are periodic leg movements associated with clinical sleep disturbance? Sleep. 1996;19:219-23.

Mignot E, Hayduk R, Black J, Grumet FC, Guilleminault C. HLA DQB1*0602 is associated with cataplexy in 509 narcoleptic patients. Sleep. 1997;20:1012-20.

Mistberger R, Rusak B. Mechanisms and models of the circadian timekeeping system. In: Kryger M, Roth T, Dement WC, editors. Principles and practice of sleep medicine. Philadelphia: WB Saunders Company; 1989. p. 141-52.

Moore T, Rabben T, Wiklund U, Franklin KA, Eriksson P. Sleep-disordered breathing in men with coronary artery disease. Chest. 1996;109:659-63.

Nicolas A, Lespérance P, Montplaisir J. Is excessive daytime sleepiness with periodic leg movements during sleep a specific diagnostic category? Eur Neurol. 1988;40:22-6.

Nieto FJ, Young TB, Lind BK, Shahar E, Samet JM, Redline S, et al. Association of sleep-disordered breathing, sleep apnea, and hypertension in a large community-based study: Sleep Heart Health Study. JAMA. 2000;283:1829-36. Erratum in JAMA. 2002;288:1985.

Oakson G, Steriade M. Slow rhythmic oscillations of EEG slow-wave amplitudes and their relations to midbrain reticular discharge. Brain Res. 1983;269:386-90.

Ohayon MM, Zulley J, Guilleminault C, Smirne S. Prevalence and pathologic associations of sleep paralysis in the general population. Neurology. 1999;52:1194-200.

O'Keeffe ST, Gavin K, Lavan JN. Iron status and restless legs syndrome in the elderly. Age Ageing. 1994;23:200-3.

Olson EJ, Boeve BF, Silber MH. Rapid eye movement sleep behaviour disorder: demographic, clinical and laboratory findings in 93 cases. Brain. 2000;123:331-9.

Peppard PE, Young T, Palta M, Skatrud J. Prospective study of the association between sleep-disordered breathing and hypertension. N Engl J Med. 2000;342:1378-84.

Pevernagie DA, Boon PA, Mariman AN, Verhaeghen DB, Pauwels RA. Vocalization during episodes of prolonged expiration: a parasomnia related to REM sleep. Sleep Med. 2001;2:19-30.

Peyron C, Tighe DK, van den Pol AN, de Lecea L, Heller HC, Sutcliffe JG, et al. Neurons containing hypocretin (orexin) project to multiple neuronal systems. J Neurosci. 1998;18:9996-10015.

Poceta JS, Dalessio DJ. Identification and treatment of sleep apnea in patients with chronic headache. Headache. 1995;35:586-9.

Rosenow F, Kotagal P, Cohen BH, Green C, Wyllie E. Multiple sleep latency test and polysomnography in diagnosing Kleine-Levin syndrome and periodic hypersomnia. J Clin Neurophysiol. 2000;17:519-22.

Ross JJ. Neurological findings after prolonged sleep deprivation. Arch Neurol. 1965;12:399-403.

Ruottinen HM, Partinen M, Hublin C, Bergman J, Haaparanta M, Solin O, et al. An FDOPA PET study in patients with periodic limb movement disorder and restless legs syndrome. Neurology. 2000;54:502-4.

Saito T, Yoshikawa T, Sakamoto Y, Tanaka K, Inoue T, Ogawa R. Sleep apnea in patients with acute myocardial infarction. Crit Care Med. 1991;19:938-41.

Scammell TE. The neurobiology, diagnosis, and treatment of narcolepsy. Ann Neurol. 2003;53:154-66.

Schenck CH, Boyd JL, Mahowald MW. A parasomnia overlap disorder involving sleepwalking, sleep terrors, and REM sleep behavior disorder in 33 polysomnographically confirmed cases. Sleep. 1997;20:972-81.

Schenck CH, Bundlie SR, Mahowald MW. REM behavior disorder (RBD): delayed emergence of Parkinsonism and/or dementia in 65% of older men initially diagnosed with idiopathic RBD, and an analysis of the minimum and maximum tonic and/or phasic electomyographic abnormalities found during REM sleep. Sleep. 2003;26 Suppl:A316.

Schenck CH, Mahowald MW. REM sleep parasomnias. Neurol Clin. 1996;14:697-720.

Schenck CH, Mahowald MW. REM sleep behavior disorder: clinical, developmental, and neuroscience perspectives 16 years after its formal identification in SLEEP. Sleep. 2002;25:120-38.

Schenck CH, Mahowald MW, Sack RL. Assessment and management of insomnia. JAMA. 2003;289:2475-9.

Shamsuzzaman AS, Gersh BJ, Somers VK. Obstructive sleep apnea: implications for cardiac and vascular disease. JAMA. 2003;290:1906-14.

Silber MH, Krahn LE, Morgenthaler TI. Sleep medicine in clinical practice. London: Taylor & Francis; 2004.

Silber MH, Rye DB. Solving the mysteries of narcolepsy: the hypocretin story. Neurology. 2001;56:1616-8.

Sun ER, Chen CA, Ho G, Earley CJ, Allen RP. Iron and the restless legs syndrome. Sleep. 1998;21:371-7.

Thannickal TC, Moore RY, Nienhuis R, Ramanathan L, Gulyani S, Aldrich M, et al. Reduced number of hypocretin neurons in human narcolepsy. Neuron. 2000;27:469-74.

Turjanski N, Lees AJ, Brooks DJ. Striatal dopaminergic function in restless legs syndrome: 18F-dopa and 11C-raclopride PET studies. Neurology. 1999;52:932-7.

Van Dongen HP, Maislin G, Mullington JM, Dinges DF. The cumulative cost of additional wakefulness: dose-response effects on neurobehavioral functions and sleep physiology from chronic sleep restriction and total sleep deprivation. Sleep. 2003;26:117-26. Erratum in: Sleep. 2004;27:600.

Vetrugno R, Provini F, Plazzi G, Vignatelli L, Lugaresi E, Montagna P. Catathrenia (nocturnal groaning): a new type of parasomnia. Neurology. 2001;56:681-3.

Williams JT. Synaptic and intrinsic membrane properties regulating nor-adrenergic and serotonergic neurons during sleep/wake cycles. In: Lydic R, Baghdoyan HA, editors. Handbook of behavioral state control. New York: CRC Press; 1999. p. 257-76.

Willson GN, Wilcox I, Piper AJ, Flynn WE, Grunstein RR, Sullivan CE. Treatment of central sleep apnoea in congestive heart failure with nasal venti-lation. Thorax. 1998; 53 Suppl 3:S41-6.

Yoss RE, Daly DD. Criteria for the diagnosis of the narcoleptic syndrome. Mayo Clin Proc. 1957;32:320-8.

Appendix. Common Causes of Intermittent Sleep Disturbance in Adults

	Obstructive sleep apnea	Restless legs syndrome	Periodic limb move-ment disorder	REM sleep behavior disorder
Clinical complaint of patient or bed partner	Snoring, apnea, nonrestorative sleep, excessive daytime sleepiness, fatigue	Unpleasant limb sensation (creepy-crawling) with irresistible urge to move legs > arms around bed-time, insomnia, excessive daytime sleepiness	Spontaneous leg jerking, insomnia, excessive daytime sleepiness	Active dreaming, vocalization, excessive movements with injury to self or partner
Typical demographic features	Obese males Any age	Slight female pre-dominance Increases with age	Similar to restless legs syndrome	Male predominance Age: 50+ years
Examination findings	Obesity, short thick neck, crowded air-way, craniofacial abnormalities	Normal or peripheral neuropathy Laboratory studies may show low levels of hemoglobin, ferritin, folate, vitamin B_{12}	Same as for restless legs syndrome	Examination may be normal or show evidence of parkinsonism, dementia, or autonomic insufficiency
Findings on poly-somnography	Recurrent apneas and hypopneas with frequent arousals	Frequent leg movements during wakefulness Often periodic limb movements during sleep	Rhythmic toe and ankle dorsiflexion, knee and hip flexion of one or both legs during early stages of sleep	Absence of muscle atonia and excessive motor behavior during REM sleep
Treatment	Weight loss, sleep hygiene, positional therapy, oral appli-ance, CPAP, BiPAP, rarely surgery (tonsillectomy in children, UPPP, tongue base reduc-tion, tracheostomy)	Dopamine agonists, levodopa, benzo-diazepines, gabapentin, low-potency opioids Iron replacement if ferritin low	Same as for restless legs syndrome	Bedroom safety Clonazepam, melatonin

BiPAP, bilevel positive airway pressure; CPAP, continuous positive airway pressure; UPPP, uvulopalatopharyngoplasty.

QUESTIONS

1. Which of the following is true about sleep architecture?
   a. Most dreaming occurs in the first half of the night
   b. Stage I is light sleep
   c. K complexes and sleep spindles occur in slow wave sleep
   d. Delta slowing on EEG is common in stage II sleep
   e. REM sleep represents about two-thirds of the total sleep time

2. Which of the following is true about sleep testing?
   a. Sleep latency of 4.5 minutes on the multiple sleep latency test (MSLT) is considered normal
   b. An actigraph records sleep stages
   c. Polysomnography (PSG) involves simultaneous EEG and EMG recording
   d. Continuous positive airway pressure (CPAP) should not be tried during overnight PSG
   e. MSLT should be performed after sleep deprivation

3. Which of the following is true about sleep disorders?
   a. Serum carbon dioxide levels can be normal in central sleep apnea
   b. HLA-B27 is closely associated with narcolepsy
   c. Recurrent hypersomnia primarily affects elderly women
   d. The most useful tool in diagnosing chronic insomnia is polysomnography (PSG)
   e. Patients with obstructive sleep apnea are aware of most arousals

4. A patient who continues to go to bed late at night and arise late in the morning has:
   a. Periodic limb movement disorder
   b. Pavor nocturnus
   c. Cataplexy
   d. Advanced sleep phase pattern
   e. Delayed sleep phase pattern

5. Which of the following is true about sleep-related neurologic conditions?
   a. REM sleep behavior disorder represents enhanced REM atonia
   b. The pathologic substrate of REM sleep behavior disorder is thought to be a tauopathy
   c. First-line treatment for REM sleep behavior disorder includes low-dose levodopa
   d. Epileptiform discharges arise predominantly out of NREM sleep
   e. Cluster headache arises predominantly out of NREM sleep

6. Which one of the following stimuli is most effective in synchronizing internal circadian rhythms in humans?
   a. Exercise
   b. Food
   c. Bright light
   d. Social cues
   e. Caffeine

7. A 45-year-old woman complains of an uncomfortable crawling sensation and aching in both legs in the evenings when she sits quietly and watches TV. The symptoms become even more prominent when she lies down in bed. She feels a need to move her legs and will ambulate, with temporary relief of the discomfort. Her spouse reports that her legs frequently jerk during sleep. She has a history of hypertension. What is the most likely diagnosis?
   a. Akathisia
   b. Sensory neuropathy
   c. Restless legs syndrome
   d. Anxiety disorder
   e. Fragmentary myoclonus

8. For the patient in Question 7, what should be performed next?
   a. EMG
   b. Serum electrolyte level
   c. Serum ferritin level
   d. Psychiatric evaluation
   e. Fasting serum glucose and hemoglobin A_{1c}

9. How would you initially treat the patient in Question 7?
   a. Amitriptyline
   b. Selegiline
   c. Trazodone
   d. Pramipexole
   e. Fluoxetine

10. A 20-year-old college student complains of difficulty staying awake in class. He remembers having always been sleepy during the daytime since his early teenage years. He reports getting about 7 hours of sleep nightly. He feels more alert after taking a short nap. Lately, he has developed spells of sudden leg weakness when laughing or being angry. He has fallen during such attacks but denies loss of consciousness. The patient most likely has:
   a. Complex partial seizures

b. Syncopal events
c. Narcolepsy
d. Psychogenic unresponsiveness
e. Idiopathic hypersomnia

11. Which of the following agents is *least* likely to improve the attacks of weakness in the patient in Question 10?
a. Phenytoin
b. Selective serotonin reuptake inhibitors
c. Tricyclic antidepressants
d. γ-Hydroxybutyrate

12. How should the sleepiness of the patient in Question 10 be treated?
a. Selective serotonin reuptake inhibitors
b. Stimulants
c. Tricyclic antidepressants
d. Clonazepam
e. Caffeine

13. Deficiency of which of the following neurotransmitters has been implicated in the pathogenesis of the condition diagnosed in the patient in Question 10?
a. Noradrenaline
b. Acetylcholine
c. Serotonin
d. Histamine
e. Hypocretin

14. A 4-year-old boy has frequent episodes of inconsolable crying shortly after falling asleep. His parents have noted that his pupils appear large and his heart races. He appears very scared and confused and will not react to his parents' attempts to comfort him. This child most likely has:
a. Nocturnal seizures
b. Nocturnal panic attacks
c. Sleep terrors
d. REM sleep behavior disorder
e. Sleep-onset association disorder

15. The human circadian pacemaker is located in the:
a. Locus ceruleus
b. Dorsal raphe nucleus
c. Intralaminar thalamic nuclei
d. Suprachiasmatic nucleus of hypothalamus
e. Posterolateral hypothalamus

16. A 75-year-old man with Parkinson's disease has nocturnal episodes of yelling, screaming, punching the air, and kicking his legs as if he were fighting someone. He has fallen out of bed and sustained bruises and lacerations while striking the bedside table. His wife has suffered bruises from being kicked by him. He appears asleep during the episode but, if awakened, recalls vivid dreams of being chased by somebody. He denies feeling sleepy during the daytime. The most likely diagnosis is:
a. Nightmares
b. Sleep terrors
c. Sleep talking
d. REM sleep behavior disorder
e. Nocturnal seizures

Answers

1. Answer: b.
Dreaming occurs primarily during REM sleep, with the majority occurring during the second half of the night. REM sleep occupies about one-fourth of the night. K complexes and sleep spindles are seen during stage II sleep, delta slowing in stages III and IV of sleep.

2. Answer: c.
Normal sleep latency is more than 10 minutes. Actigraphy indirectly measures sleep-wake activity. CPAP is often tried during PSG for patients with sleep-disordered breathing events. MSLT is valid only after an adequate night's sleep.

3. Answer: a.
HLA-DQB1*0602 is associated with narcolepsy. Recurrent hypersomnia, or Kleine-Levin syndrome, primarily affects teenage boys. Insomnia is diagnosed mainly on the basis of history. Patients with obstructive sleep apnea are unaware of most arousals.

4. Answer: e.
Periodic limb movements involve repetitive toe extension, foot dorsiflexion, and knee and hip flexion. Pavor nocturnus is also known as night terrors. Cataplexy is abrupt loss of skeletal muscle tone. Advanced sleep phase tendency most often affects the elderly, and patients go to bed early and complain of early awakening.

5. Answer: d.
REM sleep behavior disorder represents the absence of skeletal muscle atonia in REM sleep and is associated with synucleinopathies. It is treated with long-acting benzodiazepines such as clonazepam. Cluster headaches arise out of REM sleep.

6. Answer: c.
The other factors listed influence circadian rhythms to a lesser degree.

7. Answer: c.
Akathisia is an urge for constant, whole body movement and is often related to medication use. Sensory neuropathy can occur in various conditions and is not usually relieved by movement. An anxiety disorder typically would not be manifested only in the legs. It usually has other accompaniments such as recurrent thoughts, shortness of breath, and chest pressure. Myoclonus is a brief, repetitive movement involving certain muscle groups.

8. Answer: c.

Low serum level of ferritin is correlated with restless legs syndrome, and correction with iron supplementation can relieve the symptoms.

9. Answer: d.
Dopamine agonists are the first-line treatment for restless legs syndrome.

10. Answer: c.
Excessive daytime sleepiness and cataplexy are typical features of narcolepsy. Complex seizures are not typically provoked by mood changes. Syncopal episodes would result in impairment of consciousness. There are no major psychiatric elements to the history. Idiopathic hypersomnia does not entail cataplexy.

11. Answer: a.
Anticonvulsants have no proven role in treatment of narcolepsy with cataplexy.

12. Answer: b.
Stimulants such as modafinil or methylphenidate are effective for sleepiness. Caffeine would not be as effective, and the other medications listed might increase the degree of sleepiness in this patient.

13. Answer: e.
Hypocretin, also known as orexin, is deficient in the cerebrospinal fluid of most narcoleptics with cataplexy.

14. Answer: c.
The history is consistent with sleep terrors, and management would consist of family education and reassurance. If a question of seizure remained, EEG would be appropriate.

15. Answer: d.
The suprachiasmatic nucleus is a cluster of neurons in the hypothalamus, superior to the optic chiasm. It receives light signals from the retina via the retinohypothalamic tract to control circadian rhythms.

16. Answer: d.
The history is typical for REM sleep behavior disorder: an elderly man with an associated synucleinopathy who acts out his dreams, resulting in injury to himself and his bed partner. Patients with epilepsy do not recall dream details after a seizure, and nightmares, sleep terrors, and sleep talking do not usually result in physical injury.

20

Disorders of the Spinal Cord and Anterior Horn Cells

Nima Mowzoon, M.D.

I. SPINAL CORD ANATOMY

A. Gross Appearance

1. Longitudinal gross anatomy
   a. Spinal cord extends from rostral border of the atlas to caudal border of vertebral body L1
   b. Contains two areas of enlargement: cervical and lumbar (areas that innervate upper and lower extremities, respectively)
   c. Ends as the conus medullaris: level of L1-L2 in adults (reached by age 2), L3 by birth, L4-5 by 20 weeks' gestational age
2. Filum terminale: fine, pial remnant thread extending from end of conus medullaris to the end of the dural sac (internal filum terminale), at which point it pierces the end tail of the dural sac and extends to the first coccygeal segment as the coccygeal ligament (external filum terminale)
3. Segmental transverse gross anatomy
   a. Spinal cord has 31 segments: 8 cervical, 12 thoracic, 5 lumbar, 5 sacral, 1 coccygeal
   b. Ventral and dorsal rootlets exit the cord at each segment on each side, forming ventral and dorsal roots, respectively (which exit the cord ventrolaterally and dorsolaterally, respectively)
   c. Dorsal and ventral roots join to form spinal nerves
   d. Proximal to formation of spinal nerves are dorsal root ganglia in the intervertebral foramina; those ganglia contain cell bodies of dorsal root (sensory) axons
   e. Cervical spinal nerves C1 to C7 exit spinal column at neural foramina *above* corresponding vertebral body: herniation of intervertebral disk between C4 and C5 can affect exiting C5 nerve root
   f. Cervical spinal nerve C8 and all spinal nerves below this level exit spinal column at neural foramina at the corresponding vertebral body
      1) Spinal nerves are located immediately above intervertebral disks

2) Lumbar disk herniations tend to involve nerve roots exiting below the disk (e.g., herniation of L4-L5 intervertebral disk affects L5 nerve root)
3) Exception: extreme lateral disk extrusions involve nerve roots exiting at the level of the disk
   g. Lumbar and sacral spinal roots travel a distance to reach corresponding neural foramina: this bundle of nerve roots is termed the cauda equina
4. Ligaments and supporting structures
   a. Denticulate ligaments
      1) On lateral aspect of each side of spinal cord
      2) Attach pia mater to subarachnoid membrane and dura mater
      3) Separate dorsal and ventral roots
   b. Anterior longitudinal ligament: immediately anterior to vertebral bodies
   c. Posterior longitudinal ligament
      1) Posterior to vertebral bodies
      2) Spans entire length of spinal canal, separating vertebral bodies from the thecal sac
      3) May undergo ossification and thickening, contributing to spinal stenosis
   d. Ligamentum flavum
      1) Connects vertebral lamina and facet joints
      2) May ossify and contribute to spinal stenosis

II. SPINAL CORD PHYSIOLOGY (SEE CHAPTER 2)

III. LOCALIZATION OF SPINAL CORD LESIONS

A. Complete Transaction of Spinal Cord

1. Causes: trauma, tumor, hematoma, abscess, infectious or inflammatory transverse myelitis
2. Absence of reflexes, lower motor neuron paresis, atrophy, and fasciculations at level of the lesion

3. Early period of "spinal shock": early stage of flaccid paralysis, absence of reflexes, autonomic hypoactivity below level of the lesion
4. Spastic paraparesis or quadriparesis (depending on level of the lesion) occurs in the subacute to chronic stage following early "spinal shock" phase (rest of the discussion below refers to this chronic stage)
5. Sensory level: panmodality sensory loss at and below level of the lesion
6. Anhidrosis or hypohidrosis (as seen on thermoregulatory sweat test) and diminished piloerection below level of the lesion; hyperhidrosis above level of the lesion
7. Horner's syndrome if lesion above level of segment T1: interruption of descending sympathetic pathways
8. Preserved phrenic nerve function for lesions below segment C5 (innervation is C3-C5, "C3,4,5 keep the diaphragm alive")
9. Lesions below level of segment T1 spare upper extremities
10. Lesions above midthoracic segment, episodic autonomic dysreflexia: diaphoresis, flushing, hypertension, and reflex bradycardia induced by stimulus (e.g., bladder distention)
11. Lesions above segment T6, loss of superficial abdominal reflexes (deep abdominal reflexes are often increased)
12. Lesions below segment T12 spare upper superficial abdominal reflexes
13. Lesions at level of segment T10, Beevor's sign: intact upper abdominal reflexes and weakened lower abdominal reflexes cause cephalad pulling of umbilicus when patient's head is flexed against resistance by the examiner in attempt to contract the abdominal muscles
14. Lesion at segment L1: weakness of all lower extremity muscles and panmodality sensory loss involving entire lower extremity bilaterally; brisk patellar and Achilles reflexes
15. Lesion at segment L2, absence of cremasteric reflex
16. Lesion at segment L2, L3, or L4, reduced or absent patellar reflexes
17. Lesion at segment S1, absence of Achilles reflex
18. Lesion above sacral segments
    a. Intact reflex emptying of bladder and urinary urgency and urge incontinence
    b. Priapism
    c. Bowel function: increased rectal tone and "anal wink" reflexes, constipation, sexual dysfunction in chronic stage

B. Conus Medullaris Syndrome
1. Early sphincter dysfunction
2. Urinary retention with absence of urinary sensation, loss of voluntary initiation of micturation, urinary retention, and (later) overflow incontinence
3. Pain: uncommon, may be symmetric or vague in distribution
4. Saddle anesthesia: symmetric
5. Variable presence of reflexes

C. Cauda Equina Syndrome
1. Late sphincter dysfunction
2. Pain: common, often asymmetric, may follow dermatomal distribution
3. Exacerbation of pain with lying supine, percussion tenderness over vertebral bodies, paravertebral swelling: suggestive of malignancy or infection
4. Weakness: flaccid, hypotonic, follows multiple myotomal distribution (often asymmetric)
5. Saddle anesthesia: may be asymmetric
6. Reflexes: absence of Achilles reflex, variable presence of patellar reflex (areflexic with extensive lesions)

D. Brown-Séquard Syndrome: hemisyndrome of spinal cord
1. Contralateral loss of pain and temperature sensation: involvement of crossed lateral spinothalamic tract
2. Ipsilateral loss of pain and temperature of a short segment at level of the lesion: involvement of ipsilateral dorsal roots, dorsal horns and/or the spinothalamic tracts (before crossing)
3. Ipsilateral loss of vibration and proprioceptive sensation below level of the lesion: involvement of posterior columns caudal to level of the lesion
4. Ipsilateral pyramidal weakness (spastic weakness): involvement of corticospinal tracts below level of the lesion
5. Ipsilateral lower motor neuron paresis with atrophy, fasciculations: involvement of anterior horn cells at the level of the lesion
6. Differential diagnosis: trauma; extramedullary compression by tumor, hematoma, abscess; intramedullary processes such as vascular insult, syrinx, myelitis due to inflammatory or demyelinating disease, radiation myelopathy

E. Central (intramedullary) Spinal Cord Lesions
1. First sign: involvement of anterior commissure of spinal cord and crossing spinothalamic fibers, resulting in segmental distribution of "dissociated," selective sensory loss of pain and temperature (capelike distribution if it occurs in cervical spinal cord)

2. With expansion, ventral horns are involved, and there may be weakness and atrophy of corresponding myotomes
3. With further expansion, lateral spinothalamic tracts are involved: sacral fibers lie peripherally and are often spared until late in the course of the expansion (sacral sparing)
4. With further expansion, lateral corticospinal tracts may be involved, producing upper motor neuron signs below level of the lesion
5. Involvement of sympathetic pathways in cervical cord can produce Horner's syndrome
6. Posterior columns may be relatively preserved (especially with spinal cord infarction, most of which occurs in the distribution of anterior spinal artery)
7. Differential diagnosis: trauma, demyelination, inflammatory myelitis, intramedullary tumors, syrinx, spinal cord infarction (in the distribution of anterior spinal artery)

IV. HEREDODEGENERATIVE CONDITIONS

A. **Hereditary Spastic Paraparesis** (HSP) (also called spastic paraplegia [SPG])
1. Genetics (Table 20-1)
2. Uncomplicated ("pure"): most common form
   a. Classification of uncomplicated HSP based on inheritance
      1) Autosomal dominant variants (2/3 of cases)
         a) Most common (40% of cases): SPG4 associated with mutation of gene on chromosome 2p22-p21 encoding protein spastin (age at onset varies, may range from 2 to 75 years)
         b) Second most common (9% of cases): SPG3A linked to chromosome 14q11-q21, encoding atlastin
      2) Autosomal recessive variants (1/3 of cases): SPG11 (chromosome 15q13-q15) accounts for half of autosomal recessive cases
      3) X-linked inheritance (rare)
   b. Clinical manifestations
      1) Slowly progressive spastic paraparesis
      2) Spasticity: most common feature, more disabling than weakness, most predominant in legs, symmetric
      3) Weakness: often less prominent than spasticity, often in distal lower extremities
      4) Hyperreflexia (legs > arms), extensor plantar responses common
      5) Hypertonic urinary bladder (urgency progressing into urge incontinence): early bladder disturbance occurs with SPG19

6) Mild vibratory and sometimes joint position sensory loss (usually later in course of the disorder)
7) Skeletal deformities such as pes cavus
8) Cognitive decline described in SPG4
   c. Pathology: axonal wallerian degeneration involving corticospinal tracts, dorsal columns (fasciculus gracilis > cuneatus), and (to a lesser extent) spinocerebellar pathways
3. Complicated
   a. Classification of complicated HSP based on inheritance
      1) Autosomal dominant variants
         a) SPG9 (linked to chromosome 10q23.3-q24.1)
         b) SPG17 (linked to chromosome 11q12-q14): Silver syndrome, characterized by slowly progressive spastic paraparesis with distal amyotrophy of hands and feet and pes cavus
         c) SAX1 (linked to chromosome 12p13)
      2) Autosomal recessive variants
         a) SPG7 (linked to chromosome 16q24.3, gene encoding mitochondrial protein paraplegin): bulbar involvement (dysarthria, dysphagia), optic atrophy, cortical and cerebellar atrophy, and axonal neuropathy
         b) SPG20 (linked to chromosome 13q12.3, gene encoding spartin): Troyer syndrome, characterized by early childhood onset of mild developmental delay (motor and speech), late walking, followed by gradual worsening of learned milestones, pervasive developmental problems, progressive spastic quadriparesis, dysarthria, distal amyotrophy, and choreoathetosis (when advanced)
         c) SPG21 (linked to chromosome 15q, gene encoding maspardin protein, which localizes to intracellular vesicular system): Mast syndrome, characterized by slowly progressive young adult onset of spastic paraparesis (legs > arms), bulbar involvement (dysarthria, dysphagia), cognitive decline, psychiatric symptoms, and late cerebellar and extrapyramidal deficits; early childhood may be marked by delayed motor milestones
      3) X-linked
         a) SPG1 (linked to chromosome Xq28, encoding L1 cell adhesion molecule): characterized by spasticity, ataxia, mental retardation, and adducted thumbs; mutations of this gene can cause hydrocephalus, CRASH syndrome (corpus callosum hypoplasia, retardation, adducted thumbs, spastic paraparesis, hydrocephalus) or MASA syndrome (mental retardation, aphasia, shuffling gait, adducted thumbs)

Table 20-1. **Classification of Hereditary Spastic Paraparesis (HSP)**

Subtype	Locus	Gene product	Unique feature
Autosomal dominant: uncomplicated HSP			
SPG3A	14q11-q21	Atlastin	
SPG4	2p22-p21	Spastin	
SPG6	15q11.1		
SPG8	8q23-q24		
SPG10	12q13	Neuronal kinesin heavy chain	
SPG12	19q13		
SPG13	2q33.1	Heat shock protein	
SPG19	9q33-q34		
Autosomal recessive: uncomplicated HSP			
SPG5A	8p12-q13		
SPG11	15q13-q15		
SPG24	13q14		
Autosomal dominant: complicated HSP			
SPG9	10q23.3-q24.1		
SPG17 (Silver syndrome)	11q12-q14		Distal amyotrophy
Autosomal recessive: complicated HSP			
SPG7	16q24.3	Paraplegin	Bulbar involvement, optic atrophy, axonal neuropathy, cortical and cerebellar atrophy
SPG14	3q27-q28		
SPG15	14q22-q24		
SPG20 (Troyer syndrome)	13q12.3	Spartin	Distal amyotrophy, developmental delay, dysarthria
SPG21 (Mast syndrome)	15q21-q22	Maspardin	Bulbar involvement, cognitive decline, late cerebellar and extrapyramidal features
X-linked: complicated HSP			
SPG1	Xq28 (L1CAM)	Neuronal cell adhesion molecule L1	Ataxia, mental retardation, adducted thumbs
SPG2	Xq22 (PLP1)	Myelin proteolipid protein	Congenital nystagmus (allelic with Pelizaeus-Merzbacher disease)
SPG16	Xq11.2-q23		

SPG, spastic paraplegia.

b) SPG2 (caused by point mutation of gene on chromosome Xq22 encoding myelin proteolipid protein, allelic with Pelizaeus-Merzbacher disease): characterized by progressive paraparesis, congenital nystagmus, optic atrophy, sensory loss, delayed motor milestones, and white matter changes on magnetic resonance imaging (MRI)

b. Clinical manifestations: features of uncomplicated HSP plus optic neuropathy, retinopathy, deafness, cerebellar features, ichthyosis, amyotrophy, peripheral neuropathy, cognitive deficits, seizures, autoimmune hemolytic anemia,

thrombocytopenia (Evans syndrome), extrapyramidal dysfunction, and bladder dysfunction

4. Diagnosis: exclusion of mimicking disorders and positive family history

5. Treatment: symptomatic treatment

B. Hereditary Sensory Neuropathy With Spastic Paraparesis (Cavanagh's variant)

1. Predominantly small-fiber neuropathy

2. Spasticity

3. Mutilating acropathy of lower limbs

C. Adrenomyeloneuropathy

1. Variant of adrenoleukodystrophy
2. Inheritance: X-linked recessive (linked to chromosome Xq28)
3. Clinical phenotype milder than adrenoleukodystrophy (which afflicts young boys presenting with severely progressive cognitive and psychomotor deterioration, progressive visual loss, and adrenal insufficiency)
4. Typical presentation: slowly progressive spastic paraparesis and mild peripheral neuropathy in adult men
5. Hypogonadism: mild
6. Female carriers may be asymptomatic or develop late-onset myelopathy (may present as late as fifth decade)
7. Spasticity (spastic paraparesis) predominantly affects lower limbs
8. Sensory loss involving all modalities, including proprioceptive loss
9. Abnormalities of sphincter control
10. Pathophysiology related to increased saturated, unbranched very long-chain (>24 carbon) fatty acids (VLCFAs)
11. Diagnostic evaluation
    a. Electrodiagnostic evaluation: predominantly axonal neuropathy on electromyography (EMG) and nerve conduction studies, and abnormal brainstem auditory and somatosensory evoked potentials
    b. Increased plasma VLCFAs, confirmed by assays of VLCFA concentrations in cultured skin fibroblasts
12. Treatment: symptomatic treatment of spasticity, physical therapy, and steroid replacement for adrenal insufficiency

D. Sporadic Primary Lateral Sclerosis (PLS): adult-onset

1. Clinical presentation
    a. Slowly progressive, often symmetric, spastic paraparesis (legs before arms), may progress to involve upper limbs and cranial nerves
    b. Patients eventually develop pseudobulbar palsy (there may be some asymmetry of deficits, especially early)
    c. Important features: spasticity, hyperreflexia, extensor plantar responses, upper motor neuron pattern of weakness
    d. Patients may also have cramps, fasciculations, and (less commonly) urinary urgency
    e. No sensory loss, but somatosensory evoked potentials are not always normal
    f. By definition, no lower motor neuron signs (it is debatable whether this is a subtype of amyotrophic lateral sclerosis [ALS], and some patients with ALS have prominent

upper motor neuron signs reminiscent of PLS and later develop lower motor neuron syndrome)
    g. Progression: often quite slow, may last up to 3 decades
2. Pathology
    a. Spinal cord: rarefaction and atrophy of corticospinal tracts, with neuronal loss and gliosis (Fig. 20-1)
    b. Degenerative changes also involve precentral gyrus (Betz cells in layer V) and possibly prefrontal gyrus (sensory cortex may be involved in some cases)
    c. Anterior horn cells are spared
3. Diagnosis of exclusion: must rule out other mimicking disorders with similar presentation; cortical motor evoked potentials often demonstrate absent or prolonged latencies
4. Treatment: primarily symptomatic treatment (e.g., antispastic agents such as baclofen)

E. Progressive Muscular Atrophy (PMA)

1. Pure lower motor neuron syndrome: progressive weakness and atrophy involving upper and lower limbs and bulbar and respiratory muscles
2. Most cases evolve into ALS (eventually develop upper motor neuron manifestations): diagnosis of PMA should not be made until 3 years after onset of symptoms

F. Familial Childhood Primary Lateral Sclerosis

1. Autosomal recessive (linked to chromosome 2q33, encoding alsin protein): deletion in exon 3 or 4 causes ALS phenotype (ALS2, discussed below), whereas deletions in exons 9 and 5 cause PLS phenotype
2. Characterized by childhood onset of spastic paraparesis, bulbar involvement, and gaze paresis

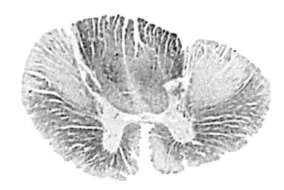

Fig. 20-1. Gross postmortem specimen from patient with primary lateral sclerosis (PLS) showing the characteristic rarefaction of the lateral and anterior corticospinal tracts because of neuronal loss.

G. Sporadic Amyotrophic Lateral Sclerosis
1. Progressive neurodegenerative disorder of motor systems
2. Prevalence: 4.09/100,000 population
3. Mean age at onset of sporadic ALS: about 56 years (mean age at onset of familial ALS, 46 years)
4. Mean duration of disease in sporadic ALS: about 3 years
5. Sporadic ALS most frequently afflicts men, with M:F=3:2 (unlike familial forms)
6. Familial in 10% of cases (discussed below)
7. Pathogenesis
   a. Excitotoxicity (induced by glutamate)
      1) Glutamate: major excitotoxic neurotransmitter
      2) Reduced sodium-dependent glutamate reuptake and increased glutamate-induced excitotoxicity (AMPA/kainate receptor) → increased permeability to calcium and increased intracellular calcium
      3) Reduced expression of excitatory amino acid transporter type 2 (EAAT2)
   b. Oxidative stress
      1) Highly reactive free radicals can injure cells through oxidation or peroxidation of proteins, lipids, and nucleic acids
      2) Superoxide radicals produced as by-products of oxidative phosphorylation
      3) *SOD1* mutations cause a toxic gain of function, enhance free radical formation as well as abnormal copper metabolism, and catalysis of tyrosine residue nitration by peroxynitrite
   c. Mitochondrial dysfunction: possibly provokes oxidative stress and mediates neuronal injury by excitotoxic and apoptotic pathways
   d. Neurofilament dysfunction and aggregation
      1) Axonal spheroidal inclusions containing aggregates of ubiquinated filaments and abnormal phosphorylated neurofilament proteins present in anterior horn cells because of oxidative stress-induced neurofilament injury
      2) Phosphorylation of neurofilaments alters their function and induces their aggregation as spheroidal inclusions
      3) Alterations in axonal transport
         a) Increased fast axonal transport
         b) Decreased retrograde slow transport
   e. Alteration in intracellular calcium levels: the common final pathway of most of the proposed mechanisms of injury
      1) Inability to handle increased intracellular calcium levels by poor expression of calcium-binding proteins parvalbumin and calbindin-D28k likely also has

important role in the pathogenesis of ALS and contributes to selective vulnerability of motor neurons in ALS
      2) Relative resistance to degeneration of subset of motor neurons (i.e., extraocular motor neurons and Onuf's nuclei) until late in disease is likely due to high expression of calbindin-D28k or parvalbumin (or both) in these motor neurons
8. Pathology (Fig. 20-2)
   a. Neuronal loss of anterior horn cells and rarefaction of ventral horns (sparing of sacral anterior horn cells in nuclei of Onuf)
   b. Bunina bodies: dense cytoplasmic granular inclusions best observed with electron microscopy to contain amorphous granular material accompanied by vesicular structures and neurofilaments
   c. Spheroids: axonal aggregations of neurofilaments
9. Clinical presentation
   a. Early symptoms of limb-onset presentation: muscle cramps, fasciculations, weight loss, fatigue
   b. Patients may present with monomelic weakness (involving multiple peripheral nerve distribution in one limb), with spread to contiguous limbs and anatomic segments
   c. Limb weakness: initial manifestations usually distal; occasionally patients may present with predominantly proximal, symmetric upper or lower limb weakness
   d. Upper limb weakness: difficulty with grip, holding or turning keys, opening bottle tops, buttoning clothes
   e. Lower limb weakness: footdrop (most common), gait instability, effort-dependent fatigue, and leg weakness with walking
   f. Bulbar involvement: dysarthria (often mixed spastic and flaccid); brisk jaw jerk; atrophied, fasciculating, weak, and spastic tongue; sialorrhea; dysphagia

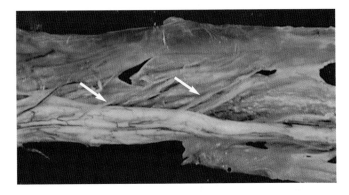

Fig. 20-2. Atrophic anterior nerve roots (*arrows*) in amyotrophic lateral sclerosis.

g. Respiratory involvement with diaphragmatic weakness presenting with dyspnea (on exertion initially, then at rest with progression)

h. Weight loss: rapidly progressive (cachexia, likely more than what can be attributed to poor caloric intake)

i. Other symptoms (indicative of upper motor neuron involvement): forced yawning, labile emotional affect

j. Some patients may have cognitive impairment in pattern consistent with frontotemporal dementia (up to 1/3 of patients, according to recent data)

k. Relative sparing of bowel and bladder function, extraocular muscles, and sensory systems

l. Examination findings
   1) Lower motor neuron signs: fasciculations (eventually develop in all patients), atrophy, weakness
   2) Upper motor neuron signs: spasticity and hyper-reflexia, including exaggerated Hoffmann sign, pathologic jaw jerk, pathologic gag reflex, extensor plantar responses (usually develop later in disease course)
   3) Hyperreflexia and spasticity of amyotrophic limb: suggestive of ALS

m. World Federation of Neurology (WFN) diagnostic criteria
   1) Clinical and electrodiagnostic evidence for upper and lower motor neuron loss (with evidence of spread within a segment or to other segments of central nervous system)
   2) Evidence of subclinical lower motor neuron involvement may be provided by electrodiagnostic studies
   3) Four segments of neuroaxis may be involved: bulbar, cervical, thoracic, and lumbosacral
   4) Definite ALS: upper and lower motor neuron clinical signs in bulbar plus two spinal segments *or* in three spinal segments
   5) Probable ALS: upper and lower motor neuron signs in at least two segments, with some upper motor neuron signs rostral to lower motor neuron signs
   6) Probable laboratory-supported ALS: upper and lower motor neuron signs in one segment *or* upper motor neuron signs in one segment and lower motor neuron signs by electrophysiologic criteria in at least two limbs
   7) Clinically possible ALS: upper and lower motor neuron clinical signs in one segment *or* upper motor neuron clinical signs in two or more regions *or* lower motor neuron clinical signs rostral to upper motor neuron clinical signs

10. Electrodiagnostic findings
    a. Performed to confirm lower motor neuron dysfunction in clinically involved segments, to detect lower motor neuron abnormalities in clinically uninvolved segments, and to exclude other diagnoses

    b. Sensory conduction studies
       1) Expected to be normal
       2) Any detected abnormality should be incidental
       3) If pronounced abnormalities, an underlying sensory axonopathy or neuronopathy may be present and diagnoses other than ALS are entertained (e.g., polyradiculoneuropathy or Kennedy's syndrome)

    c. Motor conduction studies
       1) Normal or mildly reduced (CMAP) amplitudes in early stages, with normal distal latencies and conduction velocities
       2) With ongoing uncompensated denervation and disease progression, CMAP amplitudes steadily decrease, and conduction velocities may slow down as the rapidly conducting myelinated fibers are involved
       3) Absence of conduction block (caution: phase cancellation and mild slowing of the conduction velocities may resemble partial conduction block)
       4) Reduced F wave response frequency and repeated F wave responses (due to decreased number of anterior horn cells)

    d. Repetitive stimulation
       1) May be mild decrement (often <10%)
       2) Due to impaired neuromuscular transmission between immature nerve terminals of the sprouting axonal collaterals and newly reinnervated muscle fibers
       3) Greater decrement in rapidly progressive disease

    e. Single fiber EMG: increased jitter, blocking, and increased fiber density

    f. Motor unit number estimate (MUNE)
       1) Quantitative estimate of number of functioning motor units
       2) Quantitative follow-up of progression
       3) Reduced in ALS

    g. Needle examination
       1) Signs of active denervation (fibrillation potentials, positive sharp waves, fasciculation potentials): may be limited and sparse early in disease course due to active, compensatory reinnervation
       2) Signs of chronic denervation and reinnervation: large-amplitude, long-duration motor unit potentials with reduced recruitment
       3) Increased polyphasia and instability of motor unit potentials indicate active reinnervation: impaired neuromuscular transmission of new collateral axons and slowed conduction of immature (yet unmyelinated) axon terminals are responsible for instability of motor unit potentials

4) Early in disease course: evidence of chronic, compensated reinnervation with motor unit potential remodeling and usually little uncompensated active denervation

5) With disease progression: changes of active denervation (fibrillation potentials) become more prominent, while there is ongoing, active (and uncompensated) reinnervation, latter evidenced by abundance of varying, polyphasic motor unit potentials

6) Greater occurrence of variability of motor unit potentials in rapidly progressive disease

7) Low-amplitude (sometimes short-duration) polyphasic motor unit potentials may be seen in inadequate collateral reinnervation: usually associated with rapidly progressive course; may indicate a worse prognosis when abundant

8) In most severely affected muscles, changes could be limited to severely reduced recruitment of short-duration, small-amplitude motor unit potentials: "nascent unit" potentials, indicative of early distal-to-proximal reinnervation after severe denervation axonopathy

11. Other ancillary testing
  a. Mild to moderate elevation in creatine kinase level
  b. Neuroimaging of brain and spinal cord to exclude mimicking disorders of neuraxis
  c. Anti-ganglioside autoantibodies, acetylcholine receptor antibodies, genetic testing for Kennedy's syndrome may need to be done in select situations
  d. Muscle biopsy may be needed to exclude underlying muscle disease

H. Inherited Amyotrophic Lateral Sclerosis

1. Most familial variants exhibit autosomal dominant inheritance
2. Most common of these (up to 20% of familial cases) is due to mutation of superoxide dismutase 1 (*SOD1*) gene (ALS1)
3. Often presents with weakness, atrophy, and absence of reflexes in a single limb
4. Autosomal dominant familial ALS
  a. Clinically indistinguishable from sporadic ALS
  b. More severe phenotype in homozygotes than heterozygotes
  c. ALS1: due to mutation of the *SOD1* gene on chromosome 21q22.1
    1) Most common form of familial ALS (up to 20% of familial cases)
    2) More than 100 different mutations have been identified (most are autosomal dominant inheritance, rare cases of autosomal recessive inheritance)
    3) Most common mutations: A4V (exon 1) and D90A (exon 4)

4) Up to 3% of cases of sporadic ALS have mutations in *SOD1* gene
5) SOD1 protein: cytoplasmic protein acts to detoxify oxygen radicals and prevent oxidative damage
6) *SOD1* mutation: reduced dismutase activity and toxic gain-of-function (enhanced free radical formation, abnormal copper metabolism, and catalysis of tyrosine residue nitration by peroxynitrite)
7) Mean age at onset: 46 years
8) Clinical presentation and progression closely resemble sporadic ALS

5. Autosomal recessive familial ALS: three main phenotypes
  a. Type I (designated ALS5)
    1) Linked to chromosome 15q15-q22
    2) Found in North African and European populations
    3) Age at onset: usually in second decade
    4) Predominant lower motor neuron signs
    5) Early hand involvement (sometimes for years)
    6) Pattern of weakness: distal more than proximal, arms more than legs
    7) Late bulbar involvement, absence of pseudobulbar affect as with ALS2 (discussed below)
  b. Type II
    1) Age at onset: first or second decade
    2) Involvement confined to lower limbs: usually presents with footdrop
    3) Spastic paraplegia and lower extremity amyotrophy
    4) Bulbar sparing
  c. Type III (designated ALS2)
    1) Mean age at onset: 6.5 years (up to third decade)
    2) Linked to chromosome 2q33
    3) Early onset of spastic paraplegia (presentation of juvenile primary lateral sclerosis)
    4) Mild, very slowly progressive, then amyotrophy develops: predominantly distal (legs > arms)
    5) Pseudobulbar affect
6. X-linked familial ALS
  a. Linked to chromosome Xp11-q12
  b. Rare

I. Spinal Muscular Atrophy (SMA)

1. Overview
  a. Clinically heterogenous group of disorders characterized by muscle weakness and atrophy without sensory loss or upper motor neuron findings (pure lower motor neuron syndrome) (Fig. 20-3)
  b. Pathologically due to degeneration of motor neurons (anterior horn cells) in spinal cord and brainstem
  c. Most common forms of SMA present in childhood with

symmetric proximal (more than distal) limb weakness and atrophy; show autosomal recessive inheritance

2. Genetics

a. Autosomal recessive inheritance in most cases of SMA types I to III, linked to chromosome 5 (autosomal dominant or X-linked transmission is exceedingly rare exception)

b. Autosomal recessive inheritance in 70% of adult-onset SMA (type IV), linked to chromosome 5

c. Autosomal dominant inheritance in 30% of adult-onset SMA (type IV), not linked to chromosome 5 (genetically heterogeneous)

d. Homozygous deletions of *SMN1* (telomeric survival motor neuron 1) gene are responsible for 95% to 98% of childhood SMA (rarely found in adult-onset SMA): small mutations in *SMN1* gene have been identified in other 5% of SMA patients

e. Homozygous mutations of *SMN2* (centromeric survival motor neuron 2) gene more commonly identified in adult-onset SMA

1) SMN protein is involved in messanger (m)RNA splicing

2) Motor neurons have high rate of RNA metabolism

3) Dramatic difference in phenotypic severity between SMA type I to III suggests involvement of additional genes: candidate genes include *SMN2* and *NAIP* (neuronal apoptosis inhibitory protein gene)

   a) *SMN2* is homologous to *SMN1* and is an inefficient producer of SMN protein

   b) Up to four copies of *SMN2* on each chromosome

   c) SMN protein levels determine phenotypic severity

   d) Higher number of *SMN2* copies would yield higher load of SMN protein and less severe phenotype: *SMN2* gene is modifier of disease severity in SMA

   e) Loss of *SMN2* gene occurs in 5% of normal, asymptomatic population

   f) *NAIP* is deleted in approximately 80% of patients with SMA type I, but in very few patients with SMA type II or III (more common in patients with SMA type I)

3. Electrodiagnosis

a. Reduced amplitude CMAP; normal sensory nerve action potentials

b. Needle EMG

1) Spontaneous activity: fibrillation potentials and positive waves in all subtypes

2) Voluntary activity: long-duration, large-amplitude motor unit potentials (especially with SMA types III and IV)

4. SMA type I (Werdnig-Hoffmann disease)

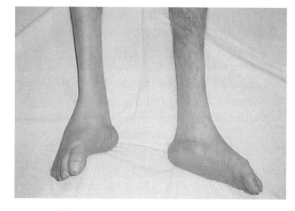

Fig. 20-3. Diffuse, severe atrophy of the lower extremities in a patient with spinal muscular atrophy.

a. Autosomal recessive inheritance

b. Presents at birth or shortly thereafter (up to 6 months of age) with hypotonia

1) In utero: mothers may experience decreased fetal movement

c. Bulbar involvement: weak cry, poor feeding, tongue atrophy and fasciculations (extraocular movements are spared)

d. Loss of cough reflex and inaudible cry with progression

e. Absence of head control ("floppy infant")

f. Severe diffuse, symmetric weakness (worse proximally); patients often in "frog-leg" position (externally rotated and abducted legs and flexed knees); patient never sits independently

g. Diffusely areflexic

h. Contractures are rare in early stages, but usually develop with advanced disease (often at knees, rarely at elbows)

i. Reduced anteroposterior diameter of thorax, pectus excavatum

j. Respiratory insufficiency due to weakness of intercostal muscles (preserved diaphragmatic function until late in disease course), causing paradoxical respirations

k. Normal intellect

l. Rapid progression; death usually before age 2 years

m. Serum creatine kinase: typically, normal levels

5. SMA type II (arrested Werdnig-Hoffmann disease, juvenile SMA)

a. Autosomal recessive inheritance

b. Most common pattern, accounting for approximately 45% of SMA cases

c. Age at onset, speed of progression, and prognosis are intermediate between SMA types I and III

d. Age at onset: before 18 months, with gradual progressive weakness and delayed motor milestone; patients never stand

e. Patients able to sit with support if positioned and eventually sit unsupported, but never stand

f. "Tremor" of hands: minipolymyoclonus (and fasciculations)

g. With progression, often contractures of knees and hips, scoliosis, and other orthopedic complications

h. Death usually after age 2 (7 months-7 years, some as late as the third or fourth decade)

i. Serum creatine kinase: typically, normal levels

6. SMA type III (Wohlfart-Kugelberg-Welander syndrome)

a. Autosomal recessive inheritance (most cases)

b. Patients normal at birth

c. Presents after 18 months of age (usually 5-15 years), usually in late childhood or adolescence

d. Many patients are able initially to achieve normal motor milestones, able to stand and walk unassisted, but later deteriorate and are usually wheelchair-bound

e. Symptoms at presentation: progressive proximal weakness and atrophy; waddling gait and exaggerated lumbar lordosis

f. With progression, patients often use Gower's maneuver to arise from supine position

g. Fasciculations and tremors are more common than in SMA type I or II

h. Deep tendon reflexes may be uniformly absent or reduced

i. *If onset before age 2*: stop walking by age 15, greater predisposition for orthopedic complications such as scoliosis, worse prognosis

j. *If onset after age 2*: better prognosis, likely ambulate into fifth decade, fewer orthopedic complications

k. Serum creatine kinase: elevated levels, up to 10 times normal (normal in SMA types I and II)

l. Normal or slightly reduced life expectancy

7. Adult-onset SMA (SMA type IV)

a. Mostly autosomal dominant or autosomal recessive inheritance

b. Adult onset: age at onset is older than 20

c. Very slow progression over decades

d. Normal life expectancy

e. Usually does not involve respiratory or bulbar muscles (unlike Kennedy's syndrome)

8. Distal hereditary motor neuronopathy

a. Group (types 1-7) of rare disorders with distal lower and upper limb weakness

b. Not formally part of SMA classification but clearly related to these disorders because of pure involvement of lower motor neurons

c. Age at onset and mode of inheritance vary

d. Previously known as the spinal form of Charcot-Marie-Tooth disease because of very similar clinical picture of slowly progressive distal atrophy and weakness: distinguishable from Charcot-Marie-Tooth disease by
1) Normal sensory examination
2) Normal sensory action potential amplitudes on nerve conduction studies
3) Axonal motor conduction studies (conduction velocity normal or reduced in proportion to amplitude loss)

9. Fazio-Londe disease

a. May be sporadic; otherwise, autosomal dominant or autosomal recessive inheritance

b. Normal at birth

c. Age at onset: 1 to 12 years

d. Motor neuron disease predominantly limited to lower cranial nerves (progressive bulbar palsy), may also include ptosis and facial weakness

e. Progression variable

10. Brown-Vialetto-van Laere syndrome

a. Progressive bulbar palsy with deafness

b. Normal early development

c. Age at onset: usually in second decade

d. Weakness is primarily bulbar (tongue atrophy and fasciculations, dysphagia) and facial

e. Bilateral sensorineural hearing loss

11. Juvenile monomelic amyotrophy

a. Also called Hirayama's disease

b. Age at onset: late teens or early twenties

c. Predilection for Asian men

d. Presenation: gradual onset and progression of painless weakness and atrophy

e. Predominantly affects muscles innervated by C7-T1 nerve roots: proximal more than distal, typically unilateral (may be bilateral)

f. Deep tendon reflexes: reduced or absent

g. Progression of weakness continues for 2 to 3 years, may stabilize within 5 years after onset

h. Progression may continue for decades (referred to as O'Sullivan-McLeod syndrome)

i. Pathophysiology may be related to mechanical distortion of cervical spinal cord and focal compression of dura mater and spinal cord against vertebrae during neck flexion

12. Hexosaminidase A deficiency

a. Autosomal recessive inheritance: mutation of *HEXA* gene on chromosome 15q23-q24, encoding protein hexosaminidase A, responsible for degrading ganglioside G_{M2}

b. Clinical phenotypes
1) Infantile hexosaminidase A deficiency (Tay-Sachs disease [TSD])

a) Complete deficiency of enzyme activity

b) Infants normal at birth

c) By 3 to 6 months of age: mild motor weakness, exaggerated startle response, myoclonus

d) By 6 to 8 months of age: developmental arrest and regression, no new motor skill is learned and the child begins to lose some acquired motor skills
    i) Reduced visual attentiveness
    ii) Cherry-red spot

e) By 8 to 10 months of age: rapid deterioration, diminution in myoclonus and spontaneous movements, deterioration in vision (cherry-red spot)

2) Juvenile hexosaminidase A deficiency

a) Heterozygotes with varying degrees of residual enzymatic activity

b) Normal early motor milestones

c) By 2 to 10 years of age: incoordination and ataxia become apparent

d) Developmental regression: cognitive decline

e) Spasticity and seizures by end of first decade

f) By 15 years of age: decerebrate rigidity, persistent vegetative state

g) Deterioration in vision: much later than the infantile form (TSD); optic atrophy and retinitis pigmentosa may be observed late in disease course

3) Chronic, adult-onset hexosaminidase A deficiency

a) Late-onset G_{M2} gangliosidosis

b) Slowly progressive symmetric proximal weakness, atrophy, fasciculations, dysarthria

c) Cerebellar ataxia

d) Some have extrapyramidal signs of dystonia, choreoathetosis

e) Some have psychiatric manifestations (without dementia), including recurrent depression, manic depression, depression with psychotic features, acute psychosis

f) Sensory neuropathy with abnormal sensory-nerve action potentials

c. Diagnosis: absent to near-absent serum hexosaminidase A enzymatic activity (or in white blood cells) in symptomatic person, in presence of normal or elevated activity of the β-hexosaminidase B isoenzyme

13. Kennedy's syndrome or X-linked spinobulbar muscular atrophy

a. Genetics

1) X-linked recessive

2) CAG trinucleotide repeat expansion in the androgen receptor gene (*AR*) on chromosome Xq11-q12

3) Longer lengths of CAG repeats: correlate with earlier age at onset

4) Genetic anticipation: larger expansion in CAG repeat number, especially with paternal transmission

b. Clinical features

1) Insidious, slowly progressive atrophy and weakness of limb and bulbar muscles beginning in the 3rd to 5th decades

2) Proximal hip and shoulder-girdle weakness: most individuals have difficulty walking up the stairs after 1 to 2 decades of symptoms

3) 1/3 of patients require a wheelchair 20 years after the onset of symptoms

4) Muscle cramps and fasciculations may precede the onset of definite weakness and wasting: characteristic facial (especially perioral) fasciculations

5) Other features: muscle atrophy, absence of reflexes

6) Tongue muscle atrophy and fasciculations

7) Dysarthria and dysphagia may occur

8) Unlike the other inherited motor neuronopathies, a mild sensory neuronopathy may also be present, related to degeneration of dorsal root ganglia: abnormal sensory potential amplitudes on nerve conduction studies do not exclude this diagnosis

9) Signs of mild androgen insensitivity

10) Gynecomastia

11) Testicular atrophy

12) Reduced fertility

13) Unlike some of the other androgen receptor mutations, sexual differentiation and development of secondary sexual characteristics are normal

c. Treatment

1) Androgen therapy is not beneficial and may be harmful: exogenous androgen therapy causes translocation of the mutant receptor-ligand complex from the cytoplasm to the nucleus where the CAG encoded polyglutamine expanded protein is more toxic

2) The role of antiandrogen treatments in Kennedy's syndrome is being evaluated

V. INTRAMEDULLARY COMPRESSIVE MYELOPATHIES

A. Neoplasms (see Chapter 16)

B. Multiple Sclerosis (see Chapter 14)

C. Syringomyelia

1. Fluid-filled cavity in spinal cord

2. May be primary, spontaneous, or secondary (latter usually posttraumatic or associated with spinal cord

intramedullary or extramedullary tumors)
3. Associated with Chiari I or II malformation
4. There may or may not be associated foramen magnum obstruction
5. Two subgroups
   a. Communicating syringomyelia
      1) Caused by primary dilatation of central canal
      2) Often associated with abnormalities of foramen magnum such as Chiari I malformations
      3) Also called hydromyelia
      4) Pure central localization
   b. Noncommunicating syringomyelia
      1) Intramedullary cyst not communicating with central canal or subarachnoid space
      2) Often due to trauma, tumor, or arachnoiditis
      3) Pure paracentral localization
6. Localization of syrinx is variable
   a. Pure central
   b. Pure paracentral
   c. Central and paracentral
7. Clinical presentation
   a. Variable depending on location and level of lesion in spinal cord
   b. Typical presentation of expanding central syrinx often starts with capelike distribution of dissociated sensory loss (preferential involvement of pain and temperature rather than vibratory or joint position sensation because of early, segmental involvement of crossing spinothalamic tracts)
   c. With further expansion of syrinx, anterior horn cells tend to be involved (causing axial and appendicular weakness and atrophy)
   d. With further expansion of syrinx, intermediolateral columns containing sympathetic pathways are involved and produce Horner's syndrome
   e. With further expansion of syrinx, corticospinal tracts and posterior columns are involved
   f. Various brainstem symptoms when associated with Chiari II malformation
   g. Asymmetric hand weakness or gait disturbance are common symptoms when associated with Chiari I malformation
   h. Extension of syrinx into brainstem is called syringobulbia
8. Diagnosis: requires neuroimaging (Fig. 20-4)
   a. MRI: most sensitive imaging
   b. Identify the syrinx, localization, and extent
   c. Provide means for radiographic follow-up
   d. Identify cause and underlying condition, particularly associated neoplasm (gadolinium must be administered)
   e. Identify associated conditions (e.g., Chiari malformations)

9. Treatment
   a. Percutaneous aspiration of syrinx, terminal ventriculostomy, shunting
   b. Posterior fossa decompression for treatment of posterior fossa abnormalities
   c. Resection of underlying causative tumor

VI. EXTRAMEDULLARY COMPRESSIVE MYELOPATHIES

A. Cause
1. May be due to combination of spondylosis, spondylolisthesis, facet joint arthropathy, ligamentum flava hypertrophy, congenital narrowing of spinal canal, degenerative osteophytosis, and vertebral disk bulging and disk herniation (extrusion)

B. Area Involved: usually lower cervical or lower lumbar segments

C. Cervical Spinal Stenosis and Myelopathy
1. Spasticity, hyperreflexia distal to level of myelopathy
2. Reduced or absent deep tendon reflexes, atrophy, and lower motor neuron pattern of weakness at level of stenosis
3. Variable degrees of sensory symptoms and possibly poorly localizing pain (central origin), but neck pain usually not prominent
4. Lhermitte's sign may be present
5. Sphincter dysfunction may occur, usually after onset of any sensory or motor (or both) symptoms
6. Clinical course may remain stable or may progress in variable fashion

D. Lumbar Spinal Stenosis: may have variable presentation
1. Asymptomatic
2. Insidious onset of neurogenic claudication: intermittent leg discomfort (pain with or without paresthesias) produced by walking or standing straight for prolonged period
3. Slow relief with rest (almost immediate relief with vascular claudication): leaning forward or sitting is required, symptoms are not relieved with rest in standing position
4. Symptoms often relieved by leaning forward (as in riding a bicycle or leaning against a grocery cart, unlike vascular claudication)
5. Variable degrees of exercise or walking distance produces

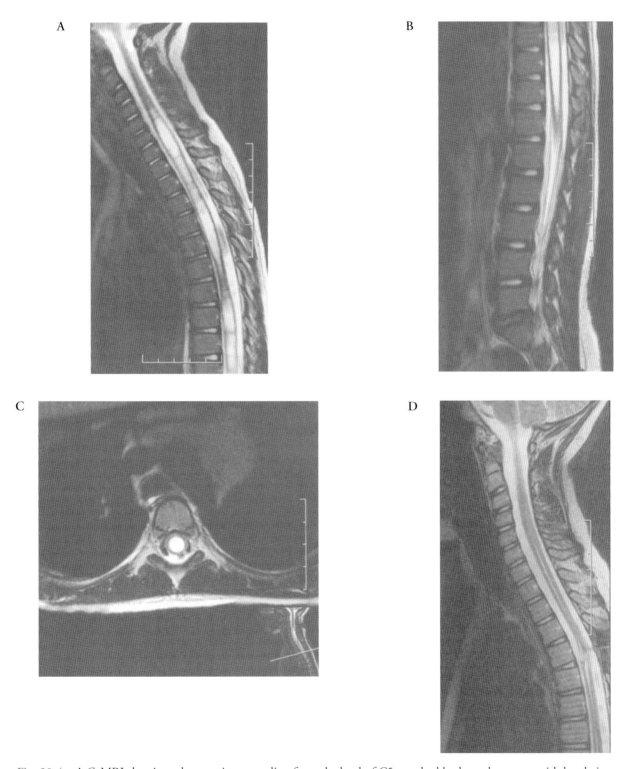

Fig. 20-4. *A-C*, MRI showing a large syrinx extending from the level of C5 vertebral body to the conus, with loculation within the upper thoracic and lower cervical syrinx. *D*, A follow-up scan after treatment with a syringopleural shunt at the level of T4 vertebral body shows marked reduction of the syrnix. Sagittal T2 (*A*, *B*, and *D*) and axial T2 (*C*) sequences.

symptoms (as opposed to vascular claudication in which fixed degree of exercise or walking distance induces symptoms)

6. Persistent, progressive back and leg pain and chronic cauda equina syndrome, often asymmetric distribution

7. May be associated with radicular symptoms

E. Epidural Lipomatosis

1. Due to nonneoplastic hypertrophy of extramedullary adipose tissue in spinal epidural space (Fig. 20-5)

2. Usually occurs at thoracic or lumbosacral segments

3. Causes
   a. Most cases associated with chronic corticosteroid use
   b. Others: Cushing's disease, Cushing's syndrome, pituitary prolactinoma, hypothyroidism, and (rarely) obesity
   c. May be idiopathic

4. Most frequently reported symptom is back pain, followed by lower limb weakness, and (rarely) sphinter dysfunction

5. Regression of compressive tissue when corticosteroids are withdrawn

6. Treatment: symptomatic measures, withdrawal of corticosteroids if possible, decompressive laminectomy with resection of epidural adipose tissue

F. Epidural Abscess

1. May develop rapidly (evolving over several days) or gradually (over several weeks)

2. Fever, back pain, local spine tenderness, and radicular pain are usually first manifestations

3. Patients may present with shock, sepsis, encephalopathy: focal spine tenderness and back pain may not be apparent

4. Weakness may evolve rapidly into paraparesis or quadriparesis

5. More than half of acute abscesses are *Staphylococcus aureus*

6. Infection in epidural space may be result of
   a. Direct extension of infection in contiguous structures (e.g., vertebral osteomyelitis, soft tissue infection, decubitus ulcer): brittle diabetes mellitus, intravenous drug abuse, and chronic alcoholism are risk factors for osteomyelitis and diskitis that may extend to epidural space
   b. Hematogenous spread from distant source (intravenous drug abuse is risk factor)
   c. Direct penetrating trauma to the back

7. Cerebrospinal fluid (CSF) examination is contraindicated: sudden shifts in CSF pressure may cause herniation of spinal cord, and passing the needle through the abscess may spread the infection to subarachnoid space

8. Diagnosis usually made with MRI

9. Treatment relies on immediate initiation of antibiotics, with or without surgical debridement or spinal decompression (or both)

G. Epidural Hematoma

1. Abrupt onset of extramedullary spinal cord compression

2. May present with sharp pain in chest or upper back

3. Should be suspected in patients receiving anticoagulation

VII. NONCOMPRESSIVE DISORDERS OF SPINAL CORD

A. Radiation-Induced Myelopathy: transient radiation myelopathy

1. Self-limiting

2. Occurs within first year after radiation

3. Usually presents with paresthesias and Lhermitte's sign

4. May be caused by transient demyelination or drop out of oligodendrocytes (or both)

B. Vascular Disease of Spinal Cord: spinal cord ischemic syndromes and vascular malformations are discussed in Chapter 11

C. Infectious Disorders of Spinal Cord

1. Tropical spastic paraparesis: human T-cell leukemia virus type 1 (HTLV-I)–associated myelopathy
   a. Transmission: vertical (mother to child), sexual, parenteral
   b. Most infected persons are asymptomatic and never develop myelopathy; only 1 in 250 develop myelopathy
   c. Age at onset: usually after 30 years (depends on mode of transmission)
   d. Chronic, slowly progressive myelopathy, primarily at thoracic segments: spastic paraparesis of lower limbs and spastic bladder
   e. Cerebellar ataxia may complicate the gait disorder
   f. May be associated with demyelinating polyneuropathy
   g. Slower progression in younger patients
   h. Intravenous drug abusers at a greater risk for acquiring infection with HTLV-I
   i. Pathology
      1) Predominantly involves middle and lower thoracic cord, extending to involve entire spinal cord
      2) Neuronal cell loss and gliosis, with microvacuolization
      3) Demyelination often accompanies long tract axonal

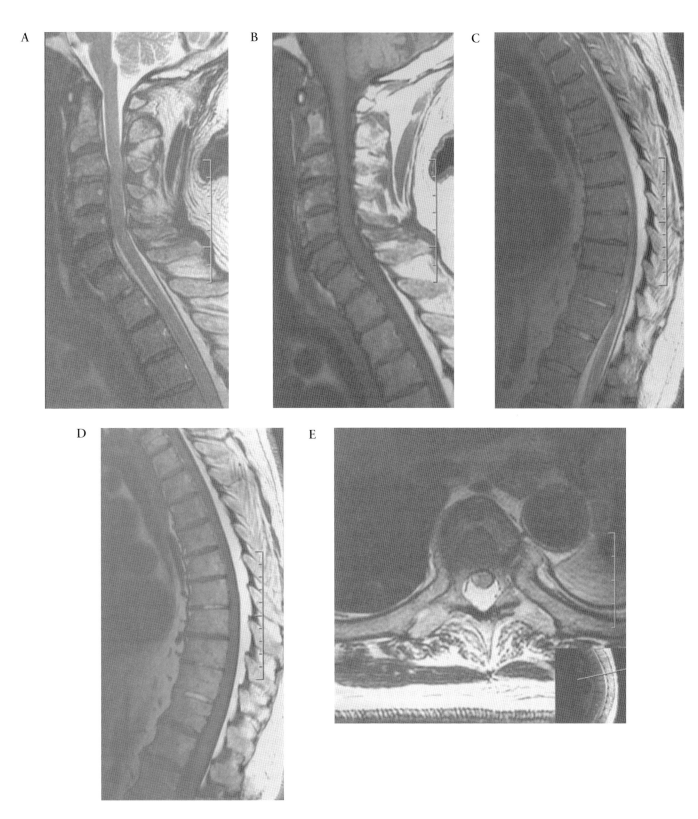

Fig. 20-5. *A-D*, Sagittal MRI sequences of a patient receiving long-term corticosteroid therapy for sarcoidosis show extensive epidural lipomatosis, extending from the lower body of C7 to T11, that resulted in severe central spinal canal stenosis. Note bright signal of the epidural lipomatosis on both the fast-spin echo T2 sequence (*A* and *C*) and T1 sequence (*B* and *D*). *E*, The marked extramedullary cord compression is best appreciated on axial fast-spin echo T2 sequences.

degeneration: involves corticospinal, spinocerebellar, and spinothalamic tracts

4) Hyalinoid thickening of media and adventitia of microvasculature, with mononuclear perivascular infiltrates

j. HTLV-I is also associated with T-cell lymphoma and leukemia

k. HTLV-II has also been associated with a progressive myelopathy (much less common than HTLV-I)

2. HIV-1–associated vacuolar myelopathy

a. Often occurs in the late stages of human immunodeficiency virus (HIV) infection

b. Often associated with acquired immunodeficiency syndrome (AIDS) dementia complex and peripheral neuropathy

c. Clinical features

1) Slowly progressive spastic paraparesis (weakness exceeding the spasticity)

2) Gait ataxia

3) Sphincter dysfunction (bowel and bladder dysfunction)

4) Paresthesias and pain in lower limbs

5) Large-fiber (posterior column) sensory loss (major small-fiber sensory loss indicates underlying concurrent peripheral neuropathy)

d. Pathology

1) Multifocal microvacuolation, spongiform degeneration

2) Loss of myelin

3) Lipid-laden macrophages

4) Pathologic changes predominantly involve dorsal and lateral tracts

5) Pathologic features resemble subacute combined degeneration

3. Herpesvirus-related myelopathy

a. Most commonly occurs in immunocompromised persons (e.g., AIDS patients or those receiving immunosuppressants after transplantation)

b. May be seen with varicella-zoster virus infection, herpes simplex virus type 2, Epstein-Barr virus, and cytomegalovirus (only rarely with herpes simplex virus type 1)

c. Varicella-zoster virus

1) Remains dormant in dorsal root ganglia

2) When reactivated, virus spreads to involve the roots and causes herpes zoster radiculitis, with severe radicular pain, sensory loss, and weakness; accompanied by vesicular rash

3) May also spread centripetally to cause necrotizing myelopathy

4) Myelopathy may be recurrent

5) CSF: varicella-zoster DNA detected with polymerase chain reaction (PCR)

6) MRI: abnormal T2 signal, contrast enhancement, and enlargement of spinal cord at affected segments

d. Herpes simplex type 2

1) Genital herpes

2) Inflammatory myelitis and radiculitis (usually lumbosacral): may be recurrent

4. Syphilis of spinal cord

a. Tabes dorsalis

1) Predominantly syndrome of dorsal columns: progressive ataxia (predominantly sensory ataxia), proprioceptive loss, rombergism, incoordination, lancinating or lightning-like pains, Lhermitte's sign

2) Genitourinary dysfunction, including atonic bladder and sexual dysfunction (impotence)

3) Loss of deep tendon reflexes

4) Pupils: irregular or unequal in most patients

5) Argyll Robertson pupils: impaired light reaction, preserved pupillary constriction to accommodation

6) Natural history and clinical progression (in sequence)

a) Tabetic pain phase: gradual onset and progression of lancinating "tabetic" pain and sphincter dysfunction

b) Ataxic phase: development of severe ataxia and trophic changes, including Charcot joints; worsening tabetic pain

c) Paralytic phase: cachexia, paralysis, and atrophy with stiffness; worsening sphincter dysfunction and other autonomic features

7) Pathology

a) Demyelination and rarefaction of posterior columns (especially fasciculus gracilis) and dorsal roots, with neuronal loss and gliosis

b) Chronic inflammatory disease of dorsal root ganglia: sparse leptomeningeal mononuclear infiltration, neuronal loss, and nodules of Nageotte (ganglion cells have degenerated)

b. Syphilitic spinal cord meningoencephalitis

1) Transverse myelitis: gradual onset and progression of limb weakness (legs > arms) with spasticity, hyperreflexia, and extensor plantar responses (mimicking cervical myelopathy), and sensory loss

2) Pathology: leptomeningeal inflammation and thickening with granulomatous arteritis of spinal cord parenchyma, predominantly involving lateral columns

c. Gummatous neurosyphilis of spinal cord: avascular gummas may be intramedullary (resembling intramedullary gliomas) or extramedullary (causing cord compression), localized form of meningeal syphilis

d. Spinal vascular syphilis: responsible for spinal cord infarction

e. Other extramedullary (compressive) syphilitic syndromes that could affect spinal cord

1) Aortitis and aortic aneurysms: cause erosion of adjacent vertebrae and compression of underlying spinal cord

2) Lesions of vertebrae: osteitis or trophic changes (Charcot vertebrae)

5. Acute poliomyelitis

a. Poliovirus infection of the nervous system, with viral affinity for anterior horn cells in brainstem and spinal cord

b. Afflicts less than 1% of patients infected with poliovirus

c. Present day: rare cases of acute poliomyelitis in U.S. because of oral poliovirus vaccine

d. Viremia follows incubation period (usually 3-6 days): about 90% of patients remain asymptomatic, other 10% develop symptoms of acute viral infection (fever, chills, nausea, malaise, headache, diarrhea)

e. 3% of patients develop aseptic meningitis (1/4 of them become afebrile for 2-3 days, followed by a second increase in temperature)

f. Aseptic meningitis tends to be self-limited in most patients; a fraction of patients develop acute paralytic poliomyelitis

g. Paralytic illness usually starts 2 to 5 days after onset of aseptic meningitis, as fever is subsiding: asymmetric paralysis mostly affecting the legs, with fasciculations, hypotonia, hypo- or areflexia, and, eventually, muscle atrophy (all lower motor neuron–type signs and symptoms)

h. CSF: pleocytosis (neutrophilic in acute phase, lymphocytic in subacute to chronic phase), increased protein, increased CSF index with increased poliovirus-specific IgM titers

6. Progressive postpoliomyelitis muscular atrophy (post-polio syndrome)

a. Typical presentation: history of paralytic poliomyelitis; partial or complete recovery of neurologic function, followed by a period of stability (usually several decades); progressive new muscle weakness and atrophy or abnormal muscle fatigability

b. Diagnosis: exclusion of other causes of new symptoms

c. Core clinical features: new weakness, muscular fatigability, general fatigue, pain

d. Progressive weakness and atrophy can occur in any muscle, including those originally seemingly spared (often

occurs in muscle groups previously affected by acute poliomyelitis, with clinical or subclinical involvement); this may include involvement of respiratory muscles

e. Examination shows lower motor neuron pattern of muscle weakness, atrophy, areflexia, fasciculations, or signs of entrapment mononeuropathies (or some combination)

f. Mechanical joint pain, especially in large weight-bearing joints

g. Predisposition to degenerative joint disease, nerve entrapment, degenerative disk disease of spine: all can cause pain

h. EMG

1) Normal to low-amplitude CMAPs

2) Needle examination: fibrillation potentials indicative of uncompensated denervation; long-duration, large-amplitude motor unit potentials indicative of extensive reinnervation

3) EMG findings: nonspecific and may occur in patients with previous history of acute poliomyelitis without progressive postpolio syndrome

4) Single fiber EMG: increased fiber density, jitter, and blocking

i. Muscle biopsy

1) Neurogenic changes: fiber-type grouping, small angulated fibers (recent and ongoing denervation)

2) Myopathic changes: muscle fiber necrosis, increased interstitial connective tissue, type I muscle fiber predominance

D. Lathyrism

1. Results from excessive consumption of the chickling pea, *Lathyrus sativus*

2. Responsible agent: thought to be glutamate agonist, β-*N*-oxalylamino-L-alanine (BOAA)

3. Acute or chronic onset of irreversible, nonprogressive spastic paraparesis associated with poorly understood degenerative changes in spinal cord

4. Associated with bladder dysfunction and sensory symptoms

5. Self-limiting, nonprogressive disease

E. Metabolic Disorders of Spinal Cord

1. Copper deficiency

a. Usually acquired: often due to chronic increased intake of zinc

b. Pathophysiology in context of hyperzincemia

1) Dietary zinc induces synthesis of metallothionein in enterocytes

2) Copper has high affinity for and tends to bind to metallothionein in enterocytes, which are sloughed

off into gastrointestinal tract and excreted

c. Clinical syndrome: myeloneuropathy

  1) Myelopathy with spastic paraparesis and posterior column dysfunction with loss of vibratory and proprioceptive sensory functions, mimicking subacute combined degeneration of vitamin B_{12} deficiency

  2) Sensorimotor peripheral neuropathy with prominent features of axonal loss on electrodiagnostic studies

d. Treatment: copper supplementation (cupric sulfate) and reduced zinc intake

2. Cobalamin (vitamin B_{12}) deficiency

a. High prevalence among elderly (15%-25%) and persons with gastrointestinal disease or malnutrion

b. Absorption of vitamin B_{12}

  1) Cobalamin binds to intrinsic factor (IF) produced by parietal cells in lower portion of stomach, forming IF-cobalamin complex

  2) IF-cobalamin complex is absorbed at ileum

c. Pathophysiology of neurologic dysfunction in vitamin B_{12} deficiency

  1) Vitamin B_{12} is important cofactor for enzyme methionine synthase (catalyzes synthesis of methionine from homocysteine) and conversion of methylmalonyl-CoA to succinyl-CoA: defect in production of methionine is likely responsible for neurologic deficits (importance of the latter reaction is unclear, may be important in fatty acid synthesis)

  2) Methionine is the precursor of S-adenosyl-L-methionine (SAM)

  3) SAM acts as methyl group donor for methylation of myelin basic protein (MBP), conferring stability on myelin structures; without SAM, deficient methylation of MBP translates into abnormal myelin structures and vacuolar myelopathy

  4) Methionine synthase also requires methyltetrahydrofolate as methyl donor for reaction catalyzed by methionine synthetase; folate deficiency may also produce subacute combined degeneration mimicking vitamin B_{12} deficiency (occurs much less frequently than with vitamin B_{12} deficiency)

  5) Nitrous oxide (NO) toxicity also mimics vitamin B_{12} deficiency: NO inhibits the production of SAM by interfering with methionine synthetase and can produce similar vacuolar myelopathy

d. Causes

  1) Absence of IF

    a) Defective IF production by parietal cells in pernicious anemia

    b) Gastrectomy

  2) Malabsorption

    a) Resection of terminal ileum

    b) Gastrointestinal disease interfering with absorption (e.g., celiac disease, Crohn's disease)

  3) Dietary insufficiency and malnutrition

e. Syndrome of subacute combined degeneration

  1) Insidious onset of paresthesias in hands and feet, Lhermitte's sign, sensation of generalized weakness and fatigue, and autonomic features (altered bowel habits, especially constipation; urinary frequency and urgency; erectile dysfunction)

  2) With progression: gait abnormalities due to combination of sensory ataxia (posterior column involvement, Romberg's sign) and spastic paraparesis (spasticity, hyperreflexia, extensor plantar responses accompanying spastic paraparesis)

  3) Weakness most prominent in legs

f. Complicating the neurologic deficits that cause gait imbalance is length-dependent peripheral neuropathy (sensory then motor involvement with progression)

g. Cognitive decline, mental slowing, personality changes, psychiatric disease (depression, psychosis)

h. Visual loss: bilateral optic atrophy, centrocecal scotoma

i. Systemic features: megaloblastic anemia (may lead to pancytopenia), hyperpigmented fingernails, diarrhea, glossitis

j. Pathology (Fig 20-6): vacuolar myelopathy (spongy white matter vacuolization in posterior and lateral columns, with loss of myelin staining)

k. Diagnosis

  1) Megaloblastic anemia

  2) Reduced serum levels of vitamin B_{12} (may be normal or borderline low)

  3) Increased serum levels of homocysteine and methylmalonic acid

  4) Hyperintense T2 abnormalities involving posterior columns, predominantly in lower cervical and upper thoracic cord

  5) Abnormal somatosensory evoked potentials

  6) Schilling test if pernicious anemia is suspected

l. Treatment

  1) Intramuscular cyanocobalamin

  2) Folate supplementation must be delayed for at least 2 weeks after initiation of cobalamin supplementation

3. Folate deficiency: neurologic deficits similar to cobalamin deficiency discussed above (much less frequently than cobalamin deficiency)

4. Nitrous oxide toxicity

a. Usually caused by nitrous oxide abuse: higher risk for those in dental profession

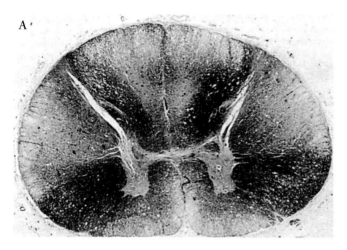
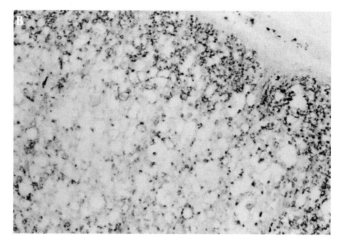

Fig. 20-6. Pathologic features of subacute combined degeneration of vitamin B$_{12}$ deficiency. *A*, Note the symmetric loss of myelin staining predominantly involving the posterior and lateral columns (Luxol fast blue stain.) *B*, Histopathologic features of vacuolar myelopathy: spongy white matter vacuolization in the posterior and lateral columns. (From Okazaki H, Scheithauer BW. Atlas of neuropathology. New York: Gower Medical Publishing; 1988, p. 255. By permission of Mayo Foundation.)

b. Nitrous oxide inhibits vitamin B$_{12}$–dependent methionine synthase
c. Clinical syndrome resembles that of vitamin B$_{12}$ deficiency: subacute combined degeneration usually beginning in thoracic segments
d. Nitrous oxide toxicity may trigger subacute combined degeneration in patients with subclinical cobalamin deficiency
e. Clinical features
　1) Sharp radicular pains
　2) Lhermitte's sign and reverse Lhermitte's sign
　3) Predominantly axonal sensorimotor peripheral neuropathy, myelopathy, optic neuropathy, and megaloblastic anemia—all resembling vitamin B$_{12}$ deficiency
f. Myelopathy is often delayed by 3 months to 5 years after exposure
g. Slow, often partial, recovery
h. Electrodiagnostic evaluation: reduced amplitude of sensory nerve action potentials, abnormal somatosensory evoked potentials
i. MRI characteristics mimic those of vitamin B$_{12}$ deficiency: high T2 signal involving posterior columns, predominantly of lower cervical and upper thoracic segments (Fig. 20-7)
j. Increased serum levels of methylmalonic acid and homocysteine
k. Treatment: cobalamin and methionine supplementation
5. Other causes of toxic myelopathies: toxicity due to organophosphates and hexocarbons

F. Transverse Myelitis Associated With Inflammatory Disorders
1. Associated with systemic inflammatory diseases: systemic lupus erythematosus, Behçet's disease, Sjögren's syndrome, and sarcoidosis
2. Associated with central nervous system inflammatory diseases: multiple sclerosis, sarcoidosis
3. Clinical features, treatment, and prognosis depend on etiology (discussed elsewhere)

G. Idiopathic, Postinfectious, and Postvaccination Transverse Myelitis
1. Due to immune-mediated neural injury, not viral infection of spinal cord
2. Same pathologic features: perivascular inflammatory exudates, edema, and hemorrhage
3. 1/3 of patients: history of viral illness or vaccination
4. Most frequently involved spinal cord segment: thoracic
5. All ages may be affected: incidence peaks between ages 10 and 19 years and again at 30 to 39 years
6. Clinical presentation
　a. Acute or subacute onset with rapid progression of symptoms in first 3 weeks of presentation (variable temporal profile)
　　1) Motor: rapidly progressive paraparesis (involving legs > arms), flaccidity followed by spasticity, and other corticospinal tract signs
　　2) Sensory: numbness, dysesthesias, or paresthesias; sensory level most often localized to thoracic segment

3) Autonomic: especially bladder dysfunction
  b. Features atypical for idiopathic transverse myelitis
    1) Mild and asymmetric: suggestive of multiple sclerosis (not idiopathic)
    2) Features of underlying inflammatory disorder (peripheral nervous system, other central nervous system, or systemic involvement): inflammatory polyradiculoneuropathy, meningitis, others
7. Laboratory evidence
  a. CSF: usually normal, but there may be lymphocytic pleocytosis and increased protein
  b. MRI: central cord T2 hyperintensity with or without enhancement or spinal cord edema
8. Treatment
  a. Intravenous high-dose corticosteroids
    1) No randomized placebo-controlled study
    2) Early treatment with high-dose corticosteroids may help reduce mortality and morbidity and improve functional outcome
  b. Plasma exchange
    1) Not shown to benefit idiopathic transverse myelitis
    2) May be tried if patient has less than adequate response to corticosteroids
9. Prognosis
  a. Up to 90% monophasic
  b. Risk factors for recurrence
    1) Multifocal central nervous system disease (especially demyelinating lesions)
    2) Serologic evidence of systemic connective tissue disease

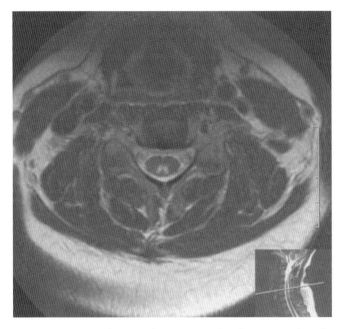

Fig. 20-7. Cervical MRI of a patient with subacute combined degeneration due to nitrous oxide toxicity shows high T2 signal involving the posterior columns (axial T2 sequences). MRI characteristics of nitrous toxicity mimic those of vitamin B_{12} deficiency.

3) CSF oligoclonal bands
4) Optic nerve involvement
5) Abnormalities on brain MRI

REFERENCES

Brooks BR, Miller RG, Swash M, Munsat TL, World Federation of Neurology Research Group on Motor Neuron Diseases. El Escorial revisited: revised criteria for the diagnosis of amyotrophic lateral sclerosis. Amyotroph Lateral Scler Other Motor Neuron Disord. 2000;1:293-9.

Cavanagh NP, Eames RA, Galvin RJ, Brett EM, Kelly RE. Hereditary sensory neuropathy with spastic paraplegia. Brain. 1979;102:79-94.

Gascon GG, Chavis P, Yaghmour A, Stigsby B, Shums A, Ozand P, et al. Familial childhood primary lateral sclerosis with associated gaze paresis. Neuropediatrics. 1995;26:313-9.

GeneTests. Seattle: University of Washington. Available from: http://www.genetests.org

Izumo S, Umehara F, Kashio N, Kubota R, Sato E, Osame M. Neuropathology of HTLV-1-associated myelopathy (HAM/TSP). Leukemia. 1997;11 Suppl 3:82-4.

Kumar N, Gross JB Jr, Ahlskog JE. Copper deficiency myelopathy produces a clinical picture like subacute combined degeneration. Neurology. 2004;63:33-9.

Naidu S, Dlouhy SR, Geraghty MT, Hodes ME. A male child with the rumpshaker mutation, X-linked spastic paraplegia/Pelizaeus-Merzbacher disease and lysinuria. J Inherit Metab Dis. 1997;20:811-6.

Pourmand R, Harati Y, editors. Advances in neurology. Vol 88: Neuromuscular disorders. Philadelphia: Lippincott Williams & Wilkins; 2002.

Rippon GA, Scarmeas N, Gordon PH, Murphy PL, Albert SM, Mitsumoto H, et al. An observational study of cognitive impairment in amyotrophic lateral sclerosis. Arch Neurol. 2006;63:345-52.

Sawa H, Nagashima T, Nagashima K, Shinohara T, Chuma T, Mano Y, et al. Clinicopathological and virological analyses of familial human T-lymphotropic virus type I—associated polyneuropathy. J Neurovirol. 2005;11:199-207.

QUESTIONS

1. A 45-year-old dentist presents with slowly progressive spasticity and paresthesias in the lower extremities. Neurologic examination shows brisk deep tendon reflexes, extensor plantar responses, and a stocking distribution pattern of sensory loss in the lower extremities. Electrodiagnostic evaluation shows decreased amplitude of motor and sensory responses, with mild fibrillation potentials distally. This patient most likely has:
   a. Amyotrophic lateral sclerosis
   b. Nitrous oxide toxicity
   c. Copper deficiency
   d. Hereditary spastic paraplegia

2. Which of the following gene products has been associated with hereditary spastic paraparesis?
   a. Parkin
   b. Neural cell adhesion molecule L1
   c. ATPase
   d. Pantothenate kinase

3. A 53-year-old man presents with a 10-year history of slowly progressive motor neuron disease, including tongue atrophy and fasciculations and facial fasciculations, and testicular atrophy. There is family history of a paternal cousin with developmental regression and a cherry-red spot. This patient most likely has:
   a. CAG trinucleotide repeat expansion, with X-linked recessive inheritance
   b. Mutation of *HEXA* gene, with autosomal recessive inheritance
   c. Deletion of the *SMN1* gene, with autosomal recessive inheritance
   d. Mutation of the *SOD1* gene, with autosomal dominant inheritance

4. A 63-year-old woman presents with gradual onset of paresthesias in the hands and feet and fatigue, followed by slow progression of spastic paraparesis. Laboratory evaluation shows anemia with macrocytosis, decreased serum level of vitamin B_{12}, and increased serum level of methylmalonic acid. The most important mechanism that accounts for this patient's neurologic dysfunction is:
   a. Defect in production of methionine
   b. Reduced conversion of methylmalonyl CoA to succinyl CoA
   c. Reduced absorption of vitamin E
   d. Increased synthesis of metallothionein in the enterocytes

5. A 60-year-old man presents 8 months after slow onset and progression of left footdrop. He has experienced progressive weakness of both lower extremities througout the 8 months before presentation. He does not have pain or sensory symptoms. There is severe weakness, atrophy, and fasciculations in the lower extremities, and spasticity and hyperreflexia in the distribution of the affected myotomes. Electrodiagnostic evaluation in this patient is most likely to show:
   a. Rapid recruitment of short-duration motor unit potentials, with minimal fibrillation potentials, and myotonic discharges
   b. Normal sensory nerve action potentials, conduction block of the peroneal nerve bilaterally, and reduced recruitment of motor unit potentials of normal morphology
   c. Low-amplitude motor and sensory responses with normal conduction velocities, long-duration motor unit potentials distally, and normal insertional activity
   d. Reduced recruitment of varying, polyphasic, long-duration motor unit potentials with fibrillation potentials and fasciculation protentials in multiple segments examined

ANSWERS

1. Answer: b.
The pattern of spastic paraplegia with an axonal sensorimotor peripheral neuropathy is highly suggestive of nitrous oxide toxicity.

2. Answer: b.
Of the listed proteins, neural cell adhesion molecule L1 (also known as L1 cell adhesion molecule, L1CAM) has been associated with X-linked familial spastic paraplegia SPG1.

3. Answer: a.
The clinical presentation is highly suggestive of X-linked spinobulbar muscular atrophy (Kennedy's syndrome). This is an X-linked recessive disorder due to CAG trinucleotide repeat expansion in the androgen receptor gene.

4. Answer: a.
This patient has the clinical syndrome of subacute combined degeneration related to vitamin B_{12} deficiency. The most important cause of the myelopathy is defective methionine production. Vitamin B_{12} acts as a coenzyme for methionine synthase, which catalyzes the synthesis of methionine from homocysteine. Methionine is the precursor of S-adenosyl-L-methionine (SAM). The latter compound is important for methylation of myelin basic protein, conferring stability on myelin structures. Defective myelination and resultant vacuolar myelopathy occurs in the absence of SAM. Vitamin B_{12} is also an important cofactor for conversion of methylmalonyl CoA to succinyl CoA, but this reaction does not seem to be important in the pathophysiology of the vacuolar myelopathy related to vitamin B_{12} deficiency.

5. Answer: d.
This patient most likely has amyotrophic lateral sclerosis with rapid progression. The typical electrodiagnostic findings are those of a rapidly progressive neurogenic process. Although active denervation may not be apparent in the early stages of motor neuron disease, electrophysiologic evidence of active denervation and reinnervation become more apparent with disease progression. The presence of varying polyphasic motor unit potentials is indicative of active reinnervation.

Disorders of the Peripheral Nervous System

Part A: Anatomy of the Peripheral Nervous System and Classification of Disorders by Localization

21

1

Dean H. Kilfoyle, M.B., Ch.B.

Lyell K. Jones, M.D.

Nima Mowzoon, M.D.

I. CLINICAL APPROACH TO DISORDERS OF THE PERIPHERAL NERVOUS SYSTEM (PNS)
(SEE APPENDIX A)

II. ANATOMY OF THE PNS AND RELATED ENTRAPMENT NEUROPATHIES

A. **Brachial Plexus:** basic neuroanatomy (Fig. 21-1)
1. Formed from spinal roots (ventral primary rami) of C5-T1
2. Dorsal scapular nerve arises from C5 nerve root and supplies the major and minor rhomboid muscles
3. Long thoracic nerve arises from C5-C7 roots and supplies the serratus anterior muscle
4. Upper trunk
   a. Formed from C5 and C6 roots
   b. Provides an anterior division to the lateral cord and posterior division to the posterior cord (contributes to all the peripheral nerves arising from the cords except the ulnar nerve)
   c. Suprascapular nerve arises from upper trunk and supplies the supraspinatus and infraspinatus muscles
   d. The nerve to the subclavius muscle also arises from the upper trunk
5. Middle trunk
   a. Formed from C7 root
   b. Provides an anterior division to the lateral cord and posterior division to the posterior cord (contributes to all peripheral nerves arising from the cords except the ulnar nerve)
6. Lower trunk: provides an anterior division to the medial cord and posterior division to the posterior cord (contributes to all peripheral nerves arising from the cords except the musculocutaneous nerve)
7. Lateral cord
   a. Gives rise to the musculocutaneous nerve and contributes to the median nerve
   b. Lateral pectoral nerve arises from the lateral cord and supplies the pectoralis major muscle
8. Posterior cord
   a. Gives rise to the axillary and radial nerves
   b. Upper scapular nerve arises from the posterior cord and supplies the subscapularis muscle
   c. Thoracodorsal nerve arises from the posterior cord and supplies the latissimus dorsi muscle
   d. Lower scapular nerve arises from the posterior cord and supplies the subscapularis and teres major muscles
9. Medial cord
   a. Gives rise to the ulnar nerve and contributes to the median nerve
   b. Medial pectoral nerve arises from the medial cord and supplies the pectoralis major and minor muscles
   c. Medial brachial cutaneous and medial antebrachial cutaneous nerves also arise from the medial cord

B. **Peripheral Nerves of the Arm and the Related Entrapment Neuropathies**
1. Treatment for all entrapment neuropathies
   a. Depends mainly on the cause
   b. Anticonvulsants and tricyclic antidepressants may be used to treat neuropathic pain
2. Axillary nerve
   a. Supplies the teres minor muscle and then deltoid muscle as it curves around the humerus
   b. Gives rise to lateral brachial cutaneous sensory nerve to lateral aspect of the arm
3. Musculocutaneous nerve
   a. Supplies the coracobrachialis, biceps brachii (short head and long head), and brachialis muscles
   b. Gives rise to lateral antebrachial cutaneous nerve
4. Median nerve
   a. Anatomic landmarks in order of occurrence
      1) In some persons, the median nerve travels inside a foramen created by a tendinous band that runs between the humerus and the medial epicondyle

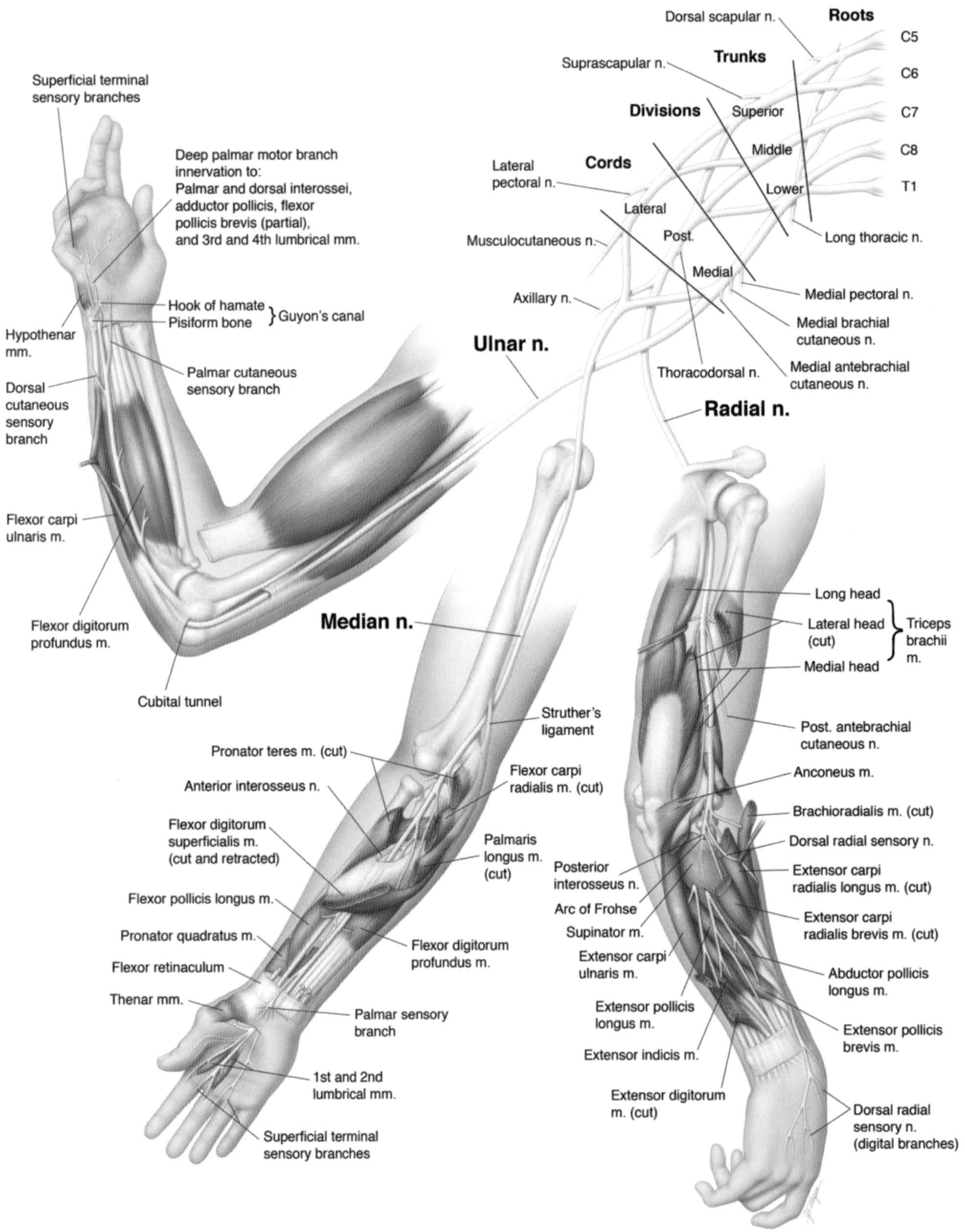

Superficial terminal
sensory branches

Deep palmar motor branch
innervation to:
Palmar and dorsal interossei,
adductor pollicis, flexor
pollicis brevis (partial),
and 3rd and 4th lumbrical mm.

Hypothenar
mm.

Hook of hamate
Pisiform bone } Guyon's canal

Dorsal
cutaneous
sensory
branch

Palmar cutaneous
sensory branch

Flexor carpi
ulnaris m.

Flexor digitorum
profundus m.

Cubital tunnel

Dorsal scapular n.   **Roots**   C5
Suprascapular n.   **Trunks**   C6
              Divisions   Superior   C7
Lateral   **Cords**   Middle   C8
pectoral n.   Lower   T1
                     Lateral
Musculocutaneous n.   Post.   Long thoracic n.
                    Medial
Axillary n.   Medial pectoral n.
                                     Medial brachial
Ulnar n.   cutaneous n.
              Thoracodorsal n.   Medial antebrachial
                                 cutaneous n.

Radial n.

Median n.

Long head
Lateral head } Triceps
(cut)   } brachii
Medial head } m.

Struther's
ligament

Pronator teres m. (cut)

Anterior interosseus n.

Flexor carpi
radialis m. (cut)

Flexor digitorum
superficialis m.
(cut and retracted)

Palmaris
longus m.
(cut)

Posterior
interosseus n.
Arc of Frohse

Post. antebrachial
cutaneous n.

Anconeus m.

Brachioradialis m. (cut)

Dorsal radial sensory n.

Extensor carpi
radialis longus m. (cut)

Flexor pollicis longus m.

Pronator quadratus m.

Flexor retinaculum

Thenar mm.

Flexor digitorum
profundus m.

Palmar sensory
branch

1st and 2nd
lumbrical mm.

Superficial terminal
sensory branches

Supinator m.

Extensor carpi
ulnaris m.

Extensor pollicis
longus m.

Extensor indicis m.

Extensor digitorum
m. (cut)

Extensor carpi
radialis brevis m. (cut)

Abductor pollicis
longus m.

Extensor pollicis
brevis m.

Dorsal radial
sensory n.
(digital branches)

Fig. 21-1. Anatomic schema of the brachial plexus and peripheral nerves of the upper extremity. Note the "claw hand" deformity of ulnar neuropathy, thenar muscle atrophy of median neuropathy at the wrist, and "wrist drop" of radial neuropathy.

(ligament of Struthers)

2) After entering the forearm, the median nerve passes underneath a fibrous aponeurotic band that runs from the tendon of the biceps brachii to forearm flexors (lacertus fibrosus)

3) Runs between the two heads of the pronator teres and innervates that muscle and the flexor carpi radialis (both C6, C7) and the palmaris longus and flexor digitorum superficialis (both primarily C8)

4) Gives rise to anterior interosseous nerve, which supplies innervation to flexor digitorum profundus I and II, flexor pollicis longus, and, most distally, pronator quadratus (all of which are primarily C8)

5) Travels in the forearm and passes deep to flexor digitorum superficialis muscle and the fibrous aponeurotic arch attached to it

6) Gives rise to the palmar cutaneous sensory branch distally to supply the area over the thenar eminence and then dives inside the flexor retinaculum (whereas the palmar sensory branch travels over the ligament)

7) Innervates abductor pollicis brevis, opponens pollicis, first and second lumbricals, and partially innervates flexor pollicis brevis (with the ulnar nerve)

b. Median neuropathy at the wrist: carpal tunnel syndrome (CTS)

1) Wrist pain and hand pain and paresthesias in median nerve distribution, sometimes radiating to the forearm and arm, episodic pain and paresthesias worse at night

2) Symptoms often provoked with extended wrist posture, such as driving or holding a book

3) Sensory fibers are affected early, motor fibers in advanced cases

4) Patients may complain of weakness of thumb abduction and opposition, followed by atrophy of thenar eminence

5) Sensation is spared over thenar eminence because the palmar cutaneous sensory branch is spared

6) Tinel's sign (induced by tapping over median nerve at the wrist) and Phalen's maneuver (passive flexion of wrist producing paresthesia)

7) Associated and predisposing conditions
   a) Hereditary neuropathy with liability to pressure palsies
   b) Diabetic neuropathy, other polyneuropathies
   c) Pregnancy
   d) Hypothyroidism
   e) Acromegaly
   f) Amyloidosis
   g) Renal failure

8) Nerve conduction studies
   a) Palmar orthodromic technique is most sensitive for demonstrating focal slowing across wrist because of shorter distance; the antidromic technique is an alternative for moderate to severe neuropathy
   b) Mild CTS: prolonged median sensory or mixed nerve action potential distal latency (orthodromic or antidromic, respectively), sensory nerve action potential (SNAP) amplitude may be reduced
   c) Moderate CTS: prolonged distal latencies of *both* median motor and sensory responses, SNAP amplitude may be reduced
   d) Severe CTS: prolonged distal latencies of *both* median motor and sensory distal latencies *and* either absent SNAP or mixed nerve action potential *or* low-amplitude thenar compound muscle action potential (CMAP)
   e) Very severe CTS: no thenar motor or sensory palmar nerve action potential

c. Anterior interosseous nerve syndrome
1) Isolated neuropathy involving anterior interosseous nerve
   a) In the setting of immune-mediated brachial plexus neuropathy (Parsonage-Turner syndrome)
   b) Less commonly, in the setting of hereditary neuropathy with liability to pressure palsy or possibly compression of anterior interosseous nerve by fibrous bands attached to flexor digitorum superficialis muscle

2) Weakness of pronation (pronator quadratus), weakness of flexion of thumb (flexor pollicis longus), and weakness of flexion of distal phalanx of the fingers (flexor digitorum profundus I and II)

3) Weakness of distal interphalangeal joints of thumb and index finger creates hyperextension at these joints when making the "OK" sign

d. Pronator syndrome
1) Compression of median nerve by the two heads of pronator teres muscle, lacertus fibrosus, and the aponeurotic fibrous arch attached to flexor digitorum superficialis muscle

2) Entrapment results from repetitive pronation

3) Variable extent of weakness (usually mild) of flexor pollicis longus, abductor pollicis brevis, and other distal median-innervated muscles

e. Entrapment at the ligament of Struthers
1) Variable degrees of weakness and sensory symptoms in distribution of median nerve

2) Paresthesias in the median nerve distribution, produced by supination of the forearm and extension at the elbow

3) Brachial artery also passes through the foramen produced by ligament of Struthers. There may be reduced radial pulses with this condition

5. Radial nerve
   a. Anatomic landmarks in order of occurrence
      1) Innervates the three heads of triceps brachii (long, medial, and lateral heads) and anconeus muscle, gives rise to posterior brachial cutaneous nerve as it passes along lateral wall of the axilla toward the spiral groove of the humerus
      2) Gives rise to lower lateral brachial cutaneous and posterior antebrachial cutaneous nerves as it passes through the spiral groove
      3) As radial nerve curves around the humerus, it supplies brachioradialis (C5, C6) and extensor carpi radialis longus (C6, C7) muscles
      4) Further down, it gives rise to superficial (dorsal) radial sensory branch
      5) Becomes the posterior interosseous nerve, which provides innervation to extensor carpi radialis brevis (C6, C7) and supinator (C5, C6) muscles and then dives into supinator muscle (arch of Frohse)
      6) Innervates rest of the digit extensors, including extensor carpi ulnaris muscle, and abductor pollicis longus muscle
   b. Lesion at the axilla
      1) May result from prolonged compression, which may occur in patients who use crutches incorrectly, applying excess pressure on the axilla
      2) Results in weakness of all radial-innervated muscles and sensory deficits involving entire radial nerve distribution (posterior arm and forearm and lateral aspect and dorsum of hand)
   c. Lesion at spiral groove at mid-arm (Fig. 21-2)
      1) "Saturday night palsy": compression at the spiral groove, as with compressing the nerve while sleeping (especially after intoxication)
      2) May also result from fracture of the humerus, multifocal motor neuropathy with conduction block, or another immune-mediated process
      3) Clinical features similar to those of axillary lesions, but with sparing of most of triceps brachii and sensation to posterior arm
   d. Posterior interosseous neuropathy
      1) Clinical features similar to those of spiral groove lesion, but also with sparing of extensor carpi radialis longus, brachioradialis, anconeus, and triceps brachii as well as any sensory deficits (purely a motor branch)
      2) Patients present with "finger drop" and supinator weakness

   e. Superficial radial sensory neuropathy (cheiralgia paresthetica)
      1) Sensory deficits involving the lateral aspect and dorsum of hands and fingers (no motor deficits)
      2) Occurs with tight handcuffs, bands, watches

6. Ulnar nerve
   a. Anatomic landmarks in order of occurrence
      1) Passes in retrocondylar groove and then in cubital tunnel formed by the medial ligament of the elbow joint and aponeurosis of flexor carpi ulnaris muscle
      2) As the ulnar nerve enters the forearm, it supplies flexor carpi ulnaris and flexor digitorum profundus III and IV and travels in forearm
      3) In distal aspect of forearm, it gives rise to dorsal ulnar cutaneous and palmar cutaneous sensory nerves responsible for sensation of hypothenar eminence

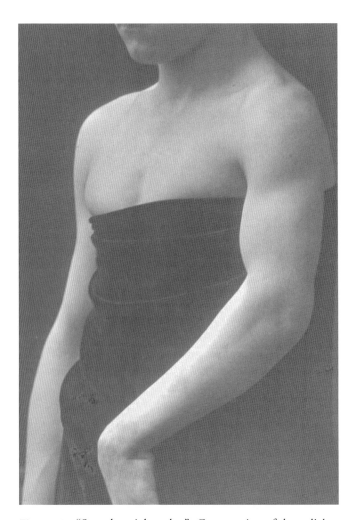

Fig. 21-2. "Saturday night palsy." Compression of the radial nerve at the spiral groove often spares most of the triceps but causes wrist drop due to weakness of digit and wrist extensors.

4) At the wrist, it gives off the digital sensory branch that supplies the fifth digit and medial half of the fourth digit

5) Supplies hypothenar muscles and immediately enters Guyon's canal formed by the pisiform bone and hook of the hamate

6) After entering Guyon's canal, the ulnar nerve ends as the deep palmar motor branch to supply interossei muscles, including first dorsal interosseous [FDI]), third and fourth lumbricals, adductor pollicis, and half the innervation to flexor pollicis brevis

b. Ulnar neuropathy at the elbow

1) Chronic mechanical compression due to repeated trauma, arthritis, and other factors causing tardive ulnar palsy

2) Ulnar palsy at the groove may also occur with mechanical compression (e.g., during general anesthesia or coma)

3) Ulnar nerve prolapse: a condition in which the ulnar nerve is displaced from the groove and predisposed to trauma

4) Ulnar compression at the cubital tunnel or the groove may occur with repeated flexion at the elbow causing chronic, minor trauma and compression

5) Some people have congenitally tight cubital tunnels and a predisposition for development of ulnar neuropathy at the cubital tunnel

6) In addition to repetitive trauma and arthritic changes, causes include tumors, fibrous bands, accessory muscles

7) Symptoms

a) Weakness of ulnar-innervated intrinsic hand muscles and atrophy in chronic cases

b) Sensory symptoms (paresthesias and dysesthesias) involve the volar and dorsal aspects of the fifth and medial aspect of the fourth digits and hand

8) Benediction posture ("clawing" of the hand): due primarily to weakness of third and fourth lumbricals causing hyperextension at metacarpophalangeal joints and flexion of proximal and distal interphalangeal joints (Fig. 21-3)

9) Wartenberg's sign: abduction of fifth digit due to weak adduction from weakness of third palmar interosseous muscle (Fig. 21-3)

10) Froment's sign:

a) Due to weakness of pinch as result of weak ulnar-innervated adductor pollicis, interossei, and flexor pollicis brevis (partially)

b) Median-innervated flexor pollicis longus and the flexor digitorum profundus I and II and superficialis are instead activated and used to pinch

11) Treatment: primarily surgical (decompression of cubital tunnel, medial epicondylectomy, and submuscular transposition of ulnar nerve) after conservative management fails (physical therapy, avoidance of leaning on elbow, or use of elbow pad)

c. Electrophysiologic evaluation for suspected ulnar neuropathy at the elbow

1) Extended elbow position may underestimate length of the nerve, and conduction velocity may seem slow across the elbow

2) More accurate measurement with the elbow flexed

3) Inching technique is often used to better localize the conduction block or slowing

4) Focal slowing

a) Abrupt drop in conduction velocities (above the elbow [AE]-to-below the elbow [BE] segment >10 m/s slower than the BE-to-wrist [W] segment)

b) Lack of adequate data in the literature for this

5) Partial conduction block or temporal dispersion (focal demyelination)

a) More than 20% decrease in amplitude of CMAP (negative peak) across elbow (10 cm), as per AAEM practice guidelines

b) This presumes absence of anomalies of innervation (i.e., Martin-Gruber anastomosis)

c) Some authorities regard more than 10% slowing across elbow as significant

d) Normal subjects may have slowing up to 10% across elbow

6) Routinely, motor conduction studies can be obtained by recording at abductor digiti minimi

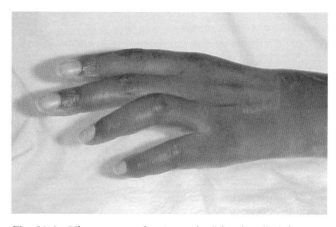

Fig. 21-3. Ulnar neuropathy. Note the "claw hand" deformity (benediction posture) due to weakness of third and fourth lumbricals, atrophy of the interossei muscles, and abduction of the fifth digit (Wartenberg's sign).

7) Because entrapment neuropathies of ulnar nerve are often fascicular, additional recording at first dorsal interosseous may increase the sensitivity

8) Dorsal ulnar cutaneous sensory conduction study may also be an important adjunct

9) Both ulnar antidromic sensory (recording at fifth digit) and dorsal ulnar cutaneous sensory studies may be abnormal in lesions at level of the elbow, whereas a dorsal ulnar cutaneous sensory study is often normal with ulnar neuropathy at the wrist because the dorsal ulnar sensory branch takes off proximal to the wrist

10) Note: ulnar neuropathies at elbow are often fascicular and may spare the dorsal sensory branch

11) Needle examination: muscles innervated by the deep palmar motor and hypothenar branches are often affected more than more proximally innervated muscles

d. Ulnar neuropathy at the wrist

   1) Motor and sensory involvement: lesion proximal to sensory and motor branches

   2) Pure sensory involvement: lesion of digital sensory branch only (rare)

   3) Pure motor involvement: lesion after the sensory branch, affecting all ulnar-innervated intrinsic hand muscles (sparing sensation of hypothenar eminence)

   4) Pure motor involvement of intrinsic hand muscles, sparing hypothenar muscles: lesion after Guyon's canal, sparing hypothenar sensory and motor function, but causing weakness of the muscles supplied by deep palmar motor branch

e. Electrophysiologic evaluation for suspected ulnar neuropathy at the wrist

   1) Nerve conduction studies must include recording at the FDI

   2) CMAP amplitudes and latencies recorded at adductor digiti minimi are expected to be normal, with lesions at Guyon's canal affecting only the deep palmar motor branch (common)

   3) Lesions distal to the dorsal ulnar cutaneous branch spare the dorsal ulnar cutaneous SNAP and cause an abnormal ulnar sensory antidromic SNAP recorded at the fifth digit

   4) If ulnar neuropathy is expected at the wrist, the distal latencies of responses obtained by stimulating ulnar and median nerves and recording at interossei and lumbrical muscles, respectively, should be performed, and inching across the wrist must be attempted

   5) Needle examination: muscles innervated by deep palmar motor branches are often most affected

C. **Lumbosacral Plexus:** basic neuroanatomy

1. Anatomically divided into lumbar plexus and sacral plexus

2. Lumbar plexus

   a. Formed within psoas major muscle

   b. L1: gives rise to ilioinguinal, iliohypogastric, and genitofemoral nerves (the latter two also receive innervation from T12 and L2)

   c. L2, L3, L4 anterior divisions: give rise to obturator nerve

   d. L2, L3, L4 posterior divisions: give rise to femoral nerve

   e. L2, L3 posterior divisions: give rise to lateral cutaneous nerve of the thigh

3. Sacral plexus

   a. Connects with lumbar plexus via lumbosacral trunk (anterior division of L4 and L5), other primary rami forming the sacral plexus are S1, S2, S3

   b. L4 to S3 anterior divisions: give rise to tibial and posterior divisions of the common peroneal portions of the sciatic nerve

   c. S1, S2, S3 anterior divisions: give rise to posterior cutaneous nerve of the thigh

   d. S2, S3, S4 anterior divisions: give rise to pudendal nerve ("S2, 3, 4 keep your pelvis off the floor")

D. **Peripheral Nerves of the Leg and Related Entrapment Neuropathies**

1. Peroneal nerve anatomy: anatomic landmarks in order of occurrence (Fig. 21-4)

   a. Common peroneal nerve travels with tibial nerve in the nerve bundle of sciatic nerve, the two nerves share a sheath but remain separated

   b. First branch of common peroneal nerve: innervation to the short head of biceps femoris muscle

   c. Common peroneal nerve then separates completely from tibial nerve

   d. Once peroneal nerve reaches popliteal fossa, it gives rise to lateral cutaneous nerve of the calf (supplying lateral proximal portion of the calf) and the sural communicating branch, which joins sural nerve (both sensory), and continues on for a short distance and wraps around the fibular neck and continues into the fibular tunnel (formed from the tendinous portion of peroneus longus and fibula)

   e. After this, it divides into superficial and deep peroneal nerves

   f. Superficial peroneal nerve gives rise to innervation to peroneus longus and brevis muscles, and then superficial peroneal sensory branch, which divides into medial and lateral branches to supply the distal aspect of lateral calf and dorsum of the foot, sparing the web space between first and second toes

g. Deep peroneal nerve is primarily motor and supplies innervation to tibialis anterior, extensor digitorum longus, extensor hallucis longus, peroneus tertius, and extensor digitorum brevis (EDB) muscles

h. Deep peroneal nerve continues on as dorsal digital cutaneous nerve to supply sensory innervation to the web space between first and second toes

2. Common peroneal neuropathy at fibular neck
   a. Predisposed to compression and nerve trauma at fibular neck

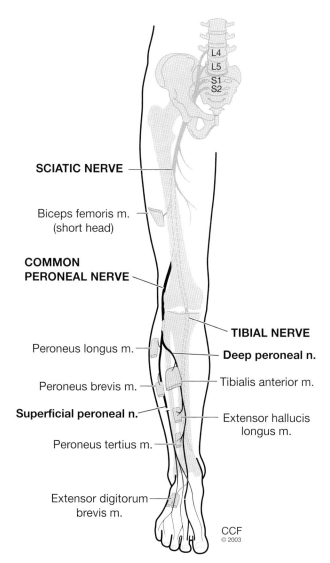

Fig. 21-4. Anatomic schema of the common peroneal nerve and its divisions. (From Katirji B, Wilbourn AJ. Mononeuropathies of the lower limb. In: Dyck PJ, Thomas PK, editors. Peripheral neuropathy. Vol 2. 4th ed. Philadelphia: Elsevier Saunders; 2005. p. 1487-510. Used with permission.)

b. Fascicles of the deep peroneal branch usually are more affected

c. Predisposing factors and etiologic circumstances: habitual leg crossing, intraoperative compression, prolonged bed rest and prolonged hospitalization, coma, casts, pneumatic compression devices, excessive weight loss with loss of supportive surrounding fat, diabetes mellitus

d. Other causes of compression may include: ganglion cysts, Baker's cyst, hematomas, tumors

e. Acute or subacute onset of partial or complete footdrop (with steppage gait), which may be related temporally to the cause (if there is one, e.g., intraoperative compression)

f. Hyperesthesia, paresthesias, and sensory deficits in peroneal nerve distribution

g. Tinel's sign at the fibular neck

h. Electrodiagnostic evaluation important to define exactly the localization, rule out other possible localization such as L5 radiculopathy, determination of prognosis, determination of presence and extent of denervation and reinnervation

i. Nerve conduction studies for suspected common peroneal neuropathy at fibular head:
   1) CMAP obtained by stimulating deep peroneal nerve at the ankle and stimulating common peroneal nerve above and below fibular head
   2) Superficial peroneal sensory conduction: often normal, but may be absent or of low amplitude if there is enough axonal injury
   3) Isolated denervation of EDB from local trauma or chronically wearing tight shoes: can cause absent responses recorded at EDB in absence of a peroneal neuropathy
   4) Otherwise, some degree of atrophy and denervation of EDB may suggest severe axonal injury in presence of a peroneal neuropathy
   5) Recording of the response at anterior tibialis muscle may reflect more accurately the degree of axonal injury and prognosis and better define the extent of the peroneal neuropathy given the commonly fascicular involvement
   6) An accessory deep peroneal nerve may be present, which should be suspected if the CMAP amplitude obtained at the knee is larger than that at the ankle
   7) Pathophysiology: primarily axonal loss
      a) Level of the lesion may not be accurately determined
      b) Sensory and motor responses may be reduced (SNAPs may be absent with severe axonal loss), and there may be mild slowing when advanced axonal injury involves the fastest fibers

8) Primarily demyelinating disease: presence of conduction block or focal slowing determines the localization

j. Needle electromyography (EMG)

1) Required for localization of peroneal neuropathy in the absence of definite, localizing conduction block

2) Short head of the biceps is the only muscle innervated by the peroneal portion of the sciatic nerve proximal to common peroneal nerve and must be examined; if abnormal, sciatic neuropathy becomes a consideration and other sciatic-innervated muscles must be examined

3. Sciatic neuropathy

a. Often occurs at hip because of proximity to hip joint

b. Most common causes: hip dislocation, fracture, perioperative associated, femur fracture, idiopathic (possibly inflammatory, less identified)

c. Other causes: external compression by prolonged sitting or lying, typically across narrow hard surfaces (including toilet seats), mass lesions in buttock (e.g., prominent vascular loop), tumors, enlargement of lesser trochanter, and, rarely, inferior gluteal venous varicosities

d. Common peroneal nerve is more predisposed to injury than the tibial portion

e. Sciatic mononeuropathy may occur with greater involvement of common peroneal portion, with subtle signs of tibial nerve involvement often present

f. Clinical signs and symptoms: variable degrees of pain, paresthesias, and weakness (often involving peroneal distribution)

g. Preferential involvement of the peroneal portion explains prominent dorsiflexion weakness and footdrop seen with milder forms

h. Prominent, concurrent weakness of tibial-innervated muscles and a flail foot may occur with severe sciatic neuropathies

i. Electrodiagnostic evaluation for suspected sciatic neuropathy

1) Nerve conduction studies: often suggest a common peroneal neuropathy (abnormal peroneal motor response)

2) Bilateral sural SNAP, H reflex, and tibial motor responses would need to be obtained for comparison

3) Asymmetry in any of these responses in addition to abnormal peroneal motor response is clue to sciatic nerve involvement

j. Tibial nerve—anatomic landmarks in order of occurrence (Fig. 21-5)

1) While in the sciatic nerve bundle, it innervates all hamstring muscles (except for short head of biceps femoris muscle) and adductor magnus (also innervated by obturator nerve)

2) First branch after separation from common peroneal nerve in the sciatic nerve bundle: sural nerve (which also receives a communicating branch from common peroneal nerve as mentioned above and supplies sensory innervation to lateral portion of the foot)

3) Dives under tendinous arch of soleus muscle and innervates soleus, gastrocnemius, tibialis posterior, flexor digitorum longus, and flexor hallucis longus muscles

4) Travels posterior to medial malleolus through tarsal tunnel to enter foot

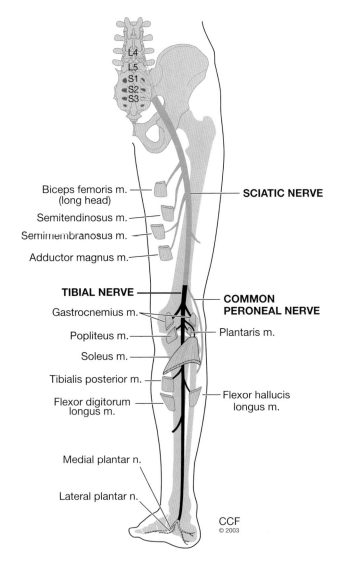

Fig. 21-5. Anatomic schema of the sciatic nerve and the tibial division. (From Katirji B, Wilbourn AJ. Mononeuropathies of the lower limb. In: Dyck PJ, Thomas PK, editors. Peripheral neuropathy. Vol 2. 4th ed. Philadelphia: Elsevier Saunders; 2005. p. 1487-510. Used with permission.)

5) Divides into three terminal branches as it runs through the tarsal tunnel underneath the flexor retinaculum
   a) First terminal branch: bundle of pure sensory nerves (calcaneal branches) supplying sensation to sole of the heel
   b) Medial plantar nerve: innervates abductor hallucis, flexor digitorum brevis, and flexor hallucis brevis muscles
   c) Lateral plantar nerve: innervates abductor digiti minimi, flexor digiti minimi, adductor hallucis, and interossei muscles

k. Tibial neuropathy proximal to the ankle
   1) May be caused by a compressive lesion (e.g., synovial cyst [Baker's cyst], fibrotic arch of soleus muscle, nerve sheath tumors)
   2) Presentation: foot pain, tenderness at the popliteal fossa or Tinel's sign, possibly weakness in more severe cases (ankle inversion, plantar flexion, and toe flexion), and absence of ankle jerks

l. Tibial neuropathy at the ankle (tarsal tunnel syndrome)
   1) Rare
   2) Caused by compression of tibial nerve or its three terminal branches as they run through the tarsal tunnel, underneath the flexor retinaculum
   3) Possible causes: idiopathic, repetitive trauma (sprains, fractures), arthritis, nerve sheath tumors, other mass lesions
   4) Possible predisposing conditions: diabetes mellitus, acromegaly, hypothyroidism
   5) Most common clinical feature: burning foot pain at the sole and ankle, often worse with weight bearing or at nighttime, and possibly paresthesias and sensory loss at sole of the foot
   6) Nerve conduction studies
      a) Tibial motor conductions recording at abductor hallucis and abductor digiti quinti may be helpful but is not sensitive (often negative)
      b) Medial and lateral plantar sensory orthodromic responses: most useful when compared with the asymptomatic side, but often normally absent
   7) Needle EMG
      a) Is used to define localization, severity
      b) Used to rule out other possibilities, such as a more proximal tibial or sciatic neuropathy
      c) Presence of occasional fibrillation potentials in intrinsic foot muscles may be normal finding and should be interpreted with caution

m. Femoral nerve—anatomic landmarks in order of occurrence (Fig. 21-6)

1) Originates predominantly from primary ventral rami of L2, L3, L4
2) Innervates psoas and iliacus muscles, runs in between these two muscles and then underneath inguinal ligament
3) Innervates all portions of quadriceps and sartorius muscles
4) Gives off three sensory branches (medial and intermediate cutaneous nerves of thigh and saphenous nerve), together supplying the medial aspect of the leg

n. Femoral neuropathy causes
   1) Most common: inflammatory (e.g., diabetic amyotrophy)

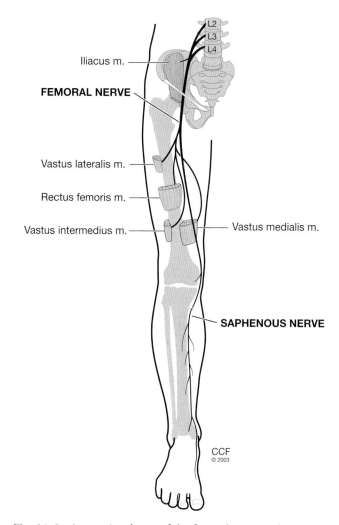

Fig. 21-6. Anatomic schema of the femoral nerve and its major sensory component, the saphenous nerve. (From Katirji B, Wilbourn AJ. Mononeuropathies of the lower limb. In: Dyck PJ, Thomas PK, editors. Peripheral neuropathy. Vol 2. 4th ed. Philadelphia: Elsevier Saunders; 2005. p. 1487-510. Used with permission.)

2) Other: isolated iatrogenic, often after abdominal and gynecologic operations, especially ones involving use of self-retracting blades, compressing the nerve between the pelvic wall and retractor

3) Lithotomy positioning, as with vaginal delivery, hysterectomy, and other surgical procedures, predisposes to unilateral or bilateral compression of femoral nerve by inguinal ligament

o. Obturator nerve—anatomic landmarks in order of occurrence

1) Originates from anterior divisions of ventral primary rami of L2, L3, L4

2) Passes in between iliacus and psoas muscles for short distance and then on the medial aspect of psoas muscle (on the edge of superior pubic ramus) and then into the obturator groove of the pubis

3) Dives into obturator foramen

4) Innervates thigh adductors (adductor magnus also has innervation from tibial division of the sciatic nerve) and gives off a sensory branch to upper medial aspect of the thigh

p. Obturator neuropathy

1) Causes: trauma, genitourinary or abdominal procedures, or vaginal delivery (especially with use of forceps)

2) Clinical features: pain in medial thigh exacerbated with exercise, weakness of thigh adduction, sometimes causing circumduction of gait

q. Lateral femoral cutaneous nerve—anatomic landmarks in order of occurrence

1) Originates from L2, 3 rami, passes over iliac crest and anterior to iliacus muscle

2) Dives under inguinal ligament (medial to anterior superior iliac spine) and enters the thigh to supply sensory innervation over lateral aspect of the thigh, not extending below the knee

r. Lateral femoral cutaneous neuropathy (*meralgia paresthetica*)

1) Usually caused by compression of the nerve by inguinal ligament

2) Predisposing factors: truncal obesity, diabetes mellitus, pregnancy

3) Clinical features: neuralgic pain, numbness, and paresthesias involving distribution of the nerve, often exacerbated with walking or standing

4) Pain may be widely distributed and may include lower back, buttock, lateral aspect of the knee, and anterolateral portion of the thigh

5) Paresthesias are usually more localized than pain to anterolateral thigh, in the distribution of lateral femoral cutaneous nerve

6) Main goal of electrodiagnosis: rule out L3 radiculopathy or femoral neuropathy, which may potentially mimic the symptoms

7) Treatment: symptomatic treatment of neuralgic pain, local corticosteroid injection, and, when intractable pain, surgical decompression of the nerve or neurolysis

s. Ilioinguinal, iliohypogastric, and genitofemoral nerves—anatomic landmarks and neuropathies

1) All predominantly arise from L1 ventral primary rami

2) Iliohypogastric and genitofemoral nerves also receive contributions from T12 and L2 rami

3) Iliohypogastric and ilioinguinal nerves pass anterior to quadratus lumborum muscle and then medial to anterior superior iliac spine and innervate lower abdominal muscles

4) Genitofemoral nerve

a) Runs over psoas muscle

b) Supplies sensory innervation over a small area on anterior aspect of proximal thigh, scrotum, and labia

c) Innervates cremasteric muscle: it is the afferent arm of the cremasteric reflex

5) Neuropathy involving these nerves

a) Most commonly the result of iatrogenic injury from genitourinary and abdominal operations (e.g., hernia repair, appendectomy)

b) Rare causes: tumors, psoas abscess (compressing genitofemoral nerve), other compressive lesions

c) Clinical features: burning pain and paresthesias in groin, scrotum, labia, and lower abdomen and bulging of lower abdomen

t. Notalgia paresthetica

1) Sensory neuropathy affecting dorsal primary rami branches of spinal nerves

2) Pain, paresthesias, hyperesthesias, pruritis in the back, sometimes resulting in well-circumscribed hyperpigmented patch in symptomatic area

3) Associated with degenerative spine disease

III. RADICULOPATHIES

A. Radiculopathy

1. Term generally applied to derangement of a ventral or dorsal spinal root or the immediate proximal spinal nerve formed by their combination

2. Synonymous with monoradiculopathy because there are alternative terms applied to disorders affecting more than one root level or more distal neural components

B. **Dermatome:** cutaneous innervation by a root segment

C. **Myotome:** muscular innervation by a root segment
1. All spinal roots have a motor component (and all but C1 have a sensory component)
2. Myotomes described in this section refer to the motor destination of each root's destination in the limbs, with emphasis on muscles easily assessed clinically or electrophysiologically
3. These muscles are innervated by ventral primary rami; dorsal primary rami innervate paraspinal muscles
   a. Cervical: Table 21-1
   b. Thoracic: except for T1, which often innervates several small muscles of the hand, ventral rami of thoracic roots primarily innervate intercostal muscles and abdominal oblique and rectus muscles according to their level in the thoracic spine
   c. Lumbosacral: Table 21-2
4. Commonly elicited muscle stretch reflexes
   a. Cervical: Table 21-3
   b. Thoracic: deep abdominal reflexes are mediated via thoracic levels T8-T12 and may be difficult to obtain in obese or multiparous patients
   c. Lumbosacral: Table 21-4

D. **Clinical Presentations**
1. Onset of symptoms may be spontaneous or associated with a precipitating event (e.g., heavy lifting)
2. Pain: most frequently the initial symptom prompting medical attention (but not always present)
   a. Pattern and progression may not be predictable
   b. Temporal profile: acute, subacute, or insidious onset
   c. Location may be variable, ranging from localized axial pain to classic radiating pain within a dermatome
   d. A specific (though not sensitive) feature of radiating pain due to a compressive lesion: worsening with cough, sneeze, or the Valsalva maneuver
   e. Cervical root pain due to compressive lesions may be alleviated with shoulder abduction and lifting hand above head

---

The suboccipital nerve (C1) usually has no sensory dermatomal innervation (pure motor) and innervates the deep muscles with insertions at the occiput (e.g., rectus capitis posterior and obliquus capitis muscles)

Table 21-1.   Cervical Myotomes: Common Root Innervations of the Most Commonly Examined Upper Limb Muscles

Muscle	C3	C4	C5	C6	C7	C8	T1
Trapezius	•	•					
Rhomboid major		•	•				
Supraspinatus			•	•			
Infraspinatus			•	•			
Deltoid			•	•			
Biceps brachii			•	•			
Triceps brachii				•	•	•	
Pronator teres				•	•		
Flexor carpi radialis				•	•		
Flexor carpi ulnaris						•	
Extensor digitorum communis					•	•	
Abductor pollicis brevis						•	•
First dorsal interosseus						•	•
Abductor digiti minimi						•	•

Table 21-2.   Lumbosacral Myotomes: Common Root Innervations of the Most Commonly Examined Lower Limb Muscles

Muscle	L2	L3	L4	L5	S1	S2	S3	S4
Iliopsoas	•	•						
Adductor longus	•	•	•					
Rectus femoris	•	•	•					
Vastus lateralis	•	•	•					
Vastus medialis	•	•	•					
Gluteus medius				•				
Gluteus maximus					•			
Biceps femoris— short head				•				
Biceps femoris— long head					•			
Anterior tibialis			•	•				
Peroneus longus				•	•			
Posterior tibialis				•				
Flexor digitorum longus				•				
Gastrocnemius					•			
Soleus						•		
Abductor hallucis					•	•		
External anal sphincter						•	•	•

Table 21-3. **Common Deep Tendon Reflexes of the Upper Limb and the Corresponding Roots**

Reflex	Root				
	C5	C6	C7	C8	T1
Biceps brachii	•	•			
Brachioradialis	•	•			
Triceps brachii			•		
Finger flexors				•	•

Table 21-4. **Common Deep Tendon Reflexes of the Lower Limb and the Corresponding Roots**

Reflex	Root				
	L2	L3	L4	L5	S1
Patellar	•	•	•		
Adductor	•	•	•		
External hamstring				•	
Achilles					•

3. Paresthesias and sensory loss
   a. Less common than pain
   b. Classically (not always): pain precedes paresthesias, paresthesias precede anesthesia
4. Weakness
   a. May develop in any radiculopathy sufficiently severe to affect motor axons
   b. May develop early or late in the course
   c. Important to recognize because of the potential for disability or prolonged convalescence after treatment of the cause
5. Recreation of compressive symptoms with
   a. Straight leg raising for lower lumbosacral radiculopathies
   b. Reverse straight leg raising for upper lumbosacral radiculopathies
   c. Spurling's maneuver: axial compression in lateral neck flexion

E. **Causes of Radiculopathy**
1. Degeneration and structural compression
   a. Spondylosis: arthropathy of facet joints and disks, associated with vertebral body osteophytes, Schmorl's nodes, synovial cysts, and extension of nucleus pulposus into the vertebral bodies
   b. Spondylolysis
      1) Separation of facet joints by a fibrous cleft at vertebral pars articularis, causing instability of facet joints, and may cause spondylolisthesis (most commonly at L4-S1 segments)
      2) May be congenital or traumatic
   c. Spondylolisthesis
      1) Anterior subluxation of one vertebral body on another, usually L5 on S1
      2) Often due to spondylotic disruption of facet joints
      3) May cause spinal stenosis if severe enough, requiring decompression surgery
   d. Disk bulges

      1) Symmetric, diffuse and circumferential bulging of disks beyond vertebral bodies
      2) Due to loss of water content from the nucleus pulposus
   e. Protrusion or extrusion of the intervertebral disk
      1) Extension of nucleus pulposus through an anular tear or fissure
      2) Most common cause of radiculopathy
      3) Collectively referred to as "disk herniation"
      4) Most common cervical roots affected: C5, C6, C7
      5) Most common lumbar roots affected: L5 and S1
      6) Location
         a) Most common: lateral and intradural (inside spinal canal)
         b) Infrequent: intradural and into nerve root sleeve or extreme lateral (transforaminal) (Fig. 21-7)
      7) Lateral protrusion of disks usually affects the nerve root exiting below the disk
         a) Example: L5-S1 disk affects the S1 root
         b) Extreme lateral protrusions may involve the root exiting above the disk, sometimes in combination with other factors such as facet arthropathy
   f. Contributing degenerative changes
      1) Facet arthropathy: enlargement of vertebral facet joints due to arthritis, which may result in dorsal encroachment on the root in the intervertebral foramen or medially
      2) Juxtafacet cysts (synovial cysts and ganglion cysts): formed by extrusion of synovial fluid or cystic degeneration of collagenous connective tissue or by other mechanisms (Fig. 21-8)
      3) Osteophytic spurs
      4) Ligamentum flavum hypertrophy
      5) Ossification of posterior longitudinal ligament
      6) Congenitally short vertebral pedicles
      7) Congenitally narrow central spinal canal
   g. Cervical spinal stenosis (cervical spondylotic myelopathy) (Fig. 21-9)

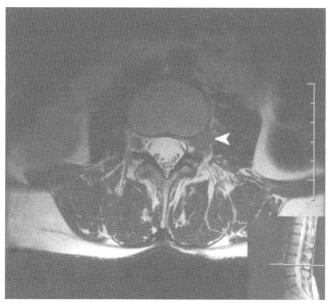

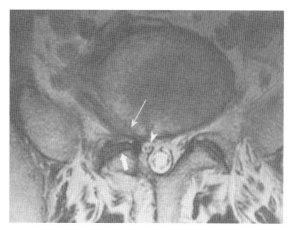

Fig. 21-8. Lateral disk protrusion (*thin arrow*), synovial cyst (*arrowhead*), and adjacent hypertrophied facet joint (*thick arrow*) together compress the traversing right S1 nerve root at the L5-S1 interspace.

Fig. 21-7. Axial T2-weighted MRI of lumbar spine demonstrates extreme lateral (transforaminal) extrusion of the nucleus pulposus of L3-L4 intervertebral disk into the neural foramen (*arrowhead*), compromising the exiting left L3 nerve root in the foramen.

1) May present with symptoms of cervical nerve root compression or irritation and/or cervical cord compression (myelopathy)
2) Usually caused by more than one aforementioned degenerative mechanism
3) Temporal profile: variable
   a) Precipitous onset (especially with trauma)
   b) Gradual onset
   c) Gradual, stepwise progression
   d) No progression, stable deficits
4) Upper motor neuron signs of spasticity and hyperreflexia below the segment of the lesion
5) Lower motor neuron findings at the segment of the lesion (reduced or absent reflexes or other sensory or motor symptoms indicative of root involvement)
6) Some patients may have Lhermitte's sign
h. Lumbar spinal stenosis
   1) May be caused by a combination of compressive lesions, including disk bulges and herniation, hypertrophy of the ligamentum flavum, facet arthropathy, and other degenerative changes discussed above
   2) Uncommon in people younger than 40 years
   3) May be asymptomatic
   4) Insidious onset of lower back pain and lower limb pain, symptoms of neurogenic claudication—

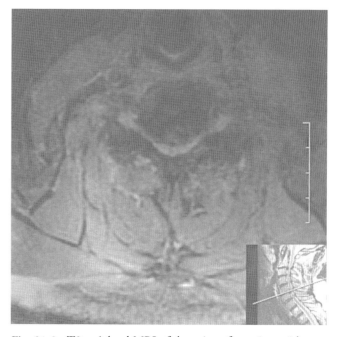

Fig. 21-9. T2-weighted MRI of the spine of a patient with severe cervical spinal stenosis (cervical spondylotic myelopathy) at level of C5-C6, with complete effacement of the subarachnoid space and marked compression and deformity of the cervical spinal cord by disk herniation and ligamentum flava hypertrophy. This patient had ligamentum flava hypertrophy throughout the entire cervical spinal canal and focal disk extrusions at multiple segments, as depicted in the sagittal T2-weighted image in the right lower corner.

important to distinguish from vascular claudication (Table 21-5)

5) Most patients do not have signs of nerve root damage
6) Bladder function often not affected
7) Lateral recess syndrome
    a) Refers to compression of nerve roots immediately before entrance into the foramina
    b) Presents with chronic, gradually progressive unilateral or bilateral symptoms of neurogenic claudication
i. Acute cauda equina syndrome (typical features)
    1) Early unilateral or asymmetric bilateral lower limb radicular pain in distribution of compressed roots
    2) With more severe involvement: asymmetric hypotonic, flaccid, areflexic weakness in myotomal distribution and sensory loss in dermatomal distribution
    3) Asymmetric saddle anesthesia
    4) Sphincter changes tend to be late in course of disease
j. Conus medullaris syndrome: typical features
    1) Symmetric flaccid weakness, areflexia, and sensory loss
    2) Symmetric saddle anesthesia
    3) Pain uncommon and not severe when present
    4) Sphincter changes tend to be early in the course of disease
k. Electrophysiologic testing (see Chapter 5)
    1) Nerve conduction studies
        a) Sensory conduction studies: normal SNAPs given the usual preganglionic localization
        b) Rare exception to the above: dorsal root ganglia in L5 and S1 segments may be located within the spinal canal and a far lateral disk herniation could potentially involve the ganglia or the postganglionic segment, and in this case, SNAPs may be affected, but this occurs much less frequently than expected
        c) CMAPs corresponding to affected nerve root may be of low amplitude
    2) Needle EMG: most useful in identifying localization and severity, and denervation in otherwise clinically asymptomatic muscles
l. MRI
    1) In normal child
        a) Very high T2 signal of both nucleus pulposus and anulus fibrosus
        b) This is gradually lost with age
    2) Anular tear: high T2 signal with or without enhancement, may be concentric, radial, or transforaminal
    3) Disk herniation: focal extension of disk material beyond the anulus, often associated with anular tear (high T2 signal in posterior anulus)

Table 21-5.   Comparison of Neurogenic Claudication From Lumbar Canal Stenosis and Vascular Claudication

Clinical feature	Neurogenic claudication (pseudo-claudication)	Vascular claudication
Sensory symptoms	May have dermatomal distribution	Never in clear dermatomal distribution (often stocking distribution)
Symptoms elicited by	Walking a variable distance or variable degree of exercise Standing for prolonged periods	Walking a fixed distance or fixed degree of exercise Prolonged standing *usually* does not provoke symptoms
Relief of symptoms with rest (cessation of walking or exercise)	Slow and variable Positional Patients often continue to have symptoms while standing, and sitting may be required	Immediate relief (within seconds) after stopping walking (including standing)
Relief of symptoms with flexing forward (e.g., holding onto grocery cart, bicycling)	Relief of symptoms	No change in symptoms
Distal lower extremity skin color and temperature and peripheral pulses	Normal (in absence of vascular disease)	Decreased

4) Facet hypertrophy and synovial cyst: variable T2 signal intensity (Fig. 21-8)
m. Treatment is determined by severity of the clinical syndrome, with more invasive therapy being appropriate in setting of refractory pain or progressing deficit
    1) Medications such as tricyclic antidepressants or anticonvulsants useful for neuropathic pain
    2) Epidural injection of anesthetics and anti-inflammatory medications
    3) Open surgical correction with laminectomy,

foraminotomy, or diskectomy, as indicated by structural derangement

2. Autoimmune and infectious inflammatory
   a. Inflammatory causes of diffuse polyradiculopathy (see below, Section IV. Polyradiculopathies and Polyradiculoneuropathies) may occasionally present with spatially restricted disease limited to a single spinal root or segment
   b. Should be considered in absence of a structural cause on imaging
   c. Varicella zoster reactivation
      1) Most common recognized cause of infectious monoradiculopathy
      2) Should be considered in presence of a dermatomal vesicular rash
   d. Diabetic monoradiculitis is likely the most common inflammatory/autoimmune monoradiculopathy

3. Traumatic
   a. Acute radiculopathy in the setting of trauma is most often associated with other injuries
   b. The force required to cause traumatic radiculopathy often injures contiguous peripheral nerves or plexi, creating difficulty in localization
   c. The most severe traumatic radiculopathies result from root avulsion, for which the prognosis of spontaneous recovery is poor (discussed below)
   d. EMG is useful in this setting
      1) Needle EMG: paraspinal muscles generally show evidence of denervation
      2) In nerve root avulsion without plexus or nerve injury, sensory nerve action potentials are preserved

4. Neoplastic
   a. Compression of nerve roots by extraneural tumors is more common than by intrinsic neural tumors
   b. Neoplastic monoradiculopathies: typically insidious in onset and progression
   c. "Intrinsic" causes of radiculopathy
      1) Schwannoma
      2) Neurofibroma
      3) Meningioma
      4) Ependymoma
      5) Paraganglioma
      6) Primitive neuroectodermal tumors
   d. Metastatic or "extrinsic" causes of radiculopathy, often from invasion of structures adjacent to the root
      1) Lymphoma
      2) Breast carcinoma
      3) Lung carcinoma
      4) Prostate carcinoma
      5) Colon carcinoma

      6) Melanoma
   e. Diagnosis: imaging characteristics, cerebrospinal fluid analysis (CSF) (nonspecifically abnormal in any leptomeningeal disease, but cytology may help identify type), ultimately biopsy

IV. POLYRADICULOPATHIES AND POLYRADICULONEUROPATHIES

A. Introduction

1. Polyradiculopathy: any disease process affecting multiple spinal roots
2. Polyradiculoneuropathy: any disease process affecting multiple spinal nerve roots and ganglionic or post-ganglionic segments of the nerves
3. Causal overlap between polyradiculoneuropathies and some causes of both radiculopathy and peripheral neuropathy
4. Severe length-dependent neuropathies that extend to proximal components of peripheral nerves may be clinically and electrophysiologically indistinguishable from polyradiculopathies; understanding the history of progression in these patients is crucial

B. Clinical Presentation

1. Sensory changes and motor dysfunction suggestive of a lower motor neuron process involving more than a single spinal nerve root, often more than a single limb
2. The following disorders may present with similar syndromes:
   a. Motor neuron disease: should not have sensory disturbance
   b. Proximal, distal, and diffuse myopathies: should not have sensory disturbance
   c. Myelopathy: associated with upper motor neuron signs and a sensory level
   d. Brachial or lumbosacral plexopathies (although there is often a clinical and pathologic overlap between plexopathies and polyradiculoneuropathies, particularly among inflammatory causes)
   e. Multiple mononeuropathies, inflammatory or noninflammatory
   f. Severe disorders of neuromuscular transmission may also present in a similar fashion: suggested by absence of sensory complaints

C. Laboratory Findings

1. Imaging
   a. Multilevel spondylotic disease readily identified with

magnetic resonance imaging (MRI) or conventional or computed tomographic (CT) myelography
   b. MRI: focal contrast enhancement of nerve roots affected by inflammatory process or diffuse leptomeningeal enhancement in meningeal metastasis
2. Serum
   a. Immune markers, suggesting multisystem or nerve-specific autoimmunity (e.g., antinuclear antibodies, antibodies to extractable nuclear antigens, rheumatoid factor, and antineutrophil cytoplasmic antibodies [ANCAs])
   b. Nerve-specific antibodies (e.g., anti-GM1 seen in multifocal motor neuropathy with conduction block, anti-GQ1b, and other ganglioside antibodies; anti-MAG (myelin-associated glycoprotein) antibodies, anti-sulfatide antibodies, and any of several paraneoplastic antibodies (particularly anti-Hu/ANNA-1 [antineuronal nuclear antibody] antibodies)
      1) Serum protein electrophoresis with immunofixation is critical for identifying nonspecific monoclonal proteins
   c. Metabolic testing for systemic disorders such as diabetes mellitus or sarcoidosis
   d. Antibodies to viruses (such as human immunodeficiency virus [HIV], cytomegalovirus [CMV], varicella-zoster virus [VZV]) and bacteria (such as *Borrelia burgdorferi*)
3. CSF
   a. A nonspecific inflammatory response consisting of elevated total protein with or without an associated cellular response
      1) Acute and chronic inflammatory polyradiculoneuropathies are notable for the "dissociated" elevation in protein without a prominent cellular response
   b. As with serum testing, antibodies suggesting infection or autoimmunity may be tested for with various degrees of sensitivity; for infections, CSF testing has added benefit of polymerase chain reaction (PCR) testing for specific entities, which may increase sensitivity in their detection
   c. Though less sensitive, cultures for viruses or atypical bacteria may be helpful if positive

D. **Electrophysiologic Findings**
1. Nerve conduction studies (NCSs)
   a. Polyradiculopathy
      1) Low-amplitude CMAPs in affected segments, with prolonged or F wave latencies
      2) Preganglionic sensory involvement: normal SNAPs
   b. Polyradiculoneuropathy
      1) Above plus slowing of conduction velocities and prolongation of distal latencies, mild in disorders primarily affecting axons and more prominent in

demyelinating processes (both motor and sensory)
      2) Temporal dispersion and focal conduction blocks in acquired demyelinating polyradiculoneuropathies
2. Needle EMG
   a. Identify degree of axonal damage
   b. Identify subclinical proximal denervation in patients presenting with clinical phenotype of length-dependent sensorimotor peripheral neuropathy
   c. Fibrillation potentials and reduced recruitment of large, complex motor unit potentials: indicative of axonal involvement
   d. Fasciculation potentials
   e. Myokymic discharges: may be seen in polyradiculopathies associated with radiation treatment or exposure (but not exclusively)
3. Normal EMG and NCS in polyradiculopathies restricted to sensory roots proximal to dorsal root ganglia (chronic immune sensory polyradiculopathy [CISP])
   a. Electrophysiologic abnormalities are noted only in somatosensory evoked potentials
   b. Spinal MRI with gadolinium contrast may be needed

E. **Causes of Polyradiculopathy and Polyradiculoneuropathy**
1. Most common causes: multilevel spondylotic disease of spine; less frequently, metastatic neoplastic disease
2. Autoimmune inflammatory (discussed below)
   a. Acute inflammatory polyradiculoneuropathy
   b. Chronic inflammatory polyradiculoneuropathy
   c. Sarcoidosis
   d. Paraproteinemias
   e. Diabetic polyradiculoneuropathies: very likely immune mediated
   f. CISP
      1) Predominantly demyelinating, immune-mediated process involving dorsal roots proximal to dorsal root ganglia
      2) Unlike in sensory polyganglionopathy, SNAPs are preserved because lesion (typically demyelinating) is preganglionic
      3) Thickened nerve roots may be demonstrated on high-resolution MRI
      4) Elevated CSF proteins
      5) Response to immune-mediated treatment: intravenous immunoglobulin, corticosteroids
3. Infectious inflammatory
   a. Viruses
      1) VZV
      2) CMV

3) HIV
4) Epstein-Barr virus (EBV)
5) Herpes simplex virus types 1 and 2
b. Bacteria
1) *Borrelia burgdorferi*
2) *Treponema pallidum*
3) *Corynebacterium diphtheriae* infection does not directly cause polyradiculoneuropathy, but exotoxin secreted by the bacteria does; may respond to antitoxin
4) In immunocompromised patients, syphilis, toxoplasmosis, or mycobacterial infections may present with polyradiculoneuropathy
5) Rarely, *Listeria monocytogenes, Chlamydia pneumoniae,* or *Brucella* species
4. Degenerative (structural): multilevel spondylotic disease of the spine
a. Likely the most common cause of polyradiculopathy
b. Usually results from multiple degenerative processes
c. May be associated with myelopathy
5. Neoplastic
a. Tumors of peripheral nerve origin: multiple and plexiform neurofibromas; less commonly, schwannomas, perineuromas
b. Metastatic disease
1) Diffuse leptomeningeal metastasis or focal involvement of individual roots
2) Sources of metastasis commonly include
a) Lymphoma (may rarely present primarily in the root)
b) Breast carcinoma
c) Lung carcinoma
d) Prostate carcinoma
e) Colon carcinoma
f) Melanoma
g) Primitive neuroectodermal tumors with intraxial metastasis

V.   SENSORY POLYGANGLIONOPATHY

A.   Overview
1. Predominant insult at level of dorsal root ganglion
2. Different causes clinically indistinguishable (serologic testing may be helpful)

B.   Etiology
1. Paraneoplastic
2. Nonmalignant inflammatory
3. Toxic: pyridoxine, cisplatin, paclitaxel
4. Idiopathic

C.   General Clinical Manifestations (heterogeneous, variable)
1. Subacute or chronic onset of sensory symptoms
2. Three different patterns of fiber type involvement
a. Patchy, painful dysesthesias becoming widespread in distribution
b. Prominent proprioceptive loss
1) Sensory ataxia (exacerbated in the dark)
2) "Pseudoathetosis" of the hands
c. Combination of the above
3. Generalized areflexia
4. Variable degree of autonomic impairment, which may be asymptomatic
5. Preserved strength unless more widespread nervous system involvement

D.   Nerve Conduction Studies
1. Widespread absence or severe reduction of SNAP amplitudes
2. Relatively normal motor conduction studies and EMG

E.   Paraneoplastic
1. Associated cancers
a. Most common: small cell lung cancer
b. Also common: breast, prostate, ovary, neuroblastoma, and germ cell tumors
2. Antibodies
a. ANNA-1 (anti-Hu) neuronal antibodies in serum ± CSF
b. Frequently occurs in association with other paraneoplastic syndromes: encephalomyelitis, autonomic neuropathy, cerebellar degeneration

F.   Nonmalignant Inflammatory
1. Associated with Sjögren's syndrome and other autoimmune disorders and paraproteinemias (Fig. 21-10)
2. Key features of Sjögren's syndrome-related cases
a. Dry eyes, dry mouth
b. Positive Schirmer's test
c. Antibodies to extractable nuclear antigens (anti-Ro/SSA or anti-La/SSB)
d. Lymphocytic infiltrates on minor salivary gland biopsy

G.   Differential Diagnosis
1. Features favoring paraneoplastic cause
a. Subacute presentation and rapidly progressive course
b. Coexistent multifocal nervous system involvement (autonomic, cerebral cortex, spinal cord, cerebellum)
c. High CSF protein and/or lymphocytosis
d. Paraneoplastic serologic tests
1) Highly associated with cancer

2) Initially, cancer may not be detectable, and specific neurologic syndrome or antibody may not predict specific primary cancer
2. Other ataxic sensory syndromes
   a. Vitamin B$_{12}$ deficiency
   b. Tabes dorsalis
   c. Spinocerebellar ataxia
   d. CISP

H. Treatment and Prognosis
1. Prognosis for recovery tends to be poor, given absence of effective regeneration of sensory ganglion cells after destruction
2. Primary aim of treatment: prevent further ganglion cell loss
3. Paraneoplastic: antitumor therapy is more effective than immune-modulating therapy
4. Inflammatory
   a. No randomized controlled data
   b. Anecdotal reports of benefit with various immune-mediated treatments

VI. BRACHIAL PLEXOPATHIES

A. Traumatic Plexopathies (and root avulsions)
1. Result of direct trauma (open or closed, shear injury to nerves), secondary to injury of surrounding structures,

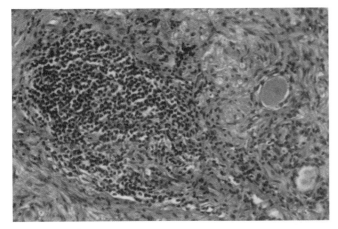

Fig. 21-10. Inflammatory sensory ganglionopathy. Microscopic examination of a dorsal root ganglion from a patient with Sjögren's syndrome shows mononuclear inflammatory infiltrates. (From Grant IA. Treatment of nonmalignant sensory ganglionopathies. In: Noseworthy JH, editor. Neurological therapeutics: principles and practice. Vol 2. New York: Martin Dunitz; 2003. p. 2070-77. By permission of Mayo Foundation.)

and iatrogenic
2. Upper plexus traumatic lesions (sometimes called Erb-Duchenne palsy)
   a. Often associated with C5 and C6 root avulsions
   b. Present with internally rotated arm, extended at elbow
3. Lower plexus traumatic lesions (sometimes called Dejerine-Klumpke palsy)
   a. Often associated with C8 and T1 root avulsions
   b. Present with intrinsic hand muscle weakness and atrophy ("claw hand" deformity)
4. Supraclavicular plexopathies: more common and more severe than infraclavicular plexopathies
5. Traction injuries occur when heavy objects fall on the shoulder or when patient falls on the shoulder, causing a supraclavicular traumatic plexopathy (more frequent than infraclavicular); upper plexus is most often damaged with closed traction injuries
6. There may be associated nerve root avulsion
   a. Worse prognosis: persistent, irreversible loss of function and intractable pain, often within 2 weeks after insult
   b. C8 and T1 roots are likely more vulnerable to avulsion injury (C5 and C6 roots are protected by fascia and bone as they exit the foramina, despite vulnerability of the upper plexus to traumatic injury)
   c. Nerve root avulsions usually cause severe deficits and pain in distribution of affected nerve
   d. Features suggestive of nerve root avulsions: complete plexopathy, intractable and severe burning pain in the hand, ipsilateral hemidiaphragm paralysis, traumatic meningocele or absence of nerve roots on neuroimaging, paraspinal fibrillation potentials and normal SNAPs, with low-amplitude or absent CMAPs
7. The primary roots are vulnerable to avulsion from traction injury because they are short and lack epineural and perineural sheaths that protect the nerves
8. Classic postoperative paralysis
   a. Often results from brachial plexus traction during surgery under general anesthesia
   b. Usually affects the upper plexus more severely
   c. Symptoms often present immediately after the operation
9. Obstetric paralysis: brachial plexus traction injuries of infants sustained during birth
   a. Occurs more frequently with complicated deliveries requiring instrumentation or those with less desirable fetal presentations (e.g., breech presentation)
   b. Predisposing risk factors: fetal macrosomia and maternal obesity and diabetes
   c. Mechanism of injury: possibly traction injury on the plexus
   d. Most often involves the upper plexus (Erb-Duchenne

palsy); less commonly, lower plexus (Dejerine-Klumpke palsy) or entire plexus

10. Burner syndrome: traumatic plexopathy caused by sudden forceful depression of shoulder and head, almost always due to certain contact sports

  a. Symptoms: acute-onset dysesthetic pain and weakness, often involving entire upper limb (unilateral), usually short duration

  b. Attacks typically resolve promptly and completely

  c. Residual weakness if attacks are unusually severe and/or numerous

  d. Almost all patients have neurogenic changes on needle EMG

  e. Clinical abnormalities are almost always restricted to upper plexus

11. Pack palsy (rucksack paralysis): weakness and paresthesias involving upper plexus, attributed to compression of upper plexus by backpack straps

B. **Neoplastic Plexopathy**

1. Secondary

  a. Lymphatic spread (most common mechanism): metastasis involving lymph nodes adjacent to the lower portion of plexus and nerves (most often lung or breast cancer)

  b. Direct extension of primary tumor (e.g., non–small cell bronchogenic carcinoma involving lung apex)

  c. Pancoast's syndrome

    1) Symptom complex referring to tumors involving lung apex

    2) These tumors most often affect lower brachial plexus (C8, T1 distribution)

    3) Presentation: pain and paresthesias in C8, T1 dermatomal distribution, Horner's syndrome, and motor involvement (weakness and atrophy of intrinsic hand muscles, thenar and hypothenar muscle groups)

  d. Treatment: often perioperative radiotherapy and resection

2. Primary: nerve sheath tumors (most common)

  a. Most often involve upper brachial plexus (C5, C6 distribution) and supraclavicular in location

  b. Primary neoplasms often cause limb pain, dysesthesias, and palpable mass; symptoms are often reproduced with palpation of the superficial tumor

  c. Most common: benign neurofibromas; more common in women (than men) and adults (than children)

  d. Next most common primary tumor: benign schwannoma

3. Radiation-induced plexopathy is main differential diagnostic consideration in patients who have received radiotherapy

C. **Radiation Plexopathy**

1. Typically, slowly progressive, long duration

2. Predominant symptom of paresthesias (much less pain than neoplastic or compressive etiology) and painless weakness

3. Primarily in distribution of upper brachial plexus

4. Features suggestive of radiation-induced plexopathy: predominance of paresthesias, slowly progressive history with presence of myokymia on EMG examination

5. Features suggestive of a cause other than radiation: rapidly progressive painful syndrome with onset of symptoms less than 6 months after radiotherapy

6. Three different presentations

  a. Onset within a few days after radiation: permanent, painless weakness and sensory loss from radiation-induced ischemic injury and occlusion of subclavian artery

  b. Reversible sensory symptoms, often paresthesias (often resolving in 6-12 months)

  c. Delayed onset of progressive and permanent motor and sensory loss from radiation-induced fibrosis (onset of symptoms may vary from several weeks to >30 years), slow progression throughout several years (radiotherapy induces primary demyelination, followed by axonal loss after several years)

7. Relative sparing of lower plexus may be explained partly by "protective" effects of the clavicle

8. Pancoast's tumor tends to involve lower brachial plexus, whereas radiation-induced plexopathy is primarily an upper brachial plexus syndrome

9. Pathophysiology: vascular endothelial thickening and resultant obliteration of microvasculature, and radiation-induced endoneural and perineural fibrosis

10. Electrophysiology

  a. Reduced SNAP and CMAP amplitudes

  b. SNAPs are usually most sensitive, show earliest abnormalities, and may be unobtainable when the process is advanced

  c. Supraclavicular stimulation may show conduction block

  d. Needle EMG examination often shows denervation, neuropathic changes, and possibly myokymic discharges

11. 3-T MRI may be helpful in differentiating infiltrative, expansile neoplastic (recurrence) plexopathy from postradiation changes: the latter often have nonexpansile, isolated T2 signal change, or may be normal

12. Poor prognosis: progressive course, no treatment

D. **Immune-Mediated Brachial Plexus Neuropathy** (also called neuralgic amyotrophy, Parsonage-Turner syndrome, idiopathic brachial plexus neuropathy)

1. Sporadic, immune-mediated (hereditary brachial plexus neuropathy is described below)
2. Males affected more frequently than females
3. Multiple episodes often occur with familial brachial plexus neuropathies, whereas sporadic brachial plexus neuropathies are often monophasic and unilateral
4. Clinical features
   a. Abrupt onset of severe pain (with tendency to occur at night and wake patient from sleep), which often lasts several days to weeks
   b. Patients tend to immobilize the arm but do not experience exacerbation of pain with the Valsalva maneuver
   c. Absence of pain (although atypical) does not rule out this diagnosis: reports of patients with painless Parsonage-Turner syndrome
   d. Pain is less frequent in pediatric patients with this condition
   e. Weakness becomes apparent after pain subsides, usually present after the third week
   f. Atrophy of affected muscle groups becomes evident later
5. Distribution of involvement
   a. Often patchy
   b. Tendency to affect pure motor nerves: long thoracic, anterior interosseous, posterior interosseous, supra-scapular, axillary nerves
   c. Also reported: fascicular involvement of musculo-cutaneous nerve
   d. Some nerves that do not arise from brachial plexus may also be involved (e.g., phrenic and spinal accessory nerves)
   e. Bilateral phrenic nerve involvement often causes dyspnea and orthopnea
6. Antecedent conditions: flulike syndrome or upper respiratory infection, postoperative (surgery at a distant site), immunization (e.g., hepatitis B vaccine), medications (interferons, lamotrigine, botulinum toxin), pregnancy, systemic vasculitis (e.g., giant cell arteritis, systemic lupus erythematosus, rheumatoid arthritis)
7. Electrodiagnosis: multifocal or patchy evidence of axonal loss on EMG and NCS
8. Pathology
   a. Not well understood
   b. Reports of epineural and endoneural mononuclear inflammatory infiltrates, microvasculitis
9. Neuroimaging (MRI)
   a. Helpful to exclude structural causes
   b. May show increased T2 signal of plexus or denervated skeletal muscles
10. CSF: often normal, may show elevated protein

11. Treatment
    a. Corticosteroids, intravenous immunoglobulin, or plasmapheresis may be tried in acute stage
    b. Improvement in pain with corticosteroids in several large open series is noted and appears dose-related
    c. Other outcomes (strength, sensory loss, length) are not established with either corticosteroids or other immune therapies
12. Prognosis
    a. Good prognosis for recovery: 89% in 3 years
    b. Resolution of pain: usually in several weeks
    c. Recovery of weakness and atrophy: depends on extent of involvement (patients with upper trunk lesions recover sooner, partly because proximal muscles are reinnervated sooner)
    d. Recovery of phrenic nerve involvement (and diaphragmatic weakness): usually late, tends to be incomplete (given the longer distance)

E. **True Neurogenic Thoracic Outlet Syndrome** (cervical rib and band syndrome)
1. Rare nontraumatic cause of supraclavicular plexopathy caused by a bony defect (a rudimentary cervical rib arising from C7 vertebra or elongated C7 transverse process)
2. Fibrous band may extend from the bony anomaly to first thoracic rib, often compressing T1 ventral primary rami or lower plexus
3. Symptoms involve lower brachial plexus: paresthesias and mild discomfort involving medial aspect of upper extremity, usually present with atrophy and weakness of thenar and intrinsic hand muscles
4. Plain film of neck: often adequate for diagnosis of the cervical rib
5. Fibrous band: usually not seen on plain films and frequently missed on CT or MRI

F. **Lumbosacral Plexopathies**
1. Neoplastic plexopathy
   a. Uncommon cause of lumbosacral plexopathy
   b. Caused by direct invasion or compression of plexus by tumor
   c. Colorectal, genitourinary (ovary, uterus, prostate), breast, lymphoma are most common types of secondary tumors to cause this condition (most common is locally invasive colorectal carcinoma)
   d. Unilateral more than bilateral plexus involvement
   e. Severe pain, followed by weakness and sensory loss
   f. Diagnosis: usually made with MRI or CT
   g. Therapy

1) Depends on lesion
2) Local radiotherapy is variably effective for pain

2. Retroperitoneal hemorrhage
   a. Often associated with therapeutic anticoagulation, trauma, or pelvic fracture
   b. Hematoma of iliacus muscle
      1) Causes intrapelvic femoral nerve compression
      2) Presents with pain in groin or lower iliac fossa radiating to anterior thigh and medial lower leg
   c. Hematoma of the psoas muscle
      1) Produces intrapelvic lumbar plexus compression
      2) Deficits in the distributions of femoral and obturator nerves
   d. Patients may assume a flexed posture to decrease pain by flexing and externally rotating the hip
   e. Diagnosis: CT of abdomen and pelvis

3. Pregnancy-related
   a. Presentation: usually postpartum from direct compression of the plexus on one or both sides by infant's head during its decent
   b. May also occur during latter part of third trimester, especially if a mass such as uterine leiomyoma compresses lumbosacral plexus
   c. Primigravida women of short stature are at risk
   d. Other risk factors: infant macrosomia, protracted labor, midpelvic forceps delivery, cephalopelvic disproportion
   e. Symptoms: commonly present with footdrop, with sensory loss often in lateral aspect of distal lower extremity and dorsum of the foot; bilateral in one-fourth of cases
   f. Prognosis: good, complete recovery is expected (usually within 3 months)

4. Radiation-induced
   a. Typically presents about 5 years (range ,1-31 years) after the radiotherapy
   b. Typical presentation: slow, progressive leg weakness (often bilateral); less often, paresthesias and numbness
   c. May be associated with *mild* pain (severe pain experienced with plexopathies related to malignant infiltration is atypical)
   d. Symptoms typically start in distal aspect of affected lower limb(s) (as compared with plexopathies due to neoplastic infiltration, which are typically proximal in distribution)

   e. Electrophysiologic characteristics mimic those of radiation-induced brachial plexopathy discussed above, including presence of myokymia
   f. CSF: protein may be elevated
   g. Imaging and potentially site-directed biopsy: may help distinguish between infiltrative and radiation-induced changes

5. Traumatic
   a. Uncommon; caused by falls or motor vehicle accidents
   b. Mostly caused by double vertical fracture-dislocations of bony pelvic ring, also with fracture-dislocation of hip joint and acetabulum
   c. May be associated with root avulsions
   d. Weakness commonly affecting lumbosacral trunk (L5- and S1-innervated muscles); may also affect obturator and superior gluteal nerves and ventral primary rami of L5 and sacral roots
   e. The weakness may be overshadowed by pelvic pain, but this diagnosis needs to be considered in patients with persistent leg weakness following pelvic fracture

6. Immune-mediated nondiabetic lumbosacral plexus neuropathy
   a. The "leg equivalent" of neuralgic brachial amyotrophy
   b. Subacute to acute onset of pain: may be anterior thigh with lumbar predominance or posterior thigh and buttock area with sacral predominance, may mimic disk because of distribution and rapidity of onset
   c. Weakness becomes apparent as pain disappears
   d. Pathology: microvasculitis and local nerve ischemic injury, similar to changes seen in diabetic amyotrophy (described below)
   e. Acute painful plexopathy with stepwise progression may be seen in systemic vasculitis
   f. There is often associated weight loss and sometimes increased erythrocyte sedimentation rate (ESR), in the absence of other rheumatologic markers
   g. Adequate data for treatment are lacking, but open trials with intravenous methylprednisolone reduced progression and helped pain
   h. Intravenous immunoglobulin may also be helpful

7. Diabetic lumbosacral plexus neuropathy (diabetic amyotrophy) (see Part B of this chapter)

Disorders of the Peripheral Nervous System

Part B: Specific Inherited and Acquired Disorders of the Peripheral Nervous System

Dean H. Kilfoyle, M.B., Ch.B.

Lyell K. Jones, M.D.

Nima Mowzoon, M.D.

I. Hereditary Neuropathies

A. Overview

1. Inherited neuropathies include disorders that primarily affect the PNS only (e.g., Charcot-Marie-Tooth disease, hereditary motor and sensory neuropathy), the PNS and CNS (e.g., spinocerebellar ataxia) and disorders that have systemic organ involvement (e.g., Fabry's disease) (Table 21-6)
2. Classification schemes

    a. Hereditary motor and sensory neuropathy (HMSN), also called Charcot-Marie-Tooth (CMT) disease: motor predominant sensory and motor-length dependent peripheral neuropathy

    b. Hereditary sensory and autonomic neuropathy (HSAN): small-fiber sensory neuropathy with variable degree of autonomic neuropathy

    c. Spinocerebellar ataxia (SCA): autosomal dominant inherited cerebellar ataxia with variable degree of peripheral neuropathy

Table 21-6. **Summary of Inherited Neuropathies**

Condition	Inheritance	Gene(s)	Nerve conduction study	Other
Motor/sensory				
HMSN I	AD	*PMP22* (Ia)	D	Onion bulbs
		MPZ (Ib)		
HMSN II	AD		A	
HMSN X	XLR	*Cx32*	D>A	
HNPP	AD	*PMP22* deletion	D	Tomaculae
Sensory/autonomic				
HSAN I	AD	*SPTLC1*	A	Onset in 2nd or later decade
HSAN II	AR	Unknown	A	Childhood onset
HSAN III	AR	*IKBKAP*	A	Autonomic
Multisystem—Metabolic				
MTLD	AR	Arylsulfatase	D	Metachromatic granules
Krabbe's disease	AR	*GALC*	D	Globoid cells in CNS
Fabry's disease	XLR	Galactosidase A	A	Angiokeratoma
Refsum's disease	AR	Phytanoyl-Co hydroxylase	D	Phytanic acid
Multisystem—other				
TTR amyloidosis	AD	Transthyretin	A	Congophilia
Kennedy's disease	XLR	Androgen receptor	A	Gynecomastia
Freidreich's ataxia	AR	Frataxin (GAA rpt)	A	

A, axonal; AD, autosomal dominant; AR, autosomal recessive; CNS, central nervous system; D, demyelinating; HMSN, hereditary motor and sensory neuropathy; HNPP, hereditary neuropathy with liability to pressure palsies; HSAN, hereditary sensory and autonomic neuropathy; MTLD, metachromatic leukodystrophy; XLR, X-linked recessive.

d. Spinal muscular atrophy (SMA), also called hereditary motor neuronopathy (HMN): autosomal recessive lower motor neuronopathy

2. Important additional individual inherited neuropathies include
   a. Hereditary neuropathy with liability to pressure palsies (HNPP)
   b. Hereditary brachial plexitis
   c. Friedreich's ataxia
   d. Kennedy's disease
   e. Transthyretin amyloidosis

3. Many inherited metabolic multisystem disorders may also cause neuropathy
   a. Lipid metabolism disorders (Krabbe's disease, metachromatic leukodystrophy)
   b. Lipoprotein deficiency (Tangier disease, cerebrotendinous xanthomatosis)
   c. Peroxisomal disorders (Fabry's disease)
   d. Mitochondrial disorders (Kearns-Sayre syndrome)
   e. Defective DNA maintenance (xeroderma pigmentosum, ataxia-telangiectasia)
   f. Porphyrias (acute intermittent)

B. General Principles

1. Most common pattern of inheritance is autosomal dominant—exceptions are
   a. X-Linked
      1) HMSN X
      2) Fabry's disease
      3) Kennedy's disease
   b. Autosomal recessive
      1) Most of the metabolic disorders
      2) HMSN IV
      3) HSAN II-V
      4) Friedreich's ataxia

2. In assessing an apparently sporadic idiopathic neuropathy: evaluation of asymptomatic family members may show subclinical neuropathy confirming the inherited etiology

3. Phenotypic variability: considerable within each condition and even within individual kinships

4. Phenotypic overlap (within and between classification schemes): an example is HMSN II and HSAN I, between which it may be difficult to distinguish

5. Clues to inherited etiology
   a. Family history
      1) May be lacking in autosomal recessive or X-linked recessive conditions
      2) May be subclinical in other family members (because of variable expression)

Molecular Genetics

Peripheral myelin protein 22 (*PMP22*)
   Compact myelin
   Duplicated in CMT 1a, deleted in HNPP

Myelin protein zero (*MPZ, P0*)
   Compact myelin
   Adhesion molecule
   Point mutation of *P0* in CMT 1B, some cases of CMT 2

Connexin 32 (*Cx32* or *GJB1*)
   Uncompacted paranodal myelin
   Gap junction protein
   CMT X

Transthyretin (*TTR*)
   Familial amyloidosis

IKBKAP
   Essentially all cases of HSAN III with full penetrance
   Important for carrier detection and egg selection

SMN1
   Commonly deleted in patients with SMA1-3
   Involvement of additional genes (*SMN2, NAIP*) responsible for variable expression

Trinucleotide repeat diseases of peripheral nerve
   Frataxin (Freidreich's ataxia) GAA
   Polyglutamine diseases (CAG)
      Androgen receptor (Kennedy's disease)
      Ataxin (SCA 1,2,3)

---

   3) Male-to-male inheritance: excludes X-linked recessive conditions (may partially manifest in females and mimic autosomal dominant pattern) and also inherited mitochondrial DNA mutations (caveat: nuclear DNA encodes some mitochondrial proteins)
   b. Pes cavus (Fig. 21-11)
   c. Insidious onset, very slow progression over years to decades
   d. Usually symmetric, length-dependent pattern
   e. General lack of positive sensory symptoms
      1) Prominent paresthesias more common in acquired neuropathy
      2) Common finding: marked sensory loss on examination to which the patient is symptomatically unaware,

Inherited Neuropathy Spot Diagnoses

History
    Abdominal pain: porphyria, MNGIE,
        MEN2B

Clinical
    Orange tonsils: Tangier disease
    Angiokeratoma: Fabry's disease
    Retinitis pigmentosa: HMSN VII, SCA 7,
        Refsum's disease, mitochondrial disease
    Hypertrophic nerves: HMSN I, Refsum's
        disease, Dejerine-Sottas disease (HMSN III)
    Hypotelorism, short stature: hereditary
        brachial plexopathy
    Absence of fungiform tongue papillae:
        HSAN IV
    Tongue nodules: MEN2B
    Tightly curled hair: giant axonal neuropathy
    Gynacomastia: Kennedy's disease
    Extensor plantars and absent ankle reflex:
        Friedreich's ataxia, but also vitamin B_{12}
        deficiency
    Cardiomyopathy: amyloidosis, Friedreich's
        ataxia, Fabry's disease

Laboratory
    Very low level of HDL cholesterol: Tangier disease
    Elevated serum phytanic acid: Refsum's disease

Electrodiagnostic
    Disproportionate prolongation of distal motor
        latencies: HNPP, but also anti-MAG–related
        neuropathy

Pathology
    Onion bulbs: HMSN I, Refsum's disease,
        Dejerine-Sottas disease, CIDP
    Tomaculae: HNPP, less prominently in
        HMSN I, CIDP
    Giant axons with dense cytoplasm: giant
        axonal neuropathy
    Brown granules in Schwann cell cytoplasm:
        metachromatic leukodystrophy
    Apple-green birefringence: TTR, gelsolin or
        Apo A-I familial amyloidosis

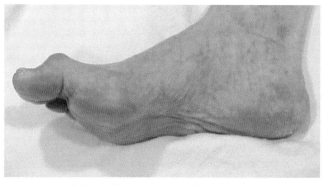

Fig. 21-11. Skeletal abnormalities of the foot of a patient with hereditary neuropathy. Note prominent pes cavus (high longitudinal arch of the foot) and hammer-toe deformity.

    a. Demyelinating motor predominant neuropathy:
        HMSN I
    b. Axonal motor predominant neuropathy: HMSN II
    c. Small-fiber sensory predominant: HSAN I
  7. Demyelinating inherited neuropathies
    a. HMSN I
    b. Dejerine-Sottas neuropathy
    c. HMSN IV
    d. HMSN X
    e. Refsum's disease
    f. Metachromatic leukodystrophy
    g. Globoid cell leukodystrophy (Krabbe's disease)
    h. Adrenomyeloneuropathy
    i. Mitochondrial neurogastrointestinal encephalopathy
        (MNGIE), also called myopathy, neuropathy, gastro-
        intestinal encephalopathy
    j. Leigh disease
    k. Caveat
        1) Many patients with a long-standing inherited
            demyelinating neuropathy develop axon loss
        2) Low-amplitude sensory and motor responses on
            NCSs and long-duration motor unit potentials on
            needle EMG are indicative of axonal loss (fibrillation
            potentials are relatively mild or absent)
  8. Inherited neuropathies with specific treatments
    a. Fabry's disease: enzyme replacement
    b. Transthyretin amyloidosis: liver transplantation
    c. Refsum's disease: phytanic acid–free diet
    d. Kennedy's disease: possible role for antiandrogen therapy

C.   Hereditary Motor and Sensory Neuropathy (HMSN)
1. Overview
    a. Genetically and phenotypically heterogeneous group of
        disorders

    sometimes with dire consequences (e.g., acral
        mutilation)
      3) Exception: spontaneous neuropathic pain of HSAN
6. Most common conditions

b. Characterized by symmetric, length-dependent, motor-predominant, sensory and motor peripheral neuropathy
c. Pathology may be predominantly axonal loss or demyelinating
d. Except for rare types V, VI, and VII, these disorders are usually restricted to PNS
2. HMSN I (CMT 1)
  a. Autosomal dominant
  b. Demyelinating neuropathy (predominantly, with late axonal changes)
  c. Pathology (Fig. 21-12)
    1) Onion bulbs: repeated cycles of demyelination and remyelination result in nerve fibers surrounded by concentric layers of Schwann cell cytoplasmic processes resembling layers of an onion
    2) Axonal loss
      a) Affects both myelinated and unmyelinated fibers
      b) Extent of axonal loss determines clinical severity: earlier axonal loss often causes slower conduction velocities on electrophysiologic testing
  d. Genetics
    1) HMSN Ia
      a) Duplication of segment of chromosome 17 (17p11.2-12) containing the peripheral myelin protein 22 gene (*PMP22*): the most commonly identified genetic abnormality in HMSN I group (approximately 75% of cases)
      b) De novo duplication of *PMP22*: approximately 10% of HMSN Ia cases
      c) Less common cause of HMSN Ia: point mutations of *PMP22*, often associated with a more severe neuropathy than patients with duplication
      d) PMP 22 is produced in Schwann cells, where it is a membrane protein in compact myelin and has a role in maintaining myelin integrity
    2) HMSN Ib
      a) Due to point mutations of gene encoding myelin protein zero (*MPZ* or *P0*)

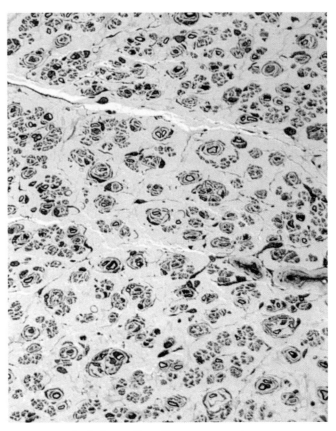

Fig. 21-12. Pathology of hereditary motor and sensory neuropathy (HMSN) I. Sural nerve biopsy specimen from a patient with autosomal recessive HMSN-Lom mutation demonstrating severe loss of myelinated fibers and a few poorly developed onion bulbs that appear as concentric encirclements of Schwann cells around axons. (From Gabreëls-Festen A, Thomas PK. Autosomal recessive hereditary motor and sensory neuropathies. In: Dyck PJ, Thomas PK, editors. Peripheral neuropathy. Vol 2. 4th ed. Philadelphia: Elsevier Saunders; 2005. p. 1769-90. Used with permission.)

      b) Accounts for approximately 5% of cases of HMSN I
      c) New mutations not uncommon, so there may be no family history
      d) MPZ is expressed by Schwann cells and is major protein of peripheral nerve myelin
      e) MPZ: a transmembrane protein; probably serves as adhesion molecule holding together adjacent myelin lamellae
      f) Almost 100 different *MPZ* mutations have been described
      g) Some of these mutations present in infancy with profound conduction slowing and a severe phenotype, others present in mid-adulthood with

---

HMSN I

Usually inherited in autosomal dominant fashion

Distinguished from HMSN II by slowed conduction velocities (normal in HMSN II)

Distinguished from CIDP by lack of temporal dispersion or conduction block

variable degrees of slowing and severity
  h) Late-onset HMSN Ib cases can be confused with chronic inflammatory demyelinating polyradiculoneuropathy (CIDP) due to sporadic onset and intermediate conduction velocities
  3) HMSN Id
  a) Due to mutations of early growth response 2 gene (*EGR2*)
  b) Unlike PMP 22, MPZ, and connexin 32 protein (Cx32) (all transmembrane myelin proteins), EGR 2 is a transcription factor and is likely responsible for activating expression of these other myelin proteins
  4) Other rare subtypes include HMSN Ic and HMSN If
  e. Clinical features: typical phenotype
  1) Age at onset varies, most typically in second decade
  2) Some patients may remain asymptomatic throughout life or present in late adulthood
  3) Insidious onset and slow progression
  4) Length-dependent symmetric pattern: feet then hands
  a) Pes cavus, hammer toes
  b) Weakness of intrinsic hand and feet muscles and peroneal-innervated muscles
  c) Distal hyporeflexia or areflexia
  d) Reduced large-fiber (vibration and touch) sensory modalities in feet and later in hands
  e) Distal atrophy with inverted "champagne bottle" legs: characteristic but relatively uncommon, late finding (Fig. 21-13)
  5) Some patients have upper limb action tremor: this group has been termed the "Roussy-Levy syndrome," but probably not a distinct genetic entity
  6) Palpable nerve hypertrophy in approximately 25% of patients
  7) Rare respiratory, cranial, and autonomic involvement
  8) HMSN Ib tends to be more severe disorder than HMSN Ia, but otherwise they are clinically and electrophysiologically indistinguishable
  f. Laboratory: normal CSF cell count and protein
  g. Electrodiagnosis
  1) NCS (primarily demyelinating pattern)
  a) Upper limb motor conduction velocity: less than 38 m/s, usually about 20 m/s
  b) Generally, conduction velocities are less than 75% of lower limit of normal
  c) In contrast to acquired demyelinating neuropathy, conduction slowing is uniform (e.g., similar conduction velocity in median and ulnar forearm segments) and not associated with conduction block or temporal dispersion

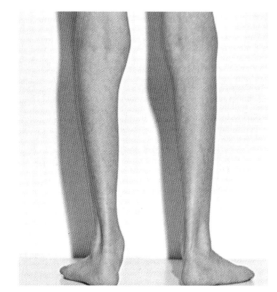

Fig. 21-13. Distal atrophy with inverted "champagne bottle" legs of a patient with hereditary motor and sensory neuropathy type I (HMSN I).

  d) Distal latencies are prolonged early in the disease
  e) Distal lower limb axonal changes: common in more advanced or long-standing cases
  f) Reduced CMAP amplitudes with advanced disease (correlates with degree of axonal loss)
  2) EMG evidence of distal reinnervation with little denervation
  h. HMSN I vs. CIDP
  1) Younger onset vs. late adulthood (exceptions—rare, early-onset CIDP and occasional late-onset sporadic cases of HMSN Ib [MPZ])
  2) Slow, steady progression over years vs. subacute or chronic relapsing
  3) Uniform conduction slowing without conduction block or temporal dispersion more common in HMSN I
  i. Treatment
  1) No specific therapy
  2) Appropriate footwear if foot deformity
  3) Ankle foot orthoses if severe footdrop
  j. Prognosis
  1) Early childhood onset often associated with severe neuropathy
  2) Later onset cases associated with normal life expectancy, many patients maintain independent ambulation because of relatively preserved proximal strength
3. HMSN II (CMT 2)
  a. Autosomal dominant

b. Axonal neuropathy

c. Genetics

   1) Heterogeneous and less well defined than HMSN I

   2) At least 6 subtypes (a-f) by linkage analysis

   3) Some specific genes identified

      a) HMSN IIa: *MFN2* and *KIF1B*

      b) HMSN IIb: *RAB7*, may also present similar to HSAN I

      c) HMSN IId: *GARS*, may also present as motor neuronopathy

      d) HMSN IIe: *NFL*

   4) Most of patients in this group do not have an identifiable or known genetic abnormality; exception is *MFN2* gene

      a) May account for up to 20% of patients with CMT 2, particularly in those presenting in childhood

      b) *MFN2* is a nuclear gene that encodes the mitochondrial protein mitofusin 2

      c) Deficient mitofusin 2 results in inability of mitochondria to fuse or move along microtubules during fast anterograde axonal transport, thus depriving the distal axon of an energy source

d. Clinical features

   1) Generally indistinguishable from HMSN I without NCSs

   2) Tendency to present later in life and develop less upper limb weakness than HMSN I

   3) Patients with this condition may be mistaken for idiopathic sensorimotor peripheral neuropathy, if careful family history and evaluation are not obtained

   4) HMSN IIb: severe sensory loss

   5) HMSN IIc: diaphragm and/or vocal cord paresis

   6) HMSN IId: upper limb involvement early in disease course

e. Electrodiagnosis

   1) NCSs (features predominantly axonal): reduced SNAPs and CMAPs, with EMG evidence of reinnervation and mild denervation

4. HMSN III (Dejerine-Sottas disease)

a. Overview

   1) Infantile onset of severe demyelinating neuropathy with profound slowing of conduction velocities

   2) Genetically heterogeneous; has been described with mutations of *PMP22*, *MPZ*, and *EGR2*

   3) HMSN III classification has been removed from modified HMSN classification, which emphasizes molecular genetic identification

b. Rare

c. Autosomal dominant or sporadic (de novo mutation)

d. NCSs (demyelinating neuropathy): markedly reduced

motor conduction velocities, usually less than 10 m/s

e. Clinical features

   1) Severe neuropathy manifesting in infancy as delayed motor milestones

   2) Progressive weakness of arms and legs

   3) Often wheelchair bound by early adulthood

   4) Generalized areflexia

   5) Palpable nerve hypertrophy

f. Laboratory

   1) Prominent onion bulbs on nerve biopsy

   2) Unlike most of the inherited neuropathies, marked CSF protein elevation is common in Dejerine-Sottas disease

5. HMSN IV

a. Autosomal recessive

b. Rare

c. No longer refers to Refsum's disease (see below)

d. Usually severe, early-onset neuropathy

e. Demyelinating pattern (discussed above) observed on NCSs

f. HMSN IVa (mutations of *GDAP1* gene of unknown function) causes basal-lamina onion bulbs, without intervening layers of Schwann cell cytoplasm

6. HMSN X (CMT X)

a. Genetics

   1) X-linked recessive: typical family history is apparently unaffected parents and/or affected brothers

   2) Gap junction beta 1 (*GJB1*) gene (encoding Cx32): Cx32 is a Schwann cell transmembrane gap junction protein located in uncompacted myelin (in contrast to MPZ and PMP 22) at paranodal region

b. Clinical features

   1) Resembles CMT 1, with onset in adolescence, early proprioceptive loss, and sensory ataxia

   2) Some with central hearing loss

   3) A subset of patients may have transient encephalopathy with exercise at altitude (usually >8,000 ft), with symmetric nonenhancing white matter abnormalities

c. Electrophysiology

   1) Mixed axonal and demyelinating features with conduction velocities intermediate between CMT 1 and CMT 2 (on electrodiagnostic evaluation)

   2) Upper limb nerve conduction velocities: typically 30 to 38 m/s

7. Other rarer forms of HMSN

a. HMSN V

   1) Autosomal dominant

   2) Associated with spastic paraplegia

b. HMSN VI

   1) Autosomal recessive

   2) Associated with optic atrophy

c. HMSN VII: associated with retinitis pigmentosa

d. Giant axonal neuropathy
   1) Rare
   2) Autosomal recessive
   3) Mutation of *GAN* gene on chromosome 16q24, encoding gigaxonin: responsible for the underlying defect of nerve axons of both PNS and CNS
   4) Onset in infancy of progressive severe sensory and motor axonal neuropathy
   5) Patients tend to walk on the inner edges of their feet
   6) Patients subsequently develop spinocerebellar degeneration
   7) Characteristic finding in some patients: tightly curled hair
   8) Death by the end of third decade
   9) MRI: abnormal signal in cerebellum and subcortical white matter
   10) Nerve biopsy: giant axonal swellings up to 50 μm (roughly 10 times average diameter of sural nerve myelinated axons) (Fig. 21-14)
      a) Swellings contain densely packed neurofilaments
      b) Often undergo secondary demyelination and may have small onion bulbs

8. Genetic testing in HMSN
   a. Commercially available "CMT panels": very expensive, includes very broad range of genetic tests
   b. Some genes that are tested are very rare or have been described only in single kindreds
   c. Insufficient testing of normal controls to establish benign polymorphisms producing indeterminant results
   d. Individual genetic tests can be selected based on clinical phenotype and nerve conduction characteristics
      1) CMT 1–like phenotype
         a) Fluorescent in situ hybridization testing for *PMP22* duplication, if negative proceed to
         b) *PMP22, Cx32, MPZ* sequencing
      2) CMT 2–like phenotype
         a) *Cx32* (unless documented male to male transmission)
         b) MPZ: although both Cx32 and MPZ are expressed in Schwann cells, they can produce intermediate range conduction velocities, thus mimicking CMT 2
         c) *MFN2*, particularly if childhood onset
         d) Consider testing *NFL*
         e) *PMP22* is very unlikely to produce this phenotype
      3) Severe/early-onset CMT 1/Dejerine-Sottas–like phenotype
         a) *PMP22* sequencing (usually not duplications)
         b) *MPZ*
         c) Consider *EGR2, GDAP1* (both rare)

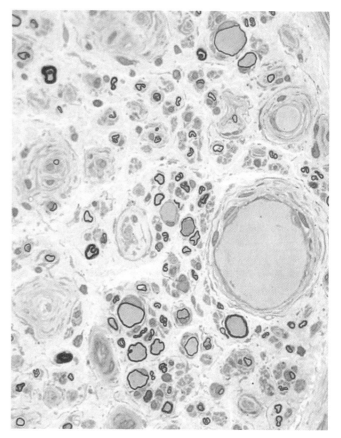

Fig. 21-14. Sural nerve biopsy specimen from patient with giant axonal neuropathy showing dense cytoplasm of many axons, some with secondary demyelination, and two enclosed by onion bulbs. Also, note concentrically arranged Schwann cells with no central fiber, suggestive of axonal loss. (From Gabreëls-Festen A, Thomas PK. Autosomal recessive hereditary motor and sensory neuropathies. In: Dyck PJ, Thomas PK, editors. Peripheral neuropathy. Vol 2. 4th ed. Philadelphia: Elsevier Saunders; 2005. p. 1769-90. Used with permission.)

D. Hereditary Neuropathy With Liability to Pressure Palsies (HNPP)
1. Outside the HMSN classification
2. Genetics
   a. Autosomal dominant
   b. Most common genetic abnormality: deletion of portion of chromosome 17 (17p11.2-p12) containing *PMP22* (this is same region duplicated in CMT 1A)
   c. Approximately 20% of cases do not have a macrodeletion: sequencing of *PMP22* in these patients may show point mutations
3. Clinical features

a. Onset: recurrent painless focal mononeuropathies at common sites of compression, often in second or third decade when patient develops
   1) Ulnar neuropathy at the elbow
   2) Peroneal neuropathy at the fibular head
   3) Radial neuropathy at the spiral groove
b. Unlike sporadic compression palsies, these patients develop palsies after relatively minor compression or trauma
c. The preceding compression may not even be apparent to patient
d. Mononeuropathy typically improves, but over days or weeks rather than minutes or hours
e. With time, some patients develop distal sensory motor neuropathy with distal sensory loss and absent ankle reflexes

4. Electrophysiology
   a. Multifocal demyelinating peripheral neuropathy
   b. Focal conduction slowing or conduction block at common sites of compression
   c. Generalized prolongation of motor and sensory distal latencies out of proportion to conduction slowing

5. Pathologic hallmark: tomaculae (Fig. 21-15)
   a. Focal areas of myelin thickening due to myelin reduplication or uncompacting of myelin lamellae
   b. Appear as focal sausage-shaped areas of teased fibers and as fibers with abnormally thick myelin for fiber diameter on methylene blue semithin sections

6. Treatment: avoid nerve trauma or compression
   a. Advise against leaning on elbows
   b. Advise against crossing legs

E. Hereditary Brachial Plexopathy
1. Genetics
   a. Autosomal dominant inheritance: a characteristic feature of the family history may be attacks in family members occurring post partum
   b. Some (not all) families show linkage to chromosome 17q24-25, the gene has not been identified

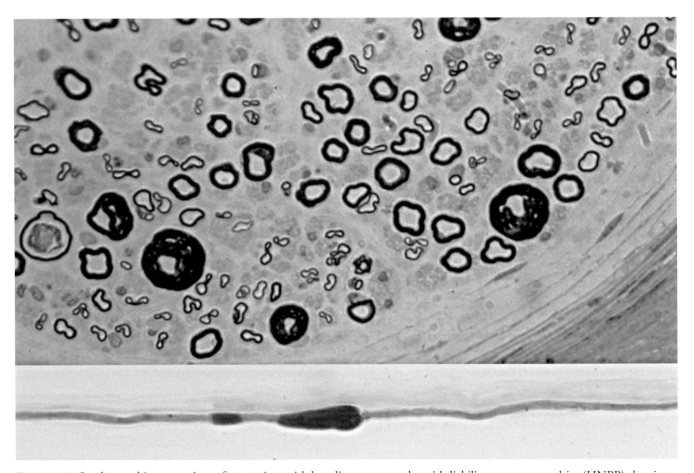

Fig. 21-15. Sural nerve biopsy specimen from patient with hereditary neuropathy with liability to pressure palsies (HNPP) showing, *top*, multiple focal thickenings of myelin sheaths, each termed a "tomaculum" and, *bottom*, the sausage-like appearance of tomaculae in a teased fiber preparation. (*Top*, methylene blue.) (*Courtesy of Guillermo A. Suarez, MD.*)

c. Minor dysmorphic features reported in some families
   1) Ocular hypotelorism (close-set eyes)
   2) Prominent epicanthal folds
   3) Short stature
2. Clinical features
   a. Recurrent attacks of painful brachial plexopathy, with onset in first to third decade
   b. Individual attacks are usually indistinguishable from idiopathic brachial plexus neuritis (Parsonage-Turner syndrome) but are recurrent
      1) Pain is severe, acute onset, precedes onset of weakness
      2) Unlike compressive radiculopathy, pain is not worse with neck movements or Valsalva maneuver but often exacerbated by arm or shoulder movement
      3) Tendency to affect muscles innervated by C5 and C6 segments, particularly shoulder girdle muscles
      4) Pattern of weakness and atrophy often suggests patchy involvement of plexus and nerve trunks (i.e., not a pure plexopathy)
   c. Pregnancy, parturition, trauma, infection, or immunization can precipitate attacks
   d. Time course is variable, but typically pain lasts for days to weeks and weakness plateaus before 1 month
3. Differential diagnosis
   a. HNPP
      1) HNPP can present with plexopathy but is usually painless
      2) Attacks are associated with minor trauma or compression rather than immune system stimulating events
      3) Patients with HNPP often have signs of generalized background neuropathy (high arches, generalized prolongation of distal motor latencies)
   b. Idiopathic brachial neuritis (Parsonage-Turner syndrome)
      1) Absence of family history
      2) Attacks are not recurrent
4. Treatment
   a. Upper limb nerve biopsy samples from small number of patients during an attack have shown prominent epineurial perivascular inflammation, providing rationale for treating acute attacks with immunotherapy
   b. Corticosteroids started at onset of an attack shorten duration of pain (anecdotal evidence)
5. Prognosis
   a. Most patients, treated or not, make good functional recovery from individual attacks: recovery may take up to 12 to 18 months
   b. Patients with frequent attacks may with time accrue some degree of permanent deficit
   c. Frequency of attacks varies greatly but tends to decrease with age

F. Hereditary Sensory and Autonomic Neuropathy (HSAN)
1. Overview
   a. Characterized by involvement of small-diameter nerve fibers (temperature and pain sensation, autonomic nerves)
   b. Genetics: less well defined than for HMSN
   c. Classification system: still based on clinical manifestations and pattern of inheritance
   d. One of the most devastating complications of HSAN: painless neuropathic ulcers, may progress to osteomyelitis and distal mutilation
   e. No specific treatment for HSAN
      1) Patient education about care of the feet is critical
      2) Advice includes following:
         a) Always wear shoes
         b) Wear comfortable shoes that are not too tight
         c) Inspect shoes for foreign bodies
         d) Inspect feet daily
         e) Avoid heavy weight bearing on feet
         f) Keep feet well moisturized to prevent cracking of the skin as a portal for infection
         g) Aggressively treat foot infections: include strict avoidance of weight bearing
2. HSAN I
   a. Most common form of HSAN: likely an underrecognized cause of adult-onset sensory neuropathy
   b. Important differences compared with other HSANs
      1) Only autosomal dominant HSAN
      2) Only adult-onset HSAN (all others are congenital)
      3) Slowly progressive (others are nonprogressive)
      4) Tendency to be restricted to lower limbs
   c. Genetics
      1) Autosomal dominant
      2) Mutation of *SPTLC1* and *RAB7* have been described in some patients
      3) Mutation of *SPTLC1* on chromosome 9q22, encoding a long-chain base 1 (LCB1) subunit of enzyme palmitoyltransferase, responsible for synthesis of sphingomyelin (found in neurilemma)
         a) Exact pathogenesis: not defined with certainty, apoptotic role of the ceramide (sphingomyelin degradation product) may contribute
         b) Phenotype of certain kindreds has included hearing loss and hyperhidrosis
      4) Full clinical and genetic spectrum of disease is probably still to be defined
   d. Clinical features of "typical" distal lower limb sensory and autonomic neuropathy and acral mutilation
      1) Onset in adult life (wide variation)

2) Slow progression but remains restricted predominantly to lower limbs

3) Distal lower limb neuropathic pain (burning, aching, lancinating) or local pain at pressure points, mostly due to plantar ulcers and other foot orthopedic complications

4) Patients gradually develop loss of small-fiber sensory modalities in length-dependent pattern

5) Loss of pain sensation predisposes to development of foot orthopedic complications such as neuropathic plantar ulcers and stress fractures: in severe cases can lead to distal mutilation from infection and osteomyelitis

6) Autonomic involvement: usually restricted to asymptomatic distal sweating loss

e. Pathology

1) Both myelinated and unmyelinated fibers of all sizes affected: small myelinated fibers may be affected more than large myelinated fibers

2) Axonal atrophy and degeneration, myelin remodeling

f. Electrophysiology

1) Features consistent with length-dependent sensory predominant sensorimotor axonal neuropathy

2) Sensory potentials may be relatively preserved early in course because of selective small-fiber involvement

3) Mild motor involvement: common finding on EMG

3. HSAN II

a. Similar clinical features: similar to HSAN I but

1) Onset in early life

2) Severe panmodality sensory loss affecting upper and lower limbs, trunk and face

3) Mutilating acropathy: distal pain insensitivity predisposes to neuropathic ulcers and mutilation of fingers and toes from early age, unrecognized fractures, and Charcot joints (Fig. 21-16)

4) Common autonomic features: distal anhidrosis, urinary sphincter disturbance, and impotence in men

b. Genetics

1) Autosomal recessive

2) Mutation of one gene at chromosome 12p13.33 may possibly be causative; no other known genetic mutations or chromosomal linkage

c. Pathology

1) Loss of myelinated fibers of all sizes (more than unmyelinated fibers)

2) Segmental demyelination and remyelination, axonal degeneration and atrophy

d. Electrophysiology: generalized loss of sensory potentials

4. HSAN III

a. Also called familial dysautonomia or Riley-Day syndrome

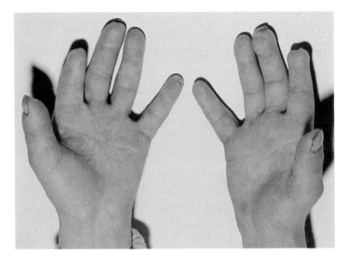

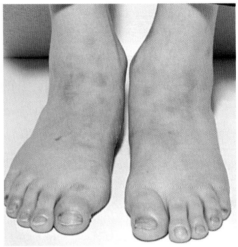

Fig. 21-16. Hands (*top*) and feet (*bottom*) of a patient with mutilating acropathy typical of hereditary sensory and autonomic neuropathy (HSAN).

b. Genetics

1) Autosomal recessive

2) Mainly reported in Ashkenazi Jews

3) Caused by mutation of *IKBKAP* located at chromosome 9q31, encoding IKAP (kinase complex-associated protein)

a) A single mutation site appears responsible for approximately 99.5% of all cases of HSAN III: this allows for reliable carrier and intrauterine detection

b) Mechanism by which this mutation causes disease is unknown

c. Clinical features

1) Presentation at birth with severe and widespread autonomic failure

a) Alacrima (absence of overflow tears)

b) Frequent respiratory infections because of dry

respiratory secretions
  c) Gastrointestinal tract dysmotility: esophageal dysmotility and megaesophagus, gastroparesis, megacolon (vomiting, poor feeding, abnormal sucking in first few years of life)
  2) Symptoms of autonomic dysregulation and overactivity, often precipitated by emotional upset
    a) Profuse sweating
    b) Skin blotching
    c) Tachycardia
    d) Hypertension
  3) Characteristic feature: absence of tongue fungiform papillae
  4) Hypotonia, hyporeflexia
  5) Kyphoscoliosis
  6) Stunted growth
  7) Decreased pain sensation at older age: distal pain sensation is relatively preserved early in disease and may become impaired later in life (in contrast to HSAN I and HSAN II)—the exception is corneal insensitivity (an early feature)
  d. Pathology
    1) Marked decrease in unmyelinated and small myelinated fibers
    2) Degeneration of neuronal cell bodies of spinal and sympathetic ganglia
  e. Prognosis: death in infancy or childhood
5. Rare HSAN subtypes
  a. HSAN IV
    1) Inheritance: autosomal recessive
    2) Mutations of *TRKA*, encoding protein tyrosine receptor kinase A (TrkA)
    3) Congenital insensitivity to pain with anhidrosis
    4) Hyperthermia due to anhidrosis
    5) Mild mental retardation in some patients (IQ in 70s)
    6) Absence of unmyelinated fibers in sural nerve biopsies
    7) Normal SNAPs
  b. HSAN V
    1) Phenotypically similar to HSAN IV, but different pathology
    2) Severe loss of small myelinated fibers, mild decrease in unmyelinated fibers
    3) Associated with mutations of *TRKA* and *NGFB*
    4) Normal SNAPs

G. **Multiple Endocrine Neoplasia 2B** (MEN 2B)
1. Genetics: autosomal dominant or sporadic mutation of *RET* proto-oncogene
2. Clinical features
  a. Dysmorphic features

    1) Diffuse irregular thickening of lips
    2) Apparent eversion of eyelids
    3) Broad nasal root
    4) Marfanoid body habitus without ectopic lens or aortic defects
    5) Tongue nodules
  b. Neoplasms
    1) Medullary thyroid carcinoma
    2) Pheochromocytoma
  c. Visceral autonomic neuropathy (ganglioneuromatosis): poor colonic motility with severe constipation and megacolon
  d. Variable degree of axonal peripheral sensorimotor neuropathy

II. Neuropathies Associated With Inborn Errors of Metabolism

A. **Overview**
1. Diverse group of disorders
2. Shared features
  a. Inheritance: autosomal recessive or X-linked recessive (e.g. Fabry's disease, adrenomyeloneuropathy)
  b. Involvement of PNS plus CNS or other organs
3. Two broad categories of presentations
  a. Demyelinating neuropathy with CNS disease
    1) Metachromatic leukodystrophy
    2) Krabbe's disease
    3) Adrenomyeloneuropathy
    4) Refsum's disease
  b. Small-fiber sensory neuropathy
    1) Fabry's disease
    2) Tangier disease

B. **Metabolic Classification** (most common conditions listed here, see Chapter 25)
1. Lysosomal enzymes
  a. Metachromatic leukodystrophy
  b. Krabbe's disease
2. Peroxisomal enzymes
  a. Adrenoleukodystrophy and adrenomyeloneuropathy
  b. Fabry's disease
  c. Refsum's disease
3. Lipoprotein deficiency: Tangier disease

C. **Metachromatic Leukodystrophy**
1. Inheritance: autosomal recessive
2. Metabolic abnormality: arylsulfatase A deficiency
  a. Lysosomal enzyme

b. Activity can be measured in leukocytes or skin fibroblasts
3. Clinical features
   a. Childhood or adult onset: early-onset disease is associated with more rapid progression
   b. PNS: distal sensorimotor peripheral neuropathy
   c. CNS
      1) Mental retardation, optic atrophy, spasticity
      2) MRI: confluent white matter plaques and atrophy
4. Electrophysiology: demyelinating features
5. Pathology: metachromatic granules
   a. Schwann cell cytoplasmic inclusions that stain differently from rest of cytoplasm (hence, metachromatic)
   b. Methylene blue preparations: normal Schwann cell cytoplasm is light blue and granules are red or black
6. Treatment: bone marrow transplantation may stabilize cognition in patients with early disease but motor dysfunction may continue to progress

D. **Globoid Cell Leukodystrophy** (Krabbe's disease)
1. Inheritance: autosomal recessive
2. Metabolic abnormality: galactosylceramidase (lysosomal enzyme)
3. Clinical features
   a. Infantile, late infantile, juvenile, and adult-onset forms
   b. PNS and CNS features similar to metachromatic leukodystrophy
4. Electrophysiology: demyelinating features
5. Pathology: globoid cells
   a. Giant multinucleated epitheloid cells in brain white matter
   b. Globoid cells are not found in peripheral nerve biopsies, which instead may show tubular clear Schwann cell cytoplasmic inclusions on electron microscopy
6. Treatment is similar to metachromatic leukodystrophy: bone marrow transplantation early in disease course may stabilize progression

E. **Adrenomyeloneuropathy** (see also Chapter 20)
1. Genetics and pathogenesis
   a. X-linked recessive
   b. Allelic with adrenoleukodystrophy
   c. Mutation of the *ABCD1* on chromosome Xq28 encoding adrenoleukodystrophy protein (ADLP), a member of the ATP-binding cassette (ABC) transporter protein family
   d. ADLP is a transmembrane protein located in the peroxisomal membrane, functions to transport very-long-chain fatty acids (VLCFAs) into peroxisome
   e. Deficiency causes accumulation of VLCFAs
2. Clinical features

a. Most common phenotype of the mutation is that of adrenoleukodystrophy (see Chapter 25)
b. Adrenomyeloneuropathy is a milder phenotype of slowly progressive spastic paraplegia in third and fourth decades, usually in adult men, sometimes with mild adrenal insufficiency
c. Female carriers may be mildly affected and present with slowly progressive spastic paraparesis
d. Mild peripheral neuropathy
e. Loss of both myelinated and unmyelinated fibers
3. Electrophysiology
   a. Mixed axonal-demyelinating peripheral neuropathy
   b. Abnormal somatosensory evoked potentials
4. Treatment: supportive

F. **Refsum's Disease**
1. Previously classified as HMSN IV
2. Inheritance: autosomal recessive
3. Metabolic deficiency: deficiency of phytanoyl-CoA hydroxylase (peroxisomal enzyme involved in oxidation of phytanic acid)
4. Clinical features
   a. Onset in second decade
   b. Initial symptom: often night blindness due to retinitis pigmentosa
   c. Distal sensory motor neuropathy
   d. Palpable nerve *hypertrophy*
   e. CNS and cranial nerve disease: ataxia, anosmia, deafness
   f. Skeletal abnormalities: short fourth metatarsal
   g. Diabetes mellitus and cardiac disease
5. Electrophysiology: demyelinating features
6. Pathology
   a. Variable hypertrophic change involving mostly brachial and lumbosacral plexi
   b. Segmental demyelination and variable loss of myelinated fibers
7. Other laboratory findings
   a. CSF protein is often very high
   b. Elevated serum phytanic acid levels
8. Treatment: dietary restriction of phytanic acid

G. **Fabry's Disease**
1. Genetics
   a. X-linked recessive
   b. Female hemizygotes can also manifest disease but typically milder severity and later onset
2. Metabolic deficiency: deficiency of α-galactosidase (a peroxisomal enzyme) resulting in accumulation of ceramide trihexoside in PNS, kidney, heart
3. Clinical features

a. Onset: usually in second decade

b. Primary manifestation of peripheral neuropathy: distal burning pain worsened by heat or physical exertion, which may occur in attacks lasting minutes to hours

c. Small-fiber sensory loss (predominantly affecting temperature sensation)

d. Autonomic neuropathy
   1) Hypohidrosis
   2) Impotence

e. Systemic manifestations
   1) Cerebrovascular disease, cardiac failure
   2) Renal failure
   3) Angiokeratomas: small raised venous skin lesions around groin
   4) Corneal opacities

4. Pathology (see Fig. 25-13): electron microscopy show accumulation of ceramide trihexoside appearing as concentric laminated cytoplasmic inclusions (likely in lysosomes)

5. Electrophysiology: may be normal (predominantly small-fiber process)

6. Treatment
   a. Symptomatic treatment of painful neuropathy: phenytoin, carbamazepine
   b. Enzyme replacement therapy is available: early work suggesting beneficial effect on neuropathy

H. **Tangier Disease**

1. Genetics
   a. Autosomal recessive
   b. Mutation of *ABCA1* encoding ABCA1 protein, member of ABC transporter family

2. Normal state: high-density lipoprotein (HDL) is responsible for
   a. Cholesterol efflux from peripheral tissues via ABCA1 transporter
   b. Esterification of free cholesterol extracted from peripheral tissue
   c. Transfer of cholesteryl esters to very-low-density lipoprotein (VLDL) and low-density lipoproteins (LDL) in exchange for triglycerol
   d. Carrying cholesteryl esters to liver to be degraded

3. Pathogenesis
   a. Defective transporter activity yields lipid-depleted HDLs, which are degraded quickly
   b. Deficient HDL results in absence of cholesteryl ester degradation, which overloads macrophages of reticuloendothelial system with deposition of cholesteryl esters
   c. Intracellular deposition of cholesteryl esters does not downregulate macrophage cholesterol scavenger receptors, and cholesterol accumulation in macrophages continues unchecked
   d. Deficient HDL also results in poor extraction of triglycerol from VLDL, resulting in elevated triglycerides and triglyceride-rich VLDLs
   e. Poor extraction of triglycerol from VLDL prevents it from becoming more dense, preventing formation of LDL

4. Clinical features
   a. Age at onset: wide range
   b. Mononeuritis multiplex-like phenotype: relapsing, asymmetric sensorimotor multiple mononeuropathies often involving individual cranial or limb nerves
   c. Distal symmetric small-fiber sensory neuropathy (slowly progressive)
   d. Pseudosyrinx phenotype: slowly progressive weakness and atrophy of face and bilateral upper limbs (and later the trunk), relative preservation of reflexes, and preferential loss of pain and temperature early in disease (other sensory modalities affected later in disease course)
   e. Enlarged orange tonsils due to lipid accumulation in reticuloendothelial system
   f. Premature coronary artery disease

5. Laboratory features (serum)
   a. Very low or absent HDL levels
   b. Low LDL levels
   c. Low or normal serum cholesterol levels
   d. Elevated VLDL levels (contain abundant triglycerides, more than cholesteryl esters)
   e. Elevated triglycerides

6. Electrophysiology: predominantly axonal but may have some demyelinating features

7. Pathology
   a. Lipid-laden vacuoles in endothelial cells of the vasa vasorum and Schwann cells (best observed with teased fiber analysis and electron microscopy)
   b. Segmental demyelination and remyelination in patients with relapsing multiple mononeuropathy presentation
   c. Axonal degeneration with loss of small myelinated and unmyelinated axons in patients with symmetric, slowly progressive peripheral neuropathy
   d. Cholesteryl ester deposits in macrophages of tonsils, spleen, lymphatic system, and other components of reticuloendothelial system

8. Treatment: supportive

I. **Porphyric Neuropathy**

1. Inheritance: usually autosomal dominant

2. Porphyrins: intermediate metabolites in synthesis of heme

3. Porphyrias: due to defects in synthesis of porphyrins
4. Neurologic manifestations probably due to accumulation of toxic precursors rather than deficiency of end product
5. Porphyric neuropathy is seen in following hepatic porphyrias:
   a. Acute intermittent porphyria: deficiency of porphobilinogen deaminase causing accumulation of mitochondrial δ-aminolevulinic acid and cytoplasmic porphobilinogen
   b. Hereditary coproporphyria: deficiency of coproporphyrinogen oxidase causing increased levels of coproporphyrinogen (including in between attacks)
   c. Variegate porphyria: deficiency of the mitochondrial protoporphyrinogen oxidase causing accumulation of protoporphyrinogen IX (cannot be measured); often normal urine porphyrin levels in between attacks (elevated fecal coproporphyrin levels)
   d. Neuropathy or other neurologic dysfunction: not a feature of erythroid porphyrias
6. Clinical features—acute intermittent porphyria, hereditary coproporphyria, variegate porphyria all share following characteristic features:
   a. Usually more severe in patients with acute intermittent porphyria
   b. Typical presentation pattern: acute abdominal pain, then psychiatric disturbance, then acute neurologic dysfunction
   c. Acute colicky abdominal pain
      1) Associated with nausea, vomiting, severe constipation
      2) May be due to acute gastrointestinal autonomic neuropathy or effect of deficiency of heme or its precursors on autonomic innervation and smooth muscle components of gastrointestinal tract
   d. Other autonomic features (usually sympathetic overactivity)
      1) Labile blood pressure
      2) Tachycardia
      3) Urinary retention
      4) Pupillary dilatation
   e. Psychiatric disturbance and CNS involvement: acute encephalopathy
      1) Agitation, restlessness, delirium, anxiety
      2) Hallucinations
      3) Psychosis
      4) Seizures
      5) May progress to coma
   f. Acute attacks of neurologic dysfunction: PNS involvement
      1) Resembles Guillain-Barré syndrome

      2) Early back or limb pain
      3) Subacute onset and progression of axonal, asymmetric generalized predominantly motor neuropathy, usually within 2 or 3 days after abdominal and psychiatric symptoms
      4) Preferential involvement of upper limbs and proximal muscle groups
      5) Distribution of weakness: may be patchy
      6) Hyporeflexia in proportion to degree of muscle weakness: reflexes are preserved early in disease course (unlike Guillain-Barré syndrome)
      7) Severe cases: flaccid quadriplegia; respiratory muscle paralysis and respiratory failure
      8) Rapidly progressive muscle atrophy: early feature, may be severe
      9) Variable sensory involvement (usually much less prominent than motor involvement): may be distal glove-stocking distribution or proximal and patchy
      10) Cranial nerve involvement is common: especially facial weakness and difficulty swallowing, other cranial nerves may be affected if more severe (causing extraocular muscle or tongue weakness)
   g. Dark urine (on exposure to light and air)
   h. Attacks precipitated by
      1) Drugs
      2) Hormonal changes
      3) Stress
   i. Cutaneous photosensitivity with variegate porphyria and hereditary coproporphyria (with hyperpigmentation and hypertrichosis of the skin)
   j. Acute intermittent porphyria clinically differs from hereditary coproporphyria and variegate porphyria by
      1) No photosensitivity
      2) Attacks are usually more severe
7. Differential diagnosis
   a. Guillain-Barré syndrome: absence of encephalopathy and reflexes
   b. Arsenic or thallium poisoning
      1) Closely mimics triad of gastrointestinal symptoms, neuropathy, encephalopathy
      2) Urinary heavy metals should be tested in all patients not known to have porphyria presenting with this triad
8. Diagnosis
   a. Electrophysiology
      1) NCS and needle EMG may be normal during first few days of acute attack
      2) Often the first abnormality is fibrillation potentials on needle EMG seen after 5 to 10 days
      3) NCS shows predominantly axonal pattern but is not otherwise specific

b. Urinary porphyrins
  1) δ-Aminolevulinic acid: severely elevated during acute attacks of acute intermittent porphyria, hereditary coproporphyria, variegate porphyria; normal or mildly elevated in between attacks
  2) Porphobilinogen
    a) Increased more than δ-aminolevulinic acid in hereditary coproporphyria and variegate porphyria
    b) Increased less than δ-aminolevulinic acid in acute intermittent porphyria
    c) Usually increased in between attacks in acute intermittent porphyria
  3) Coproporphyrin: greatly increased in both hereditary coproporphyria and variegate porphyria (even in between attacks)
    a) Increased urine excretion can be a reversible drug or heavy metal effect unrelated to disease
    b) Urine heavy metal screen may be done to rule out metal intoxication
    c) Normal fecal excretion of porphyrins if due to drug effect (urine coproporphyrins normalize 2 weeks after cessation of offending agent)
9. Treatment
  a. Patients with acute intermittent porphyria are asymptomatic in between attacks unless they have residual neuropathy from previous severe attacks
  b. Avoidance of excessive sun exposure in patients with hereditary coproporphyria and variegate porphyria
  c. Prevention of acute attacks
    1) Avoidance of known porphyrogenic drugs (many are inducers of cytochrome P-450, such as barbiturates, phenytoin, alcohol, estrogens, sulfonamides)
    2) Avoidance of prolonged starvation or excessive physical exertion without carbohydrate loading
  d. Treatment of acute attacks
    1) Careful review of current medications, cessation of any potentially exacerbating medications
    2) Acceptable acute symptomatic treatments
      a) Abdominal pain: morphine
      b) Agitation: chlorpromazine
      c) Seizures: clonazepam in small doses
    3) Identify and treat hyponatremia due to commonly associated syndrome of inappropriate antidiuretic hormone
    4) Maintain adequate carbohydrate intake: intravenous glucose if patient is vomiting
    5) Daily intravenous heme infusion until attack has abated, usually 3 to 14 days
      a) Suppresses induction of δ-aminolevulinic acid synthase

      b) If used early in attack, heme treatment can result in rapid resolution of psychiatric and autonomic symptoms
  e. Prognosis
    1) Recovery from acute neuropathy is related to severity
    2) Severe attacks associated with marked axonal degeneration: often prolonged, usually incomplete recovery

J. **Familial Amyloid Polyneuropathy** (FAP)
1. Overview
  a. Inheritance: autosomal dominant
  b. Extracellular deposition of mutant fibrillar protein that forms β-pleated structures leading to tissue infiltration and organ dysfunction
  c. Exact mechanism by which this deposition causes neuropathy is uncertain
  d. Proposed mechanisms: ischemia due to vessel occlusion by amyloid deposits in vasa nervorum, compression, or direct toxic effect
  e. Three different constituent proteins known to cause FAP
  f. Mutations of the protein's gene results in structural change of the protein that favors formation of a β-pleated structure
  g. Most cases of acquired amyloid neuropathy are AL type (immunoglobulin light chains)
2. Classification
  a. Old phenotypic classification
    1) FAP type I (transthyretin mutation): lower limb onset
    2) FAP type II (transthyretin mutation): upper limb onset (often CTS)
    3) FAP type III (apolipoprotein A-I mutation): lower limb onset, nephropathy, gastric ulcers
    4) FAP type IV (gelsolin mutation): cranial nerve involvement
  b. New genotypic classification
    1) Transthyretin (TTR) FAP
    2) Apolipoprotein A-I FAP
    3) Gelsolin FAP
3. Genetics
  a. TTR amyloidosis
    1) Autosomal dominant
    2) Most common cause of FAP
    3) Found worldwide but increased prevalence in people of Portuguese, Swedish, or Japanese descent
    4) TTR is produced in liver
    5) More than 80 known point mutations but methionine 30 (Met30) is most common
  b. Apolipoprotein A-I amyloidosis
    1) Autosomal dominant

2) Neuropathic form described in a kindred from Iowa with Gly26Arg mutation

3) Other mutations of this gene reported to cause non-neuropathic systemic amyloidosis

c. Gelsolin

   1) Autosomal dominant

   2) First described in a Finnish kindred but also reported with other genetic backgrounds

   3) Protein is expressed mainly in muscle

4. Clinical Features

a. Common features

   1) Variable age at onset, most commonly in fourth decade

   2) Painful axonal sensory more than motor neuropathy

     a) Small-fiber function affected early

     b) Motor involvement late

   3) Prominent autonomic involvement

   4) Cardiac and renal failure

b. TTR amyloidosis Met30 (formerly classified as FAP I)

   1) Most common point mutation (Val30Met)

   2) Onset of neuropathy usually in third to fifth decades

   3) Prominent autonomic symptoms (may be early and severe)

     a) Orthostatic hypotension

     b) Impotence

     c) Urinary retention

     d) Gastrointestinal dysmotility, alternating constipation, diarrhea

   4) Length-dependent sensory and motor neuropathy that usually starts in lower limbs and affects predominantly sensory small fibers

   5) With progression: eventual involvement of all sensory modalities and motor fibers later in disease course (with progressive weakness and atrophy starting in distal lower limbs and progressing to involve upper limbs)

   6) Cardiac failure more than renal failure

   7) Vitreous opacities (amyloid deposits)

   8) Rare CNS symptoms: stroke, seizures, dementia, spasticity, episodes of confusion

   9) Average survival: about 10 years

   10) Specific pathologic features of TTR amyloidosis (Fig. 21-17)

     a) Amyloid deposits in epineurium, endoneurium, perineurium

     b) Deposits often found around blood vessels

     c) Axonal loss, wallerian degeneration (initially affecting unmyelinated and small myelinated fibers, then larger myelinated fibers)

c. TTR amyloidosis Tyr 77

   1) Second most common TTR point mutation

   2) CTS very common, is often initial manifestation

   3) Absence of vitreous opacities

   4) Otherwise, clinical features identical to Met30 phenotype

d. TTR amyloidosis Ser 84 and His 58 (formerly classified as FAP II)

   1) Onset of neuropathy: usually in fourth or fifth decades with CTS

   2) Slowly progressive generalized sensory and motor peripheral neuropathy starting in upper limbs

   3) Autonomic symptoms and failure

   4) Sometimes cardiomyopathy

   5) Not associated with renal or ocular manifestations

e. Apolipoprotein A-I amyloidosis (formerly classified as FAP III)

   1) Pattern of neuropathy similar to TTR amyloidosis, but less prominent autonomic involvement

   2) High incidence of gastric ulcers and renal failure (early)

   3) Pathology: amyloid deposits throughout PNS including the dorsal root ganglia and roots, immunohistochemical characteristics of apolipoprotein A-I

f. Gelsolin amyloidosis (formerly classified as FAP IV)

   1) Presentation often in 30s with corneal lattice dystrophy due to amyloid deposition in corneal branches of trigeminal nerve

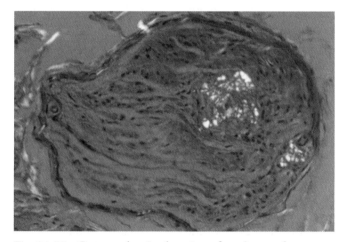

Fig. 21-17. Congo red-stained section of sural nerve from patient with familial amyloid polyneuropathy. Use of polarizing filters demonstrates the apple-green birefringence of amyloid deposits. (From Kyle RA, Dispenzieri A. Amyloidosis. In: Noseworthy JH, editor. Neurological therapeutics: principles and practice. Vol. 2. New York: Martin Dunitz; 2003. p. 2137-46. By permission of Mayo Foundation.)

2) Progressive cranial neuropathy ensues (often facial nerve involved, with facial weakness, beginning in upper facial branches supplying forehead)

3) Other cranial nerves involved: V, VIII, XII

4) Bulbar symptoms in older patients

5) Mild axonal peripheral sensory and autonomic neuropathy

6) Cardiac involvement clinically rare

7) Benign course with normal life span

8) Specific pathologic features: deposition of gelsolin amyloid in vessel walls and perineurial sheaths, nerve roots may be more severely affected than distal nerves

5. Diagnosis

a. Electrophysiology

1) Features of axonal sensorimotor length-dependent polyneuropathy and/or CTS

2) May be limited to small-fiber neuropathy (early in disease course) with normal NCS

b. Pathology: common features

1) Amyloid best demonstrated with alkaline Congo red preparations observed with polarizing filters to demonstrate the apple-green birefringence

2) Immunohistochemistry preparations (using anti-TTR, -λ, -κ, -Apo A-I monoclonal antibodies) can help determine constituent protein but are not always reliable

3) Negative anti-TTR preparation does not exclude TTR amyloid and consideration should be given to sequencing the TTR gene if patient does not have a monoclonal protein

4) Rectal or abdominal fat biopsy may provide pathologic confirmation of amyloid without need for nerve biopsy

c. Molecular genetic testing: commercially available for TTR amyloid

d. Clinical features important for staging

1) To assess severity of systemic disease

2) Electrocardiography to detect conduction block and echocardiography should be performed in all patients

3) Renal involvement (often begins as proteinuria)

6. Treatment

a. Liver transplantation for patients with TTR amyloidosis, by removing production site of mutant TTR protein, may improve cardiac and renal function but affect on neuropathy is less clear

b. Apolipoprotein A-I is produced by liver and other organs; role of liver transplantation in this condition is not defined

c. Gelsolin is produced in muscle, so liver transplantation would not be beneficial

K. **Spinal Muscular Atrophy** (see Chapter 20)

L. **Spinocerebellar Ataxias** (see Chapter 9)

M. **Friedreich's Ataxia** (see Chapter 9)

N. **Peripheral Nerve Manifestations of Mitochondrial Disorders** (see also Chapter 24)

1. Overview

a. Heterogeneous group of disorders due to mutations of mitochondrial DNA causing impaired respiratory chain function

b. Marked phenotype/genotype variability but common features include ophthalmoplegia, retinitis pigmentosa, deafness, seizures, dementia, ataxia, myopathy

c. Some respiratory chain proteins are encoded by nuclear DNA; these mutations produce phenotype similar to some mitochondrial DNA mutations and do not demonstrate mitochondrial inheritance

d. Neuropathy (usually axonal) may be found in up to 25% of patients with mitochondrial disease but is frequently overshadowed by other clinical features

e. Limited number of mitochondrial phenotypes in which neuropathy may be most prominent and/or presenting feature

2. MNGIE

a. Genetics: autosomal recessive (nuclear-encoded mitochondrial proteins)

1) Mutation of thymidine phosphorylase gene on chromosome 22

2) Abnormal cellular nucleotide pool causes multiple deletions of mitochondrial DNA with tendency to occur at certain sites

b. Clinical features

1) Onset before age 20, with death in fourth decade

2) Usually presents with gastrointestinal symptoms (abdominal pain, nausea, early satiety, diarrhea) due to visceral neuropathy

3) Demyelinating length-dependent sensorimotor neuropathy occurs in almost all patients

4) Leukoencephalopathy

3. Leigh disease

a. Genetics: heterogeneous but usually autosomal recessive with mutations of one of several nuclear genes involved in assembly of complex IV of respiratory chain

b. Clinical features

1) Devastating encephalomyopathy, with onset in infancy

2) Demyelinating neuropathy, with sometimes profound slowing of conduction velocity reported in multiple families

4. Neuropathy, ataxia, retinitis pigmentosa (NARP)
   a. Genetics: true mitochondrial DNA disease
   b. Clinical features: axonal sensory neuropathy
   c. Muscle biopsies do *not* show ragged red fibers

III. ACQUIRED PERIPHERAL POLYNEUROPATHIES

A. Acute Inflammatory Demyelinating Polyradiculo-neuropathy (AIDP), Guillain-Barré Syndrome

1. History
   a. Although recognized in the nineteenth century, the disease was characterized by and named eponymously for Guillain, Barré, and Strohl, who recognized the key cytoalbumino-logic dissociation in the CSF of affected patients
2. Clinical presentation
   a. Often preceded by illnesses ranging from nonspecific upper respiratory infections to *Campylobacter jejuni* infections, triggering autoimmune response toward root and nerve antigens
   b. Typical presentation
      1) Acute or subacute, with ascending paresthesias, sensory loss, and weakness, which may initially be distal or proximal
      2) Hyporeflexia or areflexia in early phase of disease (usually out of proportion to any weakness): Achilles tendon reflexes usually lost; biceps reflexes often spared
      3) Back pain, distal leg pain and paresthesias
      4) Cranial nerve involvement: cranial nerve VII, extraocular movements
      5) Autonomic involvement: sympathetic overactivity (transient or sustained hypertension, cardiac arrhythmias, diaphoresis), reduced sympathetic activity (orthostatism, hypotension, anhidrosis), reduced parasympathetic activity (urinary retention, ileus)
   c. Rate and extent of progression can vary widely: most patients reach the worst stage of disease within 2 to 4 weeks, and approximately one-third require ventilatory assistance at some point
   d. Most cases in North America: patchy proximal and distal demyelination with later, secondary axonal damage in many cases
3. Laboratory features
   a. CSF analysis
      1) Elevated protein (often >100 mg/dL) with normal or modest CSF leukocyte count
      2) CSF is useful in excluding clinical entities, mainly viral infections (e.g., HIV, CMV), which may mimic AIDP, but often have increased cell counts

   b. Serum studies may include assays for antibodies known to be associated with AIDP and its variants
      1) GQ_{1b} antibodies are commonly associated with Miller Fisher syndrome (also, perhaps not coincidentally, with Bickerstaff's brainstem encephalitis)
      2) GM_1 antibodies and other ganglioside antibodies associated with axonal variants
4. Electrophysiologic features
   a. Role of needle EMG and NCS: confirm diagnosis, exclude alternatives, and determine axonal damage (which may correlate roughly with prognosis)
   b. NCSs
      1) Slowing of conduction velocities and prolongation of distal latencies
      2) Temporal dispersion of CMAPs
      3) Conduction block may be present
      4) F waves may be absent or prolonged in latency
      5) Early in disease course: sensory responses often normal
      6) About 1 to 2 weeks after onset: may be relative sparing of sural response (called *sural sparing*, referring to normal sural response, in face of reduced or absent median and ulnar SNAPs); may be due to relative resistance of larger diameter myelinated fibers in sural nerve to early inflammatory attack
      7) Smaller diameter of end sensory branches of ulnar and median nerves (site of the recorded potentials from antidromic studies) are probably more predisposed to inflammatory attack
      8) Later in disease course: all sensory responses may be absent or show demyelinating changes in conduction velocity and latency
   c. Needle EMG
      1) Acute phase: may reveal only reduced recruitment of motor unit potentials in affected muscles
      2) Subacute or chronic phase: presence of fibrillation potentials and increased motor unit potential complexity or size correlates roughly with extent of axonal damage (suggesting longer, more protracted course and worse prognosis)
5. Pathology
   a. Inflammation with endoneural lymphocytic infiltration
   b. Demyelination: degradation of myelin lamellae from penetration and disruption of Schwann cell basal lamina by macrophages
   c. Axonal degeneration
6. Management
   a. Immediate management of patients with AIDP focuses on close monitoring and supportive care
      1) Serial maximal respiratory pressures and forced vital capacities (FVC)

2) Mechanical ventilation and intensive care for precipitous decrease in any measure or low respiratory values (FVC <20 mL/kg, maximal inspiratory pressure <30 mm Hg, or maximal expiratory pressure <40 mm Hg)

3) Management of autonomic instability: labile blood pressure, cardiac arrhythmias (cardiac monitoring required), urine retention, and ileus

4) Management of pain (very common symptom in acute and plateau phases of care): refractory pain may be treated with antiepileptic medications; short-term narcotics may be necessary

b. Management of disease course: immunomodulation

1) Corticosteroids have never been conclusively shown to help shorten disease course or minimize morbidity

2) Intravenous immunoglobulin and plasmapheresis are likely equally effective in mitigating disease severity and should be instituted early

B. AIDP Variants

1. Acute motor axonal neuropathy (AMAN): axonal variant

   a. Most common in China; characterized by summer epidemics, closely tied to *C. jejuni* outbreaks

   b. Primarily affects children

   c. Has been associated with various ganglioside antibodies (GM_1, GM_{1b}, and GD_{1a})

   d. Characterized by flaccid symmetric paralysis (limbs; cranial, including facial and pharyngeal muscles; respiratory muscles) developing over several weeks, without clinical or electrophysiologic sensory involvement

   e. Pathophysiology: widespread selective wallerian degeneration of motor axons

   f. Pathology

      1) Widespread wallerian-like axonal degeneration, primarily involving motor fibers (in roots and peripheral nerves)

      2) Little evidence of demyelination or lymphocytic inflammation

      3) Little, if any, involvement of sensory nerves

   g. NCSs: reduced or absent CMAPs, normal motor distal latencies and conduction velocities, normal SNAPs

   h. Needle EMG: widespread fibrillation potentials after several days

   i. Most patients experience rapid recovery, comparable to patients with prototypic demyelinating Guillain-Barré syndrome

2. Acute motor and sensory axonal neuropathy (AMSAN): axonal variant

   a. Presentation similar to AMAN but also involves sensory axons

   b. Also associated with *C. jejuni* infection

   c. Acute, severe ascending quadraparesis, atrophy, sensory loss

   d. NCSs: reduced or absent CMAPs and SNAPs, with normal conduction velocities and distal latencies, without conduction block

   e. Needle EMG: widespread fibrillation potentials

   f. Immunoglobulin and complement-mediated attack on axolemma, without much demyelination

   g. Pathology

      1) Widespread wallerian-like axonal degeneration

      2) Axonal degeneration of sensory fibers

      3) Little evidence of demyelination or lymphocytic inflammation

   h. Treatment

      1) Same as for Guillain-Barré syndrome

      2) Unlike Guillain-Barré syndrome and AMAN, patients often have incomplete and prolonged recovery

3. Miller Fisher variant

   a. Acute or subacute ataxia, areflexia, ophthalmoplegia (may also have difficulty swallowing due to craniobulbar weakness)

   b. Diplopia is usually first symptom (often from unilateral or bilateral cranial nerve VI palsy), followed by gait and limb ataxia

   c. Debatable whether Miller Fisher variant is brainstem encephalitis in clinical spectrum with Bickerstaff's brainstem encephalitis

   d. Believed to be triggered by a *C. jejuni* or *Haemophilus influenzae* infection

   e. Pathophysiology likely related to immune-mediated attack on antigens at neuromuscular junctions in somatic and extraocular muscles causing rapid, reversible defect of the acetylcholine release from presynaptic membrane, possibly due to nerve-terminal disease and conduction failure

   f. Associated with antibodies to GQ_{1b} ganglioside, probably through molecular mimicry (present in more than 85% of cases)

   g. GQ_{1b} antibodies also reported in Bickerstaff's brainstem encephalitis

   h. Elevated CSF protein

   i. Treatment: same as for Guillain-Barré syndrome

C. Chronic Inflammatory Demyelinating Polyradiculoneuropathy (CIDP)

1. History

   a. "Relapsing polyneuropathies" and "recurrent Guillain-Barré syndrome" were recognized in early twentieth century

b. CIDP was identified as a distinct entity by Dyck and colleagues in 1975
2. Clinical presentation
   a. Antecedent immune challenge such as a vaccination or infection may be seen in patients with CIDP (less common than with AIDP)
   b. Presentation in children: subacute, relatively rapid onset and progression with good response to treatment, followed by relapsing-remitting course
   c. Presentation in adults (three forms)
      1) Usually insidious onset and slow, gradual progression; may be interrupted by sequential improvements and relapses
      2) Stepwise progression
      3) Relapses: often in face of slow progressive disease course, relapsing-remitting course less common than in children
   d. Subacute or chronic presentation of weakness and sensory symptoms of large-fiber dysfunction
   e. Proximal and distal weakness: predominant feature
   f. Numbness, paresthesias, sensory ataxia
   g. Cranial nerves may be involved: most commonly, facial (VII) or oculomotor (III) cranial nerves
   h. Reflexes are reduced or absent
   i. Diagnostic criteria include disease progression longer than 8 weeks or relapses
3. Clinical variants
   a. Motor predominant CIDP
      1) Multifocal demyelinating motor neuropathy
      2) Asymmetric, predominantly motor symptoms
      3) May primarily affect upper limbs
      4) Careful electrophysiologic examination needed to exclude multifocal motor neuropathy with conduction block
   b. Sensory predominant CIDP
      1) Subacute or chronic ascending paresthesias and pain in a stocking distribution
      2) Sensory ataxia
      3) Normal strength, although some patients later develop weakness
      4) Electrophysiologic testing often shows generalized demyelinating peripheral neuropathy, including motor involvement
   c. Multifocal acquired demyelinating sensory and motor neuropathy (MADSAM), also called Lewis-Sumner syndrome or, more simply, multifocal CIDP
      1) Usually slowly progressive (sometimes relapsing-remitting) onset and progression
      2) Distribution of symptoms: asymmetric, distal more than proximal, onset in upper limbs much more frequent than lower limbs or cranial muscles

      3) Sensory symptoms of paresthesias, numbness, pain localized to distribution of single nerves: usually first manifestation
      4) Motor deficits may follow and usually involve upper limb asymmetrically
      5) Absent deep tendon reflexes
      6) Inflammatory demyelinating hypertrophy of nerves in brachial plexus (may be palpable)
      7) Pathology and electrophysiologic testing both show multifocal demyelination on background of generalized neuropathy
      8) NCSs: pattern of multiple mononeuropathies and focal (or multifocal) motor and sensory conduction block
      9) Treatment of first choice is intravenous immunoglobulin; coticosteroids shown to be effective
4. Pathology (Fig. 21-18 and 21-19)
   a. Endoneurial lymphocytic infiltration
   b. Segemental, multifocal demyelination and remyelination, with onion-bulb formation
   c. Multifocal varying degrees of interstitial edema and inflammatory cell infiltrates
   d. Axonal loss (primary or secondary) and axonal sprouting
   e. May be demyelination secondary to axonal atrophy
   f. Involvement of motor and other large fibers more than small fibers
   g. One proposed mechanism of segmental demyelination: invasion of Schwann cells and compact myelin by macrophages
5. Laboratory features
   a. CSF analysis: elevated protein, normal leukocyte count (should be <10 cells/μL); rule out infectious causes
   b. Serum studies to exclude metabolic conditions such as hypothyroidism
   c. Serum protein electrophoresis with immunofixation to exclude paraproteinemia
6. Electrophysiologic features
   a. NCSs
      1) Slowed motor and sensory conduction velocities with prolonged distal latencies
      2) Temporal dispersion and sometimes block of conduction
      3) Prolonged or absent F-wave latencies
      4) Sensory responses often absent
   b. Needle EMG
      1) May show only reduced recruitment of motor unit potentials if predominantly demyelinating lesion
      2) With secondary axonal damage (especially after years of disease), there may be fibrillation potentials and increased motor unit size and complexity

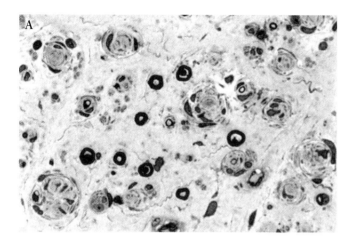

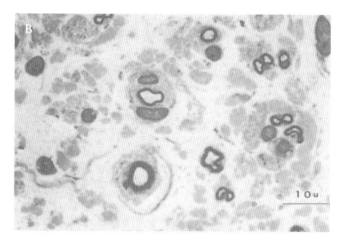

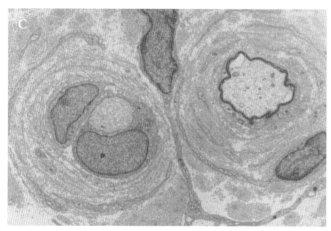

Fig. 21-18. Histopathologic characteristics of onion bulbs. *A*, Mixed pattern of onion bulbs in sural nerve of a patient with chronic inflammatory demyelinating polyradiculoneuropathy (CIDP), some with thinly myelinated central axons, most with no myelinated axons. *B*, Early onion-bulb formation, separated by marked interstitial edema in sural nerve biopsy of a different patient with CIDP. *C*, Ultrastructural appearance of onion bulbs. Note concentric proliferation of Schwann cells and the underlying basement membrane around a thinly myelinated axon (*right*) and a demyelinated axon (*left*). (*A* from Dyck PJ, Dyck PJB, Giannini C, Sahenk Z, Windebank AJ, Engelstad J. Peripheral nerves. In: Graham DI, Lantos PL, editors. Greenfield's neuropathology. Vol. 2. 7th ed. New York: Arnold; 2002. p. 551-675. Used with permission. *B* from Dyck PJ, Gutrecht JA, Bastron JA, Karnes WE, Dale AJD. Histologic and teased-fiber measurements of sural nerve in disorders of lower motor and primary sensory neurons. Mayo Clin Proc. 1968;43:81-123. *C* courtesy of Guillermo A. Suarez, MD.)

7. Treatment
   a. Unlike AIDP, parenteral and oral corticosteroids are particularly helpful in treatment and maintenance
   b. If complications of corticosteroid therapy develop, steroid-sparing agents may be used (but they may take months to become effective)
      1) Azathioprine
      2) Cyclophosphamide
      3) Mycophenolate mofetil
      4) Cyclosporine
   c. For patients with refractory disease or relapse, intravenous immunoglobulin or plasmapheresis is often effective
   d. Prognosis and response to treatment in adults: generally less favorable than in children

D. **Multifocal Motor Neuropathy With Conduction Block** (MMNCB)
1. Introduction
   a. MMNCB was recognized as distinct clinical entity by several authors in 1980s
   b. Much less common (approximately 1-2/100,000) than

disorders it may resemble clinically and electrophysiologically (e.g., motor neuron disease and CIDP)
   c. Prevalence: men more than women (2.6:1)
   d. Mean age at onset: 40 years (80% of patients are between 20 and 50 years old)
2. Clinical presentation
   a. Typical presentation: insidiously progressive (occasionally stepwise) asymmetric painless weakness in individual nerve distributions (80% of cases occur in forearm or hand muscles)
   b. Most often occurs in upper limbs initially
   c. Sensory symptoms of any type should cast doubt on this diagnosis, but they are described in a marked percentage of patients (up to 10%-20%)
   d. Presenting symptom in proximal distribution in 5% and

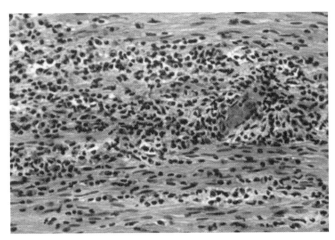

Fig. 21-19. Sural nerve biopsy specimen from patient with chronic inflammatory demyelinating polyradiculopathy (CIDP) demonstrating endoneural inflammation, with prominent mononuclear cellular endoneurial infiltration. (Hematoxylin-eosin.) (From Hahn AF, Hartung H-P, Dyck PJB. Chronic inflammatory demyelinating polyradiculoneuropathy. In: Dyck PJ, Thomas PK, editors. Peripheral neuropathy. Vol. 2. 4th ed. Philadelphia: Elsevier Saunders; 2005. p. 2221-53. Used with permission.)

in leg(s) in 10% of patients

  e. Muscle atrophy of involved muscle groups: mild in early stages

  f. Natural history: one of slow progression, which may be slowed by treatment

  g. Infrequent cranial nerve involvement (often limited to CN XII)

  h. Absent upper motor neuron signs

  i. Pathologic mechanism is poorly understood, and it is unknown if focal demyelination, axonal damage, or a combination is responsible for conduction block

3. Laboratory features

  a. Ganglioside antibodies: about half of patients with MMNCB have anti-GM_1 antibodies, which are not specific and may be seen with other neuropathies

  b. Serum and CSF tests generally serve to exclude other neuropathies

4. Electrophysiologic features (Taylor et al. 2000)

  a. One area, preferentially two areas, of persistent motor conduction block not at common sites of compression: commonly partial conduction block (definition of conduction block, see Chapter 5B)

  b. "Inching" technique is most useful for determining conduction block (definite conduction block by inching is accepted as ≥20% reduction in CMAP amplitude or area over a 10-cm segment by most authorities)

  c. No evidence of diffuse demyelination outside of segments with conduction block

  d. Normal sensory conductions in individual mixed sensory-motor nerves affected by motor conduction block

  e. Needle EMG: chronic or ongoing denervation and reinnervation in distribution affected by partial motor conduction blocks

  f. Evidence of denervation in myotomal pattern should raise specter of motor neuron disease

5. Pathology

  a. Focal areas of conduction block have *not* been definitely shown to be associated with focal demyelination

  b. No hypertrophic changes

  c. Minimal inflammation

  d. Multifocal active axonal degeneration and regeneration

6. Treatment

  a. Intravenous immunoglobulin (initial "load" followed by maintenance therapy): most patients have initial response to this treatment, but response is often transient and many relentlessly (but slowly) show progression despite maintenance therapy

  b. Only chemotherapy agent reported to have been successful: intravenous cyclophosphamide (with or without intravenous immunoglobulin)

  c. Case reports of stabilization with the use of azathioprine

E. Neuropathies Associated With Paraproteinemias

1. Introduction

  a. The presence of monoclonal immunoglobin proteins (M proteins or M spikes) is risk factor for peripheral neuropathy (conversely, patients with "idiopathic" neuropathies are more likely than controls to have a serum monoclonal protein)

  b. Direct, biologically causative links between the protein and neuropathy are often, but not always, demonstrable

  c. Characteristics of the M protein and any associated condition often dictate type and severity of neuropathy

2. Waldenström's macroglobulinemia

  a. Likely the first recognized neuropathic paraproteinemia

  b. Caused by rampant proliferation of plasma and lympho-cytoid cells that produce the M protein

  c. The M protein in these patients consists of IgM, 75% of cases are associated with a κ light chain

  d. Patients are often elderly men

  e. Presenting symptoms often nonspecific (fatigue, dyspnea, weight loss)

  f. Hyperviscosity and bleeding complications may be present

  g. Hepatomegaly, splenomegaly

h. Associated polyneuropathy
  1) Usually length-dependent sensorimotor peripheral neuropathy similar to that associated with monoclonal gammopathy of undetermined significance (MGUS) (may be predominantly demyelinating or axonal)
  2) Less often, multiple mononeuropathies associated with cryoglobulinemia and/or hyperviscosity
  3) Rarely, small-fiber neuropathy associated with amyloidosis
i. Laboratory and ancillary evaluation
  1) IgM M protein: often elevated more than 3 g/dL
  2) Monoclonal light chain is seen in urine in most cases
  3) Anti-MAG reactivity in some patients: the neuropathy tends to be predominantly demyelinating
  4) High erythrocyte sedimentation rate
  5) Moderate to severe normocytic, normochromic anemia
  6) Hyperviscosity
  7) Associated with cold agglutinins and cryoglobulinemia
  8) No lytic bone lesions
j. Treatment with plasma exchange or intravenous immunoglobulin may slow progression of neuropathy, but generally the response of IgM-associated neuropathies is less robust than with IgG-associated neuropathies
  1) Primary disease management with chemotherapy may also slow progression of the neuropathy
3. POEMS (**p**olyneuropathy, **o**rganomegaly, **e**ndocrinopathy, **M** protein, **s**kin changes) syndrome (osteosclerotic myeloma)
  a. Peak incidence in fifth to sixth decades of life
  b. Osteosclerotic myeloma is much less common than multiple myeloma (at a ratio of approximately 20:1) and are distinct entities
    1) Neuropathy is rare in multiple myeloma
    2) Neuropathy is a hallmark of osteosclerotic myeloma (occurring in 85%-90% of patients)
  c. Clinical features
    1) Polyneuropathy: often primary complaint
    2) Organomegaly: spelnomegaly, hepatomegaly, lymphadenopathy
    3) Endocrinopathy: gynecomastia, testicular atrophy, impotence in men, secondary amenorrhea in women, diabetes mellitus, hypothyroidism
    4) M protein (most often IgG or less likely IgA): usually λ light chain and α or γ heavy chain class
    5) Skin changes: hyperpigmentation, hypertrichosis, clubbing of fingers and toes, white nail beds, hemangiomas

    6) Other findings: pitting edema of lower extremities, ascites, pleural effusions, thrombocytosis, polycythemia, weight loss
  d. Most patients have radiographic evidence of sclerotic bone lesion: most commonly axial skeleton (spine, pelvis, ribs)
  e. Polyneuropathy
    1) Length-dependent
    2) Slowly progressive course with severe deficits
    3) Both sensory and motor symptoms begin in lower extremities and ascend proximally: motor predominant
    4) Often present with sensory symptoms of numbness and paresthesias, followed by symmetric weakness
    5) Motor impairment often becomes severe enough to overshadow sensory symptoms
  f. Electrodiagnosis of the neuropathy: features of demyelination (conduction block, temporal dispersion, slowing of conduction velocities, and prolongation of distal latencies) and frequently distal secondary axonal damage
  g. CSF protein is almost universally elevated (to >100 mg/dL in 50% of patients), without cellular response
  h. From 11% to 30% of patients have Castleman's syndrome (angiofollicular lymph node hyperplasia)
  i. Treatment of osteosclerotic myeloma with focused irradiation and chemotherapy may halt or slow progression of neuropathy
  j. Neuropathy may continue to respond 1 or 2 years after completion of therapy
  k. Efficacy of plasma exchange and intravenous immunoglobulin in the treatment of neuropathy: conflicting results
4. Multiple myeloma
  a. Peak incidence in seventh decade
  b. Usual presenting features: fatigue, anemia, hypercalcemia
  c. Associated with lytic lesions, osteoporosis, or fractures
  d. Most common neurologic manifestation: compressive radiculopathy (due to myelomatous infiltration and spread); in 5% of cases, myelopathy or cauda equina syndrome due to extradural spread of myeloma from vertebral body
  e. Most multiple myeloma patients have serum and urine M protein
  f. Multiple myeloma is associated with symptomatic neuropathy in less than 10% of patients (half of whom have pathologic evidence of amyloid deposition on nerve biopsy)
  g. Neuropathic presentation varies and may be length-

dependent in pattern or, less likely, polyradicular (most often features of axonal loss on electrodiagnostic evaluation)

5. Primary acquired amyloidosis
   a. Amyloid: a deposited proteinaceous material that is eosinophilic on light microscopy and appears the same regardless of origin of protein
   b. Amyloidosis can be divided loosely into acquired (primary and secondary) and familial forms (discussed above)
   c. Most cases are acquired; of these, primary amyloidosis is most commonly associated with neuropathic complications (focus of this discussion)
   d. Primary acquired amyloidosis is uncommon, occurring in fewer than 1/100,000 persons per year
   e. Presenting features: fatigue, weight loss, bruising, symptoms of associated neuropathy
   f. Serum M protein is present in about 70% of patients, reflecting plasma cell proliferative disorder; this may be
      1) Primary or
      2) Related to coexistent multiple myeloma
   g. Neuropathic manifestations of amyloidosis are protean
      1) Autonomic neuropathy: orthostatism, syncope, and impotence are common complaints
      2) Length-dependent sensorimotor peripheral neuropathy: common, manifests with predominantly painful sensory complaints and small-fiber involvement
      3) Median neuropathies at wrists: very common; are predisposed with deposition of amyloid in flexor retinaculum at the wrist
      4) Neuropathic presentation may be clouded by coexistent proximal myopathy also caused by amyloid deposition
   h. Diagnosis relies on demonstrating amyloid in tissue in appropriate clinical context: demonstration of amyloid in any affected tissue (skin, nerve, muscle, bowel, abdominal fat pad) is sufficient for diagnosis
      1) Screen for amyloid: Congo red staining (but not highly sensitive, particularly for secondary amyloid)
      2) Staining with labeled antisera to light chains may be necessary if amyloid is strongly suspected
      3) Nerve biopsies (most often performed on sural nerve) demonstrate epineurial and endoneurial deposition of amyloid, often with concomitant deposition in nerve microvasculature
      4) Amyloid appears pink with hematoxylin-eosin staining, but assumes apple-green birefringence when Congo red preparation is viewed under polarized light
   i. Electrophysiologic abnormalities may be subtle, with mild neuropathies or exclusive small-fiber involvement,

but most patients with symptomatic neuropathies have abnormal EMG findings
   1) NCSs: mild slowing, often absent compound sensory nerve action potentials
   2) Needle EMG: fibrillation potentials; large, complex motor unit potentials (and possibly features of concurrent myopathy)
   j. Survival after diagnosis of systemic amyloidosis averages approximately 1 year
   k. Multiple chemotherapy agents (melphalan, high-dose corticosteroids, alkylating agents) have been used, generally with disappointing results
   l. Possibly better success with autologous peripheral blood stem cell transplantation for patients who are candidates
   m. Treatment of amyloid neuropathy: directed at type of neuropathy and associated symptoms
      1) Symptomatic treatment of autonomic insufficiency
         a) High support stockings
         b) Cautious volume expansion with fludrocortisone or pressure support with midodrine
         c) Behavioral modification (e.g, sitting at the edge of bed) and bed tilting
      2) Symptomatic treatment of pain or dysesthesias associated with sensorimotor peripheral neuropathy
         a) Antiepileptic medications (carbamazepine or gabapentin)
         b) Tricyclic antidepressants (amitriptyline or nortriptyline)
         c) In some cases, opioids may be necessary
      3) Median neuropathies may respond to release of flexor retinaculum

6. Neuropathies associated with MGUS
   a. Hallmark: serum (or urine) M protein; serum M protein concentration less than 3 g/dL (urine M protein may be absent or present in very small amounts)
   b. No clinical or laboratory evidence of another condition associated with M proteins, systemic amyloidosis, or other lymphoproliferative disorders: absence of lytic bone lesions, hypercalcemia, anemia, renal disease, or other systemic manifestations
   c. By definition, M protein remains stable and patients do not develop other abnormalities
   d. Substantial proportion of patients originally diagnosed with MGUS ultimately develop lymphoproliferative disorders or complications of paraproteinemia
   e. Incidence: 3% of Europeans and European descendants older than 70 years
   f. Rate of progression (prorated) of these patients to marked associated comorbidity (lymphoproliferative disorder or complication of paraproteinemia): approximately

g. Size of M spike is independently predictive of this risk

h. Association of MGUS with sensorimotor peripheral neuropathy is clear, but relative risk of neuropathy in these patients varies among studies according to patient selection and definition of neuropathy

i. Features of peripheral neuropathy associated with MGUS

1) Usually insidious onset and progression

2) Generally presents as symmetric sensorimotor length-dependent neuropathy or polyradiculoneuropathy with axonal and demyelinating features

3) More common in men

4) Paresthesias and pain are often prominent features

5) CSF protein is typically elevated without an elevated cellular response

j. In MGUS patients with neuropathy, the associated M protein may be any subtype, but the protein is more likely to be IgM than in patients with MGUS and no neuropathy

1) Two-thirds of patients have κ subtype light chain

2) IgM patients also more likely to have demyelinating features on nerve biopsy and electrodiagnostic studies

3) IgM patients likely have more severe neuropathies

4) Approximately half of these patients have anti-MAG antibodies

5) MAG: minor myelin protein (noncompacted myelin), concentrated in periaxonal inner myelin membrane of Schwann cells and paranodal myelin loops

6) Antibodies to MAG likely target oligosaccharide residues of molecule and block adhesive interactions between Schwann cells and underlying axon

7) Antibodies to MAG also likely cross-react with other antigens (glycolipids and gangliosides)

k. Treatment of MGUS-associated neuropathies

1) Has included plasma exchange and chemotherapeutic agents, each with mixed success

2) As with other paraproteinemic neuropathies, patients with monoclonal IgG and IgA respond better to treatment than do those with IgM

7. Cryoglobulinemia

a. Hallmark: cryoglobulins, which precipitate on cooling and redissolve on warming (core body temperatures)

b. Type I: monoclonal immunoglobulins

1) Associated with multiple myeloma, Waldenström's macroglobulinemia, chronic leukemia, lymphoma

2) May be asymptomatic

3) Symptoms (when present): Reynaud's phenomenon, cyanosis, purpura

c. Type II: mixed polyclonal (usually IgG) and monoclonal (usually IgMκ with anti-rheumatoid factor activity)

1) Also possible: monoclonal IgG or IgA with polyclonal IgM

2) Associated with hepatitis C

3) Symptoms: purpura, cutaneous vasculitis, polyarthralgias, glomerulonephritis, Reynaud's phenomenon, peripheral neuropathy

d. Type III: mixed polyclonal IgG

e. Amount of protein present correlates poorly with severity of neuropathy (the temperature of precipitation is more predictive of symptoms than quantity)

f. Peripheral neuropathy associated with cryoglobulinemia may be asymmetric and multifocal, affecting cooler parts of body, as multiple mononeuropathies (mononeuritis multiplex) or length-dependent sensorimotor peripheral neuropathy

IV. NEUROPATHIES RELATED TO TOXIC AND METABOLIC CONDITIONS AND NUTRITIONAL DEFICIENCIES (SEE CHAPTER 17)

V. DIABETES-RELATED PERIPHERAL NERVE DISORDERS

A. Diabetic Polyneuropathy

1. Usually chronic and insidious onset; rapid onset of small-fiber–type neuropathy with dysautonomia is possible but rare

2. Predisposing factors for development of diabetes polyneuropathy: poor hyperglycemic control, male sex, long-duration of diabetes, age, and cooccurrence of hypertension

3. Pathogenesis

a. Elevated plasma glucose is directly toxic to nerve; chronic hyperglycemia induces long-term, repetitive metabolic insults to nerve

b. Rheologic effects of hyperglycemia may reduce microvascular blood flow, inducing hypoperfusion and hypoxia

c. Poorly controlled, chronic hyperglycemia predisposes to microvascular disease of small vessels of endoneurium

d. Endoneural capillaries often thickened

e. May be focal areas of axonal loss, which may be due to microinfarcts of nerve

4. Predominantly length-dependent axonal degeneration

5. Prominent demyelinating features on EMG, such as multifocal conduction block or slowing and nerve

conduction velocities less than 70% of low limit of normal are atypical

6. Presentation
   a. Slowly progressive distal sensory loss (predominantly sensory neuropathy) with feet injuries that heal poorly
   b. Neuropathic pain, paresthesias, dysesthesias
   c. Small fibers usually affected first; large-fiber sensation is affected later in course, and patients may experience sensory imbalance as a result
   d. Clinical weakness and atrophy are late signs (fibrillation potentials and neurogenic motor unit potentials may be present on needle EMG)
   e. Selective involvement of large fibers and weakness with no sensory loss are both clues that a cause other than diabetes needs to be considered
   f. Despite this, there is a less common large-fiber variant in which patients are often asymptomatic but may present with painless paresthesias, loss of joint position and vibration sensation, and gait sensory ataxia
   g. Autonomic neuropathy often complicates diabetic polyneuropathies (see below)

7. Testing
   a. Fasting blood glucose of 126 mg/dL on two or more occasions is indicative of diabetes
   b. Fasting blood glucose of more than 110 mg/dL (<126 mg/dL) is indicative of glucose intolerance and needs to be followed
   c. Hemoglobin A_{1C} reflects plasma glucose control within last 5 to 8 weeks: a negative result does not exclude diabetes
   d. Glucose tolerance test: 2-hour plasma glucose of 200 mg/dL is suggestive of diabetes
   e. EMG and NCS are important in confirming pattern and characterization of neuropathy (length-dependent axonal) and diagnosis of a superimposed process such as compression neuropathy

8. Treatment
   a. Routine foot care and inspection of feet for early abrasions or ulcers
   b. Aggressive control of blood glucose to prevent or slow progression of neuropathy
   c. Treatment of neuropathic pain with tricyclic antidepressants (amitriptyline, nortriptyline), anticonvulsive agents (gabapentin, carbamazepine, lamotrigine, topiramate)
   d. Treatment of orthostatic hypotension (usually mild)

B. Acute Diabetic Polyneuropathy
1. Also called diabetic cachexia
2. Monophasic illness lasting for more than 1 month
3. Usually precipitated by change (worsening or improving) in glycemic control
4. Acute and rapid onset, which usually follows unwanted weight loss (hence, "diabetic cachexia"), insomnia, depression, and impotence
5. Autonomic features other than impotence are rare and usually do not occur
6. Primarily involvement of small pain sensory fibers: relative sparing or mild involvement of nerve conductions, painful neuropathy (usually severe burning pain with allodynia and hypersensitivity in lower extremities), ankle jerks are present, reduced, or absent and distal weakness is very mild
7. No muscle weakness; sensory loss may be minimal

C. Insulin Neuritis
1. Acute onset of neuropathic pain and paresthesias in distal lower extremities shortly after initiating insulin therapy and obtaining glycemic control
2. Pathogenesis unclear but may be due to active regeneration

D. Autonomic Neuropathy
1. Orthostatic hypotension
2. Gastroparesis and delayed gastric emptying, constipation may be due to colonic atony, diarrhea due to involvement of small intestine autonomic innervation
3. Impotence in men: usually one of first autonomic symptoms
4. Bladder atony with urinary retention, followed by overflow incontinence
5. Sudomotor abnormalities: distal anhidrosis, hyperhidrosis of face and forehead with eating (gustatory sweating)

E. Diabetic Lumbosacral Radiculoplexus Neuropathy (DLRPN)
1. Also called proximal diabetic neuropathy or diabetic amyotrophy
2. Characteristics similar to the nondiabetic lumbosacral radiculoplexus neuropathy
3. Rare: occurs in 1% of patients
4. Usually occurs in adults with non–insulin-dependent diabetes (men more often than women)
5. Glycemic dysregulation often not severe
6. Patients often do not have many long-term complications of diabetes mellitus (e.g., retinopathy or nephropathy)
7. May occur together with diabetic thoracic radiculoplexus neuropathy
8. Abrupt and rapidly progressive onset of asymmetric, focal, predominantly proximal leg pain and weakness

a. Usually no precipitating factor can be identified
b. Pain is often severe and early, and followed by severe weakness (which then becomes a more important problem than pain)
c. Pain is usually focal, unilateral (or bilateral and asymmetric): often occurs in proximal lower limb (anterolateral thigh, hip, buttock)
d. Symptoms often quickly spread to involve both proximal and distal segments and contralateral leg and become more symmetric with early progression
e. Muscle weakness may be only proximal (e.g., involving thigh and hip) and/or distal (e.g., peroneal-innervated muscles such as anterior tibialis): distribution is usually focal and unilateral
f. Symptoms of pain and weakness may appear bilateral and symmetric at onset
9. Large, concomitant weight loss is common
10. Usually monophasic illness
11. Patients also often have sensory and autonomic symptoms
12. CSF: markedly elevated protein
13. NCSs
a. Findings indicative of axonal loss: reduced motor and sensory nerve action potential amplitudes
b. Femoral motor conduction studies may be helpful: relatively early in disease, femoral CMAP amplitude is lower on affected side than on opposite side (asymmetric), reflecting the degree of axonal loss
c. CMAP amplitudes improve with adequate reinnervation
14. Needle EMG
a. Fibrillation potentials in involved segments, including paraspinal muscles
b. With collateral sprouting and reinnervation, needle EMG shows polyphasic varying motor unit potentials of longer duration than normal
c. With adequate reinnervation, fibrillation potentials eventually disappear
15. Pathogenesis and pathology (Fig. 21-20 and 21-21)
a. Likely axonal loss due to ischemic insult to nerves as a result of microvasculitis
b. Epineurial and perineurial vasculitis and resultant ischemia and multiple foci of microinfarct, perineurial thickening, neovascularization
c. Usual clinical presentation of subacute onset of an asymmetric syndrome is typical for a vasculitic process
16. Prognosis
a. Spontaneous recovery is the rule
b. Pain may be the first manifestation to improve
c. Role of treatment is questionable and resolution of the syndrome may not be attributable to treatment, given

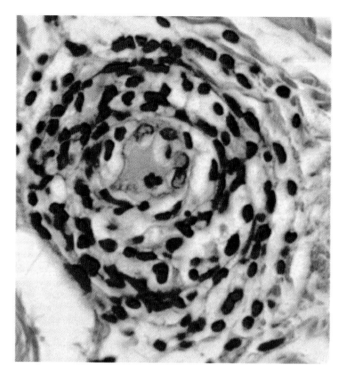

Fig. 21-20. Sural nerve biopsy specimen from patient with nondiabetic lumbosacral radiculoplexus neuropathy showing microvasculitis, with disrupted, fragmented smooth muscle layers of the tunica media, separated by mononuclear cell infiltrates. (From Dyck PJB, Windebank AJ. Diabetic and nondiabetic lumbosacral radiculoplexus neuropathies: new insights into pathophysiology and treatment. Muscle Nerve. 2002;25:477-91. Used with permission.)

the natural history of spontaneous recovery
d. Fewer long-term complications of diabetes mellitus (e.g., nephropathy) and better glycemic control than for other diabetic patients
e. Recovery usually delayed and incomplete (although usually little residua)
17. Treatment
a. Corticosteroids can produce dramatic response
b. Corticosteroids and intravenous immunogloblin may be considered for severely affected patients or those with active progression

F. Diabetic Truncal Radiculoneuropathy
1. Thoracic radiculopathy of T4-T12 segments
2. Occurs in setting of weight loss or change in the glycemic control
3. Gradual or abrupt onset
4. Thoracic dermatomal distribution sensory loss, dysesthesias, hypesthesias, focal anhidrosis (as noted on

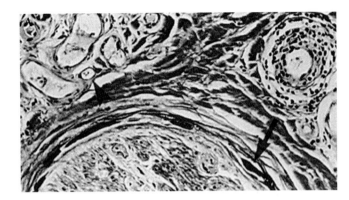

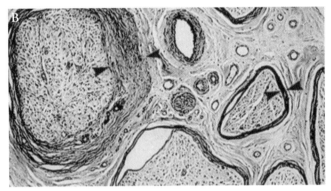

Fig. 21-21. Changes of diabetic and nondiabetic lumbosacral plexus neuropathy. *A*, Inflammatory infiltrates of an epineurial microvessel (upper right corner), fibrinoid degeneration of the perineurium (*arrow*), and a region of neovascularization (*arrowhead*). *B*, Other than neovascularization, ischemic injury also induces perineurial thickening (between two *arrowheads* on the left, as compared with the normal perineurial thickness, between two *arrowheads* on the right.)

thermoregulatory sweat test)
5. EMG: denervation and neurogenic changes in dermatomes involved, including paraspinal muscles and abdominal muscles of same dermatomal distribution
6. Natural history of several weeks to months
7. Pain persists for up to 2 months, and sensory symptoms may be lifelong

G. Diabetes-Related Mononeuropathies
1. Result of nerve infarction or entrapment
2. Nerve infarction
    a. Usually not at typical sites of compression
    b. Less common than entrapment neuropathies
    c. Marked by sudden onset of pain and weakness and development of atrophy
    d. Pathogenesis predominantly axonal loss

3. Entrapment
    a. Patients with diabetic neuropathies are more prone to compression neuropathies at usual sites of nerve compression
    b. With early, mild to moderate entrapment neuropathies, there is often focal slowing or conduction block on NCS
    c. Electrophysiologic features of axonal loss with more severe lesions that include wallerian degeneration: fibrillation potentials and reduced CMAP amplitudes
4. Cranial mononeuropathies (microvascular infarction)
    a. Most frequently affected nerves: CNs III, IV, VI; less commonly CN VII (idiopathic Bell's palsy is more common in diabetics than nondiabetics)
    b. Presentation of acute onset (often painful and associated with headache) diplopia due to unilateral cranial motor neuropathy
    c. CN III palsy is often pupil-sparing given the deep location of pupillary fibers in CN III
    d. About 72% of patients are expected to recover completely in 1 to 3 months

VI. NEUROPATHIES ASSOCIATED WITH VASCULITIS

A. General Characteristics
1. Systemic or nonsystemic vasculitis
2. Predominantly axonal neuropathies
3. Pathogenesis
    a. Humoral-mediated autoimmunity: deposition of antigen-antibody complexes formed in circulation, targeting the vessel wall antigen and complement activation; anti-endothelial antibody attack on endothelial antigenic determinants; ANCA-mediated humoral autoimmunity against cytoplasmic proteins on neutrophils and monocytes
    b. Cellular autoimmunity: direct T-cell–mediated cytotoxic effect, primarily on endothelial cells
4. Histologic tissue is often necessary for diagnosis, given potentially toxic adverse effects of treatment options
    a. Sural nerve is usually adequate for biopsy
    b. Combined muscle and nerve biopsy may have higher yield (such as superficial peroneal nerve and peroneus brevis muscle through a single incision)
5. Pathology (Fig. 21-22)
    a. Transmural or perivascular inflammation: inflammatory infiltrates within vessel wall
    b. Vascular destruction and fibrinoid necrosis
    c. Necrotizing vasculitis: segmental inflammatory necrosis and destruction of arterial wall

d. Microvasculitis: inflammatory cellular infiltration of the wall of microvessels (small arterioles and venules), causing disruption of vessel wall

e. Perivascular hemorrhage (hemosiderin deposits)

f. Thickening of vessel wall with or without intraluminal thrombus, causing narrowing or occlusion of the vessel, which can produce nerve infarcts and multifocal nerve-fiber loss

g. Vasculitis predilection for epineurial (more than endoneurial) vessels

h. Large myelinated fibers especially susceptible to ischemic injury

6. Two most common systemic vasculitic conditions: polyarteritis nodosa, rheumatoid arthritis

7. Clinical presentation

a. Rapid (acute or subacute) onset of painful multifocal sensory and motor deficits in distribution of one or more nerves: pattern of mononeuritis multiplex or asymmetric polyneuropathy

b. Relatively rapid onset of symptoms is consistent with pattern of ischemic injury

c. Most commonly affected lower extremity nerve: common peroneal nerve, followed by tibial and sural nerves

d. Most commonly affected upper extremity nerve: ulnar nerve, followed by median and radial nerves

e. Usually: asymmetric polyneuropathy due to extensive, overlapping multifocal involvement of peripheral nerves

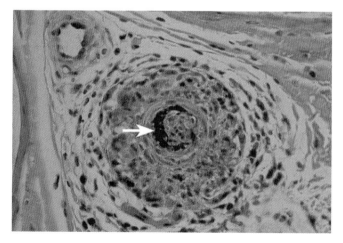

Fig. 21-22. Section through sural nerve showing necrotizing vasculitis of a small epineurial arteriole, with disruption, destruction, and thickening of the smooth muscle wall and fibrinoid degeneration (*arrow*) and luminal occlusion. (Trichrome stain.) (Courtesy of Guillermo A. Suarez, MD.)

8. Electrodiagnostic evaluation

a. Role

1) To characterize pattern and localization of disease, severity and extent of axonal loss

2) To identify suitable nerves for nerve biopsy

3) May be used to follow clinical course of patient after obtaining baseline results before treatment

b. Features predominantly of axonal loss: low-amplitude CMAP and SNAP responses, with fibrillation potentials, reduced recruitment, and chronic neurogenic changes (in chronic stage)

c. Features suggestive of mononeuritis multiplex or asymmetric polyneuropathy: predominant involvement of upper extremities and/or asymmetric findings on needle EMG between the two sides and/or between individual nerves of same dermatomal distribution in same limb

9. Generalizations about treatment options

a. Corticosteroids

1) Usually first line of treatment

2) Typical starting dose: 1 mg/kg oral prednisone (if severe, intravenous methylprednisolone)

3) Daily dose is continued for at least 2 months

4) Gradual taper and transition to alternate-day dosing and discontinuation of drug in 12 months is usual goal

5) Treatment strategy is based on underlying disease, severity at presentation, age, other factors

6) Patients should be monitored for hypertension, glucose intolerance, weight gain, glaucoma, cataracts, osteoporosis, avascular necrosis of hip, other complications related to long-term corticosteroid use

b. Cytotoxic adjuvant therapy

1) Decision to add cytotoxic agent is based on many factors: patient's response to corticosteroids, possible complications of corticosteroids in relation to underlying comorbidities, and underlying disease (e.g., all cases of Wegener's granulomatosis are treated with glucocorticoids and cyclophosphamide, as first-line agents)

2) After remission, cyclophosphamide is switched to less toxic agent such as methotrexate or azathioprine

3) Nonsystemic vasculitic neuropathy is often less aggressive and has a better prognosis than systemic vasculitic neuropathies

4) Less aggressive immunosuppressant therapy (e.g., azathioprine or methotrexte) is indicated for nonsystemic vasculitic neuropathies

5) Azathioprine is usually steroid-sparing agent of choice and is typically initiated within 6 months after initiating prednisone

B. Specific Vasculitic and Granulomatous Syndromes Associated With Peripheral Neuropathy

1. Classic polyarteritis nodosa
    a. Most common cause of systemic necrotizing vasculitis and most frequent cause of vasculitic neuropathy
    b. Focal, segmental necrotizing inflammatory vasculitis of small- and medium-size arteries
    c. Typically starts with subacute onset of constitutional symptoms, such as fever and weight loss
    d. Some cases are associated with hepatitis B virus
    e. Laboratory findings: leukocytosis, normocytic anemia, thrombocytosis, high erythrocyte sedimentation rate, antinuclear antibody (ANA), rheumatoid factor (RF), hypocomplementemia

2. Rheumatoid arthritis
    a. Systemic disease: rheumatoid arthritis, rheumatoid nodules occurring in extremities, pericarditis, pleuritis, interstitial lung disease, and systemic vasculitis causing organ infarction, glomerulonephritis, cutaneous vasculitic involvement
    b. Presentations of PNS disease
        1) Entrapment compression neuropathies
        2) Necrotizing small-vessel vasculitis causing mononeuropathy or mononeuritis multiplex (cranial nerve mononeuropathy is rare)
        3) Sensory or sensorimotor length-dependent polyneuropathy
        4) Predominantly sensory distal polyneuropathy (some patients)
    c. Laboratory findings
        1) Increased RF in 90%-95% of cases and increased erythrocyte sedimentation rate in 85% of cases
        2) C4 complement level is often low

3. Churg-Strauss syndrome
    a. ANCA-associated vasculitic syndrome of asthma, eosinophilia, systemic necrotizing vasculitis
    b. Clinical manifestations
        1) Prodromal asthma, allergic rhinitis, polyposis
        2) Intermediate stage of peripheral eosinophilia
        3) Final phase: necrotizing systemic vasculitis, including necrotizing glomerulonephritis and necrotizing neuropathy
    c. Sural nerve biopsy: epineural necrotizing vasculitis, sometimes with eosinophilic infiltrates

4. Sjögren's syndrome
    a. 90% female predominance
    b. PNS involvement in 10% to 30% of patients (also strong predilection for women)
    c. May be termed secondary Sjögren's syndrome if there are systemic signs of another connective tissue disease such as rheumatoid arthritis or systemic lupus erythematosus

    d. Sicca complex: reduced lacrimation and salivation (dry eyes, dry mouth) from lymphocytic and plasmacytic infiltration and destruction of exocrine glands (lacrimal and salivary glands)
    e. Lymphocytic infiltration of dorsal root and gasserian ganglia result in ataxic sensory neuropathy and trigeminal neuropathy, respectively
    f. Trigeminal sensory neuropathy (unilateral or bilateral) has also been associated with systemic sclerosis, mixed connective tissue disease, systemic lupus erythematosus, rheumatoid arthritis
    g. Presentations of PNS disease are as follows:
        1) Ganglionopathy
            a) Ataxic sensory neuropathy from involvement of dorsal root ganglia
            b) Large-fiber sensory loss, sensory ataxia, pseudo-athetosis, areflexia, autonomic dysfunction
            c) Trigeminal neuropathy from involvement of the gasserian ganglion: facial numbness (bilateral in half of cases) and painful paresthesias primarily involving second and third divisions of CN V (sometimes all three divisions), sparing motor fibers
        2) Mononeuritis multiplex
        3) Sensory or sensorimotor distal symmetric polyneuropathy
            a) Most common neuropathy in this setting
            b) Often presenting with slowly progressive numbness and paresthesias
            c) May be primarily sensory or there may be mild weakness
            d) Much less common: polyradiculoneuropathy, sometimes resembling CIDP
    h. Investigations
        1) Increased erythrocyte sedimentation rate, ANA (90% of cases), anti-Ro and anti-La (60%-70%), positive RF (60%-90%), hypergammaglobulinemia
        2) EMG and NCS: features of axonal loss (low sensory and motor amplitudes, fibrillation potentials)
        3) High T2 signal in dorsal columns of patients with sensory ganglionopathy
        4) Rose Bengal staining of cornea
        5) Schirmer's test (<5 mm wetting of paper strip at 5 minutes)
        6) Minor salivary gland biopsy of lower lip showing lymphocytic infiltrates
    i. Prognosis: generally good, many patients stabilize with or without treatment
    j. Treatment
        1) Corticosteroids and cytotoxic immunosuppressants
        2) Supportive treatment with artificial tears and periodic

ophthalmologic examinations are indicated for primary Sjögren's syndrome involving exocrine glands

5. Systemic lupus erythematosus
   a. Predilection for women of child-bearing age and African-American race
   b. Systemic manifestations: arthralgias, cutaneous manifestations (malar "butterfly" rash, discoid rash), photosensitivity, anemia, leukopenia, thrombocytopenia, pleuritis, pericarditis, nephropathy (proteinuria and urinary casts), Libman-Sacks endocarditis (associated with antiphospholipid antibody syndrome)
   c. CNS manifestations (see Chapter 14)
   d. Peripheral nerve manifestations
      1) Mild, distal sensorimotor neuropathy, with slow progression, may be asymmetric in onset
      2) Mononeuritis multiplex: necrotizing vasculitis of small- and medium-size arteries
      3) Polyradiculoneuropathy: sometimes inflammatory demyelinating, with subacute progression, resembling AIDP or CIDP
      4) Inflammatory brachial plexus neuropathy
      5) Cranial neuropathies: predilection for CNs III, IV, V, VII
   e. Evaluation
      1) ANA positive in 95% to 100% of cases
      2) Other markers: anti-dsDNA, Anti-Sm, anti-Ro
6. Systemic sclerosis (scleroderma)
   a. Excessive proliferation and deposition of collagen and extracellular matrix proteins and fibrosis involving skin, lungs, heart, kidneys, gastrointestinal tract, muscle, nerve
   b. Associated with CREST syndrome (**c**alcinosis, **R**aynaud's phenomenon, **e**sophageal dysmotility, **s**clerodactyly, and **t**elangiectasia)
   c. Diffuse myopathy
   d. Peripheral nerve involvement: peripheral sensorimotor neuropathy, mononeuropathy or multiple mononeuropathies (usually entrapment neuropathies due to fibrosis and calcinosis), isolated trigeminal sensory neuropathy
7. Mixed connective tissue disease
   a. Predilection for women in third and fourth decades
   b. Usual symptom at onset: Raynaud's phenomenon
   c. Laboratory data: characterized by antibodies to ribonuclear proteins (anti-U1 RNP)
   d. CNS manifestations: seizures, psychosis, aseptic meningitis
   e. Peripheral nerve involvement
      1) Trigeminal sensory neuropathy
      2) Symmetric distal sensory neuropathy
      3) Chronic polyradiculoneuropathy resembling CIDP
      4) Autonomic neuropathy

8. PNS manifestations of sarcoidosis (sarcoid neuropathy)
   a. CNS and systemic manifestations (see Chapter 14)
   b. PNS involvement: relatively rare but heterogeneous
   c. Cranial nerve involvement: CN VII is most commonly involved peripheral nerve
   d. There may be multiple cranial neuropathies with fluctuating course
   e. Multiple mononeuropathies and multifocal, asymmetric sensorimotor neuropathy
   f. Chronic symmetric distal sensorimotor peripheral neuropathy
   g. Polyradiculopathy and Guillain-Barré–like syndrome
   h. Pure motor neuropathy
   i. Pathology (Fig. 21-23)
      1) Initially: mononuclear infiltration, followed by formation of noncaseating granulomas
      2) Granuloma: collection of epithelioid cells derived from macrophages, which may form multinucleated giant cells, with fibrosis and hyalinization
      3) Epineurial and perineurial granulomatous necrotizing vasculitis
      4) CD4+ cellular proliferation in regions of active granulomatous inflammation
   j. Almost all patients with neuropathy related to sarcoid also have sarcoid myopathy
      1) A high percentage of patients with sarcoidosis have muscle involvement, although most of the patients are asymptomatic
      2) Symptomatic patients often present with proximal weakness, myalgias, tenderness of involved muscles

VII. NONVASCULITIC ISCHEMIC NEUROPATHIES

A. Ischemic Monomelic Neuropathy (IMN)

1. Rare disorder
2. Nerve damage secondary to ischemic insult resulting from insufficient perfusion inducing axonal loss
3. IMN of upper extremities
   a. Less common than IMN of lower extremities
   b. Almost always unilateral and iatrogenic
   c. Almost always secondary to arteriovenous shunt placement in upper limb for dialysis treatment in patients with end-stage renal disease
   d. Almost always in diabetics with end-stage renal disease due to diabetic nephropathy (underlying diabetic neuropathy may potentially be a predisposition)
4. IMN of lower extremities
   a. Often bilateral, noniatrogenic or iatrogenic (intra-aortic balloon pump placement, cardiopulmonary bypass

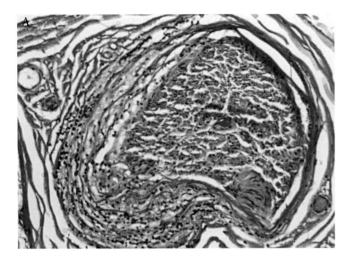

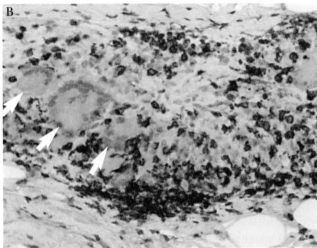

Fig. 21-23. Sural nerve biopsy specimen from patient with sarcoid neuropathy presenting with polyradiculoneuropathy. *A*, Perineurial thickening and necrotizing vasculitis with inflammatory cellular infiltration. *B*, Immunohistochemistry (CD3, T-cell marker) of a typical granulomatous necrotizing vasculitis demonstrates T-cell lymphocytic CD4+ cellular proliferation in regions of active granulomatous inflammation. Note the numerous multinucleated giant cells (*arrows*), which do not stain with CD3 immunohistochemistry. (Courtesy of P. James B. Dyck, MD.)

      cannulation)
  b. Less commonly, there may be compressive lesion such as neoplasm, hematoma, or bony anomaly that may precipitously produce limb ischemia
5. Clinical presentation
  a. Abrupt onset of deep, burning pain and paresthesias in hand or foot, with subsequent development of weakness and atrophy (after several weeks, if persistent)

  b. Despite abrupt onset, symptoms reach maximal intensity after several days
  c. Weakness is most prominent distally and there is a distal-to-proximal gradient (deficits "fade out" proximally, both clinically and electrophysiologically)
  d. This may be due to more severe nerve fiber ischemia distally; alternatively, there may be focal nerve infarctions proximally, with length-dependent axonal degeneration that accumulates along longest axons
  e. Multiple (distal-predominant axonal loss) mononeuropathies
  f. Other tissues are relatively preserved (i.e., relative absence of skin pallor, atrophic skin, or hair loss and normal pulses)
  g. Duration of the ischemic events: varies but may last as long as few minutes to hours
6. Electrodiagnostic evaluation
  a. NCS (both sensory and motor): length-dependent pattern of axonal loss (e.g., normal antebrachial conductions but motor and sensory conductions recorded at the hand tend to be abnormal)
  b. Needle EMG: fibrillation potentials and reduced recruitment noted distally, with motor unit changes noted with reinnervation
7. Treatment
  a. Shunt ligation for upper extremity IMN
  b. Carbamazepine and gabapentin for neuropathic pain
8. Prognosis
  a. Variable
  b. Spontaneous recovery may occur after several weeks to months
  c. Otherwise, symptoms may persist (including pain)

B. Acute Ischemic Mononeuropathy and Plexopathy
1. Causes
  a. Typical: large-vessel atherosclerotic occlusion or stenosis (almost always occurs in lower limbs because proximal lower limb vessels prone to atherosclerosis)
  b. Abdominal aortoiliac surgery often for treatment of ruptured aneurysms: may be due to combination of prolonged intraoperative hypotension, thromboembolism, insufficient anticoagulation, and cross-clamping of major vessels
  c. Small-vessel disease (vasculitis)
  d. Acute compartment syndrome
2. Abrupt onset of sensory loss and weakness in distribution of affected nerves
3. Changes of vascular insufficiency are often present (in contrast to IMN) and often overshadow neurologic complaints

4. Most frequently affected nerves: femoral nerve and lumbosacral plexus
5. Some patients may present with exercise-induced ischemia of lumbosacral plexus or femoral nerve
6. Neurologic examination: often normal at rest
7. With exercise, patients often experience pain (e.g., buttock pain/distribution of femoral nerve) and motor and sensory deficits in distribution of lumbosacral plexus or femoral nerve
8. Treatment: supportive
9. Prognosis: adequate data lacking, but little improvement in many cases

C. Acute Compartment Syndromes
1. Often due to trauma causing soft tissue damage, fractures, arterial compromise, burns, prolonged compression, and others
2. Often, edema and accumulation of blood, and subsequent increased intracompartmental pressure compromising tissue perfusion and predisposing to ischemia
3. Usual presentation: acute onset of deep severe pain localized to involved compartment, associated with sensory loss, paresthesias, dysesthesias, weakness—all in distribution of nerves expected to be affected
4. NCSs: may demonstrate conduction block in early phase
5. Treatment often involves urgent surgical decompression and fasciotomy
6. Volkmann's ischemic contracture (Volkmann's contracture): muscle fibrosis and resultant contractures that form as residua of severe tissue necrosis from acute compartment syndrome

D. Chronic Compartment Syndromes
1. Almost always due to overuse and exercise
2. More than one compartment often involved
3. Lower extremity compartments involved most often
4. Most commonly experience pain provoked with activity and exercise and alleviated by rest (less commonly, paresthesias and weakness)
5. Self-limited condition that responds to long periods of rest and inactivity
6. Occasionally may be acute exacerbation needing urgent treatment

VIII. Infectious Neuropathies

A. Introduction
1. Infection involving PNS may be isolated manifestation

of a primarily neurologic process or a secondary manifestation of multisystemic disease
2. Generally present in subacute or insidious fashion
3. May derange the PNS in virtually any recognized pattern

B. Leprosy
1. For decades has been recognized as leading cause of peripheral neuropathy worldwide
2. Is caused by *Mycobacterium leprae*
3. Neuropathy in leprosy classically presents in one of two forms, both of which are predominately sensory and both of which involve direct infection of peripheral nerves
   a. Tuberculoid leprosy
      1) Presents with multifocal, circumscribed areas of anesthesia
      2) Generally represents robust cell-mediated response to infection
   b. Lepromatous leprosy
      1) Presents with more widespread anesthesia (due to confluent multifocality) primarily affecting cooler areas of skin (pinnae, dorsum of forearms, etc.)
      2) Generally represents disease dissemination due to inadequate cell-mediated response
      3) Possible involvement of multiple organ systems
   c. Intermediate form (borderline leprosy) is recognized and presents with combination of tuberculoid and lepromatous findings
4. Diagnosis: based on clinical findings and characteristic neuropathologic findings
   a. Tuberculoid leprosy: destruction of peripheral nerve ultrastructure by reactive granulomas
   b. Lepromatous leprosy: diffuse infiltration of peripheral nerves, with preservation of histologic structure until late in disease
5. Treatment with multidrug therapy has become the WHO standard
   a. Dapsone
   b. Rifampin
   c. Clofazimine
   d. Minocycline
   e. Fluoroquinolones
   f. More recently, thalidomide has been used for suppression of treatment reactions

C. Lyme Disease
1. One of most common tick-borne diseases in United States
2. Caused by spirochete *Borrelia burgdorferi* and transmitted by *Ixodes dammini* and *I. pacificus*
3. Stage 1: infection is heralded at the tick site by the erythema migrans rash

4. Stage 2: disseminated infection may follow days to weeks later; there is commonly an associated lymphocytic meningitis, in the context of which several common peripheral manifestations may occur
   a. Single or multiple cranial neuropathies, most commonly CN VII (up to 10% of all patients with seropositive Lyme disease)
   b. Monoradiculopathies, polyradiculopathies, or radiculoplexopathies generally present with pain, paresthesias, and subsequently weakness in distribution of affected roots or plexi: may be widespread and fulminant, resembling AIDP
   c. Mononeuritis multiplex is a less common presentation
5. Stage 3: neurologic symptoms in late infection are usually dominated by central manifestations (encephalomyelitis), but a length-dependent sensorimotor peripheral neuropathy may develop in a few
   a. Electrophysiologic abnormalities are more common than clinical neuropathy
6. Diagnosis: made with combination of clinical (classic dermatologic findings) and serologic data
7. CSF PCR may be instructive when polyradiculoneuropathy is suspected
8. Treatment
   a. Oral doxycycline for early, limited disease
   b. Parenteral ceftriaxone for central or peripheral neurologic involvement

D. Viruses
1. HIV-related neuropathies
   a. Peripheral neurologic manifestations may occur from primary infection, any of several opportunistic infections, or potentially neurotoxic antiviral medications
   b. Peripheral nerve dysfunction varies with stage of infection
      1) Clinical syndrome resembling AIDP or CIDP may occur at seroconversion
      2) Length-dependent axonal sensory predominant peripheral neuropathy
         a) Most common peripheral manifestation of HIV infection (up to 30% of patients)
         b) Usually occurs years into infection
         c) Must often be distinguished from neuropathy associated with nucleic acid analogue antiviral medications
      3) Accompanying autonomic neuropathy may develop with sensory neuropathy
      4) Mononeuritis multiplex also occurs with chronic HIV infection, often after development of acquired immunodeficiency syndrome
   c. Neuropathic diagnosis relies on clinical assessment of

systemic stage of infection and recognition of pattern of neuropathy
   1) EMG: may help identify subclinical disease, quantify axonal damage, or identify conduction block
   2) CSF examination: may help corroborate suspected polyradiculoneuropathy
   d. Management of neuropathic complications of HIV depends largely on
      1) Optimizing antiretroviral regimen to slow progression of neuropathy
      2) Exclusion of other causes of presenting symptoms: opportunistic infections, antiviral medications (e.g., ddI)
      3) Symptomatic management of pain associated with neuropathy
2. CMV-associated neuropathies
   a. CMV: human herpesvirus with DNA-based genome
   b. Symptomatic CMV infection of CNS or PNS: rare in immunocompetent persons
   c. CMV may present with the two following typical neuropathic patterns:
      1) Painful, rapidly, or subacutely progressive polyradiculoneuropathy that may result in severe weakness
         a) Much more common in immunocompromised patients, but CMV may also present in a fashion similar to AIDP in immunologically normal patients
      2) Necrotizing microvasculitis caused by CMV may present with mononeuritis multiplex
   d. PCR for CMV in CSF: quite sensitive for most peripheral manifestations of CMV and for CNS infections (myelopathy, encephalitis, optic neuritis/retinitis)
   e. Treatment: intravenous antiviral antibiotics with activity against CMV
      1) Ganciclovir
      2) Foscarnet
   f. Optimization of any underlying immune insult (e.g., HIV infection, immunosuppression for transplantation) helps prevention and may speed recovery
3. VZV-associated neuropathies
   a. VZV: nearly ubiquitous DNA-based human herpesvirus with predilection for peripheral nerves, commonly remaining latent in sensory ganglia
   b. Typically, VZV reactivation presents in immunocompetent adults as monoradiculitis
      1) Lancinating pain in distribution of affected nerve is common harbinger of classic vesicular rash
      2) Thoracic dorsal root ganglia are most commonly affected, although any spinal or cranial level may be involved

3) Reactivation of VZV in geniculate ganglion presents with ipsilateral facial neuropathy and intra-auricular vesicles (Ramsey Hunt syndrome)

4) Reactivation in ophthalmic division (V_1) of CN V may result in delayed infectious granulomatous vasculitis of ipsilateral middle cerebral artery, producing cerebral ischemia or infarction

c. Reactivation is usually self-limited, but persistent pain (postherpetic neuralgia) is common sequela and often refractory

1) Treatment with antiviral antibiotics early in reactivation (most commonly with valacyclovir or acyclovir) may help reduce this burden

2) Symptomatic management with other medications is often necessary

   a) Gabapentin

   b) Carbamazepine

   c) Amitriptyline (and other tricyclic antidepressants)

   d) Topical lidocaine

   e) Topical ketamine

4. Herpes simplex virus (HSV)-associated neuropathies

   a. A recurrently activated neurotrophic infection

   b. Common presentation: painful eruptions around mouth or genitals, having remained latent in trigeminal or lumbosacral ganglia, respectively

   c. Typically, reactivation is not associated with peripheral nerve dysfunction

   d. Persistent neuralgia is uncommon

   e. HSV-1 and HSV-2 have been implicated in Bell's palsy and Mollaret's meningitis, prompting empiric antiviral treatment of these conditions

E. Mycobacteria

1. Mainly in immunocompromised patients, a polyradiculopathy caused by leptomeningeal infection with *Mycobacterium tuberculosis*

2. Treatment with antimycobacterial antibiotics is helpful, but patients often do poorly unless underlying immunocompromise is corrected

F. Parasites

1. Mild sensorimotor peripheral neuropathy is relatively common in patients infected with *Trypanosoma cruzi* (causative agent in Chagas' disease)

   a. Chagas' disease is also associated with severe cardiomyopathy

2. Visceral neuropathies may also be caused by *T. cruzi*, *Schistosoma* spp, and *Strongyloides stercoralis*

3. Syndrome closely resembling AIDP may develop after infection with *Plasmodium* spp (causative of malaria)

G. Toxoplasmosis

1. Rarely, polyradiculoneuropathy may develop from initial infection with *Toxoplasma gondii* or with its reactivation (most cases occur in the immunocompromised patients)

H. Syphilis

1. Historical ubiquity of syphilis has led to descriptions of most types of neuropathies associated with it

2. In antibiotic era, patients who develop peripheral nerve manifestations of syphilis often are immunosuppressed and commonly present with polyradiculoneuropathy

I. EBV

1. Polyradiculoneuropathy caused by EBV is uncommon and generally seen in immunocompromised patients in setting of multisystemic viral manifestations

J. *Corynebacterium diphtheriae*

1. Diphtheritic neuropathy generally follows subacutely after exudative pharyngitis, progressing over a period of weeks

2. Pharyngeal exudation is sometimes followed by local palatal neuropathy

3. Bulbar weakness is followed by diffuse sensory dysfunction and limb weakness and is mediated by secreted toxin rather than direct infestation of nerves

4. Neuropathy has prominent features of demyelination both pathologically and electrophysiologically, but axonal damage is not infrequent

5. 10% of patients may develop diffuse sensorimotor polyneuropathy

6. Treatment

   a. Antibiotics (often penicillin unless resistant) for infection

   b. Antitoxin for neuropathy

IX. CRITICAL ILLNESS POLYNEUROPATHY

A. **Epidemiology:** occurs in 50% to 70% of patients with systemic inflammatory response syndrome (SIRS)

B. **Possible Pathophysiologic Mechanisms**

1. Increased microvascular permeability from circulating cytokines and other mediators

2. Direct toxic effects of mediators of sepsis, including cytokines

3. Lack of autoregulation of blood vessels supplying peripheral nerves may predispose them to ischemic injury in septic shock

C. Clinical Features

1. SIRS often occurs in patients with severe infection and septic shock or evidence of severe traumatic insult
2. Usually preceded by septic encephalopathy
3. Patients: typically critically ill; have sepsis, septic shock, or evidence of multiple organ failure
4. Early indications: often difficulty in weaning patient from ventilator (even after improvement of underlying septic encephalopathy), limb weakness apparent by poor leg movements with deep painful stimulation (mild weakness to severe quadriparesis)
5. Exclusion of pulmonary or cardiac causes for difficulty weaning from ventilator
6. Tendon reflexes are preserved in up to half of patients

D. Creatine Kinase: levels often normal or near normal

E. CSF: normal or mildly elevated protein level

F. Electrophysiologic Evaluation

1. NCSs
   a. Reduced amplitude SNAPs and CMAPs, relatively preserved distal latencies and conduction velocities (in keeping with an electrophysiologic pattern of axonal polyradiculoneuropathy)
   b. Prolongation of CMAP duration: indicative of accompanying critical illness myopathy
   c. Sensory nerve responses may be normal in early stage of illness
   d. Repetitive stimulation studies may be abnormal if patient is given neuromuscular junction-blocking agents
2. Needle EMG
   a. Fibrillation potentials occur about 3 weeks after illness onset
   b. Recruitment is often reduced
   c. Motor unit potentials may appear to be short duration, low amplitude with reduced recruitment, which is likely due to dysfunction of terminal axons and not myopathy
   d. May be evidence of concurrent myopathy (critical illness myopathy) with rapidly recruited short-duration motor unit potentials

G. Pathology

1. Acute axonal degeneration of both motor and sensory fibers
2. No evidence of demyelination or inflammatory infiltrates

REFERENCES

Dyck PJ, Dyck PJB, Grant IA, Fealey RD. Ten steps in characterizing and diagnosing patients with peripheral neuropathy. Neurology. 1996;47:10-7.

Dyck PJ, Thomas PK, editors. Peripheral neuropathy. Vol. 1 and 2. 4th ed. Philadelphia: Elsevier Saunders; 2005.

Fernandez-Torre JL, Polo JM, Calleja J, Berciano J. Castleman's disease associated with chronic inflammatory demyelinating polyradiculoneuropathy: a clinical and electrophysiological follow-up study. Clin Neurophysiol. 1999;110:1133-8.

Houlden H, Blake J, Reilly MM. Hereditary sensory neuropathies. Curr Opin Neurol. 2004;17:569-77.

Kiuru-Enari S, Somer H, Seppalainen AM, Notkola IL, Haltia M. Neuromuscular pathology in hereditary gelsolin amyloidosis. J Neuropathol Exp Neurol. 2002;61:565-71.

Klein CJ, Dyck PJ. Genetic testing in inherited peripheral neuropathies. J Peripher Nerv Syst. 2005;10:77-84.

Nobile-Orazio E, Cappellari A, Priori A. Multifocal motor neuropathy: current concepts and controversies. Muscle Nerve. 2005;31:663-80.

Taylor BV, Dyck PJB, Engelstad JHT, Gruener G, Grant I, Dyck PJ. Multifocal motor neuropathy: pathologic alterations at the site of conduction block. J Neuropathol Exp Neurol. 2004;63:129-37.

Taylor BV, Wright RA, Harper CM, Dyck PJ. Natural history of 46 patients with multifocal motor neuropathy with conduction block. Muscle Nerve. 2000;23:900-8.

APPENDIX A. CLINICAL APPROACH TO PNS DISORDERS

A. Each step is presented in an order that progressively narrows the differential diagnosis and also serves to focus the evaluation of each subsequent step (Modified from Dyck PJ, Dyck PJB, Grant IA, Fealey RD. Ten steps in characterizing and diagnosing patients with peripheral neuropathy. Neurology. 1996;47:10-7. Used with permission.)

B. Step 1: characterize anatomic-pathologic pattern of involvement—"Where is the lesion?"

1. Localize to appropriate level(s) of neuraxis: Are patient's symptoms consistent with peripheral nerve disease?
   a. Some nonneurologic conditions may mimic peripheral neuropathy (e.g., plantar fasciitis)
   b. Disease of CNS may produce neuropathy-like syndromes (e.g., lower limb sensory symptoms in patients with transverse myelitis)
   c. Some conditions may affect multiple levels of neuraxis simultaneously
      1) Neuromyopathies (e.g., colchicine neuromyopathy)
      2) Myeloneuropathies (e.g., adrenomyeloneuropathy)
      3) Generalized neurologic disease as seen in some inherited metabolic disorders (e.g., Tay-Sachs disease)
2. Localize presumed pathologic site further within PNS: two critical questions achieve this
   a. What nerve fiber types are involved?
      1) Motor
      2) Sensory
         a) Small fiber: pain and temperature
         b) Large fiber: touch, vibration, joint position
      3) Autonomic
   b. What is spatial distribution?
      1) Symmetric vs. asymmetric (or multifocal) vs. focal (if focal, peripheral nerve vs. plexus vs. root?)
      2) Proximal vs. distal vs. both
      3) Spinal vs. cranial vs. both
3. Categorize neuropathy by anatomic pattern—examples of diagnostic considerations based on anatomic patterns include following:
   a. Mononeuropathy
      1) Entrapment or compressive trauma in single peripheral distribution, examples
         a) Carpal tunnel syndrome
         b) Ulnar neuropathy at elbow
         c) Radial nerve at spiral groove
         d) Common peroneal neuropathy at fibular neck
      2) Initial presentation of multiple mononeuropathy
   b. Radiculopathy
      1) Cervical and lumbar radiculopathies (most often compression due to degenerative disease)
      2) Thoracic radiculopathies
         a) Degenerative disk disease is rare
         b) Consider diskitis, malignancy, DLSRPN
   c. Multiple mononeuropathies
      1) Vasculitic neuropathy
      2) Multifocal motor neuropathy with conduction block
      3) HNPP
      4) Leprosy neuropathy
      5) Lymphoma-related neuropathies
      6) Wartenberg's migrant sensory neuritis
      7) Mononeuritis multiplex: implies inflammatory cause, does not apply to noninflammatory causes such as HNPP, and should be avoided when describing anatomic patterns
   d. Plexopathy
      1) Malignant infiltration—common examples of brachial plexus carcinomatous infiltration
         a) Breast cancer metastasis
         b) Pancoast's tumor invading brachial plexus lower trunk
      2) Radiation plexitis
      3) Idiopathic brachial plexus neuritis (Parsonage-Turner syndrome)
      4) Hereditary neuralgic amyotrophy
   e. Radiculoplexus neuropathy—examples involving lumbosacral segments
      1) Diabetic lumbosacral radiculoplexus neuropathy
      2) Nondiabetic lumbosacral radiculoplexus neuropathy
   f. Polyradiculopathy: commonly multiple compressive radiculopathies but must also consider
      1) CISP
      2) Malignant meningitis
      3) Cauda equina syndrome
   g. Polyradiculoneuropathy (proximal and distal involvement)
      1) CIDP
      2) AIDP
   h. Distal sensorimotor polyneuropathy
   i. Sensory polyganglionopathy
      1) Paraneoplastic sensory neuronopathy
      2) Nonneoplastic immune sensory neuronopathy (e.g., Sjögren's disease-related neuronopathy)
   j. Fiber types
      1) Motor neuronopathy
         a) Amyotrophic lateral sclerosis

b) Spinal muscular atrophy

c) Kennedy's disease

d) Polio, West Nile virus-related motor neuron disease

2) Motor neuropathy (e.g., multifocal motor neuropathy with conduction block)

3) Small-fiber sensory neuropathy

a) HSAN

b) Fabry's disease

c) Tangier disease

d) Amyloid neuropathy

e) Alcoholic neuropathy

4) Autonomic neuropathy

a) HSAN

b) Amyloid neuropathy

c) Diabetic neuropathies

d) Autoimmune autonomic neuropathy

e) Note: autonomic failure can also be due to central causes (e.g., multiple system atrophy)

5) Large-fiber sensory neuropathy (prominent sensory ataxia)

a) Vitamin B_{12} deficiency

b) Spinocerebellar ataxias

c) Anti-MAG–related neuropathy

d) Polyganglionopathies

4. Electrodiagnosis of NCSs

a. According to some investigators, pure small-fiber neuropathy requires normal NCSs, and needle EMG and preserved ankle reflexes

b. In clinical practice, minor abnormalities on NCS and EMG are common in patients with distal neuropathic pain and minor small-fiber sensory findings: these are better termed small-fiber–predominant

5. Although some patients with distal polyneuropathy have a treatable cause, the probability of finding a treatable or prognostically important condition rises substantially in other patterns

C. **Step 2:** confirm the inferred anatomic-pathologic pattern with appropriate tests

1. NCSs and needle EMG

a. Distinguish peripheral nerve localization from plexus or root

b. Identify subclinical multifocal or generalized neuropathy

c. Identify subclinical or asymptomatic sensory involvement

d. Distinguish motor neuropathy from myopathy or disorder of neuromuscular transmission

2. Autonomic function testing

a. Confirm presence of autonomic nervous system disease

b. Involvement of autonomic nervous system can be important clue to a specific cause or may even be the only detectable objective measure of neuropathy (as with some small-fiber neuropathies)

c. Routine clinical examination is relatively insensitive to disease of autonomic nerves

d. Noninvasive autonomic function testing can include

1) Quantitative sudomotor axon reflex test (QSART): measure of postganglionic sudomotor (sweat) function

2) Heart rate response to deep breathing: cardiovagal function

3) Blood pressure responses to Valsalva maneuver: measure of peripheral and cardiac adrenergic innervation

4) Heart rate and blood pressure response to head-up tilt: tilt table testing

e. Pattern of autonomic abnormalities can help characterize neuropathy

1) Distal absence or reduction of QSART volumes and impaired cardiovagal responses form a common pattern in length-dependent small-fiber neuropathies

3. Quantitative sensory testing

a. More sensitive for detecting subtle sensory loss

b. Characterization of pattern of involvement: small fiber, large fiber, or panmodality

c. Detect hyperalgesia (reduced pain threshold): can be early finding in some small-fiber neuropathies

4. Neuroimaging

a. May provide exact anatomic localization in focal neuropathy, for example, herniated disk, nerve sheath tumor, or compressive cauda equina syndrome (which can rarely present with sphincter disturbance and distal lower limb sensory symptoms mimicking distal polyneuropathy)

b. May also assist localization in more generalized neuropathies (e.g., abnormal nerve root signal change in inflammatory demyelinating neuropathies)

D. **Step 3:** infer mechanism of nerve fiber dysfunction

1. NCSs help determine if neuropathy is primarily axonal or demyelinating because this distinction cannot be made reliably on basis of neurologic findings

2. If predominantly demyelinating neuropathy: NCSs help determine if changes are diffuse (uniform conduction slowing) or patchy and focal (temporal dispersion, conduction block)

3. Focal conduction block, conduction slowing, and temporal dispersion strongly favor acquired process rather than inherited demyelinating neuropathy such as HMSN I

4. Mild degrees of conduction slowing are expected with

severely reduced CMAP amplitudes because this usually represents loss of large, rapidly conducting axons rather than demyelination

5. Many demyelinating conditions (particularly when chronic) are associated with some degree of axonal loss

6. Diagnostic considerations for predominantly demyelinating or axonal involvement are as follows:
   a. Uniform, predominantly demyelinating
      1) HMSN I, Dejerine-Sottas disease, Refsum's disease
      2) MNGIE, NARP
   b. Patchy, predominatly demyelinating
      1) HNPP
      2) AIDP, CIDP, MMNCB, POEMS
      3) Diphtheria
      4) Perhexiline
   c. Predominantly axonal
      1) HMSN II
      2) HSAN
      3) AMAN
      4) Vasculitic neuropathy
      5) Most metabolic, nutritional, or toxic neuropathies
   d. Either predominantly axonal or demyelinating: sarcoid neuropathy

E. **Step 4:** temporal profiles
1. Acute or Subacute
   a. Inflammatory/immune (e.g. AIDP/Guillain-Barré syndrome, vasculitic neuropathy)
   b. Infectious (e.g., neuropathy related to poliovirus, West Nile virus, Lyme disease)
   c. Inherited (e.g., acute intermittent porphyria)
   d. Toxic
2. Chronic, progressive
   a. HMSN
   b. Toxic (with ongoing exposure)
   c. Metabolic, including diabetes and nutritional deficiency
   d. Inflammatory and autoimmune: some cases of CIDP
   e. Infectious: HIV, leprosy
   f. Neoplastic and infiltrative: lymphoma, amyloidosis, malignant meningitis
3. Chronic, relapsing
   a. CIDP
   b. HNPP
   c. Hereditary neuralgic amyotrophy
   d. Intermittent toxic exposure
4. Chronic, stepwise: vasculitis (especially if restricted to PNS)
5. Subacute or chronic
   a. Inflammatory and autoimmune (e.g., sarcoid neuropathy, paraneoplastic neuropathy)

b. Neoplastic (e.g., lymphoma)
   c. Congenital or inherited
6. Assessment of temporal profile can assist in treatment decisions: temporal profile of patient's symptoms and signs is often only readily available measure of disease activity

F. **Step 5:** inherited or acquired?
1. Careful family history or family evaluation
2. Many inherited neuropathies demonstrate marked variability of expression even within single families: some family members may be severely affected and others have asymptomatic or subclinical disease (e.g., electrophysiologic abnormality only)
3. Useful family history screening questions
   a. Does anyone in family have high arches or foot deformity?
   b. Does anyone in family slap their feet when walking?
   c. Does anyone in family complain of numbness, prickling, or burning in their feet or hands?
4. If family members are not present with the patient, a telephone call can establish history of
   a. High arches
   b. Difficulty walking on heels or toes
   c. Difficulty arising from kneeling position
5. Other aspects of the history and examination can provide useful clues
   a. Acquired neuropathies: positive sensory symptoms (persistent prickling paresthesias), asymmetric distribution
   b. Inherited process
      1) Insidious onset, long duration, slow or minimal progression
      2) Patient may be unaware of relatively severe deficits
      3) Pes cavus
      4) Specific peripheral stigmata: angiokeratomas in Fabry's disease, tongue nodules in MEN 2B

G. **Step 6:** associated diseases? (neuropathy may be presenting symptom in several systemic disorders)
1. Endocrinopathy
   a. Diabetes mellitus
   b. Hypothyroidism
   c. Acromegaly
   d. MEN 2B
   e. Adrenoleukodystrophy
2. Hematologic or neoplastic
   a. Paraproteinemia (e.g., CIDP with M protein, anti-MAG–related neuropathy, AL amyloidosis, POEMS syndrome, multiple myeloma)
   b. Carcinoma (e.g., small cell lung cancer [paraneoplastic sensory neuronopathy])

c. Lymphoma
3. Organ failure
   a. Uremia
   b. Malabsorption
   c. Cardiomyopathy (Fabry's disease, Friedreich's ataxia, primary or systemic amyloidosis)
4. Infections
   a. HIV
   b. Lyme disease
   c. AIDP antecedent infections

H. Step 7: blood tests and imaging
1. No single diagnostic test for most patients with peripheral neuropathy
2. Laboratory testing is often used to exclude diagnostic considerations rather than to make specific diagnosis
3. Extent of diagnostic evaluation should be based on information gained in above steps and exclusion of potentially treatable conditions
   a. Infections (e.g., HIV)
   b. Nutritional or vitamin deficiencies (e.g., vitamin B_{12})
   c. Immune disorders (e.g., vasculitis)
   d. Systemic disease (e.g., diabetes)
4. Tests commonly performed in most patients
   a. Fasting blood glucose
   b. Serum immunofixation
   c. Vitamin B_{12}
   d. Creatinine
   e. Erythrocyte sedimentation rate
   f. Thyroid function tests
   g. NCSs and EMG
5. Genetic testing
   a. Costly, limitations
   b. Diagnostic yield depends heavily on clinical scenario
   c. High yield (85%) in setting of demyelinating CMT-like phenotype
   d. Low yield in setting of predominantly axonal CMT-like phenotype (except for screening of family members for a known mutation)

I. Step 8: evaluate kin
1. An inherited neuropathy is probably the most overlooked cause of otherwise idiopathic peripheral neuropathy; this is often compounded by three important misconceptions
   a. Inherited neuropathies present only in childhood or early adulthood: inherited neuropathy can present at any age and may be present for many years before becoming overtly symptomatic (clues: pes cavus, difficulty with school sports, etc.)
   b. Inherited neuropathy must manifest similarly within families: phenotypic heterogeneity between different family members may be dramatic
   c. Existing diagnosis of family members is correct (e.g., assuming that neuropathy in an elderly person is due to "old age" or arthritis)
2. In some cases, family neurologic examination and NCSs of family members may help detect subclinical or asymptomatic disease

J. Step 9: nerve biopsy
1. Invasive, but well tolerated in most patients; may be associated with lasting morbidity
2. Clinical usefulness
   a. Primary rationale for biopsy: detection of diagnostic interstitial abnormalities
   b. Pretest likelihood of finding such abnormalities depends on clinical situation: diagnostic yield in a patient with a chronic, slowly progressive symmetric, length-dependent neuropathy is low
   c. Nerve biopsy should *not* be performed to determine mechanism of nerve fiber function (axonal or demyelinating): less invasive NCSs and EMG may be more sensitive for answering this question
3. Conditions in which nerve biopsy may be helpful
   a. Inflammatory or immune-mediated conditions (vasculitis axonal neuropathy, inflammatory demyelination)
   b. Infiltration (e.g., lymphoma, amyloidosis)
   c. Unique pathologic finding (modern genetic and enzymatic testing may sometimes preclude need for biopsy), for example, tomaculae in HNPP, metachromatic granules in metachromatic leukodystrophy, polyglucosan bodies in polyglucosan body disease
4. Teased fiber preparations (Fig. 21-24)
5. Nerve biopsy may be normal or yield only nonspecific changes because of sampling error
6. Most commonly biopsied nerve is sural nerve because it is surgically accessible, pure sensory, produces little deficit, and commonly involved in generalized neuropathy
7. Other nerves can be considered in patients with patchy or multifocal neuropathy, particularly if sural sensory potential is preserved
   a. Superficial peroneal nerve (the peroneus brevis muscle may be biopsied at same time if condition in question is expected to also involve the muscle)
   b. Superficial radial sensory nerve
8. Patients with typical treatment-responsive CIDP do not need nerve biopsy

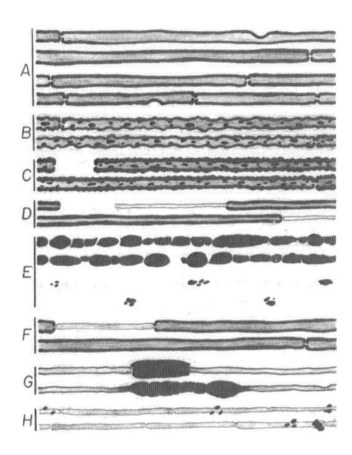

Fig. 21-24. Classification of teased fibers: drawing of consecutive lengths, from top to bottom of teased myelinated fibers. *A*, Normal fiber. *B*, Myelin wrinkling: excessively irregular myelin (not attributed to poor fixation or artifact). *C*, Paranodal or internodal segmental demyelination, with or without cytoplasmic ovoids. *D*, Segmental demyelination and remyelination. *E*, Axonal degeneration, with linear rows of myelin ovoids and balls. *F*, Segmental remyelination, with excessive variability of myelin thickness of internode segments and absence of segmental demyelination. *G*, Tomacula formation: excess variability of internodal myelin thickness with regional reduplication of myelin, and not due to excessive production of myelin. *H*, Regenerating fiber with myelin breakdown products, after axonal degeneration (regeneration of a myelinated fiber). (From Dyck PJ, Stevens JC, Mulder DW, Espinosa RE. Frequency of nerve fiber degeneration of peripheral motor and sensory neurons in amyotrophic lateral sclerosis: morphometry of deep and superficial peroneal nerves. Neurology. 1975;25:781-5. Used with permission.)

K. Step 10: therapeutic trial

1. In patients thought to have CIDP, positive response to a treatment trial (usually intravenous immunoglobulin) is useful confirmatory evidence of immune-mediated condition
2. Such trials need to be undertaken objectively with quantitative outcome measures and defined goals
   a. Patients should have at least a baseline quantitated neurologic examination (e.g., Neuropathy Impairment Score [NIS]) and NCSs
   b. These measures should be repeated in semi-blinded fashion (i.e., before taking follow-up history) after adequate time (usually 3-6 months)
   c. In some cases, first sign of treatment efficacy may be halting previously relentless progression
   d. In patients who clearly do not respond to a trial of

therapy, treatment should be discontinued (this possibility should be discussed with patient before commencing the trial)
3. Electrophysiologic variables can be compared serially using summated CMAP method

L. "The Great Mimickers"

1. Lymphoma and sarcoidosis are two great mimickers of PNS disease, being able to present in almost any temporal or anatomic pattern, as is their CNS involvement
2. Diagnosis relies on consideration of these two conditions in every neuropathy patient
3. Clues to look for
   a. Lymphoma: weight loss, elevated LDH
   b. Sarcoidosis: history of uveitis, increased serum calcium

APPENDIX B. Cutaneous Nerve Distribution of Peripheral Nerves

Anterior

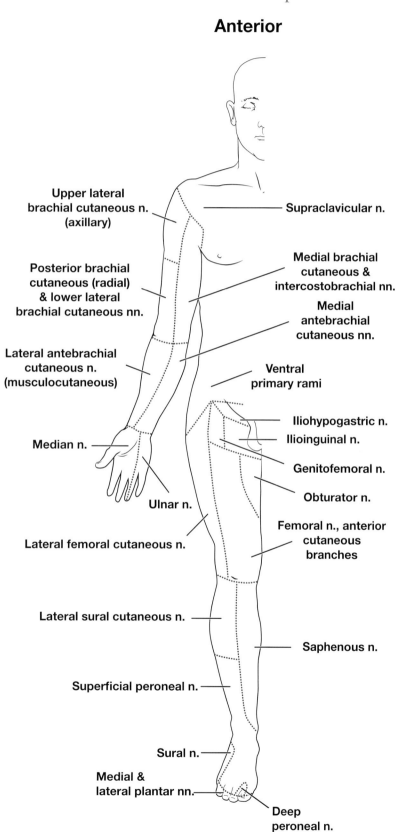

Upper lateral brachial cutaneous n. (axillary)

Supraclavicular n.

Posterior brachial cutaneous (radial) & lower lateral brachial cutaneous nn.

Medial brachial cutaneous & intercostobrachial nn.

Medial antebrachial cutaneous nn.

Lateral antebrachial cutaneous n. (musculocutaneous)

Ventral primary rami

Iliohypogastric n.

Ilioinguinal n.

Median n.

Genitofemoral n.

Obturator n.

Ulnar n.

Lateral femoral cutaneous n.

Femoral n., anterior cutaneous branches

Lateral sural cutaneous n.

Saphenous n.

Superficial peroneal n.

Sural n.

Medial & lateral plantar nn.

Deep peroneal n.

APPENDIX B. (continued)

Posterior

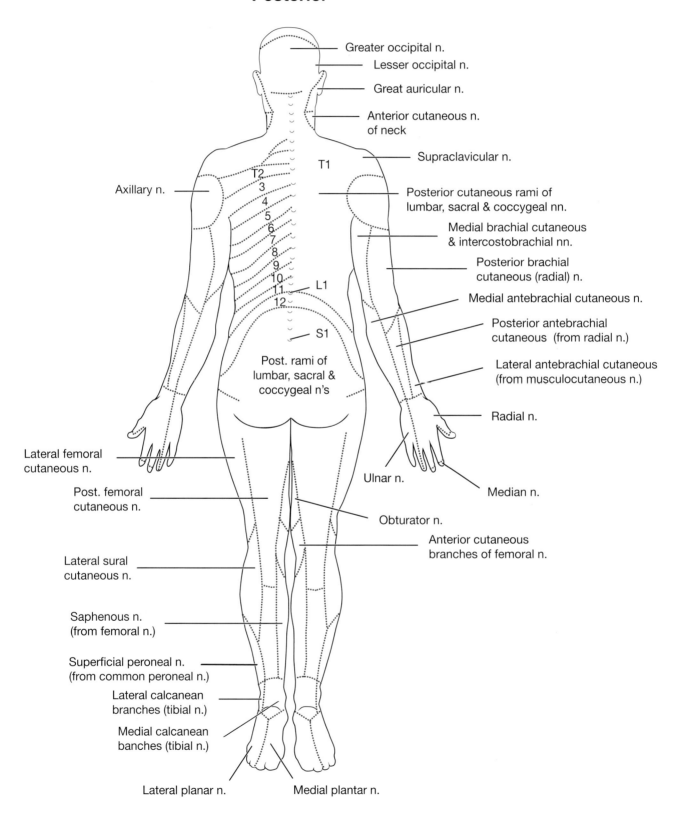

Greater occipital n.

Lesser occipital n.

Great auricular n.

Anterior cutaneous n. of neck

Supraclavicular n.

Axillary n.

Posterior cutaneous rami of lumbar, sacral & coccygeal nn.

Medial brachial cutaneous & intercostobrachial nn.

Posterior brachial cutaneous (radial) n.

Medial antebrachial cutaneous n.

Posterior antebrachial cutaneous (from radial n.)

Lateral antebrachial cutaneous (from musculocutaneous n.)

Radial n.

Post. rami of lumbar, sacral & coccygeal n's

Lateral femoral cutaneous n.

Post. femoral cutaneous n.

Ulnar n.

Median n.

Obturator n.

Anterior cutaneous branches of femoral n.

Lateral sural cutaneous n.

Saphenous n. (from femoral n.)

Superficial peroneal n. (from common peroneal n.)

Lateral calcanean branches (tibial n.)

Medial calcanean banches (tibial n.)

Lateral planar n.   Medial plantar n.

T1 T2 3 4 5 6 7 8 9 10 11 12 L1 S1

Appendix C. Dermatomal Distributions: Total Distribution of Dermatomes Are Depicted Alternatively in the Right and Left Halves to Best Illustrate Total Distribution of Innervation of Each Nerve Root

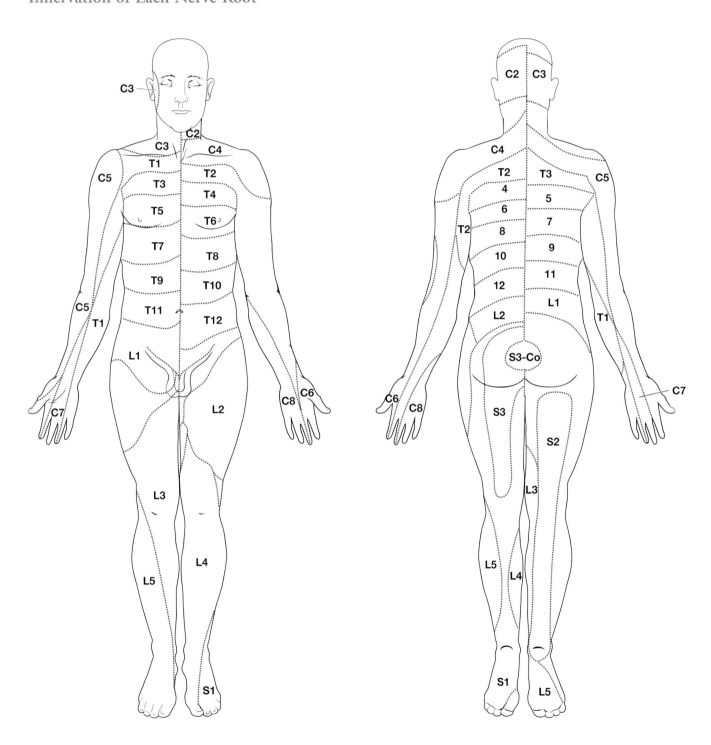

QUESTIONS

1. A 25-year-old man is evaluated for pes cavus noted by his primary care physician during a routine medical examination. The patient has no neuropathic symptoms. Examination shows mild symmetrical weakness of ankle dorsiflexion and absent ankle jerks. Light touch is impaired at the toes. His father died in a motor vehicle accident at age of 30 years but was said to have a "funny walk." Nerve conduction studies show normal compound muscle action potential amplitudes but diffuse motor conduction slowing on the order of 20 to 25 m/s without conduction block or temporal dispersion. Which of the following diagnoses is the most likely?
   a. Chronic inflammatory demyelinating polyradiculoneuropathy
   b. Hereditary neuropathy with duplication of the *PMP22* gene
   c. Hereditary neuropathy with deletion of the *PMP22* gene
   d. Hereditary neuropathy with point mutations of the *MPZ* gene
   e. Distal spinal muscular atrophy

2. A 45-year-old man has a 2-year history of intermittent paresthesias of the right hand. Nerve conduction studies confirmed the presence of a distal median neuropathy at the wrist. He now presents with slowly progressive distal upper and lower limb burning pain. He has a history of erectile dysfunction and has fainted several times after standing up. Electrocardiographic findings are abnormal. The patient's father died at age 44 years unexpectedly during sleep. An enlarged heart was found at autopsy. Which of the following diagnoses is the most likely?
   a. Hereditary sensory and autonomic neuropathy type I
   b. Fabry's disease
   c. Friedreich's ataxia
   d. Transthyretin amyloidosis
   e. Tangier disease

3. An 18-year-old woman presents with acute painless left footdrop. She had been at a concert, and on standing up from her chair, she noticed an inability to dorsiflex her left ankle. Three months earlier she had awoken with a right wristdrop that resolved after 5 days. Examination showed weakness of left toe extension, ankle dorsiflexion and eversion with preserved inversion, plantar flexion, and a normal left ankle jerk. Sensory examination was normal. The rest of the neurologic examination was normal. Nerve conduction studies showed focal motor conduction block of the peroneal nerve at the neck of the fibula. In addition, there was diffuse mild prolongation of distal motor latencies in both lower limbs. Which of the following statements is *incorrect* about this condition?
   a. A normal number of *PMP22* genes excludes this condition
   b. Sural nerve biopsy would likely show some myelinated fibers with abnormally thick myelin
   c. The prognosis for functional recovery is excellent
   d. Corticosteroid treatment is not indicated for this condition
   e. Pain is not a feature of this disorder

4. Which of the following statements is *true* regarding suprascapular neuropathy?
   a. May be caused by trauma or compression of the nerve within the suprascapular notch
   b. Compression may be caused by the suprascapular ligament
   c. Muscles that may be affected include the supraspinatus and infraspinatus
   d. Weakness of the supraspinatus muscle will cause difficulty with initiation of abduction in a fully adducted arm
   e. All the above are true regading suprascapular neuropathy

ANSWERS

1. Answer: b.
The findings presented would be most consistent with hereditary motor and sensory neuropathy (HMSN) type I (also called Charcot-Marie-Tooth type 1). The probable male-to-male transmission establishes a likely autosomal dominant inheritance pattern. The predominant features of nerve conduction studies are demyelinating, thus excluding distal spinal muscular atrophy, which has predominant features of axonal loss. The diffuse uniform slowing and absence of temporal dispersion or conduction block argue against chronic inflammatory demyelinating polyradiculoneuropathy, which can occur in young adults and even children. HMSN I can be caused by abnormalities of the *PMP22* or *MPZ* genes. The most common cause is duplication of the *PMP22* gene. Deletion of the *PMP22* gene is the most common cause of hereditary neuropathy with liability to pressure palsies. *MPZ* mutations account for a small fraction of patients with HMSN I and some patients with axonal HMSN (HMSN II).

2. Answer: d.
This patient initially presented with carpal tunnel syndrome before progressing to a more diffuse small-fiber sensory neuropathy with autonomic involvement (erectile dysfunction and orthostatic hypotension). There appears to be a family history of early cardiac disease. Selections b through d are inherited conditions associated with sensory neuropathy and cardiac disease. The neuropathy of Friedreich's ataxia predominantly affects large sensory fibers. Fabry's disease is an X-linked recessive disorder that should not, therefore, be inherited from father to son. Transthyretin amyloidosis and Tangier disease could both produce small-fiber sensory neuropathy with premature cardiac disease. Two features in this case favor transthyretin amyloidosis: prominent autonomic impairment (typical of amyloid neuropathy) and the inheritance pattern suggestive of an autosomal dominant condition (Tangier disease is an autosomal recessive condition). Inheritance patterns can be misleading, however, and it would be appropriate to test for both conditions with serum lipids for the characteristic low level of high-density lipoprotein of Tangier disease and to sequence the transthyretin gene.

3. Answer: a.
This patient has experienced two mononeuropathies that were painless and probably related to minor trauma (sitting with legs crossed, sleeping with one arm over the edge of the bed). Transient paresthesias and even mild weakness can occur in normal people in these situations, but in hereditary neuropathy with liability to pressure palsy (HNPP), the mononeuropathy is typically more severe, precipitated by minor or trivial trauma, and resolves over days or weeks rather than minutes or hours. In contrast to multiple mononeuropathies due to vasculitis, neuropathic pain is not typical and corticosteroid treatment is not indicated. Approximately 80% of patients have a deletion of one *PMP22* gene. If clinical suspicion is high, a negative deletion test should prompt sequencing the *PMP22* gene for point mutations.

4. Answer: e.
All the choices are true regarding compressive lesions of the suprascapular nerve.

<h1 style="text-align:center">DISORDERS OF THE AUTONOMIC NERVOUS SYSTEM</h1>

22

Nima Mowzoon, M.D.

I. ANATOMY OF THE AUTONOMIC NERVOUS SYSTEM

A. Central Autonomic Pathways

1. Neocortex
   a. Orbitofrontal and anterior cingulate cortex: important for regulation of genitourinary autonomic control (discussed below)
   b. Insular cortex
      1) Primary gustatory cortex (anterior insula)
      2) General visceral sensory afferent cortical region (posterior insula)
         a) Sympathetic afferents: lamina I in dorsal horn → spinothalamic tracts → ventromedial thalamus → insular cortex
         b) Parasympathetic (vagal) afferents: via nucleus solitarius (= nucleus tractus solitarius) and ventral posteromedial thalamic relay
         c) Visceral pain perception: carried primarily by sympathetic afferents
         d) Mechanical visceral sensory input (e.g., bowel distension): carried by parasympathetic input
      3) Anterior cingulate gyrus and prefrontal cortex: responsible for motivation, initiation of behavior (especially emotional behavior), and initiation of micturition response
2. Amygdala
   a. Important role in control of emotional autonomic response, including fear
   b. Responsible for integration of autonomic functions with learning, memory from previous experience, and associated emotions
   c. Projections to prefrontal cortex, hypothalamus, and brainstem
3. Hypothalamus (see Chapter 2)
   a. Paraventricular nucleus provides the major innervation of the preganglionic sympathetic neurons
4. Circumventricular organs

   a. Important in feedback control of certain autonomic functions such as feeding, body fluid balance, and cardiovascular control
   b. In proximity with the ventricles; contain fenestrated capillaries and lack intact blood-brain barrier
   c. Include subfornical organ, habenula, pineal body, subcommissural organ, area postrema, vascular organ of the lamina terminalis, median eminence, neurohypophysis
   d. Subfornical organ, area postrema, vascular organ of the lamina terminalis, and the median eminence provide humoral input to hypothalamus (vascular organ of the lamina terminalis and median eminence are located in hypothalamus)
   e. Subfornical organ and organum vasculosum: responsible for feedback control of fluid balance
   f. Area postrema: functions as emetic center
5. Brainstem reticular centers
   a. Midbrain periaqueductal gray (PAG)
      1) Responsible for visceromotor component of defensive behavior and response to stress
      2) Lateral PAG: responsible for sympathoexcitatory responses ("fight or flight")
      3) Ventrolateral PAG: initiates sympathoinhibitory responses
      4) Reciprocal connections between PAG and amydala, hypothalamus, and insular cortex
   b. Nucleus solitarius
      1) Relay for visceral sensory afferents
         a) Rostral portion of nucleus: receives taste afferents
         b) Caudal portion of nucleus: receives cardiorespiratory afferents (baroreceptors, cardiac receptors, pulmonary mechanoreceptors)
         c) Intermediate portion of nucleus receives gastrointestinal afferents (chemoreceptors)
      2) Cell bodies of neurons projecting from carotid body and sinus baroreceptors: located in inferior ganglion of cranial nerve (CN) IX (glossopharyngeal nerve)
      3) Cell bodies of neurons projecting from aortic and

visceral baroreceptors and chemoreceptors: located in inferior ganglion of CN X (vagus nerve)

c. Ventrolateral medulla, dorsal nucleus of the vagus, and nucleus ambiguus: responsible for regulating respiratory, vasomotor, and cardiomotor functions

B. **Peripheral Pathways**

1. Parasympathetic (craniosacral) division (Table 22-1, Fig. 22-1)
   a. Long preganglionic axons that synapse in ganglia close to organs
   b. Nicotinic cholinergic receptors transduce signals arriving at postganglionic neurons
   c. Postganlionic cells stimulate muscarinic cholinergic receptors on effector cells (second messenger-linked system)
2. Sympathetic (thoracolumbar) division (Fig. 22-2)

a. Sympathetic preganglionic neurons
   1) All have cell bodies in intermediolateral cell column
   2) Exit spinal cord via ventral roots
   3) Axons release acetylcholine, which acts on nicotinic cholinergic receptors on postganglionic neurons in paravertebral and prevertebral ganglia and adrenal medulla
b. Sympathetic postganglionic neurons
   1) Cell bodies are in paravertebral and prevertebral ganglia
   2) Axons project to effector organ
   3) All sympathetic postganglionic neurons are adrenergic and release norepinephrine (NE) except those innervating sweat glands and a few vasodilator neurons
c. Sympathetic postganglionic neurons innervating sweat glands: acetylcholine is major neurotransmitter, stimulates muscarinic cholinergic receptors on secretory

Table 22-1.   **Parasympathetic (Craniosacral) Autonomic Division**

Preganglionic neuron, nerve	Neurotransmitter*	Ganglion of post-ganglionic neuron	Neurotransmitter†	Effector organ (function)
Accessory oculomotor nucleus (Edinger-Westphal nucleus), oculomotor nerve (CN III)	ACh	Ciliary ganglion	ACh	Pupillary constrictors (constrict pupils)
Superior salivary nucleus, facial nerve (CN VII)	ACh	Pterygopalatine ganglion	ACh	Lacrimal gland (tearing)
		Submandibular ganglia	ACh	Submandibular and sublingual glands (salivation)
Inferior salivary nucleus, glossopharyngeal nerve (CN IX)	ACh	Otic ganglion	ACh	Parotid gland (salivation)
Dorsal motor nucleus of vagus, vagus nerve (CN X)	ACh	Thoracic and abdominal viscera ganglia	ACh	Pulmonary system (increase secretion) Gastrointestinal system (increase motility, decrease sphincter tone, increase secretions)
Ventrolateral nucleus ambiguus, vagus nerve (CN X)	ACh	Cardiac ganglia	ACh	Heart (decrease heart rate and contractility)
Intermediolateral cell column of sacral cord (S2-4), pelvic splanchnic nerves	ACh	Pelvic ganglia	ACh	Gastrointestinal and genitourinary systems (defecation, micturition, erection)

ACh, acetylcholine; CN, cranial nerve.
*Stimulate nicotinic receptors.
†Stimulate muscarinic receptors.

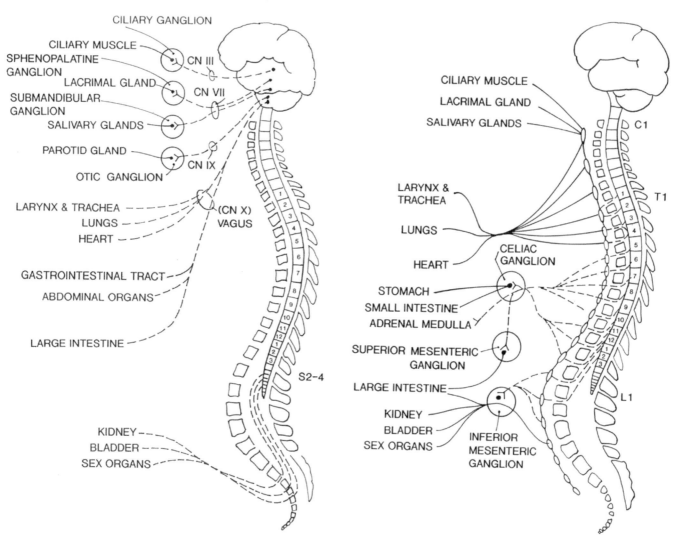

Fig. 22-1. Organization of the parasympathetic (craniosacral) division of the autonomic nervous system. CN, cranial nerve. (From Benarroch EE, Westmoreland BF, Daube JR, Reagan TJ, Sandok BA. Medical neurosciences: an approach to anatomy, pathology, and physiology by systems and levels. 4th ed. Philadelphia: Lippincott Williams & Wilkins; 1999. p. 270. By permission of Mayo Foundation.)

Fig. 22-2. Organization of the sympathetic division of the autonomic nervous system. (From Benarroch EE, Westmoreland BF, Daube JR, Reagan TJ, Sandok BA. Medical neurosciences: an approach to anatomy, pathology, and physiology by systems and levels. 4th ed. Philadelphia: Lippincott Williams & Wilkins; 1999. p. 267. By permission of Mayo Foundation.)

cells in sweat glands
  d. Sympathetic preganglionic neurons synapsing in adrenal medulla: stimulate nicotinic cholinergic receptors on adrenal chromaffin cells, which secrete epinephrine and small amounts of NE
  e. Paravertebral sympathetic ganglia chain
    1) Bilateral chains spanning entire vertebral column from C1 to conus medullaris (coccygeal segments)
    2) Afferent neurons

    a) Cell bodies in intermediolateral cell column (C8 to L1-L2)
    b) Axons pass through ventral horn to the ventral rootlets and, with the spinal nerve, exit through neural foramen
  3) Sympathetic paravertebral chain (Fig. 22-3)
    a) Located immediately adjacent to vertebral bodies
    b) Communicates with the exiting spinal nerve by two communicating nerves: white rami commu-

nicantes carry the afferent (preganglionic) input to ganglionic chain and gray rami communicantes carry efferent (postganglionic) output back to spinal nerve

4) Afferent input from the white rami communicantes may
   a) Synapse in the ganglion at the same level
   b) Travel up or down the sympathetic paravertebral chain to synapse at a different level, or
   c) Extend beyond the sympathetic paravertebral chain to synapse in a prevertebral ganglia (see below) or adrenal medulla
   d) Note: the intermediolateral column is location of all cell bodies of preganglionic sympathetic neurons (extends between C8 and L1)

5) Segmental dominance of presynaptic input: main synaptic input to a ganglion originates from a particular segment of spinal cord

6) Neurotransmitter released at the ganglionic synapse is acetylcholine (acts on nicotinic cholinergic receptors on postsynaptic cells)

f. Prevertebral sympathetic ganglia (Fig. 22-3)
   1) Include the celiac, aorticorenal, superior mesenteric, and inferior mesenteric ganglia
   2) Afferent input: neurons with cell bodies in
      a) Intermediolateral cell column

b) Axons pass from spinal nerves to white rami communicantes
c) Preganglionic axons exit white rami communicantes and form splanchnic nerves, which synapse in preverebral ganglia

C. **Autonomic Innervation of the Urinary System**
1. Cortical urinary control center (CUCC)
   a. Located in frontal lobe
      1) Possible role of prefrontal cortex and anterior cingulate cortex in initiation of micturition
      2) Left sensorimotor cortex, right lateral frontal cortex, and bilateral supplementary motor cortices may be involved in both initiation and maintenance of detrusor contraction and bladder emptying
   b. Frontal lobes: receive extensive input from other cortices, basal ganglia, and thalamus on appropriateness of micturition, emotional input, and other data to determine the timing of micturition
   c. There is also feedback from the lower (pontine) centers on the degree of bladder distension
   d. CUCC communicates with the pontine micturition center or pontine urinary control center (PUCC) and also projects directly to the pyramidal cells of the motor cortex (likely the superomedial central gyrus), which

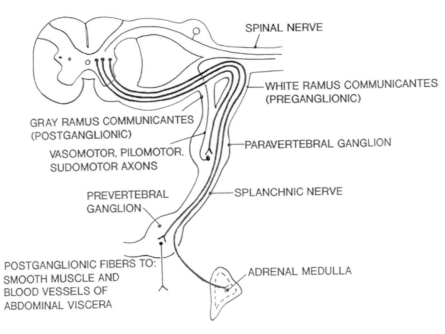

Fig. 22-3. Anatomic schema of the paravertebral and prevertebral sympathetic outflow. (From Benarroch EE, Westmoreland BF, Daube JR, Reagan TJ, Sandok BA. Medical neurosciences: an approach to anatomy, pathology, and physiology by systems and levels. 4th ed. Philadelphia: Lippincott Williams & Wilkins; 1999. p. 268. By permission of Mayo Foundation.)

then project to sacral cord to synapse on pudendal motor neurons in ventral horn (a few cross the midline to synapse on contralateral pudendal motor neurons) to provide tone in external urinary sphincter

2. Pontine urinary control center (pontine micturition center)
  a. Likely diffuse location: PAG, locus ceruleus, and pontine paramedian reticular formation have been implicated
  b. Information about the degree of bladder distension is projected to PUCC and then to CUCC
  c. PUCC also receives information from cortex and integrates this with sensory feedback information to coordinate activity of the spinal urinary control center (SpUCC)
  d. In essence, the switch from continence to micturition occurs in the pons
  e. There are also reciprocal connections with amygdala and hypothalamic preoptic area: may be important for micturition response to emotionally charged stimuli
  f. The pontine micturition center sends projections to the pelvic and pudendal nuclei in sacral cord located in conus medullaris

3. Spinal urinary control center
  a. Sympathetic autonomic innervation
    1) Sympathetic preganglionic neurons originate from intermediolateral cell column between T12 and L2, synapse in corresponding paravertebral ganglia, inferior mesenteric (prevertebral) ganglion, ganglia in pelvic plexus, vesical plexus ("vesical ganglia"), or intramural vesical ganglia (located primarily at the trigone and bladder neck)
    2) Sympathetic nerves innervate urethral smooth muscle (facilitates contraction of urethral smooth muscle) and arterial supply to bladder and not the detrusor muscle
    3) Overall effect of sympathetic innervation of the urethral smooth muscle: inhibit micturition through contraction of urethral smooth muscle and possibly inhibition of parasympathetic ganglionic transmission to detrusor muscle
  b. Parasympathetic autonomic innervation
    1) Pelvic (detrusor motor) nuclei:
      a) Located in conus medullaris (sacral cord) at S2, S3, and S4
      b) Axons form pelvic splanchnic nerves, which innervate bladder detrusor muscle, ureter, urethral smooth muscle, and prostate
    2) Overall effect of the parasympathetic pelvic splanchnic nerves: facilitation of micturition by contraction of detrusor muscle and relaxation of urethral smooth

muscle
    3) Final micturition depends on the urethral sphincter innervated by pudendal nerve (under voluntary control, not autonomic control)
  c. Somatic efferent (voluntary control, not autonomic)
    1) Pudendal nuclei in conus medullaris (segments S2-4)
    2) Axons form the pudendal nerve, which innervates urethral sphincter muscle (striated, not smooth, muscle) between the fascial layers of the urogenital diaphragm (as well as outer vagina and clitoris, penis, bulbospongiosus, ischiocavernosus, superficial transverse perineal, levator ani, and external anal sphincter muscles); striated sphincter muscle is less well-developed in females than males
  d. Sensory afferent input
    1) Information about the degree of bladder wall stretch and contractility is carried by Aδ and C fibers (free nerve endings) to dorsal horn and PUCC
    2) Pain sensation from bladder is via sympathetic nerves to dorsal horn cells, then via spinothalamic tract
    3) Information about distension of the bladder wall may be conducted via parasympathetic nerves to dorsal horn and then via spinothalamic tract and also dorsal columns
    4) Sensory input evoked by bladder distension inhibits the tonic motor excitation of pudendal motor axons innervating the external anal sphincter

D. **Autonomic Innervation of the Gastrointestinal System and Enteric Nervous System**
1. Extrinsic sympathetic innervation
  a. Preganglionic cell bodies in intermediolateral cell column between T9 and L2
    1) Preganglionic axons reach the sympathetic paravertebral chain via white rami communicantes
    2) Some axons synapse in paravertebral ganglia, and others leave the sympathetic chain as thoracic, lumbar, and sacral splanchnic nerves to synapse in prevertebral ganglia (celiac, superior, and inferior mesenteric ganglia) and inferior hypogastric (pelvic) plexus
  b. Synapses in both paravertebral and prevertebral ganglia are cholinergic (nicotinic)
  c. Prevertebral sympathetic ganglia: mediate inhibitory spinal reflexes and peripheral reflexes
  d. Postganglionic neurons
    1) Vasomotor neurons innervate submucosal blood vessels; responsible for vasoconstriction of these vessels
    2) Motility-regulating neurons innervate myenteric plexus, submucosal plexus, and smooth muscle sphincters

3) Postganglionic axons originating from celiac and superior mesenteric ganglia: innervate small intestine, appendix, and ascending and transverse colon

4) Postganglionic axons originating from inferior mesenteric ganglion: innervate descending colon, sigmoid colon, and rectum

5) Postganglionic axons originating from inferior hypogastric (pelvic) plexus: innervate lower rectum

2. Extrinsic parasympathetic innervation
   a. Consists of the vagus (CN X) and pelvic splanchnic nerves
   b. Vagus nerve efferents
      1) Cell bodies in dorsal motor nucleus of X and nucleus ambiguus; axons innervate esophagus, stomach, small intestine, appendix, and ascending and transverse colon (with a proximal-to-distal gradient of innervation, proximal gastrointestinal system receiving the bulk of the innervation)
      2) Innervate the enteric nervous system directly (myenteric plexus), releasing acetylcholine to stimulate nicotinic receptors of myenteric plexus
   c. Pelvic splanchnic (parasympathetic preganglionic) nerves
      1) Cell bodies in sacral spinal cord; axons innervate descending and sigmoid colon and rectum
      2) Axons directly innervate enteric system (myenteric plexus), as does vagus nerve
   d. Enteric nervous system acts as "postganglionic" neurons

3. Primary afferents
   a. Glutamate: primary neurotransmitter
   b. Do not penetrate the epithelium
   c. Vagus nerve afferents
      1) Cell bodies in interior ganglion of CN X
      2) Transmit information from gastrointestinal tract (from esophagus to splenic flexure) to nucleus solitarius
      3) Do not transmit information about pain
      4) Transmit information about mechanical distortion and distension of gut innervated by vagus nerve
   d. Spinal primary sensory afferents
      1) Cell bodies in dorsal root ganglia
      2) Transmit nociceptive afferent information (via sympathetic neurons and pelvic plexus and pelvic splanchnic nerves) from descending colon, sigmoid colon, and rectum to dorsal horn of the spinal cord (lamina I), from which axons project to ventromedial thalamus, which projects to insular cortex
      3) Transmit information about pain and mechanical distortion and distension of gut innervated by sacral and pelvic splanchnic nerves

4. Enteric nervous system
   a. The nervous system of the gastrointestinal tract located in the gut wall

   b. Primarily responsible for peristalsis and migrating motor complex
   c. Integrates absorptive and secretory functions of the gut with motility
   d. Enteric nervous system is essentially a semiautonomous integrative system that retains several stereotyped motility "programs" (e.g., those applied to the fasting state, postprandial state, and emesis), which are selected on the basis of input from periphery or central centers
   e. Sensory neurons consist of mechanoreceptors, chemoreceptors, and thermoreceptors
      1) Mechanoreceptors: sense mechanical changes in the gut wall and mesentery (gross movements) and information about contractile state and bowel distension
      2) Chemoreceptors: sense changes in luminal contents (including pH, osmolarity, and concentration of nutrients)
      3) Mechanoreceptor hypersensitivity in sensing distension of the bowel and contractile tension: possible explanation for pain perceived by patients with irritable bowel syndrome
   f. Interneurons
      1) Receive and integrate input from sensory neurons and central nervous system
      2) Project to enteric motor neurons
      3) Participate in reflex circuits
      4) Provide input to other interneurons
      5) Provide excitatory or inhibitory input to enteric motor neurons, which excite or inhibit the corresponding musculature
   g. Enteric motor neurons: cell bodies are in ganglia of two major plexuses—myenteric (Auerbach's) plexus and submucosal (Meissner's) plexus
      1) Myenteric plexus
         a) Located between the longitudinal and circular external muscle layers
         b) Responsible for regulation of contractility of the external muscle layers
      2) Submucosal plexus
         a) Located in the submucosal layer
         b) Responsible for regulation of the secretory and absorptive functions of the gut
         c) Innervates submucosal arteries
   h. Enteric secretomotor neurons
      1) Innervate and excite the intestinal crypts of Lieberkühn and send collaterals to surrounding blood vessels, causing them to vasodilate, thus simultaneously increasing blood flow promoting secretion
      2) Hyperactivity of these neurons observed in diarrheal illness

3) Hypoactivity of these neurons observed in constipation

i. Secretion of water, electrolytes, and mucus are followed by peristalsis and propulsive contractions of the gut

j. Peristaltic reflex in nonsphincteric regions

1) With a passing bolus, enteric excitatory musculo-motor neurons induce contraction of intestinal circular muscles orad to and longitudinal muscles caudad to the bolus (the point of activation of mechanoreceptors sensing the distension)

2) Simultaneously, enteric inhibitory musculomotor neurons inhibit contraction of (and promote relaxation of) the intestinal circular muscles caudad to and longitudinal muscles orad to the point of distension

3) This intrinsic activity of the enteric nervous system is stimulated by parasympathetic preganglionic fibers and inhibited by sympathetic innervation

k. Excitatory musculomotor neurons release acetylcholine and substance P; the predominant inhibitory neurotransmitters are adenosine triphoshate (ATP), vasoactive intestinal polypeptide, and nitric oxide

l. Destruction and absence of the inhibitory musculo-motor neurons of the myenteric plexus: continuous contraction of the self-excitable muscular syncytium of nonsphincteric regions

1) This causes failure of normal intestinal propulsion and, thus, pseudo-obstruction

2) Examples of disorders associated with pseudo-obstruction (poor or absent motility without a structural obstruction): Chagas' disease, autoimmune pandysautonomia, paraneoplastic syndrome, Hirschprung's disease, idiopathic or inherited neuropathies, achalasia (of lower esophageal sphincter)

E. **Autonomic Physiology of Sexual Function**

1. Central pathways

a. Cerebral cortex

1) Orbitofrontal cortex: associated with emotional and motivational aspects of sexual arousal

2) Anterior cingulate cortex and hypothalamus: associated with autonomic and endocrine responses

3) Head of the caudate: has been implicated by data from positron emission tomography (PET)

b. Hypothalamus: regions responsible for mediating sexual behavior are medial preoptic area in males and ventro-medial nucleus in females

c. Spinal cord: ascending fibers carry sensory input from sex organs

2. Peripheral pathways

a. Sympathetic innervation

1) Preganglionic fibers

a) Originate from intermediolateral cell column between T11 and L2

b) Exit from spinal cord in ventral roots and enter paravertebral ganglia (sympathetic chain)

c) Some synapse here and others form lumbar and sacral splanchnic nerves to synapse in prevertebral ganglia (inferior mesenteric ganglia and inferior hypogastric [pelvic] plexus)

d) Synapses are cholinergic (nicotinic) in both paravertebral and prevertebral ganglia

2) Postganglionic fibers to arteries: responsible for maintaining arterial tone

3) Postganglionic fibers to erectile tissue of penis, clitoris, and vestibular bulbs: responsible for psychogenic erection originating from cerebral cortex

4) Postganglionic fibers to smooth muscle in epididymis, vas deferens, seminal vesicles, and prostate gland: responsible for seminal emission and deposition of spermatozoa and seminal fluid

5) Postganglionic fibers to sphincter of the bladder neck: responsible for simultaneous contraction of sphincter for prevention of reflux of semen into bladder

b. Pudendal nerve

1) Originates from anterior horn cells in S2-4

2) Contains afferent input for reflexogenic penile erection, glandular secretions, seminal emission, and ejaculation

3) Contains somatic efferents for ejaculation

3. Erection

a. Penile erection is autonomically mediated increased blood flow to venous sinuses of corpora cavernosa and corpus spongiosum, accompanied by arterial dilatation and decreased venous outflow, due partly to contraction of ischiovacernosus muscle constricting the proximal corpora cavernosa

b. Occurs from

1) Local stimulation of the genitalia: reflexogenic erection (sacrospinal reflex) mediated by pudendal afferents and sacral parasympathetic efferents

2) Psychogenic stimulation: supraspinal erection mediated by cortical auditory, visual, olfactory, emotional, imaginative, or other cortical input and lumbar sympathetic efferents

4. Emission

a. Mediated by lumbar sympathetic innervation

b. Contraction of smooth muscle of epididymis, vas deferens, seminal vesicles, and prostate gland (as mentioned above)

5. Ejaculation

a. Mediated by pudendal somatic efferents (motor neurons), *not* by sympathetic innervation

b. Rhythmic contractions of bulbocavernosus, ischiocavernosus, and periurethral striated muscles are responsible for rapid and rhythmic release of semen

6. Orgasm

a. In males, mediated by pudendal sensory afferents carrying information about sensations accompanying emission and ejaculation

b. In females, mediated by pudendal sensory afferents carrying information about sensations accompanying rhythmic contraction of vagina and muscles of the pelvic floor

II. AUTONOMIC TESTING

A. Cardiovascular Autonomic Tests

1. Beat-to-beat response to Valsalva maneuver (forced expiration against resistance)

a. Beat-to-beat blood pressure and heart rate response to Valsalva maneuver

b. Four phases of Valsalva response are used to assess adrenergic function (Fig. 22-4)

c. Phase I

1) Transient increase in blood pressure and decrease in heart rate

2) Mechanical phase: due to compression of thoracic aorta and propulsion of blood into the periphery

d. Phase II

1) Early

a) Increase in heart rate and decrease in blood pressure

b) Poor venous return to the heart decreases cardiac output and, hence, blood pressure

c) This decrease in blood pressure is sensed by low-pressure aortic baroreceptors, which send signals to nucleus solitarius, eventually causing compensatory increase in heart rate

2) Late

a) Return of blood pressure to normal and continued increase in heart rate

b) Peripheral vasoconstriction due to vascular sympathetic activation causes normalization of blood pressure

3) Main mediator of late phase is vascular sympathetic innervation: this phase may be blocked by α-blockers and may be reduced or absent in conditions associated with peripheral adrenergic failure

e. Phase III: cessation of forced expiration

1) Transient decrease in blood pressure and increase in heart rate

2) Mechanical phase: release of mechanical compression on thoracic aorta causes release of resistance in the pulmonary vasculature and increase in blood flow to pulmonary vessels, hence, a decrease in cardiac output and blood pressure

f. Phase IV

1) Increase in blood pressure and decrease in heart rate

2) Sympathetically mediated overshoot increase in blood pressure is caused by increased venous return to the heart and increased cardiac output (mediated by increased myocardial contractility) in face of peripheral vasoconstriction (the latter lags behind); accompanying decrease in heart rate is baroreflex-mediated

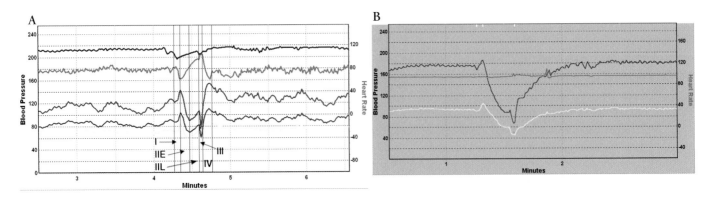

Fig. 22-4. The four phases (I-IV) of the Valsalva maneuver in a normal subject (*A*) and a patient with multiple system atrophy (*B*). Note the loss of late phase II and phase IV in the patient with multiple system atrophy. Red, systolic blood pressure; yellow, diastolic blood pressure; purple, mean blood pressure; green, heart rate; blue, respiration. IIE, early phase II; IIL, late phase II. (Courtesy of Jeanne Corfits, R.EEG.T., Mayo Clinic, Rochester, MN.)

3) Principal mediator of blood pressure overshoot: cardiac sympathetic innervation; this phase may be blocked by β-blockers

g. Phases I and III are purely mechanical, and phases II and IV are sympathetically derived and are used to assess cardiovascular adrenergic function

h. Absence of phase IV and late phase II responses and a larger decrease in blood pressure in early phase II are noted in conditions associated with generalized adrenergic failure

2. Beat-to-beat response to head-up tilting (passive standing) (Fig. 22-5)

a. Head-up tilt is passive form of standing; hence, initial decrease in blood pressure may be absent or minimal compared with response to standing

b. Normal response: initial transient decrease in blood pressure and increase in heart rate, followed by return of both heart rate and blood pressure to a new plateau (generally close to but higher than baseline)

c. Abnormal response: initial decrease in blood pressure and rise in heart rate; blood pressure continues to decrease, and heart rate does not return to a point close to baseline

d. Indicators of mild adrenergic impairment: excessive oscillations in blood pressure, transient decrease in systolic blood pressure of more than 30 mm Hg, and an increase in heart rate of more than 30 beats per minute

B. **Quantitative Sudomotor Axon Reflex Test** (Fig. 22-6 and 22-7)

1. Axonal reflex: mediated by postganglionic sympathetic axons (sudomotor axons) to eccrine sweat glands

2. Procedure

a. Nerve terminals on sweat gland stimulated by iontophoresis of acetylcholine to the skin under the stimulus compartment of the multicompartmental cell applied to the skin

b. The impulses generated travel antidromically to nearest branch point and then travel orthodromically to nearby sweat glands, stimulating muscarinic receptors on the glands to produce a sweat response that is recorded in a different compartment of the cell at a distance from the stimulus compartment

3. Interpretation of test results

a. Normal test: intact postganglionic sympathetic sudomotor axons

b. Normal test with anhidrosis on thermoregulatory sweat test: preganglionic localization of lesion

c. Abnormal test with anhidrosis on thermoregulatory sweat test: postganglionic localization of lesion (most

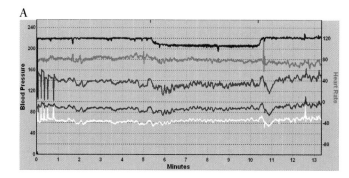

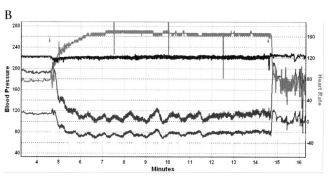

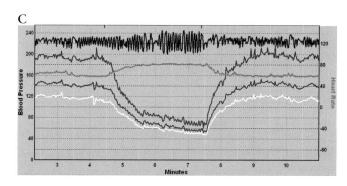

Fig. 22-5. Beat-to-beat response to head-up tilting (passive standing) in a normal subject (*A*), a patient with postural tachycardia syndrome (*B*), and a 54-year-old man with pure autonomic failure (*C*). Red, systolic blood pressure; yellow, diastolic blood pressure; purple, mean blood pressure; green, heart rate. (Courtesy of Jeanne Corfits, R.EEG.T., Mayo Clinic, Rochester, MN.)

sensitive for postganglionic autonomic neuropathy)

d. Small-fiber neuropathy

1) Reduction of sweat response distally

2) There may be persistent sweat activity in mild small-fiber neuropathies, which may be related to repetitive spontaneous firing of damaged sympathetic axon

3) Painful small-fiber neuropathies are associated with augmentation of somatosympathetic reflexes, causing markedly reduced latencies with persistent sweat

A

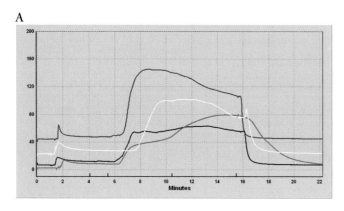

B

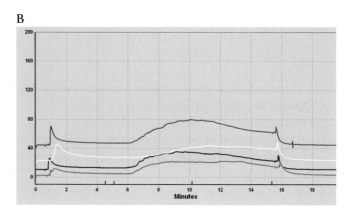

Fig. 22-6. Quantitative sudomotor axon reflex test in normal male (*A*) and female (*B*). Red, forearm; blue, proximal leg; green, distal leg; yellow, foot. (Courtesy of Jeanne Corfits, R.EEG.T., Mayo Clinic, Rochester, MN.)

A

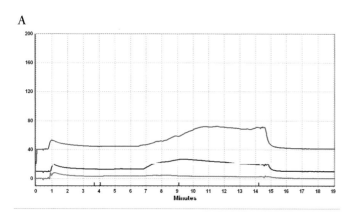

B

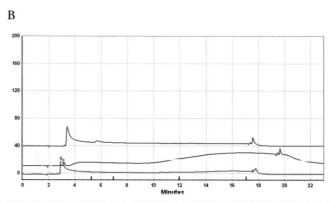

Fig. 22-7. *A*, Quantitative sudomotor axon reflex test (QSART) in a 38-year-old man with advanced, length-dependent small-fiber peripheral neuropathy. Note the decreased sweat response in the proximal leg and anhidrosis over the distal leg and foot. *B*, QSART in a 43-year-old woman with severe cholinergic autonomic neuropathy shows severe diffuse anhidrosis with minimal sweat output in the proximal leg only. Red, forearm; blue, proximal leg; green, distal leg; yellow, foot. (Courtesy of Jeanne Corfits, R.EEG.T., Mayo Clinic, Rochester, MN.)

activity
  e. Complex regional pain syndrome (CRPS): sweat activity may be reduced or exaggerated

C. **Thermoregulatory Sweat Test** (Fig. 22-8)
1. Use: evaluation of both central and peripheral efferent sudomotor pathways
2. Method
  a. Increase skin temperature and core body temperature in a sweat chamber with ambient temperature of 48°C to 50°C
  b. An indicator powder is applied to the skin before heating (often a mixture of alizarin red, cornstarch, and sodium carbonate in 50:100:50-g ratio)
  c. The powder is orange and remains orange when dry, but

turns purple when wet
3. Patterns of sweat loss
  a. Distal (length-dependent): seen with peripheral neuropathies with small-fiber involvement
  b. Focal: anhidrosis confined to a dermatome or distribution of a peripheral nerve
  c. Segmental: focal pattern, confined to a dermatome
  d. Global: diffuse anhidrosis involving more than 80% of body
4. False positive
  a. Wearing pressure wraps within 12 hours before the test may produce false-positive results, that is, anhidrosis over the distribution that was covered (there is usually straight edges)
  b. Reduced diffuse (not focal) anhidrosis with dehydration

and anticholinergic agents (should be avoided within 48 hours before the test)

  c. Elderly: there may be focal areas of anhidrosis (often affecting lower body and proximal upper limbs)

III. DISORDERS OF THE AUTONOMIC NERVOUS SYSTEM

A. Degenerative Disorders

1. Autonomic features of multiple system atrophy (see Chapter 8)
   a. Due to loss of sympathetic cells in intermediolateral cell column and paravertebral sympathetic ganglia
   b. Urogenital dysfunction: male erectile dysfunction, urinary incontinence (detrusor hyperreflexia, overflow incontinence, and urinary dyssynergia), urinary retention, and incomplete bladder emptying
   c. Cardiovascular autonomic dysfunction: orthostatic hypotension
   d. Sudomotor dysfunction: hypohidrosis or anhidrosis (caution against overheating)
   e. Selective loss of anterior horn cells in ventral horn of sacral segments (Onuf's nucleus)
   f. Other autonomic features: gastrointestinal hypomotility and sleep-related respiratory disorders (laryngeal stridor and sleep apnea)
2. Autonomic features of Parkinson's disease (see Chapter 8)
   a. Autonomic failure: well-documented; believed due to neuronal loss and degeneration of preganglionic and postganglionic neurons
   b. Lewy bodies seen in both central (substantia nigra) and peripheral neurons
   c. Cardiovascular autonomic dysfunction presenting with orthostatic hypotension (primary symptom, secondary to medications, or a combination thereof): dopaminergic drugs produce or exacerbate the symptoms
   d. Dysphagia and sialorrhea are likely due to oropharyngeal rigidity
   e. Genitourinary dysfunction: male impotence and ejaculatory dysfunction, poor libido, and bladder hyperreflexia
3. Dementia with Lewy bodies (see Chapter 7)
4. Pure autonomic failure
   a. Adult onset, sporadic, slowly progressive idiopathic degenerative condition
   b. Clinical manifestations
      1) Orthostatic hypotension, urinary and sexual dysfunction

    2) No other neurologic complaints (sparing of pyramidal, extrapyramidal, and cerebellar systems)
   c. Urinary symptoms: hesitancy, urgency, postvoiding dribbling, and incontinence
   d. Sexual dysfunction symptoms: impotence, erectile and ejaculatory dysfunction, and retrograde ejaculation
   e. Orthostatism: consciousness may be lost with or without warning
   f. Patients should be followed for at least 5 years because other neurologic symptoms may develop, and the diagnosis eventually may be changed (such as Parkinson's disease or multiple system atrophy)
   g. Laboratory findings
      1) Very low NE levels when recumbent (this is normal in patients with multiple system atrophy and Parkinson's disease)
      2) Failure of plasma NE levels to increase during upright posture (subnormal increase seen in patients with multiple system atrophy and some patients with Parkinson's disease)
      3) Neuroendocrine responses to hypotension or centrally acting adrenergic agents such as clonidine are normal in patients with pure autonomic failure or Parkinson's disease (blunted in patients with multiple system atrophy)
      4) Neuroimaging findings: normal
   h. Pathology features
      1) Presence of Lewy bodies in substantia nigra, locus ceruleus, thoracolumbar and sacral cord, sympathetic ganglia, and postganglionic nerves (may be more prominent in peripheral locations)
      2) Cell loss in intermediolateral columns and sympathetic ganglia

B. Immune-Mediated Disorders

1. Guillain-Barré syndrome (see Chapter 21)
   a. Autonomic dysfunction (hyper- or hypoactivity): relatively common
   b. Tachycardia, orthostatic hypotension (alternating with hypertension), bowel and bladder dysfunction, gastrointestinal tract dysmotility, and, less commonly, gastroparesis, pupillary dysfunction, and fecal incontinence
   c. Autonomic symptoms may be life-threatening; patients may need to be monitored closely
2. Autoimmune autonomic neuropathy
   a. May affect any age
   b. Typically subacute onset of autonomic symptoms, but a subset of patients present with more gradual onset and slow progression
   c. Diffuse autonomic dysfunction (often primarily cholinergic immune-mediated ganglionopathy) affecting both

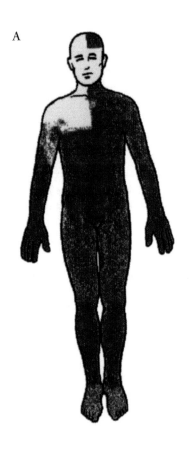

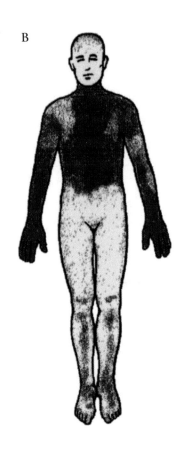

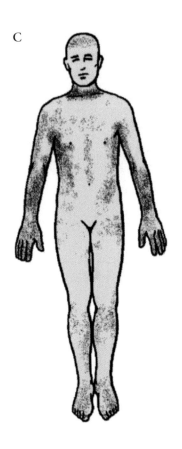

sympathetic and parasympathetic systems

d. Most patients have postural hypotension and gastro-intestinal tract dysmotility

e. Other symptoms: anhidrosis, "sicca" symptoms (dry eyes and mouth), pupillary involvement, erectile dysfunction, and urinary incontinence

f. Most patients have a monophasic exacerbation, followed by remission without recurrences

g. Serum serology

  1) Neuronal (ganglionic) nicotinic acetylcholine receptor (α_3 subunit) antibodies present in approximately 1/3 of patients

  2) Presence of this antibody has been associated with sicca complex, pupillary dysfunction, lower gastro-intestinal dysfunction, and subacute onset (temporal profile may vary)

  3) Antibody level correlates with severity of autonomic signs and symptoms

h. Cerebrospinal fluid: often has elevated protein with nor-mal cells

i. Prognosis: most patients improve spontaneously; recovery is often partial, usually slow, and may take several months to years

j. Treatment

  1) Symptomatic management

  2) Anectodal reports of response to intravenous immunoglobulin and plasma exchange (especially if given early)

3. Paraneoplastic pandysautonomia

  a. Associated with lung carcinoma, Hodgkin's lymphoma, testicular cancer, pancreatic carcinoma

  b. Associated with antineuronal nuclear (ANNA)-1 (anti-Hu) antibodies

  c. Separate from paraneoplastic ganglionopathy or Lambert-Eaton syndrome

4. Lambert-Eaton myasthenic syndrome (see Chapter 23)

  a. Usually paraneoplastic

  b. Pure cholinergic dysautonomia

  c. Autonomic failure due to defective presynaptic acetyl-choline release

5. Paraneoplastic sensory neuronopathy (see Chapters 14 and 21)

6. Sensory neuronopathy related to Sjögren's syndrome (see Chapter 21)

7. Multiple sclerosis (see Chapter 14)

  a. Related to transverse myelitis or to lesion brainstem or diencephalon

  b. Dysfunction of bowel, bladder, or sexual function is common

D 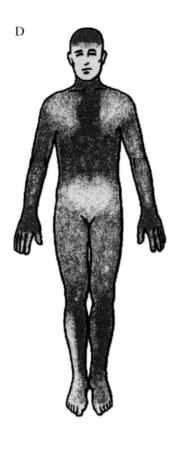 E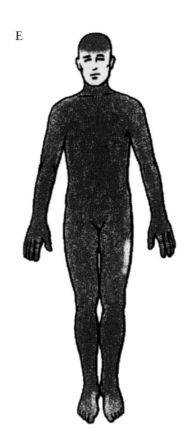

Fig. 22-8. Thermoregulatory sweat test in, *A*, patient with an apical lung (Pancoast's) tumor affecting the right sympathetic chain; *B*, patient with multiple system atrophy, note anhidrosis in much of the body below the level of a low thoracic segment; *C*, patient with pure autonomic failure, note anhidrosis over most of the body (which may also be seen with severe autonomic neuropathy, including diabetic neuropathy and multiple system atrophy); *D*, patient with small-fiber neuropathy, note distal anhidrosis affecting the right more than the left lower extremity, fingers, and abdomen; and *E*, patient with very mild small-fiber neuropathy and left lateral cutaneous neuropathy (meralgia paresthetica). Regional hypohidrosis of the proximal extremities and upper trunk in *D* is a normal finding and may represent an age-related loss of sudomotor function.

c. Bladder dysfunction is commonly detrusor hyperreflexia
8. Connective tissue disorders
   a. Rheumatoid arthritis, systemic lupus erythematosus, mixed connective tissue disease (see Chapter 14)
   b. Anhidrosis of extremities commonly occurs in rheumatoid arthritis because of damage of postganglionic sympathetic efferent fibers

C. Infectious Disorders
1. Leprosy
   a. Abnormalities range from focal anhidrosis over hypopigmented areas to more diffuse anhidrosis, postural hypotension, and cardiac denervation
2. Other infectious causes: Chagas' disease (see Chapter 15), human immunodeficiency virus (and related complications, see Chapter 15), prions (fatal familial insomnia, see Chapter 7)

D. Vascular Disorders
1. Ischemia in basilar artery distribution (e.g., lateral medullary infarction, or Wallenberg's syndrome)

E. Hereditary and Congenital Disorders (see also Chapter 21)
1. Associated with hereditary neuropathies

   a. For example, hereditary sensory and autonomic neuropathies (HSAN)
   b. Autonomic features are prominent in HSAN type III (Riley-Day syndrome)
2. Fabry's disease
   a. X-linked recessive disorder due to deficiency of α-galactosidase A
3. Tangier disease
   a. Caused by deficiency of ATP-binding cascade transporter
   b. Patients present with slowly progressive sensory small-fiber neuropathy, motor involvement (including facial diplegia), orange-yellow tonsils, enlarged liver and spleen, hypercholesterolemia, hypertriglyceridemia, reduced or absent high-density lipoproteins, and premature coronary artery disease
4. Porphyrias
5. Hereditary amyloidosis
6. Arnold-Chiari malformation (involving brainstem autonomic pathways)

F. Diabetes-Related Neuropathy (see also Chapter 21)
1. Common cause of autonomic neuropathy
2. Frequent involvement of unmyelinated fibers
3. Orthostatic hypotension, gastroparesis, impotence, retention, constipation, gustatory sweating

G. Traumatic Causes

1. Syringomyelia
   a. May also be nontraumatic, spontaneous
   b. Disruption of intermediolateral cell columns and associated projections
   c. There may be segmental autonomic deficits, including segmental hypohidrosis
2. Spinal cord transaction
   a. Supine and orthostatic hypotension (hypertension with autonomic dysreflexia)
   b. Risk of bradycardia and cardiac arrest (especially with maneuvers stimulating vasovagal reflex, such as suctioning)
   c. Enhanced role of vasopressin and the renin-angiotensin-aldosterone system in maintaining arterial blood pressure
   d. Below the lesion
      1) Lack of sudomotor and thermoregulatory responses
      2) Severe hypothermia or hyperthermia, anhidrosis
   e. Above the lesion (cervical to T5): autonomic dysreflexia
      1) Sympathetic system: reflex activation
      2) Sacral parasympathetic autonomic system: activation induced by stimulation of skin or viscera
      3) There may be vasodilatation and flushing of skin, hyperhidrosis, piloerection, pupillary dilatation, and severe hypertension (supine and orthostatic)
   f. Bladder function
      1) Complete spinal cord transaction: complete loss of voluntary control of voiding
      2) In acute phase: complete urinary retention and areflexic bladder
      3) Soon after acute phase
         a) Recovery of reflex bladder activity mediated by spinal reflex pathways
         b) Development of bladder hyperactivity due to disruption of bulbospinal inhibitory projections
   g. Spinal cord lesions above T12: preserved reflexogenic penile erection (pudendal afferents and sacral parasympathetics), but abolished psychogenic penile erection

H. Localized or Organ-Specific Autonomic Disorders

1. Adie's pupil (see Chapter 3)
2. Holmes-Adie syndrome
   a. Adie's pupil and deep tendon areflexia, the latter likely due to involvement of dorsal root ganglia
   b. Associated with autonomic neuropathy and peripheral neuropathy
   c. There may be evidence of widespread autonomic involvement such as orthostatic hypotension and sudomotor abnormalities, as noted on thermoregulatory sweat test
3. Horner's syndrome (see Chapter 3)
4. Ross syndrome
   a. Both sympathetic and parasympathetic patchy denervation (the latter is more prominent)
   b. Tonic pupils associated with hyporeflexia and segmental hypohidrosis: believed to be due to involvement of postganglionic cholinergic fibers
   c. Hyporeflexia may implicate dorsal root ganglia
   d. Tonic pupils are likely due to damage to ciliary ganglion or postganglionic cholinergic parasympathetic fibers, denervation of iris muscles, and misdirected reinnervation by parasympathetic fibers originally destined for ciliary muscle
   e. Anhidrosis likely results from damage to sympathetic ganglion cells or postganglionic projections
   f. There may be more widespread autonomic manifestations: orthostatic hypotension, Horner's syndrome
5. Harlequin syndrome
   a. Sudden onset of unilateral sweating and flushing occurring on one side of face, often induced by exercise
   b. There may be contralateral gustatory sweating
   c. Pupil may be smaller ipsilateral to nonflushing side (hypothesized to be due to sympathetic denervation supersensitivity, with partial denervation) or larger
   d. Both sympathetic and parasympathetic patchy denervation
   e. Cause: unknown, but viral infection or autoimmune mechanism has been proposed
6. Chagas' disease
   a. Infection caused by *Trypanosoma cruzi*, occurring predominantly in Latin America
   b. Combined parasympathetic and sympathetic neuropathy (predominantly parasympathetic)
   c. Acute stage: high parasitemia and widespread tissue infiltration, especially cardiac and autonomic ganglionic tissues
   d. Chronic stage
      1) Parasite leaves bloodstream, but serology tests remain positive
      2) Most of these patients with positive serology tests remain asymptomatic
      3) Approximately 1/3 of these patients develop cardiomyopathy and may develop cardiac failure and cardiac dysrhythmias
   e. Involvement of enteric nervous system: ganglionitis and destruction of Meissner's and Auerbach's plexuses, causing dilatation of esophagus (megaesophagus), stomach, or large intestine (megacolon)
   f. Involvement of parasympathetic cholinergic innervation of gastrointestinal tract

g. Other autonomic innervations affected: urinary, cardio-pulmonary (including the cardiac complications discussed above)

7. Vasospastic disorders
   a. Raynaud's phenomenon
      1) Episodes of bilateral, symmetric change in skin color, provoked by exposure to cold or emotional stimuli (pallor → cyanosis → rubor: white-blue-red)
      2) Color change is believed due to transient vasospasm of digital arteries inducing local ischemia
      3) Raynaud's *syndrome*: applies to the condition without an underlying cause
      4) Raynaud's *phenomenon*: associated with connective tissue disease (e.g., scleroderma), carpal tunnel syndrome, thoracic outlet syndrome, and drugs (amphetamines, β-blockers, ergot alkaloids, bleomycin, nitroglycerin, methysergide, bromocriptine, and cyclosporine)
   b. Acrocyanosis
      1) Benign, painless disorder
      2) Symmetric persistent cyanosis of the distal extremities that may extend to ankles and wrists, associated with hyperhydrosis and coldness of fingers and toes
      3) Results from arterial vasoconstriction
      4) Normal pulse, normal oxygen saturation on pulse oximetry
      5) Persistant cyanosis manifesting as bluish discoloration (not rubor or pallor, as with Raynaud's phenomenon)
      6) Exacerbated with exposure to cold (alleviated with exposure to heat)
   c. Livedo reticularis
      1) Mottled discoloration of extremities and trunk due to arteriolar vasospasm and obstruction or venous stasis
      2) May be benign in the absence of a systemic condition *or*
      3) May be associated with several vasculitides and connective tissue disorders, antiphospholipid antibodies (Sneddon's syndrome), hyperviscosity syndrome, thrombocythemia, drugs (e.g., amantadine)

8. Pathologic hyperhidrosis
   a. Essential (primary) hyperhidrosis
      1) Affects the palmar, plantar, and axillary regions; is often familial
      2) Evidence supports hyperactivity of sympathetic neurons in T2-4 sympathetic ganglia
      3) May be treated with β-blockers, anticholinergic agents, and surgical sympathetectomy
   b. Idiopathic postmenopausal hyperhidrosis
      1) Predominantly affects head and upper trunk
      2) Responsive to clonidine (centrally acting α_2-adrenergic receptor agonist)
   c. Facial hyperhidrosis
      1) Idiopathic hemifacial hyperhidrosis
         a) Associated with hypertrophy of sweat glands
         b) Gustatory flushing and sweating provoked by heat, emotions, and eating
         c) May be treated with stellate ganglion block
      2) Gustatory sweating
         a) May be due to damage of pre- or postganglionic sympathetic nerves (cervicothoracic sympathectomies) or local damage to autonomic innervation of the face, denervation supersensitivity, and aberrant reinnervation
         b) Autonomic denervation in the face may be followed by reinnervation of sweat glands by parasympathetics originally destined for salivary glands

9. Pathologic hypohidrosis and anhidrosis
   a. Hypohidrosis and anhidrosis cause heat intolerance, hyperthermia, dry skin, trophic skin changes, and other autonomic features, depending on extent of involvement and cause
   b. Chronic idiopathic anhidrosis
      1) Acquired widespread anhidrosis
      2) Absence of adrenergic or cardiovagal dysfunction (patients do not experience orthostatic hypotension)
      3) Some cases are associated with small-fiber neuropathy
      4) Anhidrosis may remain stable or progress
   c. Acquired focal anhidrosis
      1) Segmental radicular dermatomal, focal, or multifocal distribution of anhidrosis may be seen with diabetic truncal neuropathies and mononeuritis multiplex (as in vasculitic mononeuropathies and leprosy)
      2) Segmental anhidrosis (focal or multifocal) in distribution of sympathetic dermatomes may be seen with sympathectomies, Pancoast's tumor, and autoimmune acute pandysautonomia
      3) Cutaneous disorders causing anhidrosis (not conforming to dermatomal or single nerve distribution): local radiation injury (damaging the sweat glands), psoriasis, and hypohidrotic ectodermal dysplasia
      4) Distal (length-dependent) postganglionic anhidrosis: seen in context of peripheral neuropathies affecting sudomotor innervation; examples are diabetic peripheral neuropathy, primary systemic and familial amyloidosis, Tangier disease, Fabry's disease, and axonal neuropathies caused by drugs and toxins (e.g., chemotherapy agents and heavy metals)
   d. Hemianhidrosis
      1) Due to central lesions
      2) Brainstem lesions (infarcts, tumors, syringobulbia)

cause anhidrosis of hemibody ipsilateral to lesion (cortical infarcts may acutely cause hyperhidrosis contralateral to lesion)

    e. Global anhidrosis
        1) Inherited (e.g., hereditary sensory and autonomic neuropathy VI)
        2) Acquired ("central" disorders such as multiple system atrophy and hypothalamic tumor)

10. Erythromelalgia
    a. Painful acral erythema on cutaneous warming, associated with intense burning
    b. Mechanism believed to involve backfiring (axon reflex) of polymodal C nociceptors
    c. Often associated with small-fiber neuropathy
    d. Associated with
        1) Diabetic neuropathy, hereditary sensory neuropathy
        2) Drugs (verapamil, nicardipine, pergolide, and mercury)
        3) Vasculitis and collagen vascular diseases
        4) Pregnancy
        5) Myeloproliferative disorders
    e. Treatment
        1) Some evidence for relief with aspirin or ibuprofen
        2) Other: amitriptyline, β-blockers, capsaicin cream, clonazepam

11. Red ear syndrome
    a. Head pain and unilateral painful, burning red ear
    b. Pain may radiate to C2 and C3 dermatomes (behind and below mandible, respectively), occiput, or forehead
    c. Pain may be induced by heat, exercise, touch, chewing, coughing, sneezing, or movements of head and neck
    d. Associated with lesion of C3 root, temporomandibular joint dysfunction, and possibly migraine headaches
    e. Mechanism believed to involve backfiring (antidromic response or axon reflex) of polymodal C nociceptors

12. Cluster and migraine headaches (see Chapter 18)

13. Orthostatic intolerance
    a. Dysautonomia of upright position (symptoms relieved by lying down)
    b. Symptoms may be attributed to lack of adequate cerebral perfusion (e.g., lightheadedness and dizziness, presyncopal symptoms, disequilibrium, lower limb or overall weakness, headache, difficulty thinking, poor exercise tolerance) or autonomic overactivity (e.g., palpitations, tremulousness, nausea)
    c. Symptoms may be exacerbated by exposure to increased ambient heat, exercise, and eating
    d. May be classified as neuropathic and hyperadrenergic postural tachycardia syndrome (POTS), hypovolemia syndrome, and vasovagal syncope (the latter two are not

discussed further)

    e. Postural tachycardia syndrome
        1) Usually occurs in individuals between 15 to 50 years old
        2) Female:male = 4-5:1
        3) May be history of antecedent viral illness and/or family history
        4) Induction of symptoms upon standing and resolution of symptoms with lying down
        5) Increase in heart rate of more than 30 beats/min and/or absolute rate of more than 120 beats/min
        6) May be hyperadrenergic or neuropathic
            a) Evidence of associated autonomic neuropathy and related autonomic symptoms with neuropathic POTS, for example, distal anhidrosis on thermoregulatory sweat test or loss of late phase II with Valsalva maneuver
        7) Mild POTS is also called mild orthostatic intolerance
        8) Excessive increase in heart rate and decrease in blood pressure (pulse pressure) (Fig 22-5 *B*)
        9) Poor venous tone causes pooling of venous blood in legs and abdomen (mesenteric venous pool) with standing
        10) Differential diagnosis includes
            a) Thyrotoxicosis
            b) Dehydration and hypovolemia
            c) Medication effect
            d) Pheochromocytoma
            e) Hypoadrenalism
            f) Primary autonomic neuropathy such as amyloid neuropathy
        11) Increased supine and upright NE levels (more so with hyperadrenergic POTS than with neuropathic type)
        12) Treatment
            a) Liberal salt and fluid intake
            b) Sleep with head of bed elevated
            c) Support garments and body stocking for patients with venous pooling
            d) Use of fludrocortisone and midodrine for orthostatic hypotension intractable to simple symptomatic measures
            e) Use of α-agonist for those with loss of late phase II with Valsalva maneuver
            f) Use of low-dose β-blockers (e.g., propranolol)
            g) Use of low-dose clonidine for hyperadrenergic POTS (less effective for neuropathic POTS)

14. Complex regional pain syndrome (CRPS)
    a. Defined by International Association for the Study of Pain as follows
        1) Optional criteria: usually (not always) starts by an

inciting noxious event or cause of immobilization
   2) Mandatory criteria
      a) Continuing pain and allodynia, or hyperalgesia, disproportionate to the inciting event
      b) Pain (at some time) becomes associated with changes in the skin blood flow, edema, and/or abnormal sweating in the region of the pain
      c) No evidence of another condition to account for the symptoms
   b. Two types of CRPS are recognized by International Association for the Study of Pain
      1) Type I (formerly called reflex sympathetic dystrophy): inciting event (if it exists) spares major peripheral nerves
      2) Type II (formerly called causalgia): inciting event causes damage to a major peripheral nerve
   c. Inciting event is usually present (rarely absent) and may be trivial; if present, may be trauma with or without nerve injury, or otherwise, another insult such as hemiplegia from cerebral infarction
   d. Quality of the pain varies from deep ache to sharp, burning, and dysesthetic
   e. There may be cutaneous hyperalgesia and allodynia (increased perception of pain in response to nonnoxious stimulus)
   f. Patients may wear protective gear and clothing to avoid mechanical or thermal stimulation of painful region
   g. Abnormal vasomotor activity: skin discoloration and edema in painful region
   h. Abnormal sudomotor activity: hypohidrosis
   i. Other associated manifestations: motor dysfunction and trophic changes (atrophied skin, hair loss, and pitting nails; nails may be hypertrophied or atrophic)
   j. Stage I: pain as described above, hyperalgesia and allodynia, early vasomotor and sudomotor dysfunction (increased swelling and sweating)
   k. Stage II (after a few months): pain, sudomotor, and vasomotor dysfunction continue; often, trophic changes as described above
   l. Stage III (after a few months to years): persistent pain, sensory and trophic changes, and atrophic muscles
   m. Diagnosis
      1) Clinical diagnosis
      2) Vascular studies to rule out vascular cause
      3) Electrodiagnostic testing to rule out neuropathic process such as peripheral neuropathy or entrapment mononeuropathy
      4) Measurement of resting sudomotor activity and also with iontophoresis of acetylcholine to the skin
      5) Three-phase bone scan is very sensitive and should be performed early to detect osseous changes sooner than

with plain films
      6) Response to sympathetic blocks is often present and essential for diagnosis; however, response may not be adequate because sympathetic dysfunction may or may not be present
   n. Treatment
      1) Prevention
         a) Avoid tight casts (remove as soon as possible)
         b) Avoid procedures on patients with previous history of CRPS if possible; otherwise, sympathetic blockade of the limb undergoing procedure (surgery) may be considered
         c) Mobilize patients early
      2) Physical therapy and occupational therapy are absolutely essential
         a) Goal is to restore mobility, weight-bearing capacity, reduce swelling, and prevent osteoporosis
         b) Gentle desensitization, followed by gentle flexibility, isometric strengthening, followed by more aggressive range-of-motion exercises and strengthening as well as aerobic conditioning
      3) Corticosteroids (prednisone or methylprednisolone)
         a) Class I evidence
         b) May be most effective early on; recommended for short-term use (long-term use not usually recommended)
      4) Regional sympathetic blockade
         a) Class III evidence
         b) May be considered (especially early on) as adjunctive to corticosteroids
      5) Tricyclic antidepressants: amitriptyline, nortriptyline, and doxepin; no adequate data
      6) Anticonvulsants: gabapentin (usually ineffective as sole agent)
      7) Topical analgesics: lidocaine transdermal patches may be helpful for focal CRPS, but not for more diffuse distribution
      8) Other: epidural clonidine, transcutaneous clonidine as a patch over allodynic skin, calcium-channel blockers, oral sympathetic antagonists (e.g., terazosin or prazosin)
      9) General approach to management
         a) Treatment must be initiated as soon as possible
         b) This includes physical therapy, occupational therapy, corticosteroids, and concomitant use of nonsteroidal anti-inflammatory drugs, an anticonvulsant (e.g., gabapentin), or an antidepressant (e.g., nortriptyline)
         c) A regional sympathetic blockade may then be considered for persistent pain

References

Agarwal P, Rosenberg ML. Neurological evaluation of urinary incontinence in the female patient. Neurologist. 2003;9:110-7.

Atkins RM. Complex regional pain syndrome. J Bone Joint Surg Br. 2003;85:1100-6.

Blok BF. Brain control of the lower urinary tract. Scand J Urol Nephrol Suppl. 2002;210:11-5.

Blok BF, Sturms LM, Holstege G. A PET study on cortical and subcortical control of pelvic floor musculature in women. J Comp Neurol. 1997;389:535-44.

Blok BF, Sturms LM, Holstege G. Brain activation during micturation in women. Brain. 1998;121:2033-42.

Drummond PD. Mechanism of complex regional pain syndrome: no longer excessive sympathetic outflow? Lancet. 2001;358:168-70.

Ghai B, Dureja GP. Complex regional pain syndrome: a review. J Postgrad Med. 2004;50:300-7.

Reinders MF, Geertzen JH, Dijkstra PU. Complex regional pain syndrome type I: use of the International Association for the Study of Pain diagnostic criteria defined in 1994. Clin J Pain. 2002;18:207-15.

Rho RH, Brewer RP, Lamer TJ, Wilson PR. Complex regional pain syndrome. Mayo Clin Proc. 2002;77:174-80.

Sandroni P, Vernino S, Klein CM, Lennon VA, Benrud-Larson L, Sletten D, et al. Idiopathic autonomic neuropathy: comparison of cases seropositive and seronegative for ganglionic acetylcholine receptor antibody. Arch Neurol. 2004;61:44-8.

Shin RK, Galetta SL, Ting TY, Armstrong K, Bird SJ. Ross syndrome plus: beyond Horner, Holmes-Adie, and harlequin. Neurology. 2000;55:1841-6.

Tiihonen J, Kuikka J, Kupila J, Partanen K, Vainio P, Airaksinen J, et al. Increase in cerebral blood flow of right prefrontal cortex in man during orgasm. Neurosci Lett. 1994;170:241-3.

Wolfe GI, Galetta SL, Teener JW, Katz JS, Bird SJ. Site of autonomic dysfunction in a patient with Ross' syndrome and postganglionic Horner's syndrome. Neurology. 1995;45:2094-6.

QUESTIONS

1. Which of the following statements is *true* about the role of insular cortex?
   a. Primary gustatory cortex is located in the anterior insula
   b. Insular cortex receives visceral nociceptive input via sympathetic afferents, with a relay in ventromedial thalamus
   c. Insular cortex receives mechanical visceral input via parasympathetic (vagal) afferents via nucleus solitarius and thalamic relay
   d. All of the above

2. Sympathetic preganglionic neurons:
   a. Have cell bodies in the ventral column
   b. Receive the majority of afferent input from neocortex
   c. Release norepinephrine, which acts on postganglionic neurons
   d. Directly innervate the adrenal medulla

3. Which of the following statements is *false* about the circumventricular organs?
   a. Area postrema acts as a chemoemetic center
   b. They lack a blood-brain barrier
   c. They are anatomically close to the ventricular system
   d. They have an important role in control of emotionally charged autonomic response

4. A 26-year-old woman presents 2 years after sustaining a fall with outstretched arms, placing the majority of her weight on the right hand. Soon after the fall, progressive symptoms of burning pain, hyperalgesia, and allodynia developed in the right hand, together with skin discoloration and edema of the painful area. There has been slow progression of these symptoms, and she recently has noticed atrophic skin and nail beds in the right hand. Which of the following management strategies is *not* appropriate?
   a. Avoidance of tight casts
   b. Early mobilization, physical therapy, and occupational therapy
   c. Long-term treatment with corticosteroids
   d. Concomitant use of nonsteroidal antiinflammatory drugs and an anticonvulsant or tricyclic antidepressant
   e. Regional sympathetic blockade for intractable pain
   f. All the above are appropriate management strategies

ANSWERS

1. Answer: d.
All the statements are true about the function of the insula.

2. Answer: d.
The sympathetic preganglionic neurons have cell bodies in the intermediolateral cell column; receive major input from the paraventricular nucleus of the hypothalamus (not neocortex); release acetylcholine, which acts on nicotinic cholinergic receptors of the postganglionic neurons; and directly innervate the adrenal medulla.

3. Answer: d.
The amygdala is responsible for control of emotionally charged autonomic response. The other statements are true about circumventricular organs.

4. Answer: c.
This patient has complex regional pain syndrome. Although corticosteroids are effective early in the course of disease and often indicated for short-term treatment, they should not be considered for long-term use, especially in patients with trophic changes. Early mobilization, physical therapy, occupational therapy, and concomitant use of nonsteroidal antiinflammatory drugs and an anticonvulsant or a tricyclic antidepressant are usually the mainstay first-line treatment. Regional sympathetic blockade is often considered for intractable pain.

Sung C. Ahn, D.O.

Nima Mowzoon, M.D.

I. ANATOMY AND PHYSIOLOGY OF THE NEUROMUSCULAR JUNCTION

A. Anatomy (Fig. 23-1)

1. Motor unit: consists of a motor neuron, its axon and nerve terminals, and muscle fibers the axon innervates
2. Presynaptic nerve terminal: synthesis, storage, and release of acetylcholine (ACh)
   a. Nerve terminal does not have myelin sheath
   b. ACh is synthesized from choline and acetyl coenzyme A by action of choline acetyltransferase (ChAT)
   c. ACh is stored in synaptic vesicles
   d. One synaptic vesicle contains about 6,000 to 10,000 ACh molecules, termed a quantum of ACh
   e. Synaptic vesicles are stored in the immediate or secondary storage areas of nerve terminal

f. P/Q-type calcium channels: located on presynaptic membranes of nerve terminals
3. Synaptic space: space between nerve terminal and postsynaptic muscle membrane, about 50 nm wide
4. Postsynaptic muscle membrane, also called an end plate
   a. Has several clefts and folds, thus increasing surface area
   b. ACh receptors (AChRs): located on postsynaptic folds
   c. Acetylcholinesterase (AChE): attached to collagen fibrils of basement membrane within synaptic cleft; it breaks down ACh to choline and acetate
5. AChR: transmembrane protein of postsynaptic (muscle) membrane
   a. It consists of two α and one β, δ, and ε subunits
   b. AChRs: concentrated at end plate, directly across from nerve terminal
   c. Argin, rapsyn, and muscle-specific tyrosine kinase

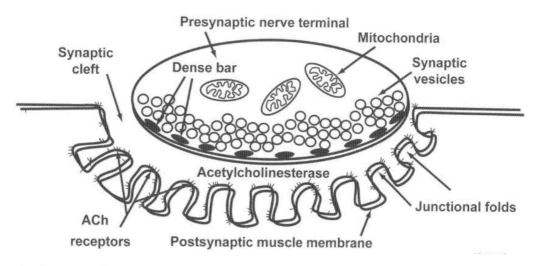

Fig. 23-1. Functional anatomy of the neuromuscular junction. (From Hermann RC Jr. Assessing the neuromuscular junction with repetitive stimulation studies. In: Daube JR, editor. Clinical neurophysiology. 2nd ed. New York: Oxford University Press; 2002. p. 268. By permission of Mayo Foundation.)

(MuSK): proteins important in clustering of AChRs at postsynaptic terminal

   d. Two molecules of ACh needed to bind to each α unit (at a site different from the immunogenic region) to open AChR channel, allowing sodium (Na^+) influx

B. Physiology of Neuromuscular Transmission

1. Release of single quantum occurs during resting state, produces postsynaptic depolarization, and is responsible for miniature end plate potential (MEPP)
2. MEPP amplitude: determined by amount of ACh released by each quantum
3. MEPP duration: determined by amount of time the AChR that receives the quantum is open
4. Action potential
   a. Generated by motor neuron
   b. Travels down axon and depolarizes nerve terminal
5. Depolarization of nerve terminal opens voltage-gated calcium (Ca^+) channel, allowing influx of Ca^+ into presynaptic nerve terminal, which triggers release of multiple quanta of ACh by exocytosis
6. Depolarization of nerve terminal allows docking and fusion of synaptic vesicles
7. Synaptic vesicles fuse with the nerve terminal (presynaptic) membrane, releasing ACh into synaptic space
8. ACh diffuses across synaptic space and binds to AChR (α subunits)
9. Binding of ACh to AChR allows influx of cations ($Na^+ \gg Ca^+$), which depolarizes end plate, generating end plate potentials (EPPs)
10. When EPP reaches threshold voltage for activating voltage-gated sodium channels, muscle fiber action potential is produced
    a. EPP: result of action potential and release of many synaptic vesicles
    b. Number of synaptic vesicles (quanta) released by action potential is called quantal content, which indicates the amount of ACh released
    c. Quantal content: $m = n \times p$ (m = amount of released quanta, n = number of quanta immediately available at nerve terminal, and p = probability of quantal release)
    d. At rest: low p and high $n \rightarrow$ low m value $\rightarrow$ small number of ACh quanta released $\rightarrow$ EPP does not reach threshold to generate muscle action potential (muscle fiber action potential is all-or-none)
    e. Generation of muscle action potential in normal subject: high p and $n \rightarrow$ high $m \rightarrow$ large number of ACh quanta released $\rightarrow$ EPP reaches threshold, generating muscle action potential
    f. Safety margin of neuromuscular transmission: defined by actual EPP amplitude produced by depolarization of nerve terminal and its difference with EPP amplitude required to trigger muscle fiber action potential (threshold)
    g. Safety margin: determined by quantal content (amount of ACh in each quantum), mechanism of quantal release, efficiency of AChE and AChRs
    h. Normal subjects: high safety margin (i.e., much higher EPP than threshold required for neuromuscular transmission)
    i. Repetitive nerve stimulation in normal subject
       1) p is high
       2) n decreases after several stimulations
       3) m gradually decreases
       4) Despite fewer molecules of ACh released, EPP is maintained above threshold to generate muscle action potential: this is due to high safety margin of neuromuscular transmission
    j. Patients with disorders of neuromuscular transmission: lower safety margin
    k. Repetitive stimulation in patient with myasthenia gravis (MG): EPP is not maintained above threshold to generate muscle action potential because of low safety margin
11. ACh is hydrolyzed by AChE
    a. 20% of released ACh hydrolyzed before binding and 80% after dissociation from AChR
    b. ACh is boken down rapidly into choline and acetate
12. Choline: taken up by presynaptic nerve terminal through sodium-dependent active transport mechanism
13. Muscle fiber action potential causes Ca^+ release from sarcoplasmic reticulum, leading to muscle contraction

II. ACQUIRED MYASTHENIA GRAVIS

A. Epidemiology

1. Incidence: 2 to 4/million annually
2. Prevalence: 50 to 400/million
3. Female:male = 3:2
4. Onset (bimodal mean age at onset) in generalized, seropositive MG
   a. Early onset
      1) Second to third decade
      2) Female predominance
      3) Associated with HLA antigens B8 and DR3
   b. Late onset
      1) Sixth to eighth decade
      2) Male predominance
      3) Associated with HLA antigens A3, B7, and DR2

5. Diseases associated with MG: connective tissue disorder, thyroid disease, insulin-dependent diabetes, Lambert-Eaton myasthenic syndrome (LEMS), pernicious anemia, multiple sclerosis, neuromyotonia, cramp-fasciculation syndrome, rippling muscle disease

B. Clinical Presentation
1. Fluctuating, intermittent symptoms sometimes with periods of spontaneous improvement, often appearing with repetitive activity and worsening as day progresses
2. Early onset
   a. Present usually after adolescence (before age 40-50 years)
   b. Female predominance
   c. Majority of patients
      1) Positive for AChR antibodies
      2) Have hyperplastic thymus glands
3. Late onset
   a. Present after age 40-50 years
   b. Slight male predominance
   c. Thymus gland usually not hyperplastic
4. Cranial symptoms
   a. Typically asymmetric, fluctuate over seconds to days
   b. Ocular
      1) More common in elderly men
      2) Evidence of subclinical generalized disease (electrophysiologic or pathologic) often present
      3) Anti-AChR antibodies present in 50% to 60% of patients (in the other patients, antibodies may be present at undetectable levels or there may be other antibodies not tested)
      4) Ocular symptoms: presenting features in about 50% of patients with MG, eventually occur in up to 90% of patients with MG
      5) 15% of patients with ocular symptoms continue to have ocular symptoms without involvement of other muscles (ocular myasthenia)
      6) Little more than 50% of patients with ocular myasthenia have generalized symptoms within the first 6 months (75% within the first year, 6% within 3 years)
      7) Pure ocular myasthenia
         a) Tends to have relatively benign course after 2 years
         b) Is only rarely associated with thymoma
         c) Is not likely to respond to thymectomy
   c. Ptosis
      1) Most common symptom
      2) Often exacerbated by fatigue, exposure to bright lights and heat
      3) Unilateral or bilateral (often asymmetric when bilateral)
      4) May or may not be associated with hyperretraction of normal eyelid; normal eyelid may then droop when examiner lifts the affected eyelid (seesaw effect)
      5) When gaze is directed upward, there may be a transient correction of the ptosis and possibly excessive elevation of the eyelid, termed Cogan's eye twitch
      6) Ptosis may improve after application of ice pack to the ptotic eyelid (ice pack test): sensitive (89%) and specific (100%) sign for diagnosis of MG
   d. Diplopia
      1) Constant or intermittent and fluctuating
      2) Worse when reading, watching television, or driving, especially in bright sunlight
      3) Extraocular muscle weakness best quantified with Lancaster red-green test
   e. Pupillary function: always spared
   f. Facial weakness: myasthenic "snarl" due to weakness of obicularis oris muscle
   g. Dysphagia: pooling in oropharynx, aspiration, nasal regurgitation (due to palatal weakness)
   h. Difficulty chewing: especially worse with prolonged chewing of solids like meat, hard candy (from weakness of muscles of mastication)
   i. Fatigable flaccid dysarthria: nasal speech due to palatal muscle weakness, may become more prominent with prolonged reading, counting, and so forth
   j. Dysphonia (rare)
5. Weakness
   a. Axial muscle weakness: neck flexors often weaker than neck extensors (may present with "dropped head" syndrome)
   b. Proximal upper and lower limbs
   c. Distal upper and lower limbs (less frequently and less severely affected than proximal involvement), more prominent in wrist and finger extensors and ankle dorsiflexors than other distal muscles
6. Respiratory involvement
   a. May be assessed by observing abdominal excursion and use of accessory respiratory muscles
   b. Measured by respiratory function tests (vital capacity and maximal inspiratory and expiratory pressures): accurate measurements rely on good effort and adequate seal of the lips around spirometer tube, which may be lacking for patients with facial weakness
   c. Symptoms of obstructive sleep apnea with bulbar involvement
   d. Initial manifestation may be exclusively respiratory muscle weakness and/or upper airway obstruction
7. Clinical course variable but progressive
8. Normal reflexes and sensory examination
9. Immune-mediated MG may be exacerbated by drugs:

aminoglycoside antibiotics, prednisone, chloroquine, quinidine, procainamide, magnesium, calcium channel blockers, and iodinated intravenous contrast agents

10. New immune-mediated MG may be drug induced (e.g., penicillamine)
11. Thymoma-associated MG: onset at any age after adolescence (peak: fourth-sixth decades)
12. Antibody-negative MG: more common with ocular MG or childhood MG
13. MuSK-antibody–associated MG
    a. More likely to have bulbar than limb weakness
    b. Majority are female (those without MuSK antibodies are more evenly distributed)
    c. Atrophy of bulbar muscles
    d. Poor response to conventional treatments, including corticosteroids and azathioprine

C. Pathophysiology
1. Increased degradation of AChRs and decreased number of functional AChRs
   a. Antibodies bind to extracellular portion of the α_1 subunit of AChR (optimal binding to ϵ subunit in ocular MG)
   b. Cross-linking of bound antibodies facilitates endocytosis
   c. Degradation of internalized AChRs
   d. Complement-mediated destruction of AChRs on postsynaptic membranes
2. Damaged postsynaptic folds
   a. Complement activation and formation of membrane attack complex (MAC) on the membrane
   b. Reduced postsynaptic folds: postsynaptic membranes appear distorted and simplified
3. "Seronegative" MG
   a. Likely also an autoimmune mechanism
   b. Improvement observed with plasma exchange
   c. Antibodies may be present but not yet identified

D. Myasthenia Gravis Foundation of America Classification
1. Class I: ocular MG
2. Class II: mild generalized MG (with or without ocular muscle weakness of any severity)
   a. Class IIa: predominately affecting limb or axial muscles (or both), may have lesser involvement of oropharyngeal muscles
   b. Class IIb: predominately affecting oropharyngeal or respiratory muscles (or both), may have lesser involvement of limb or axial muscles (or both)
3. Class III: moderate generalized MG (with or without

ocular muscle weakness of any severity)
   a. Class IIIa: predominately affecting limb or axial muscles (or both), may have lesser involvement of oropharyngeal muscles
   b. Class IIIb: predominately affecting oropharyngeal or respiratory muscles (or both), may have lesser involvement of limb or axial muscles (or both)
4. Class IV: severe generalized MG (with or without ocular muscle weakness of any severity)
   a. Class IVa: predominately affecting limb or axial muscles (or both), may have lesser involvement of oropharyngeal muscles
   b. Class IVb: predominately affecting oropharyngeal or respiratory muscles (or both), may have lesser involvement of limb or axial muscles (or both), including patients requiring use of a feeding tube without intubation
5. Class V: intubation

E. Acutely Deteriorating Patient
1. Myasthenic crisis: respiratory distress, bulbar symptoms (dysphagia, flaccid dysarthria, poor cough, reduced ability to handle oral secretions and sialorrhea), weakness, diaphoresis, improvement with edrophonium
2. Cholinergic crisis: diarrhea; fasciculations; weakness (including respiratory muscle weakness); miosis; abdominal cramps; nausea and vomiting; excessive secretions causing lacrimation, sialorrhea, and diaphoresis; worsening with edrophonium; tachycardia (immediate use of atropine and withdrawal of cholinesterase inhibitors recommended)

F. Drugs With Adverse Effects in Myasthenia Gravis and Lambert-Eaton Myasthenic Syndrome
1. Aminoglycoside antibodies (block presynaptic calcium channels): streptomycin, neomycin, gentamicin, kanamycin, others
2. Penicillamine, botulinum toxin, and interferon α are *absolutely* contraindicated
3. Neuromuscular-blocking agents such as succinylcholine or tubocurarine, vecuronium
4. Quinidine, procainamide, procaine, magnesium salts, chloroquine, prednisone
5. β-Blockers and calcium channel blockers
6. Drugs with anecdotal reports of exacerbation
   a. Erythromycin, clindamycin, ampicillin, chlorpromazine, quinine, morphine, lithium, gabapentin
   b. Contrast agents: gadolinium diethylenetriamine pentaacetic acid contrast agent used for magnetic resonance imaging (MRI) and iodine-based contrast agents

G. Drug-induced Myasthenia Gravis

1. Immune-mediated disease: associated with increased serum levels of AChR antibodies
2. Slow, insidious onset: weeks to months after initiation of offending drug
3. Penicillamine-induced myasthenia: usually mild, often restricted to ocular muscles
4. Recovery: slow and incomplete
5. Associated with penicillamine, procainamide, quinidine, chloroquine

H. Diagnostic Evaluation

1. Serologic testing
   a. Antibodies present in 80% to 85% of patients with generalized MG and 50% to 60% of those with pure ocular MG
   b. Titers vary among patients
   c. Titers may be elevated in patients with thymoma without MG or in asymptomatic family members
   d. Striational antibodies
      1) Present in 2/3 of patients before age 45 with thymoma (high predictive value for this group)
      2) Heterogeneous group of antibodies against various muscle proteins, including titin, actin, myosin, α-actinin, ryanodine receptor
      3) Titin antibodies associated with late-onset, severe MG and in association with thymoma (found in 90% of patients with MG and thymoma)
      4) Not specific for MG: may also be present in patients with LEMS, lung cancer, autoimmune liver disease, thymoma without myasthenia, drug-induced MG (e.g., penicillamine), and in bone marrow allograft recipients with graft-vs-host disease
   e. Anti-AChR–binding antibodies
      1) Highly sensitive for MG: most sensitive test, often used for screening
      2) Moderate correlation with disease severity: patients with mild or early disease are often seronegative
      3) False-positive results observed with LEMS, autoimmune liver disease, thymoma without myasthenia, and healthy relatives of patients with MG
   f. Anti-AChR–modulating antibodies
      1) Increased degradation of AChR
      2) Highly sensitive and specific for MG
      3) Performed when binding antibodies are negative (higher sensitivity when used in combination) with binding antibodies
   g. Anti-AChR–blocking antibodies
      1) Inhibits ACh and AChR binding
      2) Low sensitivity; test often does not help make diagnosis of MG
      3) When present, often correlates with disease severity
      4) False-positive results observed with LEMS
   h. Anti-MuSK antibodies
      1) Detected in up to 70% of patients with "seronegative" MG
      2) Not detected in patients with anti-AChR antibody-positive MG
      3) MuSK
         a) Receptor tyrosine kinase
         b) Muscle-specific and localized to neuromuscular junction
         c) Important in development of neuromuscular junctions
2. Chest computed tomography (CT): exclude thymoma (all patients)
3. Edrophonium test
   a. Concept
      1) Cholinesterase inhibitor: increases availability of ACh at neuromuscular junction
      2) Relatively low sensitivity (60%) compared with other tests
      3) False-positive results described in amyotrophic lateral sclerosis (ALS), LEMS, and brainstem lesions
      4) Most useful in patients with clinical weakness
      5) Most accurate in presence of ptosis or extraocular muscle weakness (examination of limb muscles is often limited to patient's maximal effort)
      6) Use in ocular MG: edrophonium may improve one of the several affected extraocular muscles, and the rest could become weaker
      7) Positive response does not predict response to other longer-acting cholinesterase inhibitors
   b. Pharmacology
      1) Mechanism: AChE inhibitor
      2) Onset of action: in 30 to 60 seconds
      3) Duration: 2 to 5 minutes
      4) Side effects (cholinergic): nausea, salivation, tearing, sweating, flushing, perioral fasciculations, bradycardia, asystole (rare), hypotension (atropine should be administered immediately)
   c. Procedure
      1) Initial test dose: 1 to 2 mg intravenously (IV); response monitored for 60 seconds
      2) If no response after 60 seconds: administer another 3 mg
      3) If no response after 60 seconds: administer additional 5 mg (for total of 10 mg IV)
      4) If clinical improvement: no further increments necessary
      5) Assessment: clinically, electrophysiologically, or Lancaster red-green test

6) If no clear response, may give 0.8 mg IV

7) Assess again for clinical change

8) Vital signs should be monitored throughout test

d. Disadvantage

    1) Lack of objective measurement of strength (best done for ptosis or extraocular muscle weakness)

    2) Short duration of action

    3) Low sensitivity (about 60%)

    4) False-positive results: may be seen in other conditions (e.g., LEMS, ALS)

4. Routine nerve conduction studies (NCSs)

    a. Motor: usually normal compound muscle action potential (CMAP), conduction velocity, and distal latency, but low CMAP may be found in severe MG

    b. Sensory: normal

5. Repetitive nerve stimulation (RNS) (see Chapter 5)

    a. Concept

        1) MG patients have low safety factor: EPPs fail to reach threshold levels at neuromuscular junction

        2) RNS: depleting the immediately available ACh produces decrement in repetitive trains of CMAPs

        3) RNS at low rates (2-5 Hz)

            a) Decrement of CMAP in weak muscles at baseline

            b) Repair of the decrement immediately after exercise, followed by worsening of the decrement for 2 to 5 minutes after exercise (postexercise exhaustion)

        4) Decrement is greatest between the first and second responses, with a smooth, continuous pattern

        5) Anticholinesterase medicines: if possible, withhold for 12 hours before test

    b. Disadvantage

        1) Abnormal RNS results may be obtained only in weak muscles

        2) May be normal in very mild disease and in ocular MG

        3) Decrement is more likely seen in proximal limb or cranial muscles

        4) RNS is technically challenging: unacceptable false-positive rate with poor technique and poor patient relaxation and discomfort

6. Concentric needle electromyography (EMG)

    a. Usually normal, may observe varying motor unit potentials (MUPs)

    b. Short-duration MUPs can be seen in severe cases

7. Single fiber EMG (SFEMG)

    a. Concept (see Chapter 5)

        1) Records two muscle fibers of same motor neuron

        2) Jitter: abnormal (increased) interpotential variability; indicative of slowed neuromuscular junction transmission (may be observed in seemingly unaffected muscles with normal strength)

        3) Blocking: complete failure of transmission; usually observed in weak muscles (significant blocking is not expected to be observed in seemingly unaffected muscle with normal strength)

        4) May be obtained when RNS and standard needle examinations are normal and MG is suspected clinically (e.g., mild generalized or ocular MG)

        5) Normal SFEMG findings in a clinically weak muscle excludes the diagnosis of MG

    b. Advantage

        1) Detection of mild generalized MG or ocular MG

        2) Most sensitive test (>95%) for detecting MG

    c. Disadvantage

        1) Not specific for MG, abnormal findings are found in certain neuropathic (e.g., ALS) or myopathic disorders with neuromuscular junction instability or other neuromuscular junction disorders

        2) Patient's tolerance and cooperation are required

        3) Time-consuming test

I.   Treatment: needs to be individualized

1. Cholinesterase inhibitors

    a. Adverse dose-dependent effects: nausea, vomiting, muscle cramps, diarrhea, excessive salivation, and lacrimation; cholinergic crisis with overdose

    b. Pyridostigmine bromide (Mestinon)

        1) Oral formulation: 60-mg regular tablets; a syrup containing 12 mg of the medicine per milliliter

        2) IV, intramuscular, or subcutaneous formulations: 2 mg

        3) Onset of action: 10 to 45 minutes

        4) Usual duration of action: 3 to 6 hours

        5) Indication: first line of treatment

        6) Dosage: 30 mg every 6 hours to 90 mg every 3 hours (total daily dose not to exceed 600 mg)

        7) Risk of cholinergic crisis with doses larger than 120 mg every 2 hours

    c. Slow-release pyridostigmine bromide (Mestinon, Timespan)

        1) Oral formulation: 90 to 180-mg slow-release tablets

        2) No IV formulation

        3) Onset of action: 1 hour

        4) Usual duration of action: 6 to 10 hours

        5) Should be limited to nighttime dose for treatment of morning symptoms, because absorption is erratic

    d. Neostigmine methylsulfate (Prostigmin)

        1) Oral formulation: 15-mg tablets

        2) Onset of action: 30 minutes

3) Usual duration of action: 2 to 3 hours (shorter than for pyridostigmine bromide)

4) Dosage (adults): 7.5 to 30 mg every 3 to 4 hours

5) More cholinergic adverse affects than with pyridostigmine bromide

e. Ambenonium chloride (Mytelase)

1) Oral formulation: 10-mg tablets

2) Duration of action: about 6 to 8 hours, greater tendency to accumulate than other cholinesterase inhibitors

2. Prednisone

a. Indication: disabling MG not responding adequately to cholinesterase inhibitors

b. Alternate-day therapy is relatively safe and effective

c. Onset: usually days to weeks, but peak is 4 to 8 weeks after initiation of therapy or change in dose

d. Adverse effect: about 10% of patients become worse initially (occurs in patients taking prednisone for first time); cushingoid features, weight gain, hypertension, myopathy, osteoporosis, aseptic necrosis of femoral head, glaucoma, cataracts, infection, diabetes mellitus, increased skin fragility, acne, sleep disturbance, psychosis, pseudotumor cerebri, adrenal suppression, peptic ulcer disease

e. Low-dose prednisone used for mild generalized MG or disabling ocular MG not responsive to cholinesterase inhibitors

1) Starting dose: generally 30 mg every other day (for 2 months)

2) Slow taper to lowest effective dose

f. High-dose prednisone used for moderate to severe generalized MG

1) Starting dose: generally 60 to 80 mg daily (usually for 1 to 2 months)

2) Slow taper over several months

g. Monitor patients carefully for exacerbation of MG while tapering prednisone

h. Blood tests (complete blood count and metabolic panel) and chest radiograph must be obtained at baseline and periodically thereafter

i. Preventive measures for complications of high-dose prednisone should be considered

1) Routine screening for osteoporosis, cataracts, glaucoma, hypertension, diabetes mellitus, hypokalemia

2) Avoidance of extra dietary salt

3) Antacids for all patients: treatment of concurrent peptic ulcer disease

4) Supplemental calcium and vitamin D

5) Prophylactic antituberculosis antibiotics for tuberculin-positive patients

6) *Pneumocystis jiroveci* (formerly *carinii*) pneumonia

prophylaxis with trimethoprim-sulfamethoxazole (Bactrim)

3. Azathioprine (Imuran)

a. Mechanism of action: decreased purine synthesis; interferes with DNA and RNA synthesis; inhibits proliferation of lymphocytes and, thus, interferes with antibody and cytokine production

b. Metabolism

1) Metabolized by oxidation or methylation in erythrocytes and liver; excreted by kidney

2) Metabolite: 6-mercaptopurine (6MP) (nonenzymatic break down), which is purine analogue acting to disrupt de novo purine synthesis

3) 6MP: eventually converted into active metabolites, 6-thioguanine nucleotides (TGNs)

4) TGNs: eventually incorporated into DNA, interfering with DNA synthesis

5) Through a different metabolic pathway, 6MP is metabolized to mercaptopurines by thiopurine methyltransferase (TPMT)

a) TPMT levels: may be used to predict and monitor efficacy and toxicity

b) Variability in TPMT levels (and metabolism of the drug): due to genetic polymorphism of TPMT; homozygous defect may lead to fatal bone marrow toxicity

6) Main pathway for detoxification of azathioprine: conversion to inactive 6-thiouric acid by xanthine oxidase (inhibited by concurrent use of allopurinol, in which case azathioprine dose has to be reduced)

c. Dose: initial dose 2.5 to 3 mg/kg; maintain dose at 1.5 to 2.5 mg/kg daily

d. Dose may be adjusted to achieve mild leukopenia and macrocytosis

e. Onset of action: slow (over 4-12 months), may be delayed further if initial dose is subtherapeutic

f. Indicated for patients with poor response to corticosteroids or limited by corticosteroid-induced side effects

g. Considered first line for patients with moderate to severe MG at high risk for corticosteroid-induced side effects (e.g., postmenopausal women and diabetics)

h. Advantage: steroid-sparing

i. Disadvantage: slow onset, expensive

j. Adverse effects: elevation in liver enzymes (reversible), dose-dependent, reversible bone marrow suppression (leukopenia, pure red cell aplasia), macrocytosis, pancreatitis, infection, possible risk of later development of malignancy (debated), infertility, teratogenic

k. Dosage should be reduced for leukocyte count $<4\times10^9$/L; held for leukocyte count $<3\times10^9$/L

4. Cyclophosphamide (Cytoxan)
   a. Interferes with DNA synthesis: alkylates and crosslinks DNA
   b. Often prescribed for disease refractory to prednisone and/or azathioprine
   c. Usual dosage: 1.0 to 1.5 mg/kg daily
   d. Adverse effects: severe bone marrow depression and cytopenias, increased risk of infection and malignancy, hemorrhagic cystitis, increased risk of bladder neoplasm, cardiomyopathy, congestive heart failure, hair loss, sterility (azoospermia, anovulation)
5. Cyclosporine
   a. Interferes with lymphocytic proliferation by reducing expression of cytokine genes required for T cell activation and proliferation
   b. Limited use because of toxicity
6. Mycophenolate mofetil (CellCept)
   a. Mechanism of action
      1) Inhibitor of de novo pathway of purine nucleotide synthesis, impairing proliferation of B and T lymphocytes
      2) Induces apoptosis of activated T cells
      3) Reduces lymphocyte attachment and mobilization by reducing synthesis of E and P selectins by endothelial cells and inhibiting interaction of lymphocytic ligands with endothelial selectin receptors (thus interfering with adhesion of lymphocytes) and by reducing glycosylation of intracellular adhesion molecules
   b. Dosage: 1 to 1.5 g every 12 hours
   c. Improvement is expected to begin 2 weeks to 2 months after initiation of treatment, but peak effect may be delayed up to 9 to 12 months
   d. Advantage: steroid-sparing, potency similar to azathioprine and cyclosporine but with lower toxicity
   e. Disadvantage: expensive
   f. Adverse effects: gastrointestinal discomfort with or without diarrhea, dose-dependent leukopenia (need to monitor blood counts, as with azathioprine)
7. Plasmapheresis
   a. Effective in all patients
   b. Proposed mechanism of action: transient removal of causative antibodies and immune mediators responsible for destruction of AChRs
   c. Three to five treatments often required for satisfactory response in setting of exacerbation
      1) Daily treatment tolerated by young patients with no other comorbidities
      2) Alternate-day treatments preferred for older patients and young patients with other comorbidities or unstable disease course

   d. May be used in myasthenic crisis and to optimize muscle function before a surgical procedure, including thymectomy
   e. Rarely used as long-term therapy (as adjunct to long-term immunosuppressive therapy)
   f. When treatment is stopped: antibody titers increase, symptoms recur, use of immunosuppressant is often needed
   g. Disadvantages: complicated (often requires placement of central venous catheter), costly, limited availability
   h. Risks and adverse effects: risks of central venous catheter (infection, pneumothorax, thrombosis), hypotension, and hypocalcemia and citrate toxicity (due to use of citrate salts)
8. Intravenous immunoglobulin (IVIg)
   a. Mechanism: unclear
   b. Used in myasthenic crisis, may be used as adjunct to long-term immunosuppressive therapy (as with plasmapheresis)
   c. Dosage: 400 mg/kg daily, usually for 5 consecutive days
   d. Advantage: easier to administer than plasmapheresis
   e. Disadvantage: costly
   f. Adverse effects
      1) Low-grade fevers, headaches, with or without aseptic meningitis
      2) Serum hyperviscosity and hyperosmolarity, sometimes inducing renal insufficiency, deep venous thrombosis, cerebral infarctions
      3) Anaphylactic reactions, especially in patients with selective IgA deficiency, agammaglobulinemia, or severe hypogammaglobulinemia
9. Thymectomy
   a. Retrospective data suggest eventual improvement in natural history of MG in up to 80% and complete remission in up to 40% of patients; improvement is often gradual (within 5-15 years)
   b. May be transient symptomatic improvement immediately postoperatively, lasting up to 2 to 3 weeks
   c. Recommended for most patients younger than 60 years
   d. Not recommended for patients older than 60 years: usually higher surgical morbidity and patients may not have adequate time to realize benefit
   e. Usually not recommended for pure ocular MG (although may prevent generalization of disease in ocular myasthenia and is sometimes recommended for young patients with relatively recent onset of symptoms)
   f. Thymoma is an absolute indication (done to cure or debulk the tumor)
   g. Thymectomy does not benefit myasthenic symptoms in patients with thymoma

h. Most effective in females with shorter duration of disease, hyperplastic glands, and high antibody titers (results equalize after 10 years, continue to be effective despite presence or absence of these factors)
i. More effective in patients who have thymectomy within 2 years after onset of symptoms
j. Preferred approach: transsternal thymectomy (ectopic thymic tissue can be missed with the transcervical approach), but data directly comparing the two surgical techniques are lacking
10. Other adjunctive measures
   a. Vaccination against influenza
   b. Immunization against pneumococcus before prednisone or other immunosuppressants are given
   c. Avoidance of drugs that can exacerbate MG: aminoglycosides, erythromycin or related antibiotics, quinine-related drugs
11. Treatment strategies
   a. Transient neonatal MG
      1) Transient disorder of infants born to mothers with MG: general weakness (floppy infants), difficulty feeding, respiratory insufficiency when severe
      2) Syndrome resolves after several weeks
      3) Anticholinesterase agents (parenteral if poor feeding)
      4) Plasma exchange or IVIg considered for severely affected infants
      5) Risk of development of neonatal MG is independent of clinical status or antibody levels of the mother
   b. MG during pregnancy
      1) MG may become worse during pregnancy or post partum
      2) Pyridostigmine and corticosteroids are relatively safe, but azathioprine and cyclosporine need to be avoided because of teratogenic effects and need to be discontinued several months before pregnancy is contemplated
      3) Dose of cholinesterase inhibitors needs to be adjusted because of altered intestinal absorption and renal excretion
      4) Changes in maternal blood volume and renal clearance affect pharmacokinetics of first-line agents
      5) One-third of infants born to mothers with MG have transient neonatal myasthenia
   c. Juvenile MG
      1) Similar approach to that for adults, with special considerations
      2) Higher rates of spontaneous remission with prepubertal onset: thymectomy is often delayed
      3) Corticosteroids inhibit growth of long bones and predispose to early osteoporosis and are best avoided

d. Ocular MG
   1) Ptosis crutches for ptosis
   2) Alternating eye patch for diplopia
   3) Treatment with cholinesterase inhibitors attempted first
   4) Treatment with alternate-day prednisone (10-30 mg every other day) may be given for disabling diplopia or ptosis not responsive to cholinesterase inhibitors (can prevent generalization because majority of patients with ocular MG eventually develop generalized disease)
e. Mild generalized MG
   1) All patients receive pyridostigmine
   2) Alternate-day prednisone is added for those without adequate response to cholinesterase inhibitors
   3) Azathioprine is often added for patients without adequate response to pyridostigmine and low doses of alternate-day prednisone
   4) Onset before age 60: thymectomy (preoperative treatment with plasmapheresis and/or high-dose prednisone to minimize risks of surgery)
f. Moderate to severe MG
   1) Alternate-day prednisone with pyridostigmine
   2) Azathioprine, myocophenolate mofetil, or cyclosporine
   3) Onset before age 60: thymectomy, as above
   4) Onset after age 60: treatment with cholinesterase inhibitors and prednisone (temporary), and immunosuppressive (steroid-sparing) agent such as azathioprine always initiated with intention to taper and discontinue prednisone
g. MG crisis or fulminant MG
   1) Usually treated initially with IVIg or plasmapheresis
   2) High-dose IV corticosteroids (methylprednisolone), followed by oral prednisone
   3) Prednisone eventually tapered off to alternate-day regimen
   4) Immunosuppressive agents may be needed as steroid-sparing agents if prednisone cannot be discontinued because of recurrence of symptoms while dose is tapered

III. LAMBERT-EATON MYASTHENIC SYNDROME

A. Epidemiology
1. Incidence: 4/1 million
2. Male > female
3. Middle age or older patients

4. About 50% of cases of LEMS are associated with malignancy (majority, small cell lung cancer [SCLC]): neoplastic-related LEMS uncommon in patients younger than 40 years
5. About 3% of cases of SCLC are associated with LEMS

B. Symptoms and Signs

1. Insidious onset
2. Fluctuating proximal muscle weakness (lower limbs > upper limbs), e.g., difficulty rising from a low chair, climbing stairs
3. Weakness elicited on examination is often less impressive than severity of symptoms reported by patient
4. Improvement in strength with repeated examinations and exercise (in contrast to MG)
5. Reflexes: markedly reduced or absent initially, but increase after a brief exercise (in contrast to MG)
6. Ocular and pharyngeal muscle weakness possible; if present, much less severe than MG
7. Sensory: may be involved, e.g., distal paresthesias
8. Metallic taste
9. Dysautonomia: dry mouth, dry eyes, impotence, constipation, blurred vision, postural hypotension
10. Lambert's sign: patient grasping the examiner's hand with maximal force has a weak grip that improves over several seconds with continued exertion

C. Pathophysiology

1. Antibodies to prejunctional P/Q-type voltage-gated calcium channel at presynaptic motor nerve terminal
2. Reduced calcium influx into presynaptic nerve terminal and reduced quantal release
3. Reduced ACh release; hence, decreased number of ACh molecules binding to AChRs
4. Reduced EPPs and activation of muscle fiber action potentials, producing clinically weak muscle contraction

D. Diagnostic Tools

1. Minimal response to edrophonium chloride (in contrast to MG)
2. Serum
   a. Antibodies to P/Q-type voltage-gated calcium channel
   b. More than 90% of patients are positive
3. Search for an underlying malignancy: CT of chest, bronchoscopy (with or without biopsy), positron emission tomography (PET) considered for chronic smokers
4. If no tumor found, a search for occult malignancy should be repeated periodically
5. NCSs

a. Motor: low CMAP amplitude, but normal conduction velocities and distal latencies
b. Sensory: normal
6. RNS
   a. LEMS has low safety factor
   b. Low-amplitude resting CMAP because of decreased release of ACh
   c. Decrement with repetitive stimulation at 2 Hz because of depletion of immediately available ACh
   d. Marked increment (more than 100%) and facilitation (more than 200%) noted immediately after rapid rates of stimulation or brief (10 seconds) exercise
      1) Due to increased calcium concentrations in presynaptic nerve terminal, allowing more ACh release, which leads to increased EPPs, increased muscle fiber activation, and improved strength on clinical examination
      2) Facilitation is noted immediately after exercise
      3) CMAP amplitudes return to baseline about 60 to 120 seconds after exercise
      4) Decrement returns about 3 to 4 minutes after exercise
7. Needle EMG: usually normal insertional activity, but motor unit potentials may be varying and/or of short duration and amplitude ("myopathic")
8. SFEMG: highly sensitive in disorders of neuromuscular transmission (not specific); abnormal jitter and blocking, less prominent when high-frequency stimulation is used

E. Treatment

1. Treatment of underlying malignancy, if present
2. Pyridostigmine bromide
3. Neostigmine methylsulfate
4. 3,4-Diaminopyridine (DAP)
   a. Mechanism of action (in sequence)
      1) Blocks voltage-gated potassium channels responsible for repolarization of action potentials, increases action potential duration and opening of P/Q-type voltage-gated calcium channels
      2) Increased duration of voltage-gated calcium channels
      3) Increased calcium influx into presynaptic nerve terminal
      4) Increased release of acetylcholine
      5) Result: improved strength
   b. Improvement seen in about 80% of patients
   c. Effective for both autonomic and neuromuscular manifestations
   d. Dose
      1) Initial: 5 to 25 mg three or four times daily
      2) Titration: gradual, by 5 mg per day

e. Effect of DAP is enhanced by concomitant use of pyridostigmine
f. Adverse effects
   1) Perioral or digital paresthesias (transient, usually with high doses)
   2) Other potential side effects (especially when given with pyridostigmine): cramps, diarrhea, nausea, and vomiting
5. Immunosuppressants considered when DAP or cholinesterase inhibitors are not effective in face of disabling symptoms, including prednisone or azathioprine
6. Plasmapheresis and IVIg: short-term improvement, less effective than with MG

IV. CONGENITAL MYASTHENIC SYNDROMES

A. General Characteristics
1. Onset: often in infancy or childhood, but may occur in adolescence or adulthood with mild phenotype, most commonly with slow-channel syndrome and familial limb-girdle myasthenia
2. Family history of similarly affected family members: autosomal dominant inheritance in slow-channel syndrome, autosomal recessive inheritance in remaining congenital myasthenic syndromes
3. Decremental response on repetitive stimulation (see below)
4. Repetitive CMAPs: AChE deficiency and slow-channel syndrome
5. Increasing weakness on sustained exertion
6. Selectively severe involvement of truncal muscles: end plate AChE deficiency
7. Selectively severe involvement of finger and wrist extensors and cervical axial muscles: end plate AChE deficiency and slow-channel syndrome
8. Mild ocular involvement: end plate AChE deficiency and slow-channel syndrome
9. Apnea episodes: ChAT deficiency (also called "congenital myasthenic syndrome with episodic apnea")
10. Negative AChR antibodies in all cases
11. Tensilon test
   a. Often positive, although a negative test does not exclude the diagnosis of a congenital myasthenic syndrome
   b. May be negative in asymptomatic patients during the time between episodes of exacerbation
   c. Always negative in patients with end plate AChE deficiency
   d. Inconsistent results in patients with slow-channel syndrome

B. Presynaptic Congenital Myasthenic Syndromes
1. End-plate ChAT deficiency
   a. Autosomal recessive; due to mutation of gene on chromosome 10q11.2 encoding ChAT protein
   b. Clinical course
     1) Marked by episodic, rapid exacerbations of bulbar and respiratory weakness
     2) Episodes of sudden, unexpected apnea, spontaneous or precipitated by concurrent infection, excitement, or exertion
   c. Recovery after each episode may be partial or complete
   d. Gradual improvement with age: reduced frequency of attacks
   e. Patients may be symptomatic at birth or in neonatal period, with poor feeding, hypotonia, bulbar and respiratory weakness (gradually improves but may be followed by attacks of apnea and bulbar weakness later in life)
   f. Patients may be normal at birth and in neonatal period, but develop ptosis, fatigable weakness, and apneic episodes during infancy or childhood; children may complain of fatigability with exertion
   g. Rare: sudden death
   h. Electrophysiologic testing
     1) Decremental response with 2-Hz repetitive stimulation; SFEMG abnormalities noted in weak muscles
     2) Decrement often not present in muscles with normal strength, especially between attacks
   i. Treatment: prophylaxis with anticholinesterase medications for patients with symptomatic weakness or frequent apneic episodes
   j. Patients with febrile illness should be hospitalized for close observation
2. Congenital myasthenic syndrome resembling LEMS
3. Congenital paucity of synaptic vesicles and reduced quantal release

C. Synaptic Congenital Myasthenic Syndrome
1. Congenital end-plate AChE deficiency
   a. Autosomal recessive inheritance
   b. Pathophysiology and microscopic morphologic features
     1) Absence of AChE
     2) Small presynaptic nerve terminals
     3) Extension of the Schwann cell processes to synaptic cleft and encasement of small nerve terminals
     4) Reduced quantal release from abnormal nerve terminals
     5) Despite restricted ACh release, there is cholinergic overloading of the synapse and prolonged exposure and desensitization of AChRs at physiologic states
     6) Cholinergic overloading is responsible for depolariza-

tion block at physiologic rates of stimulation

7) Degradation of junctional folds, with reduced number of AChRs

8) End-plate myopathy: type II muscle fiber atrophy and type I muscle fiber preponderance

c. Often presents in neonatal period with weakness

d. Lifelong history of weakness: delayed motor milestones, diffuse weakness (including facial, extraocular, proximal limb, respiratory)

e. Sluggish pupillary response

f. Slow progression

g. Spine deformities often develop

h. Electrodiagnostic evaluation: repetitive CMAP response

1) Subsides quickly with repetitive stimulation (faster than initial CMAP) in a patient not exposed to AChE inhibitors

2) Similar to slow-channel syndrome

3) Repetitive CMAP response may be absent in infancy

i. Tensilon test is always negative, may worsen clinical weakness

j. Need to avoid AChE inhibitors

D. Postsynaptic Congenital Myasthenic Syndromes

1. Slow-channel syndromes: increased response to ACh

a. Most often autosomal dominant inheritance (gain-of-function mutations)

1) Mutation of gene on chromosome 2q24-q32 encoding AChR α subunit: autosomal dominant inheritance

2) Mutation of gene on chromosome 17p13.1 encoding AChR β subunit: autosomal dominant inheritance

3) Mutation of gene on chromosome 2q33-q34 encoding AChR δ subunit: autosomal dominant inheritance

4) Mutation of gene on chromosome 17p13-p12 encoding AChR ε subunit: autosomal dominant or recessive inheritance

b. Variable clinical presentation

1) May present in early life and cause severe disability by end of first decade

2) May present later in life with little progression and disability (as late as sixth decade)

c. Selective, severe involvement of cervical axial musculature and digit and wrist extensors

d. Cranial musculature tends to be relatively spared

e. May be atrophy of severely affected muscles

f. Tensilon test: variable results

g. Electrodiagnostic evaluation

1) Decremental response with repetitive stimulation

2) Repetitive CMAP response, which subsides with

repetitive stimulation (Fig. 23-2)

h. Pathophysiology

1) Mutations often involve proteins near extracellular ACh binding sites

2) Mutations cause increased affinity of AChRs for ACh (causing channel reopening) or act to prolong open

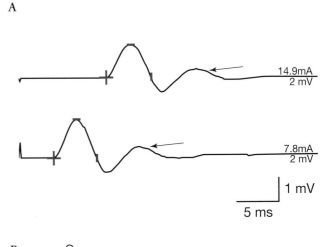

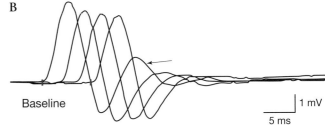

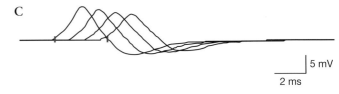

Fig. 23-2. Nerve conduction studies in a patient with slow-channel syndrome. *A,* Motor response obtained by stimulation of the peroneal nerve, with recording at the extensor digitorum brevis muscle, shows a repetitive discharge (*arrows*) immediately after the compound muscle action potential. *B,* Baseline repetitive stimulation at 2 per second shows a decremental response of both the compound muscle action potential and the repetitive discharge (*arrow*) (more rapid in the latter). *C,* The repetitive discharge disappears after rapid rates of repetitive stimulation (10 per second). (Courtesy of Brian A. Crum, MD.)

state (mutant AChR can stay open even in absence of ACh)

   3) End result: continuous cation leak into postsynaptic area is responsible for prolonged decay phase of MEPPs and EPPs

   4) Focal calcium excess may produce local excitotoxic damage and degeneration of junctional folds and reduced number of AChRs: responsible for small-amplitude MEPPs

  i. Pathology

   1) End-plate myopathy with type I fiber predominance, vacuoles in end plates, increased variation in muscle fiber size

   2) Degeneration of junctional folds

  j. Treatment

   1) Anticholinesterase inhibitors: little or no benefit

   2) Quinidine sulfate

   3) Fluoxetine: effective at relatively high doses (80 mg/day in adults)

2. Fast-channel syndromes: reduced response to ACh

  a. Autosomal recessive inheritance (loss-of-function mutations)

   1) Mutation of gene on chromosome 2q24-q32 encoding AChR α subunit

   2) Mutation of gene on chromosome 2q33-q34 encoding AChR δ subunit

   3) Mutation of gene on chromosome 17p13-p12 encoding AChR ε subunit

  b. Pathophysiology related to mutations of AChR

   1) May be decreased rates of channel opening and increased rates of channel closing

   2) Reduced gate efficiency (mild phenotype)

   3) Unstable channel kinetics (moderate phenotype)

   4) Reduced affinity of receptors for ACh (severe phenotype)

  c. Onset at birth

  d. Extraocular movement paralysis and ptosis, dysarthria, dysphagia, difficulty chewing, generalized limb weakness and fatigability, respiratory distress

  e. Definite diagnosis requires patch-clamp studies and in vitro microelectrode studies of neuromuscular junction

  f. Treatment

   1) Pyridostigmine

   2) 3,4-DAP (synergistic effect with pyridostigmine)

V. BOTULISM

A. Epidemiology

1. Caused by toxin produced by anaerobic pathogen

Clostridium botulinum

2. Pathogen produces spores (heat-resistant up to 120°C) and toxin (heat-sensitive)

3. At least eight immunologically distinct types of botulinum toxin (BTX): A, B, C1, C2, D, E, F, and G

4. BTX A: most commonly involved

5. Several clinical forms of botulism; most common are the following:

  a. Food-borne (classic) botulism

  b. Infant botulism

  c. Wound botulism (most common form of botulism in United States, usually occurs in injection drug users)

B. Pathophysiology

1. Inhibits ACh release (presynaptic blockade) from neuromuscular junction and parasympathetic and sympathetic ganglia, resulting in autonomic dysfunction and muscle weakness

2. Transfer of botulinum into cytosol: BTX binds to receptors on unmyelinated presynaptic membrane, is transferred via endocytosis into endosomes in nerve terminals, and transported to cytosol

3. In normal condition, collaboration of synaptosomal-associated protein (SNAP)-25, synaptobrevin, and syntaxin is necessary for neuroexocytosis (ACh release from presynaptic nerve terminal)

4. In botulism, BTX enters presynaptic nerve terminal and cleaves protein components of neuroexocytosis apparatus

  a. Botulinum A and E cleave SNAP-25

  b. Botulinum B, D, F, and G cleave synaptobrevin (vesicle-associated membrane protein)

  c. Botulinum C cleaves SNAP-25 and syntaxin

5. This results in impaired docking and fusion of synaptic vesicles with terminal membrane

6. This leads to impaired neuroexocytosis and fewer quanta of ACh released (*number of released quanta* is below threshold, but *size of each quantum* of ACh is normal)

C. Classic (adult) Botulism

1. Due to ingestion of preformed toxin in contaminated food

2. Initial symptoms of food-borne botulism often include nausea and vomiting, followed by neuromuscular symptoms, often after 12 to 38 hours

3. Some patients who ingest contaminated food do not become symptomatic

4. Descending weakness: involvement progressing from cranial to upper limbs to lower limbs

5. Cranial involvement: dysphagia, ptosis, diplopia,

blurred vision, dysarthria
6. Respiratory muscle weakness
7. Reduced deep tendon reflexes
8. Limb weakness: proximal more than distal
9. Normal sensory function
10. Pupillary paralysis: dilated pupils in many patients
11. Autonomic disturbance: dry mouth, urinary retention
12. Gastrointestinal autonomic involvement
    a. Nausea, vomiting
    b. Abdominal cramping
    c. Diarrhea, constipation
    d. Ileus

D. Infantile Botulism

1. Due to ingestion of pathogenic spores, with subsequent germination of spores and growth of pathogen in gastrointestinal tract and slow and steady production of small quantities of toxin
2. Sometimes due to ingestion of honey (tends to harbor type B organisms)
3. Constipation is first sign: may predispose to production of toxins
4. Listless, lethargic floppy infants (hypotonia), with reduced spontaneous movements
5. Poor sucking, drooling, and weak cry
6. Poorly reactive pupils
7. Respiratory distress

E. Diagnostic Methods

1. Tensilon test: positive in one-third of patients
2. NCSs
    a. Normal to mildly reduced CMAP with normal conduction velocity and distal latency
    b. Sensory NCS: normal
3. RNS
    a. Botulinum has low safety factor
    b. Decrement responses at rest may be seen due to reduced number of ACh quanta released because of impaired neuroexocytosis
    c. Facilitation occurs after exercise because of mobilization of stored ACh due to accumulation of calcium
    d. Facilitation is less impressive than in LEMS
4. Needle EMG
    a. Short duration, small-amplitude, varying motor unit potentials
    b. Possibly fibrillation potentials

F. Treatment

1. Mainstay: medical supportive care (including mechanical ventilation if required)
2. Botulism immune globulin
3. Antitoxin if patient presents early (must be given as early as possible, while toxin is still in bloodstream)
4. Surgical treatment of wound in wound botulism
5. Guanidine has been attempted (mixed results)

REFERENCES

Clunie GP, Lennard L. Relevance of thiopurine methyltransferase status in rheumatology patients receiving azathioprine. Rheumatology (Oxford). 2004 Jan;43:13-8. Epub 2003 Oct 17.

Drachman DB. Myasthenia gravis. N Engl J Med. 1994;330:1797-810.

Engel AG, Ohno K, Shen XM, Sine SM. Congenital myasthenic syndromes: multiple molecular targets at the neuromuscular junction. Ann N Y Acad Sci. 2003;998:138-60.

Husain AM, Massey JM, Howard JF, Sanders DB. Acetylcholine receptor antibody measurements in acquired myasthenia gravis: diagnostic sensitivity and predictive value for thymoma. Ann N Y Acad Sci. 1998;841:471-4.

Rowland LP. Prostigmine-responsiveness and the diagnosis of myasthenia gravis. Neurology. 1955;5:612-23.

Vincent A, Bowen J, Newsom-Davis J, McConville J. Seronegative generalised myasthenia gravis: clinical feaues, antibodies, and their targets. Lancet Neurol. 2003;2:99-106.

Zhou L, McConville J, Chaudhry V, Adams RN, Skolasky RL, Vincent A, et al. Clinical comparison of muscle-specific tyrosine kinase (MuSK) antibody-positive and -negative myasthenic patients. Muscle Nerve. 2004;30:55-60.

QUESTIONS

1. Which of the following is *true* about myasthenia gravis (MG) in pregnancy?
   a. Pregnant mothers with MG usually do not experience exacerbation of MG during pregnancy or the postpartum period
   b. Use of prednisone is contraindicated in pregnancy
   c. Uterine contractions during delivery are affected by the underlying disorder of neuromuscular transmission
   d. Changes in maternal blood volume and renal clearance affect the pharmacokinetic properties of some treatments used for MG

2. A 3-month-old infant is brought to the emergency department by her grandmother because of poor feeding and increasing lethargy. Physical examination shows a listless, hypotonic "floppy" baby with poorly reactive pupils, a weak cry, and drooling. The grandmother states that she has not hit or shaken the baby but says she mixed honey with the infant formula

some time before the presentation. What is the most likely diagnosis?
   a. Subdural hematoma due to shaken baby syndrome
   b. Central core myopathy
   c. Infantile botulism
   d. Tick paralysis

3. A 35-year-old woman presents with a 10-year history of asymmetric ptosis and fatigable limb weakness. Physical examination also reveals digit and wrist extensor weakness. The tensilon test was reportedly positive. Nerve conduction studies showed a repetitive compound muscle action potential, which displayed a quick decrement with repetitive stimulation. This patient most likley has:
   a. Slow-channel syndrome
   b. Fast-channel syndrome
   c. Autoimmune myasthenia gravis
   d. Congenital end-plate acetylcholinesterase deficiency

ANSWERS

1. Answer: d.
Changes in maternal blood volume and renal clearance affect the pharmacokinetic properties of first-line treatments, including pyridostigmine. Patients often experience an exacerbation of MG during pregnancy or the postpartum period. Prednisone and cholinesterase inhibitors are relatively safe in pregnancy. Uterine smooth muscle is not affected by MG.

2. Answer: c.
The presentation is that of infantile botulism, likely due to ingestion of the honey in the infant formula containing pathogenic spores.

3. Answer: a.
The repetitive compound muscle action potential response is seen in slow-channel syndrome and congenital end-plate acetylcholinesterase deficiency. The latter usually presents in the neonatal period with weakness, although it rarely may present as mild disease in childhood and become disabling in the second decade or later. The tensilon test in a patient with slow-channel syndrome produces variable results (sometimes "positive") and never results in improvement in patients with acetylcholinesterase deficiency (instead, it may worsen the clinical weakness). The most likely dignosis is slow-channel syndrome.

DISORDERS OF MUSCLE

Nima Mowzoon, M.D.

I. BASIC MUSCLE ANATOMY AND PHYSIOLOGY

A. Properties of Muscle Fibers

1. Physiologic and histochemical properties of muscle fibers are determined by the anterior horn cells innervating them
2. All muscle fibers innervated by the same anterior horn cell have similar properties
3. Denervation and degeneration of anterior horn cells prompts reinnervation of muscle fibers, which then assume the properties of the new reinnervating anterior horn cell
4. Muscle biopsy in neuropathic conditions (Fig. 24-1)
   a. Denervation atrophy with small angulated fibers and groups of atrophied fibers
   b. Denervation without reinnervation: pyknotic nuclear clumps

c. With reinnervation: grouping of muscle fibers and loss of normal "checkerboard pattern" of muscle fibers (fiber-type grouping)
   d. Grouped atrophy with little type grouping in amyotrophic lateral sclerosis (ALS)
   e. Target fibers also appear with active denervation and reinnervation (e.g., ALS): mitochondrial stains show central clear regions
5. Type I fibers (red)
   a. "Slow twitch" muscle fibers: long contraction time
   b. High oxygen consumption: dependent on aerobic metabolism
   c. More mitochondria, abundance of oxidative enzymes: lactic dehydrogenase, succinic dehydrogenase, cytochrome oxidase (stain light with adenosine triphosphatase [ATPase] stain pH 9.4, and stain dark with pH 4.3-4.6)
   d. Rich in myoglobin

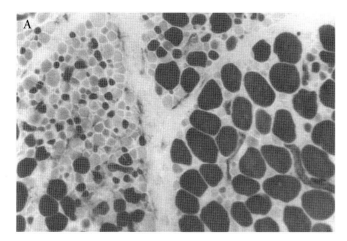
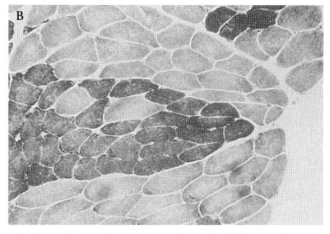

Fig. 24-1. Muscle biopsy specimens showing neuropathic conditions. *A*, Acute denervation causes small angulated fibers and groups of atrophied fibers. Note early fiber type grouping with reinnervation (*right*) and increased endomysial connective tissue. *B*, With reinnervation, there is fiber type grouping. (*A* and *B*, ATPase stain, pH 9.4, with lightly stained type I fibers and darkly stained type II fibers.) (*A*, Courtesy of Suresh Kotagal, MD. *B* from Lidov H, De Girolami U, Gherardi R. Skeletal muscle diseases. In: Gray F, De Girolami U, Poirier J, editors. Escourolle & Poirier manual of basic neurophysiology. 4th ed. Philadelphia: Butterworth-Heinemann; 2004. p. 281-314. Used with permission.)

e. Less predisposition to muscle fatigue with repeated activation

f. Respective motor neurons are small alpha motor neurons with low firing frequency

6. Type II fibers (white)
a. "Fast twitch" muscle fibers: short contraction time
b. Low oxygen consumption: dependent on anaerobic metabolism
c. Relative paucity of oxidative enzymes
d. Fewer mitochondria, abundance of glycolytic enzymes (stain dark with ATPase stain, pH 9.4, and stain light with pH 4.3-4.6)
e. Poor in myoglobin
f. Greater predispostion to muscle fatigue with repeated activation
g. Respective motor neurons are large alpha motor neurons with high firing frequency

B. **Structure of Muscle Fiber** (Fig. 24-2)
1. T tubules
a. Transverse hollow tubular structures formed by invagina-

tions of sarcolemma (plasma membrane of striated muscle)
b. Lies between two tubular portions of sarcoplasmic reticulum (forming a triad of membrane structures)
c. Depolarization of T-tubule membrane triggers release of calcium from sarcoplasmic reticulum, leading to muscle contraction

2. Myofibrils
a. Contractile elements with banded appearance
b. Composed of thick and thin filaments, constituents of the sarcomere

3. Organelles: mitochondria, sarcoplasmic reticulum, nuclei, others

C. **Structure of a Sarcomere** (Fig. 24-3)
1. Thick filaments
a. Myosin polymer admixed with nonmyosin molecules, myosin-binding proteins, which function to maintain structural integrity of thick filaments and regulate their contractile function
b. Contains a central "stem" and two globular heads

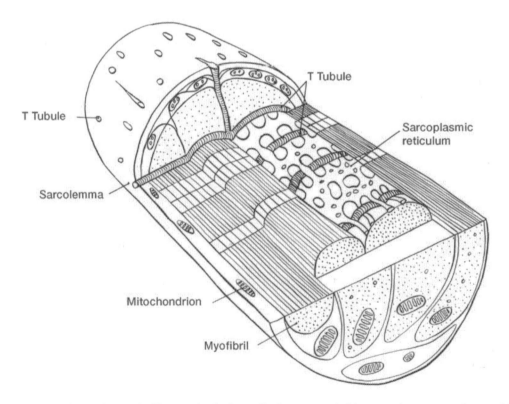

Fig. 24-2. Structure of a single muscle fiber. Individual myofibrils are encircled by sarcoplasmic reticulum and T tubules. The latter are hollow structures that are continuous with the sarcolemma and, hence, the extracellular fluid and in proximity with the sarcoplasmic reticulum. (From Benarroch EE, Westmoreland BF, Daube JR, Reagan TJ, Sandok BA. Medical neurosciences: an approach to anatomy, pathology, and physiology by systems and levels. 4th ed. Philadelphia: Lippincott Williams & Wilkins; 1999. p. 405. By permission of Mayo Foundation.)

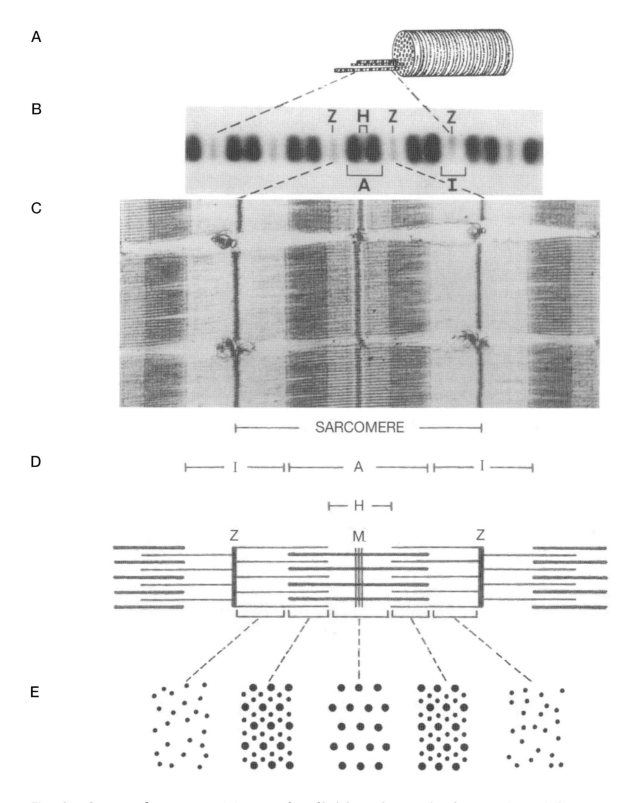

Fig. 24-3. Structure of a sarcomere. *A*, Diagram of myofibril depicted as extending from a single muscle fiber. *B*, Phase-contrast light microscopy of myofibrils showing the striations. *C*, Electron micrograph showing the striations. *D*, Basic structure of the sarcomere and the transverse striations appearing in *B* and *C*. *E*, Cross-sectional appearance of the sarcomere at different points along the sarcomere. (From Craig RW, Padrón R. Molecular structure of the sarcomere. In: Engel AG, Franzini-Armstrong C, editors. Myology: basic and clinical. Vol 1. 3rd ed. New York: McGraw-Hill; 2004. p. 129-66. Used with permission.)

c. ATPase activity of globular myosin heads: enhanced by interaction of the head with actin

2. M line
   a. Situated at center of the A band
   b. Contains protein bridges that link thick filaments together
   c. Contains creatine kinase, M protein, and myomesin
   d. Site of attachment for intermediate filaments, acting to connect subjacent myofibrils

3. Titin filaments
   a. Extends from Z disk to M line (there is overlap of adjacent titin filaments of subjacent sarcomeres)
   b. Functions
      1) Maintain structural integrity of sarcomere during both active and relaxed states
      2) Serve as structural molecular template for arrangement of different components of the sarcomere
      3) Determinant of elastic properties of muscle and passive length of muscle at rest
   c. N-terminus situated in the Z disk: binds to the titin cap (T-cap), also termed telethonin
   d. C-terminus situated at the M line: binds to myosin and myosin-binding proteins
   e. Examples of sarcomeric proteins implicated in limb-girdle muscular dystrophies (LGMDs): titin (affected in LGMD 2J) and telethonin (affected in LGMD 2G)

4. Thin filaments
   a. Components
      1) Pair of F-actin polymers arranged as a helix
      2) Tropomyosin molecules
         a) Arranged as α-helical coils of long filamentous proteins situated in grooves formed by double helical array of F-actin polymers
         b) Likely block the myosin-binding site on actin filaments at rest
         c) With activation, tropomyosin changes in configuration and exposes actin-binding sites
      3) Troponin
         a) Troponin I: inhibitory component
         b) Troponin C: calcium-binding component
         c) Troponin T: tropomyosin-binding component; binds to other troponin components (TnI and TnC) and to tropomyosin and actin—functional connection between different components of thin filaments
      4) Nebulin
         a) Spans entire structure of thin filaments
         b) C-terminus situated at the Z disk and N-terminus at the free end of thin filaments
         c) Functions: likely stabilization and length determination of thin filaments

5. A band: area of overlap of actin and myosin filaments

6. I band: area that includes only thin filaments

7. Z disk
   a. Mechanical attachment between adjacent sarcomeres
   b. Important for maintaining structural integrity of sarcomeres and arranging the sarcomeres to form myofibrils
   c. Structure: overlapping antiparallel actin and titin filaments from abutting sarcomeres connected by α-actinin
   d. Intermediate filaments encircle myofibrils at the Z lines and attach the subjacent sarcomeres together and to the sarcolemma: synemin is a component of the intermediate filament that binds α-actinin of the sarcomere

8. H zone: region containing only myosin filaments

D. Physiology of Muscle Contraction

1. Depolarization of muscle membrane and activation of muscle fibers: starts at end-plate region and propagates along the length of muscle fiber

2. At the end plate region
   a. Release of single quantum of acetylcholine (ACh) depolarizes postsynaptic membrane, called miniature end plate potential (MEPP)
   b. Arrival of an action potential at nerve terminal releases about 200 to 300 quanta of ACh to bind to the postsynaptic nicotinic cholinergic receptors
   c. This results in an aggregate potential, end plate potential (EPP), which generally exceeds the threshold for generating an action potential by activation of voltage-dependent sodium channels on the muscle membrane

3. As action potential spreads along muscle membrane (sarcolemma), depolarization extends into sarcolemmal invaginations, the transverse tubules (T tubules)

4. Depolarization of T tubules triggers rapid release of calcium from sarcoplasmic reticulum by opening the ryanodine calcium channels (termed ryanodine receptors) located at the terminal cisternae

5. With muscle fiber activation, calcium is released from sarcoplasmic reticulum, causing an increase in intracellular calcium

6. Calcium binds to troponin C

7. This triggers a change in configuration of tropomyosin
   a. At rest: tropomyosin covers the myosin-binding site of actin and inhibits this association
   b. With contraction: tropomyosin moves and uncovers the myosin-binding site, allowing interaction of actin and myosin

8. Globular myosin head then binds the actin (in a crossbridge) and undergoes configurational change (bends), allowing actin filaments to slide past thick filaments

9. Detachment of myosin from actin filaments requires adenosine triphosphate (ATP); the myosin head then reverts to original configuration

II. CLINICAL APPROACH TO DIAGNOSING MUSCLE DISORDERS

A. Define Symptoms

1. Positive symptoms: myalgias, myotonia, myoglobinuria, cramps, contractures
   a. Myoglobinuria may occur in several toxic and metabolic conditions, e.g., drugs and toxins, malignant hyperthermia associated with central core myopathy, and several inherited metabolic myopathies often cause recurrent myoglobinuria
2. Negative symptoms: weakness, atrophy, fatigue, exercise intolerance, periodic paralysis
   a. Proximal weakness is most common pattern: patients usually complain of difficulty lifting objects above the head, getting up from a low chair, or walking up steps

B. Define Pattern of Weakness

1. Proximal limb-girdle distribution
   a. Most common pattern
   b. Often symmetric weakness predominantly affecting the proximal upper and lower limbs and neck flexors and extensors; nonspecific
2. Distal distribution (most often symmetric): diagnostic considerations include
   a. Late or early adult-onset distal myopathy
   b. Facioscapulohumeral muscular dystrophy
   c. Scapuloperoneal muscular dystrophy
   d. Desmin myopathy
   e. Emery-Dreifuss muscular dystrophy
   f. Myotonic dystrophy
   g. Inclusion body myositis (often affecting finger flexors)
   h. Metabolic myopathies: debrancher deficiency, acid maltase deficiency
   i. Congenital myopathies (often cause diffuse myopathy): nemaline myopathy, central core disease, centronuclear myopathy
3. Scapuloperoneal distribution (proximal arm and distal leg, often asymmetric): diagnostic considerations include
   a. Facioscapulohumeral muscular dystrophy
   b. Scapuloperoneal muscular dystrophy
   c. Emery-Dreifuss muscular dystrophy
   d. Limb-girdle dystrophies
   e. Congenital myopathies: nemaline myopathy, central core disease
   f. Metabolic myopathies, including acid maltase deficiency
4. Distal arm and proximal leg weakness (asymmetric)
   a. Including finger and wrist flexors and quadriceps
   b. Seen with inclusion body myositis
5. Ptosis with or without ophthalmoplegia
   a. With pharyngeal involvement: oculopharyngeal dystrophy
   b. Without pharyngeal involvement: a mitochondrial cytopathy
   c. Facial weakness and ptosis, without ophthalmoplegia: facioscapulohumeral muscular dystrophy and myotonic dystrophy
6. Prominent neck extensor weakness: diagnostic considerations include
   a. Isolated neck extensor myopathy
   b. Inflammatory myopathy: dermatomyositis, polymyositis, inclusion body myositis
   c. Congenital myopathy
   d. Myotonic dystrophy
   e. Facioscapulohumeral muscular dystrophy
   f. Metabolic myopathies
   g. Entities other than myopathies (e.g., motor neuron disease, myasthenia gravis)

C. Temporal Profile

1. Age at onset
   a. Birth
      1) Congenital myopathies: central core disease, centronuclear, nemaline
      2) Congenital muscular dystrophy
      3) Congenital myotonic dystrophy
      4) Lipid storage disease: carnitine palmityltransferase deficiency
      5) Glycogen storage diseases, e.g., acid maltase deficiency
   b. Childhood
      1) Muscular dystrophies: Duchenne's, Becker's, facioscapulohumeral, Emery-Dreifuss, limb-girdle dystrophy
      2) Myopathies related to endocrine disorders
      3) Inflammatory myopathies, e.g., dermatomyositis
      4) Congenital myopathies, e.g., nemaline myopathy
      5) Mitochondrial myopathies
      6) Lipid storage diseases, e.g., carnitine palmityltransferase deficiency
      7) Glycogen storage diseases, e.g., acid maltase deficiency
   c. Adulthood
      1) Inflammatory: polymyositis, dermatomyositis, inclusion body myositis
      2) Infectious: viral
      3) Toxic-metabolic
      4) Myopathies related to endocrine disorders: thyroid, parathyroid, adrenal, pituitary
      5) Muscular dystrophies
      6) Mitochondrial myopathies

7) Lipid storage diseases and glycogen storage diseases, e.g., acid maltase deficiency

8) Congenital myopathies, e.g., nemaline myopathy

2. Temporal evolution

   a. Abrupt (acute or subacute) onset and progression/recurrent episodes: inflammatory myopathy, periodic paralysis, metabolic myopathy

   b. Chronic, slow "dystrophic" progression: muscular dystrophy

   c. Long-term, nonprogressive: congenital myopathy (some may have very slow progression later in the course)

D. Precipitating Factors That Trigger Symptoms

1. Illegal drugs, toxins, medicines (especially corticosteroids, statins)

2. Exercise, cold, or ingestion of carbohydrate-enriched meals (periodic paralysis)

E. Other Organ Involvement

1. Cardiac involvement

   a. Dysrhythmias: mitochondrial myopathies (Kearns-Sayre syndrome), Anderson's syndrome

   b. Congestive heart failure (CHF): nemaline myopathy, myofibrillar myopathy, Duchenne's and Becker's muscular dystrophies, acid maltase deficiency, carnitine palmityltransferase deficiency

   c. Both dysrhythmias and CHF: polymyositis, muscular dystrophies (myotonic; Emery-Dreifuss; limb-girdle types 1A and B, 2C-G, 2I, some distal myopathies)

2. Respiratory involvement

   a. Inflammatory: polymyositis, anti-Jo1 antibody syndrome

   b. Congenital myopathies: nemaline and centronuclear myopathies

   c. Mitochondrial myopathies

   d. Muscular dystrophies: congenital, myotonic, Emery-Dreifuss, and myofibrillar myopathy

   e. Metabolic myopathies: acid maltase deficiency, carnitine palmityltransferase deficiency

III. Congenital Myopathies

A. General Characteristics

1. Early onset with clinical manifestations present from birth

2. Prenatal course: fetal movements may be decreased or absent

3. Postnatal course: hypotonia, poor respiratory effort, complicated delivery, inability to feed, reduced muscle

bulk, diffuse or proximal weakness (nemaline myopathy may have predominantly distal weakness)

4. First year: hypotonia, weakness (may include facial weakness), flaccid speech, delayed motor milestones, failure to thrive, respiratory infections

5. Slow or nonprogressive course, but possible altered motor function and change in strength due to growth spurt, weight gain, or intercurrent illness

   a. Serial biopsy studies of nemaline myopathy may show increased connective tissue, indicating progression

6. Respiratory complications may include restrictive lung disease, sleep hypoventilation due to insidious paralysis of diaphragm

7. Orthopedic complications and skeletal deformities

B. Central Core Disease

1. Mutation in the ryanodine receptor gene (*RYR1*) on chromosome 19q13.1 (allelic with malignant hyperthermia), encoding for skeletal muscle calcium release channel

2. Autosomal dominant inheritance with variable expression and incomplete penetrance (may rarely be autosomal recessive or sporadic)

3. Proximal symmetric weakness: often mild, legs more than arms

4. Delayed motor development, unable to walk until 3 or 4 years old

5. Poor muscle bulk

6. Nonprogressive or slow progressive course

7. Normal extraocular movements, and no bulbar signs

8. May have mild facial weakness

9. Orthopedic complications such as congenital dislocation of hip (most common), scoliosis, foot deformities, ankle contractures, finger contractures

10. Severe infantile form with hypotonia and respiratory failure

11. Childhood or adult-onset cases may present with mild proximal weakness, exercise intolerance, or malignant hyperthermia with exposure to anesthetics

12. Creatine kinase: typically normal levels

13. Muscle histopathology (Fig. 24-4)

   a. Type I fiber predominance

   b. Central cores

      1) Single, well-circumscribed regions

      2) Selectively involve type I fibers

      3) Deficient in mitochondria and sarcoplasmic reticulum as well as oxidative enzymes and phosphorylase activity (detected best on sections with oxidative enzyme immunohistochemistry, as poorly stained central demarcated areas)

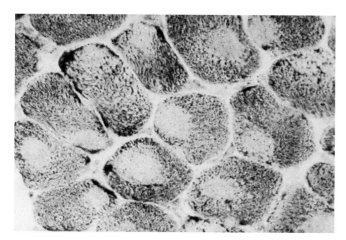

Fig. 24-4. Central core disease. The poorly stained central areas are not well demarcated from the surrounding cytoplasm. (NADH dehydrogenase stain.) (Courtesy of Andrew G. Engel, MD.)

4) Extend entire length of muscle fiber
c. Increased endomysial connective tissue
d. Often, increased number of internal nuclei
14. Treatment includes avoidance of anesthesia-induced malignant hypertension

C. Multicore (minicore) Disease
1. Congenital myopathy associated with multifocal degeneration of muscle fibers
2. Most familial cases are autosomal recessive, may also be sporadic
3. Onset in infancy or early childhood with hypotonia and delayed motor milestones
4. Weakness (usually nonprogressive) predominantly proximal → waddling gait, frequent falls, difficulty rising from chair; neck and trunk muscle involvement
5. Facial weakness (mild), bulbar weakness with hypernasal voice
6. Ptosis and extraocular muscle weakness rare
7. Cardiac manifestations uncommon (e.g., atrial and ventricular septal defects, cardiomyopathy)
8. Respiratory involvement: respiratory insufficiency or failure, sometimes with nocturnal hypoventilation (may need nocturnal ventilation)
9. Creatine kinase: normal or slightly elevated levels
10. Electromyography (EMG): normal (early on) or short-duration motor unit potentials (especially after age 4 years)
11. Muscle histopathology (Fig. 24-5)
   a. Variation in fiber size, internal nuclei, and muscle fiber splitting

b. Type I fiber predominance
c. Type I fibers may be smaller than normal; type II fibers may be hypertrophied
d. Multiple small cores in individual fibers with decreased activity on reduced form of nicotinamide adenine dinucleotide (NADH) and oxidative stains (lack of mitochondria)
e. Small cores
   1) Occur in both type I and II fibers
   2) Are short and do not extend the entire length of the muscle fiber
f. Minicores: foci of reduced sarcomeric organization with reduced mitochondrial activity
g. Lesions may represent foci of myofibrillary disintegration and collections of membraneous material and unstructured myofibrils

D. Nemaline Myopathy
1. Autosomal dominant (most families), recessive, sporadic
2. Genetic heterogeneity
   a. Mutation involving nebulin gene (*NEM2*) on chromosome 2q21-22
      1) Nebulin contributes to formation of Z disk
      2) Autosomal recessive, infantile onset
   b. Mutation involving the skeletal muscle α-actin gene (*ACTA1*) on chromosome 1q: autosomal dominant or recessive
   c. Mutation involving tropomyosin gene *TPM2* on chromosome 9p13 or *TPM3* on chromosome 1q: autosomal dominant or recessive
      1) Encoding α-tropomyosin in thin filaments of sarcomere
3. Phenotypic heterogeneity
   a. Severe neonatal congenital form
      1) Difficult delivery, cyanosis at birth, hypotonic infants with reduced muscle bulk and severe generalized weakness (few spontaneous movements), feeding difficulties (difficulties with sucking and swallowing), gastroesophageal reflux
      2) Dysmorphic features, joint contractures, foot deformities, arthrogryposis (uncommon)
      3) Recurrent pulmonary infections, high early mortality due to aspiration pneumonia or respiratory insufficiency
      4) Infants who survive respiratory failure continue to acquire motor development (delayed), with slow progressive or nonprogressive weakness
   b. Intermediate infantile congenital form
      1) Hypotonic infants with generalized weakness and

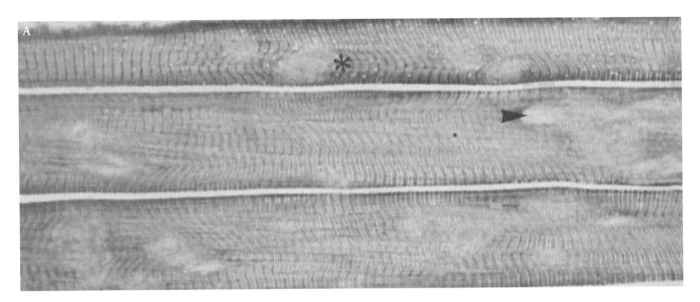

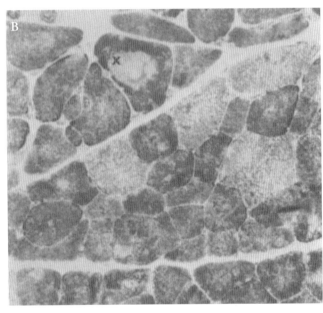

Fig. 24-5. Multicore (minicore) disease. *A*, Phase-contrast microscopy showing multiple "lesions" of loss of striations (*), arranged perpendicular to the fiber axis (*arrowhead*). *B*, Muscle biopsy specimen showing foci of reduced oxidative enzyme activity (*x*) (NADH dehydrogenase stain). (From Engle AG, Gomez MR, Groover RV. Multicore disease: a recently recognized congenital myopathy associated with multifocal degeneration of muscle fibers. Mayo Clin Proc. 1971;46:666-81.)

feeding difficulties, but often independent respiration at delivery

2) Proximal muscle weakness causing waddling gait and Gowers' sign

3) Delayed and incomplete motor development; may be wheelchair-bound by age 10 years

4) Facial and masticatory muscles severely affected: appearance of long and narrow face and open mouth

5) Narrow, high-arched palate, micrognathia, chest deformities, finger contractures

6) Nonprogressive course in many cases, but slow deterioration of motor function with time

c. Mild infantile congenital form

1) Hypotonia and feeding difficulties in first year of life

2) Respiratory involvement: mild at best or subclinical

3) Bulbar weakness: hypernasal speech, swallowing difficulties

4) Weakness usually proximal (late development of distal involvement in some patients)

d. Childhood/adolescent form

1) Motor development may be normal

2) Early distal lower extremity weakness (especially with dorsiflexion), often presenting at onset

e. Adult onset

1) Age at onset: between third and sixth decades

2) Limb-girdle proximal weakness with slow progression

3) Often no family history

4) Respiratory failure and cardiomyopathy

5) Rare adult onset of nemaline myopathy may present as cardiomyopathy or diaphragmatic muscle involvement

4. Creatine kinase: normal or mildly elevated levels

5. Cardiac involvement: rare or uncommon in all phenotypes

6. EMG
   a. Rapid recruitment of short-duration motor unit potentials
   b. Changes may be normal or very mild if study is performed very early
   c. Patients with long-standing disease or with onset at older age may show long-duration motor unit potentials
7. Muscle histopathology (Fig. 24-6)
   a. Type I fiber predominance (especially in severe cases) and atrophy
   b. Marked disproportion in fiber size, with uniformly small type I fibers and normal to large type II fibers
   c. Sarcoplasmic rods (nemaline bodies)
      1) Short, granular-appearing
      2) Subsarcolemmal and perinuclear localization in type I fibers (especially large rods)
      3) Composed of α-actinin, actin, and other Z disk proteins, and appear to arise from, are attached to, and thicken the Z disk (small rods)
   d. Intranuclear rods
      1) Observed in some patients with severe congenital or adult-onset phenotypes
      2) May be associated with more severe disease and worse prognosis

E. **Myotubular** (centronuclear) **Myopathy**
1. Inheritance: autosomal dominant, autosomal recessive, and sporadic cases reported (rare)
2. X-linked recessive (most common): chromosome Xq27.3-q28 (*MTM1* gene)
   a. Missense mutation associated with mild phenotype (variable)

   b. Severe or lethal phenotype usually seen with truncating mutations
3. Gene product: tyrosine phosphatase (myotubularin) important for signal transduction and differentiation in late myogenesis (hence, in utero onset)
4. In utero onset (common): reduced fetal movements and difficult delivery, enlarged head and polyhydramnios
5. Floppy infants (diffuse weakness and severe hypotonia), facial diplegia, bilateral ptosis, nonprogressive proximal and distal symmetric weakness, respiratory insufficiency or failure (partial or complete ventilator dependency in survivors), high mortality (usually X-linked recessive)
6. Extraocular and neck axial muscles often affected
7. Macrocephaly, narrow face, long digits
8. Carriers may have mild facial weakness
9. Associated with pyloric stenosis, spherocytosis, gallstones, kidney stones, rapid linear skeletal bone growth, and sometimes genital abnormalities (e.g., micropenis, hypospadias)
10. Autosomal forms: milder clinical course with later age of onset
11. Creatine kinase: levels may be mildly elevated
12. Electrodiagnostic evaluation
    a. Normal nerve conduction studies
    b. Needle EMG examination
       1) May be normal in mild cases and infants
       2) Rapid recruitment of short-duration polyphasic motor unit potentials, sometimes with fibrillation potentials, complex repetitive discharge, and possibly myotonic discharges
13. Muscle histopathology (Fig. 24-7)

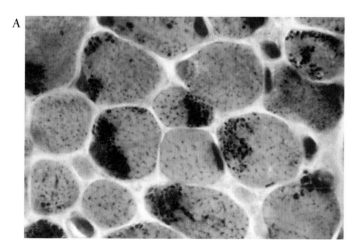
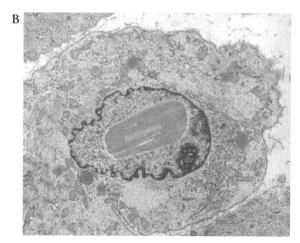

Fig. 24-6. Nemaline myopathy. *A*, Nemaline bodies (rods) (red structures) are clearly distinguished from myofibrillary background (blue-green). (Gomori trichrome stain.) *B*, Electron micrograph showing an intranuclear rod. (*A* courtesy of Andrew G. Engel, MD.)

a. Is called "centronuclear" because of predominance of small type I fibers with central nuclei

b. Type I fiber predominance (often small, atrophied)

c. Central pallor noted on ATPase staining

d. Radial distribution of sarcoplasmic strands apparent on NADH reaction

e. Interstitial connective tissue: normal or mildly increased

F. **Myofibrillar** (desmin-related) **Myopathy** (now considered a muscular dystrophy)

1. Genetic and phenotypic heterogeneity (morphologically homogeneous)

2. Mostly autosomal dominant (autosomal recessive and X-linked also described)

3. Associated chromosomes: 2q, 10q, 11q, 12q

   a. Accumulation of desmin, αB-crystallin, dystrophin, neural cell adhesion molecule, CDC2 kinase, some other proteins

4. Age at onset: may vary between early childhood and adulthood

5. Clinical features: variable

   a. Distal weakness equal to or more than proximal weakness and atrophy

   b. Peripheral neuropathy in 60% of patients (as well as myopathy)

c. Cardiomyopathy (hypertrophic and arrhythmogenic) and respiratory involvement in some patients

d. Hearing loss, palatal weakness, cataracts reported in certain subtypes

6. Muscle histopathology (morphologically homogeneous) (Fig. 24-8)

   a. Subsarcolemmal accumulation of dense granular and filamentous amorphous material: reacts intensely for actin; may contain desmin (some but not all) and other proteins such as lamin B, gelsolin, ubiquitin, dystrophin, and αB-crystallin

   b. Variation in muscle fiber size, rimmed vacuoles, centrally located nuclei, minimal fibrosis may be present

   c. Occasional perivascular or endomysial mononuclear inflammatory infiltrates in less than 10% of cases

   d. Morphologic changes typically begin at Z disk

   e. Cardiac muscle: accumulation of the intermediate filaments with disruption of myofibrils and Z disks

7. Electrophysiology

   a. Nerve conduction studies: normal or show mild axonal peripheral neuropathy

   b. Needle EMG: short-duration, low-amplitude motor unit potentials (sometimes long-duration, large-amplitude units given the chronicity); abnormal spontaneous activity, including increased insertional activity and fibrillation

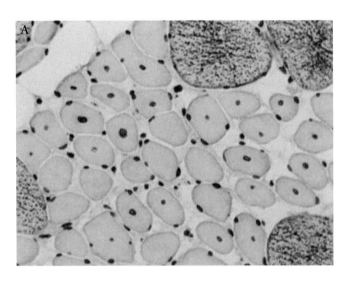 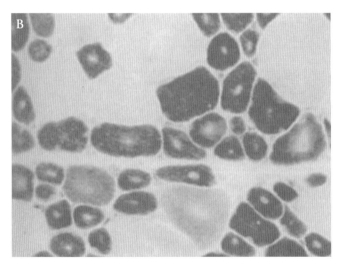

Fig. 24-7. Myotubular (centronuclear) myopathy. *A*, Centrally localized nuclei occur in almost every muscle fiber. (Hematoxylin-eosin stain.) *B*, Type I predominance and atrophy with central pallor. Note that the type I fibers appear "dark" at pH 4.6 and "light" with basic pH solutions. (ATPase stain, pH 4.65.) (*A* from Lidov H, De Girolami U, Gherardi R. Skeletal muscle diseases. In: Gray F, De Girolami U, Poirier J, editors. Escourolle & Poirier manual of basic neuropathology. 4th ed. Philadelphia: Butterworth-Heinemann; 2004. p. 281-314. Used with permission. *B* from North K. Congenital myopathies. In: Engel AG, Franzini-Armstrong C, editors. Myology: basic and clinical. Vol 2. 3rd ed. New York: McGraw-Hill; 2004. p. 1473-1533. Used with permission.)

potentials, complex repetitive discharge, and myotonic discharges

G. Congenital Fiber-Type Disproportion
1. Nonspecific histologic finding likely in congenital myopathies and other conditions
2. Diagnosis of exclusion in patient with clinical features of congenital myopathy and reduction of type I fiber size
3. Disproportion between size of type I and II fibers: type I fibers at least 12% smaller than type II fibers (normally, type I fibers may be up to 25% smaller than type II fibers in adults or infants younger than 2 months)
4. Hypotonia at birth, varying diffuse weakness that spares ocular muscles and improves with age

5. Weakness of face and neck: long thin face, fish mouth, high-arched palate, short stature
6. Contractures, kyphoscoliosis, foot deformities
7. Normal mental development (commonly)
8. Creatine kinase: normal to slightly elevated levels
9. EMG: normal or short-duration motor unit potentials

H. Treatment of Congenital Myopathies
1. Genetic counseling (when mutation has been identified)
2. Prenatal diagnosis (obtaining tissue via chorionic villus biopsy or amniocentesis)
3. Early detection and treatment of medical and orthopedic complications
4. Prevention of complications (including surgical procedures and exposure to general anesthesia)

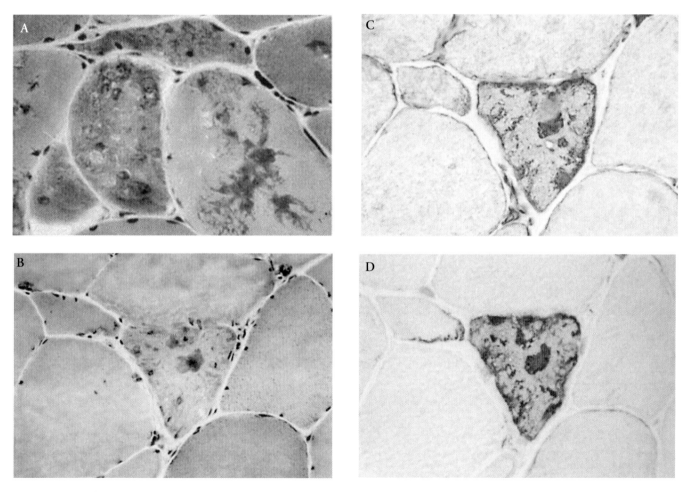

Fig. 24-8. Myofibrillar myopathy. *A* and *B*, Trichrome-stained sections show aggregates of dense granular and filamentous amorphous material and vacuolar change. Immunohistochemistry performed in sections corresponding to that in *B* demonstrates accumulation of desmin (*C*) and αB-crystallin (*D*). (*A* from Selcen D, Engel AG. Mutations in myotilin cause myofibrillar myopathy. Neurology. 2004;62:1363-71. Used with permission. *B*, *C*, and *D* from Engel AG, Franzini-Armstrong C, editors. Myology: basic and clinical. Vol 1. 3rd ed. New York: McGraw-Hill; 2004. Used with permission.)

a. Consider risk of malignant hyperthermia in patients with central core disease

b. Consider preoperative pulmonary evaluation

5. Respiratory care and physical therapy and rehabilitation

IV. MUSCULAR DYSTROPHIES

A. General Characteristics

1. Genetically determined

2. Distinguished by progressive degeneration of muscles and production of connective tissue replacing muscle fibers

3. Systemic involvement in some patients

4. Age at onset: variable

B. Dystrophin-Associated Muscle Membrane Protein Complex (Fig. 24-9)

1. Membrane-associated proteins that span sarcolemma

   a. Provide mechanical support to sarcolemma and stability between intracellular cytoskeleton and extracellular matrix

   b. May participate in signal transduction

2. Cytoplasmic complex: intracellular (subsarcolemmal) proteins associated with muscle membranes

   a. α-Dystrobrevin

      1) Binds to dystrophin

      2) Reduced or absent in subsarcolemmal space in dystrophinopathies

   b. Filamin 2

   c. Syncoilin

   d. Syntrophins

      1) Bind to dystrophin and dystrophin-related proteins such as dystrobrevin

      2) Reduced or absent in subsarcolemmal space in dystrophinopathies

   e. Dystrophin: rod-shaped cytoskeletal protein with no transmembrane regions; consists of five different domains

      1) Actin-binding domain

         a) Encoded by exons 1 to 8

         b) N-terminal domain

         c) Links dystrophin to F-actin subsarcolemmal cytoskeleton

      2) Rod domain

         a) Largest domain (2,400 amino acids), encoded by exons 9 to 62

         b) Consists of 24 triple-helical repeating units: a single repeat unit consists of one long and two shorter helices connected to next unit by short nonhelical spacer

      3) WW domain: overlaps rod domain and cysteine-rich domain

      4) Cysteine-rich domain

         a) Encoded by exons 63 to 69

         b) Responsible for attachment of subsarcolemmal complex to membrane by binding directly to the intracellular portion of β-dystroglycan

      5) C-terminal domain

         a) Encoded by exons 70 to 79

         b) Binds to syntrophins and β-dystroglycan

3. Membrane proteins

   a. Dystroglycan complex

      1) β-Dystroglycan is true membrane protein; α-dystroglycan is extracellular

      2) α- and β-Dystroglycans: encoded by same gene

      3) α-Dystroglycan protein contains laminin-binding glycoprotein that binds to extracellular laminin $\alpha2$ and provides structural link between sarcolemma and extracellular matrix

      4) α-Dystroglycan protein also binds to agrin (see below)

      5) Decrease in muscle α-dystroglycan seen in congenital muscular dystrophies

      6) β-Dystroglycan is sarcolemmal protein that binds tightly to WW domain in cysteine-rich region of dystrophin

   b. Sarcoglycan complex

      1) Group of proteins critical for sarcolemmal stability and for linking actin cytoskeleton to extracellular matrix

      2) Transmembrane proteins containing extracellular domains and a single membrane-spanning domain

      3) Types (and associated disorder)

         a) α-Sarcoglycan, adhalin (LGMD 2D)

         b) β-Sarcoglycan (LGMD 2E)

         c) γ-Sarcoglycan (LGMD 2C)

         d) δ-Sarcoglycan (LGMD 2F)

         e) ε-Sarcoglycan (myoclonus-dystonia syndrome)

         f) ζ-Sarcoglycan

   c. Other membrane proteins

      1) Sarcospan: binds to sarcoglycan complex

      2) Caveolin

         a) Integral transmembrane proteins

         b) Scaffolding proteins implicated in signal transduction

         c) Associated with caveolae (invaginations of plasma membrane)

         d) Calveolin-3 gene mutation associated with LGMD 1C (discussed below)

      3) Integrins

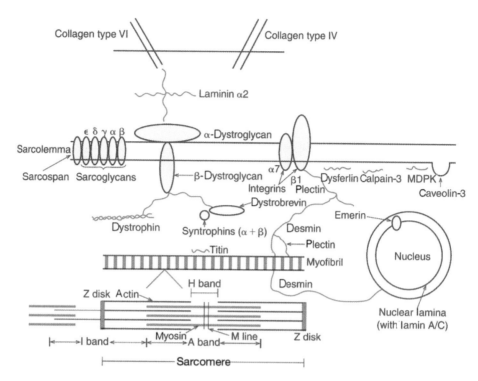

Fig. 24-9. Dystrophin-associated muscle membrane protein complex. (From Banwell BL. Muscular dystrophies. In: Noseworthy JH, editor. Neurological therapeutics: principles and practice. Vol 2. London: Martin Dunitz; 2003. p. 2312-27. By permission of Mayo Foundation.)

a) Heterodimeric membrane glycoproteins (trans-membrane adhesion molecules) that mediate wide spectrum of cell-cell and cell-matrix interactions

b) $\alpha_7\beta_1$-Integrin protein: primary integrin in sarcolemma

   i) Binds to laminin: acts as structural link between cytoskeleton and extracellular matrix

   ii) Mutation of gene on chromosome 12q13 causes a primary congenital muscular dystrophy

   iii) Levels of protein also decreased in other congenital muscular dystrophies (without mutation of gene)

4. Extracellular proteins

  a. Laminins

   1) Glycoproteins, consisting of three polypeptide chains (alpha, beta, gamma) bound to each other by disulfide bonds

   2) Cross-shaped molecules

   3) Location: extracellular, basement membranes

   4) Bind to α-dystroglycans and integrins and interact with other extracellular proteins

   5) Important role in myogenesis

   6) Implicated in congenital muscular dystrophies

  b. Agrin: component of synaptic basal lamina that induces aggregation of ACh receptors and other elements of postsynaptic membrane during synaptogenesis

  c. Collagen types IV and VI

  d. α-Dystroglycan (see above)

C. **Dystrophinopathies** (X-linked recessive inheritance)

1. Genetics

  a. X-linked recessive; Xp21

  b. Gene product is dystrophin, part of dystrophin-glyco-protein complex: deficient dystrophin may weaken sarcolemma, with subsequent muscle fiber necrosis

  c. Large deletions (65%), duplications (5%), small deletions or point mutations (30%)

  d. DNA analysis: large deletions and duplications identified with polymerase chain reaction (PCR) and Southern blot analysis

   1) Up to 65% of patients with Duchenne's muscular dystrophy have large deletions that may be identified

   2) Duplications best identified with Southern blot analysis

   3) "Negative DNA test" does not exclude the diagnosis

   4) Other methods that may be used if PCR fails:

mRNA analysis, immunoblotting, immunostaining
  e. Female carriers
    1) Usually asymptomatic (adequate sarcolemmal dystrophin is produced by the X chromosome harboring the normal dystrophin gene)
    2) 8% of female carriers may have mild to moderate myopathy, likely due to preferential inactivation of normal wild-type X chromosome and increased number of dystrophin-negative fibers (given the mosaic expression of dystrophin-positive and dystrophin-negative fibers)
2. Clinical features of Duchenne dystrophy
  a. Normal height and weight at birth, subsequent decrease in height and weight
  b. Motor developmental delay; difficulty in running, climbing, etc.
  c. Symptoms initially noted when child is observed to walk on toes, difficulty rising from floor (age at onset: about 3-5 years)
  d. Gower's sign: patient stands up by using hands pushing on knees
  e. May experience a period of apparent functional improvement due to normal increase in motor skills and strength
  f. By 5 to 6 years of age: pseudohypertrophy of the calves
  g. By 12 years: loss of ambulation, atrophy of all muscles, contractures
  h. Contracture: ankles, knees, and hips
  i. Progressive kyphoscoliosis and exaggerated lumbar lordosis: usually after loss of ambulation, possibly due to involvement of axial muscles
  j. Progression to death over 15 to 30 years (death usually due to respiratory complications)
  k. Muscle weakness (proximal more than distal), upper and lower extremities involved: "scapuloperoneal distribution," preferential involvement of proximal (more than distal) muscles and anterior tibialis and peronei muscle groups (more than gastrocnemius, soleus, and tibialis posterior muscles), neck flexors (more than neck extensors), wrist and digit extensors (more than flexors)
  l. Preservation of cranial musculature
  m. Respiratory muscle involvement
  n. At risk for malignant hyperthermia-like reactions and acute rhabdomyolysis to general anesthesia
  o. Cardiomyopathy: CHF and arrhythmias in late stages of disease
  p. Intestinal pseudo-obstruction: due to involvement of smooth muscles of gastrointestinal tract
  q. Central nervous system involvement: some with mental retardation, average IQ about one standard deviation below normal, learning disabilities

  r. Creatine kinase: markedly elevated early in the disease, but decreases with disease progression and replacement of muscle fibers with connective tissue
3. Clinical features of Becker dystrophy
  a. Later age of onset, less severe, and later progression compared with Duchenne dystrophy
  b. Usual age at onset: between 5 and 15 years (range, 3-60 years)
  c. Most patients ambulate beyond 15 years
  d. Loss of ambulation usually in the fourth decade (range, 10-78 years)
  e. Age at death: may range from 30 to 60 years
4. Muscle histopathology of dystrophinopathies (Fig. 24-10)
  a. Segmental muscle necrosis and regeneration
  b. Hypercontracted muscle fibers
  c. Abnormal variation in fiber size
  d. Muscle fiber degeneration and regeneration
  e. Macrophage invasion of the necrotic fibers, phagocytosis
  f. Progressive loss of muscle fibers and replacement with connective tissue and endomysial fibrosis with reduced regenerative capacity
  g. Absence of dystrophin in Duchenne dystrophy and reduction or altered staining patterns in Becker dystrophy
  h. Diagnosis cannot be made without immunohistochemical staining or immunoblotting
5. Electrophysiology
  a. When performed in symptomatic child: increased insertional activity, small myopathic motor unit potentials in affected muscle groups
  b. In asymptomatic phase or in patients with minimal symptoms: insertional activity may be normal
  c. With progression of disease and endomysial fibrosis: compound muscle action potential (CMAP) amplitudes may be reduced and recruitment may be reduced
6. Treatment
  a. Corticosteroids (prednisone and deflazacort) shown to be beneficial temporarily (can prolong ambulation and maintain pulmonary function)
    1) Should be started between ages 4 and 7 years
    2) Benefit best with prednisone at a daily dose of 0.75 mg/kg
    3) Benefit may be due to increased muscle mass or stabilization of sarcolemma
    4) Improvement in motor function by 10 days to 1 month and maximal within 2 to 3 months
  b. Genetic counseling, physical therapy, treatment of medical and orthopedic complications

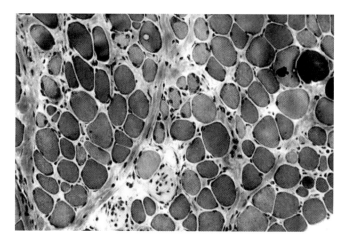

Fig. 24-10. Muscle histopathologic features of Duchenne dystrophy include endomysial and perimysial macrophage invasion of necrotic fibers undergoing phagocytosis, hypercontracted (opaque) fibers, mild endomysial fibrosis, and central fiber necrosis. (Trichrome stain.) (Courtesy of Andrew G. Engle, MD.)

D.   Emery-Dreifuss Muscular Dystrophy (EMD-1 and EMD-2)
1. Incidence 1:100,000
2. Genetics
   a. EMD-1: X-linked recessive inheritance (mutations in *STA* gene on chromosome Xq28, which encodes nuclear membrane protein emerin)
   b. EMD-2: autosomal dominant or recessive inheritance (mutations in *LMNA* gene on chromosome 1q21.23, which encodes nuclear envelope proteins, lamins A and C, not emerin)
3. Clinical features
   a. Age at onset: early to middle childhood
   b. Scapulohumeroperoneal or limb-girdle distribution, slowly progressive weakness
   c. EMD-1: early onset of joint contractures, often before notable weakness
   d. EMD-2: contractures often follow onset of notable muscle weakness
   e. Loss of ambulation more common with EMD-2
   f. Contractures: predominantly ankle, elbows, cervical spine
   g. Cardiomyopathy with conduction abnormalities: usually after second or third decades
   h. Muscle pseudohypertrophy absent
   i. Creatine kinase: normal or mildly elevated levels
4. Muscle histopathology
   a. Pattern consistent with a slowly progressive muscular

dystrophy: variation in muscle fiber size, minimal necrosis with regeneration, and increase in connective tissue
   b. Reduced or absent emerin immunostaining in muscle or skin biopsy specimens
5. Electrophysiology
   a. Chronic myopathic changes: small myopathic motor unit potentials with minimal abnormal spontaneous activity or fibrillation potentials
   b. Large motor unit potentials may be present, indicative of the chronicity of the myopathic process
6. Treatment
   a. Physical therapy with stretching exercises
   b. Prevention and screening for medical complications, including early detection of cardiac conduction abnormalities and pacemaker insertion when needed

E.   Barth's Syndrome (X-linked)
1. X-linked recessive: linked to chromosome Xp28, gene encoding Tafazzin protein
2. Onset usually in infancy
3. Mild limb-girdle myopathic weakness
4. Cardiomyopathy, short stature, neutropenia

F.   Autosomal Dominant Dystrophies
1. Facioscapulohumeral muscular dystrophy
   a. Incidence 1:20,000
   b. Genetics
      1) Autosomal dominant inheritance, with high penetrance and variable expression
      2) Chromosome 4q35 (deletion and reduced number of D4Z4 tandem repeat segments)
   c. Clinical features
      1) Usually symptomatic after age 18 (usually between second and fourth decades)
      2) Severe infantile form exists
      3) Slowly progressive (insidious onset) asymmetric weakness of facial, scapular, and proximal upper extremity muscles as well as peroneal muscles
      4) Biceps, triceps, trapezius, serratus anterior, pectoral, and scapular muscles affected; deltoid muscles spared
      5) Facial weakness causes incomplete eye closure, asymmetric defect in puckering, and flattened smile; initial symptoms often involve facial muscles
      6) Forearm muscles less involved: wrist extensors affected more than wrist flexors
      7) Ankle dorsiflexors involved early
      8) Hip flexors and quadriceps may be affected
      9) Involvement of abdominal muscles usually early and may cause protruding abdomen and Beevor's sign
      10) Symptoms often patchy and asymmetric

11) 20% of patients may eventually lose ability to ambulate
12) Slow progression over years
13) Life expectation unchanged
d. Creatine kinase: level elevated less than 5 times normal
e. Muscle histopathology
1) Dystrophic pattern: mild necrosis with regeneration, variation in muscle fiber size, increased amount of connective tissue
2) Moth-eaten appearance on oxidative enzyme stains (NADH)
2. Oculopharyngeal dystrophy
a. Genetics
1) Inheritance: mostly autosomal dominant (autosomal recessive also reported)
2) Expanded GCG repeat in *PABN1* gene on chromosome 14q11.2-q13: gene product PABPN1 (polyadenylate-binding protein nuclear 1 [previously known as PABP2]) is nuclear protein involved in polyadenylation of all mRNAs
b. Clinical features
1) Typically begins in fifth to sixth decades with progressive ptosis (bilateral and sometimes asymmetric) and dysphagia
2) Extraocular muscle involvement can occur later
3) Facial weakness in some patients
4) Weakness of proximal upper and lower extremities in some patients
5) Dysphonia from laryngeal involvement
6) Slowly progressive course
c. Creatine kinase: often normal levels
d. Electrophysiology
1) Normal nerve conduction studies (sometimes length-dependent axonal peripheral neuropathy)
2) Needle examination showing rapid recruitment of short-duration motor unit potentials, sometimes with long-duration motor unit potentials given chronicity of disorder
e. Muscle histopathology
1) Dystrophic changes: abnormal variation in fiber size, loss of muscle fibers, and increase in interstitial connective tissue and internal nuclei
2) Small angulated fibers (may be attributed to concurrent denervation or aging)
3) Autophagic (rimmed) vacuoles and intranuclear inclusions
f. Treatment
1) Prevention and treatment of medical complications (swallowing evaluation, gastrostomy as needed)
2) Lid crutches and blepharoplasty for ptosis as needed

3. Classic myotonic dystrophy type 1 (DM1): most prevalent inherited neuromuscular disease in adults
a. Genetics
1) Autosomal dominant inheritance
2) Expanded unstable CTG repeat in gene encoding myotonin protein kinase (DMPK, serine threonine protein kinase) on chromosome 19q13.3: expansion not in the coding region, not translated
3) Anticipation: average age at onset, 29 years; younger in child than in parent
4) Length of repeats correlates inversely with age at onset
b. Clinical presentation
1) Myotonia, most often affects hand grip and evoked by percussion; not seen in congenital form
2) Slowly progressive weakness and atrophy of facial muscles and distal limbs (preferentially affecting forearm and peroneal muscles)
3) With progression, proximal muscle groups may be involved
4) Frontal balding and temporal wasting
5) Cranial musculature involved (other than muscles of facial expression): tongue, palate, masseter, temporalis, neck flexors, and sternocleidomastoid muscles may be affected
6) Symmetric ptosis and reduced facial expression → characteristic facies
7) Mild and late extraocular weakness and extraocular myotonia
8) Tendon reflexes may be reduced or absent
9) Mild length-dependent peripheral neuropathy
10) Cardiac involvement
a) Conduction defects, arrhythmias, dilated cardiomyopathy
b) Sudden death may be first manifestation
11) Alimentary tract involvement due to smooth muscle involvement
a) Gastrointestinal tract dysmotility
b) Megacolon
c) Gallbladder disease (history of cholecystitis common)
d) Constipation and diarrhea
12) Cataracts, polychromatic lens opacities
13) Endocrine abnormalities
a) Testicular atrophy and secondary increase in pituitary gonadotrophic hormones (e.g., follicle-stimulating hormone)
b) Women: high rate of miscarriages; complications during pregnancy; complicated, prolonged labor and delivery
c) Hyperinsulinism and insulin resistance, abnormal

glucose tolerance test
14) Mental deficiency
   a) Abnormal verbal and nonverbal IQ scores
   b) Mental retardation in congenital myotonic dystrophy
15) Frequent miscarriages or important gestational complications in affected females who become pregnant
16) Sleep difficulties: hypoventilation, uncontrollable urge to sleep, hypercarbia due to abnormal central ventilatory response
c. Electrophysiology
   1) Nerve conduction studies: normal or length-dependent sensorimotor peripheral neuropathy
   2) Needle examination
      a) Myotonic discharges: widespread, may range from 2 to 30 seconds in duration (shorter duration of myotonic discharges in myotonia congenita, mostly <2 seconds)
      b) No myotonic discharges in congenital form
      c) Short-duration, rapidly recruiting motor unit potentials with fibrillation potentials and abnormal spontaneous activity, face and distal limbs more than proximal limbs
d. Muscle histopathology
   1) Increased internal (central) nuclei with pyknotic nuclear clumps
   2) Variation in muscle fiber size
   3) Ring fibers
   4) Small, angulated fibers
   5) Type I fiber atrophy, hypertrophy of type II fibers
   6) Occasional necrotic muscle fibers
   7) Sarcoplasmic masses
e. Ancillary testing
   1) Creatine kinase: normal to mildly elevated levels
   2) Magnetic resonance imaging (MRI): may show subcortical white matter changes
f. Diagnosis
   1) Molecular testing required to confirm the diagnosis: combination of PCR and Southern blot analysis to detect CTG expansions
   2) Prenatal testing: amniocentesis or chorionic villus sampling may identify cases of congenital myotonic dystrophy
4. Congenital myotonic dystrophy
   a. Poor fetal movements and polyhydramnios due to difficulty swallowing
   b. Usually apparent at birth
   c. Severe weakness (including facial weakness) and hypotonia
   d. Respiratory insufficiency due to intercostal and diaphrag-

matic weakness and hypoplasia
   e. Feeding difficulties due to weakness of muscles of mastication and facial expression and weakness of palatal and pharyngeal muscles
   f. Muscle histopathology: hypoplastic muscles with decreased muscle fiber size and number, absence of fiber type differentiation, presence of central nuclei, satellite cells
   g. Delayed motor development
   h. Mental retardation
   i. Clinical or electrophysiologic myotonia absent in first few years of life
5. Proximal myotonic myopathy (PROMM): type 2 myotonic dystrophy (DM2)
   a. Genetics
      1) Autosomal dominant inheritance
      2) Normal size DM1 gene
      3) Most families show linkage to DM2 markers on chromosome 3q
      4) CCTG expansion producing long repeat RNA and abnormal splicing of muscle chloride channel RNA
      5) DM2 is due to a CCTG expansion in intron 1 of the *ZNF9* gene on chromosome 3, encoding ZNF9 protein (zinc finger protein 9)
      6) Anticipation: mild, less prominent than DM1
   b. Age at onset: varies widely between 8 and 60 years
   c. Weakness: primarily proximal, severity variable
   d. Facial weakness: minimal or absent
   e. Myalgias: frequent
   f. Myotonia: clinically minimal or absent, usually detected with EMG (diagnosis is not excluded by absence of myotonia)
   g. Cataracts: eventually occur in all patients
   h. Other systemic manifestations present to lesser degree than in DM1: cardiac arrhythmias, diabetes mellitus, hearing loss
   i. No congenital form
   j. High level follicle-stimulating hormone
   k. Reduced IgG
   l. Creatine kinase: normal or mildly elevated levels
   m. Muscle histopathology: nonspecific, similar to that of DM1

G. Limb-Girdle Muscular Dystrophies (Table 24-1)
1. Clinical manifestation
   a. Clinically and genetically heterogeneous
   b. Progressive proximal muscle weakness and atrophy
   c. Face and neck muscles generally spared
   d. Distal muscles could be affected in later stages of disease
   e. Congenital and infantile onset may have hypotonia and

Table 24-1. **Classification of the Limb-Girdle Dystrophies (LGMD)**

Type	Chromosome (gene product)	Distinguishing clinical features
Autosomal dominant		
LGMD 1A	5q31 (myotilin)	Dysarthria
		Some with ankle contractures
LGMD 1B	1q (lamin A/C)	Cardiomyopathy, arrhythmias
LGMD 1C	3p25 (caveolin-3)	Onset in childhood
		Calf muscle hypertrophy
		Rippling muscle disease (variant)
LGMD 1D	7q	Cardiac arrhythmias
LGMD 1E	7q32	
Bethlem myopathy	21q, 2q (collagen type VI)	Flexion contractures, skeletal deformities
Autosomal recessive		
LGMD 2A	15q15.1-q21.1 (calpain-3)	Calf muscle hypertrophy
LGMD 2B	2p13 (dysferlin)	Weakness preferentially involving gastrocnemius, biceps brachii, pelvic-girdle muscles
LGMD 2C	13q12 (γ-sarcoglycan)	
LGMD 2D	17q12 (α-sarcoglycan)	
LGMD 2E	4q12 (β-sarcoglycan)	
LGMD 2F	5q33-34 (δ-sarcoglycan)	
LGMD 2G	17q11-12 (telethonin)	
LGMD 2H	9q31	
LGMD 2I	19q13.3 (FKRP)	Macroglossia, dilated cardiomyopathy, diaphragmatic weakness

FKRP, fukutin-related protein.

generalized weakness
f. Other features in older children and adults: ankle contractures, calf hypertrophy, exertional myalgias, lumbar lordosis
2. Muscle histopathology
  a. Nonspecific: degeneration of muscle fibers with regeneration and variable necrosis and fiber splitting, variable muscle fiber size, central nuclei
  b. Immunostaining and Western blot analysis helpful in detecting known protein deficiencies
  c. Deficiency of one sarcoglycan protein affects others → specific diagnosis of sarcoglycanopathies is difficult
3. Electrophysiology
  a. Findings correlate with severity of myopathy and timing of the study
  b. More severe forms associated with fibrillation potentials and highly polyphasic myopathic motor unit potentials
  c. Decreased insertional activity and large motor unit potentials may be seen late in disease course
4. LGMD 1: autosomal dominant inheritance
  a. Usually presents in adulthood with slowly progressive proximal weakness and atrophy, including scapular winging, calf hypertrophy, nearly normal or mildly elevated

creatine kinase levels, less severe clinical course and less common than the recessive form
  b. LGMD 1A: myotilinopathy
    1) Mutation in *MYOT* gene on chromosme 5q31-q34 encoding myotilin
    2) Myotilin mutations may also cause phenotype of myofibrillar myopathy
    3) Myotilin interacts with components of Z disk, including α-actinin
    4) Young adult onset with anticipation
    5) Proximal upper and lower extremity weakness, with later progression to distal muscles
    6) Dysarthria with hypernasal speech
    7) Joint contractures at ankles
    8) Slow progression with late loss of ambulation
    9) Creatine kinase: elevated levels
    10) Muscle histopathology: rimmed autophagic vacuoles, sarcomeric disorganization, rod-like inclusions (Z-band streaming noted on electron microscopy)
  c. LGMD 1B: laminopathy
    1) Mutation in *LMNA* gene encoding lamin A/C, associated with the nuclear envelope
    2) Allelic with autosomal dominant Emery-Dreifuss

muscular dystrophy (EMD-2)

3) Age at onset: late teens, early adulthood

4) Most common symptom at onset: difficulty with running, followed by more obvious pelvic girdle weakness

5) Slow progression to involve arms in next 10 to 20 years

6) Creatine kinase: normal or mildly elevated levels

7) Muscle contractures may develop late; are usually milder than those of Emery-Dreifuss muscular dystrophy

8) Cardiac manifestations (up to 60% of patients): conduction blocks, arrhythmias (may present with syncope or sudden death), or dilated cardiomyopathy

d. LGMD 1C: caveolinopathy

1) *CAV3* mutations on chromosome 3p25 encoding caveolin-3; cause severe depletion of caveolin-3 from sarcolemma

a) Caveolin-3: transmembrane protein of skeletal muscle; associated with invaginations of plasma membrane involved in vesicle trafficking and signal transduction (Fig. 24-9)

b) Variants: mutations in caveolin-3 may cause asymptomatic elevation of creatine kinase (hyper CK-emia), a distal myopathy, or rippling muscle disease

2) Typical phenotype

a) Early childhood onset

b) Mild to moderate proximal weakness and calf hypertrophy

c) Cramps (often experienced after exercise)

d) Calf hypertrophy

3) Intrafamilial variability

4) Creatine kinase: levels elevated 4- to 25-fold

5) Rippling muscle disease variant

a) Autosomal dominant inhieritance: linked to chromosome 1q41

b) Muscle pain and stiffness

c) Myoedema

d) Wave of involuntary contraction of muscle (electrically silent) spreading from one region to another, precipitated by percussion

6) Muscle histopathology: characterized by decreased caveolin-3 staining of muscle fiber sarcolemma

e. LGMD 1D

1) Linked to chromosome 6q

2) Mild, predominantly proximal and slowly progressive weakness

3) Cardiac manifestations: arrhythmias are common; later, cardiomyopathy

f. Bethlem myopathy

1) Autosomal dominant inheritance: many mutations identified (linked to chromosomes 21q and 2q); affected protein is collagen type VI

2) Age at onset: variable, usually congenital or childhood onset (adult onset reported)

3) Congenital onset: hypotonia (floppy infant), arthrogryposis, fetal movements may be decreased

4) Childhood onset: delayed motor milestones, "clumsy" gait, difficulty with running or other sports activities, difficulty rising from squatting position

5) Slow progression, some wheelchair use may be needed by 2/3 of patients older than 50 (range, 12-82 years)

6) Weakness: limb-girdle, later affecting anterior compartment (more than posterior compartment) muscles and extensors (more than flexors)

7) Flexion contractures at lateral four fingers, elbows, and ankles eventually present in all patients; usually apparent by end of first or second decade (there may be congenital contractures that resolve early)

8) Skeletal deformities: pectus excavatum, scoliosis, hypermobility of wrists and fingers evolving into contractures

9) Normal life expectancy

5. LGMD 2: autosomal recessive inheritance

a. LGMD 2A: calpainopathy

1) Mutation of calpain-3 protein (*CAPN3* gene on chromosome 15q15.1-q21.1): calcium-activated intracellular protease that may be involved in regulation of transcription and expression of genes involved in cell survival

a) Mutation may cause apoptosis, with altered activity of the transcription factor NF-κB (nuclear factor κB) involved in cell survival

2) Age at onset: usually between ages 8 and 15 years (range, 2-40 years)

3) Delayed walking, "toe-walking" may be noted early on in disease

4) Slow progression, some wheelchair use usually needed

5) Symmetric weakness of proximal limb-girdle and trunk muscles, including rectus abdominis, periscapular muscles, proximal arm and leg muscles; later involvement of ankle dorsiflexion and wrist extension

6) Selective atrophy of hip extensors and adductors

7) Quadriceps may be relatively spared until more advanced disease stage

8) Facial and bulbar muscles spared

9) Minimal neck involvement

10) Cardiac function normal

11) Calf hypertrophy

12) Contractures around ankles, hips, knees, elbows mild and usually more prominent later with disease progression

13) Creatine kinase: levels may be elevated 10 to 100 times normal

14) Muscle histopathology: necrosis and regeneration, muscle fiber size variability, internal nuclei, type I muscle fiber predominance, lobulation of type I muscle fibers

b. LGMD 2B: dysferlinopathy

  1) Mutations in dysferlin gene (*DYSF*) lead to either LGMD 2B or Miyoshi myopathy

  2) Age at onset: usually second to third decade of life

  3) Mild phenotype, but phenotypic heterogeneity: typically pelvic-girdle weakness in legs (waddling gait), followed by involvement of arm

  4) Relatively early involvement of distal muscles (relatively early involvement of gastrocnemius and soleus before tibialis anterior muscles)

  5) Upper extremity muscles primarily affected include biceps brachii, with relative preservation of shoulder-girdle muscle groups and periscapular muscles

  6) With progression, most leg muscles may be affected

  7) Loss of ambulation in the fourth decade

  8) Creatine kinase: typically very high levels

  9) Muscle histopathology: dystrophic changes (muscle fiber size variation, degeneration, necrosis with fiber splitting, increased endomysial connective tissue) and dysferlin staining absent or reduced

c. Sarcoglycanopathies (LGMD 2C-2F)

  1) Phenotype similar to Duchenne's and Becker's muscular dystrophies: similar pattern of weakness, associated with calf hypertrophy

  2) Age at onset: generally earlier in life than other forms of LGMD; median age, 6 to 8 years (milder course of disease with adult onset)

  3) Weakness initially detectable in pelvic girdle, proximal leg, followed by shoulder muscle groups (particularly deltoid, biceps, and infraspinatus muscles)

  4) Progression to involve distal muscle groups (preferentially anterior compartment muscles such as tibialis anterior muscle) and trunk

  5) Calf hypertrophy common

  6) Early lordosis common because of early axial and trunk muscle involvement

  7) Macroglossia

  8) Creatine kinase: severely elevated levels early in disease course, later levels decrease

  9) Cardiac involvement common (often subclinical) in β- and δ-sarcoglycanopathies, rare in γ- and α-sarco-

glycanopathies

d. LGMD 2G: telethoninopathy

  1) Phenotypic heterogeneity

  2) Atrophic myopathy: proximal and distal (predominantly anterior compartment) muscle groups

  3) Childhood onset with progression noticed in the second or third decade and wheelchair-bound by 30s or 40s

  4) Creatine kinase: mildly elevated levels

  5) Rimmed vacuoles seen on muscle biopsy and telethonin absent from muscle

e. LGMD 2I: fukutin-related proteinopathy

  1) Mutation of the *FKRP* gene on chromosome 19q13.3, encoding fukutin-related protein

  2) Phenotypic heterogeneity

  3) Mutation of *FKRP* gene also causes congenital muscular dystrophy with muscle hypertrophy and congenital merosin-deficient muscular dystrophy

  4) Age at onset: may be infantile (with hypotonia and delayed motor milestones), childhood, or young adulthood (normal early motor milestones)

  5) Weakness: predominantly pelvic girdle (also proximal upper extremities)

  6) Facial weakness: rare

  7) Macroglossia (most apparent in early-onset disease), calf hypertrophy

  8) Normal intelligence

  9) Dilated cardiomyopathy

  10) Respiratory insufficiency due to diaphragmatic weakness

  11) Creatine kinase: high

f. LGMD 2J: titinopathy

  1) Genetics: mutation of gene coding for titin, on chromosome 2q31

  2) Clinical phenotype of proximal limb-girdle weakness

  3) Onset: usually in childhood, wheelchair-bound by second decade

  4) Creatine kinase: high levels

H. Distal Myopathies

1. Late adult-onset hereditary distal myopathies

  a. Welander's (late onset type I) distal myopathy

    1) Late-onset distal myopathy

    2) Autosomal dominant inheritance, linked to chromosome 2p13 (same locus for Miyoshi distal myopathy and LGMD 2B)

    3) Mean age at onset: 47 years (range, 20-77 years)

    4) Distal weakness: upper extremities more than lower extremities

    5) Intrinsic hand muscles and finger extensors affected

first; initial symptoms at onset include clumsiness of fine-finger movements

6) Distal lower extremity weakness affecting mainly anterior compartment; toe and ankle extensors (develops with progression)

7) Slow progression with normal life span

8) Mild sensory neuropathy, may be subclinical

9) Creatine kinase: normal or mildly elevated levels

10) Muscle histopathology: dystrophic changes consisting of increased variation in muscle fiber size, increased endomysial connective tissue, central nuclei, fiber splitting, rimmed vacuoles

b. Tibial (Finnish) muscular dystrophy (Udd myopathy, late adult-onset IIa)

1) Late-onset distal myopathy

2) Autosomal dominant inheritance, linked to chromosome 2q31

3) Age at onset: fourth decade or later (childhood onset in homozygotes)

4) Selective involvement of distal lower extremity anterior compartment (anterior tibialis); later, proximal lower extremity

5) Slow progression: footdrop becomes more prominent

6) Creatine kinase: normal or mildly elevated levels

7) Muscle histopathology: dystrophic changes with rimmed vacuoles

c. Markesbery-Griggs (late adult-onset type IIb) distal myopathy

1) Late-onset distal myopathy

2) Autosomal dominant inheritance, linked to chromosome 10q

3) Affected protein: ZASP protein (Z band alternatively spliced PDZ motif-containing protein)

4) With progression: proximal arm and leg weakness

5) Age at onset: after age 40

6) Distal weakness beginning in anterior compartment of legs

7) Cardiomyopathy in some patients

8) Creatine kinase: normal or mildly elevated levels

9) Muscle histopathology: dystrophic changes with rimmed vacuoles

10) Allelic variant: ZASP-related myofibrillar myopathy

2. Early adult-onset hereditary distal myopathies

a. Nonaka distal myopathy (hereditary inclusion body myopathy)

1) Early adult-onset distal myopathy

2) Autosomal recessive inheritance, due to mutation of gene *GNE* on chromosome 9p (to date, 40 different mutations identified, most of which are missense mutations)

3) Original descriptions in Japan and Iranian Jewish families

4) Age at onset: usually second or third decade

5) Initial symptoms: gait disturbance and footdrop

6) Weakness with early and preferential involvement of distal anterior compartment muscles (ankle dorsiflexors and toe extensors), followed by proximal limb-girdle muscles with sparing of quadriceps muscles (even with advanced disease)

7) Weakness in upper extremities: shoulder-girdle muscles, wrist extensors, and intrinsic hand muscles; relative sparing of deltoid muscles

8) Sparing of bulbar muscles

9) Neck flexor weakness

10) Usually wheelchair-bound about 20 years after onset

11) Creatine kinase: mildly elevated levels

12) Muscle histopathology: rimmed autophagic vacuoles

b. Distal dysferlinopathy (Miyoshi myopathy)

1) Early adult-onset distal myopathy (type II)

2) Autosomal recessive inheritance, due to mutation of gene *DYSF* on chromosome 2p13 (coding for dysferlin)

3) Allelic with LGMD 2B

4) Asymptomatic patients may have mild muscular wasting

5) Age at onset: usually early adulthood (ages 15-30); mean age, 19 years

6) Slowly progressive weakness and atrophy of distal lower extremities, preferentially affecting posterior compartment muscle groups, with prominent involvement of gastrocnemius muscles (may be asymmetric)

7) Anterior compartment muscles, forearm muscles, proximal upper and lower extremities may be affected as disease progresses; relative sparing of intrinsic hand muscles

8) Variable progression

9) 1/3 of patients may require wheelchair after 10 years

10) Proximal pelvic girdle weakness at onset is suggestive of allelic condition LGMD 2B

11) Creatine kinase: markedly elevated levels (20-150 times normal)

12) Muscle histopathology: dystrophic changes with evidence of necrosis and degeneration, regeneration, increased endomysial connective tissue, abnormal variation in size, and perimysial and perivascular inflammatory infiltrates observed in some

c. Laing distal myopathy

1) Early adult-onset distal myopathy (type III)

2) Autosomal dominant inheritance; due to mutation of

MHC7 gene encoding protein myosin heavy chain 7, linked to chromosome 14q

   3) Other mutations of *MHC7* can cause isolated hypertrophic cardiomyopathy

   4) Age at onset: between 4 and 35 years

   5) Distal weakness at onset, preferentially affecting distal anterior compartment muscles (tibialis anterior), sternocleidomastoid muscle, and neck flexors

   6) With progression: finger extensor weakness; later, hip and shoulder-girdle weakness; relative preservation of intrinsic hand muscles

   7) Some patients have dilated cardiomyopathy

   8) Muscle histopathology: nonspecific changes

3. Distal myopathy with vocal cord and pharyngeal weakness

  a. Autosomal dominant inheritance, linked to chromosome 5q31, same locus as LGMD 1A

  b. Age at onset: fourth to sixth decades

  c. Distal upper and lower extremities (asymmetric early on), vocal cord, and pharyngeal weakness

  d. Lower extremity weakness usually starts in anterior compartment

  e. Onset of vocal cord weakness (hypophonic, hypernasal speech) usually after limb weakness

  f. Creatine kinase: normal or mildly elevated levels

  g. Muscle histopathology: rimmed vacuoles

I. Congenital Muscular Dystrophies

1. Autosomal recessive inheritance

2. Usually discovered at birth

3. Clinical course: variable (benign to death within first decade)

4. Diffuse weakness and hypotonia on presentation at birth

5. Associated with dysgenesis of brain and eye, especially type II lissencephaly (neuronal overmigration into leptomeninges)

6. Fukuyama congenital muscular dystrophy (FMDC)

  a. Autosomal recessive inheritance; caused by mutation of *fukutin* gene on chromosome 9q31

  b. Gene product (fukutin) expressed in brain, skeletal and cardiac muscle, pancreas, fetal Cajal-Retzius cells, and fetal cerebellum

  c. Clinical course: marked by diffuse weakness, ocular manifestations, and central nervous system (CNS) involvement (mental retardation and seizures)

  d. In utero: fetal movements may be poor

  e. Usually normal at birth, some have hypotonia, lack of head control with "myopathic facies" (with open, inverted V-shaped mouth) due to facial diplegia

  f. Presentation: typically in infancy, with severe weakness

and delayed development; never learn to walk, bedridden before age 10 (some may be able only to sit with support)

  g. Mean life expectancy: 15 years

  h. Joint contractures develop during first year, initially affecting ankles and knees

  i. Macroglossia by age 5 to 6 years

  j. Ocular manifestations: cataracts, strabismus, severe myopia, abnormal extraocular movements, optic pallor and atrophy, retinal detachment

  k. CNS manifestations

   1) Mental retardation (usually severe)

   2) Progressive hydrocephalus

   3) Microcephaly

   4) Seizures before age 3 years

  l. CNS anatomic changes

   1) Type II lissencephaly: pachygyria-agyria (overmigration of neuroblasts into leptomeninges, with occasional absence of gray matter lamination)

   2) Ventriculomegaly

   3) White matter: hypomyelination, diffuse lucencies

   4) Hypoplasia of corticospinal tracts

  m. Cardiac manifestations: dialted cardimyopathy, myocardial fibrosis, CHF may develop (usually in second decade)

  n. Creatinc kinasc: usually markedly elevated levels

  o. Muscle histopathology: dystrophic changes (internal nuclei, variability in fiber size, and fibrosis), with reduced expression of laminin α2, and severely reduced or absent glycosylated α-dystroglycan

7. Congenital muscular dystrophy with laminin α2 (merosin) deficiency (MDC 1A)

  a. Autosomal recessive inheritance; mutation of *LAMA2* gene on chromosome 6q2, encoding laminin α2 protein

  b. Laminins

   1) Extracellular proteins that bind to α-dystroglycans and integrins and interact with other extracellular proteins

   2) Responsible for anchoring dystroglycan complex to extracellular matrix (discussed above)

  c. In utero: fetal movements may be reduced

  d. At birth or infancy: hypotonia, poor feeding (poor swallowing, difficulty chewing, gastroesophageal reflux); persists to some degree, leading to poor nutrition

  e. Delayed motor development and contractures of feet and hips

  f. Diffuse, symmetric, nonprogressive weakness affecting both proximal and distal limb muscle groups and facial muscles (distributed evenly)

  g. Severity: variable (delayed onset and mild weakness in

mild forms, floppy infants with respiratory insufficiency in severe forms)

   h. Normal mentation in most patients (some with learning disabilities, some with mental retardation)

   i. MRI of head

     1) Diffuse abnormal white matter signal, most severe in frontal U fibers and periventricular area

     2) Migration defects: cortical dysplasia, agyria, polymicrogyria

   j. Creatine kinase: usually elevated levels

   k. Deficiency of laminin α2 demonstrated on immuno-histochemical staining of muscle or skin punch biopsy specimens

8. Santavuori congenital muscular dystrophy (muscle-eye-brain disease)

   a. Autosomal recessive inheritance; mutation of *POMGnT1* gene on chromosome 1p32-p34

   b. Gene product is glycosyltransferase O-mannose β1,2-*N*-acetylglucosaminyltransferase 1, enzyme responsible for O-mannosyl glycosylation (mannosylation) of α-dystroglycan, required for binding between α-dystroglycan and laminin

   c. Pathophysiology: related to deficient glycosylated α-dystroglycan and deficient laminin α2 binding

   d. Affected protein may also have role in neuronal migration, accounting for migration defects observed in this disorder

   e. Phenotypic heterogeneity

   f. Neonatal hypotonia, visual dysfunction, moderate to severe mental retardation

   g. Ocular manifestations and visual dysfunction causing poor visual contact and recognition of relatives: severe myopia, cataracts, glaucoma, retinal dysplasia or detachment, optic colobomas

   h. CNS structural malformations

     1) Polymicrogyria and pachygyria-agyria

     2) Features of dysmyelination: absent or partially absent corpus callosum and septum pellucidum

     3) Ventriculomegaly

     4) Hypoplastic corticospinal tracts

9. Walker-Warburg syndrome (WWS)

   a. Autosomal recessive inheritance; often due to mutation of *POMT1* gene on chromosome 9q34

   b. Mutation of *POMT2* gene on chromosome 14q24.3 has also been identified, with similar phenotype

   c. Gene product is an O-mannosyltransferase, important for mannosylation of α-dystroglycan, together with O-mannose β1,2-*N*-acetylglucosaminyltransferase noted above (the latter is deficient in muscle-eye-brain disease)

   d. Pathophysiology: related to deficient glycosylated α-

dystroglycan and deficient laminin α2 binding, as in muscle-eye-brain disease

   e. Syndrome of brain malformations, cerebellar malformations, retinal malformations, and congenital muscular dystrophy

   f. Severe mental retardation and seizures

   g. Ocular malformations: unilateral or bilateral microphthalmia, cataracts, glaucoma, retinal detachment, ocular coloboma, hypoplastic or absent optic nerve

   h. Muscular dystrophy usually present at birth: poor feeding and hypotonia

   i. Creatine kinase: severely elevated levels

   j. CNS structural malformations: similar to those of other congenital muscular dystrophies but more severe

     1) Severe hydrocephalus

     2) Encephaloceles (not reported in muscle-eye-brain disease or Fukuyama congenital muscular dystrophy)

     3) Complete type II lissencephaly (overmigration into leptomeninges) with pontocerebellar hypoplasia

V. CHANNELOPATHIES

A. General Characteristics of Periodic Paralysis (Table 24-2)

1. Autosomal dominant inheritance, with complete penetrance in men (about 50% in women)

2. Clinical manifestation: mainly periodic paralysis (intermittent weakness), muscle stiffness, and paramyotonia

3. Respiratory and cranial musculature relatively spared (exception: some hyperkalemic patients have facial muscle myotonia)

4. Clinical heterogeneity depends on

   a. The ion involved

   b. Properties of the ion channel (Table 24-3)

   c. Increased (myotonia) or decreased muscle excitability

5. In patients with sporadic periodic paralysis but no family history, other causes must be excluded (Table 24-4)

6. Serum potassium level during an attack may be normal, serial measurements may be needed

B. Periodic Paralysis Without Myotonia

1. Familial hypokalemic periodic paralysis (HypoPP)

   a. HypoPP type I

     1) Mutation of *CACNL1AS* gene on chromosome 1q31-32, encoding α1 subunit of dihydropyridine-sensitive L-type calcium channel (substitution of positively charged arginine residues in voltage-sensitive S4 segment of domains II and IV)

     2) Autosomal dominant inheritance

b. Possible mechanism of action
  1) Reduced extracellular potassium concentration causes prolonged depolarization in affected muscle (instead of normal hyperpolarization), triggering inactivation of sodium channels
  2) Reduction of calcium influx into muscle, decreased activation of ryanodine receptors, decreased calcium release from sarcoplasmic reticulum stores, muscle hypoexcitability, and reduced muscle contraction
c. HypoPP type II: mutation of *SCN4A* gene on chromosome 17q13, encoding α subunit of sodium channel, mutation causes enhancement of sodium channel slow inactivation and delay of recovery after repolarization
d. HypoPP type III: mutation of *KCNE3* gene on chromo-

some 11q13-14, encoding voltage-gated potassium channel β subunit
e. Similar phenotype observed with different genetic mutations
f. Age at onset
  1) Usually adolescence or young adulthood (usually fewer attacks after third decade)
  2) Severe cases have onset in childhood; mild cases, later age at onset (as late as third decade)
g. Precipitating factors for attacks: heavy carbohydrate meal, heavy exercise followed by period of rest, local anesthetic, fasting, dehydration, exposure to cold, administration of insulin, or other causes of increased insulin secretion
h. Characteristics of attacks

Table 24-2. **Clinical and Electrophysiologic Features of Myotonic and Periodic Paralysis (PP) Disorders**

Feature	Myotonic dystrophy	Myotonia congenita		Paramyotonia	HyperPP	HypoPP
Inheritance	Dominant	Dominant	Recessive	Dominant	Dominant	Dominant
Age at onset	2nd-3rd decades	Infancy	Early childhood	Infancy	Infancy-early childhood	Early teens
Duration of PP	No PP	No PP	Minutes	Minutes-days	Minutes-days	Hours-days
Provocative factors	None	Cold	Cold	Cold	Cold	Cold
		Exercise after rest	Exercise after rest	Fasting	Rest after exercise	Rest after exercise
					Fasting	Carbohydrate-enriched meals
Alleviating factors	None	Repeated exercise	Repeated exercise	Warming	---	Potassium
CMAP						
Amplitude after brief exercise	↓	↓	↓↓	↓ (with muscle cooling)	No change	No change
Amplitude after cooling	No change	No change	No change	↓↓	No change	No change
Decrement at rest after 2-Hz repetitive stimulation	+	+	++	None	None	None
Motor unit potentials (duration)	Myopathic (↓)	Normal	Normal, may be myopathic	Normal	Normal, myopathic late in course	Normal, myopathic late in course
Myotonia	Long, slow	Brief, rapid	Brief, rapid	Long, slow (rare)	Long, slow	None

CMAP, compound muscle action potential; HyperPP, hyperkalemic periodic paralysis; HypoPP, hypokalemic periodic paralysis; ↓, decrease; ↓↓, greater decrease.

Table 24-3. Classification of Channelopathies Associated With Periodic Paralysis

Chloride channelopathies
  Autosomal dominant myotonia congenita (Thomsen's disease)
  Autosomal recessive myotonia congenita (Becker dystrophy)
Sodium channelopathies (with or without paralysis)
  Potassium-aggravated myotonias
  Hyperkalemic periodic paralysis
  Paramyotonia congenita
  Hypokalemic periodic paralysis type II
Calcium channelopathies
  Hypokalemic periodic paralysis, type I

Table 24-4. Differential Diagnosis of Periodic Paralysis

Calcium abnormalities other than channelopathies
Potassium abnormalities other than channelopathies
Hypophosphatemia
Hypermagnesemia
Thyrotoxicosis
Rhabdomyolysis
Myasthenia gravis
Lambert-Eaton myasthenic syndrome

1) Attack usually begins with sensation of heaviness or aching fatigue and progresses to weakness (proximal > distal); begins in most recently exercised muscles
2) Attacks are more severe and last longer (but less frequent) than hyperkalemic form
3) Weakness usually lasts several hours, but mild residual weakness may last for up to 3 to 4 days
4) Diurnal fluctuation: weakest during the night and early morning, best in midday
5) Attack may be severe and patient unable to move; the muscle may be electrically and mechanically inexcitable and reflexes lost at height of weakness
6) Respiratory function not usually compromised
7) Cranial musculature rarely affected
8) Affected muscle may feel swollen
  i. Frequency of attacks
    1) Typically occur once or twice weekly (less frequent with increasing age)
    2) Severe cases: attacks may be daily; may not be full recovery between attacks
  k. Most patients develop permanent myopathy of variable

severity
  l. Diagnosis based on demonstration of weakness caused by low levels of potassium (poor correlation between potassium level and clinical syndrome)
  m. Potassium is released from muscle at end of an attack
  n. Low potassium levels between attacks suggest secondary HypoPP
  o. Provocative maneuvers may be helpful (including oral glucose load), continuous electrocardiographic (ECG) monitoring required
  p. Genetic testing: preferred method of diagnosis
  q. Secondary causes of HypoPP: thyrotoxicosis, primary hyperaldosteronism, potassium-depleting diuretics, gastrointestinal potassium wasting (diarrhea), renal potassium wasting, corticosteroid use, alcoholism, lithium
  r. Muscle histopathology
    1) May be normal or show minimal myopathic changes
    2) Few vacuoles may be seen if permanent weakness
  s. Treatment
    1) Acute treatment with oral potassium
    2) Prophylaxis with acetazolamide (prevention of attack recurrence and improvement of weakness during each attack)
    3) Dichlorphenamide (another carbonic anhydrase inhibitor)
    4) Triamterene and spironolactone as adjunctive agents
    5) Low sodium or low carbohydrate diets may be helpful
  t. Prognosis and chances of permanent weakness: depends on frequency of episodic weakness
2. Thyrotoxic periodic paralysis
  a. Age at onset: usually between third and fifth decades
  b. Predisposition for Asians
  c. A secondary hypokalemic periodic paralysis
  d. Tendency to develop weakness with thyrotoxicosis may be inherited as autosomal dominant
  e. Thyrotoxicosis usually precedes or occurs with the attack
  f. Symmetric proximal weakness most often affects legs during attack
  g. Maximal weakness upon awakening
  h. Muscle stiffness and cramps precede weakness
  i. Respiratory and bulbar muscles relatively spared
  j. Symptoms of thyrotoxicosis
  k. Treatment
    1) Acute attacks: replace potassium, avoid rebound hyperkalemia
    2) Treat underlying thyroid disorder; propranolol for associated symptoms
3. Andersen's syndrome
  a. Syndrome of periodic paralysis, cardiac arrhythmias, dysmorphic features

b. Autosomal dominant inheritance, mutation of *KCNJ2* gene on chromosome 17q23, encoding an inwardly rectifying potassium channel (Kir2.1)

c. Age at onset: usually childhood

d. Some with permanent muscle weakness

e. Cardiac dysrrhythmias: long QT syndrome, ventricular extrasystoles

f. Dysmorphic features: may include hypertelorism, broad nose, low-set ears, short index finger, clinodactyly of fifth finger, syndactyly of toes, scoliosis, cryptorchidism

C. Sodium Channel Myotonias

1. Genetics and pathophysiology

   a. Autosomal dominant inheritance with high penetrance in both sexes

   b. Missense mutation affecting *SCN4A* gene (chromosome 17q23-25) encoding for α-subunit of the skeletal muscle sodium channel (SkM1, Nav1.4)

   c. Four phenotypes (sodium channel myotonias): hyperkalemic periodic paralysis, paramyotonia congenita, potassium-aggravated sodium channel myotonias, and HypoPP type II

   d. Potential mechanism: spontaneous reopening of mutant sodium channels after normal depolarization, causing increased sodium influx

      1) Slight depolarization can cause hyperexitability and myotonia

      2) More prolonged depolarization causes paralysis and inexcitability of muscle fiber

2. Familial hyperkalemic periodic paralysis (HyperPP)

   a. Rest-induced or potassium-induced paralysis

   b. Age at onset: usually in childhood, but patients may show signs and symptoms as early as first year of life

   c. Infantile onset: attacks may consist of a sudden change in infant's cry or infant may develop unusual stare with exposure to cold

   d. First attack: usually in childhood, may be provoked by enforced sitting in school

   e. Attacks

      1) Usually frequent, focal, short duration (usually 15 minutes to 1-2 hours, up to 4-5 hours); may occur several times daily

      2) Increase in frequency and severity with time

      3) Milder and shorter duration than HypoPP

      4) May be aborted by exercise early in episode

      5) May be precipitated by exposure to cold, rest after exercise or oral intake of potassium, emotional stress, pregnancy

      6) May occur during sleep; may not be a precipitating factor

   f. Episodes more frequent when poor oral intake and high potassium diet

   g. Severity of attacks may range from mild weakness (usually) and fatigue to severe paralysis

   h. Myotonia may or may not be present: generalized distribution if present

   i. Serum potassium measured during an attack: not reliable; often normal but may be high or even low

   j. Creatine kinase: normal or slightly elevated levels

   k. Diagnosis by provocative testing: demonstration of potassium sensitivity to potassium loading (infusion)

      1) Potassium is administered shortly after exercise, and patient is instructed to rest

      2) Potassium levels are closely monitored

      3) Generalized weakness occurs usually within 1 hour, may last up to an hour, and may involve respiratory muscles

      4) Must be avoided in patients with renal insufficiency

      5) Continuous ECG monitoring is necessary for the load

      6) If negative, loading may be repeated

   l. Muscle histopathology: usually normal, but vacuolar changes may eventually occur

   m. Electrodiagnostic evaluation

      1) CMAPs

         a) Normal amplitude, with no decrement at slow or fast rates of repetitive stimulation

         b) No change with cooling

      2) Needle EMG

         a) Myotonic discharges: long and slow discharges

   n. Secondary causes of HyperPP: renal failure, adrenal failure, potassium-sparing diuretics, hypoaldosteronism

   o. Treatment

      1) Acute treatment may not be needed because of brevity of attacks

      2) Ingestion of carbohydrates and sugars may prevent or abort attack

      3) Prophylaxis with hydrochlorothiazide and carbonic anhydrase inhibitors (acetazolamide and dichlorphenamide)

3. Potassium-aggravated myotonia congenita (delayed myotonias): myotonia fluctuans and myotonia permanens

   a. Muscle stiffness provoked by exercise; has distinguishing feature of initial nonmyotonic interval, unlike paradoxical myotonia (paramyotonia, discussed below)

   b. "Warm-up phenomenon": alleviation of muscle stiffness with continued muscle contraction and exercise (unlike paramyotonia)

   c. Myotonia: variation in intensity, may be severe and cause patient to fall or to be unable to rise from a seated position

d. Stiffness occurs during rest after a period of exercise (delayed)

e. Exacerbation of myotonia when given potassium, and improvement with administration of carbonic anhydrase inhibitors

f. Stiffness may affect rested muscles with quick movements such as quick saccades or forceful biting

g. Myotonic discharges on needle examination, not aggravated with cooling

h. Treatment: mexiletine and acetazolamide

4. Paramyotonia congenita

a. Autosomal dominant inheritance

b. Mutation of gene *SCN4A*, encoding α-subunit of voltage-gated sodium channel

c. Mutation affects fast inactivation and deactivation of sodium channels, responsible for persistant membrane depolarization from cumulative increase of sodium flux during activation

d. Paradoxical myotonia: muscle stiffness or persistent involuntary muscle contraction after brief voluntary contraction that worsens with repeated muscle contraction or exercise (vs. true myotonia, in which repeated muscle contraction and exercise decrease muscle stiffness)

e. Muscle stiffness is extremely cold sensitive

f. Age at onset: infancy or childhood

g. Persistent eye closure or facial grimacing in infants after crying or exposure to cold washcloth

h. Weakness especially noted with exposure to cold

i. Delayed opening of eyelids after repeated eyelid closure

j. Action or percussion myotonia after limb cooling

k. Electrodiagnostic evaluation

1) Nerve conduction studies

a) Normal nerve conduction

b) Decrement to slow repetitive stimulation when muscles are cooled (uncommon at rest)

c) Short exercise test when muscle is cooled: sudden decrease in amplitude with slow subsequent recovery on warming (unlike myotonic syndromes or periodic paralysis)

2) Needle examination

a) Rare myotonic discharges: long, slow discharges, as with myotonic dystrophy

b) Small motor unit potentials with fibrillation potentials may be observed late in disease course, likely reflect pathologic changes described below

c) Response to cooling (in sequence): increase in fibrillation potentials (disappear below 28ºC), disappearance of myotonic discharges, and electrical silence (below 20ºC)

d) Rewarming: slow return of voluntary and spontaneous activity

e) Single fiber EMG: increased jitter, with blocking

l. Muscle histopathology: unremarkable; possibly nonspecific changes such as central nuclei, fiber size variation, and hypertrophic, atrophic, or regenerative fibers

m. Treatment

1) Avoidance of precipitating factors such as cold or exercise

2) Patients may become weak with potassium depletion

3) Prophylactic treatment with sodium channel blockers such as mexiletine or tocainide

D. Chloride Channel Myotonias: *myotonia congenita*

1. General characteristics

a. Genetics and pathophysiology

1) Due to mutations of gene *CLCN1* on chromosome 7q, encoding sarcolemmal voltage-gated chloride channel

2) Chloride channels: responsible for chloride current that is activated by depolarization

3) About 70% of conductance in resting muscle is due to chloride ion currents

4) Chloride channels act as buffer and cause large chloride current flow when there is any deviation from the resting muscle membrane potential; this avoids any spontaneous discharges that could be produced by increased muscle excitability from accumulation of potassium ions in T tubules; this duration of depolarization of T tubules is limited by resting chloride current

5) Mutation affecting chloride channel can reduce chloride conductance and cause myotonic activity

6) Autosomal *recessive* myotonia congenita (Becker dystrophy): usually caused by loss of functional channel proteins (due to several different mutations, including deletions and missense mutations)

7) Autosomal *dominant* myotonia congenita (Thomsen's disease): usually caused by loss of function (dominant negative effect) or gain of abnormal function (such as increasing sodium conductance)

b. Thomsen's disease: autosomal dominant myotonia congenita

1) Painless myotonia may be present in infancy (more severe in males)

2) Age at onset: usually first apparent in early adolescence

3) Nearly normal strength, with normal or mildly increased muscle bulk

4) Milder than recessive form

5) Family members may be asymptomatic or have mild symptoms
6) Clinical course: constant, nonprogressive, but may be variable
7) Repetitive muscle use and exercise restores strength
8) Creatine kinase: levels occasionally may be mildly elevated

c. Becker's disease: autosomal recessive myotonia congenita
  1) Weakness, possibly muscle wasting
  2) Both myotonia and weakness can improve with repetitive muscle contraction and exercise
  3) Myotonia presents later and is more severe and disabling than in Thomsen's disease
  4) Myotonia often presents early in the second decade (often between 10 and 14 years), may be slowly progressive
  5) Creatine kinase: higher levels than in Thomsen's disease
  6) Muscle hypertrophy in upper and lower limbs

d. Clinical features
  1) Myotonic muscle stiffness: most prominent with forceful contraction, often after a period of rest, subsides after exercise
  2) Delayed opening of eyelids after forceful contractions
  3) Lid-lag phenomenon: observed with sudden downward gaze, immediately after sustained upward gaze
  4) Delayed opening of fist after forceful contractions
  5) Percussion myotonia
  6) "Warm-up phenomenon": strength returns to normal; myotonia (and accompanying stiffness) is reduced with repetitive activity and exercise
  7) Myotonia may be painless or painful
  8) Myotonia may be subjectively exacerbated by cold (not electrophysiologically) and may be found in face, tongue, and limbs
  9) Muscle hypertrophy
    a) Apparent bulking of muscles with repetitive severe myotonic contractions ("work hypertrophy")
    b) Muscles usually well developed despite weakness

e. Electrophysiology
  1) Slow repetitive stimulation causes small decrement in CMAP amplitude
    a) After brief forceful contraction (exercise), decrement disappears (but CMAP amplitude diminished) and later reappears and is exaggerated progressively
  2) Fast repetitive stimulation also causes decrement in CMAP amplitude; there may be a late facilitation
  3) No decrease in CMAP amplitude after cooling
  4) Needle examination

  a) Myotonic discharges: higher frequencies and shorter durations than those of myotonic dystrophy or paramyotonia congenita
  b) Normal motor unit potentials
  c) During period of transient weakness after brief forceful contraction: decrease in amplitude of motor unit potentials, there may be electrical silence

VI. METABOLIC MYOPATHIES

A. **Disorders of Glycogen Metabolism:** glycogen storage disorders (GSDs)
  1. Type II glycogenosis (acid maltase deficiency)
    a. Genetics and pathophysiology
      1) Autosomal recessive inheritance: deficiency of lysosomal acid maltase (α-1,4-glucosidase), gene locus on chromosome 17q21-23
      2) Residual enzyme activity inversely correlates with disease severity and age at onset
      3) A small amount of glycogen is normally present, continuously degraded to glucose by lysosomal acid maltase
      4) With deficient acid maltase, glycogen accumulates in lysosomes and cytoplasm
      5) Muscle fiber damage secondary to intracellular glycogen accumulation and possibly lysosomal rupture and release of lysosomal enzymes
    b. Pompe's disease (severe infantile form)
      1) Age at onset: within first few months of life
      2) Cardiomegaly, macroglossia, hepatomegaly
      3) Progressive weakness and hypotonia within first 3 months of life (including feeding and neuromuscular respiratory difficulties)
      4) Death: usually within first month, generally from respiratory failure
    c. Childhood acid maltase deficiency
      1) Age at onset: first decade of life
      2) Delayed motor development
      3) Slowly progressive proximal muscle weakness (more than distal), respiratory muscle weakness, calf hypertrophy
      4) Cardiomegaly and hepatomegaly uncommon
      5) Associated with basilar artery aneurysms, possibly because of glycogen deposition in arterial smooth wall
      6) Cause of death usually respiratory complications, respiratory failure
    d. Adult-onset form of acid maltase deficiency
      1) Age at onset: variable, usually in the third or fourth

decade

    2) Partially deficient enzyme

    3) Proximal muscle weakness and atrophy, with possible involvement of face and tongue

    4) Hip adductors and pectoralis major muscles (sternal head) may be selectively affected more severely

    5) Respiratory involvement: one-third present with respiratory insufficiency, almost all eventually have respiratory involvement (usual cause of death)

    6) Possible macroglossia

    7) Cadiomegaly or hepatomegaly not seen

  e. Laboratory tests

    1) Creatine kinase: mildly elevated levels (more prominent in the infantile form)

    2) Liver enzymes may be elevated in children

    3) Acid maltase activity may be measured in muscle, cultured fibroblasts, lymphocytes, urine

    4) Cultured fibroblasts as confirmatory test for patients with low leukocyte activity

    5) Acid maltase enzyme activity on cultured amniotic fluid cells for prenatal diagnosis

    6) Electrophysiology

      a) Low-amplitude CMAPs in atrophic muscles

      b) Rapidly recruiting short-duration motor unit potentials with increased insertional activity, fibrillation potentials, and possibly myotonic discharges seen more often in proximal muscles and diaphragm

  f. Muscle histopathology: autophagic vacuolar myopathy (strongly acid phosphatase positive) with accumulation of glycogen in vacuoles (Fig. 24-11)

2. Type V glycogenosis (McArdle's disease): myophosphorylase deficiency

  a. Autosomal recessive inheritance

  b. Pathophysiology

    1) Myophosphorylase initiates muscle glycogen breakdown (encoding gene is on chromosome 11q13)

    2) Glycogen phosphorylase cleaves α-1,4 glycosidic bonds between glycosyl residues and degrades glycogen chains until four glycosyl residues remain before a branch point; debranching enzyme then removes branches, simplifying glycogen chain complex

    3) Different mutations of the gene identified; all essentially cause reduced enzyme activity

    4) Symptoms of exercise-induced fatigue and contractures may not be due to depleted ATP stores (there may be increased calcium sensitivity, increased extracellular potassium causing depolarization of muscle membrane, and increased intracellular adenosine diphosphate [ADP], inhibiting ADP dissociation

from actin-myosin cross-bridges)

  c. Age at onset: usually first decade

  d. Male predominance

  e. Presents with exercise intolerance

  f. Symptoms (usually noted with high-intensity activities such as weight lifting): exercise intolerance, myalgia, cramps

  g. Sensation of "hitting a barrier," followed by muscle pain, cramps, possibly contractures (electrical silence on EMG) if exercise continues

  h. "Second wind" phenomenon with low-intensity activities: reduced level of exercise after brief rest period following onset of muscle pain or cramps

    1) Likely due to use of metabolism of fatty acids, instead of glycogen metabolism, for source of acetyl-CoA

  i. Myoglobinuria, rhabdomyolysis, possibly renal failure

  j. Some patients may develop progressive proximal weakness in adulthood as presentation

  k. One-third may have fixed weakness after age 40 (possibly due to collective muscle damage)

  l. Laboratory tests

    1) Creatine kinase: elevated levels (variable)

    2) Hyperuricemia

    3) Ischemic forearm exercise test

      a) Intravenous catheter placed

      b) Baseline lactate and ammonia levels determined

      c) Blood pressure cuff placed (proximal to the catheter) and inflated to approximately 20 mm Hg above systolic blood pressure

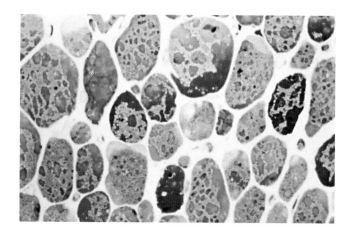

Fig. 24-11. Muscle histopathologic features of infantile acid maltase deficiency. PAS–methylene blue staining demonstrates glycogen accumulation in skeletal muscle fibers. Note vacuoles of various sizes and shapes and filled with PAS–positive material. (Courtesy of Andrew G. Engel, MD.)

d) Exercise for 1 minute by rapid opening and closing of hand

e) Blood pressure cuff removed and serum lactate and ammonia levels measured at 1, 2, 4, 6, and 10 minutes

f) Normal response: 3- to 5-fold increase in lactate and ammonia levels

g) If neither level increases: test is inadequate and needs to be repeated

h) 3- to 5-fold increase in ammonia level without an increase in lactate level: suggests glycogen metabolism disorder

i) In glycolytic disorders, increase in ammonia level is often exaggerated

j) If the ischemic forearm test is abnormal, muscle biochemical analysis may be performed

4) Electrophysiologic studies

a) Motor and sensory nerve conduction studies: usually normal interictally

b) With permanent weakness, CMAP amplitude may be reduced, may be myopathic small motor unit potentials

c) Electrical silence of severe muscle cramps and contractures

d) Decremental response after brief exercise or rapid stimulation (20 Hz for 50 seconds) because of energy failure and electrical silence in some muscle fibers

5) Muscle histopathology

a) Subsarcolemmal and intermyofibrillary accumulation of glycogen and vacuoles

b) Type I fiber atrophy

c) Occasionally, muscle necrosis and regeneration

m. Treatment

1) High protein diet for most patients

2) Better exercise tolerance may be achieved with administration of oral glucose or fructose loads or glucagon administration

3. Glycogenosis type III: Cori disease (debrancher deficiency)

a. Genetics and molecular biochemistry

1) Autosomal recessive inheritance (chromosome 1p)

2) Glycogen branches are removed as follows:

a) Oligo-(α1,4-α1,4)-glucantransferase (glycosyl 4:4 transferase): removes outer three of four glycosyl units at end of each branch

b) Amylo-α-(1,6)-glucosidase activity removes remaining glycosyl unit that has α-1,6 linkage to glycogen complex

3) Debranching enzyme complex is responsible for removing branches and simplifying glycogen chain complex, so ongoing glycogen myophosphorylase activity can further decrease glycogen chain

4) Deficiency of enzyme causes glycogen accumulation in muscle and, to some degree, in peripheral nerves

b. Clinical features

1) Disease types

a) GSD type IIIa (85%)

i) Deficiency of the debrancher enzyme in both liver and muscle

ii) Slowly progressive weakness

iii) Age at onset: usually third or fourth decade

b) GSD type IIIb (15%): liver involvement only

i) Benign disease, presenting in infancy and childhood with hepatomegaly, failure to thrive, fasting hypoglycemia

ii) Some patients with liver failure

2) Infantile onset

a) Recurrent hypoglycemia, seizures, predominant liver dysfunction and hepatomegaly, severe cardiomegaly

b) Death before age 5 years

3) Childhood onset

a) Liver dysfunction and hepatomegaly, seizures, recurrent hypoglycemia, growth retardation

b) Transient muscle weakness, resolves by puberty

4) Adult onset

a) Age at onset: after third decade

b) Slowly progressive muscle weakness and atrophy (distal or proximal)

c) Liver dysfunction and mild cardiomyopathy may be seen

d) 50% of patients: myalgias, muscle cramps, stiffness, and exercise intolerance

e) Associated with distal sensorimotor polyneuropathy

c. Laboratory features

1) Muscle, fibroblasts, or lymphocyte biochemical assays

2) Creatine kinase: elevated levels at rest, 5 to 45 times normal

3) ECG: may show conduction defects and arrhythmias (echocardiography may show ventricular hypertrophy)

4) Electrophysiology

a) Nerve conduction studies: may show axonal neuropathy (caused by glycogen accumulating in peripheral nerves)

b) Needle examination

i) May show combination of denervation and myopathic features distally

ii) Myopathic features with fibrillation potentials, complex repetitive discharges, and myotonic discharges

5) Muscle histopathology: vacuolar myopathy with abnormal subsarcolemmal and intermyofibrillary glycogen accumulation; similar to acid maltase deficiency except for poor acid phosphatase staining, suggesting glycogen accumulation is not primarily lysosomal

4. Glycogenosis type IV: Andersen's disease (branching enzyme deficiency)
   a. Pathophysiology and genetics
      1) Autosomal recessive inheritance (linked to chromosome 3)
      2) Mutation of 1,4-α-glucan branching enzyme (responsible for production of branched glycogen molecule)
      3) Result: accumulation of abnormal linear glycogen chains with few branch points
   b. Phenotypic heterogeneity
   c. Liver disease predominates clinical picture
   d. Infantile and childhood onset: rapidly progressive disorder with splenomegaly, hepatomegaly (with cirrhosis and liver failure), and sometimes muscle weakness and atrophy with hypotonia
   e. Death: usually before age 4 years, usually from liver failure or gastrointestinal tract bleeding
   f. Hydrops fetalis may occur if congenital
   g. Cardiomegaly in some patients
   h. Primarily CNS involvement: polyglucosan body disease phenotype; adults with progressive upper and lower motor neuron weakness, sensory neuropathy, cerebellar ataxia, and dementia
   i. Laboratory features
      1) Creatine kinase: levels sometimes elevated
      2) Electrodiagnostic evaluation may show features of axonal sensorimotor peripheral neuropathy in adults
      3) Muscle histopathology: polyglucosan bodies (PAS-positive filamentous polysaccharide deposition) in CNS, peripheral nerves, muscle, skin, liver
   j. Treatment: liver transplantation may be beneficial, especially for children with liver cirrhosis and portal hypertension

5. Glycogenosis type VII: phosphofructokinase deficiency (Tarui's disease)
   a. Autosomal recessive inheritance
   b. Absence or reduced phosphofructokinase levels in muscle or red blood cells
   c. Several mutations identified in gene for M isoform of phosphofructokinase on chromosome 1
   d. Clinical features similar to McArdle's disease (exercise intolerance with muscle pain, cramps, contractures)
   e. Male predominance (9:1)
   f. Age at onset: usually second to fourth decades
   g. Exercise intolerance, with muscle pain, cramps, contractures, "second wind phenomenon," and myoglobinuria, similar to McArdle's disease but less severe and less frequent
   h. Exercise intolerance may be exacerbated with high carbohydrate meals, which may reduce serum free fatty acid levels
   i. Late onset: fixed proximal (occasionally scapuloperoneal) myopathy, usually with exercise intolerance when younger
   j. Other features: hemolytic anemia, hyperuricemia and gout, hyperbilirubinemia, gastric ulcers, hepatomegaly
   k. Other variants
      1) Severe infantile form with fixed weakness, respiratory failure, cardiomyopathy
         a) Some with arthrogryposis, corneal clouding, seizures, cortical blindness
      2) Hemolytic anemia without myopathy
   l. Laboratory features
      1) Creatine kinase: high levels
      2) Hyperbilirubinemia
      3) Hyperuricemia (due to degradation of ATP to adenosine monophosphate [AMP], which is metabolized to uric acid and other purine metabolites)
      4) No lactate level increase on ischemic exercise test
      5) Diagnosis: biochemical and histochemical analysis demonstrating phosphofructokinase deficiency and reduced activity and staining
   m. Muscle histopathology
      1) Subsarcolemmal glycogen accumulation and vacuoles
      2) Glycogen content may be normal or high
      3) Myopathic dystrophic changes
      4) PAS-positive polysaccharide bodies possible

B. **Lipid Metabolism and Related Disorders**
1. Physiology of lipid metabolism
   a. Mobilization of fatty acids
      1) Free fatty acids (FFAs) move through adipocyte cell membranes and are bound immediately by albumin
      2) Albumin-bound FFAs are transported to muscle and other tissues, where they are oxidized for ATP generation
   b. Transport of FFAs across inner mitochondrial membrane
      1) First, FFAs must be transferred across inner mitochondrial membrane to be oxidized
      2) Long-chain FFAs do not readily pass mitochondrial membranes and must be modified (unlike short-

chain and medium-chain FFAs)

3) Long-chain FFAs first combine with coenzyme (CoA) in reaction catalyzed by acyl CoA synthetase to make fatty acyl CoA

4) Fatty acyl CoA combines with cytosolic carnitine in reaction catalyzed by carnitine palmitoyltransferase 1 (CPT1) located on outer mitochondrial membrane, producing free CoA released into cytosol and fatty acyl carnitine

5) Fatty acyl carnitine complex is transported across inner mitochondrial membrane in exchange for carnitine, the latter being transported out of mitochondrion in opposite direction to combine with another fatty acyl CoA

6) Fatty acyl carnitine complex (now inside mitochondrion) combines with free CoA in reaction catalyzed by carnitine palmitoyltransferase 2 (CPT2) located on inner mitochondrial membrane, producing fatty acyl CoA and free carnitine, which is transported outside mitochondrion in exchange for another fatty acyl carnitine complex

c. β-Oxidation of FFAs

1) Repetitive series of enzymatic reactions to eventually break down fatty acyl CoA to acetyl CoA

2) Occurs inside mitochondrial matrix

3) Each acetyl CoA provides 12 ATP molecules when converted into carbon dioxide and water by Krebs' cycle

4) Reactions of β-oxidation also yield NADH and reduced form of flavin adenine dinucleotide ($FADH_2$), which provide ATP when oxidized by electron transport chain

2. General characteristics of disorders of fatty acid metabolism

a. Failure of FFA oxidation to meet increased metabolic demand

b. Failure of long-chain FFA transfer across mitochondrial membrane makes this unavailable for use by affected tissue; may cause abnormal accumulation of excess FFAs and chronic myopathy (lipid storage myopathy) or cause rhabdomyolysis and myoglobinuria when metabolic demand increases

c. Defective long-chain FFA metabolism: more severe presentation than lipid storage diseases involving short- or medium-chain FFAs

d. Symptomatic hypoglycemia: reduced synthesis of acetyl CoA reduces ketogenesis (reduced ketones in times of increased metabolic demand), causing increased use of peripheral glucose

e. Cardiac and skeletal muscles depend on metabolism of long-chain FFAs for energy: dysfunction produces myopathy and cardiomyopathy

f. With exercise (increased metabolic demand), glycogen stores and plasma glucose are depleted, rhabdomyolysis may occur

g. Symptoms are induced by

1) Exercise

2) Fasting (in which predominant energy source is ketones)

3) Exposure to cold and body's natural response to increase core temperature, including shivering (muscle metabolism highly dependent on oxidation of long-chain FFAs); rhabdomyolysis may occur

4) Infection

3. Carnitine deficiency

a. Secondary carnitine deficiency: organic acidurias, mitochondrial respiratory chain defects, malnutrition, renal failure, medications (including valproate)

b. Primary carnitine deficiency: primary defect of carnitine transport system (two phenotypes: primary systemic carnitine deficiency, primary muscle carnitine deficiency)

c. Autosomal recessive inheritance (primary carnitine deficiency)

d. Primary muscle carnitine deficiency

1) Slowly progressive cardiomyopathy (dilated or hypertrophic)

2) Myopathy: progressive proximal weakness with atrophy, worsens during pregnancy

3) Not associated with encephalopathy

e. Primary systemic carnitine deficiency (age at onset: 3 months-2 years)

1) Recurrent episodes of encephalopathy related to hypoglycemia and hypoketonemia

2) Hepatomegaly

3) Muscle involvement: progressive proximal myopathy, not a prominent feature

f. Reduced plasma and tissue carnitine levels in primary systemic and secondary carnitine deficiency (only muscle carnitine levels decreased in primary muscle carnitine deficiency)

g. Creatine kinase: normal or elevated (especially with fasting) levels

h. Urine ketones are elevated with fasting

i. Treatment: oral carnitine supplementation

4. CPT2 deficiency

a. Autosomal recessive inheritance

b. CPT2 deficiency type 1

1) Most common disorder of lipid metabolism

2) Juvenile-adult onset

3) Myoglobinuria (induced by exercise, fever, exposure

to cold, fasting, low carbohydrate/high fat diet, concurrent treatment with valproate)
4) Muscular pain and stiffness induced by exertion and exercise, may be followed by myoglobinuria and weakness if continued presence of precipitating factor
5) Severe myoglobinuria may cause acute tubular necrosis
6) Malignant hyperthermia induced by general anesthesia or postoperative myoglobinuria reported: may be prevented by intravenous glucose before and during general anesthesia
7) Creatine kinase
   a) Normal or mildly elevated (50%) levels between episodes
   b) High levels with rhabdomyolysis
c. CPT2 deficiency type 2
   1) Infantile onset
   2) Severely affected phenotype (often fatal): may present with seizures, coma, respiratory distress
   3) Static encephalopathy may result from hypoglycemic episodes
   4) Psychomotor developmental delay
   5) Hepatomegaly
   6) Cardiomegaly, cardiac arrhythmias
   7) Laboratory analysis: hypoketotic hypoglycemia, elevated liver enzymes, increased plasma creatine kinase, and often low plasma levels of carnitine
d. CPT2 deficiency type 3
   1) Neonatal onset
   2) Most severe CPT deficiency phenotype
   3) Hyporeflexia, hypotonia, seizures, respiratory distress, generalized seizures, lethargy
   4) Laboratory findings: hypoketotic hypoglycemia, hyperammonemia, metabolic acidosis

VII. MITOCHONDRIAL MYOPATHIES

A. Mitochondrial Genetics
1. Maternal inheritance of disorders linked to mutations of mitochondrial DNA (mtDNA), with minor exception of paternal transmission of mtDNA in skeletal muscle
2. Most mitochondrial proteins encoded by nuclear DNA
3. Mutations in mtDNA are more likely to cause mitochondrial phenotypic disease than mutations of nuclear mtDNA because mtDNA
   a. Lacks introns
   b. Some lack termination codon
   c. Rapid replication with lack of proofreading and mutation rate greater than nuclear DNA

d. Poor repair mechanisms
4. Mutant mitochondrial genomes passed on randomly to daughter cells during mitosis or meiosis
   a. Normal homoplasty: daughter cells contain no mutant mitochondrial genomes
   b. Mutant homoplasty: daughter cells contain predominantly mutant mitochondrial genomes
   c. Heteroplasty: daughter cells contain some mutant genome (variable distribution of mtDNA mutations in different cells or tissues)
5. Variability of phenotypic expression depends on
   a. Proportion of mutant mitochondria within each cell
   b. Threshold effect
      1) Proportion of mutant genome needs to be above a certain threshold to cause clinical manifestation
      2) Tissue-specific thresholds
   c. Segregation: during cell division, relative cellular proportion of mutant mtDNA may shift between generations
   d. Genetic and phenotypic heterogeneity within individual and families with identical mutations

B. Pathology
1. Abnormal mitochondria seen with modified Gomori trichrome staining: subsarcolemmal accumulation of abnormal mitochondria, "ragged red" appearance (hence, "ragged red fibers" [RRFs])
2. Cytochrome oxidase (COX) stain: affected by mtDNA mutations, unstained muscle fibers indicate mitochondrial disease
3. Succinate dehydrogenase (SDH) stain: affected by nuclear DNA mutations, dark staining of muscle fibers with mitochondrial accumulation ("ragged blue fibers," SDH equivalents of RRFs)

C. Myoclonic Epilepsy With Ragged Red Fibers (MERRF)
1. Genetics
   a. Mitochondrial inheritance
   b. Most affected individuals have point mutations of mitochondrial genome (mtDNA) affecting the transfer RNA gene
2. Clinical features (variable phenotypic expression)
   a. Age at onset: late adolescence to early adulthood
   b. Proximal muscular weakness
   c. Myoclonus, at rest or stimulus-sensitive
   d. Generalized seizure disorder (including myoclonic and generalized tonic-clonic seizures), may be photosensitive
   e. Ataxia, dementia, hearing loss (40% of patients), optic atrophy (20%)
   f. Distal sensorimotor peripheral neuropathy

g. Other: short stature (10% of patients), multiple lipomatoses, cardiomyopathy

h. No ptosis or ophthalmoplegia

3. Laboratory features
   a. Creatine kinase: normal or slightly elevated levels
   b. Serum lactate: elevated levels
   c. Epileptiform activity on electroencephalography (EEG)
   d. Pathology: also includes neuronal loss and gliosis of red nucleus, substantia nigra, inferior olivary nuclei, optic nerves
   e. Neuroimaging evidence of cerebral or cerebellar atrophy, with latter corresponding with degenerative changes in cerebellar hemispheres and dentate nucleus

4. Muscle histopathology
   a. RRF on modified Gomori trichrome stain
   b. Reduced or absent COX staining

D. **Mitochondrial Encephalomyopathy, Lactic Acidosis, and Stroke-Like Episodes** (MELAS)

1. Associated with several mtDNA point mutations (genetic heterogeneity)

2. Clinical features (phenotypic heterogeneity)
   a. Age at onset: usually in childhood (range, 3-40 years)
   b. Proximal muscle weakness (87% of patients) and atrophy (Fig. 24-12)
   c. Easy fatiguability (15%-18% of patients)
   d. Episodic encephalopathy (nonfocal) characterized by headaches, vomiting, seizures, loss of consciousness
   e. Stroke-like focal episodes
      1) Focal events that do not conform to arterial vascular territory
      2) May represent neuronal hyperexcitability
   f. Recurrent headaches
   g. Seizures
   h. Short stature
   i. Normal early developmental milestones with eventual dementia in some cases
   j. Other features (less common): myoclonus, hearing loss, optic atrophy, pigmentary retinopathy, cardiomyopathy with CHF, progressive external ophthalmoplegia, diabetes mellitus

3. Neuroimaging characteristics
   a. Basal ganglia calcification
   b. Cerebral, cerebellar, and brainstem atrophy
   c. MRI
      1) Multifocal laminar cortical areas of high T2 signal with some involvement of juxtacortical white matter and relative sparing of deep white matter
      2) Normal or increased signal on apparent diffusion coefficient maps in region of acute stroke-like event

(in contrast to ischemic infarction): supports a metabolic insult as the underlying pathophysiology

d. Proton magnetic resonance spectroscopy: region of acute stroke-like event may have increased lactate/creatine ratio and decreased N-acetylaspartate/creatine ratio

4. Muscle histopathology (Fig. 24-12)
   a. RRFs on modified Gomori trichrome stain
   b. Unlike other disorders caused by mtDNA, RRFs react with COX staining

5. Management
   a. Treatment strategies
      1) Supplementation of respiratory chain components
      2) Removal of noxious metabolites
      3) Administration of artificial electron acceptors
   b. Coenzyme Q_{10}
      1) Theoretically may help in transference of electrons from complexes I and II to III
      2) Possible decrease in lactate and pyruvate levels in cerebrospinal fluid (CSF)
   c. Dichloroacetate
      1) Targets the lactate accumulating in tissues
      2) Inhibits phosphorylation of pyruvate dehydrogenase complex, leaving active form free to oxidize pyruvate to acetyl CoA
      3) Acts to decrease levels of pyruvate available for conversion into lactate
   d. Genetic counseling

E. **Kearns-Sayre Syndrome**

1. Molecular genetics
   a. Single large mtDNA mutations of varying size
   b. Usually sporadic (rarely inherited)

2. Clinical features
   a. Age at onset: 20 years or younger
   b. Progressive external ophthalmoplegia
   c. Retinitis pigmentosa
   d. Heart block and arrhythmias
   e. Proximal muscle weakness
   f. Short stature
   g. Sensorineural hearing loss
   h. Dementia
   i. Ataxia
   j. Endocrinopathies (e.g., diabetes mellitus)
   k. Potential for respiratory insufficiency and decreased ventilatory drive with CNS depressants, surgery, and infection

3. Laboratory features
   a. Elevated levels of serum lactate and pyruvate and CSF protein
   b. Nerve conduction studies: normal, rarely axonal

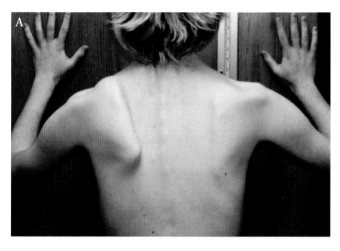
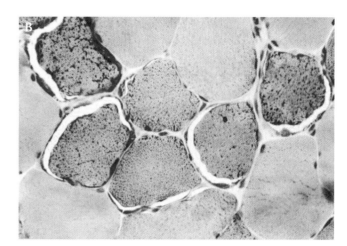
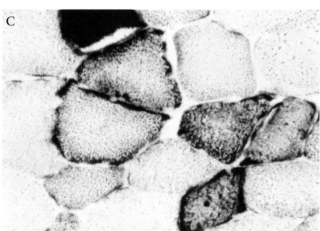
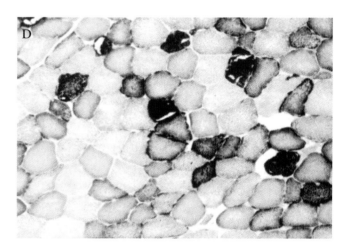

Fig. 24-12. Mitochondrial encephalomyopathy, lactic acidosis, and stroke-like episodes (MELAS). *A*, 19-year-old patient with long-standing proximal weakness and atrophy presented with stroke-like episodes and lactic acidosis. Note marked atrophy of the periscapular and paraspinal muscles. *B*, Muscle biopsy showed ragged red fibers and mitochondrial aggregates with ragged red appearance on modified Gomori trichrome staining. *C* and *D*, With SDH staining, the aggregates in *B* appear as ragged blue fibers. (Courtesy of Andrew G. Engel, MD.)

polyneuropathy
  c. EMG: may show myopathic motor unit potentials
4. Muscle histopathology
  a. RRFs seen on modified Gomori trichrome stain
  b. COX-stained fibers are reduced or absent
5. Treatment
  a. Specific treatment for complications, e.g., hormone replacement for endocrinopathies, pacemaker insertion for cardiac conduction defects
  b. Poor prognosis

F. Progressive External Ophthalmoplegia
1. Clinical features
  a. Genetically heterogeneous: may have autosomal domi-

nant and maternally inherited forms; sporadic subtype may be variant of Kearns-Sayre syndrome
  b. Age at onset: childhood or adolescence
  c. Gradual progression
  d. Ptosis and external ophthalmoplegia with or without muscle weakness
  e. No systemic manifestation, including cardiac involvement, endocrinopathy, retinopathy
  f. Potential for respiratory insufficiency and decreased ventilatory drive with CNS depressants, surgery, and infection
2. Laboratory features
  a. Creatine kinase and lactate: normal or elevated levels
  b. CSF protein: concentration may be increased

c. EMG: may show myopathic motor unit potentials

3. Treatment: treat complications

G. Autosomal Recessive Cardiomyopathy and Ophthalmoplegia

1. Autosomal recessive inheritance; mutation may involve nuclear genes regulating mitochondrial genome
2. Childhood-onset progressive external ophthalmoplegia
3. Facial and proximal limb muscle weakness
4. Cardiomyopathy
5. No other systemic manifestations
6. Myopathic motor unit potentials and RRFs

H. Mitochondrial DNA Depletion Syndrome

1. Autosomal recessive involving nuclear genes responsible for regulating mitochondrial genome
2. Fatal infantile myopathy
   a. Severe early-onset form
   b. Begins at birth with generalized hypotonia, proximal more than distal progressive weakness, feeding difficulties, respiratory failure, and death (usually within first year of life)
   c. Other features may include ptosis, ophthalmoplegia, peripheral neuropathy, renal tubular necrosis, seizures, liver failure, cardiomyopathy
3. Benign infantile myopathy
   a. Severe early onset of weakness, hypotonia, and respiratory and feeding difficulties
   b. Improvement in strength during first year, with some possible delay in motor development
   c. Usually normal life expectancy

I. Focal Mitochondrial Depletion

1. Autosomal recessive inheritance
2. Phenotypic heterogeneity
3. Clinical presentation can range from infantile onset hypotonia, weakness, developmental delay to adolescent to adult onset of proximal muscle weakness and myoglobinuria and fatigue

J. Mitochondrial Neurogastrointestinal Encephalomyopathy (MNGIE)

1. Mutations in mtDNA and chromomosome 22
2. Age at onset: usually before 20 years
3. Earliest sign referable to gastrointestinal dysmotility
4. Generalized weakness and atrophy most prominent distally
5. Sensory neuropathy
6. Ophthalmoplegia, ptosis, retinal degeneration
7. Hearing loss, facial weakness, dysarthria, hoarseness
8. Mental retardation

9. Ataxia
10. MRI: leukoencephalopathy involving cerebral and cerebellar white matter
11. EMG: neuropathic and myopathic motor unit potentials
12. Muscle biopsy: RRFs with increased NADH and SDH staining
13. Abnormal mitochondria with paracrystalline inclusions in muscle fibers and Schwann cells
14. Neuronal loss and fibrosis in autonomic ganglia and celiac, myenteric, and Auerbach's plexuses

VIII. INFLAMMATORY MYOPATHIES

A. General Concepts

1. Epidemiology
   a. Dermatomyositis affects children and adults (more frequently females)
   b. Polymyositis affects adults and rarely children
   c. Inclusion body myositis occurs more frequently in adults older than 50 (three times more frequent in men than women, more common in whites than African Americans)
2. Proximal weakness with subacute monophasic or polyphasic clinical presentation
   a. Weakness of neck flexor, limb-girdle, and proximal muscles
   b. Inclusion body myositis may present insidiously, involving predominantly finger flexors, hip flexors, quadriceps (latter spared in familial form, Nonaka distal myopathy); may be asymmetric
3. Progression: subacute (over weeks or months) for polymyositis and dermatomyositis, slow for inclusion body myositis
4. Facial muscles normal in polymyositis and dermatomyositis (except for advanced cases); mild facial weakness may be seen in up to 60% of cases of sporadic inclusion body myositis
   a. Marked facial weakness is not expected and raises possibility of another diagnosis
5. Esophageal dysmotility and dysphagia (due to involvement of striated muscle of pharynx and upper esophagus) observed in up to 30% of patients with polymyositis and dermatomyositis and up to 60% of those with inclusion body myositis
6. Muscular atrophy and wasting and reduced deep tendon reflexes, with severe weakness and prolonged progression
7. Other associated features

a. Respiratory involvement: generalized respiratory muscle weakness and interstitial lung disease (anti-tRNA synthetase [Anti-Jo-1] antibody present in up to 50% of patients with interstitial lung disease)

b. Cardiac involvement (nonspecific ST-T changes, bundle branch block, and arrhythmias)

8. Creatine kinase: usually elevated levels but may be normal or mildly elevated in long-standing cases such as inclusion body myositis

9. Antibodies associated with primary myositis syndromes

a. Anti-Jo-1 (anti-histidyl-ERNA synthetase) antibodies: observed in 20% of patients with dermatomyositis and polymyositis, associated with interstitial lung disease, associated with relatively severe disease phenotype

b. Anti-signal recognition particle: observed in 5% of patients (specificity of 93% when present)

c. Anti-Mi-2: associated with 15% to 35% of patients with dermatomyositis and 5% to 9% of those with polymyositis; associated with relatively mild disease phenotype

10. Antibodies associated with overlap syndromes

a. Anti-PM/Scl (IgG) antibody: observed in 24% of patients with polymyositis/scleroderma overlap syndrome; up to 88% of seropositive patients have this overlap syndrome

b. Anti-Ro/SSA antibodies and anti-La/SSB: associated with Sjögren's syndrome and corresponding overlap syndrome

c. Anti-U1 snRNP: nonspecific antibody associated with overlap syndromes of systemic lupus erythematosus, systemic scleroderma, rheumatoid arthritis, or mixed connective tissue disease

d. Anti-U2 snRNP: associated with scleroderma

11. Immunopathogenesis

a. Polymyositis and inclusion body myositis

1) Cytotoxicity mediated by cytotoxic $CD8^+$ T cells: release perforins and granzyme granules, causing muscle fiber necrosis

2) Cell death by apoptosis has a small role, given strong anti-apoptotic mechanisms

3) Nonimmune degenerative processes in inclusion body myositis

a) Presence of amyloid deposits in some vacuolated muscle fibers

b) Accompanied by β-amyloid precursor protein, chymotrypsin, apolipoprotein E, and phosphorylated tau

c) Mitochondrial abnormalities and mitochondrial deletions in 70% of muscles affected by inclusion body myositis (importance unclear)

b. Dermatomyositis

1) Humoral attack on endomysial blood vessels and capillaries, causing early changes in endothelial cells (obliteration, necrosis, thrombi)

2) Changes mediated primarily by activation of complement and deposition of C5b-9 complement membrane attack complex on small blood vessels, followed by induction of cytokines and endothelial expression of cell adhesion molecules

3) Vascular endothelial injury leads to destruction of capillaries, microinfarctions, muscle fiber destruction, and perifascicular atrophy

12. Risk of malignancy

a. Highest risk in adults with dermatomyositis

b. 30% to 40%: overall risk of developing malignancy with dermatomyositis (most commonly, ovarian and lung)

c. 15%: overall risk of developing malignancy with polymyositis (most commonly, lymphoma [non-Hodgkin's] and lung)

13. Treatment of inflammatory myopathies

a. Corticosteroids (first-line treatment, usually prednisone): weakness usually improves after the creatine kinase normalizes; patients initially may receive high-dose methylprednisolone or dexamethasone

b. Second-line treatment: azathioprine, methotrexate, mycophenolate mofetil

c. Third-line treatment: cyclosporine, cyclophosphamide, intravenous immunoglobulin, and plasma exchange

d. Same approach can be taken for treating inclusion body myositis: treatment has been shown to provide benefit or to slow disease progression

B. **Polymyositis**

1. Idiopathic

a. Symmetrical proximal weakness, including neck muscles

b. Associated with myalgias and elevated creatine kinase levels

c. Oculopharyngeal and esophageal involvement: dysphagia

d. Cardiac involvement

e. Respiratory involvement

f. EMG: positive sharp waves, fibrillation potentials, rapid recruitment of short-duration polyphasic motor unit potentials

2. Overlap syndromes

a. Myositis secondary to systemic inflammatory illness and not as a consequence of disuse atrophy or chronic corticosteroid use

b. Younger age at onset (mean, 35 years)

c. Predominantly females

d. Treatment may be modified according to underlying

condition

    e. Prognosis depends on underlying condition

    f. Scleroderma-myositis

      1) Systemic features: Raynaud's phenomenon, thick shiny skin, gastrointestinal tract dysmotility, cardiac involvement (pericarditis, myocardial fibrosis), sensorimotor peripheral neuropathy

      2) Localized or systemic

      3) Mild, nonprogressive weakness

      4) Creatine kinase: normal or mildly elevated levels

      5) Positive antinuclear antibody (ANA) and anti-PM/Scl (IgG) antibody

    g. Mixed connective tissue disease

      1) Clinical features of dermatomyositis with systemic lupus erythematosus and scleroderma

      2) Edema of hands

      3) Lupus-like erythematous rash

      4) Raynaud's phenomenon

      5) Hepatosplenomegaly, lymphadenopathy

      6) Synovitis

      7) Myositis (often severe), myalgias

      8) Pulmonary involvement common

    h. Other associated inflammatory conditions: mixed connective tissue disease, systemic lupus erythematosus, Sjögren's syndrome, rheumatoid arthritis

3. Anti-Jo-1 antibody syndrome (anti-synthetase syndrome)

    a. Polymyositis associated with anti-Jo-1 antibodies (IgG1 antibodies targeted at histidyl tRNA synthetase)

    b. 20% to 25% of patients with polymyositis have anti-Jo-1 antibodies

    c. Patients with polymyositis and interstitial lung disease: antibodies positive in 50% to 75%, negative in 20% to 25%

    d. Predominantly females

    e. Proximal symmetric myopathic weakness with myalgias, systemic features including seronegative, nonerosive arthritis and Raynaud's phenomenon (associated with relatively severe muscle and systemic disease)

    f. "Mechanic's hands": thickening of skin over hands and fingers

    g. Pulmonary involvement: interstitial lung disease

    h. Other laboratory markers: elevated creatine kinase level, erythrocyte sedimentation rate, and ANA and anti-Ro52 titers

    i. Linked to DR3, DRw52, DQA1*0501 HLA haplotypes

    j. Pulmonary disease may be responsive to corticosteroids

4. Muscle histopathology of polymyositis (Fig. 24-13)

    a. Invasion and destruction of nonnecrotic muscle fibers by endomysial, perimysial, and perivascular mononuclear inflammatory cell aggregates (T cells and macrophages) with characteristic autoaggressive behavior (as compared with perivascular inflammation in dermatomyositis)

    b. Nonspecific findings: necrotic and regenerating muscle fibers, increase in central nuclei, muscle fiber size variation

    c. Lack of perifascicular atrophy, microvascular injury, microvascular deposition of membrane attack complexes, and endothelial hyperplasia and inclusions (microtubules)

C. **Dermatomyositis**

1. Characteristic heliotrope rash accompanying or preceding weakness

    a. Primarily involves periorbital regions (associated with periorbital edema), anterior neck and upper chest (V sign), shoulders (shawl sign), buttocks, and extensor surfaces of fingers (Gottron's sign), knuckles (Fig. 24-14), elbows, and knees

    b. Erythematous, scaly periungual regions

    c. Calcinosis: subcutaneous calcifications in up to 50% of children affected

    d. Rash may occur without muscle involvement

2. Proximal pattern of muscle weakness and myalgias

3. Other organs involved

    a. Cardiac involvement: pericarditis, myocarditis, cardiomyopathy with CHF

    b. Pulmonary involvement: interstitial lung disease associated with antibodies to histidyl tRNA synthetase (Jo-1)

    c. Other systemic vasculitic manifestations may include gastrointestinal involvement, renal involvement, or other systemic features (e.g., arthralgias)

4. Laboratory features

    a. Creatine kinase: usually elevated levels, poor correlation with severity of weakness

    b. Other markers that potentially may be elevated: aldolase, myoglobin, lactate dehydrogenase, erythrocyte sedimentation rate, ANA, myositis-specific antibodies (specific HLA haplotypes), anti-Jo-1 antibodies (often with interstitial lung disease)

5. Muscle histopathology of dermatomyositis (Fig. 24-15)

    a. Characteristic perifasicular atrophy, microvascular injury, microvascular deposition of membrane attack complex, endothelial microtubular inclusions and hyperplasia (arterioles and capillaries), ongoing endothelial injury and regeneration

    b. Perimysial inflammatory cell aggregates (least prominent in endomysial region) consist of B and CD4$^+$ T lymphocytes

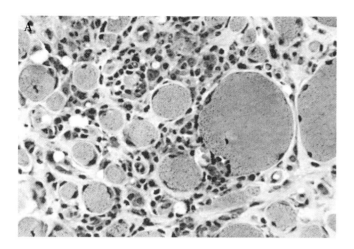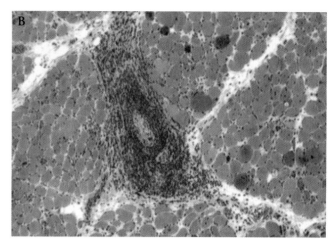

Fig. 24-13. Characteristic muscle histopathologic features of polymyositis include endomysial (*A*) and perivascular and perimysial (*B*) collections of mononuclear cellular infiltrates, increased variation in muscle fiber diameter, and muscle fiber necrosis. (*A* courtesy of Andrew G. Engel, MD. *B* from Lidov H, De Girolami U, Gherardi R. Skeletal muscle diseases. In: Gray F, De Girolami U, Poirier J, editors. Escourolle & Poirier manual of basic neurophysiology. 4th ed. Philadelphia: Butterworth-Heinemann; 2004. p. 281-314. Used with permission.)

D. Inclusion Body Myositis

1. Clinical features
   a. Age at onset: typically older than 30 years
   b. Common presentation: slowly progressive painless weakness (variable distribution)
   c. Weakness involves both proximal and distal muscles, with characteristic distribution of weakness affecting finger and wrist flexors (more than wrist extensors) and quadriceps muscles
   d. Muscle atrophy may be proportional to weakness (Fig. 24-16)
   e. Duration of illness: usually more than 6 months, slowly progressive course
2. Laboratory features
   a. Creatine kinase: normal or mildly elevated levels (80% of patients)
   b. Erythrocyte sedimentation rate and autoantibodies may be increased in 10% to 20% of patients
   c. Monoclonal gammopathy (23% of patients)
   d. EMG
      1) Usually nonspecific myopathic features with increased insertional activity, short-duration low-amplitude motor unit potentials; long-duration high-amplitude motor unit potentials in 1/3 of cases, complex repetitive discharges
      2) Long-duration high-amplitude motor unit potentials may reflect chronicity of disease rather than neurogenic involvement
      3) Nerve conduction studies: usually normal (alterna-

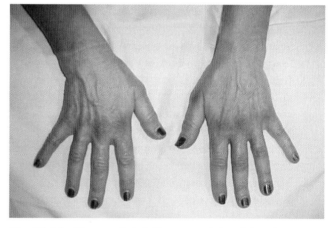

Fig. 24-14. Characteristic heliotrope rash involving the extensor surfaces of the fingers of a patient with dermatomyositis.

tively, mild peripheral neuropathy or mononeuropathy in 10%-30% of patients)
      4) In advanced cases, CMAP amplitudes may be reduced
   e. Muscle histopathology of inclusion body myositis (Fig. 24-17)
      1) Vacuoles within muscle fibers rimmed with granular material and filaments
         a) May contain paired helical filaments containing phosphorylated tau protein
         b) Intracellular β-amyloid deposition in vacuoles (visualized with polarized light)

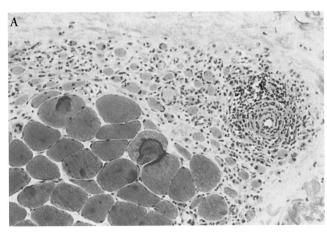 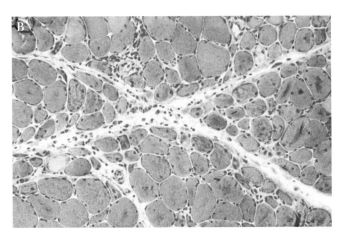

Fig. 24-15. Perivascular clusters of inflammatory cells (*A*) and perifascicular atrophy (*A* and *B*) are characteristic histopathologic features of dermatomyositis. The atrophy is most prominent in the perifascicular muscle fibers bordering the enlarged connective tissue septa, indicative of muscle fiber necrosis and insufficient regeneration. (*A*, Hematoxylin and eosin; *B*, modified Gomori trichrome stain.) (Courtesy of Andrew G. Engel, MD.)

2) Focal invasion of nonnecrotic muscle fibers
3) Endomysial inflammatory infiltrates (predominantly CD8$^+$ cells)
4) Inflammatory response potentially may be secondary to degenerative process
f. Treatment: prednisone, methotrexate, azathioprine usually not beneficial
g. Variants
1) *IBM2* (Nonaka myopathy, hereditary inclusion body myopathy linked to chromosome 9p) (see above)
2) *IBM3*, caused by missense mutation in gene encoding myosin heavy chain IIa (chromosome 17p)
3) Inclusion body myopathy with dementia and Paget's disease of bone
a) Autosomal dominant inheritance, linked to chromosome 9p
b) Age at onset: third and fourth decades
c) Proximal and distal weakness of arms and legs, including scapular winging; cranial nerve involvement
d) Slow progression
e) Paget's disease of bone (mean age at onset, 35 years): affects spine, hip and pelvis, skull
f) Dementia: frontotemporal dementia with features of aphasia and personality changes
g) Cardiomyopathy late in disease course
h) Creatine kinase: normal to mildly elevated levels

E. Sarcoid Myopathy
1. Systemic, multiorgan disorder of unknown cause, characterized by granulomatous lesions often involving pul-

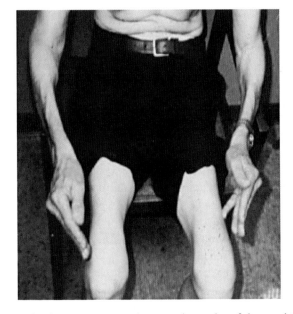

Fig. 24-16. Prominent weakness and atrophy of the quadriceps and finger flexors in a patient with sporadic inclusion body myositis. (From Engel WK, Askanas V. Inclusion-body myositis: clinical, diagnostic, and pathologic aspects. Neurology. 2006;66 Suppl 1:S20-9. Used with permission.)

monary and lymphatic systems
2. Epidemiology: 10 to 20 times more frequent in African Americans than whites, F > M (slightly)
3. Usual presenting symptoms of arthritis and erythema nodosum

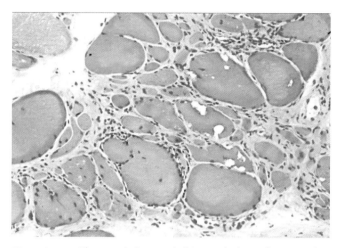

Fig. 24-17. Characteristic muscle histopathologic features of inclusion body myositis include vacuoles rimmed by small granules, endomysial inflammatory cells, and focal invasion of muscle fibers by inflammatory infiltrates. (Courtesy of Andrew G. Engel, MD.)

4. Large percentage of patients have muscle involvement (presence of granulomas), most of whom are asymptomatic
5. Presentations of muscle disease
   a. Asymptomatic: most patients do not have signs or symptoms of muscle involvement (presence of granulomas)
   b. Chronic myositis: muscle weakness and atrophy (proximal > distal); may be myalgias, cramps, contractures
   c. Acute myositis: painful myalgias common, with proximal weakness
   d. Nodular myositis: granulomatous nodules may be palpated or found on biopsy even if asymptomatic
6. Painful myalgias common
7. Skeletal muscle is often involved, and there is often muscle lesion even in absence of symptoms
8. Diagnostic investigation to include chest films (to examine for hilar adenopathy); serum angiotensin-converting enzyme, calcium, and creatine kinase (may be normal or mildly elevated); muscle biopsy
9. Muscle histopathology consistent with noncaseating granulomas with giant cells, epithelioid cells, and lymphocytes, often perivascular distribution (Fig. 24-18)
10. Treatment and prognosis
    a. Frequent spontaneous remissions are the rule
    b. Corticosteroids (prednisone) often provide best relief
    c. Corticosteroid-refractory patients may benefit from methotrexate

F. Myositis Related to Vasculitis
1. Polyarteritis nodosa: symmetric or asymmetric weakness and myalgias in context of fevers, arthralgias, glomerulosclerosis, distal peripheral neuropathy, and mononeuritis multiplex (Fig. 24-19)
2. Churg-Strauss syndrome: necrotizing granulomatous arteritis, fever, vasculitic myositis, eosinophilia, asthma
3. Wegener's granulomatosis: necrotizing granulomatous arteritis, glomerulonephritis, cranial mononeuropathies, mononeuritis multiplex, vasulitic myositis

IX. INFECTIOUS DISEASES OF MUSCLE

A. Bacterial Infections
1. Clostridial myonecrosis
   a. Caused by *Clostridium perfringens*
   b. Acute onset of myalgias, local tenderness, myofascial edema, and serosanguinous, malodorous discharge
   c. Inciting event: often trauma, sepsis, abdominal surgery
2. Streptococcal myonecrosis
   a. Caused by group A β-hemolytic streptococci
   b. Bacterial invasion of the trauma sites
   c. Erythema, sloughing of skin, myofascial necrosis; may be followed by bacteremia, sepsis, death
3. Legionnaires' disease
   a. Caused by *Legionella pneumophila* (gram-negative aerobic bacillus)
   b. Polymyositis (necrotizing myopathy): painful proximal weakness, elevated creatine kinase levels, rhabdomyolysis, myoglobinuria
4. Neuroborreliosis (Lyme disease)
   a. Caused by *Borrelia burgdorferi*
   b. Diffuse inflammatory myositis with diffuse weakness, myalgias, muscle tenderness, cramps

B. Viral Infections
1. Orthomyxoviruses: influenza A and B (rarely C)
   a. Abrupt onset of myalgias (especially in calves and thighs), generalized weakness, muscle tenderness, myoedema
   b. Myoglobinuria (may cause acute tubular necrosis), elevated levels of creatine kinase and aldolase, elevated liver function enzymes
   c. Natural history of myositis: self-limited course, resolves within 2 to 3 months after onset
   d. Muscle biopsy usually not indicated
   e. Muscle histopathology: necrotizing myositis
2. Acute coxsackie-related myositis: symptoms are pre-

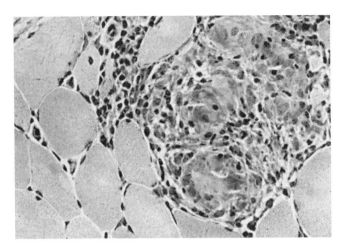

Fig. 24-18. Sarcoid myopathy. Characteristic focal invasion and replacement of muscle fibers by noncaseating granulomas with giant cells, epithelioid cells, and lymphocytes. (Courtesy of Andrew G. Engel, MD.)

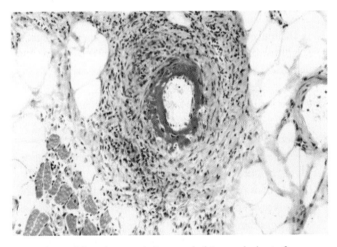

Fig. 24-19. The characteristic muscle histopathologic feature of necrotizing myositis related to polyarteritis nodosa is fibrinoid necrosis of the wall of small-sized arteries. Note the expansion of the surrounding connective tissue and invasion of the wall of the small-sized artery by the inflammatory cells, with spread into the adjacent thickened connective tissue. (Courtesy of Andrew G. Engel, MD.)

dominantly fatigue and muscle pains, occurring up to 10 days after initial phase of viral illness, which may or may not be accompanied by diffuse myositis (generalized weakness), myoglobinuria, and myoedema

3. Myositis related to human immunodeficiency virus (HIV)
   a. Commonly a complication of fully developed acquired immunodeficiency syndrome (AIDS); may present early in course of HIV infection
   b. Symmetric, painless proximal muscle weakness, myalgias, with or without atrophy
   c. Creatine kinase: elevated levels
   d. Pathologic features of HIV-1–associated inflammatory myositis
      1) HIV polymyositis: involves endomysial inflammation
      2) HIV inclusion body myositis: inflammatory myopathy associated with vacuolated fibers
      3) HIV necrotizing myopathy: minimal inflammation and predominant features of muscle fiber necrosis
      4) HIV myopathy with nemaline rod bodies: rare
   e. HIV wasting syndrome
      1) Severe fatigue, myalgias, diffuse muscle atrophy
      2) Normal muscle enzyme levels
      3) Strength: normal or may be mild weakness disproportional to degree of atrophy

X. ACQUIRED TOXIC AND METABOLIC DISORDERS OF MUSCLE

A. Acquired Metabolic Myopathies

1. Disorders of glucocorticoid excess: corticosteroid myopathy
   a. Due to exogenous (corticosteroid intake) or endogenous (Cushing's disease) glucocorticoid excess
   b. Exogenous and endogenous causes of steroid myopathy produce similar clinical and histopathologic features
   c. Corticosteroids likely to induce steroid myopathy: triamcinolone (most likely), dexamethasone, betamethasone
   d. Likely due to increased muscle protein catabolism
   e. Preferential type II fiber atrophy
   f. Myopathy may occur several weeks after onset of steroid therapy, but typically occurs after chronic administration of high-dose oral corticosteroids
   g. Severe acute quadriplegic myopathy rarely occurs with administration of high-dose intravenous corticosteroids, marked by generalized muscle weakness with or without respiratory involvement and severe elevation of the serum creatine kinase level
   h. Chronic corticosteroid myopathy (most common presentation of corticosteroid myopathy): proximal muscle weakness with some atrophy in patients given high-dose corticosteroids for prolonged periods
   i. Gradual onset of proximal muscle weakness and atrophy, myalgias (legs > arms)

j. Cranial and sphincter muscles spared

k. Clinical course worsened with fasting and inactivity

l. Other stigmata of glucocorticoid excess: "moon facies," fragile skin, osteoporosis, weight gain, hypertension, glucose intolerance, hirsutism, growth retardation in children

m. Creatine kinase: normal levels

n. EMG: often normal, may show mild proximal myopathic motor unit potentials

o. Muscle histopathology: type II fiber atrophy

p. Treatment
   1) Reduce dose of exogenous corticosteroid to lowest possible dose (alternate-day regimen preferred)
   2) Change to a nonfluorinated preparation if possible
   3) Physical therapy and exercise to prevent disuse atrophy (also type IIB fiber atrophy)
   4) Adequate nutrition to avoid protein deprivation
   5) Treatment of underlying Cushing's syndrome (endogenous source): removal of the corticosteroid- or corticotropin (ACTH)-producing tumor (e.g., adrenal adenoma, ACTH-producing pituitary adenoma, or ectopic ACTH source)

2. Thyrotoxic myopathy
   a. Myopathic weakness: proximal weakness, disproportional to degree of atrophy; present in most patients, but presenting complaint of only 5%
   b. Distal weakness may occur
   c. Common complaints: myalgias, fatigue, exercise intolerance
   d. Respiratory insufficiency
   e. Tendon reflexes appear brisk because of shortened relaxation times
   f. Other features of thyrotoxicosis: weight loss, palpitations, tachycardia, anxiety, insomnia, tremors, heat intolerance, warm skin
   g. Creatine kinase: normal levels
   h. With treatment of the underlying hyperthyroidism, muscle strength improves gradually over several months

3. Thyrotoxic periodic paralysis: secondary form of HypoPP (see above)

4. Hypothyroid myopathy
   a. Proximal weakness, myalgias, cramps, fatigue
   b. Myoedema and enlargement of muscles
   c. Slow movements: slow muscle contractions with delayed relaxation
   d. Associated with polyneuropathy and entrapment neuropathies (most often median nerve at the wrist)
   e. Elevated creatine kinase level (in symptomatic patients, often tenfold more than normal) and myoglobin

5. Hyperparathyroidism-related myopathy

a. May be primary (due to parathyroid adenoma or hyperplasia) or secondary (renal failure and impaired kidney production of 1,25-dihydroxyvitamin D)

b. Most patients experience generalized weakness, fatigue, and muscle stiffness

c. Myopathy occurs in 2% to 10% of patients

d. Proximal symmetric weakness and atrophy (affect legs > arms)

e. Relative sparing of bulbar muscles and sphincter function

f. Myalgias

g. Increased tendon reflexes

h. May be a concomitant polyneuropathy

i. Creatine kinase: normal levels

6. Critical illness myopathy
   a. Risk factors include: renal failure, concomitant presence of critical illness neuropathy, administration of corticosteroids and neuromuscular junction blocking agents
   b. Often occurs in context of multiorgan failure, including renal failure, sepsis, systemic inflammatory response syndrome
   c. Diffuse flaccid paresis, including weakness of bulbar and respiratory muscles (difficulty weaning from ventilator when intubated, ventilator dependence)
   d. Often concomitant occurrence of critical illness neuropathy
   e. Electrodiagnostic evaluation
      1) Nerve conduction studies: low-amplitude, broadened, long-duration CMAPs; relative preservation of the sensory responses; low-amplitude or absent sensory nerve action potentials may indicate concomitant neuropathy
      2) Needle EMG: increased insertional activity with fibrillation potentials and positive sharp waves may be present
      3) Muscle-evoked CMAP (responses obtained with direct muscle stimulation) may be compared with nerve-evoked CMAP to help differentiate critical illness neuropathy from myopathy (but both may be present)

B. **Toxic Myopathies**

1. Exogenous corticosteroid myopathy (see above)

2. Colchicine myopathy
   a. Most often affects men older than 50
   b. Renal insufficiency: a risk factor
   c. Subacute onset of proximal weakness
   d. Clinical and electrophysiologic myotonia may be present
   e. Creatine kinase: elevated levels
   f. Muscle weakness and elevated creatine kinase levels

resolve within 4 to 6 weeks after discontinuation of offending agent

g. Pathophysiology

1) Colchicine interacts with tubulin, inhibiting polymerization of microtubules

2) Causes disruption of muscle microtubule-dependent cytoskeletal network, which leads to deficient transport and intracellular accumulation of lysosomes and autophagic vacuoles (vacuolar myopathy)

3. Zidovudine (AZT) myopathy

a. Toxic mitochondrial myopathy (accompanied by T cell–mediated inflammatory response)

b. Clinical presentation mimics HIV-1–associated inflammatory myositis (see above)

c. Muscle weakness in patients infected with HIV is often multifactorial

d. Progressive proximal weakness, fatigue, myalgias, elevated creatine kinase levels

e. Clinical presentation variable: range from mild myalgias with no weakness to severe proximal weakness

f. Creatine kinase: normal to moderately increased levels

g. Often, recovery several months after discontinuation of AZT

h. Histopathology: mitochondrial changes

1) RRFs

2) Mitochondrial abnormalities seen on electron microscopy

3) Scattered interstitial lymphocytic infiltrates (possibly T cell–mediated inflammatory response)

4. Myopathy related to HMG-CoA reductase inhibitors (e.g., lovastatin, simvastatin)

a. "Statin myopathy" refers to spectrum of phenotypes

b. Clinical phenotype may be predominantly that of myalgias (muscle pain) without true myositis and elevated creatine kinase levels or there may be myositis with elevated creatine kinase levels and rhabdomyolysis

c. Myalgias without true myositis commonly occur transiently with initiation of therapy, without progression to myositis

d. Onset of symptoms: usually about 2 to 3 months after initiation of statin therapy (up to 2 years)

e. Incidence of myalgias, as high as 20%; incidence of true myositis, 0.2%

f. Risk factors: female sex, old age, short stature, hypothyroidism, renal insufficiency, severe hepatobiliary disease, perioperative period, high dose of offending statin, polypharmacy and concomitant use of gemfibrozil, nicotinic acid, cyclosporine, colchicine, calcium-channel blockers, nefazodone, or erythromycin

g. Statin-induced myositis has been associated with reduced concentrations of coenzyme Q_{10}

h. Histopathology of statin-induced myositis: muscle fiber necrosis, regeneration, mononuclear cell infiltration

i. Treatment: discontinuation of the offending drug

j. Persistence of symptoms several months after discontinuation of the drug indicates different diagnosis

5. Myopathy related to fibric acid derivatives (e.g., clofibrate, gemfibrozil)

a. Necrotizing myopathy often occurring within 2 to 3 months after starting the drug

b. Generalized cramps, weakness, muscle tenderness

c. Associated with elevated creatine kinase levels and myoglobinuria

6. Alcohol-induced myopathy

a. Acute alcoholic myopathy

1) Necrotizing myopathy in setting of chronic heavy alcohol use, with or without episodes of binge drinking

2) Painful diffuse weakness accompanied by myoedema and myonecrosis, with variable severity

3) Myoglobinuria, which may be followed by acute tubular necrosis and renal failure

4) Patients who develop an attack are predisposed to have another episode if alcohol abuse continues

b. Acute hypokalemic alcoholic myopathy

1) Observed with chronic alcoholism and alcohol withdrawal

2) Acute-onset vacuolar myopathy

3) Acute, painless muscle weakness without myoedema or muscle tenderness

4) Hypokalemia

5) Creatine kinase: markedly elevated levels

6) Muscle histopathology: vacuolar myonecrosis

7) Reversible with repletion of potassium: response noted within first week, complete recovery expected by 2 weeks

c. Chronic alcoholic myopathy

1) Debated entity

2) Myalgias, cramps, proximal weakness

3) Creatine kinase: elevated levels

4) Myoglobinuria

5) Often associated with other alcohol-related complications, including dilated cardiomyopathy and peripheral neuropathy

6) Muscle histopathology: type II fiber atrophy, variation of fiber size, subsarcolemmal nuclei, sparse muscle fiber necrosis and regeneration, "moth-eaten" fibers

REFERENCES

Amato AA. Acid maltase deficiency and related myopathies. Neurol Clin. 2000;18:151-65.

Aoki M, Liu J, Richard I, Bashir R, Britton S, Keers SM, et al. Genomic organization of the dysferlin gene and novel mutations in Miyoshi myopathy. Neurology. 2001;57:271-8.

Argov Z, Sadeh M, Mazor K, Soffer D, Kahana E, Eisenberg I, et al. Muscular dystrophy due to dysferlin deficiency in Libyan Jews: clinical and genetic features. Brain. 2000;123:1229-37.

Benarroch EE, Westmoreland BF, Daube JR, Reagan TJ, Sandok BA. Medical neurosciences: an approach to anatomy, pathology, and physiology by systems and levels. 4th ed. Philadelphia: Lippincott Williams & Wilkins; 1999.

Chariot P, Gherardi R. Myopathy and HIV infection. Curr Opin Rheumatol. 1995;7:497-502.

Crum NF. Bacterial pyomyositis in the United States. Am J Med. 2004;117:420-8.

Dalakas MC, Rowland LP, DiMauro S. Inflammatory myopathies. In: Vinken PJ, Bruyn GW, Klawans HL, editors. Handbook of clinical neurology. Vol 62 (Revised Series 18). Amsterdam: Elsevier Science Publishers; 1992. p. 369-90.

Demaugre F, Bonnefont JP, Colonna M, Cepanec C, Leroux JP, Saudubray JM. Infantile form of carnitine palmitoyltransferase II deficiency with hepatomuscular symptoms and sudden death: physiopathological approach to carnitine palmitoyltransferse II deficiencies. J Clin Invest. 1991;87:859-64.

DiMauro S, Lamperti C. Muscle glycogenoses. Muscle Nerve. 2001;24:984-99.

Engel AG, Franzini-Armstrong C, editors. Myology. 3rd ed. New York: McGraw-Hill; 2004.

Engel AG, Gomez MR, Groover RV. Multicore disease: a recently recognized congenital myopathy associated with multifocal degeneration of muscle fibers. Mayo Clin Proc. 1971;46:666-81.

Engel WK, Askanas V. Inclusion-body myositis: clinical, diagnostic, and pathologic aspects. Neurology. 2006;66 Suppl 1:S20-9.

Felice KJ, North WA. Inclusion body myositis in Connecticut: observations in 35 patients during an 8-year period. Medicine (Baltimore). 2001;80:320-7.

Rowland LP. Polymyositis, inclusion body myositis, and related myopathies. In: Rowland LP, editor. Merritt's neurology. 10th ed. Philadelphia: Lippincott Williams & Wilkins; 2000. p. 765-9.

Selcen D, Engel AG. Mutations in myotilin cause myofibrillar myopathy. Neurology. 2004;62:1363-71. Erratum in: Neurology. 2004; 63:405.

Selcen D, Engel AG. Mutations in ZASP define a novel form of muscular dystrophy in humans. Ann Neurol. 2005;57:269-76.

Simpson DM, Citak KA, Godfrey E, Godbold J, Wolfe DE. Myopathies associated with human immunodeficiency virus and zidovudine: can their effects be distinguished? Neurology. 1993;43:971-6.

Stephan DA, Buist NR, Chittenden AB, Ricker K, Zhou J, Hoffman EP. A rippling muscle disease gene is localized to 1q41: evidence for multiple genes. Neurology. 1994;44:1915-20.

QUESTIONS

1. Which of the following is *not* true about nemaline myopathy?
   a. The most common presentation is congenital hypotonia
   b. Motor development may be normal
   c. Extraocular muscles are often involved and there may be partial or complete ophthalmoplegia
   d. Patients are intelligent and have no psychomotor retardation
   e. Patients with infantile-onset nemaline myopathy present with an open mouth appearance due to facial diplegia

MATCHING. Toxic myopathies. Match the appropriate myopathic syndrome in the right column with the corresponding cause in the left column.

2. Prednisone   a. Vacuolar myopathy
3. Colchicine   b. Type II fiber atrophy
4. Zidovudine (AZT)   c. Mitochondrial myopathy with ragged red fibers

5. Which of the following is *not* a typical histopathologic feature of myotonic dystrophy?
   a. Central nuclei
   b. Preferential atrophy of type I muscle fibers
   c. Variation in muscle fiber size
   d. Ragged red fibers
   e. All the above are typical histopathologic features of myotonic dystrophy

TRUE or FALSE
6. Patients with McArdle's disease and phosphofructo-kinase deficiency do not have a normal increase in serum lactate level with the ischemic exercise test.

7. The muscle biopsy specimen from a 60-year-old man who presents with 1-year history of progressive, painless weakness predominantly involving the flexors of the fingers, wrist, and hip and the quadriceps muscles most likely shows:
   a. Perifascicular muscle fiber atrophy and perivascular inflammatory infiltrates
   b. Ragged red fibers
   c. Nemaline rods
   d. Rimmed vacuoles, intracellular β-amyloid deposition in vacuoles

8. Mutations producing deficiency of calpain-3 produce which of the following conditions:
   a. Limb-girdle muscular dystrophy 2A (LGMD 2A)
   b. Limb-girdle muscular dystrophy 2B (LGMD 2B)
   c. Sarcoglycanopathies
   d. Myotonic dystrophy

9. A 23-year-old man presents with progressive external ophthalmoplegia, retinitis pigmentosa, and heart block. The genetic abnormality is most likely that of:
   a. Mutation of nuclear DNA encoding mitochondrial proteins
   b. Expanded, unstable CTG repeat on chromosome 19q
   c. Mutation of mitochondrial DNA
   d. Mutation of the *LMNA* gene on chromosome 1q

ANSWERS

1. **Answer: c.**
Extraocular muscles are often spared in nemaline myopathy.

2. **Answer: b.**

3. **Answer: a.**

4. **Answer: c.**

5. **Answer: d.**
Ragged red fibers are characteristic of mitochondrial myopathies.

6. **Answer: True.**

7. **Answer: d.**
The presentation is highly suggestive of inclusion body myositis. Vacuoles within muscle fibers rimmed with granular material and filaments and intracellular β-amyloid deposition in vacuoles are characteristic histopathologic findings in inclusion body myositis.

8. **Answer a.**
Mutation of the gene encoding calpain-3 is responsible for LGMD 2A (calpainopathy).

9. **Answer c.**
The presentation is that of a mitochondrial myopathy such as Kearns-Sayre syndrome, most of which occur with mitochondrial inheritance.

Inborn Errors of Metabolism   25

Hema R. Murali, M.B.B.S.

Deborah L. Renaud, M.D.

I. Overview

A. Incidence: overall, 1 in 1,000 to 1 in 3,000 live births

B. Inheritance
1. Generally autosomal recessive
2. Few are autosomal dominant, X-linked recessive or X-linked dominant
3. Mitochondrial disorders may be maternally inherited

C. Pathophysiology
1. Excessive metabolite causing toxic effects
2. Inadequate metabolite required for normal cellular activity
3. Secondary disruption of essential metabolic pathway

D. Onset According to Age
1. Neonatal: urea cycle disorders, organic acidurias, aminoacidurias, nonketotic hyperglycinemias, galactosemia, pyridoxine dependency, peroxisomal disorders
2. Infantile: medium-chain acyl-CoA dehydrogenase deficiency, lysosomal storage disorders, mitochondrial disorders, peroxisomal disorders
3. Childhood: lysosomal storage disorders, peroxisomal disorders, congenital disorders of glycosylation, mitochondrial disorders, fatty acid disorders
4. Adolescence: neuronal ceroid lipofuscinosis, fatty acid disorders, certain glycogen storage disorders, porphyria, certain lysosomal storage disorders
5. Adulthood: late-onset lysosomal disorders, fatty acid disorders, certain glycogen storage disorders, porphyria

E. Clinical Features
1. May be primarily neurologic or involve multiple organ systems
2. Clinical features depend on the following:
   a. Type of molecule involved

1) Disorders of small molecules: aminoacidurias, organic acidurias, urea cycle defects, neurotransmitter defects, and disorders of purine, pyrimidine, and fatty acid metabolism
2) Disorders of large molecules: lysosomal storage disorders, peroxisomal disorders, congenital disorders of glycosylation, cholesterol biosynthetic disorders
   b. Cellular energy metabolism affected: glycogen storage diseases, fatty acid disorders, mitochondrial disorders
   c. Isolated seizures with inborn errors of metabolism
1) Folinic acid dependency
2) Multiple carboxylase and biotinidase deficiencies
3) Nonketotic hyperglycinemias
4) Sulfite oxidase and molybdenum cofactor deficiencies
5) Pyridoxine deficiency
   d. Abnormal urine odor
1) Maple syrup urine disease: maple syrup
2) Isovalericacidemia: sweaty feet
3) Glutaricacidemia type II: sweaty feet
4) Hypermethioninemia: boiled cabbage
5) Multiple carboxylase deficiency: tomcat urine
6) Phenylketonuria: mousy or musty
   e. Recurrent hypoglycemia
1) Galactosemia
2) Hereditary fructose intolerance
3) Glycogen storage diseases
4) Fatty acid oxidation disorders
5) Endocrinopathy
   f. Abnormal ophthalmologic findings
1) Cataracts
   a) Galactosemia
   b) Menkes' syndrome
   c) Mucopolysaccharidosis
   d) Peroxisomal disorders
2) Cherry-red spot
   a) GM_1 gangliosidosis (infantile form only)
   b) GM_2 gangliosidosis
   c) Niemann-Pick disease type A

d) Sialidosis type I
3) Lens dislocation
   a) Homocystinuria
   b) Molybdenum cofactor deficiency
   c) Sulfite oxidase deficiency
4) Retinopathy
   a) Congenital disorders of glycosylation
   b) Neuronal ceroid lipofuscinosis
   c) Mitochondrial disorders
   d) Peroxisomal disorders
g. Hepatosplenomegaly/hepatocellular dysfunction
1) Lysosomal storage disorders
2) Galactosemia
3) Hereditary fructose intolerance
4) Congenital disorders of glycosylation
5) Glycogen storage diseases
6) Fatty acid oxidation disorders
7) Peroxisomal biogenesis disorders

F. Diagnosis
1. Blood tests: newborn screening by tandem mass spectrometry—glucose, lactate, pyruvate, ammonia, pH, amino acids, carnitines, acylcarnitines (Fig. 25-1 and 25-2)
2. Urine tests: organic acids, mucopolysaccharides, sulfatides, oligosaccharides, purines and pyrimidines, acylglycines, ketoacids
3. Cerebrospinal fluid (CSF): glucose, neurotransmitters, pyruvate, lactate, serine, glycine, 5-methyltetrahydrofolate
4. Electromyography (EMG): nerve conduction velocity in metachromatic leukodystrophy, Krabbe's disease
5. Magnetic resonance imaging (MRI): white matter and gray matter degenerative disorders
6. Magnetic resonance spectroscopy (MRS): Canavan's disease, mitochondrial disorders, disorders of gluconeogenesis, creatine deficiency syndromes
7. Enzyme assays for specific disorders: leukocytes, fibroblasts, tissues
8. Molecular genetics: common mutations and full gene sequencing available for many disorders

G. Management
1. Decrease substrate
2. Decrease levels of toxic metabolites
3. Replenish depleted metabolites
4. Provide alternate source of energy
5. Replace enzyme
6. Replace enzyme-producing cells through bone marrow or liver transplantation

H. Diagnosis Suspected at Time of Death—the following samples should be collected:
1. Frozen plasma
2. Frozen urine
3. Skin biopsy specimens stored at room temperature
4. Skin sample placed in glutaraldehyde for electron microscopic studies
5. Frozen tissues (−80°C) for enzymatic assays, including muscle, heart, liver as indicated by clinical presentation

II. DISORDERS OF CARBOHYDRATE METABOLISM

A. Galactosemia
1. Inheritance: autosomal recessive
2. Epidemiology: panethnic, approximately 1 in 30,000 live births
3. Pathophysiology
  a. Buildup of galactose, galactitol
  b. Galactose-1-phosphate accumulates in galactose-1-phosphate uridyltransferase (GALT) deficiency but not galactokinase deficiency
  c. Galactitol accumulation causes cataracts
  d. Endogenous galactose production in diet-restricted patients leads to continuing features of disease
  e. Uridine diphosphate galactose 4'-epimerase deficiency usually occurs only in erythrocytes
4. Clinical features
  a. GALT deficiency: severe (classic galactosemia)
    1) Presents in first weeks of life, with poor feeding, jaundice, vomiting, diarrhea, lethargy, hypotonia
    2) Liver dysfunction, cataracts, and *E. coli* septicemia may be found on examination

---

Classic Galactosemia

Neonatal onset

After onset of milk feeds

Vomiting

Diarrhea

Jaundice

E. coli sepsis

Bilateral cataracts

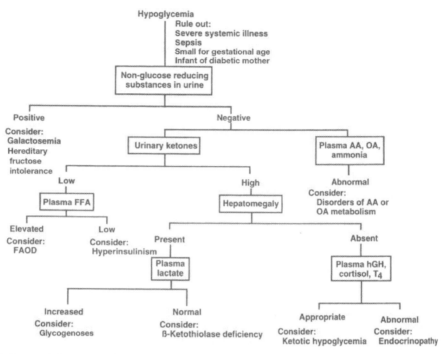

Fig. 25-1. Approach to differential diagnosis of hypoglycemia. AA, amino acids; FAOD, fatty acid oxidation defect; FFA, free fatty acids; hGH, human growth hormone; OA, organic acids; T_4, thyroxine. (Modified from Clarke JTR. A clinical guide to inherited metabolic diseases. 2nd ed. Cambridge: Cambridge University Press; 2002. p. 102. Used with permission.)

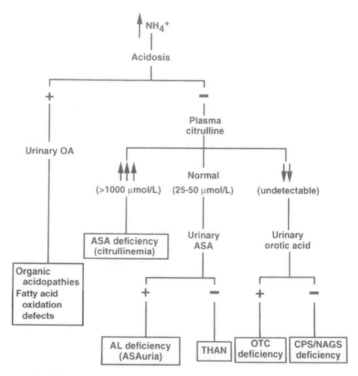

Fig. 25-2. Differential diagnosis of urea cycle defects in the newborn. AL, argininosuccinic acid lyase; ASA, argininosuccinic acid synthetase; CPS, carbamoylphosphate synthetase I; NAGS, *N*-acetylglutamate synthetase; OA, organic acids; OTC, ornithine trans-carbamoylase; THAN, transient hyperammonemia of the newborn. (Modified from Clarke JTR. A clinical guide to inherited metabolic diseases. 2nd ed. Cambridge: Cambridge University Press; 2002. p. 177. Used with permission.)

3) Less often, patients present with persistent poor feeding and vomiting, failure to thrive, developmental delay
   b. Galactokinase deficiency: bilateral cataracts occur by about 4 weeks of life; pseudotumor cerebri occurs rarely
   c. Uridine diphosphate galactose 4'-epimerase deficiency: usually normal growth and development; rarely, a generalized severe form of enzyme deficiency occurs with clinical features similar to classic galactosemia
5. Diagnosis
   a. Hypoglycemia, reducing substances in urine, and galactosuria should suggest diagnosis
   b. Enzyme defect in plasma and peripheral erythrocytes is confirmatory
   c. Fluorescent spot test available for diagnosis of galactosemia
   d. Computed tomographic (CT) and MRI findings in classic galactosemia with late neurologic disease: abnormal white matter, ventricular enlargement, diffuse cortical atrophy with basal ganglia and brainstem involvement, and cerebellar atrophy
   e. Newborn screening available
6. Management
   a. Strict removal of lactose and galactose from diet leads to resolution of features, including cataracts
   b. Regular slit-lamp examination is advised
7. Prognosis
   a. Strict galactose restriction early in life can reverse cataracts and prevent neurologic deficits
   b. Late effects: learning disabilities, developmental verbal dyspraxia, ovarian failure, and ataxia may occur despite early diagnosis and treatment of classic galactosemia
8. Prenatal diagnosis: DNA analysis and enzyme analysis in cultured amniocytes and chorionic villi

B. **Pyruvate Dehydrogenase Deficiency**
1. Inheritance
   a. Multienzyme complex
   b. E_1 defects are X-linked dominant
   c. Other defects are autosomal recessive
2. Epidemiology: panethnic
3. Pathophysiology
   a. It may be due to defective E_1 pyruvate decarboxylase α and β subunits, E_2 transacetylase, E_3 dihydrolipoamide dehydrogenase, E_3 binding protein (protein X), or pyruvate dehydrogenase phosphatase component of pyruvate dehydrogenase complex
   b. Most common defect is in the E_1 component
   c. Pyruvate dehydrogenase complex activity is rate-limiting step in aerobic oxidation of glucose by the brain

4. Clinical features
   a. Degree of lactic acidemia determines severity of the disease: fatal infantile lactic acidosis > Leigh disease > psychomotor retardation > ataxia > muscular weakness/retinal degeneration
   b. Dysmorphism similar to fetal alcohol syndrome occurs in one-third of cases
   c. Most severe form: severe lactic acidosis at birth, death in neonatal period
   d. Infantile form: moderate lactic acidemia, but progressive profound psychomotor retardation, with death in infancy
5. Diagnosis
   a. Increased lactic and pyruvic acid levels
      1) Lactate:pyruvate ratio <25 suggests defect in pyruvate dehydrogenase pathway or in one of the gluconeogenic enzymes
      2) A persistently increased lactate:pyruvate ratio, >30, suggests pyruvate carboxylase (type A) deficiency, nuclear or mtDNA respiratory chain defect, or Krebs cycle defect
      3) Patients with E3 deficiency also have biochemical features of maple syrup urine disease
   b. Basic measurements required: blood lactate, pyruvate, 3-hydroxybutyrate, acetoacetate; quantitative serum amino acids; urine organic acids by gas chromatography/mass spectrometry; fasting blood glucose, lactate, 3-hydroxybutyrate; in some cases, muscle biopsy
   c. Decreased enzyme activity in leukocytes, cultured skin fibroblasts, or muscle or liver biopsy (depending on suspected defect) is confirmatory
6. Pathology
   a. Leigh disease-like features of cystic lesions in basal ganglia and brainstem, cerebral atrophy, cerebral cysts
   b. Some neonatal cases have had agenesis of the corpus callosum

Pyruvate Dehydrogenase Deficiency
Fatal infantile lactic acidosis

Leigh disease

Psychomotor retardation

Ataxia

Muscular weakness

Retinal degeneration

7. Management
   a. Thiamine
   b. High fat, low carbohydrate (ketogenic) diet
   c. Dichloroacetate lowers lactate but has no clear effect on neurologic symptoms
   d. Carnitine to correct deficiency
8. Prognosis
   a. Poor
   b. Even prospectively treated infants before onset of neonatal symptoms are at high risk for neurologic deficits

C. Disorders of Creatine Metabolism

1. Inheritance: 3 disorders
   a. Errors of creatine biosynthesis—autosomal recessive
      1) Guanidinoacetate methyltransferase (GAMT) deficiency
      2) Arginine:glycine amidinotransferase (AGAT) deficiency
   b. Creatine transporter defect: X-linked, milder phenotype in females
2. Epidemiology: panethnic
3. Pathophysiology: very low creatine levels present in the brain in all forms
4. Clinical features: hypotonia, developmental delay, autism, movement disorder, seizures
5. Diagnosis
   a. MRI: may show abnormalities of globus pallidus
   b. MRS: absence of creatine peak (improves with supplementation in synthesis defects)
   c. Electroencephalography (EEG): slow background with multifocal independent spikes
   d. Blood and urine analysis of creatine and guanidinoacetate (GUAC) (Table 25-1)
6. Management
   a. Oral creatine monohydrate supplementation
   b. Good response in AGAT deficiency
   c. Incomplete response to creatine supplementation in GAMT deficiency may be due to increased GUAC
   d. MRS creatine peak is absent and does not respond to treatment in creatine transporter deficiency
7. Prognosis: patients with synthesis defects treated with creatine show improvement in development, extrapyramidal symptoms, and seizures

D. Glucose Transporter (GLUT)-1 Deficiency

1. Inheritance
   a. Autosomal dominant
   b. Homozygous mutations produce very severe phenotype or are lethal to embryo
2. Epidemiology: panethnic
3. Pathophysiology: defect in glucose transport across blood-brain barrier because of decreased GLUT-1 activity
4. Clinical features
   a. Infantile-onset seizures with epileptic encephalopathy

Disorders of Creatine Metabolism

Hypotonia

Developmental delay

Autism

Movement disorder

Seizures

Absent peak on MRS

Table 25-1. **Diagnosis of Disorders of Creatine Metabolism**

Disorder	Brain creatine	Plasma and urine GUAC	24-Hour urine creatinine
GMAT	Very low	Increased	Low
AGAT	Very low	Decreased	May be low
CRTR	Very low	Normal	May be low (creatine elevated)

AGAT, arginine:glycine amidinotransferase; GAMT, guanidinoacetate methyltransferase; GUAC, guanidinoacetate.

GLUT-1 Deficiency

Infantile-onset seizures

Epileptic encephalopathy

Developmental delay

Acquired microcephaly

Low CSF glucose

Low CSF lactate

Ketogenic diet

    b. Developmental delay

    c. Deceleration of head growth with acquired microcephaly

    d. Abnormal involuntary movements and spasticity

    e. Milder phenotypes can occur from increased residual GLUT-1 activity

5. Diagnosis

    a. Low CSF glucose (<40 mg/dL) and lactate with normal blood glucose is suggestive

    b. 3-*O*-methyl-D-glucose uptake studies in erythrocytes and molecular analysis are confirmatory

6. Management: ketogenic diet

7. Prognosis: treatment with ketogenic diet improves seizures and other paroxysmal events but is not as effective for improving cognitive deficits

E. Congenital Disorders of Glycosylation (CDG)

1. Glycosylation is synthesis and attachment of glycans

2. Glycans have many important roles; about 50% of proteins are glycosylated

3. 500 genes are involved in glycosylation

4. Protein glycosylation: *O*-linked to serine or threonine or *N*-linked to asparaginine

5. Disorders of *N*-glycosylation

    a. Two types of inborn errors of metabolism pattern

      1) Type 1: absence of glycans

      2) Type 2: increased number of bands because of abnormal structure of glycans

    b. CDG-I

      1) Assembly defects

      2) Cytosol and endoplasmic reticulum

      3) Sialotransferrin type 1 pattern

      4) Eight known genes: 1a →1h

    c. CDG-II

      1) Processing defects

      2) Endoplasmic reticulum and Golgi body

      3) Type 2 pattern

      4) Four known genes: 2a →2d

    d. Acquired disorders

      1) Galactosemia

      2) Fructosemia

      3) Chronic alcoholism

      4) Hemolytic uremic syndrome

    e. CDG-Ia

      1) >350 patients have been described, autosomal recessive, panethnic

      2) *PMM2* gene

      3) Multisystem involvement with dysmorphic features and organ involvement, including inverted nipples, buttock fat pads, developmental delay, hypogonadism

      4) Central nervous system (CNS) and peripheral nervous system (PNS) abnormalities include hypoplastic cerebellum and peripheral neuropathy

      5) Stroke-like episodes with febrile illnesses but no neuroradiologic correlate

      6) Lysosomal inclusions in liver and brain

      7) Treatment: symptomatic, antiepileptic drugs, aspirin, possibly mannose

    f. CDG-Ib

      1) From nondisease to fatal condition with recurrent vomiting, diarrhea, hypoglycemia, liver dysfunction

      2) No CNS sequelae

      3) Treatment: mannose

    g. CDG-Ic

      1) Milder than CDG-Ia

      2) Hypotonia, seizures, developmental delay, strabismus

      3) No cerebellar hypoplasia

      4) Albumin normal; cholesterol and factor XI low

    h. CDG-Id: macrocephaly, seizures, lack of development

    i. CDG-Ie: developmental delay, seizures, hypotonia, failure to thrive, mild dysmorphy

    j. CDG-If: developmental delay, seizures, poor vision, ichthyosis, dwarfism, contractures

    k. CDG-Ig: dysmorphic features, hypotonia, progressive microcephaly, developmental delay

    l. CDG-Ih

      1) Protein-losing enteropathy, moderate hepatomegaly

      2) No CNS symptoms

    m. CDG-IIa

      1) Dysmorphic features, developmental delay, behavioral disturbance, seizures

      2) May have abnormal liver enzymes

    n. CDG-IIb: dysmorphic features, hypotonia, seizures, early death

    o. CDG-IIc (4 patients)

      1) Severe neurologic symptoms, failure to thrive, dysmorphic features

      2) Recurrent infections (leukocyte adhesion defect type II)

    p. CDG-IId (1 patient): Dandy-Walker malformation, myopathy, developmental delay

6. Disorders of *O*-glycosylation

    a. Assembly disorders in Golgi body

    b. Two defects

      1) Galactosyltransferase I deficiency: Ehlers-Danlos phenotype vs. progeroid variant

      2) *N*-acetylhexosaminyltransferase deficiency: multiple exostoses

7. Disorder of combined *O*- and *N*-glycosylation: hereditary inclusion body myopathy

III. AMINOACIDURIAS

A. Phenylketonuria (PKU)
1. Inheritance: autosomal recessive
2. Phenylalanine hydroxylase deficiency
3. Epidemiology: incidence, 1 in 10,000
4. Pathophysiology (Fig. 25-3)
   a. Phenylalanine hydroxylase deficiency leading to inability to metabolize and breakdown phenylalanine
   b. Enzyme converts phenylalanine to tyrosine
   c. Tetrahydrobiopterin (BH4) required as cofactor

d. Phenylalanine and phenylketones (phenyllactate, phenylacetate) accumulate in urine
e. Toxic effects of phenylalanine, including inhibition of protein and neurotransmitter synthesis, cause symptoms
f. Impaired myelination during development

5. Clinical features
   a. Normal at birth
   b. If untreated: developmental delay evident at 2 months
   c. Severe mental retardation in untreated cases
   d. Common features: small stature, hypopigmentation, microcephaly

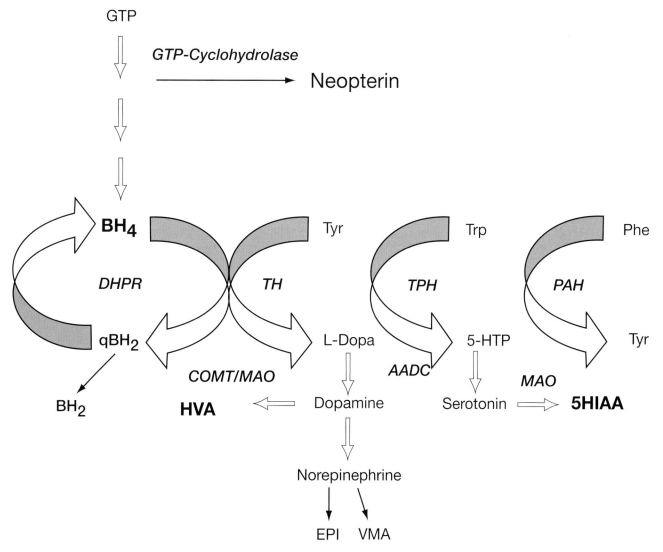

Fig. 25-3. Metabolic pathways of catecholamines, serotonin, and tyrosine synthesis. AADC, amino acid decarboxylase; BH4, tetrahydrobiopterin; COMT, catechol O-methyltransferase; DHPR, dihydrobiopterin reductase; EPI, epinephrine; GTP, guanosine triphosphate; HVA, homovanillic acid; 5-HTP, 5-hydroxytryptamine (serotonin); MAO, monoamine oxidase; PAH, phenylalanine hydroxylase; Phe, phenylalanine; qBH2, quinonoid dihydrobiopterin; TH, tyrosine hydroxylase; TPH, tryptophan hydroxylase; Trp, tryptophan; Tyr, tyrosine; VMA, vanillylmandelic acid. (Modified from Hyland K. The lumbar puncture for diagnosis of pediatric neurotransmitter diseases. Ann Neurol. 2003;54 Suppl 6:S13-7. Used with permission.)

e. Musty odor due to phenylketone accumulation

f. Other associated features: seizure, spasticity, hypotonia, tremor, severe behavioral disturbances

g. Children treated from neonatal period with phenylalanine-restricted diet have normal intelligence

h. Infants of mothers with inadequately treated PKU are usually born with microcephaly and mental retardation

6. Diagnosis

   a. Increased blood level of phenylalanine; decreased blood level of tyrosine

   b. Phenylalanine response to BH_4 and measurement of pterins and neurotransmitters in blood and urine are used to screen for BH_4-deficient forms of PKU

   c. Multiple PKU screening tests available at birth and are routine in most states

7. Pathology: dysmyelination evident on MRI

8. Management

   a. Dietary restriction of phenylalanine to maintain low blood levels of phenylalanine throughout childhood, preferably throughout life, and especially during pregnancy

   b. This requires frequent blood level monitoring

   c. BH_4 deficiency must be excluded before treatment

   d. BH_4-deficient forms of PKU are treated with phenylalanine-restricted diet, L-dopa, 5-hydroxytryptophan, and folinic acid

9. Prognosis

   a. Untreated: severe mental retardation

   b. Early treatment: normal or near-normal intelligence

   c. Diet should be life-long to prevent late neurologic sequelae

10. Prenatal diagnosis: when feasible, DNA analysis, enzyme assay, and measurement of metabolites in amniotic fluid are available

11. PKU variant: dihydropteridine reductase deficiency results

in hyperphenylalaninemia, monoamine deficiency, and defective folate metabolism due to impaired BH_4 recycling

B. **Homocystinuria** (Fig. 25-4)

1. Inheritance

   a. Autosomal recessive

   b. Classic homocystinuria is due to cystathionine β-synthase (CBS) deficiency

   c. Disorders of the remethylation cycle affecting conversion of homocysteine to methionine include 5-methylene-tetrahydrofolate reductase deficiency and disorders of cobalamin metabolism

   d. Methylmalonic aciduria is also present in Cbl C, Cbl D and Cbl F diseases

2. Epidemiology: panethnic

3. Pathophysiology

   a. Homocysteine accumulates intracellularly, then is exported to plasma

   b. Increased methylation of homocysteine to methionine leads to increased plasma and CSF levels of methionine in classic homocystinuria

   c. Vitamin B_{12} is required to methylate homocysteine and thus synthesize methionine

   d. Damage to fibrillin purportedly leads to both ectopia lentis and bony abnormalities

   e. Increased thromboembolism is related to increased effects on endothelial cells and possibly is due to effects on factor V, protein C, lipoprotein (a), platelets and nonendothelial vascular cells

   f. Pyridoxine responsiveness suggests presence of a small amount of residual activity of mutant cystathionine β-synthase

4. Clinical features

   a. Major organs involved: eye, skeleton, vascular system, CNS

Phenylketonuria (PKU)

Most common inborn error of metabolism

Phenylalanine hydroxylase deficiency

Severe mental retardation

Seizures

Hypopigmentation

Microcephaly

Musty odor

Homocystinuria

Marfanoid habitus

Epilepsy

Mental retardation

Downward dislocation of lens

Stroke

Osteoporosis

Psychiatric disturbance

Homocystinuria

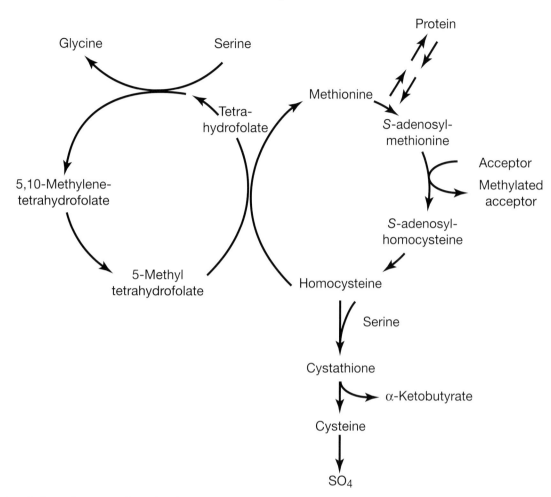

Fig. 25-4. Metabolic pathways implicated in homocystinuria.

b. Most common finding: ectopia lentis with downward dislocation of lens, starting by age 2 years

c. Osteoporosis of the spine, followed by long bones, by about age 20 years

d. Patients develop marfanoid habitus with thin and long bones, with pectus carinatum, pes cavus, genu valgum

e. Thromboembolism: most common cause of death, with occlusion of any vessel at any age

f. CNS

   1) Mental retardation presents with developmental delay in first 2 years of life and is most common CNS abnormality

   2) Seizures: one-fifth of untreated patients

   3) Psychiatric illnesses: approximately one-half of patients

   4) Strokes can occur at any age

5. Diagnosis

a. Homocystinuria presents with increased plasma homocysteine and presence of homocystine in urine

b. Decreased plasma cystine levels and increased plasma methionine levels are present in the classic form of homocystinuria

c. Low methionine level is present in remethylation disorders because of impaired conversion of homocysteine to methionine

d. Methylmalonic aciduria may be present in disorders of cobalamin metabolism

e. A decreased enzyme level in hepatocytes or skin fibroblasts is definitive

f. Pyridoxine responsiveness in CBS deficiency is established with presence of decreased homocysteine levels following adequate doses of pyridoxine for a few weeks

g. Newborn screening usually only diagnoses CBS-deficient

patients because increased methionine levels are detected

6. Management
   a. Low methionine, cystine-supplemented diet only for CBS patients
   b. Pyridoxine may be used and continued in patients responsive to it
   c. Betaine lowers total plasma homocysteine by converting to methionine
   d. Folate may be needed to allow adequate pyridoxine response, with adequate care to supplement vitamin B_{12} in such cases
   e. Folate and vitamin B_{12} in large doses are required for treatment of remethylation disorders
   f. Some groups use dipyridamole or aspirin for stroke prevention

7. Prognosis
   a. Ectopia lentis can lead to acute angle-closure glaucoma, myopia, retinal degeneration, and other conditions
   b. Increased risk for thromboembolism postoperatively and in postpartum period
   c. Outcome improved by aggressive treatment to decrease total plasma homocysteine level

8. Prenatal diagnosis: enzyme activity can be tested in amniocytes and chorionic villi cells

C. **Maple Syrup Urine Disease** (branched-chain ketoaciduria)

1. Inheritance: autosomal recessive
2. Due to branched chain α-keto acid dehydrogenase (BCKAD) complex deficiency: the E3 form has combined BCKAD, pyruvate dehydrogenase, and α-ketoglutarate dehydrogenase deficiency
3. Epidemiology: more common among Mennonites
4. Pathophysiology: branched-chain amino acids (leucine, isoleucine, valine) and their keto acids accumulate in blood
5. These are both ketogenic and glucogenic
6. Clinical features: multiple phenotypes
   a. Classic
      1) Most common and most severe form, with neonatal onset
      2) Patients present in neonatal period with altered sensorium and poor feeding, followed by seizures, alternating hypotonia and hypertonia, decerebrate posturing as a dystonic manifestation, coma, death
      3) Maple syrup odor is evident during a crisis
      4) Heterotopia occurs
   b. Intermediate: patients present in late infancy with developmental delay and/or seizures
   c. Intermittent: patients are normal until they suddenly

decompensate during illness, with altered sensorium, ataxia, abnormal odor
   d. Thiamine-responsive: patients present with developmental delay and periodic crises during illnesses
   e. Dihydrolipoyl dehydrogenase deficient: lactic acidosis accompanied by failure to thrive, hypotonia, developmental delay, movement disorder

7. Diagnosis
   a. Branched-chain amino acids, particularly leucine, are increased in plasma and urine
   b. Presence of alloisoleucine is diagnostic
   c. Decreased enzyme level in hepatocytes and skin fibroblasts is definitive
   d. Newborn screening is available

8. Management
   a. In classic type, life-long treatment with branched-chain amino acid–restricted diet must be instituted within 2 weeks after birth to achieve normal IQ levels
   b. Trial of thiamine to determine responsiveness
   c. Aggressive intervention during metabolic crises and infections
   d. Liver transplantation for classic maple syrup urine disease is experimental

9. Prognosis
   a. Untreated patients with classic disease die within few months after birth with progressive encephalopathy and recurrent metabolic crises
   b. Survivors have severe mental retardation, spasticity, and occasionally, cortical blindness
   c. Prognosis improves substantially with early treatment, particularly for milder forms

10. Prenatal diagnosis: enzyme activity can be tested in amniocytes and chorionic villi cells

D. **Nonketotic Hyperglycinemia**
1. Inheritance: autosomal recessive

Maple Syrup Urine Disease
Branched chain α-ketoacid dehydrogenase deficiency

Neonatal encephalopathy

Maple syrup odor

Developmental delay

Seizures

Ataxia

2. Glycine encephalopathy
3. Epidemiology: onset in newborn period, most common in Finland
4. Pathophysiology
   a. Error in glycine degradation
   b. Four proteins are involved in glycine cleavage system: P (pyridoxal phosphate-dependent glycine decarboxylase), H (hydrogen carrier), T (tetrahydrofolate-dependent protein), M (lipoamide dehydrogenase)
   c. Enzyme most commonly defective is P
   d. Glycine accumulates and is an excitatory neurotransmitter, acting through NMDA-type glutamate receptors in brain and is inhibitory neurotransmitter in spinal cord and brainstem
   e. There is relative serine deficiency
5. Clinical features
   a. Usually presents in early newborn period with progressive lethargy, hypotonia, hiccups, myoclonic jerks, apnea; rapidly progresses to coma with ventilator dependence
   b. If child survives, then profound mental retardation and intractable seizures
   c. Atypical presentations occur in later infancy and childhood with developmental delay and psychomotor retardation, seizures, hyperactivity, spinocerebellar degeneration, vertical gaze palsy, optic atrophy, chorea, pulmonary hypertension
   d. Transient neonatal deficiency with classic symptoms also occurs in some instances
6. Diagnosis
   a. Measurement of glycine cleavage system activity and activity of individual components on open liver biopsy showing deficiency is confirmatory
   b. Increased CSF:plasma glycine ratio >0.08 (normal <0.04) is suggestive
   c. Plasma glycine levels are also high, except in atypical cases
   d. Hyperglycinemia may also occur in
      1) Methylmalonic, propionic, and isovaleric acidemias,

with ketosis and no CSF hyperglycinosis
      2) Starvation
      3) Kwashiorkor
      4) Valproic acid therapy
      5) Hypoxic ischemic encephalopathy
      6) Other rare inborn errors of metabolism
   e. Mutation analysis is difficult because of inadequate knowledge of mutations involved and many private mutations
7. Management: symptomatic treatments marginally effective
   a. Sodium benzoate (depletes glycine)
   b. Dextromethorphan (NMDA receptor antagonist)
   c. Treatment of seizures
8. Prenatal diagnosis: glycine cleavage system activity can be tested in chorionic villi cells

E. Urea Cycle Disorders (Fig. 25-5)
1. Inheritance: autosomal recessive except for ornithine transcarbamoylase (OTC) deficiency, which is X-linked
2. Epidemiology
   a. Panethnic
   b. Incidence: 1 in 8,000 live births
   c. OTC deficiency is most common form and accounts for almost two-thirds of all cases
   d. Arginase deficiency: extremely rare
3. Pathophysiology: hyperammonemia leads to astrocyte swelling from glutamine accumulation, leading to brain edema acutely
4. Clinical features (Table 25-2)
   a. Neonatal onset of OTC, carbamoylphosphate synthetase (CPS), argininosuccinic acid synthetase (AS), and argininosuccinic acid lyase (AL) deficiencies cannot be differentiated by clinical symptoms
   b. Symptoms are due to hyperammonemia and hyperglutaminemia
   c. Triad of hyperammonemia, encephalopathy, and respiratory alkalosis occurs and is due to hyperventilation
   d. Symptoms usually present between 24 and 72 hours of life, usually in term infant
      1) Vomiting, poor feeding, apnea, hypothermia and lethargy are followed by coma and then seizures
      2) Severity of encephalopathy correlates with ammonia levels
      3) AL deficiency has severe hepatomegaly in early-onset form and trichorrhexis nodosa in late-onset form
   e. Late onset of OTC, CPS, AS, and AL deficiencies can present any time in life and symptoms are often associated with infections and high protein meals
      1) They are characterized by features of hyperammonemia

---

Nonketotic Hyperglycinemia

Neonatal encephalopathy

Profound mental retardation

Intractable seizures

Chorea

CSF:plasma glycine ratio: >0.8

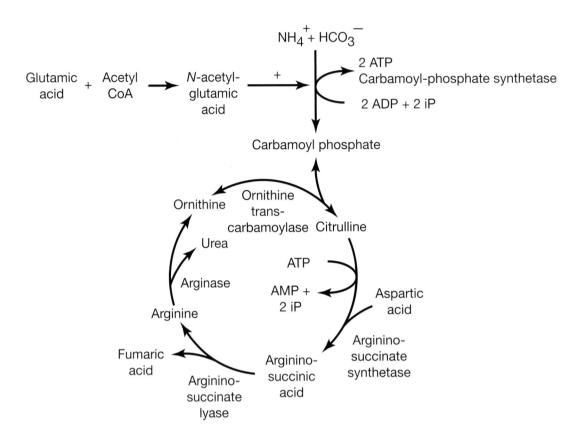

Fig. 25-5. Urea cycle. ADP, adenosine diphosphate; AMP, adenosine monophosphate; ATP, adenosine triphosphate; iP, inorganic phosphorus.

such as vomiting, altered mental status, ataxia, amblyopia
2) Seizures, developmental delay, and growth retardation occur
3) Female carriers of OTC deficiency may present post partum with hyperammonemic encephalopathy
f. Arginase deficiency does not cause symptoms in newborn
g. Progressive spastic quadriplegia, seizures, mental retardation, hyperactivity and growth failure occur
h. Hyperammonemia is less severe and infrequent
i. Episodic encephalopathy can occur in newborns with partial deficiency of CPS and in female carriers of OTC deficiency
5. Diagnosis
  a. In newborns: hyperammonemia without organic acidemia should suggest a urea cycle disorder
  b. Diagnosis can be determined by analysis of quantitative amino acids in plasma and urine and measurement of organic acids and orotic acid
  c. Enzyme defect in peripheral leukocytes or hepatocytes is confirmatory
  d. Respiratory alkalosis with hyperammonemia suggests urea cycle defect
  e. Imaging shows cerebral edema during acute encephalopathy
  f. Liver function tests are normal, unlike in Reye's syndrome
6. Pathology: cerebral edema with astrocyte swelling and Alzheimer type II cells occur in neonatal encephalopathies
7. Management
  a. Acute hyperammonemia
    1) All dietary and parenteral nitrogen intake must be discontinued
    2) Intravenous sodium benzoate, sodium phenylacetate, and 10% arginine hydrochloride should be commenced immediately in CPS, OTC, and AS with a priming dose
    3) AL requires intravenous infusion of 10% arginine hydrochloride
    4) Hemodialysis or peritoneal dialysis is indicated in acute phase if hyperammonemia lasts more than 8 hours
  b. Raised intracranial tension should be treated with mannitol

Table 25-2. **Urea Cycle Disorders**

Urea cycle disorder	Clinical features	Diagnosis	Management
Carbamoylphosphate synthetase (CPS) deficiency	Neonatal encephalopathy or intermittent vomiting, lethargy, unusual eye movements	Hyperammonemia, low plasma citruline No orotic acid Low CPS levels in hepatocytes	Hemodialysis for hyperammonemia Sodium benzoate, phenylbutyrate Citrulline and arginine to bypass block in urea cycle Low protein diet
Ornithine transcarbamoylase (OTC) deficiency	Males: neonatal encephalopathy, respiratory alkalosis, mental retardation, death Females: normal or intermittent headache, vomiting, ophthalmoplegia	Hyperammonemia, respiratory alkalosis, high urinary orotic acid (orotic aciduria) Low plasma citrulline	
Arginosuccinic acid synthetase (AS) deficiency	Neonatal encephalopathy, mental retardation, seizures, ataxia, vomiting	Hyperammonemia, very high levels of plasma citrulline, citrullinuria	
Arginosuccinic acid lyase (AL) deficiency	Neonatal encephalopathy, mental retardation, seizures, trichorrhexis nodosa, ataxia, vomiting ± hepatomegaly	Hyperammonemia, mildly elevated plasma citrulline, arginosuccinate aciduria	
Arginase deficiency	Mental retardation, seizures, spastic tetraplegia, growth failure	Hyperammonemia, hyperargininemia, diaminoaciduria (arginine, ornithine, cystine, and lysine), may have mild orotic aciduria	

c. Hyperventilation is inadvisable because of decreased blood flow due to hypocapnia in presence of hyperammonemia

d. Long term

1) Low protein diet, essential amino acid mixture, citrulline supplementation for CPS and OTC, and arginine supplementation for AS and AL deficiency, with the intention to allow growth while preventing hyperammonemia

2) Arginase deficiency is similarly treated with protein restriction and possibly sodium benzoate and phenylacetate

e. Liver transplantation for neonatal-onset OTC deficiency and CPS deficiency

8. Prognosis

a. All infants, including those prospectively treated before onset of neonatal symptoms, are at high risk for neurologic deficits

b. Late-onset disease stabilizes at level of neurologic function at time of therapy initiation

9. Prenatal diagnosis: consists of DNA analysis and enzyme analysis in cultured amniocytes and chorionic villi cells

IV. ORGANIC ACIDURIAS

A. Propionic Acidemia

1. Inheritance: autosomal recessive

2. Propionyl-CoA carboxylase deficiency

3. Previously called ketotic hyperglycinemia

4. Epidemiology: rare

5. Pathophysiology: propionyl-CoA carboxylase (biotin-dependent) has α and β subunits encoded by chromosomes 13 and 3

6. Clinical features: three different presentations that range in severity

a. Severe metabolic acidosis of newborn with feeding refusal, vomiting, lethargy, hypotonia, seizures and dehydration, with hepatomegaly occurring less often

b. Infantile onset of episodic encephalopathy, vomiting, ketoacidosis, dehydration

c. Later onset of mental retardation or dementia, chorea, dystonia

d. Common to see thrombocytopenia, neutropenia, basal ganglia abnormalities

e. Attacks often precipitated by infection or protein ingestion

7. Diagnosis

a. Anion gap acidosis with ketonemia and ketonuria with propionic acid and its metabolites in blood and urine is suggestive

b. Propionate also accumulates in disorders of methylmalonate metabolism, which should be ruled out

c. Confirmation is by measuring propionyl-CoA carboxylase activity in leukocyte or fibroblast extracts

8. Management

a. Supportive care

b. Low protein diet with frequent feeding

c. Ketoacidosis crises must be treated with protein restriction, sodium bicarbonate, carnitine, and glucose

d. Peritoneal dialysis may be required; carnitine and biotin supplementation

e. Metronidazole decreases propionate production by gut bacteria

9. Prognosis: treatment is difficult and neurologic sequelae are common

10. Prenatal diagnosis

a. Propionyl-CoA carboxylase activity in cultured amniocytes and chorionic villi can be measured

b. Methylcitrate level can be measured in amniotic fluid

B. **Methylmalonic Acidemia** (MMA)

1. Inheritance: autosomal recessive

2. Epidemiology: rare

3. Pathophysiology

a. Several metabolic types: methylmalonyl-CoA mutase deficiency (complete or partial) is major form

b. This enzyme converts L-methylmalonyl-CoA to succinyl-CoA, which enters Krebs cycle

c. Vitamin B_{12} (adenosylcobalamin) required as coenzyme

d. Errors in cobalamin metabolism account for other forms of methylmalonic acidemia alone (Cbl A, Cbl B) and MMA with homocystinuria (Cbl C, Cbl D, Cbl F)

e. Bone marrow suppression may occur in mutase-deficient forms

4. Clinical features

a. Mutase deficiency (*mut0*), Cbl A, and Cbl B present in a similar fashion with profound neonatal or infantile methylmalonic acidosis

b. Episodic encephalopathy, vomiting, failure to thrive, and hypotonia occur in neonatal period

c. Seizures

d. Pancytopenia and immune dysfunction may occur

e. Developmental delay, hepatomegaly, and coma occur in some patients

f. *cblC*, *cblD*, *cblF* mutations present with combined homocystinuria and methylmalonic acidemia

g. No ketoacidosis

h. Usually have less severe acidemia (hyperglycinemia, hyperammonemia less common) and more common hematologic manifestations

i. Patients with later onset of disease present with acute neurologic findings of dementia, delirium, tremor, myelopathy

5. Diagnosis

a. Anion gap acidosis with increased methylmalonic acid,

Propionic Acidemia

Propionyl-CoA carboxylase deficiency

Catastrophic neonatal metabolic acidosis

Neonatal encephalopathy

Infantile episodic encephalopathy

Mental retardation

Dementia

Thrombocytopenia

Neutropenia

Methylmalonic Acidemia

Methylmalonyl-CoA mutase deficiency

Vitamin B_{12} coenzyme

Bone marrow suppression

Profound neonatal or infantile acidosis

Episodic neonatal encephalopathy

Developmental retardation

Hepatomegaly

3-OH propionic acid, and methyl citric acid in urine, ketonemia and ketonuria in 80%, and hyperammonemia in 70% during acute presentation

b. Increased urine homocystine with low serum levels of methionine and normal leves of cobalamin occur in cobalamin disorders (Cbl C, Cbl D, and Cbl F)

c. Hypoglycemia occurs in some

6. Management
   a. Acutely: management of metabolic acidosis, hyperammonemia, and hypoglycemia with high rate of glucose infusion and discontinuation of protein intake
   b. Long term
      1) Protein restriction, at least to restrict amino acid precursors of methylmalonic acid for disorders presenting with MMA alone
      2) Hydroxocobalamin supplementation
      3) Carnitine supplementation
      4) Betaine for treatment of homocystinuria
      5) Metronidazole therapy may help if methylmalonate and propionate metabolites are persistently increased
   c. Prenatal therapy with cobalamin has been tried
   d. Gene therapy and liver transplant are experimental

7. Prognosis
   a. *mut0* group has worst prognosis for survival and development
   b. Strokes and chronic renal failure have been known in long-term survivors

8. Prenatal diagnosis
   a. Mutase activity in cultured amniocytes can be measured
   b. Methylmalonic acid level can be measured in amniotic fluid and maternal urine

C. Disorders of Biotin Metabolism

1. Multiple carboxylase deficiency
   a. Inheritance: autosomal recessive
   b. Holocarboxylase synthetase deficiency: early-onset (neonatal) multiple carboxylase deficiency
   c. Epidemiology: rare
   d. Pathophysiology
      1) Manifests due to defective function of several biotin-dependent enzymes: acetyl-CoA carboxylase, propionyl-CoA carboxylase, 3-methylcrotonyl-CoA carboxylase, and pyruvate carboxylase leading to buildup of branched-chain amino acids and organic acidemia
      2) These enzymes have important roles in gluconeogenesis, fatty acid synthesis, and amino acid catabolism
      3) A disorder of biotinylation
   e. Clinical features
      1) Often present in neonatal period, with feeding and

breathing difficulties, lethargy, and seizures, followed by skin rash, alopecia, glossitis, hypotonia, recurrent infection

      2) Sometimes progresses to developmental delay or coma
      3) Tomcat urine odor
   f. Diagnosis
      1) Metabolic acidosis, organic aciduria in characteristic pattern, and mild to moderate hyperammonemia
      2) Enzyme assay in leukocytes and fibroblasts is diagnostic
   g. Management: biotin 10-40 mg/d
   h. Prognosis: excellent with biotin replacement
   i. Prenatal diagnosis: by measuring abnormal organic acids in amniotic fluid and/or by assaying mitochondrial carboxylase activities in amniocytes cultured with and without biotin; mutation analysis possible

2. Biotinidase deficiency
   a. Also known as late-onset (juvenile) multiple carboxylase deficiency
   b. Inheritance: autosomal recessive
   c. Epidemiology
      1) Approximately 1 in 60,000 to 100,000
      2) Onset at different ages with different severity
   d. Pathophysiology
      1) Disorder of biotin recycling
      2) Decreased biotin in brain may lead to decreased pyruvate carboxylase activity and, thus, lactic acid accumulation in brain
   e. Clinical features
      1) Age at onset varies from infancy to childhood
      2) Seizures, hypotonia, ataxia, breathing problems, hearing loss, optic atrophy, developmental delay, rash, and alopecia are common
   f. Diagnosis
      1) Children have lactic acidosis, ketosis, hyperammonemia, and characteristic organic aciduria
      2) Decreased levels of biotinidase in serum and leukocytes
      3) Clinical features are similar to holocarboxylase synthetase deficiency, although biotinidase deficiency presents a little later in infancy
   g. Pathology: chronic cerebellar degeneration and atrophy
   h. Management: newborn screening is offered in most states; oral biotin replacement is effective
   i. Prognosis
      1) Untreated disease leads to marked neurodegeneration
      2) Prognosis improved substantially by early treatment with biotin
   j. Prenatal diagnosis: consists of analysis of biotinidase enzyme activity in amniocytes or chorionic villi
   k. Partial biotinidase enzyme deficiency also occurs

D. **Glutaric Acidemia Type I**

1. Inheritance: autosomal recessive
2. Epidemiology: 1 in 30,000; more frequent incidence in Old Order Amish
3. Pathophysiology
   a. Glutaryl-CoA dehydrogenase deficiency
   b. Increased glutaric acid and relative deficiency of γ-aminobutyric acid (GABA) because of inhibition of glutamate decarboxylase
4. Clinical features
   a. Macrocephaly, usually at birth
   b. Rapid onset childhood dystonia, hypotonia, and choreoathetosis occur following acute encephalopathic episode with an illness in first few years of life
   c. This is followed by progressive extrapyramidal syndrome with incomplete recovery from initial illness
   d. Some patients present with gradual extrapyramidal symptoms with no acute onset
   e. Wide range in severity
   f. Some patients have episodic encephalopathy during illnesses
   g. Relative preservation of intellect
5. Diagnosis
   a. Increased glutaric acid and 3-hydroxyglutaric acid in urine and deficiency of glutaryl-CoA dehydrogenase in cultured fibroblasts are diagnostic; glutaric acid may be normal or only slightly elevated when patient is well
   b. Neuroimaging (Fig. 25-6)
      1) Collection of fluid over frontal lobes and base of brain; may be present at birth
      2) Subdural hematomas may occur spontaneously and can be confused with child abuse
      3) Frontotemporal atrophy and arachnoid cysts may predate degeneration of caudate and putamen
      4) Widening of sylvian fissure is common
      5) Thalamus and globus pallidus usually not affected
6. Pathology: striatal degeneration, especially caudate and putamen

7. Management
   a. Protein-restricted diet with special formula limiting lysine and tryptophan intake to essential levels
   b. Riboflavin supplementation
   c. Early supplementation with L-carnitine, and vigorous fluid, glucose, and insulin repletion during intercurrent infections
   d. Baclofen, valproic acid, and vigabatrin have been tried to increase GABA levels in brain
8. Prognosis: death in first decade during acute intercurrent illnesses or survival into adulthood
9. Prenatal diagnosis: glutaryl-CoA dehydrogenase deficiency in cultured amniocytes and increased glutaric acid level in amniotic fluid are diagnostic

E. **Glutaric Acidemia Type II** (multiple acyl-CoA dehydrogenase deficiency)

1. Inheritance: autosomal recessive
2. Epidemiology: rare

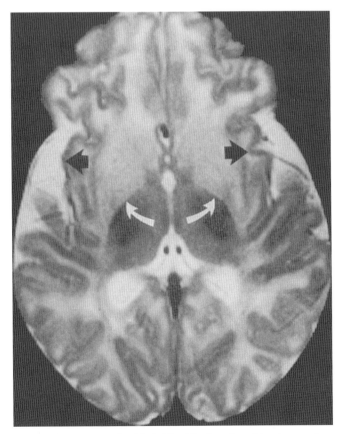

Fig. 25-6. A 3-month-old child with glutaric acidemia type I. T2-weighted MRI shows enlargement of the sylvian fissures (*black arrows*) and diffuse hyperintensity of basal ganglia bilaterally (*white arrows*). (From Osborn AG. Diagnostic neuroradiology. St. Louis: Mosby; 1994. p. 716-47. Used with permission.)

Glutaric Acidemia Type I

Macrocephaly

Acute encephalopathic crisis

Movement disorder

Dystonia

Spontaneous subdural hematoma

3. Pathophysiology
   a. Defect in electron transfer from flavoprotein dehydrogenases to respiratory chain resulting in functional deficiency of multiple enzymes
   b. Electron transfer flavoprotein (ETF) and ETF-ubiquinone oxidoreductase (ETF-QO) are nuclear-encoded proteins through which electrons are transferred to ubiquinone in the respiratory chain
   c. Inherited defects of either protein cause glutaric acidemia type II
4. Clinical features
   a. Common features: hypoketotic hypoglycemia and metabolic acidosis
   b. Complete enzyme defects, especially of ETF-QO, are often associated with multiple congenital anomalies, including renal cystic dysplasia
   c. Neonatal onset with congenital anomalies
      1) Often born premature and present during first 24 to 48 hours of life with hypotonia, hepatomegaly, severe hypoglycemia and metabolic acidosis, and odor of sweaty feet
      2) Enlarged kidneys, facial dysmorphism, rocker-bottom feet, anterior abdominal wall defects, and hypospadias and chordee occur
   d. Neonatal onset without anomalies
      1) Present with hypotonia, metabolic acidosis, hepatomegaly, hypoglycemia, and "sweaty feet" odor within first few days of life
      2) Some have Reye syndrome-like episodes later in life
      3) Hypertrophic cardiomyopathy may develop
   e. Mild and/or later onset: at any age, with episodic vomiting, hypoglycemia, hepatomegaly, and proximal myopathy; also known as ethylmalonic-adipic aciduria
5. Diagnosis
   a. Increased levels of organic acids in characteristic pattern in serum, urine, and CSF in setting of hypoketotic hypoglycemia and metabolic acidosis
   b. Metabolic acidosis may be absent in late-onset cases and organic acid findings may be intermittent
   c. Specific diagnosis is by fibroblast analysis of ETF and ETF-QO activity
   d. MRI may show hypoplastic temporal lobes, as in glutaryl-CoA dehydrogenase deficiency
   e. Abdominal ultrasound or CT may show renal cysts
   f. Generalized aminoaciduria and increased urinary acylcarnitines occur in neonatal-onset patients
6. Pathology: fatty infiltration of liver, heart, kidneys
7. Management
   a. No effective treatment for patients who present in early infancy

   b. Fat and protein restriction, and treatment with riboflavin, and L-carnitine may help in less severely affected patients
8. Prognosis: neonatal patients die within first week of life or rarely later because of cardiomyopathy
9. Prenatal diagnosis: possible in some cases by demonstrating increased concentrations of glutaric acid in amniotic fluid, acylcarnitine esters in maternal urine, or impaired substrate oxidation in amniocytes

V. DISORDERS OF NUCLEIC ACID METABOLISM (PURINES AND PYRIMIDINES)

A. Lesch-Nyhan Disease
1. Deficiency of hypoxanthine-guanine phosphoribosyltransferase at the rate-limiting step in the "salvage pathway" of purine degradation
2. Inheritance: X-linked recessive
3. Epidemiology
   a. Panethnic
   b. Occurs in 1 in 380,000 live births
4. Pathophysiology: accumulations of uric acid, purines, hypoxanthine, and xanthine from changes in regulation of purine synthesis and degradation
5. Clinical features
   a. Presentation in infancy with variable developmental retardation leading to debilitating neurologic disability, dystonia, choreoathetosis, dysphagia, dysarthria, spasticity, seizures
   b. Characteristic severe self-mutilation behavior
   c. Uric acid stones
6. Diagnosis
   a. Hyperuricemia is suggestive of diagnosis in appropriate clinical setting
   b. Hypoxanthine guanine phosphoribosyl transferase (HGPRT) activity in peripheral lymphocytes or cultured fibroblasts is confirmatory
7. Pathology: Nonspecific findings, including cerebral atrophy of varying severity
8. Management
   a. Purine-restricted diet
   b. Maintain adequate hydration to prevent uric acid stones
   c. Allopurinol blocks overproduction of uric acid to reduce risk of nephrolithiasis and gout with no efficacy against CNS features
   d. Supportive care needs to be intensive, including padded wheelchairs with protective straps with no access to any potentially injurious object
   e. Self-biting may need drastic measures such as edentulation

> **Lesch-Nyhan Disease**
>
> X-linked recessive
>
> Hypoxanthine-guanine phosphoribosyltransferase deficiency
>
> Developmental retardation
>
> Dystonia
>
> Choreoathetosis
>
> Spasticity
>
> Seizures
>
> Severe self-mutilation behavior
>
> Severe gout

    f. Dopamine receptor antagonists, selective serotonin reuptake inhibitors (SSRIs), hypoxanthine, and magnesium have been tried with variable success for dystonia and behavioral problems

    g. Spasticity responds to baclofen and benzodiazepines

9. Prognosis

    a. Cervical spine injury and myelopathy can occur secondary to dystonia

    b. Self-mutilation can lead to amputation of digits

    c. Patients are wheelchair-bound by second year of life

10. Prenatal diagnosis: DNA analysis and enzyme analysis in cultured amniocytes and chorionic villi cells

11. Note: patients with 1.5% to 8% of residual HGPRT activity have variable CNS features of minor clumsiness to debilitating extrapyramidal and pyramidal motor dysfunction; those with more than 8% residual activity have no neurologic symptoms

B. Dihydropyrimidine Dehydrogenase Deficiency

1. Inheritance: autosomal recessive
2. Epidemiology
    a. Panethnic
    b. Rare
3. Pathophysiology: rate-limiting step in degradation of the pyrimidines uracil and thymidine
4. Clinical features
    a. Variable degree of developmental delay, seizures, macrocephaly, hypotonia
    b. Toxicity associated with treatment with fluorouracil (5-FU)
5. Diagnosis

    a. Urinary excretion of thymidine and uracil
    b. Enzyme assay for dihydropyrimidine dehydrogenase deficiency is confirmatory
6. Management
    a. Symptomatic
    b. Avoidance of 5-FU
7. Prognosis: variable, ranging from severe childhood neurologic syndrome to CNS toxicity in adults with 5-FU
8. Other pyrimidine disorders with neurologic symptoms
    a. Ureidopropionase deficiency with choreoathetosis, hypotonia, and microcephaly
    b. Thymidine phosphorylase deficiency with mitochondrial neurogastrointestinal encephalomyopathy (MNGIE)

VI. PORPHYRIAS

A. Inheritance

1. Autosomal recessive: 5-aminolevulinic acid dehydratase-deficient porphyria (ADP)
2. Autosomal dominant: acute intermittent porphyria (AIP), hereditary coproporphyria (HCP), and variegate porphyria (VP)

B. Epidemiology

1. AIP may be more common in northern European countries
2. Prevalence of AIP is about 5 in 100,000
3. VP is especially common in South Africa
4. The four acute hepatic porphyrias (ADP, AIP, HCP and VP) cause neurologic disease

C. Pathophysiology

1. Heme biosynthetic pathway consists of eight enzymes that sequentially convert glycine and succinyl CoA to heme
2. Rate of aminolevulinic acid synthesis is important controlling step for heme formation, especially in liver
3. Hepatic porphyrias are pharmacogenetic or ecogenetic conditions, i.e., drugs, hormones, and nutritional alterations influence rate of heme biosynthesis in the liver and precipitate clinical expression of the underlying genetic trait
4. Accumulation of aminolevulinic acid occurs in the liver in AIP, ADP, HCP, VP; aminolevulinic acid may be neurotoxic

D. Clinical Features

1. Porphyria attacks usually occur after puberty, generally

in third or fourth decade

2. All acute porphyrias (ADP, HCP, and VP) have the same clinical features as AIP

3. Precipitating factors that incite attacks are most often drugs: barbiturates, sulfonamides, analgesics, nonbarbiturate hypnotics, anticonvulsants, female sex hormones

4. Fasting or malnutrition, stress, infection, smoking, alcohol consumption may also precipitate attack

5. Photosensitivity and skin manifestations: main clinical features of other types of porphyria (Table 25-3)

6. ADP
   a. Very rare
   b. Variable presentation
   c. Abdominal pain, peripheral neuropathy in teens, and syndrome of inappropriate secretion of antidiuretic hormone (SIADH), with increased susceptibility to lead poisoning in heterozygotes

7. AIP
   a. An acute hepatic porphyria
   b. Most common of acute porphyrias
   c. Visceral, autonomic, PNS, CNS involvement
   d. Wide variety of manifestations that are usually intermittent and nonspecific
   e. Acute attacks
      1) Most common presenting symptom: severe abdominal pain
      2) Other gastrointestinal symptoms such as nausea, vomiting, severe constipation, and signs of ileus, or diarrhea may occur
      3) Urinary retention may occur; urine is often dark red or color of port wine
      4) Marked absence of tenderness, fever, leukocytosis

Porphyria

Drug-induced crises

Infection- and stress-induced crises

Abdominal pain

Peripheral neuropathy

Psychiatric symptoms

Porphyrias With CNS Symptoms

5-Aminolevulinic acid dehydratase-deficient porphyria (ADP)

Acute intermittent porphyria (AIP)

Hereditary coproporphyria (HCP)

Variegate porphyria (VP)

Table 25-3. **Porphyrias**

Name of disease	Deficient enzyme	Inheritance	Clinical features	Diagnosis
5-Aminolevulinic acid dehydratase-deficient porphyria (ADP)	5-Aminolevulinic acid dehydratase	Autosomal recessive	Abdominal pain, peripheral neuropathy, increased susceptibility to lead poisoning	Normal urinary PBG in the presence of increased urinary ALA and coproporphyrin Markedly decreased erythrocyte ALAD activity
Acute intermittent porphyria (AIP)	Porphobilinogen deaminase partial deficiency	Autosomal dominant	Abdominal pain, acute neuropathy, seizures, autonomic dysfunction	Marked increase in PBG Markedly increased urinary excretion of ALA and PBG
Hereditary coproporphyria (HCP)	Coproporphyrinogen oxidase partial deficiency	Autosomal dominant	Same as for AIP	Marked increase in urinary and fecal coproporphyrin III
Variegate porphyria (VP)	Protoporphyrinogen oxidase deficiency	Autosomal dominant	Same as for AIP	Fecal protoporphyrin, coproporphyrin III, and urinary coproporphyrin III are markedly increased during active disease Increased urinary ALA and PBG

ALA, aminolevulinic acid; ALAD, 5-aminolevulinic acid dehydrase; PBG, porphobilinogen.

5) Seizures are common, particularly in association with hyponatremia

6) Features of sympathetic overactivity may occur; autonomic neuropathy may present with postural hypotension

7) Diffuse pain, muscle weakness, sensory loss can occur

8) Extremity pain may be manifestation of early peripheral neuropathy

9) Recurrent attacks tend to be similar in a given patient

f. Neurologic features

1) Primarily motor axonal peripheral neuropathy, symmetric proximal muscle weakness, cranial nerve (CN) VII and CN X neuropathy

2) Rare optic neuropathy or cortical blindness and sensory involvement occur

g. CNS involvement

1) Common and highly variable

2) Severe anxiety, insomnia, depression, disorientation, hallucinations, and paranoia during acute attacks

3) Chronic depression and psychiatric symptoms may occur

h. Seizures

1) May be manifestation of porphyria itself or secondary to hyponatremia

2) Almost all antiseizure drugs can exacerbate acute porphyria

i. Metabolic: hyponatremia, hypercalcemia, hypomagnesemia may occur

8. HCP

a. Same clinical features as AIP

b. Cutaneous photosensitivity occurs

9. VP

a. Can present with neurologic manifestations and/or cutaneous photosensitivity

b. Homozygous dominant patients can present with growth retardation and severe neurologic manifestations in infancy or childhood, with no acute attacks

E. Diagnosis

1. Inquiry about abdominal pains, severe constipation and vomiting, color of urine and skin lesions is important in patients with epilepsy

2. Neurologic manifestations correlate with levels of δ-aminolevulinic acid and porphobilinogen

3. Marked increase in urinary porphobilinogen is found only in AIP, HCP, and VP

4. Urinary porphyrins are unreliable because they are increased in liver or bone marrow dysfunction

5. Stool porphyrins and blood aminolevulinic acid levels are helpful

6. Enzyme analysis is diagnostic

7. AIP: partially deficient porphobilinogen deaminase activity in erythrocytes in patients with symptoms of AIP is suggestive; detecting the specific *PBGD* mutation in each family makes the definitive diagnosis of AIP

8. HCP

a. Marked increase in urinary and fecal coproporphyrin III

b. Urinary aminolevulinic acid, porphobilinogen, and uroporphyrin are increased during acute attacks

9. VP: fecal protoporphyrin and coproporphyrin III and urinary coproporphyrin III are markedly increased during active disease; increased urinary aminolevulinic acid and porphobilinogen

F. **Pathology:** nonspecific findings, including cerebral atrophy of varying severity

G. Management

1. AIP, HCP, VP

a. Adequate nutritional intake

b. Prompt treatment of intercurrent illnesses

c. Avoidance of drugs known to precipitate attacks

d. Gabapentin and clonazepam are useful for seizures

e. Heme therapy (hematin, heme albumin or heme arginate) and carbohydrate loading repress hepatic δ-aminolevulinate 1 and reduce urinary aminolevulinic acid and porphobilinogen and are considered specific therapies

f. Monitor for hyponatremia and signs of SIADH

g. Narcotic analgesics for abdominal and extremity pain and phenothiazine for nausea, vomiting, anxiety, and restlessness are effective

2. ADP: not known

3. Photosensitivity

a. Protection from sunlight is mandatory

b. Increasing the amount of skin pigment by exposure to short-wavelength ultraviolet light may help

H. Prognosis

1. Advanced motor neuropathy, respiratory and bulbar paralysis, and death due to porphyria occur only if disease is unrecognized

2. Acute attacks of porphyria may resolve quite rapidly, with abdominal pain disappearing within a few hours and paresis within a few days

3. Advanced motor neuropathy is potentially reversible, unless recurrent

I. Prenatal Diagnosis

1. DNA analysis and enzyme analysis in cultured amnio-

cytes and chorionic villi cells

2. Because of variable expressivity of heterozygous state, porphyria is not generally considered an indication for pregnancy termination

VII. Lipid Disorders

A. Abetalipoproteinemia (Bassen-Kornzweig syndrome)

1. Inheritance: autosomal recessive
2. Epidemiology: panethnic
3. Pathophysiology
   a. Most cases are due to defects of one or more proteins involved in processing apolipoprotein B through the secretory pathway for very low-density lipoprotein (VLDL) and chylomicrons
   b. Absence of activity of microsomal triglyceride transfer protein leads to lack of lipidation of B proteins
   c. Absence of apolipoprotein B causes severe fat malabsorption that is central feature of this disease
   d. Most clinical symptoms appear to be secondary to defects of transport of tocopherol (vitamin E) in blood
4. Clinical features
   a. Neonatal onset of fat malabsorption with failure to thrive and subsequent onset in early childhood of severe anemia, degenerative pigmentary retinopathy, and progressive neurologic disease
   b. Most cases present in early childhood, unless diarrhea is absent, in which case it is recognized later
5. Neurologic features
   a. First signs: decreased tendon reflexes in early childhood; next, vibratory sense and proprioception are progressively lost, with features of cerebellar dysfunction appearing later, suggesting spinocerebellar ataxia
   b. Demyelinating peripheral neuropathy and cardiomyopathy may occur
   c. Muscle contractions are common, leading to pes cavus, pes equinovarus, kyphoscoliosis
   d. Occasionally Babinski response and mental retardation have been described
6. Diagnosis
   a. Acanthocytosis on peripheral blood smear and low total cholesterol
   b. Lipid analysis: absence of plasma VLDL, chylomicrons with very low low-density lipoprotein (LDL)
   c. Markedly decreased plasma vitamin E levels
   d. Diminution in amplitude of sensory potentials in tibial and sural nerves, with slowing of conduction velocity, may be present in patients with peripheral neuropathy
7. Pathology

   a. Degeneration of fasciculi cuneatus and gracilis
   b. Demyelination and axonopathy in peripheral nerves
8. Management
   a. Restriction of triglycerides containing long chain fatty acids
   b. Vitamin E supplementation in large doses and vitamin A, D, and K supplementation needed
9. Prognosis
   a. By third decade, untreated patients are often unable to stand unaided
   b. Tocopherol supplementation inhibits progression of neurologic disease and retinopathy and probably leads to some improvement of symptoms
10. Note: familial hypobetalipoproteinemia has the same clinical features in the homozygous form and similar but milder neurologic features alone in the heterozygous form

B. Familial Analphalipoproteinemia: Tangier disease

1. Inheritance
   a. Autosomal recessive
   b. Caused by mutations in the gene of the ATP-binding cassette transporter 1 (ABC1), on 9q31
2. Epidemiology
   a. Rare
   b. Panethnic
3. Pathophysiology
   a. ABC1 has pivotal role in secretion of cellular lipids and formation of mature high-density lipoprotein (HDL)
   b. Defective HDL maturation seems to lead to enhanced catabolism of apolipoprotein A-I and apolipoprotein A-II, resulting in HDL deficiency
   c. Severely decreased level or absence of plasma HDLs and accumulation of cholesteryl esters in many tissues, including tonsils, peripheral nerves, intestinal mucosa, spleen, liver, bone marrow, lymph nodes, thymus, skin, cornea
4. Clinical features
   a. Major clinical signs: hyperplastic orange tonsils, hepatosplenomegaly, relapsing neuropathy
   b. Neuropathy may be asymmetric mononeuropathy, symmetric polyneuropathy, or syringomyelia-type sensory loss
   c. Children usually are identified on basis of large, yellow-orange tonsils; adult patients have neuropathy
   d. Other features may include premature myocardial infarction or stroke, thrombocytopenia, anemia, gastrointestinal problems, corneal clouding
5. Diagnosis
   a. Plasma concentration of apolipoprotein A-I is extremely low (<3% that of controls)

b. Cholesterol profile: HDL deficiency, low plasma cholesterol concentration, normal or increased triglyceride levels

c. Characteristic cholesterol profile in clinical presence of hyperplastic orange-yellow tonsils and adenoidal tissue is pathognomonic for familial analphalipoproteinemia

6. Pathology

a. Tangier histiocytes appear as foam cells with sudanophilic lipid droplets and occasionally as crystalline material

b. Most droplets within the cytoplasm are not membrane-bound and contain cholesteryl esters

c. Demyelination and remyelination of peripheral nerves in the mononeuropathic form

d. Axonal degeneration of small myelinated and unmyelinated fibers and small dorsal root ganglion cells in the syringomyelia-like neuropathy

7. Management: no specific treatment available

8. Note: heterozygotes present with no clinical symptoms but with half-normal levels of HDL cholesterol and apolipoprotein A-I

VIII. Neurotransmitter Disorders

A. Dopamine β-Hydroxylase Deficiency

1. Inheritance

a. Autosomal recessive

b. Glycine encephalopathy

c. Chromosome 9q34

2. Epidemiology: onset in newborn period

3. Pathophysiology (Fig. 25-3)

a. Congenital deficiency of dopamine β-hydroxylase (final enzyme in conversion of dopamine to norepinephrine), resulting in norepinephrine deficiency and orthostatic hypotension

b. Dopamine in sympathetic terminals instead of norepinephrine leads to hypotension

c. Supine hypertension and nocturia occur from reversal of circadian rhythm of blood pressure

d. Requires BH4 as cofactor and deficiency of that can lead to similar symptoms

4. Clinical features

a. Congenital cause of severe orthostatic hypotension, ptosis, noradrenergic failure

b. Noradrenergic failure presents with hypothermia, hypoglycemia, prolonged or retrograde ejaculation, and reduced exercise tolerance

c. Other features: hypotonia, hypomagnesemia, atrial fibrillation, decreased duration of rapid eye movement sleep

d. There may be a more severe form that leads to death in utero or in early infancy

5. Diagnosis

a. Plasma catecholamine levels, autonomic function tests, therapeutic effect of dihydroxyphenylserine are used for diagnosis

b. Activity of dopamine β-hydroxylase is not reliable because 3% to 4 % of normal population has low activity

6. Management

a. D,L-threodihydroxyphenylserine (DL-threodops) is converted to norepinephrine via dopa decarboxylase, bypassing dopamine β-hydroxylase enzyme

b. Very effective

IX. Lysosomal Disorders

A. Sphingolipidoses: Gaucher's disease

1. Inheritance

a. Autosomal recessive

b. Acid β-glucosidase (glucocerebrosidase) deficiency

c. Rarely due to deficiency of saposin C, an activator protein

d. More common in Ashkenazi Jews

2. Epidemiology (onset at different ages)

a. Type I: most common form, does not affect CNS

b. Type II: acute infantile form (1-2 years)

c. Type III: juvenile form affects brain

3. Pathophysiology

a. Glucocerebrosidase is needed for degradation of glucosylceramide, a glycosphingolipid

b. Deficiency of glucocerebrosidase or a proteolytic product of prosaposin leads to accumulation of glucocerebroside (glucosylceramide)

4. Clinical features

a. Type I

1) No CNS involvement

Dopamine β-Hydroxylase Deficiency

Norepinephrine deficiency

Severe orthostatic hypotension

Nocturia

DL-threodihydroxyphenylserine (DL-threodops) is therapeutic

2) Mild hepatomegaly, splenomegaly
3) Skeletal and pulmonary involvement
b. Type II
  1) Acute neuronopathic form
  2) Infantile onset of motor regression; cranial nerve dysfunction including horizontal supranuclear gaze palsy, choreoathetosis, with initial hypotonia followed by spasticity
  3) Convulsions are rare
  4) Mild hepatomegaly and marked splenomegaly occur with attendant complications of hypersplenism
  5) May present at birth with hydrops
c. Type III
  1) Onset in late first decade, with slow progression
  2) Initial hepatosplenomegaly, followed by seizures and regression characterized by varying degree of memory problems, spasticity, ataxia, and cranial nerve dysfunction, including supranuclear horizontal gaze palsy
  3) Skeletal involvement is common
5. Diagnosis: deficiency of glucocerebrosidase in leukocytes, hepatocytes, or cultured fibroblasts is confirmatory
6. Pathology
   a. Gaucher cells are present in several tissues, including spleen, lymph nodes, and bone marrow; may be detected on bone marrow aspiration
   b. Gaucher cells are macrophages filled with insoluble glycolipids derived from phagocytosis of erythrocytes and leukocytes
   c. Perivascular clusters of elongated Gaucher cells may be seen in the subcortical white matter (Fig. 25-7), cerebral cortex and cerebellum
7. Management: enzyme replacement therapy effective for systemic symptoms, but does not affect the neurologic symptoms
8. Prognosis: rapid deterioration occurs in type II and causes death by age 2 years
9. Prenatal diagnosis: analysis of acid β-glucosidase in amniocytes or chorionic villus sample (CVS)

Gaucher's Disease

Glucocerebrosidase deficiency

Hepatosplenomegaly

Tone abnormalities

Developmental regression

---

10. Comments: human saposin C deficiency, transmitted as autosomal recessive trait, results in a clinical picture similar to type III Gaucher's disease

B. Sphingolipidoses: GM$_1$ gangliosidosis
1. Inheritance: autosomal recessive, deficiency of β-galactosidase
2. Epidemiology
   a. Panethnic
   b. Onset at different ages: classic infantile form, late-infantile/juvenile form, and adult forms
3. Clinical features (depend on age at onset)
   a. Infantile: onset between 3 and 6 months, with developmental plateau and then regression, seizures, spasticity, encephalopathy; cherry-red spot may be seen in infantile form but not usually in other forms
   b. Late infantile and juvenile
      1) Variable age at onset and rate of progression of CNS symptoms, including developmental regression, seizures, pyramidal signs
      2) Cherry-red spot, dysmorphic features, skeletal dysplasia and hepatosplenomegaly usually not present, but vertebral dysplasia has been described
   c. Adult
      1) Slowly progressive dystonia, gait, speech disturbance
      2) Pyramidal signs are present but cognitive decline is not remarkable
4. Diagnosis
   a. Deficiency of β-galactosidase in leukocytes or cultured fibroblasts is confirmatory; there is relative deficiency in juvenile and adult forms

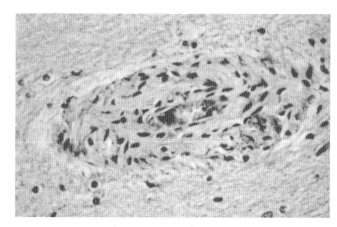

Fig. 25-7. Perivascular collections of Gaucher cells in subcortical white matter. (From Okazaki H. Fundamentals of neuropathology: morphologic basis of neurologic disorders. 2nd ed. New York: Igaku-Shoin; 1989. p. 183-202. By permission of Mayo Foundation.)

b. Keratan sulfate and abnormal oligosaccharides may be detected in urine

c. MRI: in early-onset patients, diffuse cortical atrophy is associated with myelin loss in cerebral white matter

5. Pathology
   a. Macroscopic: marked atrophy
   b. Electron microscopy: characteristic inclusion bodies similar to those in Tay-Sachs disease

6. Management: supportive treatment for seizures, spasticity, motor impairments

7. Prognosis: infantile onset has the worst prognosis, with death between 2 and 5 years

8. Prenatal diagnosis: analysis of β-galactosidase in CVS and cultured amniocytes

C. **Sphingolipidoses:** GM$_2$ gangliosidosis

1. Inheritance
   a. Autosomal recessive
   b. Deficiency of α subunit of β-hexosaminidase A in Tay-Sachs disease and of both β-hexoaminidase A and B in Sandhoff's disease
   c. Highest carrier rates in Ashkenazi Jews

2. Epidemiology (onset at different ages): classic infantile form (1-2 years), juvenile form (3-15 years), adult form

3. Pathophysiology: hexosaminidase defect results in metabolic block leading to abnormal accumulation of GM$_2$ ganglioside in brain

4. Clinical features of Tay-Sachs disease (depend on age at onset)
   a. Classic infantile (onset between ages 2 and 6 months)
      1) Progressive weakness, motor regression, decreased social interaction, exaggerated startle response, progressive blindness, seizures, spasticity, encephalopathy
      2) Cherry-red spot (Fig. 25-8) and macrocephaly
   b. Late infantile and juvenile (onset between ages 3 and 6)
      1) Triad of psychiatric illness, ataxia, motor neuron disease (upper or lower)
      2) Psychiatric disease includes schizophrenia, psychosis, mood disorder, and, later, dementia
      3) Dysarthria, blindness, seizures, weakness may occur
      4) No cherry-red spot
   c. Adult: slowly progressive motor neuron disease similar to spinocerebellar degeneration, with proximal muscle weakness, poor coordination, dysarthria, dystonia, tremor, and, in some patients, intermittent psychosis

5. Clinical features of Sandhoff's disease
   a. Similar to Tay-Sachs disease
   b. In contrast to Tay-Sachs, hepatosplenomegaly may be present
   c. Classic form, like Tay-Sachs disease, is the infantile form

6. Diagnosis
   a. Deficiency of hexosaminidase A or both A and B in leukocytes, serum, or cultured fibroblasts is confirmatory
   b. Relative deficiency in juvenile and adult forms
   c. DNA mutation analysis
   d. Pathology
      1) Prolonged survival in infantile forms leads to megalencephaly
      2) Ballooned cortical neurons with foamy cytoplasm and displaced nuclei (Fig. 25-9)
      3) Electron microscopy: characteristic inclusion bodies, "membranous cytoplasmic bodies," are visible
      4) In adults, the inclusions are located preferentially in anterior horn cells and cerebellum, accounting for amyotrophic lateral sclerosis–like presentation

7. Management

Tay-Sachs Disease (Infantile Form)
Deficiency of α subunit of β-hexosaminidase A

Progressive blindness

Seizures

Spasticity

Cherry-red spot

Macrocephaly

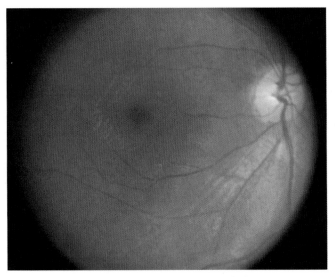

Fig. 25-8. Cherry-red spot observed on ophthalmoscopic examination of patient with Tay-Sachs disease. (Courtesy of Brian R. Younge, MD.)

a. Symptomatic treatment for spasticity and seizures

b. Bone marrow transplant, enzyme replacement therapy, substrate deprivation, stem cell transplant are in investigative phase

8. Prognosis

a. Infantile onset has worst prognosis, with death between 2 and 5 years

b. Juvenile-onset patients die during their teens

9. Prenatal diagnosis

a. In Ashkenazi Jews, carrier testing is performed with enzyme assay and DNA mutation analysis because carrier frequency is 1 in 30

b. Analysis of hexosaminidase A in amniocytes is performed when mutation is unidentified

10. Comments: deficiency of GM_2 activator of hexosaminidase A can give similar clinical picture

D. **Sphingolipidoses:** Niemann-Pick disease types A and B

1. Inheritance

a. Autosomal recessive

b. High carrier rates of type A disease in Ashkenazi Jews

2. Epidemiology (onset at different ages): acute infantile onset (1-2 years) in type A; type B diagnosed in childhood because of hepatosplenomegaly

3. Pathophysiology: types A and B have deficient acid sphingomyelinase due to mutations in *ASM* gene, which results in accumulation of sphingomyelin and other lipids in monocyte-macrophage system

4. Clinical features

a. Type A

1) Severe neurovisceral disease with onset between 2 and 6 months, with failure to thrive, progressive hepatosplenomegaly, liver dysfunction

2) Developmental delay in infancy, followed by regression associated with ataxia, hypotonia, vertical gaze apraxia between age 1 and 3 years

3) Cherry-red spot and organomegaly

b. Type B

1) Pure visceral form, with liver, spleen, lung involvement

2) Milder course than type A

5. Diagnosis

a. Deficiency of sphingomyelinase in leukocytes or cultured fibroblasts is confirmatory

b. Patients with type A generally have less than 5% activity; those with type B have 5% to 10% of normal residual activity

6. Pathology: Niemann-Pick cells are lipid-laden histiocytes (foam cells) located in clinically involved tissues; in bone marrow, they are described as "sea-blue histiocytes"

7. Management

a. Symptomatic

b. Bone marrow transplant and enzyme replacement therapy are experimental

8. Prognosis

a. Type A has the worse prognosis, with death between 2 and 5 years

b. Patients with type B survive into adulthood

c. More severely affected patients with type B may have progressive pulmonary infiltration

9. Prenatal diagnosis

a. Biochemical carrier testing is not reliable

b. Sphingomyelinase assay can be performed on chorionic villi cells in types A and B

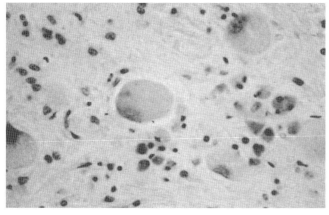

Fig. 25-9. Ballooned cortical neurons with displaced nuclei and Nissl substance in a patient with Tay-Sachs disease. (From Okazaki H. Fundamentals of neuropathology: morphologic basis of neurologic disorders. 2nd ed. New York: Igaku-Shoin; 1989. p. 183-202. By permission of Mayo Foundation.)

Niemann-Pick Disease Types A and B

Failure to thrive

Progressive hepatosplenomegaly

Developmental regression

Ataxia

Hypotonia

Cherry-red spot

E. Sphingolipidoses: Niemann-Pick disease type C
1. Inheritance: autosomal recessive
2. Epidemiology
   a. Incidence: approximately 1 in 150,000
   b. Much more common in isolated Acadian populations in Nova Scotia
   c. Onset at different ages from fetal life to late adulthood
3. Pathophysiology
   a. Type C is a cellular lipid-trafficking disorder in which LDL-derived cholesterol is sequestered in lysosomes, and there is a block or delay in esterification of LDL-derived cholesterol
   b. In type C, sphingomyelinase deficiency is not seen in liver, spleen, or leukocytes, but is secondarily present in cultured fibroblasts
   c. Mutations in two genes have been identified: *NPC1* and *NPC2*; result in similar phenotypes; most patients have mutations in *NPC1*
4. Clinical features
   a. Ataxia or dystonia occur, followed by apraxia of vertical gaze and cognitive difficulties
   b. Gelastic cataplexy, spasticity, seizures, dementia, horizontal gaze palsy occur with progression
   c. Hepatosplenomegaly and severe neonatal jaundice may occur
   d. May present at any age: acute forms occur in infancy, with death by 2 years of age, and in adult forms, with onset in seventh decade
5. Diagnosis: cultured fibroblasts have increased perinuclear filipin-positive stain suggestive of increased free cholesterol and demonstrate decreased cholesterol esterification
6. Pathology
   a. Macroscopic
      1) Hepatosplenomegaly is frequently present in childhood but may regress or be absent in older patients
      2) Cerebellar vermis and brainstem atrophy: occur early in disease course
      3) Cortical atrophy and ventricular enlargement occur later
   b. Microscopic
      1) Cholesterol and lipid-laden cells (foam cells) in liver and bone marrow biopsy specimens
      2) Sea-blue histiocytes may be seen in bone marrow
      3) CNS: ectopic dendritogenesis, axonal spheroids, neurofibrillary tangles, and ballooned neurons containing finely granular storage bodies (Fig. 25-10)
   c. Electron microscopy: characteristic finding in neurons, skin, conjunctiva, and rectum is "polymorphous cytoplasmic bodies" or "zebra bodies"
7. Management

   a. Symptomatic treatment for seizures, cataplexy, spasticity, dystonia
   b. Physical, occupational, and speech therapy
8. Prognosis: gradual progressive neurodegeneration leading to death
9. Prenatal diagnosis
   a. Biochemical carrier testing is not reliable
   b. Mutation analysis for *NPC1* and *NPC2* genes can be performed and is preferred method

F. Sphingolipidoses: metachromatic leukodystrophy
1. Inheritance
   a. Autosomal recessive
   b. Due to deficiency of arylsulfatase A, saposin B (activator) deficiency, or multiple sulfatase deficiency
2. Epidemiology
   a. Incidence: 1 in 50,000 to 100,000
   b. Onset at different ages: late infantile form (1-2 years), juvenile form (3-15 years), adult form (>16 years)
3. Pathophysiology
   a. Arylsulfatase enzyme is needed for degradation of cerebroside sulfate (galactosyl sulfatide), a glycolipid found mainly in myelin membrane
   b. Deficiency of arylsulfatase A or its activator, saposin B, leads to accumulation of cerebroside sulfate, which causes progressive demyelination both in CNS and PNS
4. Clinical features (depend on age at onset)
   a. Late infantile
      1) Gait disturbance with weakness, ataxia, developmental delay, aphasia, optic atrophy, progressive spastic paraplegia
      2) Fatal outcome
      3) Most common form of disease
   b. Juvenile

Niemann-Pick Disease Type C
Lipid-trafficking disorder

Ataxia

Dystonia

Apraxia of vertical gaze

Cataplexy

Spasticity

Seizures

Dementia

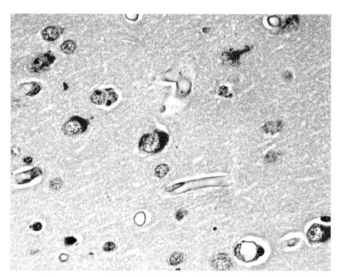

Fig. 25-10. Niemann-Pick disease type C. Finely granular storage bodies in neurons are best demonstrated with PAS staining.

1) Developmental regression, speech disturbances, ataxia, gait clumsiness may progress slowly or occasionally rapidly to a vegetative state
2) Seizures occur in most and spastic quadriparesis is final outcome
c. Adult
1) Slowly progressive course of behavioral abnormalities, dementia, peripheral neuropathy, pyramidal signs, seizures, ataxia
2) Symptoms of acute cholecystitis due to sulfatide accumulation in mucosa of gallbladder may occur
5. Diagnosis
a. Deficiency of arylsulfatase A in leukocytes or cultured fibroblasts is confirmatory
b. Accumulation of sulfatides in urine is supportive
c. Electrophysiology: nerve conduction velocities are uniformly slowed
d. Evoked potentials: prolongation of interpeak latencies and subsequent loss of wave components on brainstem auditory evoked potentials, similar findings on somatosensory and visual evoked potentials
e. MRI
1) Diffuse hyperintense signal in both periventricular and subcortical white matter on T2-weighted images sparing U fibers (arcuate fibers) and cerebellum
2) With progression, there is often involvement of arcuate fibers and cerebellar white matter, with diffuse secondary cortical atrophy
6. Pathology (Fig. 25-11)
a. Diffuse loss of myelin in subcortical white matter, sparing U fibers

Metachromatic Leukodystrophy
Arylsulfatase A deficiency

Ataxia

Developmental delay

Spastic paraparesis

Peripheral neuropathy

b. Ballooned macrophages with "metachromatic" brown-purple sulfatide deposits best observed with basic dyes (acidified cresyl violet or thionin staining of frozen tissue)
c. Peripheral nerve
1) Sulfatide deposits may be present in Schwann cells and large perivascular macrophages
2) Often, segmental demyelination and remyelination with slight onion-bulb formation and reduced myelinated fiber density
7. Management
a. Treatment may be necessary to control spasticity
b. Antiepileptic medication may be needed
c. Bone marrow transplant may arrest fatal progression of disease
d. Bone marrow transplant should be considered in presymptomatic children with late infantile metachromatic leukodystrophy or early in course of juvenile or adult metachromatic leukodystrophy
8. Prognosis: generally, earlier the onset, worse the prognosis
9. Prenatal diagnosis: analysis of arylsulfatase A in amniocytes
10. Comments
a. Human saposin B deficiency, transmitted as autosomal recessive trait, results in tissue accumulation of cerebroside sulfate and clinical features resembling metachromatic leukodystrophy (activator-deficient metachromatic leukodystrophy); normal arylsulfatase A levels but increased urinary sulfatides
b. Pseudodeficiency of arylsulfatase A occurs in 2% of healthy people; enzyme activity in vitro is 5% to 10% of normal, but people are asymptomatic; sulfatides are not present in urine and metachromatic granules not present in peripheral nerve tissues; this should be confirmed or excluded by DNA analysis
c. Patients with multiple sulfatase deficiency have features of metachromatic leukodystrophy, mucopolysaccharidosis, and ichthyosis

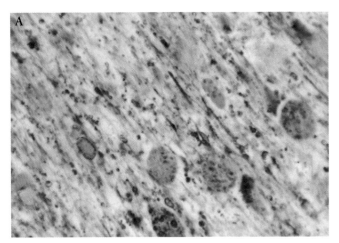 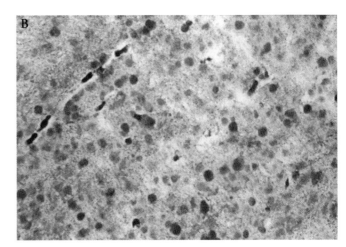

Fig. 25-11. Metachromatic leukodystrophy. *A*, Subcortical white matter with severe loss of myelin and ballooned macrophages interspersed among the remaining myelinated fibers. *B*, Frozen section stained with acidified cresyl violet demonstrates the metachromatic brown-purple appearance of macrophages containing stored sulfatide. (From Ellison D, Love S, Chimelli L, Harding B, Lowe J, Roberts GW, et al. Neuropathology: a reference text of CNS pathology. London: Mosby; 1998. p. 23.14. Used with permission.)

G. Sphingolipidoses: Krabbe's disease

1. Inheritance: autosomal recessive
2. Epidemiology
   a. Incidence: 1 in 100,000 to 200,000
   b. Onset at different ages: classic infantile white matter degenerative form, slowly progressive late infantile form, juvenile form, adult form
3. Pathophysiology
   a. Galactocerebroside β-galactosidase (β-galactocerebrosidase, galactosylceramidase) deficiency
   b. Deficiency of saposin A, activator protein, may lead to late-onset slowly progressive disease
   c. Galactocerebroside from catabolized myelin elicits globoid cell (altered macrophages) formation
   d. Because galactocerebroside cannot be degraded, globoid cells are permanent
   e. Psychosine, degraded by same enzyme that breaks down galactosylceramide, accumulates and possibly causes myelin degeneration and oligodendrocyte death, leading to astrocytic gliosis
4. Clinical features
   a. Infantile
      1) CNS involvement is more severe than PNS
      2) Irritability, hypersensitivity to stimuli, recurrent fevers of unknown origin are followed by seizures, spasticity, opisthotonos, optic atrophy, severe psychomotor retardation
      3) Late in disease course: the infant becomes decerebrate and blind
      4) Demyelinating peripheral neuropathy with absence of

   reflexes also possible
   b. Late infantile
      1) Onset between 6 months and 3 years of age, with irritability, hypertonia, psychomotor regression, ataxia, blindness
      2) Death 2 to 3 years after onset
   c. Juvenile
      1) Onset in late first decade, with slow progression
      2) Vision loss, hemiparesis, ataxia, psychomotor regression
   d. Adult: slowly progressive spastic paraparesis or ataxia
5. Diagnosis
   a. Deficiency of galactocerebroside β-galactosidase in leukocytes or cultured fibroblasts is confirmatory
   b. EMG: slowed conduction velocities, increased distal latency
   c. CSF: increased protein in acute infantile form occurs early, may be normal in juvenile and adult forms
6. Pathology (Fig. 25-12)
   a. Macroscopic appearance
      1) White matter very firm (normal consistency of cerebral cortex) to palpation
      2) Diffuse atrophy, often severe
      3) U fibers often spared
   b. Microscopic CNS appearance
      1) Widespread demyelination with axonal loss throughout white matter, often sparing U fibers
      2) Globoid binucleated or multinucleated macrophages with PAS-positive ballooned cytoplasm due to cerebroside accumulation, often appearing as perivascular clusters

Krabbe's Disease (Infantile Onset)
Galactocerebroside β-galactosidase deficiency

Seizures

Spasticity

Optic atrophy

Severe psychomotor retardation

Peripheral neuropathy

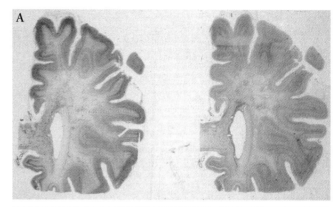

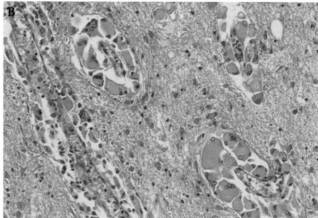

Fig. 25-12. Krabbe's globoid cell leukodystrophy. *A,* Diffuse pallor of white matter with sparing the U fibers (*left,* Luxol fast blue stain; *right,* Bodian stain). *B,* Perivascular clusters of mult-inucleated globoid macrophages. (Hematoxylin-eosin stain.) (From Okazaki H, Scheithauer BS. Atlas of neuropathology. New York: Gower Medical Publishing; 1988. p. 245. By permission of Mayo Foundation.)

   c. PNS pathology
     1) Thickened, pale peripheral nerves
     2) Globoid cells (multiple nucleated macrophages) abound in perivascular regions, with attendant demyelination
     3) Endomysial fibrosis of peripheral nerves, with segmental demyelination
     4) PAS-positive tubular inclusions in globoid cells, endomysial macrophages, Schwann cells
7. Management: stem cell transplant and bone marrow transplant are experimental
8. Prognosis: rapid deterioration occurs in classic infantile type to cause death by age 2 years
9. Prenatal diagnosis: analysis of galactocerebroside β-galactosidase activity in amniocytes or chorionic villi cells; if mutations are known, then DNA analysis

H. Sphingolipidoses: Fabry's disease (Anderson-Fabry disease or angiokeratoma corporis diffusum universale)
1. α-Galactosidase A deficiency
2. Inheritance
   a. X-linked recessive
   b. Female carriers can have later onset and milder disease
3. Epidemiology: onset in late childhood or adolescence, males
4. Pathophysiology
   a. α-Galactosidase A is responsible for breakdown of globotriaosylceramide (ceramide trihexosamide) and related glycosphingolipids, which are components of cell membrane
   b. α-Galactosidase A deficiency leads to progressive accumulation of globotriaosylceramide in plasma and lysosomes of most cells in the body and accumulation in vascular endothelium leads to ischemia and infarction
5. Clinical features
   a. Hemizygous males
     1) Normal intelligence
     2) Severe episodic pain crises, chronic acroparesthias in extremities, hypohidrosis, and angiokeratomas
     3) Mild to severe gastrointestinal disturbances, including diarrhea, nausea, vomiting
     4) Angiokeratomas: small, slightly raised, purplish red, nonblanching telangiectases in lower abdomen and lower legs but can occur anywhere
     5) Characteristic whorled corneal opacity seen on slit-lamp microscopy; retarded growth; delayed puberty; and sparse, fine facial and body hair
     6) Nephropathy with proteinuria and eventual renal failure leads to hypertension and uremia
   b. Variant: isolated cardiomyopathy with residual enzyme activity

> **Fabry's Disease**
> α-Galactosidase A deficiency
>
> Severe episodic limb pain crises
>
> Angiokeratomas
>
> Cardiomyopathy
>
> Nephropathy
>
> Stroke
>
> Normal IQ

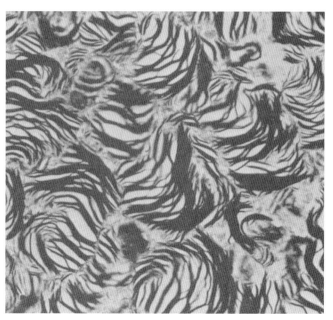

Fig. 25-13. Electron micrograph of a spinal ganglion of a patient with Fabry's disease shows tightly packed lamellated inclusions in the cytoplasm of the cell bodies. (From Onishi A, Dyck PJ. Loss of small peripheral sensory neurons in Fabry disease: histologic and morphometric evaluation of cutaneous nerves, spinal ganglia, and posterior columns. Arch Neurol. 1974;31:120-7. Used with permission.)

    c. Heterozygous females
      1) May be asymptomatic or have presentations as severe as in males
      2) Early-onset stroke and myocardial infarction, whorl-like corneal epithelial dystrophy, distal interphalangeal joint arthritis
6. Diagnosis
    a. Deficiency of α-galactosidase in leukocytes or fibroblasts is confirmatory
    b. Female carriers may have normal or low enzyme activity
    c. Ceramide trihexoside accumulates in urine
    d. EMG: likely normal, because it is small-fiber peripheral neuropathy
7. Pathology
    a. Widespread deposition of glycosphingolipids, with birefringence and Maltese crosses seen with polarized light microscopy
    b. Electron microscopy: cytoplasmic lamellated inclusions may be tightly packed (Fig. 25-13) or stacked in loose arrangement
    c. In PNS, this deposition may be observed in spinal ganglia, vasa nervorum, and perineurium of peripheral nerves
8. Management
    a. Enzyme replacement therapy is effective
    b. Supportive care: regular monitoring of renal function, cardiac function, hematology, electrolytes, urinalysis
    c. Bone marrow transplant, substrate depletion and deprivation, and gene therapy are all experimental
9. Prognosis
    a. Death occurs with enzyme replacement by fifth or sixth decade
    b. Acute renal failure usually occurs in fourth decade but can occur as early as second decade

10. Prenatal diagnosis
    a. Analysis of α-galactosidase activity in amniocytes or chorionic villi cells
    b. If the mutations are known, then DNA analysis can be done

I. Mucopolysaccharidosis
1. Definition: lysosomal storage disorders due to deficiency of enzymes needed to break down glycosaminoglycans, including heparan sulfate, dermatan sulfate, keratan sulfate, chondroitin sulfate, hyaluronan
2. Inheritance: all are autosomal recessive, except Hunter's syndrome, which is X-linked recessive
3. Epidemiology
    a. Rare
    b. Most of the children are normal at birth and present with developmental plateau between 6 months and 4 years, followed by developmental regression
4. Pathophysiology
    a. Accumulation of glycosaminoglycans in lysosomes leads to multisystem dysfunction

b. Tissues involved: bone, cartilage, cornea, leptomeninges, connective tissue; mucopolysaccharides are stored in all these tissues

c. Gangliosides are stored in neurons, and this occurs in all types that manifest with mental retardation

5. Clinical features

a. Hurler's syndrome and Sanfilippo's syndrome: onset in infancy

b. Hunter's syndrome and Sly's syndrome: onset in childhood

c. Sly's syndrome: may present with hydrops fetalis

d. Multiple common clinical features; few that are distinctive (Table 25-4)

e. Insidious onset and chronic progressive course of multiple-organ involvement, hepatosplenomegaly, dysostosis multiplex, coarse facies

f. Dysostosis multiplex occurs in various storage disorders and is characterized by following radiologic features: thickened calvarium, large skull, shallow orbits, enlarged sella turcica, abnormally shaped teeth, anterior beaking of lumbar vertebrae, enlarged diaphysis of long bones, small femoral heads, poorly formed pelvis with coxa valga, shallow acetabulum, thick irregular clavicles, oar-shaped ribs, shortened trapezoid phalanges

g. Corneal clouding
   1) Occurs in following syndromes: Hurler's, Scheie's, Morquio's type A, and Maroteaux-Lamy
   2) Chacteristically, does not occur in Hunter's syndrome and may be absent in Sly's syndrome

h. Deafness may occur in Hunter's, Hurler's, Hurler-Scheie, and Morquio's syndromes

i. Hurler-Scheie, Scheie's, Maroteaux-Lamy, and Morquio's syndromes, mucopolysaccharidosis type IX, and milder form of Hunter's syndrome: all have normal IQ

j. Coarse facies may be absent in Sanfilippo's syndrome, which usually has primary CNS involvement with no somatic features

k. Atlantoaxial joint is often unstable (most commonly in Morquio's, Hurler's, Hunter's and Maroteaux-Lamy syndromes)

6. Diagnosis

a. Deficiency of specific enzymes in leukocytes, hepatocytes, or cultured fibroblasts is confirmatory

b. Urinary mucopolysaccharides as a screening test have high false-negative rate

c. Quantitative glycosaminoglycans in urine with electrophoresis is now preferred

d. Radiologic findings of dysostosis multiplex are characteristic

7. Pathology

Normal IQ in Mucopolysaccharidosis
Hurler-Scheie syndrome

Scheie's syndrome

Maroteaux-Lamy syndrome

Morquio's syndromes

Mucopolysaccharidosis type IX

Milder form of Hunter's syndrome

Dysostosis multiplex
Thickened calvarium

Large skull

Abnormally shaped teeth

Anterior beaking of lumbar vertebrae

Enlarged diaphysis of long bones

Oar-shaped ribs

Shallow acetabulum

Conditions With Dysostosis Multiplex
Mucopolysaccharidosis

Mucolipidosis

α-Mannosidosis

Fucosidosis

Sialidosis type II

Galactosialidosis

Corneal Clouding
Hurler's syndrome

Scheie's syndrome

Morquio's syndrome type A

Maroteaux-Lamy syndrome

Not in Hunter's syndrome

Table 25-4. **Mucopolysaccharidoses**

Eponym	Number	Enzyme deficient	Glycoaminoglycan affected	Clinical features
Hurler's syndrome (untreated)	MPS IH	α-L-Iduronidase	Dermatan sulfate Heparan sulfate	Corneal clouding, progressive psychomotor retardation, dysostosis multiplex, dwarfism, valvular heart disease, hernias, macroglossia, hearing loss, chronic hydrocephalus and myelopathy Death in childhood
Scheie's syndrome	MPS IS	α-L-Iduronidase	Dermatan sulfate Heparan sulfate	Normal intelligence and life span Corneal clouding, valvular disease, coarse features, stiff joints
Hurler-Scheie syndrome	MPS IH/S	α-L-Iduronidase	Dermatan sulfate Heparan sulfate	Intermediate phenotype between Hurler's and Scheie's syndromes
Hunter's syndrome (severe)	MPS II (severe)	Iduronate sulfatase	Dermatan sulfate Heparan sulfate	Mental retardation of slower progression than Hurler's syndrome Deafness, dysostosis multiplex and organomegaly, ivory-colored nodules in shawl-like distribution, chronic hydrocephalus, joint stifffness, nerve entrapments occur Death in second decade
Hunter's syndrome (mild)	MPS II (mild)	Iduronate sulfatase	Dermatan sulfate Heparan sulfate	Normal intelligence, short stature, normal life span
Sanfilippo's syndrome A	MPS III A	Heparan *N*-sulfatase	Heparan sulfate	Relatively mild somatic features Profound mental retardation, sleep disorders, hyperactivity, aggressiveness Hirsutism and synophrys Speech delay, severe hearing loss and seizures may occur Death by age 20
Sanfilippo's syndrome B	MPS III B	α-*N*-acetyl glucosaminidase	Heparan sulfate	Similar phenotype in Sanfilippo's syndrome A
Sanfilippo's syndrome C	MPS III C	Acetyl CoA:α-glucosaminidine acetyltransferase	Heparan sulfate	Similar phenotype to Sanfilippo's syndrome A
Sanfilippo's syndrome D	MPS III D	*N*-acetylglucosamine-6-sulfatase	Heparan sulfate	Similar phenotype to Sanfilippo's syndrome A
Morquio's syndrome A	MPS IV A	*N*-acetylglucosamine-6-sulfatase	Keratan sulfate	Preserved intelligence, short-trunk dwarfism, corneal deposits, spondyloepiphyseal dysplasia, odontoid hypoplasia causing atlantoaxial subluxation, valvular heart disease, deafness, coarse facies
Morquio's syndrome B	MPS IV B	β-Galactosidase	Keratan sulfate	Similar spectrum as Morquio's syndrome A

Table 25-4. (continued)

Eponym	Number	Enzyme deficient	Glycoaminoglycan affected	Clinical features
Maroteaux-Lamy syndrome	MPS VI	*N*-acetylgalactosamine-4-sulfatase (arylsulfatase B)	Dermatan sulfate	Normal intelligence Dysostosis multiplex, corneal clouding, myelopathy, hepatomegaly Mild-severe forms with similar somatic features as Hurler's syndrome
Sly's syndrome	MPS VII	β-Glucuronidase	Dermatan sulfate Heparan sulfate Chondroitin 4-, 6-sulfates	Variable Typical Hurler's syndrome somatic features Neonatal presentation as hydrops Corneal clouding is variably present May have normal intelligence
	MPS IX	Hyaluronidase	Hyaluronan	Single patient: periarticular soft tissue masses, normal IQ

a. Vacuolated (Gasser) lymphocytes with refringent inclusions may be seen on microscopy
b. Other cytologic abnormalities that can be seen in these conditions: Buhot cells (vacuolated plasma cells seen on bone marrow smears), peripheral blood neutrophils with Alder-Reilly anomaly
c. Zebra bodies on electron microscopy in neurons in Hurler's syndrome are possibly inclusion bodies containing glycolipids

8. Management
   a. Enzyme replacement therapy and bone marrow transplant are effective for Hurler's syndrome and have had variable success in other types of mucopolysaccharidosis
   b. Stem cell transplant may be the treatment of choice for child younger than 2 years with Hurler's syndrome and no CNS manifestations
   c. Supportive care
      1) Ventriculoperitoneal shunt
      2) Routine EMG and nerve conduction velocity studies to diagnose carpal tunnel syndrome
      3) Atlantoaxial joint stabilization
      4) Routine echocardiograms to diagnose valvular heart disease
      5) Vision and hearing screening
      6) Regular MRI of cervical spine to diagnose myelopathy

9. Prognosis

a. Sly's syndrome can cause death in infancy
b. Most of other severe disorders cause death in second decade from respiratory and cardiac problems
c. Others survive to third to seventh decade variably
d. Early treatment of Hurler's syndrome has changed the course of this disease

10. Prenatal diagnosis
    a. Analysis of enzymes in amniocytes or chorionic villi cells
    b. Carrier testing can be performed if mutation is known

J. Mucolipidosis

1. Inheritance: all are autosomal recessive
2. Epidemiology
   a. Rare
   b. Mucolipidosis type IV is relatively common among Ashkenazi Jews
3. Pathophysiology
   a. Abnormal lysosomal enzyme transport occurs in cells of mesenchymal origin
   b. Defective packaging of enzymes into lysosomes: enzymes are released into extracellular fluid instead
   c. Multiple lysosomal enzyme deficiencies result
4. Clinical features (Table 25-5)
   a. Mucolipidosis type I is sialidosis (see below)
   b. Mucolipidosis type II
      1) More severe disease, but clinical features similar to Hurler's syndrome

2) Severe gingival hyperplasia is characteristic
c. Mucolipidosis type III
1) Milder and later onset than Hurler's syndrome
2) No organomegaly or mucopolysacchariduria
d. Mucolipidosis type IV
1) Severe psychomotor delay, corneal clouding, retinal dystrophy, and optic atrophy may be first noticeable signs of disease in infancy
2) Hypotonia occurs and progresses to spasticity
3) Nonprogressive psychomotor delay, but regression can occur
4) No dysmorphic features, hepatosplenomegaly, or skeletal abnormalities
5. Diagnosis
a. Mucolipidosis types II and III
1) Deficiency of specific enzymes in leukocytes, hepatocytes, or cultured fibroblasts is confirmatory
2) Ratio of extracellular to intracellular lysosomal enzyme levels can also be used because the serum enzyme levels are high
b. Mucolipidosis type IV
1) No characteristic enzyme abnormality
2) Gastric achlorhydria with increased serum gastrin
3) MRI: thin corpus callosum with dysplasia of splenium
4) Mutations in *MCOLN1* (mucolipidin 1) gene

Table 25-5. Mucolipidoses

Name	Type	Enzyme deficiency	Characteristic features
I-cell disease	ML-II	*N*-acetylglucos-aminephos-photransferase	Hurler's phenotype, earlier onset, severe gingival hyperplasia
Pseudo-Hurler poly-dystrophy	ML-III	Partial deficiency of *N*-acetyl-glucosamine-phosphotrans-ferase	Milder and later onset with Hurler's phenotype. No organomegaly
	ML-IV		No dysmorphism, skeletal abnormalities or organomegaly. Psychomotor delay, visual abnormalities, hypotonia, and spasticity occur. Corneal clouding

ML, mucolipidosis.

6. Pathology
a. Mucolipidosis types II and III: prominent cytoplasmic inclusions consisting of membrane-bound vacuoles
b. Mucolipidosis type IV: biopsy findings are similar to Tay-Sachs disease with cytoplasmic inclusions and lamellar concentric bodies seen on electron microscopy
7. Management
a. Supportive care similar to that needed in mucopolysaccharidosis
b. Bone marrow transplant is experimental
8. Prognosis: death can occur by age 5 in mucolipidosis type II
9. Prenatal diagnosis
a. Analysis of enzymes in amniocytes or chorionic villi cells
b. Carrier testing can be performed if mutation is known

K. **Oligosaccharidoses** (disorders of glycoprotein metabolism)
1. α-Mannosidosis
a. Inheritance: autosomal recessive; α-mannosidase deficiency
b. Epidemiology (onset at different ages)
1) Severe infantile (type I) form
2) Slowly progressive juvenile-adult (type II) form
c. Pathophysiology: progressive accumulation of partially degraded oligosaccharides in brain and visceral tissue produces clinical features of other lysosomal storage disorders such as mucopolysaccharidosis
d. Clinical features: similar to mucopolysaccharidosis
1) Infantile: rapidly progressive mental retardation, hepatosplenomegaly, and severe dysostosis multiplex, hearing loss, speech problems, ataxia; recurrent bacterial infection has been noted
2) Juvenile-adult
a) Milder features than above and more slowly progressive course
b) Sensorineural hearing loss is more prominent
d. Diagnosis
1) Deficiency of α-mannosidase in fibroblasts or leukocytes is confirmatory
2) Abnormal urinary excretion of oligosaccharides in a characteristic pattern
e. Pathology
1) Granular or foamy cytoplasm in hepatocytes
2) Electron microscopy: vacuoles in hepatocytes and neurons
f. Management: Hematopoietic stem cell transplant is experimental
g. Prognosis
1) Death occurs in type I between 3 and 12 years

2) Type II patients survive into adulthood
h. Prenatal diagnosis: analysis of α-mannosidase activity in amniocytes or chorionic villi cells

2. β-Mannosidosis
   a. Inheritance: autosomal recessive; β-mannosidase deficiency
   b. Pathophysiology: progressive accumulation of partially degraded oligosaccharides in brain and visceral tissue produces the clinical features
   c. Clinical features
      1) No dysmorphism, organomegaly, or dysostosis multiplex
      2) Onset at various ages, with seizures, quadriplegia, behavioral abnormalities at severe end of spectrum and angiokeratomas at the mild end
      3) Sensorineural hearing loss is prominent
   d. Diagnosis
      1) Deficiency of β-mannosidase in fibroblasts or leukocytes is confirmatory
      2) Abnormal urinary excretion of oligosaccharides in a characteristic pattern
   e. Pathology: not well characterized
   f. Management: supportive
   g. Prognosis
      1) Death occurs earlier in more severe forms
      2) Patients with milder forms have relatively benign course
   h. Prenatal diagnosis: analysis of β-mannosidase activity in amniocytes or chorionic villi cells

3. Fucosidosis
   a. Inheritance: autosomal recessive; α-L-fucosidase deficiency
   b. Epidemiology
      1) Rare
      2) Onset at different ages: severe infantile form (type I) and slowly progressive milder form (type II)
   c. Pathophysiology: progressive accumulation of partially degraded oligosaccharides in brain and visceral tissue produces clinical features of other lysosomal storage disorders like mucopolysaccharidosis
   d. Clinical features
      1) Type I
         a) Similar to mucopolysaccharidosis, with onset of psychomotor retardation in infancy
         b) May be hepatosplenomegaly, cardiomegaly, seizures, recurrent infections
      2) Type II
         a) Milder features than type I, with onset of retardation by age 1 or 2 years
         b) Characteristic angiokeratomas similar to those of

Fabry's disease
   e. Diagnosis
      1) Deficiency of α-fucosidase in fibroblasts or leukocytes is confirmatory
      2) Abnormal urinary excretion of oligosaccharides in characteristic pattern
      3) Sweat chloride is increased in type I
   f. Pathology
      1) Granular or foamy cytoplasm in hepatocytes
      2) Electron microscopy: vacuoles in hepatocytes and neurons
   g. Management: hematopoietic stem cell transplant is experimental
   h. Prognosis
      1) Type I: death between 3 and 12 years
      2) Type II: death by second decade
   i. Prenatal diagnosis: analysis of α-fucosidase activity in amniocytes or chorionic villi cells

4. Sialidosis
   a. Inheritance: autosomal recessive
   b. Both types I and II have neuraminidase (sialidase) deficiency
   c. Type I: "Cherry-red spot–myoclonus syndrome"
   d. Epidemiology (onset at different ages with different severity)
      1) Type I: adult onset
      2) Type II: congenital and infantile forms
   e. Pathophysiology: progressive accumulation of partially degraded oligosaccharides in brain and visceral tissue produces clinical features
   f. Type I clinical features
      1) No dysmorphism
      2) Usually presents in second to fourth decade with gait abnormalities, myoclonus, visual disturbance
      3) Ataxia, hyperreflexia, nystagmus, dysarthria, seizures have been described
      4) Decreased color vision, decreased visual acuity; there may be night blindness in addition to cherry-red spot
   g. Type II clinical features: classic mucopolysaccharidosis phenotype
      1) Congenital: hydrops fetalis, hepatosplenomegaly, hernias, facial edema may be present at birth
      2) Infantile
         a) Rapidly progressive mental retardation, hepatosplenomegaly, severe dysostosis multiplex, hearing loss, speech problems, ataxia
         b) Cherry-red spots and myoclonus have been noted
   h. Diagnosis
      1) Deficiency of neuraminidase in fibroblasts is confirmatory

2) Abnormal urinary excretion of oligosaccharides in a characteristic pattern

3) Type II is clinically indistinguishable from galacto-sialidosis, which has both neuraminidase and β-galactosidase

i. Pathology

   1) Type II has foamy cytoplasm in lymphocytes and bone marrow

   2) Electron microscopy: membrane-bound vacuoles in hepatocytes and neurons

j. Management: hematopoietic stem cell transplant is experimental

k. Prognosis

   1) Death occurs in type II congenital form in utero or in infancy

   2) Infantile-onset patients with type II may survive to second decade

l. Prenatal diagnosis: analysis of enzyme activity in amnio-cytes or chorionic villi cells

5. Galactosialidosis

a. Inheritance

   1) Autosomal recessive

   2) Combined β-galactosidase and neuraminidase defi-ciency secondary to deficiency of protective protein/cathepsin A protein

b. Epidemiology (onset at different ages with different severity): early infantile, late infantile, and juvenile-adult–onset forms

c. Pathophysiology: progressive accumulation of partially degraded sialyloligosaccharides in brain and visceral tissues

d. Clinical features

   1) Types I and II are similar to other lysosomal disorders and clinically indistinguishable from sialidosis type II

   2) Most reported patients have the juvenile-adult–onset form

   3) Type I (early infantile): fetal hydrops, edema, ascites, hepatosplenomegaly, skeletal dysplasia

   4) Type II (infantile)

     a) Classic mucopolysaccharidosis phenotype

     b) Significant neurologic symptoms are rare

   5) Type III (juvenile-adult)

     a) Slowly progressive dementia, myoclonus, ataxia and angiokeratomas

     b) No visceromegaly

e. Diagnosis

   1) Deficiency of neuraminidase and β-galactosidase in fibroblasts is confirmatory

   2) Abnormal urinary excretion of oligosaccharides in a characteristic pattern

3) Types I and II are clinically indistinguishable from sialidosis, which has only neuraminidase deficiency and is associated with mutation of a different gene

f. Pathology: electron microscopy shows membrane-bound vacuoles in multiple tissues

g. Management: hematopoietic stem cell transplant is experimental

h. Prognosis

   1) Death occurs in type II congenital form in utero or in infancy

   2) Type III survives late into adulthood

i. Prenatal diagnosis: analysis of neuraminidase and β-galactosidase enzyme activity in amniocytes or chorionic villi cells

L. **Neuronal Ceroid Lipofuscinosis** (NCL) (see Chapter 8)

1. Inheritance: autosomal recessive (except CLN4, auto-somal dominant)

2. Epidemiology

a. Most common lysosomal storage disorders

b. Onset at different ages with different severity: infantile, classic late infantile, and juvenile-onset forms, also a few adult and variant late infantile forms

3. Pathophysiology

a. Clinical syndrome due to progressive accumulation of autofluorescent storage material in brain and visceral tissue

b. Eight genes have been described (*CLN1-CLN8*) with defects in palmitoyl protein thioesterase (*CLN1*), tripep-tidyl peptidase (*CLN2*), and battenin (*CLN3*) being the most common; each defect shows clinical heterogeneity with severe and later onset forms

4. Clinical features (see Chapter 8)

a. Major features are those of gray matter degenerative dis-order, with seizures, developmental regression, blindness

b. No abnormalities outside CNS

c. Infantile NCL (Santavuori-Haltia disease): normal development in early infancy, followed by developmental

---

Neuronal Ceroid Lipofuscinosis

Seizures

Blindness

Developmental regression

Psychiatric features in juvenile form

plateau and then regression, hypotonia, ataxia, microcephaly, myoclonus, and progressive blindness; repetitive
hand movements reminiscent of Rett syndrome are present for a few months; profound degeneration with nonreactive EEG by age 3 years

    d. Classic late-infantile NCL (Jansky-Bielschowsky disease):
others are Finnish variant and other unnamed variants;
severe myoclonic seizures with onset between 2 and 4
years, developmental regression, ataxia, and gradually
progressive blindness

    e. Juvenile NCL (Batten-Vogt-Spielmeyer disease): most
common form; progressive blindness between 4 and 9
years of age, followed by gradual psychomotor regression;
psychiatric symptoms and seizures may be present

    f. Adult-onset NCL (Kufs' disease): dementia, psychosis,
pyramidal or extrapyramidal symptoms, and seizures
with no visual symptoms, with onset in the fourth
decade but may occur earlier

5. Diagnosis

    a. Electron microscopy: recognition of storage material in
rectal mucosa, skin or conjunctival biopsy specimens, or
leukocytes

    b. Diagnostic enzyme assays are available for *CLN1* and
CLN2; DNA mutation testing is currently available for
CLN1, CLN2, CLN3, CLN6

    c. Electroretinogram: usually abnormal early in course of
visual loss

    d. MRI: various degrees of cerebral and cerebellar atrophy
with evidence of demyelination proportionate to clinical
deterioration

6. Pathology (Fig. 25-14)

    a. Diffuse cortical atrophy with thin cortical ribbon

    b. Neuronal storage material often strongly staining with
PAS

    c. Electron microscopy: characteristic storage material

       1) Infantile form: granular osmiophilic deposits

       2) Classic late infantile form: curvilinear profiles

       3) Juvenile form: fingerprint profiles

7. Management

**Electron Microscopy in Neuronal Ceroid
Lipofuscinosis**

Infantile form: granular osmiophilic deposits

Classic late infantile form: curvilinear profiles

Juvenile-onset form: fingerprint profiles

---

    a. Supportive care

    b. Bone marrow transplant has been ineffective

8. Prognosis (dependent on age at onset)

    a. Infantile forms: death usually in the first decade

    b. Late infantile forms: survive into second decade

    c. Juvenile and adult forms: death in the third to fifth
decades

9. Prenatal diagnosis

    a. Analysis of enzyme activity in amniocytes or chorionic
villi cells

    b. DNA testing can be performed if mutation is known

X. PEROXISOMAL DISORDERS

A. Peroxisomal Biogenesis Disorders

1. Inheritance: autosomal recessive

2. Epidemiology: panethnic

3. Pathophysiology

    a. Peroxisomal biosynthesis defects include Zellweger spec-
trum disorders, of which Zellweger syndrome, Refsum's
disease, and neonatal adrenoleukodystrophy (ALD) are
variants

    b. Zellweger syndrome is most severe form and infantile
Refsum's disease is mildest

    c. Most patients synthesize peroxisomal membranes and
peroxisomal membrane proteins, but are defective in
import of peroxisomal matrix proteins

    d. Accumulation of saturated very long-chain fatty acids
(VLCFAs) such as tetracosanoic (C24:0) and hexacosanoic (C26:0) acid in brain and plasma

    e. Deficiency of multiple peroxisomal enzymes

4. Clinical features

    a. Zellweger syndrome (cerebrohepatorenal syndrome)

       1) Characteristic facies: high forehead, large fontanelle,
shallow orbital ridges, epicanthic folds, micrognathia,
broad nasal bridge, pinna deformity, high arched
palate

       2) Eye abnormalities: Brushfield's spots, cataracts, glau-
coma, corneal clouding

       3) Severe hypotonia, weakness and neonatal seizures

       4) Profound mental retardation

       5) Progressive liver and renal dysfunction

       6) Neuronal migration defects

    b. Neonatal ALD: less dysmorphic than Zellweger syn-
drome, with later onset disease and regression leading to
mental retardation, seizures, retinopathy, hearing loss of
variable severity

    c. Infantile Refsum's disease

       1) Features similar to neonatal ALD, with hepatomegaly,

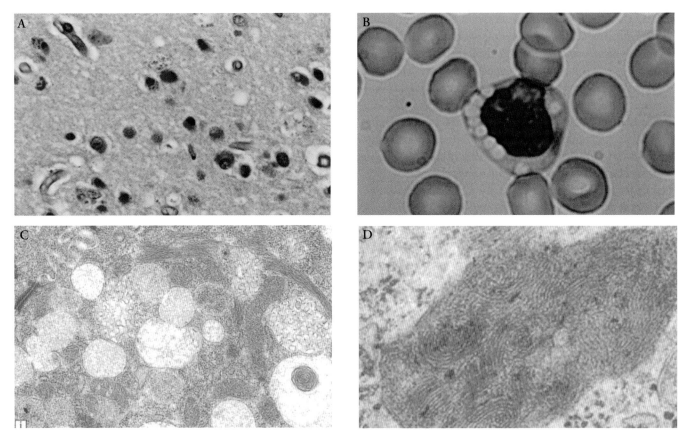

Fig. 25-14. Neuronal ceroid lipofuscinosis. *A*, Neuronal storage material reacting strongly with PAS stain. *B*, The blood smear of an affected patient shows a vacuolated lymphocyte. Electron microscopy demonstrates curvilinear bodies within a sweat gland epithelial cell in a patient with late-infantile disease (*C*) and fingerprint bodies in a patient with the juvenile form (*D*). (*C*, from Ellison D, Love S, Chimelli L, Harding B, Lowe J, Roberts GW, et al. Neuropathology: a reference text of CNS pathology. London: Mosby; 1998. p. 23.5. Used with permission. *D*, from Anthony DC, Goebel H, Mikol J. Hereditary metabolic diseases. In: Gray F, De Girolami U, Poirier J, editors. Escourolle & Poirier manual of basic neuropathology. 4th ed. Philadelphia: Butterworth-Heinemann; 2004. p. 219-48. Used with permission.)

       sensorineural deafness, retinal degeneration, dysmorphism
    2) Anosmia
    3) Mental retardation
5. Diagnosis
   a. Increase in plasma VLCFAs, pipecolic acid, and bile acid intermediates: suggestive
   b. VLCFA levels are highest in Zellweger syndrome
   c. Phytanic acid levels are increased in all varieties of the spectrum that survive beyond 40 weeks
   d. Reduced plasmalogen levels
   e. Calcific stippling of patella and epiphyses of long bones in Zellweger syndrome
   f. Definitive diagnosis: through demonstration of multiple peroxisomal enzyme deficiencies in skin fibroblast culture

   g. Mutation analysis is available
   h. Adrenal insufficiency possible
6. Pathology: electron microscopy shows absence of normal peroxisomes and presence of peroxisome ghosts consisting of peroxisomal membranes devoid of their contents
7. Management
   a. Supportive care
   b. Some milder forms may respond to docahexanoic acid supplementation with improvement in tone, vision, development
8. Prognosis: Zellweger patients rarely survive beyond early infancy, but patients with milder forms may survive for months to years
9. Prenatal diagnosis: mutation analysis and VLCFA levels in cultured amniocytes and chorionic villi cells

Peroxisomal Biogenesis Defects

Zellweger syndrome

Infantile Refsum's disease

Neonatal adrenoleukodystrophy

Peroxisomal Disorders: Clinical Features

Encephalopathy

Seizures

Hypotonia

Deafness

Rentinopathy

Dysmorphism

B. X-linked ALD (X-ALD)
1. Inheritance: X-ALD occurs in boys, females with lyonization or Turner's syndrome, and 20% of heterozygotes
2. Epidemiology: panethnic
3. Pathophysiology
   a. Gene for ALD codes for a peroxisomal membrane protein with homology to ATP-binding cassette transporter superfamily of proteins
   b. Accumulation of saturated VLCFAs such as tetracosanoic (C24:0) and hexacosanoic (C26:0) acid in brain, adrenal glands, plasma
   c. Mechanism for VLCFA accumulation is not known, but it leads to membrane instability
   d. Cerebral forms are associated with rapidly progressive, intensely inflammatory myelinopathy that usually begins in parieto-occipital region and may involve autoimmune mechanisms
   e. Adrenomyeloneuropathy: noninflammatory distal axonopathy of spinal cord tracts and, to some extent, peripheral nerves
4. Clinical features (age at onset varies from infancy to childhood)
   a. Childhood cerebral X-ALD: childhood onset
      1) Normal development until 4 to 8 years of age, followed by progressive neurodegeneration, with behavioral and cognitive deficits, spasticity, impaired vision and hearing

2) Adrenal insufficiency in most patients, with hyperpigmentation of skin and mucosa
   b. Adolescent cerebral X-ALD: features similar to childhood onset with onset in second decade
   c. Adrenomyeloneuropathy
      1) Slowly progressive paraparesis in adulthood, with long tract signs, upper motor neuron bowel and bladder disturbances, distal sensory loss
      2) Adrenal insufficiency in two-thirds of patients
      3) Impotence, hypogonadism, depression often occur
   d. Other phenotypes
      1) Pure adrenal insufficiency (Addison's disease)
      2) Progressive cerebral dysfunction in adults, with dementia and behavioral deficits (adult cerebral ALD)
      3) Asymptomatic
5. Diagnosis
   a. Increase in plasma VLCFAs: suggestive
   b. Definitive diagnosis is through enzyme assay in skin fibroblasts and mutation analysis
   c. MRI
      1) Symmetric demyelination in parieto-occipital region and connecting corpus callosum
      2) Central necrotic zone appears as a highly hyperintense region on T2-weighted images and is surrounded by zone of active demyelination, which enhances with gadolinium (Fig. 25-15)
   d. MRS alterations may precede MRI changes and show decreased N-acetylaspartic acid peaks and increased choline peaks
   e. Increased ACTH levels are often seen
   f. Abnormal evoked potentials
6. Pathology
   a. X-ALD
      1) Macroscopic: confluent symmetric demyelination, most prominent in parieto-occipital region, milder cerebellar demyelination
      2) Microscopic: marked loss of myelinated axons and oligodendrocytes with reactive astrocytosis; lymphocytic perivascular collection
      3) Electron microscopy: lamellar cytoplasmic inclusions
   b. Adrenomyeloneuropathy
      1) Myelinated axon and some oligodendroglial loss in long ascending and descending tracts in spinal cord
      2) Fasciculus gracilis and lateral corticospinal tracts are affected most
      3) Minimal involvement of cerebral or cerebellar white matter
      4) Peripheral nerves: loss of large and small myelinated fibers
7. Management

X-linked Adrenoleukodystrophy

Childhood-onset degeneration

Behavioral abnormalities

Adrenal insufficiency

Spasticity

(Adrenomyeloneuropathy in adults)

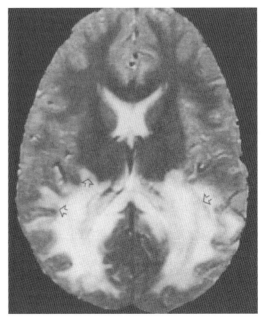

Fig. 25-15. X-linked adrenoleukodystrophy. T2-weighted MRI of the brain shows symmetric, confluent demyelination bilaterally of occipital white matter and splenium of corpus callosum. *Arrows*, intermediate zones of active demyelination. (From Osborn AG. Diagnostic neuroradiology. St. Louis: Mosby; 1994. p. 716-47. Used with permission.)

a. Adrenal hormone therapy needed for all patients with adrenal insufficiency
b. Bone marrow transplant benefits patients with early brain involvement, defined by clinical features and changes noted on MRI screening at 6 to 12–month intervals
c. Lorenzo's oil (4:1 mixture of glyceryl trioleate and glyceryl trierucate) appears to have preventive effect in boys who are younger than 6 years, neurologically asymptomatic, and have normal MRI; recommended for this group (but thrombocytopenia can be important adverse effect)
d. Supportive treatment
e. Experimental strategies: lovastatin, intravenous arginine butyrate, gene therapy
8. Prognosis
   a. MRS and MRI changes: good prognostic correlation
   b. 34-Point X-ALD MRI Severity Score (Loes score): useful for prognostication
   c. Enhancement on MRI: poor prognostic indicator
9. Prenatal diagnosis: mutation analysis and VLCFA levels in cultured amniocytes and chorionic villi cells

XI. OTHER DISORDERS PRIMARILY AFFECTING WHITE MATTER

A. Pelizaeus-Merzbacher Disease

1. Inheritance: X-linked recessive
2. Pathophysiology
   a. Poor formation of myelin
   b. Due to mutation of proteolipid protein 1 gene (*PLP1*) located on X chromosome (Xq22.2): often point mutations or duplications (latter being most common type of mutation)
   c. Allelic to spastic paraplegia type 2: Mutation of *PLP1* gene may also cause spastic paraplegia type 2

d. *PLP1* gene encodes compact myelin proteins PLP1 and DM20 (produced by alternate splicing of mRNA)
e. Fluorescence in situ hybridization (FISH) and polymerase chain reaction (PCR) confirmation of *PLP* gene mutation has been developed
3. Pathologic features
   a. Absence of or reduced myelin sheaths in white matter (especially in periventricular white matter), with relative preservation of axons
   b. Patchy areas of residual myelin islets with a "tigroid" appearance and tendency for perivascular locations
   c. Marked astrocytosis
   d. Sparing of subcortical U fibers
   e. Sparing of myelin in peripheral nerves, including cranial nerves
   f. Normal cerebral cortex
4. Clinical features
   a. Early manifestations usually noted in the first 3 months of life: delayed motor milestones, hypotonia, nystagmus
   b. Ataxia and other movement disorders such as choreoathetosis by 6 to 18 months
   c. Progressive spasticity usually after age 4 years
   d. Despite symptoms, motor development continues slowly,

reaches a plateau in second decade of life, followed by psychomotor deterioration

5. MRI
   a. Lack of normal high T1 signal of white matter
   b. No clear demarcation between white and gray matter
   c. Persistently high T2 signal present diffusely in white matter (relatively sparing of subcortical U fibers) (Fig. 25-16)
   d. No change on repeated MRI studies despite clinical progression

B. **Alexander's Disease**
1. Sporadic, may also be inherited, but the mode of inheritance is not known
2. Pathophysiology
   a. Mutation of the *GFAP* gene encoding protein glial fibrillary acidic protein (GFAP) may be responsible for most cases
   b. Pathophysiology of demyelination not understood
   c. Not due to enzyme deficiency
   d. Demyelination may be result of a gain of function of abnormal function of GFAP; mechanism not clear
3. Pathologic features (Fig. 25-17)
   a. Brain size and mass may be increased from deposition of Rosenthal fibers
   b. Cystic and cavitary white matter degeneration
   c. Rosenthal fibers
      1) Cytoplasmic inclusions in astrocytes, containing GFAP associated with α- and β-crystallin and heat shock proteins
      2) Located primarily in periventricular, subependymal, and subpial white matter
4. Clinical features
   a. Infantile onset
      1) Megalencephaly and slow enlargement of the head, irritability, progressive psychomotor retardation, pyramidal involvement, seizures, and rigidity and opisthotonos in terminal stages
      2) Usual age at onset: by 6 months
   b. Juvenile onset: ataxia, spasticity, bulbar symptoms, relatively preserved cognition, slower progression
   c. Adult onset
      1) Heterogeneous phenotype
      2) Slowly progressive or relapsing-remitting course
5. MRI: diffuse high T2 signal in white matter, with predilection for frontal lobes; best appreciated in early stages
6. Treatment: supportive, no specific treatment

C. **Canavan's disease** (spongiform leukodystrophy)
1. Inheritance: autosomal recessive

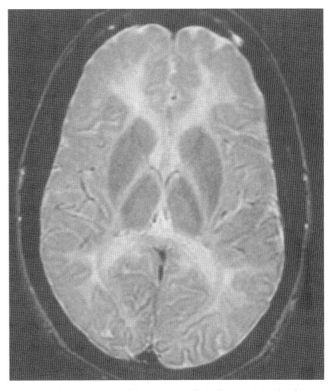

Fig. 25-16. A 20-year-old patient with Pelizaeus-Merzbacher disease. T2-weighted MRI of the brain shows diffuse high signal in white matter with sparing of subcortical U fibers. (From Koeppen AH, Robitaille Y. Pelizaeus-Merzbacher disease. J Neuropathol Exp Neurol. 2002;61:747-59. Used with permission.)

2. Pathogenesis
   a. Mutation of aspartoacylase gene on short arm of chromosome 17 (17p13)
   b. Aspartoacylase deficiency causing accumulation of *N*-acetylaspartic acid in brain
3. Pathology
   a. Megalencephaly with increased brain weight and volume
   b. Diffuse demyelination preferentially affects subcortical U fibers
   c. Progression of demyelination: initially involves subcortical white matter and then deep white matter with more advanced disease
   d. Microscopic appearance: rarefaction and vacuolation of white matter with gliosis
4. Clinical features
   a. Infantile onset with developmental delay, hypotonia, poor head control, poor visual tracking
   b. During first year: irritability, megalencephaly, head lag, developmental delay more obvious

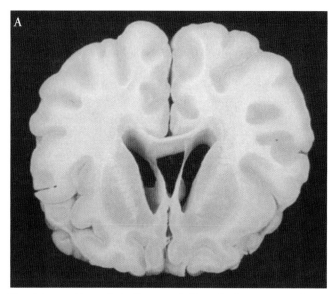
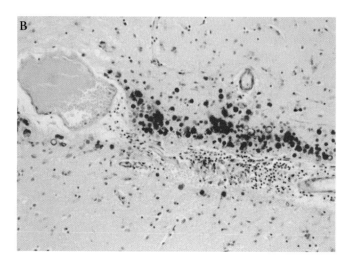

Fig. 25-17. Alexander's disease. *A*, Gross brain specimen shows diffuse discoloration of the white matter. *B*, A characteristic microscopic feature is Rosenthal fibers, which are often deposited around blood vessels, as shown here.

c. Children never develop ability to sit or stand

d. Older children: spasticity replaces hypotonia

5. Diagnosis

   a. Increased urine level of *N*-acetylaspartic acid

   b. MRI: symmetric diffuse high T2 and low T1 signal in involved white matter

   c. MRS: increased peak of *N*-acetylaspartic acid

6. Treatment

   a. Prevention by carrier detection and genetic counseling

   b. Prenatal diagnosis: measurement of amniotic fluid concentration of *N*-acetylaspartic acid; assay for aspartoacylase activity in chorionic villi likely unreliable

   c. Symptomatic treatment, no specific treatment available

D. Childhood Ataxia With CNS Hypomyelination (see Chapter 9)

E. Megalencephalic Leukoencephalopathy With Subcortical Cysts

1. Inheritance: autosomal recessive

2. Associated with mutation of *MLC1* gene on chromosome 22q

3. Clinical features

   a. Macrocephaly

   b. Slowly progressive deterioration of motor functions, ataxia, spasticity; cognitive decline

   c. Occasional seizures

REFERENCES

Altarescu G, Sun M, Moore DF, Smith JA, Wiggs EA, Solomon BI, et al. The neurogenetics of mucolipidosis type IV. Neurology. 2002;59:306-13.

Anderson KE, Sassa S, Bishop DF, Desnick RJ. Disorders of heme biosynthesis: X-linked sideroblastic anemia and the porphyrias. In: Scriver CR, Beaudet AL, Valle D, Sly WS, Vogelstein B, Childs B, et al, editors. The metabolic and molecular bases of inherited disease [online edition]. The McGraw-Hill Companies; c2001-2005 [updated 2002 Jun 24; cited 2005 Oct 12]. Available from http://genetics.accessmedicine.com/server-java/Arknoid/amed/mmbid/co_chapters/ch124/ch124_p01.htm.

Assmann G, von Eckardstein A, Brewer HB Jr. Familial analphalipoproteinemia: Tangier disease. In: Scriver CR, Beaudet AL, Valle D, Sly WS, Vogelstein B, Childs B, et al, editors. The metabolic and molecular bases of inherited disease [online edition]. The McGraw-Hill Companies; c2001-2005 [updated 2002 Jun 24; cited 2005 Oct 14]. Available from http://genetics.accessmedicine.com/server-java/Arknoid/amed/mmbid/co_chapters/ch122/ch122_p01.htm.

Baumann N, Masson M, Carreau V, Lefevre M, Herschkowitz N, Turpin JC. Adult forms of metachromatic leukodystrophy: clinical and biochemical approach. Dev Neurosci. 1991;13:211-5.

Blau N, Thöny B, Cotton RGH, Hyland K. Disorders of tetrahydrobiopterin and related biogenic amines. In: Scriver CR, Beaudet AL, Sly WS, Valle D, editors. The metabolic and molecular bases of inherited disease. 8th ed. New York: McGraw-Hill; 2001. p. 1725-76.

Brusilow SW, Horwich AL. Urea cycle enzymes. In: Scriver CR, Beaudet AL, Sly WS, Valle D, editors. The metabolic and molecular bases of inherited disease. 8th ed. New York: McGraw-Hill; 2001. p. 1909-63.

Clarke JTR, editor. A clinical guide to inherited metabolic diseases. 2nd ed. Cambridge: Cambridge University Press; 2002. p. 102, 177.

d'Azzo A, Andria G, Strisciuglio P, Galjaard H. Galactosialidosis. In: Scriver CR, Beaudet AL, Sly WS, Valle D, editors. The metabolic and molecular bases of inherited disease. 8th ed. New York: McGraw-Hill; 2001. p. 3911-26.

Desnick RJ, Brady RO. Fabry disease in childhood. J Pediatr. 2004;144 (5 Suppl):S20-6.

Fenton WA, Gravel RA, Rosenblatt DS. Disorders of propionate and methylmalonate metabolism. In: Scriver CR, Beaudet AL, Sly WS, Valle D, editors. The metabolic and molecular bases of inherited disease. 8th ed. New York: McGraw-Hill; 2001. p. 2165-93.

Fernandes Filho JA, Shapiro BE. Tay-Sachs disease. Arch Neurol. 2004;61:1466-8.

Frerman FE, Goodman SI. Defects of electron transfer flavoprotein and electron transfer flavoprotein-ubiquinone oxidoreductase: glutaric acidemia type

II. In: Scriver CR, Beaudet AL, Sly WS, Valle D, editors. The metabolic and molecular bases of inherited disease. 8th ed. New York: McGraw-Hill; 2001. p. 2357-65.

Germain DP. Gaucher's disease: a paradigm for interventional genetics. Clin Genet. 2004;65:77-86.

Girodon F, Faivre L, Devillier N, Carli PM, Maynadie M. Atypical large granular lymphocytes in a child. Br J Haematol. 2003;123:192.

Godra A, Kim DU, D'Cruz C. Pathologic quiz case: a 5-day-old boy with hydrops fetalis: mucolipidoses I (sialidosis III). Arch Pathol Lab Med. 2003;127:1051-2.

Goebel HH, Wisniewski KE. Current state of clinical and morphological features in human NCL. Brain Pathol. 2004;14:61-9.

Goodman SI, Frerman FE. Organic acidemias due to defects in lysine oxidation: 2-ketoadipic acidemia and Glutaric acidemia. In: Scriver CR, Beaudet AL, Sly WS, Valle D, editors. The metabolic and molecular bases of inherited disease. 8th ed. New York: McGraw-Hill; 2001. p. 2195-2204.

Gordon N. Alexander disease. Eur J Paediatr Neurol. 2003;7:395-9.

Gravel RA, Kaback MM, Proia RL, Sandhoff K, Suzuki K, Suzuki K. The GM2 gangliosidosis. In: Scriver CR, Beaudet AL, Valle D, Sly WS, Vogelstein B, Childs B, et al, editors. The metabolic and molecular bases of inherited disease [online edition]. The McGraw-Hill Companies; c2001-2005 [updated 2002 Jun 6; cited 2005 Oct 12]. Available from http://genetics.accessmedicine.com/server-java/Arknoid/amed/mmbid/co_chapters/ ch153/ch153_p01.htm.

Grewal SS, Shapiro EG, Krivit W, Charnas L, Lockman LA, Delaney KA, et al. Effective treatment of alpha-mannosidosis by allogeneic hematopoietic stem cell transplantation. J Pediatr. 2004;144:569-73.

Hageman AT, Gabreels FJ, de Jong JG, Gabreels-Festen AA, van den Berg CJ, van Oost BA, et al. Clinical symptoms of adult metachromatic leukodystrophy and arysulfatase A pseudodeficiency. Arch Neurol. 1995;52:408-13.

Haltia T, Palo J, Haltia M, Icen A. Juvenile metachromatic leukodystrophy: clinical, biochemical, and neuropathologic studies in nine new cases. Arch Neurol. 1980;37:42-6.

Hanefeld FA. Alexander disease: past and present. Cell Mol Life Sci. 2004;61:2750-2.

Hoffmann SL, Peltonen L. The neuronal ceroid lipofuscinosis. In: Scriver CR, Beaudet AL, Sly WS, Valle D, editors. The metabolic and molecular bases of inherited disease. 8th ed. New York: McGraw-Hill; 2001. p. 3877-94.

Hyland K. The lumbar puncture for diagnosis of pediatric neurotransmitter diseases. Ann Neurol. 2003;54 Suppl 6:S13-7.

Jaeken J. Komrower Lecture. Congenital disorders of glycosylation (CDG): it's all in it! J Inherit Metab Dis. 2003;26:99-118.

Jinnah HA, Friedmann T. Lesch-Nyhan disease and its variants. In: Scriver CR, Beaudet AL, Valle D, Sly WS, Vogelstein B, Childs B, et al, editors. The metabolic and molecular bases of inherited disease [online edition]. The McGraw-Hill Companies; c2001-2005 [updated 2002 Jun 24; cited 2005 Oct 12]. Available from http://genetics.accessmedicine.com/server-java/Arknoid/amed/mmbid/co_chapters/ch107/ch107_p01.htm.

Johnson AB. Alexander disease: a review and the gene. Int J Dev Neurosci. 2002;20:391-4.

Kane JP, Havel RJ. Disorders of the biogenesis and secretion of lipoproteins containing the B apolipoproteins. In: Scriver CR, Beaudet AL, Valle D, Sly WS, Vogelstein B, Childs B, et al, editors. The metabolic and molecular bases of inherited disease [online edition]. The McGraw-Hill Companies; c2001-2005 [updated 2002 Jun 24; cited 2005 Oct 12]. Available from http://genetics.accessmedicine.com/server-java/Arknoid/amed/mmbid/co_chapters/ch115/ch115_p01.htm.

Koeppen AH, Robitaille Y. Pelizaeus-Merzbacher disease. J Neuropathol Exp Neurol. 2002;61:747-59.

Kolodny EH. Niemann-Pick disease. Curr Opin Hematol. 2000;7:48-52.

Korman SH, Gutman A. Pitfalls in the diagnosis of glycine encephalopathy (non-ketotic hyperglycinemia). Dev Med Child Neurol. 2002;44:712-20.

Kornfeld S, Sly WS. I-cell disease and pseudo-hurler polydystrophy: disorders of lysosomal enzyme phosphorylation and localization. In: Scriver CR, Beaudet AL, Sly WS, Valle D, editors. The metabolic and molecular bases of inherited disease. 8th ed. New York: McGraw-Hill; 2001. p. 3469-82.

Kretz KA, Carson GS, Morimoto S, Kishimoto Y, Fluharty AL, O'Brien JS. Characterization of a mutation in a family with saposin B deficiency: a glycosylation site defect. Proc Natl Acad Sci U S A. 1990;87:2541-4.

MacFaul R, Cavanaugh N, Lake BD, Stephens R, Whitfield AE. Metachromatic leucodystrophy: review of 38 cases. Arch Dis Child. 1982;57:168-75.

Moser H, Dubey P, Fatemi A. Progress in X-linked adrenoleukodystrophy. Curr Opin Neurol. 2004;17:263-9.

Moser HW, Smith KD, Watkins PA, Powers J, Moser AB. X-linked adrenoleukodystrophy. In: Scriver CR, Beaudet AL, Sly WS, Valle D, editors. The metabolic and molecular bases of inherited disease. 8th ed. New York: McGraw-Hill; 2001. p. 3257-301.

Mudd SH, Levy HL, Kraus JP. Disorders of transsulfuration. In: Scriver CR, Beaudet AL, Sly WS, Valle D, editors. The metabolic and molecular bases of inherited disease. 8th ed. New York: McGraw-Hill; 2001. p. 2007-56.

Muenzer J, Fisher A. Advances in the treatment of mucopolysaccharidosis type I. N Engl J Med. 2004;350:1932-4.

National Institutes of Health Consensus Development Panel. National Institutes of Health Consensus Development Conference Statement: phenylketonuria: screening and management, October 16-18, 2000. Pediatrics 2001;108:972-82.

Neufeld EF, Muenzer J. The mucopolysaccharidoses. In: Scriver CR, Beaudet AL, Sly WS, Valle D, editors. The metabolic and molecular bases of inherited disease. 8th ed. New York: McGraw-Hill; 2001. p. 3421-52.

Pampols T, Pineda M, Giros ML, Ferrer I, Cusi V, Chabas A, et al. Neuronopathic juvenile glucosylceramidosis due to sap-C deficiency: clinical course, neuropathology and brain lipid composition in this Gaucher disease variant. Acta Neuropathol (Berl). 1999;97:91-7.

Pastores GM, Kolodny EH. Inborn errors of metabolism of the nervous system. In: Bradley GW, Daroff RB, Fenichel GM, Jankovic J, editors. Neurology in clinical practice: the neurological disorders. Vol 2. 4th ed. Philadelphia: Butterworth-Heinemann; 2004. p. 1811-32.

Patterson MC. A riddle wrapped in a mystery: understanding Niemann-Pick disease, type C. Neurologist. 2003;9:301-10.

Raas-Rothschild A, Cormier-Daire V, Bao M, Genin E, Salomon R, Brewer K, et al. Molecular basis of variant pseudo-Hurler polydystrophy (mucolipidosis IIIC). J Clin Invest. 2000;105:673-81.

Rezvani I, Rosenblatt DS. An approach to inborn errors. In: Behrman RE, Kliegman RM, Jenson HB, editors. Nelson textbook of pediatrics. 16th ed. Philadelphia: WB Saunders; 2000. p. 343-4.

Robinson BH. Lactic acidemia: disorders of pyruvate carboxylase and pyruvate dehydrogenase. In: Scriver CR, Beaudet AL, Valle D, Sly WS, Vogelstein B, Childs B, et al, editors. The metabolic and molecular bases of inherited disease [online edition]. The McGraw-Hill Companies; c2001-2005 [updated 2002 Jun 24; cited 2005 Oct 12]. Available from http://genetics.accessmedicine.com/server-java/Arknoid/amed/mmbid/co_chapters/ch100/ch100_p01.htm.

Shintaku H, Kure S, Ohura T, Okano Y, Ohwada M, Sugiyama N, et al. Long-term treatment and diagnosis of tetrahydrobiopterin-responsive hyperphenylalaninemia with a mutant phenylalanine hydroxylase gene. Pediatr Res. 2004 Mar;55:425-30. Epub 2003 Dec 17.

Stromberger C, Bodamer OA, Stockler-Ipsiroglu S. Clinical characteristics and diagnostic clues in inborn errors of creatine metabolism. J Inherit Metab Dis. 2003;26:299-308.

Surendran S, Michals-Matalon K, Quast MJ, Tyring SK, Wei J, Ezell EL, et al. Canavan disease: a monogenic trait with complex genomic interaction. Mol Genet Metab. 2003;80:74-80.

Sutton VR. Tay-Sachs disease screening and counseling families at risk for metabolic disease. Obstet Gynecol Clin North Am. 2002;29:287-96.

Suzuki K, Suzuki Y. Globoid cell leucodystrophy (Krabbe's disease): deficiency of galactocerebroside beta-galactosidase. Proc Natl Acad Sci U S A. 1970;66:302-9.

Thomas GH. Disorders of glycoprotein degradation: α-mannosidosis, β-mannosidosis, fucosidosis, and sialidosis. In: Scriver CR, Beaudet AL, Sly WS, Valle D, editors. The metabolic and molecular bases of inherited disease. 8th ed. New York: McGraw-Hill; 2001. p. 3507-33.

Vanier MT. Prenatal diagnosis of Niemann-Pick diseases types A, B and C. Prenat Diagn. 2002;22:630-2.

Walter JH, Tyfield LA. Galactosemia. In: Scriver CR, Beaudet AL, Valle D, Sly WS, Vogelstein B, Childs B, et al, editors. The metabolic and molecular bases of inherited disease [online edition]. The McGraw-Hill Companies; c2001-2005 [updated 2004 Oct 29; cited 2005 Oct 12]. Available from http://genetics.accessmedicine.com/server-java/Arknoid/amed/mmbid/co_chapters/ch072/ch072_p01.htm.

Wang D, Pascual JM, Yang H, Engelstad K, Jhung S, Sun RP, et al. Glut-1 deficiency syndrome: clinical, genetic, and therapeutic aspects. Ann Neurol. 2005;57:111-8.

Webster DR, Becroft DMO, van Gennip AH, Van Kuilenburg ABP. Hereditary orotic aciduria and other disorders of pyrimidine metabolism. In: Scriver CR, Beaudet AL, Valle D, Sly WS, Vogelstein B, Childs B, et al, editors. The metabolic and molecular bases of inherited disease [online edition]. The McGraw-Hill Companies; c2001-2005 [updated 2002 Jun 24; cited 2005 Oct 12]. Available from http://genetics.accessmedicine.com/server-java/Arknoid/amed/mmbid/co_chapters/ch113/ch113_p01.htm.

Wolf B. Disorders of biotin metabolism. In: Scriver CR, Beaudet AL, Sly WS, Valle D, editors. The metabolic and molecular bases of inherited disease. 8th ed. New York: McGraw-Hill; 2001. p. 3935-62.

Zafeiriou DI, Knotopoulos EE, Michelakakis HM, Anastasiou AL, Gombakis NP. Neurophysiology and MRI in late-infantile metachromatic leukodystrophy. Pediatr Neurol. 1999;21:843-6.

QUESTIONS

1. A 9-month-old baby girl presents with history of intractable seizures since age 3 months. She has a history of developmental delay and microcephaly, but otherwise no dysmorphism. Neurologic examination findings are remarkable only for tremors. Electroencephalography shows generalized atypical spike-and-waves. On cerebrospinal fluid (CSF) analysis, glucose is 10 mg/dL; plasma glucose is normal at 72 mg/dL. CSF lactate is reported to be the lower end of normal range. What medication is likely to be effective for management of this patient's seizures?
   a. Valproic acid
   b. Lamotrigine
   c. Felbamate
   d. Ketogenic diet

2. You are called to the newborn nursery to evaluate a hypotonic term baby boy who is ventilator-dependent. He also has feeding difficulties. On examination, he appears dysmorphic, with a large forehead and flattening of the midface. The head circumference is increased for age. On neurologic examination, the baby appears alert. He has very few movements of the extremities, despite normal extraocular movements. MRI of his brain shows features of a migrational disorder. Which of the following tests will be confirmatory?
   a. Ammonia
   b. Fibroblast culture for peroxisomal enzymes
   c. Electroencephalography
   d. Chromosomes

3. Magnetic resonance spectroscopy would be diagnostic in which of the following disorders, which manifests with developmental retardation and epilepsy?
   a. Hurler's syndrome
   b. Krabbe's disease
   c. Tuberous sclerosis
   d. Creatine deficiency

4. A 6-month-old baby presents with regression of milestones and seizures. The general physical examination is normal. No abnormality is detected on ophthalmoscopy. T1- and T2-weighted magnetic resonance images show diffuse abnormality of the white matter. What is the likely diagnosis?
   a. Tuberous sclerosis
   b. Neurofibromatosis type I

   c. Globoid cell leukodystrophy
   d. Fabry's disease

5. A 10-year-old boy presents with a history of developmental regression, visual symptoms, and "heart disease." His sister is similarly affected. On examination, he has coarse facies, with kyphosis and short stature. He has global developmental delay. Which of the following diagnoses is *least* likely?
   a. Mucolipidosis
   b. Fucosidosis
   c. Mucopolysaccharidosis
   d. Medium-chain acyl-CoA dehydrogenase deficiency

6. A 14-year-old boy presents with an acute ischemic infarct in the territory of the left middle cerebral artery. He is tall, has long fingers, and complains of long-standing visual symptoms and progressive myopia. What single blood test is likely to be of diagnostic use in this patient?
   a. Peripheral blood smear
   b. Thyroid-stimulating hormone
   c. Lactic acid
   d. Homocysteine

7. A 4-day-old male child presents to the emergency department with poor feeding and lethargy. There is no history of trauma or respiratory symptoms. He is mildly hypothermic, with a respiratory rate of 60 breaths/min. His heart rate is normal, with good peripheral pulses. Examination shows a profoundly lethargic child with bulging anterior fontanelle and normally reactive pupils. Laboratory evaluation demonstrates a normal complete blood count, electrolytes and glucose. Respiratory alkalosis was present. Results of blood culture and cerebrospinal fluid analysis are pending. Computed tomography shows decreased gray matter–white matter differentiation and small brain ventricles. As the neurologist on call, what other test would you order on an urgent basis?
   a. Magnetic resonance imaging of the head
   b. Urine organic acids
   c. Plasma ammonia
   d. Chromosomes

8-11. Match the deficient enzyme (a-d) with the disease (8-11):

8. Metachromatic leukodystrophy

9. Krabbe's disease

10. Homocystinuria

11. Pompe's disease

a. Cystathionine β-synthetase

b. Arylsulfatase A

c. α-Glucosidase

d. Galactocerebroside β-galactosidase

12-15. Match the disease (12-15) with the pathologic finding (a-d):

12. Alexander's disease

13. Niemann-Pick disease

14. Neuronal ceroid lipofuscinosis

15. Zellweger syndrome

a. Sea-blue histiocytes

b. Fingerprint inclusions

c. Peroxisome ghosts

d. Rosenthal fibers

ANSWERS

1. Answer d.
Glucose transporter type I deficiency may present with intractable seizures associated with low CSF glucose and low or low-normal CSF lactate in infancy. Patients respond to an alternative fuel source in the form of ketone bodies, as supplied by the ketogenic diet.

2. Answer: b.
Zellweger cerebrohepatorenal syndrome presents in infancy with hypotonia and craniofacial dysmorphic features. There is widespread neuronal migration defects, especially pachygyria and cerebellar abnormalities. Some of the characteristic facial features include a high forehead, shallow supraorbital ridges, epicanthic folds, broad nasal bridge, and midface hypoplasia. Eye abnormalities include Brushfield's spots, cataracts, glaucoma, and corneal clouding. Severe weakness, hypotonia, and seizures are common. Diagnosis is suggested by increased levels of saturated and unsaturated very long-chain fatty acids in body fluids. Definitive diagnosis is through demonstration of multiple peroxisomal enzyme deficiencies in skin fibroblast culture.

3. Answer: d.
Creatine deficiency syndromes are a newly described group of inborn errors of creatine synthesis (arginine:glycine amidino-transferase [AGAT] deficiency), creatine transport (creatine transporter [CRTR] deficiency), and guanidinoacetate methyl-transferase (GAMT) deficiency. The common clinical features of creatine deficiency syndromes are mental retardation and epilepsy. Patients with GAMT deficiency may have a more complex clinical phenotype, with a movement disorder and intractable epilepsy. The common biochemical finding in creatine deficiency syndromes is cerebral creatine deficiency, which is demonstrated by in vivo magnetic resonance spectroscopy.

4. Answer: c.
Krabbe's disease (or globoid cell leukodystrophy) manifests in infancy with regression of milestones, increased muscle tone, and loss of tendon reflexes due to peripheral neuropathy. There is demyelination of the brain, spinal cord, and peripheral nerves due to deficiency of galactosylceramidase. Cerebrospinal fluid protein level is elevated. Nerve conduction velocities are slowed.

5. Answer: d.
Coarse facies, developmental regression, and dysostosis multiplex can be a manifestation of multiple lysosomal disorders. Medium-chain acyl-CoA dehydrogenase deficiency usually presents with altered sensorium after fasting. These children can have developmental delays and muscle weakness. They do not have features of skeletal dysplasia.

6. Answer: d.
Homocystinuria is inherited as an autosomal recessive disorder and is due to deficiency of various enzymes, including cystathionine β-synthase. Patients have a marfanoid appearance, with long limbs, arachnodactyly, and ectopia lentis with downward dislocation of the lens. Approximately 50% of the patients have mental retardation. Most neurologic features result from cerebral thromboembolic disease. Approximately 40% of the patients with cystathionine β-synthase deficiency respond to pyridoxine.

7. Answer: c.
Urea cycle disorders present in the neonatal period with clinical features as described above. Marked hyperammonemia in the presence of metabolic acidosis suggests the diagnosis. Ornithine transcarbamoylase deficiency is an X-linked disorder that has a poor neurologic outcome if the hyperammonemia remains untreated for a long time. For the hyperammonemia, discontinue protein intake and treat with hemodialysis, sodium benzoate, sodium phenylacetate, and arginine hydrochloride.

8. Answer: b.

9. Answer: d.

10. Answer: a.

11. Answer: c.

12. Answer: d.

13. Answer: a.

14. Answer: b.

15. Answer: c.

INDEX

('b' indicates boxed material; 'i' indicates an illustration; 't' indicates a table)

Protoplasmic astrocytomas, 629
Pseudo-Hurler polydystrophy, 966t
Pseudotumor cerebri, 105, 122, 124-125
    headache, 710-712
Pseudoxanthoma elasticum, 528t, 531t,
    541t, 546-547
    stroke, 466
Psychiatry
    anxiety disorders, 237-243
    mood disorders, 232-237
    personality disorders, 258-262
    psychopharmacology, 262-271
    psychotherapy, 271-272
    psychotic disorders, 225-232
    substance-related disorders, 243-258,
        244t-246t
    terms and definitions, 227t
Psychoanalysis, 271
Psychopharmacology, 262-271
Psychophysiologic insomnia, 731-732
Psychotherapy, 271-272
Psychotic disorders, 225-232
Ptosis, 118
Pufferfish poisoning, 685-686
Pupil, autonomic innervation, 113i
Pupillary disorders, 111-115
Pupillary light reflex, 111-112, 112i
Pure autonomic failure, 855i, 857
Purine bases, 72b
Purine metabolism disorder, 949-950
Purkinje cell migration, 14
Pyridoxine-dependent seizures, 490
Pyrimidine bases, 72b
Pyrimidines, metabolism disorder, 950
Pyruvate dehydrogenase deficiency,
    936-937, 936b

Q

Quadrantic defects, 85i, 89-90, 286
Quantitative sudomotor axon reflex test
    (QSART), 855-856, 856i
Quetiapine (Seroquel), 267

R

Rabies virus, central nervous system
    effects, 607-608
Radial glial cells, 14
Radial nerve, 778i, 780
Radial neuropathy, 778i, 780
Radiation-induced myelopathy, 766
Radiation-induced plexopathy, 795, 796
Radiculopathies, 788-791

Radiculopathy
    definition, 786
    infectious, 791
    sensory nerve action potential, 192,
        210
Radiotherapy, seizures, 510-511
Ramsay Hunt syndrome, 138, 140, 604
Rapid eye movement (REM) sleep, 47i,
    48-49, 52i, 167b, 170i, 719,
    720, 721-722, 721b, 724i
    parasomnias, 738-740, 741i
Rapid eye movement (REM) sleep
    behavior disorder (RBD),
    729, 738-739, 739b, 741i,
    744
Rasmussen's encephalitis, 497
Raynaud's phenomenon, 861
Rebound headache, 702
Recurrent hypersomnia, 730-731
Red ear syndrome, 862
Reelin, 14, 22, 23
Referential montage, EEG, 165-166
Reflex seizures, 498
Reflexive saccades, 97
Refsum's disease, 388, 799t, 801b, 809,
    810
    infantile, 969-970
Relapsing-remitting multiple sclerosis,
    559
Relative afferent pupillary defect
    (RAPD), 105
Renal failure, neurologic impact,
    687-688
Repetitive nerve stimulation technique,
    199-200, 200i, 201i
Resting membrane potential (RMP), 37
Restless legs syndrome, 367, 733-734,
    734b
Reticular nucleus, thalamus, 67
Retina, 83, 84i, 85i
Retinal migraine, 103, 105
Retinal nerve fiber layer, 83, 86-87, 86i
Retinal receptors, 55, 56i
Retinoic acid, 3
Retroperitoneal hemorrhage, 797
Rett syndrome, 328, 328b
Reversible posterior leukoencephalopathy
    (RPLE), 688
Rheumatoid arthritis, 576t, 580
    autonomic dysfunction, 859
    peripheral neuropathy, 838
Rhodopsin, 83
RhoGTPase, 27, 28
Rhombencephalon, 3, 4i, 14

Rhombomeres, 3
Rhythmic movement disorder, 734
Rickettsial infective meningitis, 599-600
Ring scotoma, 86-87
Risk factors, neural tube defects, 3
Risperidone (Risperdal), 266
Rivastigmine (Exelon), 304
Rocky Mountain spotted fever, 599-600
Rods, 55-56, 56i, 86i
Rolandic epilepsy, 178b
Rosenthal fibers, 973, 974i
Ross syndrome, 114, 860
Rostrocaudal defects, 3b
Roussy-Levy syndrome, 803
Rowland Payne syndrome, 112
Rubella, polymicrogyria, 16
Rubrospinal tract, 64
Rucksack paralysis, 795
Ruffini ending, 55t, 58
"Rule of the pupil," 94

S

Saccadic system, 97-101, 97i
Sacral plexus, 782
Sandhoff's disease, 955
Sanfilippo's syndrome, 963, 964t
Santavuori congenital muscular
    dystrophy, 907
Saphenous nerve, 785i
Saposin A, 960
Saposin B, 958, 959
Sarcocanopathies (LGMD 2C-2F), 904
Sarcoid myopathy, 924-925, 926i
Sarcoid neuropathy, 829, 830i
Sarcoidosis
    peripheral nervous system disease
        mimicker, 840
    polyradiculopathy, 792
    transverse myelitis, 771
Sarcomere, structure, 886-888, 887i
"Saturday night palsy," 780, 780i
Schaffer collateral pathway, 290
Scheie's syndrome, 963, 964t
Schizencephaly, 8, 15b, 18i
Schizoaffective disorder, 230, 230b, 274,
    276
Schizoid personality disorder, 259
Schizophrenia, 225-229, 225b, 227b,
    274, 276
    epidemiology, 227
    genetics, 228
    neurologic manifestations, 229b